Occupational Therapy

Overcoming Human Performance Deficits

Occupational Therapy
Overcoming Human Performance Deficits

Edited by

Charles Christiansen

Charles Christiansen, EdD, OTR, OT(C), FAOTA
Director of the School of Rehabilitation Medicine
Professor, Division of Occupational Therapy
Faculty of Medicine
University of British Columbia
Vancouver, British Columbia, CANADA

Carolyn Baum

Carolyn Baum, MA, OTR, FAOTA
Elias Michael Director, Program in Occupational Therapy
Director of Clinical Services, Irene Walter Johnson Institute of Rehabilitation
Assistant Professor, Occupational Therapy and Neurology
Washington University School of Medicine
St. Louis, Missouri, USA

SLACK Incorporated, 6900 Grove Road, Thorofare, NJ 08086-9447

SLACK International Book Distributors

In Japan
  Igaku-Shoin, Ltd.
  Tokyo International P.O. Box 5063
  1-28-36 Hongo, Bunkyo-Ku
  Tokyo 113
  Japan

In Canada
  McGraw-Hill Ryerson Limited
  300 Water Street
  Whitby, Ontario
  L1N 9B6

In all other regions throughout the world, SLACK professional reference books are available through offices and affiliates of McGraw-Hill, Inc. For the name and address of the office serving your area, please correspond to

McGraw-Hill, Inc.
Medical Publishing Group
Attn: International Marketing Director
1221 Avenue of the Americas —28th Floor
New York, NY 10020
(212)-512-3955 (phone)
(212)-512-4717 (fax)

Executive Editor: Cheryl D. Willoughby
Publisher: Harry C. Benson

Cover Artwork: Reproduction of *Eros* by Paul Klée is with permission of the estate of Paul Klée; Rosengart Galerie, Lucerne, Switzerland; CosmoPress, Geneva, Switzerland; and the Artists' Rights Society, New York.

Printed in the United States of America

Library of Congress Catalog Card Number: 86-60419

ISBN: 1-55642-180-X

Published by: SLACK Incorporated
                6900 Grove Road
                Thorofare, NJ 08086-9447

Last digit is print number: 10 9 8 7 6 5 4 3 2

This book is dedicated
to Pamela, Erik, Kalle and Carrie Christiansen;
to Kirstin Baum;
and to our friends, colleagues
and students throughout the world.

Contents

Expanded Contents

Contributing Authors

Karin J. Barnes is an Associate Professor of Occupational Therapy at the University of Texas Health Science Center at San Antonio, where she has held a faculty appointment since 1980. Professor Barnes earned her undergraduate degree in occupational therapy from the University of Kansas, and later completed a Master of Science degree in Special Education at the same institution. As a highly experienced developmental therapist, she has conducted funded research and published several papers in the area of the development of prehension skills in children with cerebral palsy. An accomplished practitioner, she is certified in the administration of the *Southern California Sensory Integration Tests* and has completed the eight week neurodevelopmental treatment certification course. Ms. Barnes has an avid interest in the effects of physical barriers on performance and independence.

Carolyn Baum is Assistant Professor and Elias Michael Director of the Occupational Therapy Program at Washington University School of Medicine in St. Louis, Missouri, and Director of Occupational Therapy Clinical Services at the Irene Walter Johnson Institute of Rehabilitation at Washington University Medical School. She earned her undergraduate degree in occupational therapy at the University of Kansas, holds an M.A. in Health Management, and is currently pursuing a doctorate in Social Policy and Gerontology at Washington University. Ms. Baum has held a number of positions in professional organizations, including President of the American Occupational Therapy Association, member of the Board of Directors of the American Occupational Therapy Foundation, and President of the American Occupational Therapy Certification Board. As a Fellow of the American Occupational Therapy Association, she was invited to present the Eleanor Clarke Slagle Lecture in 1980 and has received other prestigious awards, including the Award of Merit and *Who's Who in American Women*. Ms. Baum is the coauthor of a monograph on the prospective payment system, and has published extensively in the rehabilitation literature.

James E. Berger holds a B.S. in Pharmacy from the University of Cincinnati College, an M.S. in Microbiology from the University of Cincinnati, and a Ph.D. in Pharmacology from the University of Florida. He is currently Coordinator of Student Services and Professor of Pharmacology in the College of Pharmacy at Butler University. Dr. Berger has published widely in professional journals such as *Indiana Pharmacist, Pharmacology*, and the *Journal of Pharmacy and Pharmacology*, as well as in various textbooks and monographs. He has presented major seminars and is extensively involved in community and civic experiences. Since 1968, Dr. Berger has served as a frequent consultant and expert witness in pharmacology.

Barbara Borg holds a B.S. degree in Occupational Therapy from Colorado State University and an M.A. in Counseling Psychology from the University of Northern Colorado. She is currently in private practice, providing counseling and occupational therapy services in psychosocial dysfunction. She also works as a consultant and seminar leader in the areas of cognitive dysfunction and cognitive retraining, coping skills, stress management, grief work and chronic depression. Ms. Borg has served on the faculty of Colorado State University and has held the position of Director of Occupational Therapy at Bethesda Hospital, Denver. Her professional affiliations include membership in the American Occupational Therapy Association, the Colorado Occupational Therapy Association, and the Colorado Council on Basic Education. Barbara Borg's articles have appeared in *The American Journal of Occupational Therapy*, and she is the coauthor of two books (with Mary Ann Bruce) in the area of psychosocial occupational therapy: The *Group System: The Therapeutic Activity Group in Occupational Therapy* (1991) and *Frames of Reference in Psychosocial Occupational Therapy* (1987).

Caroline R. Brayley is Associate Professor and Chair of the Department of Occupational Therapy, School of Health Related Professions at the University of Pittsburgh. Dr. Brayley completed her undergraduate degree in Occupational Therapy at the University of New Hampshire, and later earned the M.Ed. degree from the State University of New York at Buffalo. Her Ph.D. in Higher Education was earned at the University of Pittsburgh. Dr. Brayley has been on the faculties of Cleveland State University, The State University of New York at Buffalo, and two community colleges. As a practicing therapist she has worked with persons who have physical disabilities, psychosocial deficits and problems related to aging. She is a Fellow of the American Occupational Therapy Association and has served as President of the Ohio Occupational Therapy Association and Secretary of the American Occupational Therapy Foundation. The recipient of many recognitions and awards, Dr. Brayley is widely published and serves on the Editorial Board of *The Occupational Therapy Journal of Research*.

Mary Ann Bruce is currently an occupational therapy consultant and doctoral student. She earned her B.S. in Occupational Therapy at Colorado State University and later completed an M.S. in Counseling Psychology. Mrs. Bruce has a distinguished career in occupational therapy education, having held senior faculty and administrative appointments at Quinnipiac College in Connecticut and at the University of Texas Health Science Center at San Antonio. Her interests are in mental health, gerontology and education. She is the co-author of *Frames of Reference in Psychosocial Occupational Therapy* and *The Group System: The Therapeutic Activity Group in Occupational Therapy* , both published by Slack, Inc. Mrs. Bruce holds membership in several health-related organizations.

Charles Christiansen is Professor and Director of the School of Rehabilitation Medicine, Faculty of Medicine, at The University of British Columbia. Prior to his present position, he held appointments in the Schools of Medicine and Allied Health Sciences at the University of Texas Health Science Center at San Antonio, and as Chairman/Director of Occupational Therapy at the University of Texas Medical Branch at Galveston. Dr. Christiansen earned his undergraduate degree in Occupational Therapy at the University of North Dakota, later completing an M.A. in Counseling Psychology and earning a Doctorate in Education at the University of Houston. He is a Fellow of the American Occupational Therapy Association and has held many elected and appointed positions of distinction in that organization, including Chairmanship of the Accreditation Committee and Fiscal Advisory Committee. He was elected Treasurer of the Association in 1986, and became Chair of the Research Advisory Council of the American Occupational Therapy Foundation in 1989. He is the founding editor of *The Occupational Therapy Journal of Research*, serving from 1981-1986. Widely published, Dr. Chris-

tiansen serves on the review panels of several publications and granting agencies. As an active consultant, his assignments have taken him throughout the United States and to various foreign countries. Dr. Christiansen is a member of the Canadian Association of Occupational Therapists. He also holds elected membership in the American Congress of Rehabilitation Medicine, Sigma Xi, and the Human Factors Society.

Harriett Davidson is Assistant Professor and Administrative Coordinator of the School of Occupational Therapy at Texas Woman's University in Houston. She holds a B.A., B.S. in Occupational Therapy from Texas Women's University, and an M.A. in Occupational Therapy from the University of Southern California. Ms. Davidson has an extensive background in education, having taught at both the technical and professional levels. She is extensively involved in committee responsibilities at national, state, local, university and departmental levels and has received several professional honors such as selection for inclusion in Marquis' *Who's Who in Rehabilitation*. Ms. Davidson was named Occupational Therapist of the Year in 1986 by the Texas Occupational Therapy Association. She has presented many papers and holds several publications to her credit. She is interested in various aspects of rehabilitation, including the use of therapy as a socialization process.

Elizabeth DePoy received her B.S.O.T. from the State University of New York at Buffalo in 1972, and then practiced occupational therapy in mental health until her entrance into graduate studies in social welfare at the University of Pennsylvania. After receiving her M.S.W., Dr. DePoy directed and taught in an Occupational Therapy Assisting Program at a community college in New Jersey and then returned to direct practice working with catastrophically injured adults in their homes. Later, she accepted a faculty position in the Department of Occupational Therapy at Thomas Jefferson University, where she began her research career. She completed her Ph.D. at the University of Pennsylvania in the Graduate School of Education where she studied philosophical foundations of knowledge and research methodology. Currently, she is an assistant professor in the Department of Social Work at the University of Maine where she teaches courses in adult development and research methods, and conducts research in the areas of adult health and productivity.

Elizabeth Devereaux is Associate Professor in the Department of Psychiatry, School of Medicine, Marshall University in Huntington, West Virginia. She earned her B.S. in Occupational Therapy at Ohio State University and her Master of Social Work degree at the West Virginia

University. Ms. Devereaux practiced extensively in community mental health prior to beginning her career in academic medicine. A Fellow of the American Occupational Therapy Association, she has held a number of key positions in that organization, including Chair of the Accreditation Committee and Chair of the Fiscal Advisory Committee. Ms. Devereaux is a member of the American College of Social Work and has published widely in the rehabilitation literature. She currently serves as the President of the American Occupational Therapy Foundation. Ms. Devereaux has a strong interest in pharmacology and was a member of the research team at Marshall University that conducted a five year clinical trial of mood disorders under the direction of Dr. Donald S. Robinson, an internationally recognized pharmacologist.

Janet Duchek is Assistant Professor in the Program in Occupational Therapy and the Department of Neurology at Washington University in St. Louis. She holds a B.A. in Psychology from the University of Missouri at St. Louis, and both an M.A. and Ph.D. in Experimental Psychology from the University of South Carolina. Dr. Duchek's past professional and teaching experiences include work in Cognitive Research at the University of Massachusetts, and positions as Research Instructor in the Departments of Neurology/Psychology at Washington University and Project Coordinator of the Memory and Aging Project at Washington University. Dr. Duchek has written many articles that have been published in professional journals such as *Developmental Psychology, Psychology and Aging,* and *Archives of Neurology.* Dr. Duchek has also presented numerous papers at professional meetings within and outside the United States. Her research interests include aging and cognitive processes; memory deficits in Alzheimer Disease; and other aspects of memory as a cognitive function.

Winnie Dunn is Professor and Chairperson of the Occupational Therapy Program at Kansas University Medical Center. Dr. Dunn earned a B.S. in Occupational Therapy and an M.S. in Education/Learning Disabilities from the University of Missouri, and holds a Doctor of Philosophy degree in Neuroscience from the University of Kansas. She has held various positions in developmental rehabilitation, including service with the University Affiliated Facility at the University of Missouri, Coordinator of Postgraduate Education and Professional Development, and Coordinator of Pediatric Outreach Programs at St. Luke's Hospital of Kansas City. Dr. Dunn has received several honors and awards for her professional service. She is a Fellow of the American Occupational Therapy Association and an active member of Sensory Integration International. Dr. Dunn has published widely in professional journals, has

served on the editorial boards for various publications, and is the editor of a book on pediatric occupational therapy practice, entitled *Pediatric Occupational Therapy: Facilitating Effective Service Provision.*

Shereen D. Farber is Assistant Director and Associate Professor in the Occupational Therapy Program at Indiana University School of Medicine and also a consultant in private practice to Neurorehabilitation Services. Dr. Farber holds a B.S. in Occupational Therapy from Ohio State University, an M.S. in Learning Disabilities and Special Education from Butler University, a Ph.D. in Anatomy (Neuroanatomy) from Indiana University, and post-doctoral training in Neurophysiology and Neurotransplantation at Indiana University. Dr. Farber has wide experience as a clinician and an educator. She has held membership in a wide variety of professional societies, and has served on the editorial board of three journals. Dr. Farber has presented over 250 invited lectures on neurorehabilitation, neuroanatomy, and neurophysiology throughout North America. Her honors include The Eleanor Clark Slagle Lectureship for 1989 and the Award for Scientific Excellence in the area of Sensory Integration. She has published widely in the area of neurological therapy, and her book *Neurorehabilitation: A Multisensory Approach*, is widely cited.

Ellen Kolodner is Assistant Professor and Fieldwork Coordinator at Thomas Jefferson University, College of Allied Health Sciences, Department of Occupational Therapy. She received a B.S. in Occupational Therapy from the University of Pennsylvania, and a Master of Social Services from Bryn Mawr College. She has had extensive experience as a practitioner, administrator and consultant in psychosocial rehabilitation. She has served on many professional committees and has gained recognition in both professional and community organizations. The author of a number of papers, Ms. Kolodner is a Fellow of the American Occupational Therapy Association, and was elected Secretary of that organization in 1989.

Laura H. Krefting is an Associate Professor and Career Scientist in the School of Rehabilitation Therapy at Queen's University in Kingston, Ontario, Canada. She received her undergraduate degree in occupational therapy from the University of Alberta and a Masters degree in the area of gerontology from the University of British Columbia. She earned her Ph.D. in rehabilitation and anthropology at the University of Arizona, where her studies built on her long-standing interest in culture and disability. Dr. Krefting's practical experience is varied and includes mental health, psychogeriatrics, vocational rehabilitation and community rehabilitation of brain-injured persons. Prior to assuming her present position, she chaired the graduate program in Occupational Therapy at the University of Alberta. She is active in the American Anthropology Association (disability studies group) as well as a number of rehabilitation organizations.

Douglas V. Krefting is a graduate student in the anthropology program at the University of Alberta. His research interests include the transmission of culture and health and healing as a reflection of the larger culture. His studies in anthropology are complemented by many years of international experience, most recently in community-based rehabilitation in Indonesia. Recently, he has been working with his wife, Laura Krefting, on joint projects focusing on two cultural groups—rural disabled persons in Indonesia and Native Indians in Canada.

Ruth E. Levine is presently Professor and Chairman of the Department of Occupational Therapy, College of Allied Health Sciences at Thomas Jefferson University in Philadelphia. She received her Occupational Therapy degree from the University of Pennsylvania, and also holds the M.Ed. in Psychoeducational Processes and Doctor of Education degree from Temple University. She has held a number of professional and community positions, among which are the 1989-90 Research Fellow of St. Loye's School of Occupational Therapy at Exeter University in Devon, England, the founder of Community Occupational Therapy Consultants, a Fellow of the American Occupational Therapy Association, and President of the Pennsylvania Occupation Therapy Association. Widely published, Dr. Levine serves on the editorial boards of three journals, has presented numerous papers and workshops, received grants and awards for her dedication to the profession of Occupational Therapy, and has served as consultant for numerous facilities.

Lela A. Llorens is Chair of the Department of Occupational Therapy, and Graduate Coordinator and Professor, at San Jose State University. She received a B.S. in Occupational Therapy from Western Michigan University, an M.A. in Vocational Rehabilitation from Wayne State University, and earned a Ph.D. from Walden University. Dr. Llorens has an extensive amount of professional and academic experience. She served as Chair of the Department of Occupational Therapy at the University of Florida prior to assuming her current appointment. Dr. Llorens is very active and widely known for her Eleanor Clarke Slagle lecture, which provided a developmental model for occupational therapy practice. She has been awarded numerous grants and for work in various areas of rehabilitation. Her list of publications is extensive, and includes many papers, chapters, and books. Her service as the first Chair of the Research Advisory Council, a collaborative body of the American Occupational Therapy

Association and American Occupational Therapy Foundation, was instrumental in advancing occupational therapy research. Dr. Llorens has received numerous honors and awards during her distinguished career in occupational therapy.

Marian A. Minor has a B.S. in Physical Therapy from the University of Kansas, an M.S.P.H. in Community Health Education from the University of Missouri, and a Doctorate in Human Performance from the University of Missouri. Her professional employment includes positions as Clinical Instructor for the Department of Medicine, Assistant Professor for the School of Health Related Professions at the University of Missouri School of Medicine, and Associate Director of the Central Missouri Regional Arthritis Center. Dr. Minor has given numerous scientific presentations and is published in various professional journals such as the *Journal of Rheumatology and Arthritis and Rheumatism*.

Karin Joann Opacich is Assistant Professor, Section of Occupational Therapy, Department of Related Health Programs at Rush University and a contract therapist in various Chicago home health agencies. She holds a B.S. in Occupational Therapy from the University of Kansas, and a Masters degree in Health Professions Education from the University of Illinois Medical Center. She has also had past experience in the area of pediatrics. Ms. Opacich is currently affiliated with various professional organizations and many committees at professional, departmental, and college levels. As an investigator, she has worked on various research projects and has been a primary advisor to students with graduate and clinical experiences. Ms. Opacich has contributed to or published articles and chapters in books. She has also given numerous major professional presentations and has a diverse background in continuing education.

Barbara Boyt Schell has held various administrative positions in occupational therapy, including Director of Occupational Therapy Services at the Harmarville Rehabilitation Center in Pittsburgh, PA. She earned her undergraduate degree in Occupational Therapy from the University of Florida and holds an M.S. in Business Management from the University of South Florida. Ms. Schell has developed extensive community networks for setting up new programs such as re-entry for head injury and spinal cord injury populations, meal groups for stroke patients, and pain management programs. Her development and implementation of productivity, quality assurance, and personnel management systems have earned her wide recognition and she is a frequent consultant to rehabilitation facilities. Ms. Schell has been extensively involved in professional activities, committees, and associations, and has numerous presentations and publications to her credit.

Richard K. Schwartz is Associate Professor and Director of the Occupational Therapy Program at The University of Texas Health Science Center in San Antonio. He received his B.S. in Occupational Therapy from Washington University School of Medicine in 1972, his M.S. in Occupational Therapy from Sargent College of Boston University in 1976, and is currently completing a Ph.D. in Educational Psychology at the University of Texas at Austin. He is a co-founder of The Freedom Center, a service delivery center to provide access to technology for disabled persons, and is Software/Technology Editor for the *American Journal of Occupational Therapy*. The author of the text, *Therapy As Learning*, he received a Presidential Award for Excellence in Teaching from the University of Texas Health Science Center at San Antonio. For the past three years his research and publications have focused on industrial accident and injury prevention. He has a special interest in how cognitive processes influence behaviors which prevent accidents and injury.

Roger O. Smith is Associate Director, Trace Research and Development Center at the University of Wisconsin-Madison. He is also a research/lecturer in the Occupational Therapy Program at the University of Wisconsin and a doctoral student in Human Factors Engineering/Health Systems Engineering in the Department of Industrial Engineering. Mr. Smith earned his B.A. degree in Psychology at Goshen College in Indiana and a Master of Occupational Therapy Degree at the University of Washington in Seattle. His career in rehabilitation has included a broad array of responsible positions in direct care and administration with a wide spectrum of disabilities. He is a recognized expert in the applications of technology to rehabilitation, and he has been involved in developing assessments, adaptive devices, and documentation systems. He is widely published, and has served in a number of capacities with national rehabilitation organizations, including RESNA and the American Occupational Therapy Association.

Jean Cole Spencer holds a doctorate in anthropology from Rice University and an M.O.T. degree from Texas Woman's University. Before becoming an occupational therapist, Dr. Spencer worked for ten years for a medical rehabilitation facility where she conducted research and managed independent living and transitional living programs. After becoming an occupational therapist, she worked clinically with neurology patients (primarily persons with head injury, spinal cord

injury, and stroke) at Hermann Hospital in Houston, Texas. She is currently an Associate Professor and Occupational Therapy Research Coordinator at the Houston Campus of Texas Woman's University. Dr. Spencer's publications deal primarily with independent living and community adaptation. Her current research interests center on community functioning of elderly persons, cultural issues in adaptation, and transitional adaptive periods of persons who are leaving treatment facilities and returning to community living environments.

Mary Sladky Struthers attended Southern Methodist University in Dallas and later earned a B.S. in Occupational Therapy from the University of Wisconsin and an M.S. in Higher Education Administration from the University of Pennsylvania. She has held clinical and adjunct appointments with various universities, including the University of Texas Medical Branch, Texas Woman's University, Temple University, and Boston University. She has also served as a lecturer in the Department of Physical Medicine and Rehabilitation at the University of Pennsylvania School of Medicine. Her clinical experiences have been in the area of pediatric developmental disabilities, and she has been affiliated with the Austin (Texas) Independent School District, the Shriner's Burn Institute in Galveston, Texas, Austin State Hospital, and more recently as Director of Occupational Therapy for the Hospital of the University of Pennsylvania. Ms. Struthers is an active member in many professional and scientific societies, including the American Occupational Therapy Association, the American Society of Allied Health Professionals, and RESNA, the Association for the Advancement of Rehabilitation Technology. Currently a Ph.D. candidate in Regional Planning Health Policy at the University of Pennsylvania, Ms. Struthers has a private consulting practice.

Mary Warren is Assistant Director of Occupational Therapy at the Rehabilitation Institute in Kansas City, MO. She has a B.S. in Occupational Therapy and an M.S. in Education, both obtained from the University of Kansas. She has been a teaching consultant to various universities in the Missouri area. Ms. Warren has published articles in the *American Journal of Occupational Therapy* and has also been a member of its Editorial Board. She is now a reviewer for that professional journal. Ms. Warren also has given over 25 lectures and/or presentations at various workshops.

Foreword

The health care industry, which accounts for nearly 12% of the gross national product in the United States and sizeable proportions in other countries, has become an object of close scrutiny by government and consumers alike. There is concern that the cost increases occurring over the past two decades are not wholly justified by either improvements in service or statistical evidence of improved health status. Part of the increases have been due to a dramatic growth in the number of physicians and other health care providers, many of whom have emerged in response to new technologies that have developed over the period.

The cost of maintaining health, whether funded by increased taxes or higher premiums for fees and health insurance, focuses even more attention on accountability and raises more questions about the benefits associated with higher costs. In those areas where progress by medicine has been less dramatic, such as with congenital disabilities, chronic diseases, permanent injuries and the aging process, there is even greater dissatisfaction about medicine's neglect of the real issue of illness or disease—how it impacts on the daily lives of individuals. As a result, functional assessment and functional outcome are likely to be keywords of the nineties.

Certainly, those professionals who possess the knowledge and skills to reduce the impact of disabling conditions on life performance will be in a favorable position to gain increased public support and attention. As we move toward the twenty-first century, occupational therapy, with its long-standing concern for the ability of an individual to perform those life tasks that bring meaning to existence, may very well have a competitive advantage within such a functionally-oriented health care system.

If occupational therapy is to take full advantage of this opportunity, it must assure that its practitioners have a *bona fide* claim to the knowledge base underlying human performance. Heretofore, there has existed no single text in the field that focuses specifically on human performance. Other occupational therapy texts, which are largely modeled after the disease/diagnosis/intervention approach to care, address the issues of human performance either indirectly or incompletely. In contrast, this text organizes information based upon the useful person/environment/performance framework.

The central tenet of this book is that occupational therapists are concerned with overcoming performance deficits. To do this, they must first be able to identify those factors that interfere with performance, both those that are extrinsic to the individual (environmental) or those that are intrinsic (psychological or somatic). They must also be able to address performance deficits through assessment. Complete assessment of any set of performance deficits must be based on a knowledge of a wide range of factors and how those factors interfere with successful performance. This information gained from assessment leads logically to invervention. Since performance deficits have meaning only in relation to the specific occupational requirements of each individual receiving services, it is useful to organize intervention strategies by general category rather than by deficit area. Knowledge of these categories and principles is in keeping with a professional rather than technical approach to performance intervention.

This book is unique for two reasons. First, it assembles important information about occupational performance, much of which has not been found in occupational therapy textbooks before. Second, it organizes the information in a manner that avoids the ambiguity of most previous textbooks in the field, in which organization has been based partly on the medical model and partly on a social intervention model. There should be little doubt in the reader's mind that this book has been written about human performance deficits and how they can be assessed and ameliorated. In my view, it represents an important step forward in consolidating the rich and diverse knowledge base upon which we must draw for competent practice.

Wilma L. West, MA, OTR, FAOTA
President Emerita, American Occupational
Therapy Foundation
Reston, Virginia

Preface

Writing a textbook is always a difficult task. It is made infinitely more difficult if one attempts to organize information in a manner different from traditional approaches. Despite a widespread recognition of the limitations of doing so, knowledge relevant to practice in occupational therapy has continued to be viewed and disseminated according to medical taxonomies. Given that prominent information retrieval systems perpetuate such methods of classification, it is perhaps understandable why this should be so.

In this text, however, the reader will find that information has been organized around a performance-oriented framework for occupational therapy practice. Using this framework, this text analyzes the factors important to the performance of life tasks, reviews how such factors can be assessed, and presents strategies for overcoming performance deficits. No specific frame of reference used in current practice has been embraced, but rather, an attempt has been made to draw from aspects of several contemporary frames of reference as their elements are relevant to the topic under discussion.

In order to practice effectively, therapists must consider three major domains. First, they must have a knowledge of the persons they treat. Second, they must have a knowledge of the environments in which their patients or clients live or hope to live. Finally, they must have at least a basic understanding of the performance dimensions that underlie the tasks of living to be performed by the individual receiving occupational therapy services, whether these tasks are related to work, play, or self-maintenance.

These three crucial elements of person, environment, and performance, comprise the framework we have used to organize information in this text. The framework recognizes that effective intervention requires that therapists draw upon knowledge from several disciplines and conceptual frames of reference.

Because performance is a complex phenomenon involving many components, systems theory has been used as a means of explaining the relationships between the various performance elements in the framework. Moreover, because of the biosocial nature of the framework, a great deal of additional information relevant to the field has been included that traditionally has not been found in occupational therapy texts.

Section I focuses on the person/environment/performance framework and attempts to provide a transactional context within which the information presented in the book can be organized. Section II addresses the many determinants of occupational performance, ranging from physiological factors to sociocultural and political influences. Section III addresses assessment from the broadest possible perspective, and Section IV gives detailed reviews of intervention strategies.

We have assumed that persons using this text have completed those basic and clinical sciences necessary for understanding occupational therapy concepts, including anatomy, physiology, neuroanatomy, and kinesiology. We also trust that being professionally-minded, readers will avail themselves of the many references provided in each chapter and consult the recommended readings for further in-depth information. A great number of these sources are from disciplines outside the field. As a result, many of the concepts introduced in the various sections contain new material that has been missing from traditional textbooks aimed at the practice of occupational therapy.

We offer this book as a useful, and hopefully aesthetic portrait of the profession. When viewed through the eyes of the profession's scholars and master clinicians, the image revealed should be one of a defined and emerging body of knowledge organized with the intent of helping individuals overcome performance deficits related to the activities, tasks and roles required in everyday living.

During the extended development of this book, the Editors experienced many of life's significant events—two children were born, another finished college, both Editors undertook new professional roles, one Editor's family moved to Canada, and new friendships were formed. It was a great time for us. The process of preparing this book for publication was a long one. We found that there were many people with important things to say. For what they said and their patience, we thank them.

We are grateful to Wilma West for her vision, continued support and energy; to Ellie Gilfoyle for introducing us to the project and to each other; to Harry Benson for having an open mind and taking a risk; to Cheryl Willoughby for her talent and drive; to Elaine Schultz for her tenacity and kindness as a messenger; and most of all to our families who were forgiving of late night phone calls, visitors for weekends, and endless "I'm sorry, not now's."

Charles Christiansen and Carolyn Baum

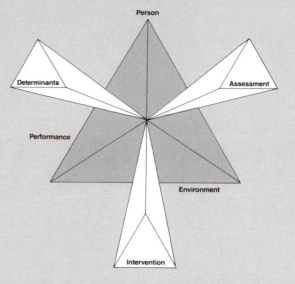

Section One

Person—Environment—Performance as a Perspective for Practice

CHAPTER CONTENT OUTLINE

KEY TERMS

Achievement

Adaptation

Autonomy

Competence

Disability

General systems theory

Handicap

Helplessness

Holistic

Impairment

Occupation

Occupational performance

Self-actualization

Skill

ABSTRACT

This chapter provides an overview of occupational therapy, beginning with the historical and philosophical ideas that formed the roots of the profession, to the present day rationale for using systems theory as an instrumental concept. The person-environment-performance framework is used as an approach for organizing practice-related information. This framework emphasizes the importance of considering the individual, the environment and the occupations relevant to an individual's life in order to understand what motivates and facilitates performance capabilities. The occupational therapy process is reviewed in terms of a problem-solving model for planning assessment and intervention. Major strategies for intervention are identified, along with basic principles of patient/client management.

Occupational Therapy
Intervention for Life Performance

Charles Christiansen

"Humans are healthy or diseased in terms of the activities or functions open to them or denied them."

—H. Tristram Englehardt, Jr., 1977

OBJECTIVES

The information in this chapter is intended to help the reader—

1. appreciate the historical and philosophical influences on contemporary occupational therapy practice.

2. define technology and science, and distinguish between the various terms used to describe conceptual tools.

3. appreciate the usefulness of general systems theory as a means for organizing concepts relevant to occupational therapy practice.

4. understand the person-environment-performance framework as an approach to viewing occupational performance.

5. review approaches for classifying occupational performance.

6. understand the complexities and challenges of a problem-solving approach for identifying performance deficits and planning effective intervention.

7. identify major categories of occupational therapy intervention and general principles for effective performance-oriented practice.

THE EVOLUTION OF AN IDENTITY

The nineteenth century Austrian philosopher Ludwig Wittgenstein once noted that "the aspects of things that are most important for us are hidden because of their simplicity and familiarity." Similarly, life satisfaction is not determined by the momentous events that make significant marks in our memories (weddings, graduations, promotions, etc.), but rather from our everyday tasks of living or occupations, which we take for granted until their accomplishment becomes difficult or improbable.

Whether the reason for a disruption in a person's ability to perform daily activities is temporary (e.g., a broken arm) or permanent (e.g., paralysis), overcoming a limitation in task performance assumes great importance. This is because life itself is defined by occupation. It is clear also that while performance deficits are frequently imposed by physical conditions, they can also result from emotional difficulties or environmental circumstances with equally devastating effect. Thus, as H. Tristram Englehardt's opening quotation for this chapter suggests, health and illness must be measured in terms of their impact on engagement in life.

Viewing health in the context of life performance has been a distinguishing characteristic of occupational therapy since its inception early in the twentieth century. While history has influenced the settings and modalities,

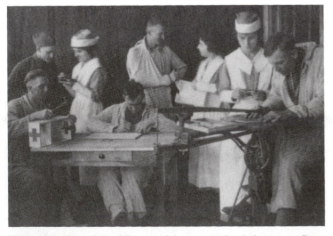

Figure 1-1. Wounded soldiers receiving occupational therapy at Camp Grant, Illinois, 1919. *From Stattel, F., Occupational therapy: A sense of the past—focus on the present. American Journal of Occupational Therapy 31 (10), 649. Copyright 1977 by the American Occupational Therapy Association. Reprinted with permission.*

occupational therapy has remained committed to its original purpose, that of helping people cope with the challenges of everyday living imposed by congenital anomalies, physical and emotional illnesses, accidents, the aging process, or environmental restrictions.

Medicine and Occupational Therapy

Occupational therapy is described as a *health* discipline rather than a *medical* discipline. This is because occupational therapy's focus on the effects of disease or injury on *everyday living* is a uniquely non-medical focus. Medicine, at least that practiced in the western hemisphere, has been traditionally organized around a mechanistic cause and effect model of scientific thought.

This view had its roots in the seventeenth century work of the French philosopher and scientist, Rene Descartes, who believed that the mind and body should be viewed as separate. He emphasized a scientific approach based on reducing structures to their component parts and subjecting the parts to careful analysis. This approach led to the development of the germ theory of disease, advanced by the work of Koch and Pasteur, which further solidified a view of medical practice based on diagnosis and treatment. Today, the idea persists that the human being, like a machine, can be taken apart and reassembled if its structure and function are sufficiently well understood. It is commonly believed that simple cause and effect relationships can be used to explain most disease processes.

It is true that this tendency to explain by reducing the body to parts, such as bones, organs, and cells, has been useful in helping medical science to explain the cause and identify the cure of many diseases and physical disorders. However, an English bioscientist, Thomas McKeown (1978) has argued convincingly that many other factors unrelated to medical intervention can also be used to explain the dramatic improvement in life expectancy over the past 150 years. Specifically, improved sanitation, nutrition, and birth control have each been identified as having played an important role in improving health status and life expectancy. Perhaps these factors are less well appreciated than "miracle drugs" or vaccines because they are behavioral rather than mechanistic in nature and thus do not fit well within the orientation of contemporary medicine.

This preoccupation with component parts is frequently referred to as *reductionism*, and is reflected in the everyday use of medical terminology. Consider the word *function*, for example. If used by an occupational therapist, function would likely describe some behavior related to task performance. However, in medicine, function is most often interpreted in its reductionistic sense in relation to the function of human organs, such as pulmonary function or liver function.

Paradoxically, the successes of reductionistic medicine have also revealed its weaknesses (Fabrega, 1975). For example, it has been noted that developments in medicine and surgery during the past 50 years have prevented the deaths of thousands of persons who were critically ill, including many casualties from both World Wars. However, a large number of these individuals were left with disabilities, such as paralysis and amputations, and required rehabilitation. West (1978) has observed that the provision of services for disabled soldiers in military and veterans hospitals, in which many occupational therapists have traditionally been employed, has played an important role in establishing some of the key principles underlying rehabilitation, thereby also influencing the development of occupational therapy.

Historical Influences of Medicine

Medicine's successes with the reductionistic approach have also influenced the history of occupational therapy practice. Over several decades beginning in the 1930s, the ideas influencing practice gradually changed. What began as a view of human function that was **holistic** and occupation-centered, changed to an emphasis on techniques and components of function, such as muscle strength, range of motion, or disturbed thought processes, with little consideration given to how these components affected performance in day-to-day living. The reductionistic influences of medicine persisted until the late 1970's, when several occupational therapy scholars published articles expressing concern for this state of affairs and encouraging a return to the occupation-centered philosophy upon which the profession was first established.

Prominent among these was Phillip Shannon. In his article entitled ''The Derailment of Occupational Therapy,'' Shannon (1977, p. 233) lamented that

'' . . . a new hypothesis has emerged that views man not as a creative being, capable of making choices and directing his own future, but as a mechanistic creature susceptible to manipulation and control via the application of techniques. The technique hypothesis, inspired by the principles of reductionism, subverts the occupational therapy hypothesis of man using his hands to influence the state of his own health .''

Later in the same year, Kielhofner and Burke (1977) provided a detailed account of various bases influencing

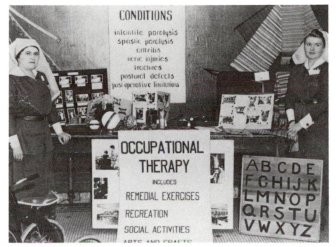

Figure 1-2. Medicine's early influence on occupational therapy is evident in this photo of an occupational therapy display at the Canadian National Exhibition, Toronto, Ontario in the early 1930's. *Photo courtesy Canadian Association of Occupational Therapists.*

practice during the first 60 years of occupational therapy in the United States. They traced the evolution of guiding principles from their humanistic roots to the competing ideas of the 1970s, noting that the paradigm of reductionism was reflected in three dominant treatment models that continued to influence practice: the kinesiological model, the psychoanalytic or interpersonal model, and the sensory integrative or neurological model.[1] The authors concluded that advancement of the field would require a theoretical approach that went ''beyond reductionism'' and allowed an understanding of human adaptation or ''social man within a holistic theoretical framework.'' (Kielhofner & Burke, 1977, p. 686).

In further emphasizing the distinction between occupational therapy and medicine, Rogers (1982a) examined the two disciplines according to their views of the concepts of order, disorder, and control. In her analysis, the concept of *order* refers to a desired state of affairs. In medicine, this is the absence of disease, but in occupational therapy order is competence in the performance of work, play, or self-care **''occupations.''** *Disorder* is defined in medicine as disease, but in occupational therapy it is seen as performance dysfunction. Since access to occupational therapy services is greatly influenced by medical decisions, individuals who experience **occupational performance** problems that are

---

1. The term *model* as used in this excerpt, refers to a framework for organizing information relevent to practice. Although the terms model, paradigm and frame of reference are often used interchangeably, they have distinct definitions, as elaborated later in this chapter. These terms should not be confused with the term *theory*, which rightly deserves more precise attention to its definition and can evolve from models, paradigms and frames of reference.

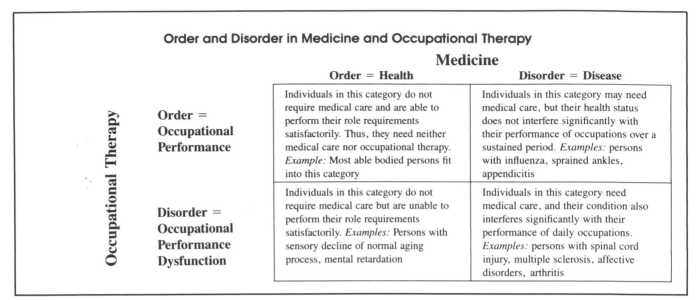

Figure 1-3. Order and Disorder in Medicine and Occupational Therapy. *Adapted from Rogers, J. (1982). Order and disorder in medicine and occupational therapy. American Journal of Occupational Therapy, 36(1), 29-35.*

not accompanied by disease, frequently have difficulty gaining access to occupational therapy services. On the other hand, there exists a category of individuals who require medical care but not occupational therapy because their conditions do not result in occupational performance dysfunction. Finally, many categories of illness and disease can result in impairment which influences performance. According to Rogers, persons in this category constitute the group for whom occupational therapy services are most likely to be provided (See Figure 1-3). In her comparative analysis, Rogers argued convincingly that the biomedical influences on traditional health care have been a limiting factor in the development of occupational therapy because of their emphasis on disease and functional deficit rather than emphasis on occupational performance and competence.

Philosophical Influences on Practice

The values, beliefs, and principles of a discipline have a major influence on its identity and development, and are known collectively as its philosophy. Shannon (1986) points out that philosophical issues fall into three dimensions: (1) those that address the nature of humankind (metaphysics), (2) the process by which we come to know (epistemology), and (3) values (axiology), which include beliefs about what is desirable and how we should conduct ourselves.

Bockhoven (1971) and others have argued that the philosophical roots of occupational therapy practice can be traced to the moral treatment movement reflected in practices of some early nineteenth century mental hospitals. These approaches were designed to promote accommodation or **adaptation** through involving patients[2] in various activities which would promote the establishment of cultural values and mores.

Adolph Meyer, a neuropathologist who taught at Johns Hopkins University and a proponent of occupational therapy during its early years, is credited widely for having made the most important contribution to the development of a philosophy for the field. In an address given at the fifth annual meeting of the National Society for the Promotion of Occupation Therapy in 1921 in Baltimore, Meyer suggested (1922, p. 6) that occupational therapy represented an important manifestation of human philosophy, namely "the valuation of time and work" and the role of performance and completion in bringing meaning to life.

Meyer wrote that *"man learns to organize time and he does it in terms of doing things,"* thus emphasizing his view of the importance of doing to achieving self-fulfillment. Elsewhere in his address, Meyer suggested that the view of mental illness as a problem of living rather than a structural, toxic, or constitutional disorder, was an important characteristic of the field, and that occupational therapists could

---

2. Throughout this chapter, the term *patient* or *individual* is used in preference to the term *client*. While it is recognized that for therapists working in some settings (such as public schools), use of the term patient can seem inappropriate; Reilly (1984) and Yerxa & Sharrot (1985) have argued convincingly that retention of the term "patient" is an ethical issue, since its use reflects many of the basic values upon which the profession was founded.

provide opportunities "*. . . to work, to do and to plan and create, and to learn to use material.*" Meyer thought such opportunities would assist patients in gaining pleasure and pride in achievement. He said, "*Performance and completion form also the backbone and essence of what Pierre Janet has so well described as the 'fonction du real'—the realization of reality, bringing the very soul of man out of dreams of eternity to the full sense and appreciation of actuality.*"

In summarizing Meyer's address, we can observe that he viewed the individual and health in a holistic rather than structural sense and believed that engagement in occupations or doing provided a sense of reality, **achievement**, and temporal organization. Meyer perceived occupational therapy as providing opportunities for engagement which would contribute to learning and improve one's sense of fulfillment and self-esteem. In doing so, he was proclaiming occupational therapy's concern for quality of life and suggesting a clear relationship between our ability to perform daily occupations and our life satisfaction.

Meyer's themes have been repeated in more recent contributions by scholars reflecting on the unique characteristics of the field. For example, Yerxa (1967) in her Eleanor Clarke Slagle address, emphasized the role of occupational therapy in providing opportunities for fulfillment in doing when she wrote:

"In occupational therapy, the patient experiences the reality of his physical environment and his capacity to function within it. Our clinics may be chambers of horror for some individuals as they confront their physical disability for the first time by trying to do something, perhaps as simple as self-feeding. Yet, if the individual is to function with self actualization, he must discover both his limitations and his possibilities. We meet our responsibilities to the client when we provide him with opportunities to readjust his value system through the development of both new capacities and the ability to substitute for some lost capacities. We are like mirrors which can reflect, without the distortion of wish-fulfillment or self-deprecation, a true image of the client's potential" (p. 5).

Fidler and Fidler (1978) also emphasized the role of occupation or doing in gaining **self-actualization**:

"The ability to adapt, to cope with the problems of everyday living, and to fulfill age-specific life roles requires a rich reservoir of experiences gathered from direct engagement with both human and non-human objects in one's environment. Doing is a process of investigating, trying out, and gaining evidence of one's capacities for experiencing, responding, managing, creating, and controlling. It is through such action with feedback from both non-human and human objects that an individual comes to know the potential and limitations of self and the environment and

achieves a sense of competence and intrinsic worth" (p. 306).

While both Yerxa and the Fidlers reaffirmed Meyer's beliefs and values that occupational therapy affords opportunities for self-actualization, they also emphasized the role of the therapist in assisting the individual to cope with problems of everyday living and to adapt to limitations that interfere with competent role performance.

These philosophical cornerstones of practice must also be viewed in the wider context of important cultural values. For example, Americans have tended to value activity and self-reliance over passivity and dependence. Bockhoven (1971) points out that moral treatment was influenced by cultural attitudes of communities in the Northeastern United States in the early nineteenth century. An important characteristic of this culture, derived from political and religious beliefs, was a respect for human individuality and rights of independent self-expression. To be sure, the widespread belief in the virtues of independence and self-reliance continue within Western cultures. Perhaps because of this, there has been support for goals of rehabilitation when

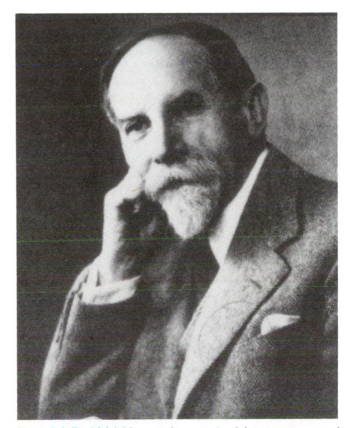

Figure 1-4. Dr. Adolph Meyer, early occupational therapy proponent and philosopher. (Fabian Bachrach Photo.) *Courtesy of the Archives of the American Psychiatric Association.*

Views of Occupational Therapy as Reflected in Definitions of Practice

YEAR	DEFINITION	SOURCE
1922	Any activity, mental or physical, definitely prescribed and guided for the distinct purpose of contributing to, and hastening recovery from disease or injury.	Pattison, H.A. (1922). The trend of occupational therapy for tuberculosis. *Archives of Occupational Therapy, 1,* 19-24.
1947	Any activity, mental or physical, medically prescribed and professionally guided to aid a patient in recovery from disease or injury.	McNary, H. (1947). The scope of occupational therapy. In Willard, H.S. and Spackman, C.S. (Eds.). *Occupational therapy.* Philadelphia, J.B. Lippincott, p.10
1962	Occupational therapy is the art and science of directing man's response to selected activity to promote and maintain health, to prevent disability, to evaluate behavior and to treat or train patients with physical or psychosocial dysfunction.	Official definition adopted by the Executive Board of the American Occupational Therapy Association, January, 1969.
1972	The art and science of directing man's participation in selected tasks to restore, reinforce, and enhance performance, facilitate learning of the skills and functions essential for adaptation and productivity, diminish or correct pathology, and to promote and maintain health.	Council of Standards, AOTA. (1972). Occupational Therapy: Its definition and functions. *American Journal of Occupational Therapy, 26,* 204-5.
1977	Occupational therapy is the application of occupation, any activity in which one engages for evaluation, diagnosis, and treatment of problems interfering with functional performance in persons impaired by physical illness or injury, emotional disorder, congenital or developmental disability, or the aging process in order to achieve optimum functioning and for prevention and health maintenance.	AOTA Representative Assembly: Minutes. (1977). *American Journal of Occupational Therapy, 31,* 599.
1981	Occupational therapy is the use of purposeful activity with individuals who are limited by physical injury or illness, psychosocial dysfunction, developmental or learning disabilities, poverty and cultural differences, or the aging process in order to maximize independence, prevent disability, and maintain health. The practice encompasses evaluation, treatment and consultation. Specific occupational therapy services include: teaching daily living skills, developing perceptual motor skills and sensory integrative functioning, developing play skills and prevocational and leisure capacities; designing and fabricating or applying selected orthotic and prosthetic devices and equipment; using specifically designed crafts and exercises to enable functional performance; administering and interpreting tests such as manual muscle and range of motion; and adapting environments for the handicapped. These services are provided individually, in groups, or through social systems.	Official Definition for Licensure. (1981). Adopted by the AOTA Representative Assembly. *American Journal of Occupational Therapy, 35,* 798.
1986	Therapeutic use of self-care work and play activities to increase independent function, enhance development, and prevent disability. May include adaptation of task or environment to achieve maximum independence and to enhance the quality of life.	AOTA. (1986). Representative assembly, Minutes. *American Journal of Occupational Therapy, 40,* 852.

Figure 1-5. Views of Occupational Therapy as Reflected in Definitions of Practice.

expressed in terms of increasing the patient's independence. As a rehabilitation discipline, occupational therapy has also inculcated this value, as reflected in some definitions of the field. See Figure 1-5.

Rogers (1982b) has maintained that "functional independence is not just a core concept of occupational therapy theory, it is the goal of the occupational therapy process." Noting that the requirements for independence are **competence** and **autonomy,** she suggested that autonomy is reflected in the ability to make choices and have control over the environment. The opportunities afforded within occupational therapy practice for developing competence and teaching strategies for exerting autonomy make it unique among the rehabilitation disciplines.

This uniqueness led Englehardt, a physician and philosopher, to describe occupational therapy as reflecting a "praxial," rather than a somatic, psychological, or even social work model of practice. Praxial, derived from the Greek word praxis meaning an action or transaction, connotes the adaptive nature of engagement in occupations. Englehardt noted that:

> "In viewing humans as engaged in activities, realizing themselves through their occupation, occupational therapy supports a view of the whole person in function and adaptation often absent in somatic medicine, the psychological health care professions, and social work as well. The virtue of occupational therapy is engagement in the world" (p. 672).

Thus in summary, we can list the following as the important beliefs and values which continue to influence occupational therapy practice:

1. Engagement in occupation is of value because it provides opportunities for individuals to influence their well-being by gaining fulfillment in living.
2. Through the experience of occupation or doing, the individual is able to achieve mastery and competence by learning skills and strategies necessary for coping with problems and adapting to limitations.
3. As competence is gained and autonomy can be expressed, independence is achieved.
4. Autonomy implies choice and control over environmental circumstances, thus opportunities for exerting self-determination should be reflected in intervention strategies.
5. An individual's choice and control extend to decisions about intervention, thus occupational therapy is identified as a collaborative process between the therapist and recipient of care, whose values are respected.
6. Because of occupational therapy's focus on life performance, it is neither somatic, nor psychological, but concerned with the unity of body and mind in doing.

Early Occupational Therapy Leader
Eleanor Clarke Slagle
1876-1942

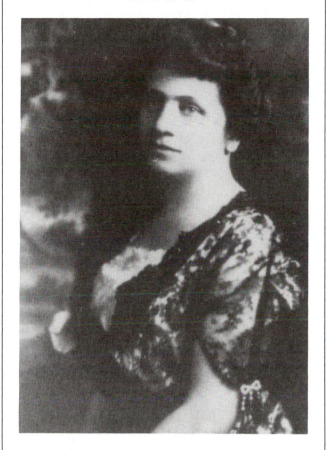

Figure 1-6. Eleanor Clarke Slagle: 1876-1942, the daughter of a prominent architect, was a founder of the Society for the Promotion of Occupation Therapy, now known as the American Occupational Therapy Association (AOTA). As an associate of Adolph Meyer and William Rush Dunton, she developed an appreciation for the importance of occupation to health and well-being, and served as the founding director for the Henry P. Favill School of Occupations in Chicago, the first organized school for occupational therapists in the United States. Later, she became the Director of Occupational Therapy for the New York State Department of Mental Hygiene, a position she held from 1921 until 1942. A strong leader and organizing influence of the AOTA, Mrs. Slagle was named honorary president in 1937 at a ceremony attended by Eleanor Roosevelt. Today, her legacy of strong leadership and devotion to challenge lives on in the Eleanor Clarke Slagle lectureship, one of the most prestigious honors awarded by the American Occupational Therapy Association. *From Bing, RK, Eleanor Clarke Slagle lectureship— 1981—Occupational Therapy revisited: a paraphrastic journey. American Journal of Occupational Therapy, 35(8), 511. Copyright 1981 by the American Occupational Therapy Association. Reprinted with permission.*

Occupational Therapy Code of Ethics: American Occupational Therapy Association (AOTA)

The American Occupational Therapy Association and its component members are committed to furthering people's abilities to function fully within their total environments. To this end the occupational therapist renders service to clients in all stages of health and illness, to institutions, to other professionals and colleagues, to students, and to the general public.

In furthering this commitment, the American Occupational Therapy Association has established the Occupational Therapy Code of Ethics. This code is intended to be used as a guide to promoting and maintaining the highest standards of ethical behavior.

This Code of Ethics shall apply to all occupational therapy personnel. The term *occupational therapy personnel* shall include individuals who are registered occupational therapists, certified occupational therapy assistants, and occupational therapy students. The roles of practitioner, educator, manager, researcher, and consultant are assumed.

Principle 1 (Beneficence/Autonomy)

Occupational therapy personnel shall demonstrate a concern for the welfare and dignity of the recipient of their services.

A. The individual is responsible for providing services without regard to race, creed, national origin, sex, age, handicap, disease entity, social status, financial status, or religious affiliation.

B. The individual shall inform those people served of the nature and potential outcomes of treatment and shall respect the right of potential recipients of service to refuse treatment.

C. The individual shall inform subjects involved in education or research activities of the potential outcome of those activities.

D. The individual shall include those people served in the treatment planning process.

E. The individual shall maintain goal-directed and objective relationships with all people served.

F. The individual shall protect the confidential nature of information gained from educational, practice, and investigational activities unless sharing such information could be deemed necessary to protect the well-being of a third party.

G. The individual shall take all reasonable precautions to avoid harm to the recipient of services or detriment to the recipient's property.

H. The individual shall establish fees, based on cost analysis, that are commensurate with services rendered.

Principle 2 (Competence)

Occupational therapy personnel shall actively maintain high standards of professional competence.

A. The individual shall hold the appropriate credential for providing service.

B. The individual shall recognize the need for competence and shall participate in continuing professional development.

C. The individual shall function within the parameters of his or her competence and the standards of the profession.

D. The individual shall refer clients to other service providers or consult with other service providers when additional knowledge and expertise is required.

Principle 3 (Compliance With Laws and Regulations)

Occupational therapy personnel shall comply with laws and Association policies guiding the profession of occupational therapy.

A. The individual shall be acquainted with applicable local, state, federal, and institutional rules and Association policies and shall function accordingly.

B. The individual shall inform employers, employees, and colleagues about those laws and policies that apply to the profession of occupational therapy.

C. The individual shall require those whom they supervise to adhere to the Code of Ethics.

D. The individual shall accurately record and report information.

Principle 4 (Public Information)

Occupational therapy personnel shall provide accurate information concerning occupational therapy services.

A. The individual shall accurately represent his or her competence and training.

B. The individual shall not use or participate in the use of any form of communication that contains a false, fraudulent, deceptive, or unfair statement or claim.

Principle 5 (Professional Relationships)

Occupational therapy personnel shall function with discretion and integrity in relations with colleagues and other professionals, and shall be concerned with the quality of their services.

A. The individual shall report illegal, incompetent, and/or unethical practice to the appropriate authority.

B. The individual shall not disclose privileged information when participating in reviews of peers, programs, or systems.

C. The individual who employs or supervises colleagues shall provide appropriate supervision, as defined in AOTA guidelines or state laws, regulations, and institutional policies.

D. The individual shall recognize the contributions of colleagues when disseminating professional information.

Principle 6 (Professional Conduct)

Occupational therapy personnel shall not engage in any form of conduct that constitutes a conflict of interest or that adversely reflects on the profession.

Figure 1-8. Occupational Therapy Code of Ethics. This document was approved by the Representative Assembly of the AOTA in April 1988; it replaces the (1977/1979) "Principles of Occupational Therapy Ethics." (See Appendix F for the ethics approved by the Canadian Association of Occupational Therapists. *From AOTA, Occupational Therapy Code of Ethics, American Journal of Occupational Therapy, 42(12), 795-796. Copyright 1988 by The American Occupational Therapy Association, Inc. Reprinted with permission.*

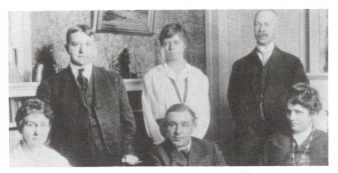

Figure 1-7. Founders of the American Occupational Therapy Association pictured in 1917. *Front row:* (L-R) Susan C. Johnson, George E. Barton, Eleanor Clarke Slagle. *Back row:* William R. Dunton, Jr., Isabel G. Newton, Thomas B. Kidner. *From Stattel, F, Occupational therapy: sense of the past—Focus on the present. Photo courtesy Archives of the American Occupational Therapy Association. Reprinted with permission.*

Reflecting Philosophical Values in Practice: Occupational Therapy Ethics

Ethics are philosophical stands on the rightness or appropriateness of various voluntary actions. The ethics of a profession flow from its philosophical underpinnings. The adoption of ethical principles is one characteristic often used to distinguish professions from other occupations.

Ethical principles form the basis for judgments and actions in practice. In acknowledging this, Rogers (1983) writes: ''The ultimate question we, as clinicians, are challenged to answer is: What, among the many things that could be done for this patient, ought to be done? This is an ethical question.'' (p. 602).

This view has been substantiated by Hansen (1984, 1988) who studied the ethical dilemmas faced by occupational therapists in their daily practice. She found that deciding which type of treatment would be most effective was the most common dilemma. Other common ethical dilemmas faced by therapists included deciding whether to receive and act on referrals that are inappropriate, being unable to provide adequate therapy because of constraints in the work setting, and resolving disagreements between the therapist and patient or patient and family regarding treatment goals.

These ethical dilemmas are not unlike those being experienced in other rehabilitation professions. Caplan and associates (1987) have noted that pressures for cost containment and changes in public attitudes toward disability have contributed to an increased interest in ethical issues surrounding rehabilitation practices. Relationships among caregivers, patients, and families are frequently complicated by difficult choices which concern the need to balance efficiency and accountability with a concern for maintaining patient autonomy and quality of life. As these difficult situations continue to affect practice, the benefit of having principles to guide behavior becomes more apparent.

The most recent (1988) ethical document approved by the American Occupational Therapy Association identifies six principles of ethical responsibility ranging from concern for the welfare and dignity of the recipient of service to avoiding conflicts of interest (See Figure 1-8). Ethical principles have meaning only to the extent that they are reflected in the day-to-day practices of those who subscribe to them. However, ethical practices serve not only to guide professional behavior, but also as an important source of continuity of professional ideals, since they embody the philosophical values of the profession.

CONCEPTUAL SYSTEMS FOR GUIDING PRACTICE

While philosophical values and beliefs have an important and enduring influence on a profession's activities, they are not a sufficient basis for practice. There must also be systems for generating, organizing, and applying knowledge that is useful to practice.

Knowledge about the nature of things is typically derived from scientific *disciplines* in the form of theories. These abstract truths about nature may or may not be useful to scientific *professions*, which are concerned with the application of knowledge to the conditions in the real world. Occupational therapy is a scientific profession which draws much of its knowledge from other scientific disciplines and applies it in day-to-day practice.

Technology and Science

Before proceeding with our discussion, it is important to distinguish between science and *technology*. Most scholars would agree that technology constitutes the procedures and products that are developed to deal with real world problems. Thus, examples of the technology of occupational therapy would include neuromuscular facilitation techniques as well as adaptive devices. *Science*, on the other hand, consists of pure knowledge derived from theory in the scientific disciplines for the purposes of explanation and prediction. Many examples of scientific knowledge used regularly in occupational therapy can be provided from anatomy, physiology, and psychology.

Not all technology is derived from science. Some procedures and techniques in occupational therapy and other practice disciplines emanate from trial and error, observation and intuition, and chance occurrences. One unfortunate example of this was the wide use of electroconvulsive therapy (known to the general public as shock therapy), a technique which was not derived from science. Henderson (1988) argues that the aim of research in a profession is to increase the proportion of technology

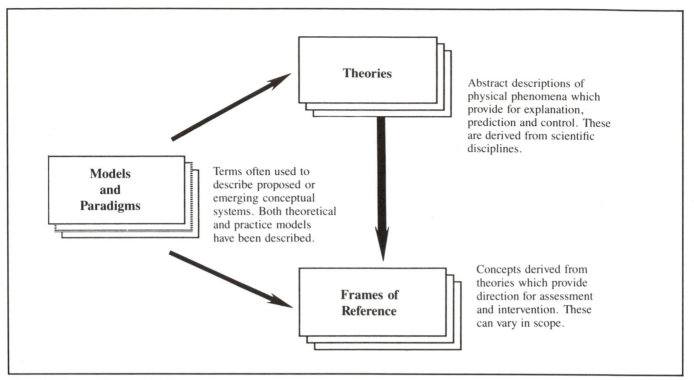

Figure 1-9. Types of Conceptual Tools.

derived from science or scientific methods, and thus decrease the number of techniques and procedures which are not scientifically derived.

It can be argued that because of the history and nature of the field, nearly all of the unique knowledge generated in occupational therapy has been devoted to technology. In recent years, however, there has been growing concern about the need for development of a science for occupational therapy, from which theoretical knowledge about the nature of human occupation would emanate (AOTA, 1987; Christiansen, 1981, 1986; Mosey, 1985; Tanguay, 1985; Yerxa, 1983, 1987).

Theories, Models, and Frames of Reference

A review of the scholarly literature in occupational therapy quickly will reveal that there is little agreement among writers about how to describe organized knowledge in the field. The terms *theory, model, frame of reference,* and *paradigm* have been variously used to describe subsets of the profession's knowledge. Parham (1987) describes theory as a "tool for thinking." This apt description applies equally well to the other terms listed. However, while each of the terms describes a conceptual tool, they should not be viewed as interchangeable. In fact, as suggested by Reed (1984), they can be viewed in a hierarchy as reflected in Figure 1-9.

Theories are principles and statements of relationship which permit prediction of phenomena under specified circumstances. Theories are usually thought to be the product of scientific disciplines in their attempt to explain natural phenomena.

Paradigms are often described as new ideas or novel ways of thinking about old problems. The term paradigm has been made popular by the work of Thomas Kuhn, who described them in the context of the emergence of controversial new ideas in science which often meet with resistance from those holding established views. According to Kuhn (1970), the struggle between old and new paradigms can be likened to scientific revolutions.

The term *model* refers to any of a variety of ways of structuring or organizing knowledge for the purpose of guiding thinking. Models differ in their scope and level of abstraction, but share a common purpose of helping us analyze situations, determine methodologies, or conceive alternatives. In this way, they can be useful in building theories.

Frames of reference can be viewed as those portions of models which are methodological in focus. As described by Mosey (1985, 1989) *frames of reference* are appropriately viewed as mechanisms for linking theory to practice. There are many frames of reference in occupational therapy which vary widely in their scope and utility. Mosey (1989) has suggested that in order to be maximally useful, frames of reference should provide the following: (1) information on their domain of concern, (2) the theories upon which their assertions are based, (3) the nature of function and dysfunction, (4) behaviors which reflect these states, and (5) the principles regarding intervention or how one can change from a dysfunctional to a functional state.

Figure 1-10 provides an overview of selected frames of reference which guide occupational therapy practice and have been developed from within the field. No attempt has been made here to be comprehensive, since individual elements of these frames of reference, particularly assessment and intervention approaches, are introduced and addressed throughout the text. Some of these frames of reference, which serve as the basis for selected intervention strategies, emanated from other professions. Examples include the psychoanalytic and behavioral frames of reference, which are addressed, as appropriate, in later sections. The reader is encouraged to consult the many excellent references which elaborate the bases for these various frames of reference, many of which are identified in the recommended readings section at the end of the chapter.

Over the years, several writers have proposed that occupational therapy should adopt a single conceptual framework which is broad enough to provide a basis for unifying the diverse elements of practice (Christiansen, 1981, 1990; Howe and Briggs, 1982; Kielhofner, 1982; King, 1978, Llorens, 1976; Reilly, 1966). However, Mosey (1985) contends that the profession has a tradition of multiple frames of reference (*pluralism*), and therefore the selection of one unifying framework (*monism*) could be unnecessarily restrictive.

Contemporary Frames of Reference

Occupational therapy draws its knowledge from many sciences, thus it is not surprising that many frames of reference guide its practice. These frames of reference vary in scope and development. However, if they are to be used in practice, they should be consistent with the philosophical assumptions of the profession.

To the student, beginning therapist, and outside observer, the multiple frames of reference and broad scope of practice in occupational therapy are often viewed as confusing. This complexity of practice has been identified as one reason why some reductionistic approaches to treatment persist in occupational therapy clinics. By reducing complex problems into simpler parts which can be controlled or more readily understood, an illusion of mastery is achieved. But the cost of the illusion is dear. When complex therapeutic problems are oversimplified, the goals of occupational therapy are seldom attained, and individuals are not helped to attain the levels of performance necessary to gain a sense

of competence and satisfaction within their unique environmental contexts.

Yerxa has described this tendency to oversimplify in occupational therapy as "the hobgoblin" of theory and practice and recommends that, "An essential quality of occupational therapy needs to be made more visible to the eye. That quality is the complexity of occupational therapy practice and the knowledge upon which it is based" (1988, p. 2). Yerxa suggests that viewing the person as a hierarchically-arranged, complex open system with interrelated levels of function can assist the therapist in understanding the complexities of occupational therapy practice. This view of the person requires an understanding of **general systems theory**[3] which is a manner of thinking about natural phenomena that will be discussed in the following section.

SYSTEMS THEORY AS AN INSTRUMENTAL CONCEPT

General systems theory can best be described as a means for organizing seemingly disparate categories and levels of information. It is useful to describe the systems perspective as a means of looking at the same phenomenon from several different perspectives simultaneously. (Berrien, 1968; von Bertalanffy, 1968).

A system can be described as a whole consisting of numerous interdependent and related parts. Systems have important properties which make them different from other entities. For example, if the organization of a system's parts or subcomponents is altered, the function of the system will change, even though the components remain unchanged. Conversely, subcomponents can be replaced with similar elements without altering the system's function.

Each living system can be viewed as a component (or subsystem) of a yet larger system. For example, the liver is composed of cellular components and is a system; but it is a subsystem of the human body, which can be viewed as a subsystem of some social group. As one moves up this hierarchy of living systems, greater complexity is found, and with that complexity a greater flexibility is found in the system's response to environmental change. (See Figure 1-11.)

Open Systems

Living systems are open systems. Open systems can exist only if they maintain certain kinds of transactions with their environment that produce changes in the systems themselves

---

3. Reilly (1969) and Kielhofner (1977) deserve extraordinary credit for drawing the attention of the field to the importance of general systems theory in organizing the complexities of occupational therapy practice.

Summary of Selected Frames of Reference

PRINCIPAL AUTHOR(S)	FRAME OF REFERENCE	WHAT IS THE NATURE OF THERAPY?	FOR WHOM IS IT DONE?	WHAT IS THE EXPECTED OUTCOME?
Allen, Claudia	Cognition & Activity	Providing activity compensations	Physically and cognitively impaired persons	To improve performance in requested activities
Ayres, A. Jean	Sensory Integration	Eliciting adaptive responses	Persons with neurophysiological deficits	To improve sensory integrative function, performance
Gilfoyle, Elnora & Grady, Ann	Spatio-temporal Adaptation	Using activities to develop sensorimotor skills.	Children with developmental deficits	To improve independent functioning, adapatation
Kielhofner, Gary & Burke, Janice	Human Occupation	Providing opportunities for directed experiences (participation in life tasks)	Persons with occupational dysfunction	To improve organization, function, and adaptation, as reflected in occupational performance
King, Lorna J.	Adaptive Responses	Eliciting adaptive responses	Persons with developmental or life challenges, impairment	To permit functional patterns that meet life's demands
Llorens, Lela	Facilitating Growth & Development	Facilitating mastery of developmental tasks or stages	Persons with developmental deficits	To permit mastery of developmental requirements
Mosey, Anne	Role Acquisition	Using activities and relationships to learn role skills	Persons in role transition or those with unmet role requirements	To acquire competence in social roles
Reilly, Mary	Occupational Behavior	Using occupation to promote life satisfaction	Persons for whom attainment of competence is thwarted by disease or injury	To permit successful role performance

Figure 1-10. Summary of Selected Frames of Reference.

Summary of Selected Frames of Reference *(continued)*

HOW IS THE PURPOSE ACHIEVED?	SELECTED MAJOR IDEAS	MAJOR REFERENCE(S)
Through evaluation, activity analysis, modification, and treatment of underlying factors	• Activity analysis consists of identifying the physical and/or cognitive abilities required to improve performance in the requested activities. • Therapists compensate for disability by removing obstacles to satisfactory performance and by using the person's available capacities.	Allen, C. (1987). Activity: occupational therapy's treatment method. *AJOT, 41,* 563-575.
Controlled sensory input	• Controlled sensory input can elicit an adaptive response. • Adaptive responses require that sensation be organized, situations be appraised accurately and responses be executed competently. • Situations which combine challenge with success are most therapeutic.	Ayres, A.J. (1979) *Sensory Integration and the Child.* Los Angeles: Western Psychological Services
Via movement patterns which require new responses	• Movement puts children in a relationship with their surroundings, providing opportunities for interaction and perception during goal accomplishment. • Environmental challenges present stress situations, which require linking of lower level functions to purposes of new experiences. • Adaptation spirals through primitive, transitional and mature phases of development	Gilfoyle, E. & Grady, A. (1989). *Children Adapt.* (2nd Edition). Thorofare, NJ: Slack.
Through changes in self-image, skill development, new habits, acquired roles and environmental changes.	• Human occupation is governed by three subsystems which influence occupation: volition, habituation, and performance. • Occupation is central to human adaptation. Therefore its absence or disruption is a threat to health and well-being. • Guided participation in life tasks influences the integrity and organization of structures and functions in the individual.	Kielhofner, G. & Burke, J. (1980). A model of human occupation: Framework and content. *AJOT, 34,* 572-581
Through graded, purposeful activity	• The adult nervous system is capable of change. • Adaptive responses are most efficiently organized at the subcortical level, and when elicited, are self-reinforcing. • Activities used in occupational therapy should require an active response by the patient, based on a specific environmental demand. • Purposeful activity can facilitate development of more normal neurological patterns.	King, L.J. (1978). Toward a science of adaptive response. *AJOT, 32* 429-436.
Through skilled application of carefully selected tasks, activities, and relationships	• Individuals develop simultaneously in the areas of neurophysiological, physical, psychosocial, and psychodynamic growth and mature in these areas as they age. • Mastery of skills and abilities and relationships is necessary for achieving satisfactory coping behavior and adaptive relationships. • Physical and psychological trauma can interrupt the developmental process.	Llorens, L.A. (1976). *Application of developmental theory for health and rehabilitation.* Rockville, MD: AOTA
Through learning the task skills and interpersonal skills necessary for social roles and temporal adaptation	• Individuals have an inherent need to explore the environment. From this need arises a desire to be competent and exert mastery. • Successful adaptation implies skillful role performances in a variety of roles, including family interaction, ADL, play, recreation and leisure, and work.	Mosey, A.C. (1986). *Psychosocial components of occupational therapy.* New York: Raven Press
Active engagement in tasks that will develop work skills for life roles	• Humans have a need to master their environments and occupation is vital to this mastery. • Mastery occurs primarily through the continuum of play and work. Play is the practice arena for work. • Through the continuum of work and play, individuals learn the roles needed to become competent in mastery.	Reilly, M. (1974). *Play as exploratory learning.* Los Angeles: Sage.

Figure 1-10. (Continued).

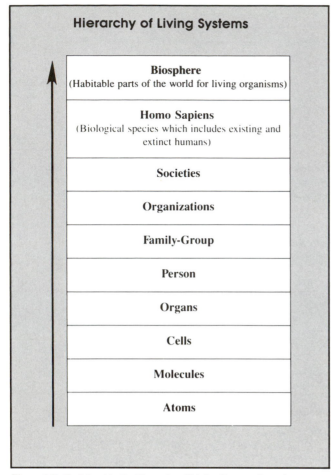

Figure 1-11. Each level in the Hierarchy of Living Systems is a subsystem or component of the next higher level with increasing complexity as one ascends the hierarchy.

and the environment. Because of this relationship with the environment, the subsystems of an open system are constantly processing energy and information.

One characteristic of the human system that distinguishes it from lower level living systems is its capacity to reflect. This unique capacity allows us to delay our responses to events requiring action; to think, evaluate, and choose a course of action. Through this ability, we are able to shape our future through behaviors that are carefully considered and self-directed.

Disruption and Resonation

It should be clear that because of the hierarchical and interdependent characteristics of systems, a disruption at one level affects other system levels or components. Moss (1973) refers to this tendency for disruption and change to affect all components of an open system as *resonation*. In the human, this concept can be understood readily using a widely known disease process, rheumatoid arthritis. The

inflamed joints and pain characteristic of arthritis can easily result in a reduced level of activity. This illustrates how a component of a system (the joints) can affect the functioning of the system as a whole (the human organism). To illustrate the concept further, reduced levels of activity, in turn, can affect metabolism, resulting in weight gain. Other systems, such as the heart and lungs, are now affected since they must work harder and the person tends to reduce activities further because energy is diminished. Since many of these activities typically involve other people, social interaction is reduced.

While there can be numerous other consequences of arthritis, these examples illustrate that disruptions can impact components at the same level or at higher and lower levels of the systems hierarchy. This makes it a particularly good example of a disease process which must be viewed in a systems context in order to be fully understood in terms of its impact on the individual. Unfortunately, arthritis is often viewed only in terms of its physiological consequences in producing pain or limiting joint motion.

Some Principles of System Dynamics

Returning to the discussion of systems, it is important to review some principles which describe the relationships of system components (subsystems) with each other. One important characteristic of an open system is its hierarchy of structures and functions, which means that some components or subsystems are governed by others. Thus, higher order systems may determine if and when a lower order system functions, but at the same time can be limited by those functions.

An example here may help illustrate the relationships described. If a man chooses not to wear a necktie, it does not matter that he has the bilateral muscular coordination or ability to fashion the knot. The tie will not be worn because a higher order systems component (motivation) governs a lower system (muscles and nerves comprising the neuromotor system). However, if the man desires to wear a necktie, the presence of motor incoordination may constrain the end result and require the man to wear a pre-knotted tie. The limiting effects of lower systems and the governing effects of higher order systems are sometimes referred to respectively as *constraining* and *commanding* (Weiss, 1971).

It has been observed that living systems, as open systems, must interact with their environments in order to survive. The constant flow of matter, energy, and information being exchanged between open systems and their surroundings occurs as a cycle and requires that open systems continually change or adapt to different conditions. It is this property of living systems that underlies the ''systems view'' of health, which has been defined as *''the ability of a system to respond adaptively to a wide array of environmental challenges''* (Brody & Sobel, 1979, p. 93). The late Rene Dubos (1965) was a particularly articulate spokesperson for this point of view.

Person-Environment Transactions

The interplay between the human organism (as an open system) and its environment can be described as a transaction. Transactions between individuals and their surroundings occur at multiple levels of the system's hierarchy as information (or energy) is fed into the system (input), processed (throughput), and output. At the level of the individual, output takes the form of behavior, the results of which influence the cycle through a feedback loop. This feedback portion of the cycle consists of information about one's performance which has been derived from the self and others (Figure 1-12).

It is within the context of performance transactions that individuals, as open systems, encounter the objects, people, conditions, and events which provide for development or maturation. Although change is not always grossly apparent, experiences accumulate which reinforce or modify individual characteristics (Kielhofner, 1985, p. 41). Over time, changes become more evident, although the overall trend may be characterized by periods of varying organization or advancement. As the life cycle progresses, the desired course is one of greater satisfaction within one's environmental circumstances and an increasing sense of fulfillment through life's activities.

Performance is described as a *transaction* because individuals and their environments influence each other in a reciprocal manner.[4] Transaction is the term suggested by Dewey and Bentley (1949) for processes involving object relationships within a system and has been traditionally used by scientists using the transactional model for several decades. The use of the term *transaction* not only suggests mutual influence, but implies a dynamic situation in which individuals alter their performance based on their perceptions of changing conditions in the environment.

A daily routine may help to illustrate this point. While the morning task of dressing is almost habitual for most of us, it is undoubtedly influenced by our expectations of environmental encounter each day. For example, we select our best clothes if we anticipate having lunch with the boss. If we have houseguests, we might alter our usual morning habit of putting on the ragged old robe and wear something else that will give a more favorable impression. In either case, our behavior has been changed as the result of changes

---

4. As we discussed, the individual is a component of a larger system in a potentially infinite hierarchy. Thus, the distinction between the individual and the environment is a convenient abstraction, since one is a subsystem of the other. Technically, to speak of a person-environment transaction is to describe relationships which occur between hierarchical levels of systems. As Llorens (1984) noted succinctly, ''the individual is the first level environment'' (p. 29).

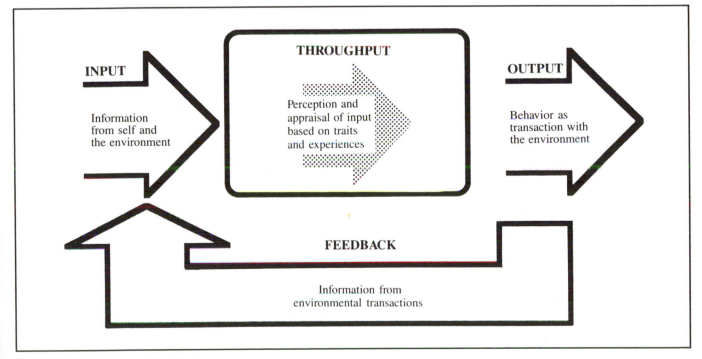

Figure 1-12. The Human as an Open System.

in our environment and our perception of the meaning of those changes as they affect our well-being.

People spend most of their waking hours engaged in occupations that include productive and leisure pursuits. Thus, to speak of performance in an occupational context is to refer to occupational performance. Viewing *occupational performance* as a transaction between the individual as an open system and the environment provides a useful framework for viewing occupational therapy practice. Consistent with West's (1984) recommendation, this approach defines occupational therapy's domain of concern as occupational performance dysfunction, and reaffirms its commitment to what she eloquently describes as the ''mind-body environment interrelationships activated through occupation'' (p. 22). In this volume, we will refer to this approach as the *Person-Environment-Performance Framework*.

PERSON-ENVIRONMENT-PERFORMANCE AS A CONCEPTUAL FRAMEWORK FOR PRACTICE

Organizing knowledge for occupational therapy practice using a person-environment-performance framework offers several advantages over less complete and reductionistic approaches. (1) It facilitates consideration of the multiple factors that influence occupational performance, including the characteristics of individuals, the unique environments in which they function, and the nature and meaning of the activities, tasks and roles they perform. (2) It permits assimilation of existing technologies in practice within a framework that is conceptually sound and readily understood. (3) It reflects an established framework for viewing and studying human behavior within the social sciences, which facilitates the importing of information from other professions and disciplines.

The major ideas underlying the person-environment performance framework are not new. It embraces concepts that are included in models proposed by Howe and Briggs (1982), Clark (1979a, 1979b), Kielhofner and Burke (1980), and Reed (1984). It also includes concepts addressed by Engel (1977), Mosey (1974, 1985), and Reilly (1974). These major ideas are as follows:

1. Performance is the result of complex relationships between the individual as an open system and the specific environments in which tasks and roles occur,
2. Stages of development influence motivation, skills and roles, and thus affect occupational performance,
3. Performance is a biopsychosocial phenomenon; that is, it is determined by biological, psychological and social factors, and

4. Occupational therapy is viewed as a means for facilitating an individual's adaptation (in the broadest sense) when performance deficits are identified.

However, the person-environment-performance framework identifies additional individual and environmental factors which impact performance. Moreover, in this framework, intervention includes an array of active efforts designed to facilitate, maintain, or restore role performance. These efforts may or may not involve the use of occupation, since in some cases (e.g., environmental modification), the patient's active involvement may be limited to a collaborative determination of goals and strategies.

The principal components of a person-environment-performance framework will be reviewed and major concepts relevant to each component will be identified and discussed, including the nature of the person as an occupational being, an analysis of the context (environment) in which performance takes place, and examination of occupational performance, how it can be classified, and the nature of occupational performance dysfunction. Figure 1-13 provides an overview of the person-environment-performance framework.

The Person as Doer: Human Factors Influencing Performance

Because of the nature and complexity of open systems, occupational performance can be viewed as the collective product of all human subsystems. These subsystems or factors make greater or lesser contributions to occupational performance depending upon the nature of the tasks involved. In this text, we will refer to the human subsystems underlying performance as *intrinsic enablers of performance*. To facilitate learning and understanding, these enablers are organized into psychological, cognitive, neuromotor, sensory, and physiological areas. It is again stressed that within a systems perspective, no element should be viewed as working in isolation from other intrinsic factors nor from elements in the environment (extrinsic factors).

In keeping with a systems perspective, the consideration of individual characteristics that influence performance should begin with an examination of higher order factors first. Thus one would evaluate factors affecting motivation and view of self (psychological and cognitive factors), proceed to factors that constrain and limit performance by interfering with one's ability to process information from the environment (sensory and perceptual factors), and then to consider factors that might inhibit one's ability to act on that information (neuromotor and physiological factors). An additional chapter is included in this text which relates to the performance effects of pharmacological agents introduced into the body. Since a large percentage of the persons seen by occupational therapists are taking prescribed medications, a consideration of the known effects of these agents on performance seems especially relevant to occupational therapy practice.

Competence. There is considerable agreement that the single characteristic of the individual which has the greatest influence on performance is one's sense of competence. The concept of competence is based on an important assumption about human organisms: that the human organism has an innate drive toward environmental mastery which can be met only through occupation.

White (1959, 1964, 1971) has defined competence as efficacy in meeting environmental demands. He noted that

there is an intrinsic drive in humans to influence the environment. This drive provides the motivation for exploring, manipulating, and acting, and is thus an important component in developmental learning. By observing the results of actions, individuals are provided with feedback which allows them to determine the effectiveness of their actions within the environment.

This feedback permits adaptations, as the individual modifies and adjusts to environmental circumstances. While the environment is a source of restriction, it is also a source of satisfaction and learning, allowing for the development of flexibility and strength in dealing with the varied circumstances of living. The extent to which individuals are able to develop a positive sense of self and belief in their autonomy is largely based on their successes in dealing with

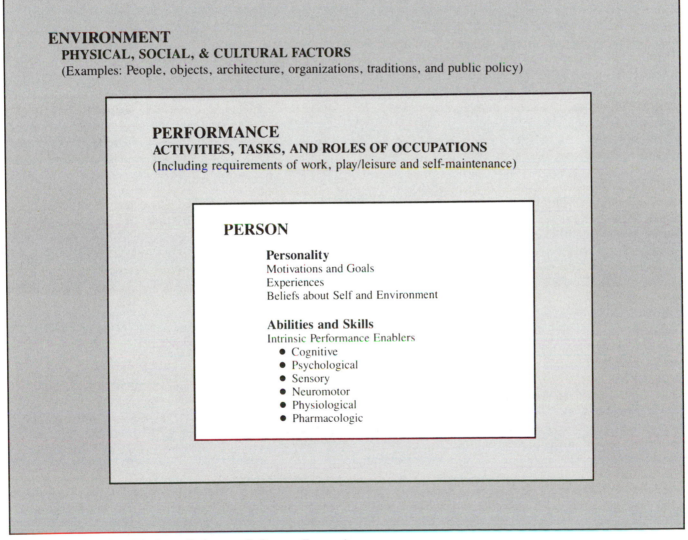

Figure 1-13. An Overview of the Person-Environment-Performance Framework.

environmental challenges and the repertoire of behaviors they have developed through those successful transactions.

Albert Bandura (1977) has been especially interested in how successes shape behavior. His work has indicated that being successful in one's transactions with the environment leads to expectations (*expectancies*) about the probability of being successful in the future. These expectancies are viewed by Bandura and others as an important component of motivation, because if one expects success, one is more likely to attempt new activities.

Locus of Control. The concept of *locus of control* as introduced by Rotter (1966) is closely related to the notion of expectancy. Rotter believed that behavior is influenced by a person's expectation of a successful outcome and also recognized the influence of the individual's perception of the importance of the outcome. But Rotter included an additional characteristic that he believed greatly influenced people's actions, that of their belief in their personal responsibility for the outcome of an action or *locus of control*. He observed that people with an *external locus of control* attributed success or failure in given situations to events or situations outside themselves or unrelated to their own actions, while persons with an *internal locus of control* attributed their success or failure in those situations to their own actions.

Personal Causation. The work of Heider (1958) and DeCharms (1968) is also important to an understanding of competence or feelings about mastery over the environment. While locus of control addresses one's sense of responsibility for the outcome of an event, Heider was interested in the individuals' perceptions of why they acted or the cause of their behavior. He used the term *locus of causality* to distinguish between whether the perceived origin or cause of behaviors was external or internal to the individual.

In later work, DeCharms used the term personal causation to refer to *"the initiation by the individual of behavior intended to produce a change in his environment."* He believed personal causation accounted for the motivation of individuals in complex social environments.

DeCharms described behaviors in terms of two dominant themes, *the pawn* and *the origin*. Persons with pawnlike behaviors are described as driven by the belief that they are controlled by the environment, and therefore have little motivation for personal choice and feel victimized. In contrast, originlike behaviors are characterized by an internal locus of control and a belief in one's ability to control one's own destiny. It is important to note that these characteristics are related to specific situations, so that most individuals exhibit both types of behaviors at different times.

Persons who consistently experience negative outcomes and experiences in their undertakings fail to develop feelings of personal causation and perceive that they are controlled by the environment. This negative view of self and one's ability to influence events is termed **helplessness.** A severe traumatic event which renders one dependent, such as spinal cord injury or stroke, can engender feelings of helplessness. Helplessness is frequently accompanied by depression, a pessimistic outlook toward the future, and considerable anxiety.

In an excellent summary of the various dimensions of personal causation and their clinical implications for occupational therapists, Burke (1977) noted that expectancies, internal/external orientation, sense of efficacy, and belief in **skill** can individually or collectively provide useful information for clinical planning. These dimensions provide insights regarding both the motives and methods underlying goal-directed behaviors and have obvious implications for performance.

Such performance effects were demonstrated in a controlled study of patients with spinal cord injury. A group receiving training designed to improve their sense of competence through task-related successes showed significantly greater success in subsequent performance on experimental tasks than those in comparison groups (Wool, Siegal & Fine, 1980). These findings were similar to those found in a study of patients with depression (Kilpatrick-Tubak & Roth, 1978).

No discussion of competence would be complete without mention of the cumulative impact of one's successes or failures in meeting environmental challenges. Psychologist M. Brewster Smith (1974) noted that attitudes toward self form the motivational core of competence and can result in benign or vicious cycles of adaptation. Smith noted that

"The crucial attitude toward the self is self-respect as a significant and efficacious person. Complementary to self-respect is an attitude of hopefulness toward the world as the sort of place where one can be efficacious. These paired attitudes provide the basis for an active, coping orientation that involves the person in a benign spiral of increasing competence and fulfillment. In the converse, unfavorable case we find the combination of helplessness and hopelessness that is at once the root problem requiring therapeutic assistance and the chief obstacle to its solution" (p. 14).

Abilities and Skills. The sense of self-respect and efficacy that define competence are gained through engagement in the tasks and roles required of daily living. Underlying the performance of life tasks are requisite abilities and skills.

Definitions for Ability Categories

1. **Oral Comprehension** is the ability to understand spoken English words and sentences.
2. **Written Comprehension** is the ability to understand written sentences and paragraphs.
3. **Oral Expression** is the ability to use English words or sentences in speaking so others will understand.
4. **Written Expression** is the ability to use English words or sentences in writing so others will understand.
5. **Fluency of Ideas** is the ability to produce a number of ideas about a given topic.
6. **Originality** is the ability to produce unusual or clever ideas about a given topic or situation. It is the ability to invent creative solutions to problems or to develop new procedures to situations in which standard operating procedures do not apply.
7. **Memorization** is the ability to remember information, such as words, numbers, pictures, and procedures. Pieces of information can be remembered by themselves or with other pieces of information.
8. **Problem Sensitivity** is the ability to tell when something is wrong or is likely to go wrong. It includes being able to identify the whole problem as well as the elements of the problem.
9. **Mathematical Reasoning** is the ability to understand and organize a problem and then to select a mathematical method or formula to solve the problem. It encompasses reasoning through mathematical problems to determine appropriate operations that can be performed to solve problems. It also includes the understanding or structuring of mathematical problems. The actual manipulation of numbers is not included in this ability.
10. **Number Facility** involves the degree to which adding, subtracting, multiplying, and dividing can be done quickly and correctly. These can be steps in other operations like finding percentages and taking square roots.
11. **Deductive Reasoning** is the ability to apply general rules to specific problems to come up with logical answers. It involves deciding if an answer makes sense.
12. **Inductive Reasoning** is the ability to combine separate pieces of information, or specific answers to problems, to form general rules or conclusions. It involves the ability to think of possible reasons for why things go together.
13. **Information Ordering** is the ability to follow correctly a rule or set of rules to arrange things or actions in a certain order. The rule or set of rules used must be given. The things or actions to be put in order can include numbers, letters, words, pictures, procedures, sentences, and mathematical or logical operations.
14. **Category Flexibility** is the ability to produce many rules so that each rule tells how to group a set of things in a different way. Each different group must contain at least two things from the original set of things.
15. **Speed of Closure** involves the degree to which different pieces of information can be combined and organized into one meaningful pattern quickly. It is not known beforehand what the pattern will be. The material may be visual or auditory.
16. **Flexibility of Closure** is the ability to identify or detect a known pattern (like a figure, word, or object) that is hidden in other material. The task is to pick out the disguised pattern from the background material.
17. **Spatial Orientation** is the ability to tell where you are in relation to the location of some object or to tell where the object is in relation to you.
18. **Visualization** is the ability to imagine how something will look when it is moved around or when its parts are moved or rearranged. It requires the forming of mental images of how patterns or objects would look after certain changes, such as unfolding or rotation. One has to predict how an object, set of objects, or pattern will appear after the changes are carried out.
19. **Perceptual Speed** involves the degree to which one can compare letters, numbers, objects, pictures, or patterns, quickly and accurately. The things to be compared may be presented at the same time or one after the other. This ability also includes comparing a presented object with a remembered object.
20. **Control Precision** is the ability to move controls of a machine or vehicle. This involves the degree to which these controls can be moved quickly and repeatedly to exact position.
21. **Multilimb Coordination** is the ability to coordinate movements of two or more limbs (for example, two arms, two legs, or one leg and one arm, such as in moving equipment controls. Two or more limbs are in motion while the individual is sitting, standing, or lying down.
22. **Response Orientation** is the ability to choose between two or more movements quickly and accurately when two or more different signals (lights, sounds, pictures) are given. The ability is concerned with the speed with which the right response can be started with the hand, foot, or other parts of the body.
23. **Rate Control** is the ability to adjust an equipment control in response to changes in the speed and/or directions of a continuously moving object or scene. The ability involves timing these adjustments in anticipating these changes. This ability does not extend to situations in which both the speed and direction of the object are perfectly predictable.

continued

Figure 1-14. Definitions for Ability Categories. *Reprinted with permission from Fleishman, E. & Quaintance, M. (1984). Taxonomies of human performance: the description of human tasks. pp. 461-464. Orlando, FL: Academic Press.*

24. **Reaction Time** is the ability to give one fast response to one signal (sound, light, picture) when it appears. This ability is concerned with the speed with which the movement can be started with the hand, foot, or other parts of the body.

25. **Arm-Hand Steadiness** is the ability to keep the hand and arm steady. It includes steadiness while making an arm movement as well as while holding the arm and hand in one position. This ability does not involve strength or speed.

26. **Manual Dexterity** is the ability to make skillful coordinated movements of one hand, a hand together with its arm, or two hands to grasp, place, move, or assemble objects like hand tools or blocks. This ability involves the degree to which these arm-hand movements can be carried out quickly. It does not involve moving machine or equipment controls like levers.

27. **Finger Dexterity** is the ability to make skillful, coordinated movements of the fingers of one or both hands and to grasp, place, or move small objects. This ability involves the degree to which these finger movements can be carried out quickly.

28. **Wrist-Finger Speed** is the ability to make fast, simple repeated movements of the fingers, hands, and wrists. It involves little, if any, accuracy, careful control, or coordination of movement.

29. **Speed of Limb Movement** involves the speed with which a single movement of the arms and legs can be made. This ability does not include accuracy careful control, or coordination of movement.

30. **Selective Attention** is the ability to concentrate on a task one is doing. This ability involves concentrating while performing a boring task and not being distracted.

31. **Time Sharing** is the ability to shift back and forth between two or more sources of information.

32. **Static Strength** is the ability to use muscle force in order to lift, push, pull, or carry objects. It is the maximum force that one can exert for a brief period of time.

33. **Explosive Strength** is the ability to use short bursts of muscle force to propel oneself or an object. It requires gathering energy for bursts of muscle effort over a very short time period.

34. **Dynamic Strength** is the ability of the muscles to exert force repeatedly or continuously over a long time period. This is the ability to support, hold up, or move the body's own weight and/or objects repeatedly over time. It represents muscular endurance and emphasizes the resistance of the muscles to fatigue.

35. **Trunk Strength** involves the degree to which one's stomach and lower back muscles can support part of the body repeatedly or continuously over time. The ability involves the degree to which these trunk muscles do not fatigue when they are put under such repeated or continuous strain.

36. **Extent Flexibility** is the ability to bend, stretch, twist, or reach out with the body, arms, and/or legs, both quickly and repeatedly.

37. **Dynamic Flexibility** is the ability to bend, stretch, twist, or reach out with the body, arms and/or legs, both quickly and repeatedly.

38. **Gross Body Coordination** is the ability to coordinate the movement of the arms, legs, and torso together in activities in which the whole body is in motion.

39. **Gross Body Equilibrium** is the ability to keep or regain one's body balance or to stay upright when in an unstable position. This ability includes maintaining one's balance when changing direction while moving or standing motionless.

40. **Stamina** is the ability of the lungs and circulatory systems of the body to perform efficiently over long time periods. This is the ability to exert oneself physically without getting out of breath.

41. **Near Vision** is the capacity to see close environmental surroundings.

42. **Far Vision** is the capacity to see distant environmental surroundings.

43. **Visual Color Discrimination** is the capacity to match or discriminate between colors. This capacity also includes detecting differences in color purity (saturation) and brightness (brilliance).

44. **Night Vision** is the ability to see under low light conditions.

45. **Peripheral Vision** is the ability to perceive objects or movement towards the edges of the visual field.

46. **Depth Perception** is the ability to distinguish which of several objects is more distant from or nearer to the observer, or to judge the distance of an object from the observer.

47. **Glare Sensitivity** is the ability to see objects in the presence of glare or bright ambient lighting.

48. **General Hearing** is the ability to detect and to discriminate among sounds that vary over broad ranges of pitch and/or loudness.

49. **Auditory Attention** is the ability to focus on a single source of auditory information in the presence of other distracting and irrelevant auditory stimuli.

50. **Sound Localization** is the ability to identify the direction from which an auditory stimulus originated relative to the observer.

51. **Speech Hearing** is the ability to learn and understand the speech of another person.

52. **Speech Clarity** is the ability to communicate orally in a clear fashion understandable to a listener.

Figure 1-14. Continued.

Although the terms ability and skill have often been used interchangeably in occupational therapy,[5] it is useful to view them as distinct concepts.

Definitions provided by Fleishman (1975), a human factors scientist, are useful here. He defines *abilities* as general traits which are a product of genetic make-up and learning, much of which occurs during childhood and adolescence. Abilities are brought forth when one begins to learn a new task. As general factors, abilities may relate to performance on a variety of diverse tasks. For example, an ability called *spatial orientation* is necessary for success at reading a road map and finding your way through a familiar room when the lights are out. *Reaction time*, another ability, is necessary for us to avoid snowballs hurled at us, return slams in a ping-pong match, and apply the brakes quickly when a dog suddenly decides to cross the road in front of our car. These examples are from a list of 52 abilities which have been derived from empirical studies over a number of years (Fleishman and Quaintance, 1984). A comprehensive list of these abilities with accompanying definitions can be found in Figure 1-14.

In contrast, the term *skill* pertains to the level of proficiency in a specific task. The assumption is that skill in complex tasks can be explained by the presence of various underlying general abilities, for example, a professional race car driver has much more driving skill than the average person. This level of skill is determined by

reaction time, perceptual speed, rate control, and other abilities, such as peripheral vision.

It is presumed that there is a relationship between learning and abilities (Fleishman, 1972). An individual with a high number of abilities is more readily able to learn the skills necessary to become proficient at a variety of specific tasks. However, studies have shown that the combinations of abilities influencing proficiency change as an individual gains experience at a particular task. For example, if one is engaged in a visual discrimination reaction task that requires moving a lever quickly on the basis of visual cues as in an arcade game, spatial abilities may influence performance more during early learning of the task, but motor abilities could assume increased importance with greater practice.

These findings have important implications for predicting performance and for training to improve skills in complex tasks. If the abilities required for different levels of task proficiency change during the course of learning, methods designed to predict performance should be based on the abilities required at final proficiency rather than during learning. Further, emphasizing the abilities required for final proficiency in a task during training should increase the efficiency of task learning. In fact, experiments in training pilots have shown that this principle is valid (Parker & Fleishman, 1960).

It has taken a great deal of methodical research to demonstrate that a relatively small number of underlying general abilities can explain proficiency in a large number of tasks. Research has shown that knowledge of these abilities and how to measure them can be linked with knowledge about the nature of tasks to predict performance and design efficient training programs. This approach to understanding the dimensions underlying task proficiency is known as the *ability requirements approach* and seems to hold considerable promise for those concerned with human performance.

---

5. Kielhofner and Burke (1985), drawing from the work of Jerome Bruner and others, seemingly equate skills with abilities and identify three types of skills: perceptual motor, process and communications/interaction. These broad skill areas are supported by combinations of the 52 discrete abilities identified in empirical research by Fleishman and colleagues, as detailed in Figure 1-14.

Intrinsic Enablers of Performance

Pharmacologic Factors (Chemical Agents)	Physiological Factors	Sensory Factors	Neuromotor Factors	Cognitive Factors	Psychological Factors
Includes the performance oriented effects of chemical agents introduced into the body	Includes cardiac and pulmonary factors necessary for sustained productive activity	Includes factors related to the reception, transmission, and perception of environmental information	Includes factors related to central and peripheral control and coordination of motor behavior	Includes abilities to receive, process, and store information necessary for competent behavior	Includes personality trait and state (emotional) factors affecting behavior and social interaction

Figure 1-15. Intrinsic Enablers of Performance.

Development of Abilities and Skills. It was noted earlier that abilities are the product of genetic factors and learning. Piaget and others have contributed immeasurably to our understanding of the processes through which cognitive and motor learning take place during early childhood. We know, for example, that abilities are developed very rapidly during the first years of life and that skill is attained in various age-related tasks in a complex spiral of maturation and interaction with the environment as the individual matures.

Exploration can be viewed as a developmental step toward the attainment of competent performance. Reilly (1974) and others (Robinson, 1977) have noted the exploratory nature of play and its contribution to the acquisition of knowledge and skills necessary for competent performance. Through their interactions with people and things, individuals form sets of internal rules which govern future actions. Learning these internal rules is instrumental to the development of competence (Bruner, 1973).

While abilities can be developed throughout the lifespan, most ability development occurs during childhood and adolescence. In adulthood, existing abilities are called on in the mastery of new tasks. In Chapter 2, Llorens summarizes the complexities of this developmental process as it influences occupational performance throughout the lifespan.

Intrinsic Enablers of Performance. Underlying general abilities are various supporting elements, which are referred to as performance enablers.[6] As described earlier, intrinsic factors contributing to performance are organized into psychological, cognitive, sensory, neuromotor, and physiological categories. These categories are consistent with, but not identical to, categories outlined in the uniform terminology practice documents developed by the American Occupational Therapy Association (1979, 1989) and referred to there as performance components (See Appendix A). Figure 1-15 provides a summary of the major elements of these intrinsic performance categories. In later chapters, each of these categories is explored in detail, including structural and functional considerations of relevance to occupational performance, as well as methods for assessing function.

---

6. This term is derived from the work of Nelson (1988) who provided the helpful observation that use of the term "performance components" is misleading in that it implies that these phenomena collectively account for performance.

ENVIRONMENTAL FACTORS: THE CONTEXT OF PERFORMANCE

We have observed that because of its reciprocal nature, occupational performance is always influenced by the characteristics of the environment in which it occurs. In noting this, Rogers (1983, p. 604) described the qualities of the environment as important "enablers of human performance." Perhaps because of the influence of medicine and its orientation toward the internal workings of the body, occupational therapists have given insufficient attention in the past to environmental factors and their influence on performance.

Barris (1982, Barris, Kielhofner, Levine & Neville 1985) was one of the first writers in the field to attempt to organize dimensions of the environment within a conceptual framework. Barris' work views the environment as consisting of progressively inclusive layers, which include object, task, social, and cultural dimensions. She emphasizes that the characteristics of the environment at every layer influence persons' decisions to interact with their surroundings and have an impact on the quality of their performance.

The following is a brief review of a few key concepts related to environments as they affect occupational performance: the physical environment and the social, cultural, and political dimensions of the environment. These will be discussed in more detail in later chapters.

The Physical Environment

The physical properties of environments are the most obvious, and thus the most likely to be given consideration when environmental influences on performance are discussed. For many years, therapists have been doing pre-discharge home assessments, or surveying worksites in order to identify modifications necessary to accommodate persons with mobility limitations or other types of **disability,** such as sensory deficits. Clearly, design is an important characteristic of the physical environment and one that is deserving of even greater attention than it has received in the past.

For example, space and furnishings must support the fundamental types of activities people do in various environments, a concept described by Spivak (1973) as *archetypal places.* Hall (1966) has similarly identified the importance of space as it affects human interaction in various types of settings, using the term *proxemics* to describe those interactive distances. Other dimensions of the physical environment that influence behavior include the availability of objects, the design of tools, and the symbolic meaning of objects and places. These characteristics frequently interact in complex ways with social and cultural aspects of the environment.

Social Dimensions

The social dimensions of environments have profound implications for occupational performance. For example, the size and function of groups, their entry requirements, and their complexity can affect the development of roles. Large groups create expectations for specialized roles, while smaller groups may demand that individuals assume multiple responsibilities.

Cross-cultural social attitudes and values can also influence behaviors. This is especially relevant for persons with disabilities, since they must learn to recognize and contend with the stigma that accompanies their conditions (Goffman, 1963). An important goal for occupational therapy with some individuals is to help them to manage the impressions of others in social interaction.

Finally, mention should be made of the dimension of social support. Research has shown that the presence or absence of social networks which provide support and information is a salient factor in the coping process. The value of these networks for persons with performance deficits is suggested by the large numbers of self-help groups organized around specific disability types.

Cultural Influences

Culture refers to the values, beliefs, customs, and behaviors that are passed on from one generation to the next. Culture affects performance in many ways, including prescribing norms for the use of time and space, influencing beliefs regarding the importance of various tasks, and transmitting attitudes and values regarding work and play (Altman & Chelmers, 1980; Hall, 1973).

It has been suggested that the beliefs, values, and customs derived from cultural influences are the most influential of the environmental factors affecting performance, because of their powerful influence over the behaviors in which people engage and the settings in which they occur. For example, in a later chapter it will be shown that cultural beliefs about health care can have a profound influence on individuals' motivation to participate in their treatment programs as well as their preferences for various types of intervention strategies.

Arousal and Press

Through a process identified by Berlyne (1960) as *arousal*, environments can influence our inclination to interact with or explore our surroundings. Arousal has both physiological and psychological characteristics related to one's level of alertness and has its most obvious effect on performance when persons are bored and inattentive (underaroused)[7] or anxious (overaroused). Three groups of environmental variables are associated with arousal: (1) psychophysical characteristics, such as loud noises and bright lights; (2) ecological events which are related to one's well-being, such as a severe storm; and (3) situations viewed as novel, surprising, or ambiguous (*collative characteristics*). The degree of match between the characteristics of the environment and our interests and values may have an influence on our inclination to explore or interact within that setting. Barris notes that the characteristics of settings which influence arousal must be carefully considered, so that an optimal level (producing neither boredom nor anxiety) is attained (Barris, 1982, p. 638).

The personality theorist Murray (Murray, Barrett & Hamburger, 1938) was one of the first to recognize that characteristics of environments influence behavior by creating demands or expectations, either objectively or as perceived by the individual. He referred to this as *press*. The concept of press has been refined and extended by other investigators, including Lawton (1980), and given prominence in the occupational therapy literature by Barris (1982; Barris, Kielhofner, Levine & Neville, 1985). Waiting rooms demonstrate press inasmuch as their occupants are expected to sit patiently and quietly until their names are called. Evidence of press can be observed in the differences in behavior expected at a coffee shop versus an elegant restaurant. In an elegant restaurant, there may even be overt demonstrations of press, such as an enforced dress code or the disapproving glances of other customers.

An individual's reaction to press is dependent upon both their abilities and their experiences. As experiences with new settings increases, an individual learns those behaviors which are expected, thus feeling competent within the chosen environment. This may encourage the individual to seek new settings which will provide novelty or challenge, thus providing motivation to acquire new skills.

Occupational behaviors involve interactions with other individuals and with objects. The presence or absence of objects within the environment, termed *availability*, influences both arousal and press. For example, a playground is much more likely to attract teens if it is equipped with basketball hoops. Similarly, if necessary tools are not available, the quality of one's task performance can be diminished.

Objects have various dimensions which contribute to their symbolic meaning and can convey status, prestige, or

---

7. Parent (1978) in an article in the *American Journal of Occupational Therapy*, provided an excellent overview of the effects of low stimulus environments on behavior.

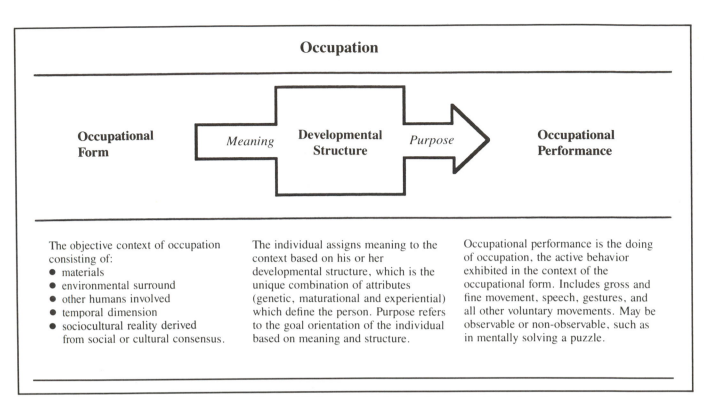

Occupation

Occupational Form	Meaning → Developmental Structure → Purpose	Occupational Performance

The objective context of occupation consisting of:
- materials
- environmental surround
- other humans involved
- temporal dimension
- sociocultural reality derived from social or cultural consensus.

The individual assigns meaning to the context based on his or her developmental structure, which is the unique combination of attributes (genetic, maturational and experiential) which define the person. Purpose refers to the goal orientation of the individual based on meaning and structure.

Occupational performance is the doing of occupation, the active behavior exhibited in the context of the occupational form. Includes gross and fine movement, speech, gestures, and all other voluntary movements. May be observable or non-observable, such as in mentally solving a puzzle.

Figure 1-16. Occupation as the Relationship Between Form and Performance. *Adapted from Nelson, DL. Occupation: Form and performance. American Journal of Occupational Therapy 42, (10), 633 - 641. Copyright 1988 by the American Occupational Therapy association, Inc. Reprinted with permission.*

independence. For example, having a car can be a symbol of independence. The complexity of objects can often convey prestige; for example, in health care, the use of highly sophisticated and technical equipment is often viewed as a sign of prestige.

Public Policy

Public policy influences performance in subtle ways and can have a significant effect on the success of intervention. While it is recognized that policy is a social phenomenon, it transcends the traditional concept of social group and culture and therefore seems worthy of attention as a unique environmental factor in its own right.

Public policies determine funding for social services and transportation, and establish criteria for access to such services. As a result of public policy, many communities now have standards in place for assuring that buildings and streets do not deny community access to persons with disabilities. Unfortunately, public policy can also contribute to the phenomenon of excess disability (Kahn, 1965). The term *excess disability* refers to the discrepancy which exists when a person's functional incapacity is greater than that warranted by the objective degree of impairment. The presence of other physical disorders and social and psychological factors have a cumulative impact

on function which goes beyond that which can be explained by physical impairment alone. Thus, when public policy creates disincentives to employment, ignores architectural accessibility issues, or unintentionally fosters stereotypical or prejudicial attitudes toward persons with disabilities, it limits full social participation by disabled persons and thus contributes to excess disability.

CLASSIFYING OCCUPATIONAL PERFORMANCE

Occupation is a general term that refers to engagement in activities, tasks, and roles for the purpose of productive pursuit (such as work and education), maintaining oneself in the environment, and for purposes of relaxation, entertainment, creativity, and celebration. The position taken here is that all goal-oriented behavior related to daily living is occupational in nature. This differs from earlier assertions made by Reilly (1962) and Kielhofner (1988) that some activities are not occupational in nature, such as some survival, sexual, social, and spiritual pursuits. However, since such pursuits are often requirements of social roles, it seems inconsistent to exclude them from the general consideration of occupational performance.

When we speak of occupational performance, we refer to the day-to-day engagement in occupations that organize our lives and meet our needs to maintain ourselves, to be productive, and to derive enjoyment and satisfaction within our environments. Occupational performance includes engagement in tasks as routine and necessary as bathing and dressing and those more involved and complex that are related to one's work requirements.

It has been conventional within occupational therapy to categorize performance within three areas: self-maintenance,[8] work, and play/leisure. However, it is not always possible to classify occupation based on a knowledge of a specific activity alone. For example, writing could be classified as a leisure activity, as a work-related or educational activity, or an act necessary for self-maintenance, such as in writing a check to pay household expenses. It is only by knowing the context or form of an occupation that one can discern into which domain a given activity falls.

Purpose and Meaning in Occupation

Many scholars have contributed to our understanding of the issues of meaning and purpose in occupation. However, the recent work of Nelson (1988) has been especially useful and will be drawn from extensively here. Nelson has proposed a means of viewing occupation in terms of elements which reduce the ambiguity of terminology and serve to clarify concepts. A depiction of Nelson's schema is presented in Figure 1-16. In his schema, occupation is defined as the relationship between an *occupational form* and *occupational performance*. All the elements comprising the context of the occupation are what Nelson (1988) terms *the form* of occupation. Occupational performance consists of *the doing* of occupation.

The occupational form consists of the objective elements of the occupation, that is the human elements, the environment, the temporal context, and the materials used. It also includes a social and cultural reality that includes performance norms or expectations as reflected in values, roles, symbols, and sanctions for interpreting the physical elements. These aspects of the social and cultural environment are unlikely to be recognized by the casual observer.

Historically, practitioners have been inclined to attempt

to classify activities as purposeful or non-purposeful. However, as Lyons (1983) has suggested, it is pointless to consider a unit of behavior as having an intrinsic purpose, since the act can be interpreted only in the context of the individual and environment in which it is being performed. Thus, if we were to view a short videotape segment depicting a pair of gloved hands using scissors to make one straight cut across a sheet of paper, we would be unable to discern whether we were watching a seven-year-old girl making paper dolls or a skilled Japanese artisan practicing the ancient and delicate art of origami. The ultimate goals or purposes can be determined only through knowing more about the individual using the scissors and the environment in which the cutting is being performed. That is, interpretation can be made only in terms of all the elements comprising the context of the occupation.

As observers, however, our interpretation cannot always discern the meaning or purpose of an occupation to the performer. Nelson (1988) has suggested that occupations have meaning only insofar as their forms are interpreted by individuals. An occupational form can have a social or cultural meaning, an individual or idiosyncratic meaning, or little meaning at all (Fidler, 1981; Nelson, 1988).

In this regard, Kielhofner (1985) has noted that individuals find meaning in occupations based on their association with past experiences and the feelings they engender, such as having a calming or arousing effect. These meanings are most likely dynamic, in that they change with additional experiences as one matures. For example, the act of driving may mean status and independence to an adolescent or

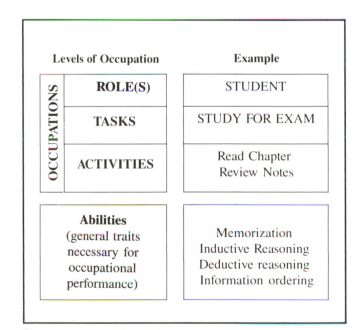

Figure 1-17. Levels of Occupation.

freedom to a person with spinal cord injury. Within a culture in which most people cannot afford cars, driving one can symbolize wealth. Thus the tools and objects associated with the physical form can contribute to its meaning. In addition to the influences of its physical and sociocultural dimensions, the same occupational form can have different meanings to different individuals depending upon their backgrounds and other factors which bear upon their developmental make-up (Cynkin, 1979). As used here, the term *developmental make-up* refers to the sum total of experiences and attributes that influence a person's behavior at any point in time.

Similarly, the purpose of the occupation to the performer is also related to his or her developmental make-up. Nelson (1988) compares the concepts of meaning and purpose in activity in a useful way. He suggests that *the meaning* of occupation is retrospective, while *the purpose* of occupation is prospective. That is, the meaning a person derives from engagement in doing comes from reflecting on past experiences, while the purpose in doing is based on an expectation or goal(s). As Nelson states:

> "In performing a particular occupation, an individual may simultaneously be seeking (a) specific changes in the occupational forms materials (a product), (b) the praise of a supervisor, (c) money, (d) the tactile sensations of handling the materials, and (e) satisfaction of the need to be productive, leading to confirmation of personal efficacy" (1988, p. 637).

While some conventions have been established for classifying occupation on the areas related to purpose (i.e., work, play, self-maintenance), little progress has been made toward classifying occupation in terms of its level of complexity. As a result, many terms have been used interchangeably, resulting in great ambiguity. Examples of such terms include activity, task, and occupation. However, in this text, terms relating to occupational performance will have specific meanings within the framework of a hierarchy of occupational performance.

Occupational Performance Hierarchy

The occupational hierarchy or levels of occupation to be used in this text are illustrated in Figure 1-17; they range from activities to roles. Using this hierarchy, the basic unit of occupational performance is *the activity*, which consists of specific goal-oriented behaviors. Tasks are defined as sets of activities sharing some purpose recognized by the task performer (Miller, 1967). *Roles* are the third and highest level and are defined as distinctive positions in society, each having a defined status and specific expectations for behavior. Roles can be occupational, familial, or sexual, and a person can have multiple roles at the same time, such as therapist and mother. Note that although roles are occupied by persons, they define performance expectations and are viewed here as attributes of performance and not of individuals. Stated in another way, in the absence of social context and specified behaviors, the concept of role has no meaning. Thus, it is appropriately classified in the performance hierarchy and discussed in this section.

Performance Requirements

The performance requirements at each level of the functional hierarchy are of interest to the occupational therapist, because each provides specific information which can be useful in the assessment and intervention process. For example, successful performance in the role of parent is a societal expectation. As a parent, one may be expected to work at gainful employment, assist in child rearing, provide household maintenance, and participate in family recreation. These expectations cut across all the occupational performance areas of work, play/leisure, and self-maintenance.

Within these performance areas, requirements are organized according to specific tasks. Thus, within the performance area of self-maintenance one is required to maintain personal hygiene through regular bathing. Bathing, in turn, requires a specific set of activities, such as filling the tub, getting undressed, climbing into the bathtub, and washing.

The requirements of each of these activities can be further analyzed according to steps. Thus, the activity of filling the tub could be broken down into such steps as plugging the drain, reaching for the handle, turning the faucet on, monitoring the water level, and turning the faucet off. Further, these steps can be analyzed in terms of their requisite abilities, such as near vision, extent flexibility, or manual dexterity. Underlying these abilities are performance enablers, such as physiological, cognitive, sensory, and neuromotor factors. The specific levels of analysis required by the occupational therapist will depend upon the nature of the clinical problem, a matter that will be given detailed examination in later chapters.

Activity

It has been traditional in occupational therapy to use the term activity in a general way to refer to all purposeful behaviors. Unfortunately, this general use does not lend itself to an appreciation of the varying complexities of occupation. As defined earlier, an activity is the basic unit of occupational performance, consisting of specific goal-oriented behavior directed toward the performance of a task. Activities consist of steps and can be analyzed according to requisite abilities. In general, it is not useful to speak of activity skill, because it would be difficult to distinguish levels of proficiency at this level of performance.

World Health Organization Dysfunctional Hierarchy		
Handicap	Disadvantage for a given individual, resulting from an impairment or a disability, that limits or prevents the fulfilment of a role that is normal (depending on age, sex, and social and cultural factors) for that individual	**System Level = Social** (Society, organization, family-group)
Disability	Restriction or lack (resulting from impairment) of ability to perform an activity in the manner or within the range considered normal for a human being	**System Level = Person**
Impairment	Loss or abnormality of psychological, physiological, or anatomical structure or function.	**System Level = Performance Enablers** (organs, tissues)

Figure 1-18. World Health Organization Dysfunctional Hierarchy. *From World Health Organization (1980). International Classification of impairments, disabilities and handicaps: A manual of classification relating to consequences of disease. Geneva: (pp. 47, 143, 183)*

Tasks

A task has been defined earlier as a set of activities sharing some purpose recognized by the task performer. Tasks have dimensions related to their complexity, their degree of structure (specific methods or flexibility and creativity), and their purposes (e.g., for work, for pleasure, or for self-maintenance). These characteristics of tasks, along with social dimensions, such as whether they entail cooperation or competition and whether they are public or private, have a vital influence on performance.

An important characteristic of tasks is their temporal dimension. This pertains to how long they last and at which time(s) they are performed. Adolph Meyer observed that occupations provide a necessary structure to our existence and noted that many persons in mental institutions at the time had lost the temporal order in their daily lives. Kielhofner (1977) has provided a useful analysis of the temporal properties of occupation and remarked that physical and mental illnesses frequently interfere with an individual's abilities to manage time, either because their sense of time is distorted or because of changes in the amount of time required to accomplish necessary tasks. He further suggested that role changes require a corresponding adjustment in the manner in which one organizes time. This phenomenon can be observed in retired persons who have not prepared for the increased amount of leisure time available in their lives. The term *temporal adaptation* has been used to describe the process of adjusting to changing temporal requirements in daily life or throughout the lifespan.

The nature of tasks can provide the motivation and context for learning skills and roles necessary for competent life performance. The performance of tasks also can reveal important information about the nature of emotional and cognitive disorders. A knowledge of the various characteristics of tasks is essential for the occupational therapist, who can use these dimensions in the selection of approaches to intervention.

Role: Acquisition, Performance, and Transition

Role responsibilities define the nature of occupational performance at various points in one's lifespan. Thus, it can be asserted that performance deficits have meaning principally in the context of an individual's role responsibilities. To speak of occupational dysfunction, then, is to refer to one's inadequate performance of social roles. In this section, social roles are examined from the standpoint of their organizing properties and changing nature over the lifespan.

As we have seen, role occupies the highest level of the occupational performance hierarchy. As such, it is one of the most important concepts for occupational therapists to understand, because roles organize occupational behavior by defining performance expectations.

The concept of role emanates from social psychology and the symbolic interactionist school of thought, advanced

Continuum of Occupational Function/Dysfunction—Model of Human Occupation

Occupational Function			Occupational Dysfunction		
Achievement Demonstrated in role performance beyond the standards expected.	**Competence** Demonstrated in performance that is adequate to the demands of the situation.	**Exploration** Demonstrated in circumstances allowing for discovery of characteristics and potentials.	**Inefficacy** Demonstrated in situations where performance does not meet standards allowing for personal satisfaction.	**Incompetence** Demonstrated in circumstances where one's performance becomes consistently inadequate.	**Helplessness** Demonstrated in circumstances where one is totally unable to act on one's environment.
← Progressive development of skills and habits into satisfactory role performance accompanied by an increased sense of personal causation			Progressive reduction of skills and habits which preclude role performance and lead to a diminished sense of personal causation →		

Figure 1-19. Continuum of Occupational Function/Dysfunction—Model of Human Occupation. *Adapted from Kielhofner, G. (1985). Occupational Function and Dysfunction (pp. 63-75). In Kielhofner, G. (Ed): A model of human occupation: Theory and application. Baltimore, MD: Williams & Wilkins.*

principally by George Herbert Mead (1934) and Harry Stack Sullivan (1953). This view proposes that roles, defined as positions in society having expected responsibilities and privileges, form the very nucleus of social interaction. Smooth social interaction requires *role-reciprocity*, or the effective role performance of each member in a group. Roles affect development and personality both through strong social approval when roles are enacted successfully or through equally strong sanctions when role expectations are not met. Socialization is thus the process of learning role behaviors.

Sarbin & Allen (1968) noted that within the boundaries of each role, expectations are formed by both society and the role occupant. Thus, one's satisfaction with the performance of valued roles is based on internal as well as external appraisals. This external influence is reflected in exemptions granted by society to persons who are experiencing difficult life events. One example of society's exemptions is the *sick role* described by Parsons (1975). The sick role excuses persons from fulfilling role responsibilities during illness, as long as certain conditions are met, including seeking and complying with medical advice. Unfortunately, when the sick role is adopted by or ascribed to individuals with disabling conditions, the passivity and compliance expected in the sick role may conflict with the goals of the rehabilitation process. This is especially likely in situations in which occupational therapy is appropriately practiced, because active participation and independence are valued (Burke, Miyake, Kielhofner, & Barris, 1983).

Roles are dynamic as they are acquired or replaced throughout the lifespan. For example, during adolescence, a major concern is occupational choice or determining the specific nature of one's worker role. Later, parental roles may be acquired, but these parental roles are replaced again when one's children leave home. These developmental transitions are especially important because they involve the development of new skills or the integration of skills previously learned.

Dysfunction is present when persons cannot perform roles to satisfaction, either because of deficits in abilities and skills due to disease or disability, the conflicting demands of multiple roles (*role conflict*), or because of unclear role expectations. Such disruption in the roles of daily living is termed *occupational performance dysfunction* (Rogers, 1983) and constitutes the appropriate type of problem for occupational therapy intervention.

Taxonomies of Performance Dysfunction

The profession of occupational therapy lacks a means of classifying occupational performance dysfunction according to an appropriate taxonomy. The Cartesian or traditional view of medicine has had an influence on terminology related to disrupted performance. For many years, words reflecting the impact of disease on daily living were used interchangeably, and there was virtually no distinction between how the terms **impairment,** disability, and **handicap** were used. Although classification systems had been developed to promote the precise use of terminology for diseases, there was no perceived need to be concerned with terms relating to rehabilitation.

In 1980, the World Health Organization (Wood, 1980) undertook the task of addressing this problem in a manner consistent with its *International Classification of Diseases* (ICD). This work was subsequently incorporated into a document called the *International Classification of*

Impairment, Disability, and Handicap (ICIDH). The dysfunctional hierarchy is depicted in Figure 1-18.

As suggested by the title, the terms impairment, disability, and handicap have distinct meanings which correspond to the impact of a condition on daily living from the point of view of systems theory. **Impairment** is defined as, "any loss or abnormality of psychological, physiological or anatomical structure or function" (p. 47). An impairment may be permanent or temporary.

The next level of dysfunction called *disability*, is at the level of the person. "A disability is any restriction or lack (resulting from an impairment) of ability to perform an activity in the manner or within the range considered normal for a human being" (p. 143). The performance can reflect a deficit or an excess that may be permanent or temporary, reversible or progressive. Attention is given to the person's ability to perform in daily life and to fulfill his or her roles in life.

"A **handicap** is a disadvantage for a given individual, resulting from an impairment or a disability, that limits or prevents the fulfillment of a role that is normal (depending on age, sex, and social and cultural factors for that individual" (p. 183). Handicaps result when a person cannot meet his/her own standards of performance nor those of the groups of which he/she is a member. This discord has social, cultural, economical, and environmental consequences for the individual.

While this dysfunctional hierarchy reflects a systems orientation and hence a promising awareness of the effects of disease and disability on role performance, it does not provide a delineation of the extent of such disruption. Consequently, it is not practical as a means for organizing knowledge which could guide occupational therapy intervention.

According to Rogers (1983), what is needed is an approach to classifying performance dysfunction. She argues that such a taxonomy is necessary for the advancement of the field because it identifies concepts relevant to practice, facilitates communication between practitioners and scholars, and clarifies the nature and scope of occupational therapy services to the general public. By having such a taxonomy, therapists would be able to characterize the nature of performance dysfunction in terms of a *diagnostic statement*, which can be defined as a conclusion about the status of a patient after considering biological, psychological, and social data relevant to occupational performance.

Kielhofner (1985) has proposed a continuum of occupational function and dysfunction which incorporates the concepts of competence, efficacy, and helplessness. In this six stage continuum depicted in Figure 1-19, the optimal level of occupational function is *achievement*. The concept of achievement derives from the work of McClelland (1961) and represents a stage, typically reflected in vocational pursuits, during which the individual strives to enhance existing levels of performance. At the next level, *competence*, performance is at a level which is satisfactory to the demands of a given task. The third level of *exploration* is one in which individuals discover the limits of their abilities and skills and their capacity to act on the environment. An example of the exploration level is that which is found in childhood play and requires an environment viewed as risk-free and supportive. Exploration is driven by the curiosity reflected in environmental observation and manipulation.

Kielhofner notes that normal development is characterized by a progression from exploration to achievement which may recur during adulthood as individuals make changes in their careers or lifestyles. This continuum of occupational function applies to all areas, so that individuals may be at different stages within different domains. For example, an individual could be at the exploration level in leisure pursuits but at the competence stage in their career.

At the maladaptive end of the continuum, Kielhofner proposes that the stages include inefficacy, incompetence,

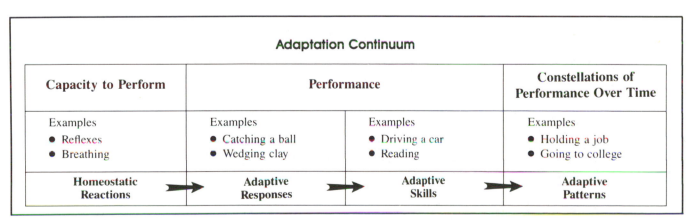

Adaptation Continuum			
Capacity to Perform	**Performance**		**Constellations of Performance Over Time**
Examples • Reflexes • Breathing	Examples • Catching a ball • Wedging clay	Examples • Driving a car • Reading	Examples • Holding a job • Going to college
Homeostatic Reactions →	**Adaptive Responses** →	**Adaptive Skills** →	**Adaptive Patterns**

Figure 1-20. Adaptation Continuum. *Adapted from Kleinman, B.L. & Bulkley, B.L. Some implications of a science of adaptive responses. American Journal of Occupational Therapy, 36(1), 16. Copyright 1982 by the American Occupational Therapy Association, Inc. Reprinted with permission.*

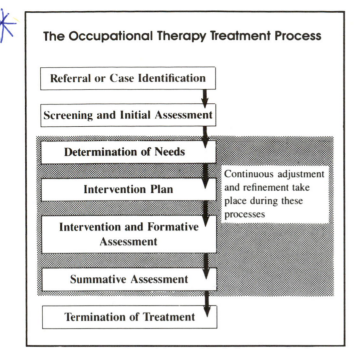

Figure 1-21. A problem-solving model of the occupational therapy treatment process. *Adapted from Pelland, M.J. (1987). American Journal of Occupational Therapy, 41: 351-359.*

and helplessness. *Inefficacy* is defined as a stage in which there is interference with performance caused by environmental or individual constraints which leads to dissatisfaction. *Incompetence*, the next lower stage, is characterized by a major loss or limitation of skills. Persons in this category are unable to adequately perform tasks of everyday living, either due to disease or injury, environmental deprivation, or other life circumstances. At this level, role performance is compromised. *Helplessness* is the most dysfunctional level of occupational performance on the continuum. This level is characterized by feelings of ineffectiveness and alienation and frequently accompanied by depression. Fulfillment of the requirements of life roles at this level of performance is seldom possible.

Performance and Adaptation

Few concepts have been as widely embraced within occupational therapy as that of adaptation. The term *adaptation* as used in occupational therapy has typically referred to any adjustment or change of behavior in response to the challenges or demands of living. Behaviors are described as adaptive if they result in an improvement in the *fit* between the individual and environment.

Lorna Jean King (1978), in her Eleanor Clarke Slagle lecture, suggested that adaptation could serve as an important unifying concept in the field, noting that the term had been used in 1922 by Adolph Meyer in his influential essay, *The*

Philosophy of Occupation Therapy. She identified characteristics of a process she termed, *individual adaptation*, and suggested that the essential purpose of occupational therapy is to stimulate and guide the adaptive process through "eliciting an adaptive response." An analysis and extension of King's concept of adaptation was later provided by Kleinman and Bulkley (1982) as a proposal for mapping the domain of occupational therapy practice. Their essay suggested that adaptation could best be viewed as a continuum ranging from homeostatic reactions, which include reflexes and autonomic functions outside of conscious control, to adaptive patterns, which were defined as representing "a constellation of skills that contribute to an adaptive lifestyle" (p. 17). Occupational therapy's primary concern, from the viewpoint of Kleinman and Bulkley, should be eliciting adaptive responses as a precursor to skill learning (See Figure 1-20).

It is interesting to note that Kleinman and Bulkley used descriptors of performance to parallel the stages of their adaptive continuum. In doing so, they equated homeostatic reactions with one's capacity to perform, adaptive responses and adaptive skills as *performance*, and adaptive patterns as *constellations of performance* over time. Because of the dynamic nature of the individual as an open system and the changing nature of environments, it can be asserted that life itself represents a continuous process of adaptation. This is reflected in performance changes that range from the subtle to the pronounced, and these performance variations are influenced by various levels of the system. Collectively and over time, these performance patterns represent a trajectory or growth, hesitation, or decline.

It has been claimed that satisfactory occupational performance leads to adaptation. A theme in this chapter and throughout this book is that *occupational therapy assists patients in overcoming performance deficits related to living*. Therapists devise strategies which enable patients to acquire the physical, psychological, and social abilities and skills necessary to meet the requirements and cope with the demands of daily life. To the extent that these strategies contribute to the patient's mastery of existing or future environmental challenges, adaptation is facilitated.

Although the term adaptation has appeared with regularity in the occupational therapy literature, the concept of coping has received relatively little attention. This may reflect that scholars in the field have not considered that the terms have distinct meanings. It is necessary to make a distinction, however, in recognition that much work has been done in psychology which may be valuable to our understanding of human behavior under various conditions of stress.

When one encounters situational demands which cannot be met through one's existing repertoire of skills, a special response is necessary. These situational responses have been labeled *coping*. One must be successful in coping for adaptation to occur. A great deal of research has been conducted by psychologists in attempts to explain the nature of these coping mechanisms. Of special interest to occupational therapy is the work aimed at identifying the process through which individuals evaluate demanding situations and select behavioral responses. This research is particularly signicant to occupational therapy because it can be argued that performance deficits themselves are situations of considerable stress, particularly when they are substantial enough to threaten independent function. A review of coping research as it pertains to occupational therapy can be found in Chapter 3, Performance Deficits as Sources of Stress.

OCCUPATIONAL THERAPY: OVERCOMING LIFE PERFORMANCE DEFICITS

The goal of occupational therapy is to prevent, remediate, or reduce dysfunction relating to occupational performance. In addressing occupational performance needs, therapists work with the individual and other professional disciplines to characterize the nature of the problem, develop an intervention plan, and deliver services. The success of intervention strategies must be determined through evaluation during and following the delivery of services. These events together constitute the approach taken in a *problem-oriented process model*. The model presented is based substantially on ideas elaborated by Pelland (1987). See Figure 1-21.

Although the individual elements of the occupational therapy process are discussed sequentially in the following sections, it is important to realize that the problem-oriented approach is not a linear process. Rather, it is a conceptual process during which the therapist continually moves back and forth between elements in attempts to craft an approach that is tailored to the unique needs of a given patient. In doing so, the therapist is engaged in a process of analyzing cues which confirm or refute tentative hypotheses regarding the nature of a patient's occupational performance deficits.

Although an approximate treatment plan may be conceived during the initial phases of treatment based on early hypotheses, it is adjusted and refined in a series of successive therapeutic encounters which yield additional information regarding the profile of a given patient. A patient may have several performance deficits, each requiring a separate process of validation on the part of the therapist during the assessment stages. The validation of hypotheses concerning the nature of a patient's deficits is viewed as critical to the determination of intervention strategies. Even after

intervention has begun, the therapist will be alert to cues which suggest refinement of hypotheses and appropriate adjustment in intervention strategies, thus the processes of assessment and intervention continue throughout the therapeutic encounter.

Regardless of whether the patient is referred for occupational therapy because of a performance deficit resulting from a developmental condition, disease, or injury or for the purpose of maintaining or improving one's current occupational performance, the problem-solving approach is appropriate.

Assessment

Following referral, (if appropriate) or case identification, an initial phase in providing service involves the identification of appropriate frames of reference. Using these frameworks which guide thinking about treatment, the gathering of performance-related information proceeds. In collecting information, the therapist attempts to characterize the nature of a patient's occupational performance status.

Assessment data should include details about the individual's assets and deficits and should always reflect the environmental context in which the individual typically performs the activities, tasks, and roles of daily living. Information on the patient's past performance and environmental demands are relevant and should provide a sense of the patient's interests, values, and use of time. Analysis of these data will permit the identification of strengths and weaknesses. Based on this analysis, the therapist is able to make an informed decision about the types of intervention which will be most effective in a given instance.

Assessment is a process of collecting information in order to become fully informed about a patient. It may include formalized approaches, such as standardized tests and structured interviews, and less obtrusive techniques gained through informal interaction and skillful observation. In recognition that there are limitations in existing quantitative and qualitative approaches to gathering information about performance, clinical assessment has become one of the most vital issues confronting researchers in occupational therapy.

It would be ideal if all assessment information could be gathered prior to developing a treatment plan and beginning intervention. However, in nearly every instance, intervention begins before the therapist gains a complete picture of the individual. In fact, it is misleading to characterize the assessment process as a discrete event which precedes intervention. In actual practice, experienced clinicians tend to make tentative inferences about patients before formalized assessment is completed. This process, termed reflection-in-action by Schön (1983), is viewed as instrumental to achieving the purpose of assessment, which is to frame the problem. These inferences represent informed guesses about what the individual is like and are based on experiences with similar patients. As the therapist gains more experience (and thus more assessment information) with a particular patient, earlier inferences may be discarded or refined. Thus, information about the patient is gathered throughout the intervention process.

In medical settings, a diagnosis has frequently been made on the patient prior to referral to occupational therapy. In such cases, this medical diagnosis may guide the therapist toward specific assessment tools and provide tentative expectations about the nature of performance deficits. But the medical diagnosis is a totally inadequate basis for planning intervention, because it usually fails to provide any insight into those factors which most influence occupational performance. Furthermore, it says nothing about the assets of the patient, which are critical to forming a complete picture of the patient's occupational performance status.

The diagnosis may also be accompanied by information on the physician's plan for medical management. This will be relevant to occupational therapy if it involves planned surgery, chemotherapy, or other types of treatment which will create anxiety, influence attentional states, or otherwise diminish the patient's physical or mental capacity to participate in treatment.

There are scores of existing tools for assisting the therapist in gaining a complete picture of the patient and those factors underlying his/her occupational performance. Some provide information on specific enabling components, such as sensory, cognitive, or psychological areas; while others are more global in their approach to describing or measuring occupational performance. Because the objective is to select that combination of data collection approaches that will provide the clearest and most complete picture of the individual's level of occupational performance with the least expenditure of time, energy, and cost, the determination of utility and validity of these approaches is of great import to occupational therapists. Developing a sound approach to assessment requires a basic understanding of various concepts, including the selection of a framework for organizing and interpreting information. These issues are addressed in later chapters on assessment, particularly Chapter 14, Assessment and Informed Decision-making.

Planning Intervention Strategies

In addressing the needs of patients, competent occupational therapists draw upon their knowledge of the individual and the environment and the assets and limitations which affect the quality of occupational performance. A careful consideration of this information and the possible treatment alternatives permits the selection of various strategies for meeting identified goals. In each case, the particular application of an intervention process should be unique, since individuals and their circumstances are unique. Rogers (1983) sums this up by stating, "*The occupational therapy treatment plan details what a particular patient should do to enhance occupational role performance. The therapeutic action must be the right action for this individual. This implies that it must be as congruent as possible with the patient's concept of the good life. Treatment should be in concert with the patient's needs, goals, lifestyle, and personal and cultural values. A therapeutic program that is right for one patient is not necessarily right for another.*" (p. 602)

Rogers (1983, p. 602) has suggested that clinical inquiry focuses on the following three questions:

1. What is the patient's current status in occupational role performance?
2. What could be done to enhance the patient's performance?
3. What ought to be done to enhance occupational performance?

For example, consider the performance challenges created by spinal cord injury. Even if two men of the same age from the same hometown were to sustain the same degree of quadriplegic paralysis, it is likely that their occupational therapy would vary considerably. There would be substantial differences in many individual and environmental factors which could affect their performance, ranging from the physical characteristics of their usual living environment to their family and work roles, leisure interests, and personalities. Thus, in competent practice, the same strategy will never be repeated in exactly the same manner with different individuals, since each will have a different configuration of intrinsic and extrinsic circumstances (See Figure 1-22).

It is this critical analysis of performance deficits and planning of intervention for the unique constellation of circumstances of each patient which makes occupational therapy an immensely complex undertaking. Because of this complexity, treatment planning is one of the most challenging and critical skills for therapists to master. In fact, one recent study revealed that practicing therapists find it difficult to articulate the logic underlying their clinical plans (Rogers & Masagatani, 1982). Despite its complexities, effective treatment planning can be accomplished if careful attention is devoted to the following elements of the process:

1. *Summarizing the assessment data.* In this initial component of the process, it is necessary to review

Spinal Cord Injury: A Case Comparison of Occupational Therapy Intervention

Spinal cord injury (SCI) represents one of the major causes of death and disability among young adults. For those surviving, over half must contend with paralysis affecting sensation and voluntary motor control in all four extremities (quadriplegia). Acute medical intervention is designed to prevent further injury to the spinal cord and stabilize the body systems to assure satisfactory respiration, circulation and metabolism.

Once stabilization has occurred, the patient is ready for rehabilitation. Interdisciplinary teams, including the occupational therapist, strive to help the patient achieve as much independence as possible in all dimensions of life.

Patients with injuries at the level of the sixth cervical vertebra (C-6) are quadriplegic, maintaining only limited muscular control of their head and neck, upper trunk, and arms. However, they can attain high levels of independence. The following case summaries describe the circumstances and occupational therapy treatment of two 28-year-old men. The reader will find that although the diagnoses and ages of the patients may be the same, their therapeutic regimens are likely to vary significantly, based on their personalities, experiences, interests, motivations, social situations, and views of self.

Eric M.

Background: Eric was a 28-year-old law school graduate when he sustained his level C-6 spinal cord injury in an automobile accident on the way home from a family shopping trip. His wife, pregnant at the time, suffered a fractured arm, but recovered and delivered a healthy baby girl, their first child, three months later. Eric has worked as a staff assistant in the office of the county district attorney since receiving his law degree. As a child, he was an avid reader, who excelled in school. In his leisure time, he participated in team sports. He excelled in college and was active in student governance. Eric has remained very close to his parents and siblings. His father is a high school principal, and his mother is an English teacher. His three brothers and sisters live within a 50 mile radius of the old house Eric and his wife had begun restoring just months before their accident.

Intervention: During the early phases of treatment, Eric's occupational therapist provided passive range of motion of his joints to prevent deformities and introduced some activities to increase strength and endurance. Later, when he had gained the ability to sit upright without dizziness, he began learning how to pull himself to a sitting position without assistance. At first using a device called a mobile arm support, he was taught to eat and drink with a cuff designed to help him hold utensils. Once he gained sufficient strength, he began learning how to get into his wheelchair and propel it around the facility. He learned quickly because he was anxious to try new challenges, less afraid of failure because of the many experiences in his life where he had experienced success and mastery over challenges.

Eric's therapy team quickly involved his family in planning treatment and learning to provide needed assistance. A home visit by a member of the staff suggested that because of the nature of the old house they owned, it would be best to begin looking for a newer home without as many steps and architectural barriers.

After learning to use a special flexor hinge splint to allow independent grasp, he was quickly able to resume his professional activities on a part-time basis. Later, he was given training to drive a specially modified car, in which he can transport himself to work. Despite his impairment and disability, Eric has been able to return to active participation in the roles he previously occupied.

John R.

Background: John was also 28 when he crashed his motorcycle on the way home from a construction site where he worked as a house framer. John was living alone at the time of accident, saving money to attend a local technical school, where he intended to learn auto repair. He had previously attended a junior college for two years, but his academic performance suffered because he was unsure of his goals. His mother, a widow, died of cancer during this period. As an only child, John was not encouraged to be independent. He was an average student, who became interested in carpentry and mechanics during high school. He enjoyed working on his motorcycle and going on cross-country motorcycle outings as hobbies. John had a girlfriend at the time of his accident whom he had been dating for nearly twelve months, but had few other close friends.

Intervention: John's occupational therapists also provided passive range of motion of his joints to prevent contractures and introduced some activities to help build strength and endurance in his shoulders and arms for later parts of his therapy. John's acceptance of his condition was slow to develop. He was hostile toward staff and non-compliant. Although the nature of his work had provided him with sufficient strength in his upper arms to easily learn to transfer and propel his wheelchair, his progress was slow. He was depressed—especially after his girlfriend ended their relationship after learning of his permanent paralysis. He was fearful of attempting new skills and failing. Soon, he began attending group outings organized by the occupational therapy staff. His mood and interest in participating in his rehabilitation program improved somewhat after he began socializing with other patients who participated in these outings.

Nevertheless, John's progress was slow. His mechanical interests made him curious about the devices demonstrated by his occupational therapist to help him attain independence in self-care, but he remained reluctant to attempt new skills. Because of his physical limitations, pursuit of his previous vocational ambitions was not possible. After a series of tests, the vocational counselor recommended he study mechanical engineering, which he is now considering. He has become independent enough to be discharged to a group living facility, in which several former patients share attended apartments.

Figure 1-22. Spinal Cord Injury: A Case Comparison of Occupational Therapy Intervention.

Major Intervention Categories in Occupational Therapy

Use of Occupation as a Therapeutic Medium	Education and Training Strategies	Strategies for Sensory and Neuromotor Remediation	Modification of the Physical Environment	Application of Technological Aids and Devices
Includes those strategies in which occupation, as activity, task, or role, is devised with therapeutic intent	Includes those strategies which employ education or training to enable acquisition of abilities or skills necessary for the performance of tasks or roles or use of remaining abilities to compenstate for skill deficits	Includes strategies directed toward remediation of sensory and/or motor deficits. Frequently employs principles of reflex maturation and neurophysiology	Includes those strategies aimed at modifying aspects of the physical environment, either through attention to press or arousal or through changing physical and social properties	Includes the use of various devices and equipment which enable performance of tasks and roles despite limitations in ability or skill. Includes both low technology and high technology aids and equipment
Example: Group shopping trip to purchase party supplies by residents of nursing home	*Example:* A woman with multiple sclerosis learns energy conservation techniques	*Example:* Neuromotor techniques are used with a man who has left-sided paralysis following stroke	*Example:* Doors are widened in the home of a person who has paralysis due to spinal cord injury	*Example:* A child with cerebral palsy learns to communicate using a microcomputer with a special input device.

Figure 1-23. Major Intervention Categories in Occupational Therapy.

the patient's strengths and weaknesses from the perspective of engagement in daily living activities, biopsychosocial status, and physical and social environments.

2. *Goal identification.* Based upon the summary of strengths and weaknesses, a list of goals is developed. These should directly relate from each identified problem or need. Short-term goals will often relate to problems identified in intrinsic enabling components, while long-term goals generally relate to the performance of functional daily living tasks related to role performance.

3. *Selecting intervention plans and methods.* In this process, specific methods and techniques for achieving goals must be determined. In achieving short-term goals, the emphasis is often on restoring ability and skills, thus techniques will be remedial in nature, such as developing strength or balance. Longer term goals may be more adaptive in nature, because tasks may need to be performed with abilities and skill that

are restricted. As a consequence, compensatory techniques, special equipment, and environmental modification may be necessary to accommodate residual disability. Pelland (1987) has observed that effective treatment plans are balanced, addressing both remedial and adaptive goals within and across treatment sessions. For example, in treatment of a grandmother who is recovering from stroke, one might devote time to reducing spasticity in an affected arm and learning one-handed baking skills if the patient likes to bake.

4. *Planning for further data collection.* Pelland also notes the importance of planning for further data collection and documenting these intentions. By including assessment intentions within the overall intervention plan, the therapist assures that this important aspect of treatment is not neglected.

5. *Developing Priorities.* Once each problem has an accompanying goal and plan, the vital task of determining priorities must take place. While the frames of reference selected by the therapist can provide guid-

ance, those interventions which are directed at reducing pain or preventing complications or deformities must be given first priority. Another principle is that assessment must take precedence over intervention, since effective treatment is contingent on complete information. Principles of therapeutic management also apply to this, such that trunk stability and arm positioning must be given attention before fine motor skill. Simultaneously, the therapist can give early attention to goals and strategies which have clear implications for motivation and patient compliance.

Treatment planning includes a logical flow from identified problems to goals to intervention strategies. In essence, the treatment planning process when performed by the master clinician can be likened to weaving. There is a clear design and guiding principles. The challenge is to combine the warp and weft in a way that captures opportunities for creativity and yet yields a satisfactory outcome.

Implementing Treatment

Intervention strategies for addressing identified performance deficits tend to fall into five major categories, all of which are addressed in this text, including *(1) use of occupation as a therapeutic medium, (2) education and training strategies, (3) strategies for sensory and neuromotor remediation, (4) modification of the physical environment, and (5) application of technological aids and devices* (See Figure 1-23). Intervention with a given patient will typically involve a combination of strategies from among several categories. The categories emphasized in this text provide a means of organizing intervention-related information in a manner consistent with a performance-oriented approach to occupational therapy. The therapist will be able to select and apply intervention strategies consistent with general principles of occupational therapy treatment as elaborated in the following section.

General Principles

Several general principles relevant to the spectrum of occupational therapy intervention have evolved over the years. These pertain to the patient, the therapist, and the setting and are summarized as follows:

Principle 1. *The patient is an agent of change.* One characteristic of occupational therapy that makes it different from medicine and most other health disciplines is its collaborative, cooperative orientation to intervention. The patient is not a passive recipient of care; rather active involvement of the patient is necessary throughout the intervention process, beginning with the establishment of treatment goals and concluding with decision-making on the termination of treatment or discharge. The abilities to be developed, the skills and approaches to be learned, and

ultimate performance in the non-treatment environment are all dependent upon the will and determination of the patient.

Principle 2. *The occupational therapist serves as a teacher-facilitator.* Effective intervention requires that the therapist possess not only an adequate knowledge of the abilities, skills, and conditions influencing occupational performance, but also the ability to develop a special relationship with the patient, characterized by effective communication, trust, and confidence. Devereaux (1984) suggested that in addition to effective communication, the essentials of an effective therapeutic relationship include the following practitioner characteristics: belief in the dignity and worth of the patient; belief that the patient has the potential for change and growth; clear values, a sense of humor, and the ability to use touch as a gesture of caring. Additionally, Mosey (1981) notes that the ability of the therapist to understand meanings and values of occupation from the patient's perspective (i.e., exhibiting role-taking or empathic skills) is essential to an effective therapeutic relationship.

This therapeutic relationship facilitates a level of interaction which helps the therapist identify interpersonal barriers to progress and discover interests and experiences of the patient which can be used in planning strategies. In its ideal form, the relationship is one which fosters an understanding of the patient in terms of past and present with the purpose of planning for the future. It should be characterized by a sense of professionalism which compels the therapist to maintain objectivity and recognize that the goals of treatment are paramount; even though that may require that the patient experience emotional or physical discomfort or that the therapist become a target of rejection or anger.

Peloquin (1989) has provided one of the few essays on the art of occupational therapy practice, which she describes as being centered on the relationship between the therapist and patient, on the qualities that make relationships meaningful, and on the meaning of occupation in life. Noting that use of the word *art* in official definitions of occupational therapy was deleted in the period between 1972 and 1981 (see Figure 1-5), she maintains that despite the implication that *relationships* are no longer perceived to be as important a dimension of practice as in earlier times, they are just as necessary today for competent practice.

Principle 3. *The treatment setting is an environment for developing life performance skills.* Each treatment session, viewed as a Gestalt, represents an opportunity for making progress toward treatment goals. Through careful planning, the setting can be organized to impose a level of press which promotes involvement and maximum performance by providing opportunities for choice, challenge, and success. Moreover, it must be reasonably representative of the setting(s) and sequences in which occupational performance is to occur in the patient's life. In this manner, it is perceived as relevant by the patient and generalization of skills and techniques is assured.

Principle 4. *Occupation is the preferred intervention medium.* Occupation is both the concern of occupational therapy and preferred medium of intervention. Much has been written about the importance of meaning in occupation and debates have continued regarding the use of exercise versus *purposeful* activity. It is maintained here that no medium of intervention offers the richness of diversity, the flexibility of adaptation, the potential for meaning, the opportunity for developing abilities and learning skills, or the relevance for everyday living, that occupation provides. When occupation is analyzed with expertise and selected with knowledge of the patient's level of ability, skill, interests, and treatment goals, it offers the most effective intervention strategy available to the occupational therapist.

However, it should be noted that as a vehicle for change, occupation becomes an element of the environment and therefore influences press and arousal. Its characteristics can facilitate social interaction and necessitate modifications in the physical environment. Thus, it is often used in conjunction with other intervention strategies.

Reassessment

Reassessment is often viewed as a sequential step that follows intervention. However, because intervention is dynamic rather than sequential, both planned and spontaneous reassessment during intervention provide information which results in changes in the therapeutic process. Thus, reassessment provides both *formative* or ongoing information and *summative* or outcome-oriented information.

This means that reassessment contributes corrective information or feedback during the intervention process, which permits alterations in strategy. In short, it tells the professional whether or not she/he is headed in the right direction. Once intervention is terminated, it also provides a retrospective appraisal of the extent to which strategies were successful. In this sense, it provides evaluation information on process and outcome.

Since treatment plans typically include intermediate and long-term goals, more frequent assessment (whether formal or informal) provides greater opportunity to adjust strategies and obtain the best fit between the strategies selected and the characteristics of a particular patient. However, as the therapist becomes more familiar with the patient, there is an inherent danger of losing the degree of objectivity that existed during initial assessment activities. As a consequence, the therapist must be alert to subjective influences which can bias her/his interpretation of information gained during reassessment.

Summary: The Occupational Therapy Process

Occupational therapy can be described as a dynamic process of determining the occupational performance needs of patients and designing and implementing plans of intervention that are uniquely suited to their life circumstances and which are sensitive to their interests and values, their roles, and their aspirations. While goal-oriented and systematic in nature, the treatment process is also opportunistic. The most effective intervention strategies are those which offer meaning through choice and success, while simultaneously enabling improvement in those abilities and skills which will contribute to satisfying life performance. Recognizing that the environment has profound influences on eliciting performance and determining its success, the therapist regularly analyzes its various dimensions and modifies or designs them as appropriate to enable successful occupational performance transactions.

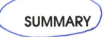

SUMMARY

In order to understand the current nature of the occupational therapy profession, one must understand the history and philosophy that shaped its beginning. The reductionistic and analytic orientation of medicine has not been consistent with the ideals and original tenets of the field of occupational therapy, which emphasize a more holistic approach. Effective occupational therapy views occupational performance as a central concern of practice and an important mechanism for adaptation, with the belief that by engaging in occupations or in doing, one can gain a sense of reality, achievement and temporal organization which ultimately contribute to one's sense of fulfillment and self-esteem.

General systems theory is described as an important structure for viewing the knowledge underlying occupational therapy. This perspective, which embodies various principles governing the relationships between and within systems, helps to organize and facilitate an understanding of the complexities underlying occupational performance. The person/environment/performance framework was presented as a means for organizing information useful to occupational therapy practice and establishes occupation as a transaction between the person and the environment. This framework highlights the necessity of considering the environment, the individual, and the occupations relevant to an individual's life when trying to understand what motivates and facilitates performance capabilities.

There are many aspects which influence one's

occupational performance, including both human and environmental factors. Of the human factors, many believe an individual's sense of competence to be perhaps the most important influence on one's ability to satisfactorily meet role demands over time. This sense of competency is developed through successful attempts to deal with environmental challenges throughout one's lifespan. There are other human factors at work during this process which can be described as intrinsic enablers of performance. These include psychological, cognitive, sensory, neuromotor, and physiological subsystems, as well as pharmacologic agents that can act on these subsystems.

In addition to the human factors, there are environmental factors that influence occupational performance. These include the physical, social, cultural, and political dimensions which must be considered by the occupational therapist in considering performance capabilities. Some factors, such as cultural beliefs and traditions, have an organizing influence on behavior, while others, such as conditions in the physical environment, can constrain performance through limiting access to settings or objects. Collectively, these human and environmental factors work together in complex ways to contribute to the general properties of the environment known as arousal and press, which have an important impact on human behavior.

Various taxonomies for classifying occupational performance exist. The levels of the performance hierarchy include activities, tasks, and roles, whereby there are required skills and abilities that underlie the tasks and roles necessary for successful occupational performance. The World Health Organization has developed a method for categorizing the consequences of disease which makes distinctions among the classifications of impairment, disability, and handicap.

Use of a problem-solving model for intervention results in the selection and use of one or more strategies from occupational therapy's major intervention categories. These include (1) environmental strategies, such as the use of technological devices and modification of the physical environment (2) person-oriented approaches such as education and training, (3) intrinsic performance approaches that are principally aimed at neuromotor and sensory reeducation and developing compensatory abilities and skills, and (4) the use of therapeutic occupation. Regardless of the strategies used, the relationship between the therapist and patient is vital, and must reflect collaborative goal-setting and effective communication if intervention is to be successful.

Study Questions

1. Identify several influences of medicine on the development of occupational therapy as a health profession. Discuss the values, benefits, and limitations of these influences.

2. Cite at least four philosophical beliefs and values that affect occupational therapy practice today. To what extent do you feel these values are shared by the general public?

3. Cite examples of patients with impairments who would not require occupational therapy. Can you cite an example of a person without disease or injury who might require occupational therapy services?

4. Review the principles underlying general systems theory. Identify the characteristics of an open system and relate these characteristics to the behavior of an individual in an environment. (For example, identify the characteristics of input, throughput, and output for a person playing tennis.)

5. Review White's definition of competence. Identify examples of situations or challenges in your own life which exemplify the attainment of competence. Is there a point at which competence is attained as an occupational therapist?

6. Consider the concept of environmental press as discussed in the chapter. Can you identify examples of press in your personal environment?

7. Identify various intrinsic enablers of performance. Can these components of performance be arranged in a systems hierarchy? Explain.

8. Distinguish between activity, task, and role. What individual characteristics provide the foundations for competent performance in these levels of occupational performance?

9. Define and provide examples of the terms impairment, disability, and handicap. Which organization is responsible for providing the definitions which embody the dysfunctional hierarchy?

10. Consider the practice of occupational therapy . Is the process best described as linear, circular, or interactive? Explain.

Acknowledgment

The Person-Environment-Performance framework described in this chapter, and which forms the organizational basis for this book, was developed by the author in collaboration with Carolyn Baum, MA, OTR, FAOTA. Her contributions to its evolution are acknowledged with warm appreciation. I also thank Wilma West, MA, OTR, FAOTA and Pamela Christiansen, MS, OTR, OT(C) for their thoughtful comments regarding early drafts of this chapter.

Recommended Readings

Brody, H. & Sobel, D.S. (1979). A systems view of health and disease. In Sobel, D.S. (Ed.). *Ways of health.* New York: Harcourt Brace Jovanovich.

Dubos, R. (1965). *Man adapting.* New Haven: Yale University Press.

Englehardt, H.T. (1977). Defining occupational therapy: The meaning of therapy and the virtues of occupation. *American Journal of Occupational Therapy, 31*(10), 675-690.

Hamburg, D.A., Coelho, C.V., & Adams, J.E. (Eds.). *Coping and adaptation.* New York: Basic Books.

Hansen, R. (Ed.). (1988). Special Issue on Ethics. *American Journal of Occupational Therapy, 42,*(5).

Kielhofner, G. & Burke, J.P. (1977). Occupational therapy after 60 years: An account of changing identity and knowledge. *American Journal of Occupational Therapy, 31*(10), 675-690.

Meyer, A. (1922). The philosophy of occupation therapy. Archives of Occupational Therapy, 1, 1-10. Reprinted in the *American Journal of Occupational Therapy, 1977, 31*(10), 639-642.

Sarbin, T.L. & Allen, V.L. (1968). Role theory. In Lindsey, G. and Aronson, E. (Eds.). *Handbook of social psychology (2nd edition).* Reading, MA: Addison-Wesley

Shannon, P.D. (1977). The derailment of occupational therapy. *American Journal of Occupational Therapy, 31*(4),229-234.

White, R.W. (1959). Motivation reconsidered: The concept of competence. *Psychological Review, 66,* 297-233.

References

Allen, C.K. (1987). Activity: Occupational therapy's treatment method. *American Journal of Occupational Therapy, 41*(9), 563-575.

Alton, I. &. Chelmers, M. (1980). *Culture and environ-ment.* Monterey, CA: Brooks/Cole.

American Occupational Therapy Association (1979). *Occupational therapy output reporting system and uniform terminology for reporting occupational therapy services.* Rockville, MD: American Occupational Therapy Association.

American Occupational Therapy Association (1987). *Occupational therapy: Directions for the future.* Rockville, Maryland: American Occupational Therapy Association.

American Occupational Therapy Association (1988). Occupational Therapy Code of Ethics. *American Journal of Occupational Therapy, 42*(12), 795-796.

American Occupational Therapy Association (1989). *Uniform terminology for occupational therapy (2nd edition).* Rockville, MD: American Occupational Therapy Association.

Bandura, A. (1977). Self-efficacy: Toward a unifying theory of behavioral change. *Psychological Review, 84,* 191-215.

Bandura, A. (1982). Self-efficacy mechanisms in human agency. *American Psychologist, 37,* 122-147.

Barris, R. (1982). Environmental interactions: An extension of the model of occupation. *American Journal of Occupational Therapy, 36*(10), 637-644.

Barris, R., Kielhofner, G., Levine, R.E., & Neville, A.M. (1985). Occupation as interaction with the environment (pp. 42-62). In Kielhofner, G. (Ed.). *A model of human occupation: Theory and application.* Baltimore: Williams & Wilkins.

Berlyne, D.E. (1960). *Conflict, arousal and curiosity.* New York: McGraw-Hill.

Berrien, F.K. (1968). *General and social systems.* New Brunswick, NJ: Rutgers University Press.

Bing, R.K. (1981). Occupational therapy revisited: A paraphrastic journey. *American Journal of Occupational Therapy, 35,* 499-518.

Bockhoven, J.S. (1971). Legacy of moral treatment-1800s to 1910. *American Journal of Occupational Therapy, 25,* 223-225.

Brody, E.M., Kleban, M.H., Lawton, M.P., & Silverman, H.A. (1971). Excess disabilities of mentally impaired aged: Impact of individualized treatment. *The Gerontologist,* 124-133.

Brody, H. & Sobel, D.S. (1979). A systems view of health and disease. In Sobel, D.S. (Ed.). *Ways of health.* New York: Harcourt Brace Jovanovich.

Bruner, J.S. (1973). Organization of early skilled action. *Child Development, 44,* 1-11.

Burke, J.P. (1977). A clinical perspective on motivation: Pawn versus origin. *American Journal of Occupational Therapy, 31*(4), 254-258.

Burke, J., Miyake, S., Kielhofner, G., & Barris R. (1983).

The demystification of health care and demise of the sick role: implications for occupational therapy (pp. 197-210). In Kielhofner, G. (Ed.). *Health through occupation: theory and practice in occupational therapy.* Philadelphia: F.A. Davis.

Caplan, A.L., Callahan, D., & Haas, J. (1987). Ethical and policy issues in rehabilitation medicine. *Hastings Center Report, 17*(4) special supplement, 1-20.

Cheng, S. & Rogers, J.C. (1989). Changes in occupational role performance after a severe burn: A retrospective study. *American Journal of Occupational Therapy, 43*(1), 17-24.

Christiansen, C.H. (1981). Toward resolution of crisis: Research requisites in occupational therapy. *Occupational Therapy Journal of Research, 1*(2), 115-124.

Christiansen, C.H. (1986). Research as reclamation. *Occupational Therapy Journal of Research, 6*, 323-326.

Christiansen, C.H. (1991). The perils of plurality. *Occupational Therapy Journal of Research, 10*(5), 259-265..

Christiansen, C., Schwartz, R., & Barnes, K. (1988). Self care: Evaluation and management (pp. 95-115). In DeLisa, J. (Ed.). *Rehabilitation medicine: Principles and practice.* Philadelphia: J.B. Lippincott.

Clark, P. (1979a). Human development through occupation: theoretical framework in contemporary occupational therapy practice. Part 1. *American Journal of Occupational Therapy, 33*, 505-514.

Clark, P. (1979b). Human development through occupation: A philosophy and conceptual model for practice. Part 2. *American Journal of Occupational Therapy, 33*, 577-585.

Cynkin, S. (1979). *Occupational therapy: Toward health through activities.* Boston: Little, Brown and Co.

DeCharms, R. (1968). *Personal causation: The internal affective determinants of behavior.* New York: Academic Press.

Devereaux, E.B. (1984). Occupational therapy's challenge: The caring relationship. *American Journal of Occupational Therapy, 38*, 791-798.

Dewey, J. & Bentley, A.F. (1949). *Knowing and the known.* Boston: Beacon.

Dubos, R. (1965). *Man adapting.* New Haven: Yale University Press.

Engel, G. (1977). The need for a new medical model: A challenge for biomedicine. *Science, 196*, 129-136.

Englehardt, H.T. (1977). Defining occupational therapy: The meaning of therapy and the virtues of occupation. *American Journal of Occupational Therapy, 31*(10), 666-672.

Fabrega, H. (1975). The need for an ethnomedical science. *Science, 189*, 969-975.

Fidler, G.S. (1981). From crafts to competence. *American Journal of Occupational Therapy, 35*, 567-573.

Fidler, G.S. & Fidler, J.W. (1978). Doing and becoming: Purposeful action and self-actualization. *American Journal of Occupational Therapy, 32*, 305-310.

Fleishman, E.A. (1972). On the relation between abilities, learning and human performance. *American Psychologist, 27*, 1017-1032.

Fleishman, E.A. (1975). Toward a taxonomy of human performance. *American Psychologist, 30*(12), 11-27-1149.

Fleishman, E.A. & Quaintance, M.K. (1984). *Taxonomies of human performance: The description of human tasks.* Orlando: Academic Press.

Goffman, I. (1963). *Stigma: Notes on the management of a spoiled identity.* Englewood Cliffs, NJ: Prentice-Hall.

Hall, E. (1966). *The hidden dimension.* Garden City, NY: Anchor Books.

Hall, E.T. (1973). *The silent language.* Garden City, NY: Anchor Books.

Hansen, R.A. (1984). Moral reasoning of occupational therapists: Implications for education and practice. Unpublished Doctoral Dissertation, Wayne State University, Detroit, MI.

Hansen, R.A. (1988). Ethics is the issue. *American Journal of Occupational Therapy, 42*(5), 279-281.

Heard, C. (1977). Occupational role acquisition: A perspective on the chronically disabled. *American Journal of Occupational Therapy, 31*(4), 243-247.

Heider, F. (1958). *The psychology of interpersonal relations.* New York: Wiley.

Henderson, A. (1988). Occupational therapy knowledge: From practice to theory. *American Journal of Occupational Therapy, 42*(9), 567-576.

Howe, M.C. & Briggs, A.K. (1982). Ecological systems model for occupational therapy. *American Journal of Occupational Therapy, 36*, 322-327.

Kahn, R.S. (1965). Comments. In *Proceedings of the York House Institute on the Mentally Impaired Aged.* Philadelphia: Philadelphia Geriatric Center.

Kielhofner, G. (1977). Temporal adaptation: A conceptual framework for occupational therapy. *American Journal of Occupational Therapy, 31*(4), 235-242.

Kielhofner, G. (1978). General system theory: Implications for the theory and action in occupational therapy. *American Journal of Occupational Therapy, 32*, 637-645.

Kielhofner, G. (1982). A heritage of activity: Development of theory. *American Journal of Occupational Therapy, 36*(11), 723-730.

Kielhofner, G. (1985). *A model of human occupation: Theory and application.* Baltimore: Williams and Wilkins.

Kielhofner, G. (1988). Occupational therapy-base in occupation (pp. 84-92). In Hopkins, H. & Smith, H. (Ed.). *Willard & Spackman's Occupational Therapy*. Philadelphia: J.B. Lippincott.

Kielhofner, G. & Burke, J.P. (1977). Occupational therapy after 60 years: An account of changing identity and knowledge. *American Journal of Occupational Therapy, 31*, 675-689.

Kielhofner, G. & Burke, J.P. (1980). A model of human occupation. Part 1. Conceptual framework and content. *American Journal of Occupational Therapy, 34*, 572-581.

Kielhofner, G. & Burke, J.P. (1985). Components and Determinants of Human Occupation (pp. 12-36). In Kielhofner, G.W. (Ed.). *A model of human occupation: Theory and application*. Baltimore: Williams & Wilkins.

Kilpatrick-Tubak, B. & Roth, S. (1978). Attempt to reverse performance deficits associated with depression and experimentally induced helplessness. *Journal of Abnormal Psychology, 87*, 141-154.

King, L.J. (1978). Toward a science of adaptive responses. *American Journal of Occupational Therapy, 32*, 429-437.

Kleinman, B.L. & Bulkley, B.L. (1982). Some implications of a science of adaptive responses. *American Journal of Occupational Therapy, 36*(1), 15-19.

Kuhn, T. (1970). *The structure of scientific revolutions (2nd edition)*. Chicago: University of Chicago Press.

Lawton, M.P. (1980). *Environment and aging*. Monterey, CA: Brooks-Cole.

Llorens, L.A. (1970). Facilitating growth and development: The promise of occupational therapy. *American Journal of Occupational Therapy, 24*, 93-101.

Llorens, L.A. (1976). *Application of developmental theory for health and rehabilitation*. Rockville, MD: American Occupational Therapy Association.

Llorens, L.A. (1984). Changing balance: Environment and individuals. *American Journal of Occupational Therapy, 38*, 575-584.

Lyons, B.G. (1983). Purposeful versus human activity. *American Journal of Occupational Therapy, 37*(7), 493-498.

Mayer, N.H., Keating, D.J., & Rapp, D. (1986). Skills, routines and activity patterns of living: A functional nested approach (pp. 205-224). In B.P. Uzzell & Y. Gross (Eds.). *Clinical neuropsychology of intervention*. Boston: Martinus Nijhoff Publishing.

McClelland, C.D. (1961). *The achieving society*. Princeton, NJ: Van Nostrand.

McKeown, T. (1976). *The role of medicine, dream, mirage or nemesis?* London: Nuffield Provincial Hospital Trust.

McKeown, T. (1978). Determinants of health. *Human Nature, 1*(4), 60-67.

Mead, G.H. (1934). *Mind, self and society*. Chicago: University of Chicago Press.

Meyer, A. (1922). The philosophy of occupation therapy. *Archives of Occupational Therapy, 1*(1), 1-10.

Miller, R.B. (1967). Task taxonomy: Science or technology? In Singleton, W.T., Easterly, R.S., & Whitfield, D.C. (Eds.). *The human operator in complex systems*. London: Taylor & Francis.

Mosey, A.C. (1974). An alternative: The biopsychosocial model. *American Journal of Occupational Therapy, 28*(3), 137-140.

Mosey, A.C. (1981). *Occupational Therapy: Configuration of a profession*. New York: Raven Press.

Mosey, A.C. (1985). A monistic or pluralistic approach to professional identity. *American Journal of Occupational Therapy, 39*(8), 504-509.

Mosey, A.C. (1989). The proper focus of scientific inquiry in occupational therapy: Frames of reference (Editorial). *Occupational Therapy Journal of Research, 9*(4), 195-201.

Moss, G. (1973). *Illness, immunity and social interactions*. New York: Wiley.

Murray, H.A., Barrett, W.G., & Hamburger, E. (1938). *Explorations in personality*. New York: Oxford University Press.

Nelson, D.L. (1988). Occupation: Form and performance. *American Journal of Occupational Therapy, 42*(10), 633-641.

Parent, L.H. (1978). Effects of a low stimulus environment on behavior. *American Journal of Occupational Therapy, 32*, 19-25.

Parham, L.D. (1987). Toward professionalism: The reflective therapist. *American Journal of Occupational Therapy, 41*, 555-561.

Parker, J.R., Jr. & Fleishman, E.A. (1961). Use of analytical information concerning task requirements to increase the effectiveness of skill training. *Journal of Applied Psychology, 45*, 295-302.

Parsons, T. (1975). The sick role and the role of the physician reconsidered. *Health and Society*, 257-278, 257-278.

Pelland, M.J. (1987). A conceptual model for the instruction and supervision of treatment planning. *American Journal of Occupational Therapy, 41*(6), 351-359.

Peloquin, S.M. (1989). Sustaining the art of practice in occupational therapy. *American Journal of Occupational Therapy, 43*(4), 219-226.

Pervin, L.A. (1968). Performance and satisfaction as a function of individual-environment fit. *Psychological Bulletin, 69*, 56-68.

Reed, K.L. (1984). *Models of practice in occupational therapy*. Baltimore: Williams & Wilkins.

Reilly, M. (1962). Occupational therapy can be one of the great ideas of 20th century medicine. *American Journal of Occupational Therapy, 16*, 300-308.

Reilly, M. (1966). A psychiatric occupational therapy program as a teaching model. *American Journal of Occupational Therapy, 20*, 61-67.

Reilly, M. (1974). Preface. In Reilly, M. (Ed.). *Play as exploratory learning.* Beverly Hills: Sage.

Reilly, M. (1984). The importance of the client versus patient issue for occupational therapy. *American Journal of Occupational Therapy, 38*(6), 404-406.

Robinson, A.L. (1977). Play: The arena for acquisition of rules for competent behavior. *American Journal of Occupational Therapy, 31*(4), 248-253.

Rogers, J.C. (1982a). Order and disorder in medicine and occupational therapy. *American Journal of Occupational Therapy, 36*, 29-35.

Rogers, J.C. (1982b). The spirit of independence: The evolution of a philosophy. *American Journal of Occupational Therapy, 36*, 709-715.

Rogers, J.C. (1983). Clinical reasoning: The ethics, science and art. *American Journal of Occupational Therapy, 37,* 601-616.

Rogers, J. & Masagatani, G. (1982). Clinical reasoning of occupational therapists during the initial assessment of physically disabled patients. *Occupational Therapy Journal of Research, 2*(4), 195-219.

Rotter, J.B. (1966). Generalized expectancies for internal versus external control of reinforcement. *Psychological Monographs 80,* (Whole No. 609).

Sarbin, T.R. & Allen, V.L. (1968). Role theory. In Lindsey, G. & Aronson, E. (Eds.). *Handbook of social psychology (2nd edition).* Reading, MA: Addison-Wesley.

Schon, D. (1983). *The reflective practitioner: How professionals think in action.* New York: Basic Books.

Shannon, P.D. (1977). The derailment of occupational therapy. *American Journal of Occupational Therapy, 31*(4), 229-234.

Shannon, P.D. (1986). Philosophical considerations for the practice of occupational therapy. In Ryan, S.E. (Ed.). *The certified occupational therapy assistant: Roles and responsibilities* (pp. 38-44). Thorofare, NJ: Slack.

Sharrott, G.W. & Yerxa, E.J. (1985). Promises to keep: Implications of the referent "patient" versus "client" for those served by occupational therapy. *American Journal of Occupational Therapy, 39*(6), 401-406.

Smith, M.B. (1974). Competence and adaptation: A perspective on therapeutic ends and means. *American Journal of Occupational Therapy, 28*(1), 11-15.

Spivak, M. (1973). Archetypal places. *Architectural Forum, 140,* 43-48.

Sullivan, H.S. (1953). *Conceptions of modern psychiatry.* New York: W.W. Norton.

Tanguay, P.E. (1985). The issue is: Does occupational therapy belong in the university? *American Journal of Occupational Therapy, 39*, 466-468.

von Bertalanffy, L. (1968). General system theory — a critical review (pp. 11-30). In Buckley, W. (Ed.). *Modern system's research for the behavioral scientist.* Chicago: Aldine.

Weiss, P.S. (1971). *Hierarchically organized systems in theory and practice.* New York: Hafner.

West, W.L. (1978). Reflections at retirement. *American Journal of Occupational Therapy, 32*(1), 9-12.

West, W.L. (1984). A reaffirmed philosophy and practice of occupational therapy for the 1980s. *American Journal of Occupational Therapy, 38*(1), 15-23.

White, R.W. (1959). Motivation reconsidered: The concept of competence. *Psychological Review, 66,* 297-333.

White, R.W. (1964). Sense of interpersonal competence. In White, R. (Ed.), *The study of lives.* New York: Atherton Press.

White, R.W. (1971). The urge toward competence. *American Journal of Occupational Therapy, 25,* 271-274.

Wood, P.H.N. (1980). Appreciating the consequences of disease: the International Classification of Impairments, Disabilities and Handicaps. *World Health Organization Chronicle, 34,* 376-380.

Wool, R.N., Siegel, D., & Fine, P.R. (1980). Task performance in spinal cord injury: Effect of helplessness training. *Archives of Physical Medicine and Rehabilitation, 61,* 321-325.

World Health Organization. (1980). *International Classification of impairments, disabilities and handicaps: A manual of classification relating to the consequences of disease.* Geneva: World Health Organization.

Yerxa, E. (1967). Authentic occupational therapy. *American Journal of Occupational Therapy, 21,* 1-9.

Yerxa, E. (1983). Research priorities. *American Journal of Occupational Therapy, 37*(10), 699.

Yerxa, E. (1987). Research: the key to the development of occupational therapy as an academic discipline? *American Journal of Occupational Therapy, 41,* 415-419.

Yerxa, E. (1988). Oversimplification: The hobgoblin of theory and practice in occupational therapy. *Canadian Journal of Occupational Therapy, 55*(1), 5-6.

Yoder, R.M., Nelson, D.L., & Smith, D.A. (1989). Added purpose versus rote exercise in female nursing home residents. *American Journal of Occupational Therapy, 43*(9), 581-595.

CHAPTER CONTENT OUTLINE

KEY TERMS

Activity

Adaptation

Competence

Extrinsic Motivation

Intrinsic motivation

Life roles

Mastery

Self-care/self-maintenance

Work/education

ABSTRACT

This chapter identifies the development of various occupational tasks and roles at specific ages and stages throughout the life span. It investigates the role of human development in relation to functional adaptation from infancy to old age. By engaging in valued activities, tasks, roles, and interpersonal interactions at each of these life stages, individuals can achieve a sense of competence and mastery which allows adaptation to occur. The achievement of competence, mastery, and adaptation are viewed as central to occupational performance.

Performance Tasks and Roles Throughout the Life Span

2

Lela A. Llorens

"Humanization, becoming part of human society . . . [is] the process whereby the individual, beginning life as a biologic organism, becomes a person whose primitive actions are gradually transformed into behavior that . . . satisfies needs . . . [and] contributes to societal development."

—Fidler & Fidler, 1978

OBJECTIVES

The information in this chapter is intended to help the reader—

1. recognize the role of human development in relation to functional adaptation.

2. identify occupational roles at specific ages and stages over the life span.

3. describe areas of occupational performance from infancy through old-old age.

4. describe the component behaviors of occupational performance from infancy through old-old age.

5. identify levels of mastery for successful adaptation.

6. recognize the influence of activity on task performance and role competence.

7. describe the role of family relationships in development and maturation.

8. describe role competence and adaptation in occupational performance.

INTRODUCTION

Engagement in **activities,** tasks, and interpersonal interactions assists in the development of skills and abilities that support occupational performance in **self-care/self-maintenance,** work/education, play/leisure, and rest/relaxation. Such engagement is motivated by **intrinsic** and **extrinsic** forces, is purposeful, and is valued by the task performer. Through engagement in valued activities, tasks, and interpersonal interactions, achievement of **competence, mastery, and adaptation** occurs. The achievement of competence, mastery, and adaptation is central to occupational performance.

Occupational performance, defined here as the accomplishment of tasks related to self-care/self-maintenance, work/education, play/leisure, and rest/relaxation, is critical to the assumption of social or **life roles,** the functional positions that people hold in the society—worker, parent, mate, peer, etc. Successful performance in these areas is demanded by the environment, consistent with cultural requirements at specific ages and stages across the life span. **Self-care/self-maintenance** refers to independence in physical daily-living skills. It includes, but is not limited to, grooming and hygiene, feeding and eating, dressing, and functional mobility. Ability to manipulate objects is a necessary skill for independence in self-care/self-maintenance (AOTA, 1981/1989). **Work/education** refers to skill and performance in purposeful and productive activities in the home, in employment, in school, and in the community. Play/leisure refers to ''skill and performance in choosing, performing, and engaging in activities for amusement, relaxation, spontaneous enjoyment, and/or self-expression'' (AOTA, 1981/1989, p. 13). Rest/relaxation refers to performance during time not devoted to other activity and during time devoted to sleep.

The accomplishment of tasks is predicated on the ability to achieve mastery of skills. **Mastery** of skills, in turn, depends on efficient neurophysiological and neuromuscular functioning. This is manifested in occupational performance components or subskills: sensory perception, sensory integration, motor coordination, psychosocial (affective) and psychodynamic responses, sociocultural development, social language responses, and cognition (Llorens, 1976).

Intact neurophysiological development is the foundation for occupational performance. Neurophysiological as used here refers to nervous system control of bodily functions and processes, specifically brain function. Neuromuscular refers to nervous system control of muscle functions. Sensory functions include tactile (relating to touch), visual, auditory, vestibular (relating to orientation), gustatory (relating to taste), olfactory (relating to smell), proprioceptive (relating to position), and kinesthetic (relating to movement). Sensory integration refers to the brain's ability to process stimuli presented to the senses. The result of sensory integration can be observed in physical motor movement and psychological (affective) responses. Further, sensory integration influences occupational role adaptation and the development of social behavior, social language, and learning. Sociocultural refers to behavior required by the learner within the culture for social interaction (Llorens, 1976).

Adaptation results from the interaction of the individual with the environment through purposeful activity (American Occupational Therapy Association, 1979). Levels of mastery for successful adaptation are illustrated in Figure 2-1. Mastery of Level 1, occupational performance enablers, provides a foundation for Level 2, occupational performance. Levels 1 and 2 together provide a foundation for Level 3, occupational roles.

When deficits occur in adaptive functioning and in developmental expectations, behaviors, and needs, efficient functioning for adaptation can be facilitated by engagement in prescribed activities, tasks, and interpersonal interactions. Table 2-1 illustrates this process. Deficits in areas listed in Section 1 of the schematic can be corrected or offset by use of the activities identified in Section 2. These will assist in the development of behavior and performance in the daily-life activities identified in Section 3.

Figure 2-2, a schematic representation of the influence of activity on life task performance, depicts the role of activities, tasks, and interpersonal interactions in adaptation. Activities, tasks, and interpersonal interactions provide stimulation to the tactile, visual, auditory, vestibular, gustatory, olfactory, proprioceptive, and kinesthetic systems. The stimulation influences the sensory systems, and elicits behavior that results in the development of occupational performance enablers (subskills). Activities, tasks, and interpersonal interactions also assist in the development of occupational performance skills, which support occupational role behavior (Clark & Allen, 1989; Llorens, 1981; Llorens & Burris, 1981).

Successful performance in self-care/self-maintenance, work/education, play/leisure, and rest/relaxation is demanded by the environment, consistent with cultural requirements at specific ages and stages across the life span. Growth and development continue throughout the life span; however, decline in some aspects of functioning may decline as the individual ages. Even so, adaptation continues until death.

Gesell, Freud, Erikson, Maslow, Piaget, Havighurst, Kohlberg, and Peck have provided background knowledge on the biological and behavioral bases for human development through the life cycle (Erikson, 1985; Hall, 1979; Havighurst, 1979; Knoblock & Pasamanick, 1974; Maier, 1978; Papalia & Olds, 1986). Table 2-2 summarizes this knowledge. Occupational therapy theorists Ayres (1972, 1979), Reilly (1974), Mosey (1968, 1971), Llorens (1970, 1976), Clark and Allen (1985), and Gilfoyle, Grady, and Moore (1980) have described applications of developmental and neurophysiological theory relevant to understanding the role of mastery, growth and development across the life span. Table 2-3 summarizes these applications.

In the following sections, developmental stages and occupational performance skills are described relative to occupational and social role expectations and the adaptive behaviors required to function in roles associated with each developmental stage. Occupational performance areas of self-care/self-maintenance, work/education, play/leisure, and rest/relaxation are explained for each stage, along with the components that support their development and maintenance. Occupational performance enablers, in turn, are supported by the developmental integrity of the human system.

Examples of adaptation are presented in the discussion of developmental stages. Developmental theorists describe the acquisition and the expression of occupational performance skills and skill components in greater detail for infants and children than for adults. Therefore, beginning with the section on middle adulthood, vignettes are used to illustrate the expression of achieved skills and skill components in occupational roles.

INFANCY AND TODDLERHOOD

Occupational Performance

This age group spans newborn to age two. Social and occupational roles that may be associated with infancy and

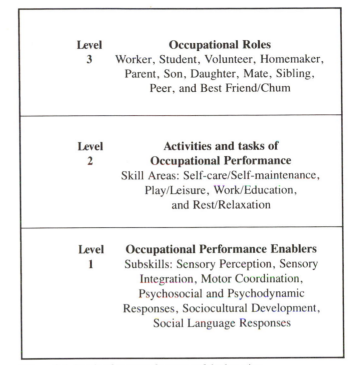

Figure 2-1. Levels of mastery for successful adaptation.

toddlerhood include son, daughter, brother, sister, grandson, and granddaughter. Adaptive behaviors required to function in these roles range from responding to nurturing and taking nourishment, to talking, walking, and controlling elimination. Emotional bonding facilitates the relationship with the primary caregivers and family members.

Self-care/self-maintenance activities are focused on nurturance and competence. Specific milestones include recognition of the source of food (the breast or the bottle) and response in the feeding situation by expectancy and readiness. As the infant moves toward toddlerhood, more self-sufficiency develops. The child is able to hold a cup, hold a spoon, feed himself or herself neatly, and control elimination.

Play/leisure activities assist the infant in developing skills through engagement with objects and through interaction with caregivers and family members. The infant and the toddler practice and achieve mastery of the skills of motor planning and problem solving using rattles, pots and pans, and other objects. The infant develops form and space perception, equilibrium (balance), and postural flexibility in reaction to the environment.

Rest/relaxation takes the form of sleep, which occupies considerable time in the first year of life—11 to 16 hours or more per day. The child usually begins to sleep completely through the night between four and six months of age,

Table 2-1
Facilitation of Growth and Development

Section 1
Developmental Expectations, Behaviors and Needs

Neuropsychological Sensorimotor (Ayres)	Physical-Motor (Gesell)	Psychosocial (Erikson)	Psychodynamic (Grant/Freud)	Sociocultural (Gesell)	Social Language (Gesell)	Activity of Daily Living (Gesell)
0-2 yrs. Sensorimotor — Tactile, vestibular, visual, auditory, olfactory, gustatory functions	0-2 yrs — Head sags, Fisting, Gross motion, Walking, Climbing	Basic Trust vs. Mistrust/Oral Sensory — Ease of feeding, Depth of sleep, Relax. of bowels	0-4 yrs. Oral — Dependency, Init. aggress.	Oral erotic activity — Individual mothering person most important; Immediate family group important	Small sounds, Coos, Vocalizes, Listens, Speaks	Recognizes bottle, Holds spoon, Holds glass, Controls bowel
6 mo.–4 yrs. Integration of Body Sides — Gross motor plan, Form & space, Balance, Post. and bilateral integration, Body scheme-develop.	2-3 yrs. — Runs, Balances, Hand preference, Coordination	Autonomy vs. Shame & Doubt/ Muscular-Anal — Conflict between holding on & letting go	0-4 yrs. Independence, Resistiveness, Self-assertiveness, Narcissism, Ambivalence	Parallel play, Often alone, Recognizes extended family	Identifies objects verb., Asks "why?", Short sentences	Feeds self, Helps undress, Recognizes simple tunes, No longer wets at night
3-7 Discrimination — Refined tactile, kinesth, visual, auditory, olfact., gustatory functions	3-6 yrs. — Coordination more graceful, Muscles develop, Skills develop	Initiative vs. Guilt/ Locomotor-Genital — Aggressiveness, Manipulation, Coercion	3-6 yrs Genital-Oedipal — Genital interest, Poss. of opp. parent, Antag. to same parent, Castration fears	Seeks companionship, Makes decisions, Plays with other children, Takes turns	Combines talking and eating, Complete sentences, Imaginative, Dramatic	Laces shoes, Cuts with scissors, Toilets independently, Helps set table
3- Abstract Thinking — Conceptualization, Complex relations, Read, write, numbers	6-11 yrs. — Energy development, Skill practice to attain proficiency	Industry vs. Inferiority/ Latency — Wins recognition thru productivity, Learns skills & tools	6-11 yrs Latency — Prim. struggles quiescent, Init. in mastery of skills, Strong defenses	Group play & team activities, Independence of adults, Gang interests	Language major form of communication	Enjoys dressing up, Learns value of money, Responsible for grooming
Continue to develop Conceptualization, Complex relations, Read, write, numbers	11-13 yrs. — Rapid growth, Poor posture, Awkwardness	Identity vs. Role Confusion/Puberty & Adolescence — Identification, Social roles	11- Adolescence — Emancip. from parents, Occup. decisions, Role experiment, Re-exam of values	Team games, Organization important, Interest in opposite sex	Verbal language predominates	Interest in earning money
Development presumably maintained	Growth established and maintained	Intimacy vs. Isolation/Young Adulthood — Commitments, Body & ego mastery	Outgrow need for parent validation, Identify with others	Group affiliation, Family, social, civic, interest	Non-verbal behavior used	Concern for personal grooming, mate, family
Alterations begin to occur in sensory functions conceptualization, and memory	Alterations begin to occur in motor behavior, strength, and endurance	Generativity vs. Stagnation/ Adulthood — Guiding next generation, Creative, productive	Emotional responsibilities may lessen, Phys. and econ. independ. accepted, Shift from survival to enjoyment			Accepting and adjusting to changes of middle age
Alterations in sensory functions, conceptualization, and memory	Alterations in motor behavior, strength, and endurance	Ego Integrity vs. Despair/Maturity — Acceptance of own life cycle	Continued growth after middle age, Inner trend toward survival			Adjusting to changes after middle age

Table 2-1
Facilitation of Growth and Development (continued)

Section 2 — Facilitating Activities and Relationships (Selected)					Section 3 — Behavior Expectations and Adaptive Skills		
Sensorimotor Activities	**Developmental Activities**	**Symbolic Activities**	**Daily Life Tasks**	**Interpersonal Activities**	**Developmental Tasks (Havighurst)**	**Ego-Adaptive Skills—(Mosey, Pearce & Newton)**	**Intellectual Development (Piaget)**
Tactile, visual, aud., olfact., gust., Stimulation	Dolls Animals Sand Water Excursions	Biting Chewing Eating Blowing Cuddling	Recog. food Hold feed. equip. Use feed. equip.	Individual Interaction	Learning to walk, talk, take solids Elimination,	Ability to respond to mothering Mastering of gross motor responses	Motor skills Integrated
Phys. exercise Balancing Motor planning	Pull toys Playground Clay Crayons Chalk	Throwing Dropping Messing Collecting Destroying	Feeding Toileting	Individual Interaction Parallel play	Sex difference Form concepts of soc. & physical reality Relate emotionally to others Right vs. wrong Develop a conscience	Ability to respond to routines of daily living Mastery of 3 dimen. space Sense of body image	Investigative Imitative Ecocentric
Listening Learning Skilled tasks & games	Being read to Coloring Drawing Painting	Destroying Exhibiting	Feeding Dressing Toileting Simple chores	Individual Interaction Play small groups		Ability to respond to routines of daily living Mastery of 3 dimen. space Tolerate frustrations Sit still Delay gratification	Egocentrism reduced, social increased Lang. Rep. motor
Reading Writing Numbers	Scooters Wagons Collections Puppets Bldg.	Controlling Mastery	Feeding Dressing Grooming Spending	Individual Interaction Groups Teams Clubs	Learn phys. skills Getting along Reading, writing Values Social attitudes	Ability to perceive, sort, organize & utilize stimuli Work in groups Master inanimate obj.	Orders exper. Relates parts to wholes Deduct.
All of the above available to be recycled	Weaving Machinery tasks Carving Modeling	All of the above available to be recycled	Feeding Dressing Grooming Pre-voc. skills	Individual Interaction Groups Teams	More mature relationships Social roles Select occupation Achieving emot. independence	Ability to accept & discharge respn. Capacity for love	Systematic approach to problems Sense of equality
	Arts Crafts Sports Club & interest groups Education Work		Feeding Dressing Grooming Life role skills	Individual Interaction Groups	Selecting a mate Starting family Marriage, home Congenial social group	Ability to function indep Control drives Plan & execute Purposeful motions Obtain org. & use knowledge Part. in primary group Part. in variety of relationships Exp. self as accept. Part. in mutually satisfying heterosexual relations	Development established and maintained
					Civic & social responsibility Econ. standard of living Dev. adult leisure activities Adjust to aging parents Adjust to decr. phys. health, retire., death Age group affiliations Meeting social obligations		Alterations in other areas may affect

From: Lorens, L.A. (1976). *Application of developmental theory for health and rehabilitation.* Rockville, MD: American Occupational Therapy Association.

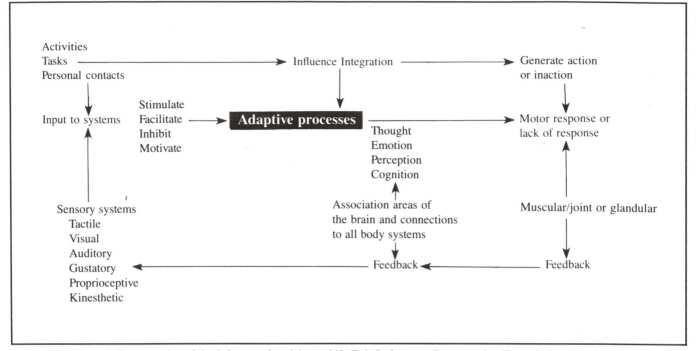

Figure 2-2. Schematic Representation of the Influence of Activity on Life Task Performance Demonstrating Theoretical Assumptions Regarding Why Occupational Therapists Use Occupation. *Reproduced with permission of Lela A. Llorens. See also Llorens, L.A.: Occupational therapy: state of the art—potential for development, Proceedings of New Zealand Association of Occupational Therapists Annual Conference, Auckland, N.Z., 1981; and Llorens, L.A., and Burris, B.B.: Development of sensory integration in learning disabilities, Baltimore, 1981, University Park Press.*

although night wakefulness is common. Sleep patterns differ with each infant.

Occupational Performance Enablers

Sensory development is key to the developing neurophysiological integrity of the infant and the child. The tactile, vestibular, visual, auditory, olfactory, gustatory, proprioceptive, and kinesthetic systems receive stimuli through the interaction of the infant and the child with the environment. Self-care, play, and interpersonal interaction provide the activities to nurture the development of these systems.

Physical motor development includes the ability to suck, to achieve head and trunk flexibility and stability, to make a fist, and to follow objects visually. Development progresses to standing, walking with assistance, and lowering to a seated position. Gross movements for purposeful and more complex activity such as climbing stairs (first by holding on, later independently) and walking while carrying objects develop next. Activities that facilitate physical motor learning must be mastered to form the foundation for occupational performance. Gross motor activities employ environmental objects such as kitchen cupboards, furniture, and toys. They also involve interaction with others.

Psychological/social development requires engagement in activities that elicit a positive response to nurturing and to an interactive empathetic relationship. Social trust is created in the bond that develops between the child and the caregiver through feeding, through the environmental response to sleep needs, providing consistency and continuity, and through habit training associated with elimination. Responsiveness to attention provided by a nurturing caregiver can be observed in smiles, muscle tone, and emotional disposition. Psychological/social development is also achieved in interaction with other members of the family as the infant and the toddler share in family activities.

Psychodynamic development is focused on oral and anal activities; mastery of eating and elimination skills is significant at this stage.

Social language development in infants and toddlers proceeds from the utterance of small throaty sounds, coos, and laughs; to vocalizing and listening to their own vocalizations; to understanding simple statements and speaking a few words; to attaching words to objects in the possessive; to speaking simple phrases and following simple requests, such as that they put their toys away.

Activities that contribute to sociocultural development are centered on the child's interactions with his or her responsible caregiver and the immediate family. They assist in forming the trust relationships that are important to future performance and achievement. Caregivers' differentiation between the child's "soiled diaper cry" and his or her "hunger cry" contributes to development in this area, as does the inclusion of the child in social events of the family.

Cognitive development at this stage is promoted through the repetitive use of primitive reflexes and tasks, which combine with physical and neurological maturation to form habits. Movement and toys that elicit it, stimulate sensorimotor functioning and encourage both solitary play and interactive play, which contribute to cognitive development. Spontaneous repetition, provided by play activities and stimulated by internal drives for competence and external environmental stimuli, offers experiences in which maturation of cognitive skills can occur.

EARLY CHILDHOOD

Occupational Performance

The roles of early childhood, from ages two to five, again include son, daughter, brother, sister, grandson, granddaughter, and a new role of peer. At ages three to five, the role of student may be added. Adaptive behavior associated with these roles is focused on refinement and mastery of abilities that had their rudimentary development in the first two years of life.

Self-care/self-maintenance activities are primarily related to developing self-sufficiency in eating, dressing, and washing. Children in this age group may wet the bed at night occasionally, but for the most part have reached dryness by age three. Independence in dressing is attained through the stages of assisting with undressing, then assisting with dressing. Eating without spilling is also achieved.

Play/leisure activities are focused on continual exploration and investigation of the environment. Engagement in repetitive activity and imitative behavior characterizes the activities. Use of language as play is common, and self-absorption is expected. Between two and three years of age, children may engage in parallel play with peers, although children at this stage often play alone. Extended-family members and others contribute to the achievement of skills through play. Capacity for organized group play and taking turns develops at this time, as does the ability to follow directions and to concentrate on a given task for reasonable periods. Items and activities that are useful for development are pull toys; playground equipment; plastic media such as clay, silly putty, and Play-Doh; paints, crayons, and chalk; and listening activities.

Work/education activities may begin in the form of preschool or nursery school involvement as soon as elimination is mastered. The environment will require skills for social interaction and should support positive growth and development.

In the rest/relaxation area, children in this age group usually sleep through the night. However, wakefulness is common at two and three years of age or in response to stressful situations. Older children will often prolong the bedtime ritual by requesting water or other attention. Three-year-olds or older children may need a night light (Papalia & Olds, 1986).

Occupational Performance Enablers

Sensory development to refine the tactile, visual, auditory, vestibular, olfactory, gustatory, proprioceptive, and kinesthetic functions is effected by occupational performance activities and is supportive of mastery and competence in social and occupational roles. Touching, grasping, having questions answered about the environment, and playing interactive games that require attention and cooperation are developmental activities of this age group (2-5 years).

For physical motor development, running, climbing, digging, balancing, skipping, jumping, stair climbing, and walking—all smoothly executed gross motor movements—are characteristic of the age group. Fine motor development and eye-hand coordination are demonstrated in activities such as copying geometric figures. Coordination is generally more graceful, hand preference is established, arms and legs lengthen, and a full set of baby teeth is completed. For physically limited children, positioning in an appropriate conveyance may be of paramount importance in facilitating the development of skills needed for adaptation.

Psychological/social development is focused on achieving a balance between "holding on" and "letting go" and developing autonomy through engagement in activities that permit choice. The child develops the ability to separate from caregivers as he or she observes and participates in leave-taking in which caregivers go away and return without abandonment. Being given opportunity for choice in food, play activities, and color of clothing builds children's confidence in their abilities to make decisions and to become autonomous.

Psychodynamic development is focused on the transition from oral and anal to genital activities. Genital interest and initial interest in sexual differences are evident. Answering questions that stem from sexual curiosity matter-of-factly and at the level of the child's understanding is important.

**Table 2-2
Developmental Theorists and Theoretical Orientations**

Arnold Gesell

Described a biological and behavioral foundation for development in five major fields of behavior (Knobloch & Pasamanick, 1974). Included the zone of preterm viability, in which fetal development is influenced in utero.

Field I. Adaptive Behavior

The ''organization of stimuli, the perception of relationships, the dissection of wholes into component parts and the reintegration of these parts in a meaningful fashion'' (p. 4).

Field II. Gross Motor Behavior

Postural control, head balance, and muscle tone underlying the development of coordinated motor behavior for turning, sitting, standing, walking, and so on.

Field III. Fine Motor Behavior

Hand and finger use in prehension, grasp, and object manipulation.

Field IV. Language Behavior

Social language, from babbling and cooing to articulation, vocabulary, adaptive use of verbal symbols and nonverbal gestures, and comprehension. Follows a developmental sequence.

Field V. Personal Social Behavior

''The child's personal reactions to the social culture in which he lives'' (p. 5). These responses interact with neurophysiological functioning, which serves as the biological basis for development of adaptive, personal social behavior.

Jean Piaget

Described four major stages of cognitive development (Papalia & Olds, 1986).

Stage I. Sensorimotor Stage (birth to 2 years)

Infants mature from primarily reflexive beings to more neurophysiologically organized beings through play experiences and interpersonal interaction. Children learn the existence of the world outside themselves.

Stage II. Preoperational Stage (2-7 years)

The child ''develops a representational system and uses symbols such as words to represent people, places, and events'' (p. 15). Egocentrism is a factor in this stage.

Stage III. Concrete Operations Stage (7-11 years)

The child begins to ''understand and use concepts [to] ... deal with the immediate environment'' (p. 15) and solve problems logically when related to actual events and objects. Conservation is a major cognitive skill achieved in this stage. Conservation is the notion that objects remain the same in different contexts as long as nothing is added or taken away.

Stage IV. Formal Operations Stage (12-15 years through adulthood)

Competence is achieved in abstract thinking and the ability to handle hypothetical situations, consider multiple possibilities, and systematically solve complex problems.

Sigmund Freud

Presented a psychoanalytic perspective that characterizes development as the struggle between natural instincts and the constraints imposed by society (Papalia & Olds, 1986). Development occurs in five stages relative to shifts in the instinctual energy of the body zone considered primary:

Stage I. Oral Stage (birth to 12-18 months)

Body zone of the mouth perceived to be primary area of gratificaiton, for survival and for pleasure.

Stage II. Anal Stage (12-18 months to 3 years)

Body zone of the anal area perceived to be primary area of gratification. Toilet training, particularly withholding and expelling feces, considered important aspect of this stage.

Stage III. Phallic Stage (3 to 5-6 years)

Body zone of the genital area perceived to be primary area of gratification. Erotic feelings toward parent of the opposite sex are a conflict to be resolved in this period. Repression of erotic feelings for the opposite-sex parent and identification with same-sex parent are considered to be a satisfactory result of the stage. Conscience, in the form of superego, develops.

Stage IV. Latency Stage (5-6 years to puberty)

A time of relative sexual calm between Stages III and V.

Stage V. Genital Stage (from puberty on)

Body zone of the genital area perceived to be the primary area of gratification. Hormonal changes signaling mature adult sexuality and the development of satisfying sexual relationships outside the family are characteristic of this stage.

Abraham Maslow

Focused on a hierarchy of needs that motivate human behavior (Papalia & Olds, 1986, p. 20). Specified the fulfillment of needs at each level as the foundation for the next level. Recognized complete self-actualization as a goal toward which individuals strive.

Level I. Physiological Needs

Hunger, thirst, emotional sustenance, and so forth.

Level II. Safety Needs

The need to feel secure and out of danger.

Level III. Affiliation Needs

Needs for belonging, love, and acceptance.

Level IV. Esteem Needs

Strivings for achievement, competence, approval, and recognition.

Level V. Cognitive Needs

The quest for knowledge and understanding, the push toward exploration.

Level VI. Aesthetic Needs

The search for symmetry, order, and beauty.

Level VII. Self-Actualization Needs

The drive toward self-fulfillment and realization of one's potential.

Table 2-2 (continued)
Developmental Theorists and Theoretical Orientations

Erik Erikson

Extended Freud's psychoanalytic view of ego development to include the influence of the social and cultural environment on the individual (Maier, 1978; Papalia & Olds, 1986). Outlined eight stages of psychosocial development, each dependent on successful resolution of crises of development in preceding stages.

Crisis I. Basic Trust Versus Mistrust (birth to 18 months)

To mature, the infant must acquire a sense of basic trust and overcome a sense of basic mistrust. Affective (socioemotional) development dependent on building a solid foundation in this period.

Crisis II. Autonomy Versus Shame and Doubt (18 months to 3 years)

As infants gain trust in the caretaker and the environment, they discover that they can exert control. Thus they acquire a sense of autonomy, and develop will.

Crisis III. Initiative Versus Guilt (3-5 years)

Conscious control of the environment enhances mastery and competence, resulting in acquiring a sense of initiative. A balance between initiative and passivity develops.

Crisis IV. Industry Versus Inferiority (6-11 years)

The determination to achieve mastery is a major theme of this phase of development. Acquiring a sense of industry overcomes a sense of inferiority.

Crisis V. Identity Versus Role Confusion (12-17 years)

A sense of identity in adolescence signals mastery of childhood crises. Identity development is closely linked to mastery of skills and achievement of competence. Acquiring identity overcomes role confusion.

Crisis VI. Intimacy Versus Isolation (Young Adulthood)

Acquiring a sense of intimacy in relationships reinforces affiliation and reduces isolation. Differentiation occurs in men's and women's patterns of development by choice, influenced by sociocultural expectations.

Crisis VII. Generativity Versus Stagnation (Maturity)

Acquiring a sense of generativity forestalls a sense of self-absorption, stagnation. Generativity refers to society at large and the contribution that the mature adult can offer the next generation in terms of "hope, virtue, and wisdom" (Maier, 1978, p. 121).

Crisis VIII. Ego Integrity Versus Despair (Old Age)

Acquiring a sense of integrity forestalls a sense of despair. The cycle is complete. Acceptance of one's life cycle and inevitable death is a developmental task of this stage.

Lawrence Kohlberg (Morality)

Expanded "Piaget's concept that moral development is related to cognitive development and . . . proceeds in a definite sequential pattern" (Papalia & Olds, 1986, p. 16). Was primarily concerned with thinking rather than behavior. Did not include concepts of "morality such as compassion and integrity" (p. 16).

Specified three levels of moral reasoning (Papalia & Olds, 1986, p. 251):

Level I. Preconventional Morality (4-10 years)

Emphasis on external control, standards of others. The individual seeks to avoid punishment and receive rewards.

Level II. Morality of Conventional Role Conformity (10-13 years)

Beginning internalization of environmental standards. The individual starts to exercise judgment about what is considered "good" and to identify with roles of authority figures who are judged to be good.

Level III. Morality of Autonomous Moral Principles (13, young adulthood, or never). True morality achieved at this level, if at all. Control of conduct is internalized as to standards and reasoning.

Robert J. Havighurst

Presented developmental tasks as behavior mediated by societal demands and individual needs (Havighurst, 1979). Perceived the learner as an "active doer" in an active social ennvironment. Interpreted developmental tasks to include socioeconomic and sociocultural aspects, and described developmental tasks for six developmental stages:

Stage I. Infancy and Early Childhood (birth to 6 or 7 years)

Learning to walk, talk, eat, and control elimination; learning sex differences and modesty; forming concepts, social language, and physical reality; preparing to read; learning to distinguish right from wrong; and beginning to develop a conscience.

Stage II. Middle Childhood (6-12 years)

Learning physical skills for achieving competency in games and activities; building wholesome attitudes about self; getting along with peers; learning appropriate social and sexual roles; developing skills of reading, writing, and calculating; developing perceptions of everyday life and incorporating abstract concepts; developing a sense of conscience, morality, and values; achieving personal independence; and developing social attitudes toward groups and institutions.

Stage III. Adolescence (12-18 years)

Achieving more mature relations with peers of both sexes and social and sexual roles; learning to accept one's body and protect it effectively and satisfactorily; achieving emotional independence of parents and other adults; preparing for adult life and economic independence; acquiring a set of values and ethics; and developing an ideology and socially responsible behavior.

Stage IV. Early Adulthood (19-30 years)

Selecting and learning to live with a mate; deciding to begin or not to begin a family; managing a home; beginning employment; taking on civic responsibility; and engaging in congenial social group activities.

Stage V. Middle Age (30-60 years)

Assisting adolescents in becoming responsible, productive adults; achieving adult social and civic responsibility; reaching and maintaining satisfactory career performance; developing adult leisure activities; committing oneself to an intimate relationship; accepting and adjusting to physiological changes in midlife; and adjusting to aging parents.

Stage VI. Later Maturity (over 60 years)

Adjusting to decreasing physical strength and health, retirement and reduced income, and the death of one's spouse; establishing explicit affiliations with peers; adopting/adapting social roles in a flexible way; and establishing satisfactory physical living arrangements.

Robert F. Peck

Stressed circumstance versus age or stage as the issue of concern in evaluating critical elements of adult development. Expanded Erikson's concepts to specify four psychological developments as critical to successful adaptation in middle age:

I. Recognizing the value of wisdom as compensation for diminishing physical strength, stamina, and youthfulness

II. Developing a preference for socializing or sexualizing in interpersonal relationships and recognizing companionship and friendship as increasingly valuable

III. Developing the ability to use emotional flexibility as a strategy for adaptation to compensate for exigencies of midlife, such as disruptions in relationships, death of parents, and independence of children

IV. Developing mental flexibility to use past and present experiences to solve problems and plan for future requirements.

Table 2-3
Occupational Therapy Theorists'
Conceptualizations of Developmental Theory

A. Jean Ayres

Described concepts of central nervous system function, and dysfunction and purposeful activity (Llorens, 1984). Conceptualized neurobehavioral theory for understanding intersensory processing of internal and external stimuli (Ayres, 1972). Described sensory integration theory, emphasizing the ''importance of adequate sensory integration as a foundation for normal learning and emotional behavior'' (Clark & Allen, 1989).

Mary Reilly

Organized theoretical concepts of Vickers, Berlyne, Buhler, White, and McClelland into a theory of the role of work and play in adaptation. Proposed general systems theory as a concept for organizing the complex phenomena relating to acquisition of competency behaviors for adaptation. Proposed play as a system for learning. Described a hierarchy of play behavior that includes exploration, competence, and achievement (Clark & Allen, 1985).

Ann C. Mosey

Proposed a developmental frame of reference for evaluation and treatment, deriving the theoretical base from personality and developmental theories described by Sullivan, Piaget, Bruner, A. Freud, S. Freud, Llorens, Schilder, Searles, Secheheye, Ayres, and Hartman (Miller et al., 1988).

Lela A. Llorens

Described a theory of facilitating growth and development (chronologically and simultaneously) that synthe-

sized developmental theories of Gesell, Freud, Erikson, Havighurst, Mosey, Pearce and Newton, and Piaget. Described the role of activities, the role of the individual, and the role of interpersonal interaction in the maturation process and the achievement of mastery (Clark & Allen, 1985; Llorens, 1970, 1976).

Proposed 10 premises for understanding the developmental nature of the acquisition of skill for mastery, the role of trauma in disrupting the developmental cycle, and the reinstitution of the cycle using activity, tasks, and interpersonal interactions (Llorens, 1970, 1976, 1981).

Pat N. Clark & Anne S. Allen

Classified selected developmental theories from biological and behavioral theorists and occupational therapy theorists on a continuum of developmental stages.

Described theoretical schools of thought according to the theorist's view of the control of developmental behavior by internal processes and/or external forces (Clark & Allen, 1985, p. 21).

Elnora Gilfoyle, Ann Grady, & Josephine Moore

Described a spatiotemporal model using a spiralling continuum to express concepts of development based on nervous system maturation. Viewed adaptation as a function of resolving crises of spatiotemporal distress that provoke dysfunction. The resolution occurs through engagement in purposeful developmental activities and behaviors providing stimulation to enhance maturation (Gilfoyle, Grady, & Moore, 1980).

The use of social language increases at this age. Children identify objects and are often embarrassingly direct in the comments and the questions that they direct to strangers. They use complete sentences, and their imaginations are apparent. Many children are very dramatic in their language use. Responsiveness of the environment to the child's use of language ensures its continuance and further development.

Activities that facilitate sociocultural development include finding companionship, playing in organized groups, and imitating adult behavior. The child's status in the family is important; each child's receiving special attention helps develop his or her self-esteem. Cooperative

behavior, such as sharing and taking turns, and delay of gratification for reasonable periods are key sociocultural achievements.

Cognitive development at this stage occurs through repeated contact with others, which reduces self-absorption and increases social skills. Thinking and reasoning are developed. Thinking occurs in parts as well as wholes. Words are used in thinking. Language replaces motor behavior. The foundations for reading, writing, and calculating develop. Attention and concentration lengthen as the child moves from early childhood into childhood (sometimes called middle childhood).

CHILDHOOD

Occupational Performance

Childhood spans ages 6 to 12. Roles include son, daughter, brother, sister, grandson, granddaughter, peer, and added new role of best friend/chum, and student. The role of worker may be initiated as the child begins to take on jobs at home and in the community.

Adaptive behavior associated with these roles is focused on refining perception and organization, learning appropriate social skills, acquiring skills for everyday living, and developing healthy attitudes toward self and others. Higher-level mastery of reading, writing, calculation, and conceptual thinking is achieved. The sensory functions continue to be used and adapted as the child grows and develops.

Self-care/self-maintenance skills mastered earlier continue to be practiced. As the child matures, he or she enjoys dressing up, as portrayed in this description of a student: *She arrived at school dressed neatly in a pink dress and white tights. Her dark hair was carefully tied with a ribbon. Her slender body had good muscle tone and reflected conscientious personal hygiene.*

Responsibility for personal needs in dress and grooming is assumed to a greater extent as the child grows older. Peer influence and peer acceptance become more important. Children also begin to learn the value of money and to identify ways of earning it.

Play/leisure is focused on group and team activities. Peer recognition and competition are important. Play activities include social clubs, secret societies, and sports and games with and without rules. Games with rules require that the rules be followed, such as not stepping over the line or taking only a designated turn.

Work/education takes the form of primary and middle school activities, which begin at and continue throughout this stage of development. Mastery of reading, writing, calculation, decision making, and problem solving is fostered in school and initial work activities. Responsibility for preparing for social roles is a focus. Socializing may be viewed by the older child as a main activity in the school environment.

Rest/relaxation is important. Balance among the four areas of occupational performance is controlled to some extent by the environment. As the child ages, propensities for early or late rising and early or late bedtime manifest themselves.

Occupational Performance Enablers

Tactile, visual, auditory, vestibular, olfactory, gustatory, and proprioceptive-kinesthetic functions are refined. This foundation of development will be used throughout life, can be adapted, and will change as the person ages. Sensory integration continues for and through task engagement. Disuse can lead to atrophy, dysfunction, and decreased efficiency.

The development of physical motor skill, musculature, and coordination advances through practice of activities and tasks that are required to attain efficiency in this area. In the average child, smooth, coordinated fine and gross motor movement should be occurring. Physical activity such as walking, running, jumping, and playing with bicycles, balls, and other toys is common. Hand and foot preferences form and can be observed in play activities. Eye-hand coordination for pencil-and-paper activities is refined. Children who are physically limited may require adaptation to assist them in growing and developing.

Psychological/social development is focused on mastery of interpersonal skills. This includes demonstrating initiative, creating with arts and crafts, and playing with scooters, jump ropes, and skateboards alone and with others. The child in this age group also strives to achieve recognition by producing objects and learning to use tools and materials skillfully.

Psychodynamic development results in a period of ''sexual quiet'' between the struggles with initial sexual interest and discovery, and adolescence, with its challenges for establishing sexual identity. The period is called latency. The activities that contribute to development in this component are those that reinforce reality, encourage mastery of skills, and permit constructive competitiveness.

Language is developed for communication. Communication with peers is preferred over communication with adults. The companionship of peers contributes to language development. Use of complete sentences, questioning, and talking even though no one is listening are characteristic of this stage.

Play is a key element in sociocultural development, which is fostered through group activity and team sports. Peer group interests are important, and group standards take preference over adult standards. Social clubs and secret societies contribute to the development of sociocultural skills. Children learn to work in groups while achieving personal independence. The child starts to develop social values, a sense of morality, and a conscience. Interest in the affairs of the community, the state, and the country begins.

Moral development occurs, initially through external control as the child observes the standards of others to avoid punishment or reap rewards. This learning is facilitated by family and social groups. Rules are learned in games, sports and club activities, and in the home around such expectations as completing homework, caring for belongings, and performing chores. These standards are internalized by children as they age (Papalia & Olds, 1986).

In cognitive development, acquisition of the capacity to understand and achieve complex adaptive relationships, to read, to write, and to calculate is facilitated by formal schooling, intrinsic motivation, and environmental expectations. Demands for competence require the use of active mental processes. Memory lengthens, the ability to attend and to withstand frustration increases, and the shift from inductive to deductive reasoning occurs.

ADOLESCENCE

Occupational Performance

Adolescence, 13 to 19 years of age, is a period of budding independence and developing identity. Adolescent roles include son, daughter, brother, sister, grandson, granddaughter, peer, best friend/chum (very important at this age), and new roles include employed worker, and volunteer. Adolescents may become parents. Membership in civic, social, and spiritual groups begins.

Adaptive behavior is associated with building relationships, defining occupational and social roles, and achieving emotional independence of parents and other adults. Adolescents start to achieve the skills needed for financial independence as they select and begin training for a vocation or a profession. Adolescence is a time of preparation for adult life. Development of intellectual skills and concepts to live in the world and achieve socially responsible behavior is a function of this stage. Adolescence is also a time for acquisition of values and ethics.

Exercising independence in dressing, feeding, grooming, and hygiene, and accepting and carrying out responsibility for themselves are key self-care/self-maintenance activities for adolescents. Individual tastes in clothes, food, and friends develop as distinct from the perceived tastes of parents. Interest in financial matters, in having and earning money, is important. Developmental skills achieved earlier are practiced for mastery.

Play/leisure activities in adolescence focus on the desire for attention and recognition. Enjoyment is also important. Team participation is characteristic. Interests may include artistic, literary, social, and intellectual pursuits as well as sports and more physically demanding activities. Spending time in solitary activities is as important as spending time in groups.

Work/education activities for the adolescent primarily relate to schooling. Engagement in paid work such as sales, delivery, and child care or in volunteer jobs in schools or hospitals may signal the adolescent's entry into the workplace. In these roles, the adolescent learns the ability to accept and discharge responsibility and practices this ability for mastery. Consideration of vocational possibilities occurs, with serious pursuit of various options beginning in late adolescence and continuing into adulthood. Accomplishment of chores such as laundry, vacuuming, housecleaning, and yard work also assists the adolescent in demonstrating the ability to carry out work activities.

Rest/relaxation is more controlled by the individual in this period than it is at earlier stages of development. The needs associated with balance between rest and other activities vary. Engagement in presleep fantasies serves the adolescent as a mechanism for role experimentation.

Occupational Performance Enablers

The level of development of sensory (perceptual) functions achieved in earlier stages is presumably maintained, and the functions are constantly used for growth and adaptation. Sensory integration continues to occur through task engagement, and competence is achieved through practice. The ability to conceptualize, to reason, is manifest.

Rapid physical growth occurs during this period. Arms, legs, and trunk lengthen. Most adolescents achieve their adult height. As physical maturation occurs, discomfort may be experienced, and poor posture and motor awkwardness may be observed. Engagement in activities and tasks in which competence is achieved may assist in a smooth developmental transition. Physical activities such as sports, or academic endeavors that focus attention on areas of greater comfort can ease the strain of this period.

In psychological/social development, adolescence is a time of struggle to achieve identity (Erikson, 1985). The integration of attitudes, social roles, and personal identity strengthens the functioning of the ego, but not without associated role confusion. The major ego-adaptive task of adolescence is developing one's identity. Learning to love, to live, and to share with others is a function of the resolution of the identity crisis.

Psychodynamic development focuses on becoming independent, emancipated, and inner-directed. Sexual identity is integrated with social roles. Emotional intensity is characteristic, with difficulty observed in compromise. Typically in this stage, close examination of adult and societal values occurs.

In social language development, adolescents may use peer buzz words, slang, and secret codes to isolate themselves from adults. Sociocultural development is driven by group consciousness and team play, the need for attention, and the importance of having space of one's own. Sexual preference develops. Time spent with friends is highly valued. Adolescents identify best with other adolescents because they share similar bodily and emotional changes (Papalia & Olds, 1986).

True moral development is achieved in this stage. Resolution of conflicting social standards occurs. Control of conduct is internalized, both in standards and in reasoning right and wrong (Papalia & Olds, 1986). Today's adolescents may be influenced in their moral development by television viewing and movie attendance. Young people have cited life on television situation comedies, soap operas, and family-oriented shows as a source of their emerging concepts of morality.

Cognitive development is demonstrated in the adolescent's capacity to think beyond his or her individual world and own beliefs. The ability to solve problems, reason by hypotheses, and consider "what if?" grows. Self-centered behavior lessens and a sense of equality gradually replaces the previous submissiveness to adult authority. Demonstrating curiosity about other people and writing stories and letters are behaviors and activities that support this stage of development.

YOUNG ADULTHOOD

Occupational Performance

Young adulthood, between ages 20 and 35, is focused on the assumption of increasing responsibility in the roles of son, daughter, grandson, granddaughter, parent, friend, colleague, worker, student, and volunteer. Characteristic of this period is adaptive behavior associated with mastery of personal grooming and hygiene skills, the development of financial independence, the ability to manage a home, commitment to an intimate relationship, and possibly the beginning of a family.

Independence in self-care, home management, and home maintenance is achieved. Experimentation with dress and with life-style can lead to greater confidence and increased quality in self-care. Home-management skills include financial management. Competence in skills, such as maintaining and balancing a checking account, is important.

Engagement in social games, parties, and group activities, including sports and hobbies, is characteristic of this stage. Play/leisure activities may include education to update knowledge and skills or to change positions or careers.

Performance in work/education involves committing oneself to the responsibility of a job or a position, functioning as a member of a work group, operating independently, and organizing, planning, and carrying out purposeful activities. Developing financial independence through paid work is typical of this period. Volunteer experience may assist in achievement of life satisfaction.

Maintaining balance among self-care/self-maintenance, work/education, play/leisure, and rest/relaxation is important. It serves as a foil for stress that may accompany career achievement and the multiple roles associated with this stage.

Occupational Performance Enablers

Sensory development and sensory integration skills already achieved are presumably maintained and refined. Mastery in physical motor development attained to this point also continues to be used for occupational performance.

Psychological/social development is focused on commitment to partnerships and affiliations. Mastery of ego functions is associated with this stage. Independence, control of drives, participation in mutually satisfying sexual relationships, and satisfaction of needs are key goals.

Psychodynamic development involves the assumption of responsibility for emotional growth. Independence, separation from home and the primary family, usually occurs during this period.

Social language is predominantly verbal. Nonverbal behavior—body language—is also used to communicate socially.

Sociocultural development occurs in interactions with family members and others in social, interest, civic, and other groups. Cognitive development is maintained; higher levels of conceptualization may be achieved.

MIDDLE ADULTHOOD

Occupational Performance

Midlife occurs between 35 and 50 years of age. The roles may include son, daughter, parent, grandparent, grandson, granddaughter, friend, colleague, and perhaps caregiver. Worker roles may occur in a hierarchy, as with supervisor and supervisee, or on a peer basis. Student and volunteer roles may also be a part of this stage.

Adaptive behaviors associated with the roles are focused on achieving civic and social responsibility; maintaining financial responsibility; assisting family members, children, and aging parents; and achieving satisfying relationships with friends. Acceptance of and adjustment to physiological changes that occur in middle age and changes in interests and work roles are major tasks of this period.

Independence in self-care is maintained, while home-management skills and those associated with the care of others are refined. Care of others may find the adult in the later years of midlife "sandwiched" between the demands of adolescent children who are becoming adults and the needs of parents or grandparents who are aging (Sheehy, 1976). Financial independence continues, along with deepening or destruction of intimate relationships.

Hobby interests, social games, sports, and travel are play/leisure activities associated with this stage of life. Play/leisure interests are established for the present and for the future.

Maintaining responsibility and commitment in work activities is important for independent functioning. Work includes organizing, planning, and carrying out purposeful activities and continuing to function effectively in a primary group. This stage may include a career or job change. Choice of work may reflect childhood play interests.

Balance among self-care/self-maintenance, work/education, play/leisure, and rest/relaxation is important for maintaining adaptation.

Occupational Performance Enablers

Sensory development and sensory integration achieved to this point begin to change, with some decline in acuity of tactile, visual, auditory, vestibular, olfactory, gustatory, and proprioceptive-kinesthetic functions. Disparity between motor planning and execution may begin to occur toward age 50. Form and space perception, postural flexibility, and perception of body scheme may also change. Corrective devices may be required for vision and hearing.

Physical motor development may also begin to decline. Arm and leg coordination, trunk control, muscle strength, physical endurance, and muscle tone may be affected.

Psychological/social development is focused on generativity (guiding the next generation), creativity, and productivity. Continued independent functioning, control of drives, and the selection of appropriate sexual partners are functions of psychological/social development. The ability to organize, plan, and use purposeful activities is important. The ability to obtain, organize, and use knowledge for participation in a variety of social relationships and the capacity to perceive oneself as a holistic, acceptable person continue.

Psychodynamic development centers on changes in emotional responsibilities for parents as their children leave home and for other adults as they adjust to choices made earlier in life. Financial responsibility becomes finite and predictable. Coping with the lost capacity to bear children is a developmental task for women. Accepting and adjusting to changes in physical status are also tasks of the stage.

Social language development is primarily verbal. However, nonverbal language is also used to communicate socially. Sociocultural development focuses on group relationships; the family; social, interest, and civic groups; and others.

Moral development matures through experience. Judgment is shaped through reasoning. Adults in this stage of development act according to an internalized set of beliefs regardless of the opinions of others. This is consistent with Kohlberg's stage of morality of autonomous moral principles (Papalia & Olds, 1986).

Cognitive development is presumably maintained at this point. Information processing through sensory integration may begin to alter. Memory and conceptualization may be affected.

Case Studies 2-1 and 2-2 illustrate occupational role performance of women at midlife.

Case Study 2-1

Alice at Midlife: As a 37-year-old woman, Alice fulfills roles of worker, spouse, student, daughter, sibling, and friend. She is experiencing a transition in terms of career choice. Having been a practicing professional for 10 years, she is beginning to feel dissatisfaction with her career. Her current work is ''boring, one-dimensional, requiring too much mental discipline, and too demanding.'' To gain greater work satisfaction, Alice is turning to her craft business, with which she is more content than she is with her profession. She describes it as ''tactile, visual, colorful, and creative.'' Alice is continuing her professional practice part-time. As the craft business increases, she expects to pursue it full-time.

Alice was attracted to creative, imaginative, and self-expressive types of activities as a child. She is using these same interests and talents in her business. They have not been reflected in her profession.

Other aspects of Alice's occupational performance are satisfying. She balances work, leisure, self-care, and rest well. With regard to occupational performance components, her verbal responses and the interviewer's observations of her behavior during the interview indicate intact sensory, motor, psychological, social, and cognitive development. Her language use is articulate. Her ability to produce intricate designs in needlepoint reflects functional tactile, visual, and motor coordination abilities.

Note. Adapted from an interview by Alison H. George, Department of Occupational Therapy, San Jose State University, 1987.

Case Study 2-2

Carolyn at Midlife: Carolyn, a 46-year-old woman, is beginning to show physical alterations in motor strength and endurance, but her conceptualization and memory are intact. She requires corrective lenses for sight. Carolyn exemplifies generativity (Erikson, 1985), has mastered the stage of formal operations (Piaget, as cited in Papalia & Olds, 1986), and is engaging in appropriate developmental tasks (Havighurst, 1972). She guides the next generation and is productive. Her leisure activities are civic and social. She is functionally independent, uses knowledge for adaptation, participates in groups, and maintains a variety of relationships. Also consistent with her level of development, Carolyn accepts herself; that is, she accepts her past and her present as part of the person she is.

The norm for this developmental stage is fewer demands for material acquisition, more available personal freedom, and less evident economic concerns. For Carolyn, however, a divorced mother of three teenagers, this middle-adulthood achievement will be somewhat delayed. There is increased demand for material acquisition, little personal freedom, decreased opportunity for leisure pursuits, and considerable economic stress.

Carolyn's occupational roles include sibling, parent, daughter, and worker. As a sibling, Carolyn offers psychological support to her sister and brothers, who live a distance away. As a parent, she is emotionally, physically, and financially supportive of her children. As a daughter, she is warm, caring, and understanding of her mother's perception of life. As a worker, she is flexible and uses experience and understanding, rather than rigidity of thought, to approach problems.

Given the demanding, very busy roles of her life, Carolyn's occupational performance is remarkably well balanced among work, leisure, self-care, and rest. Carolyn not only manages her home, family, and full-time employment, but also makes time for leisure and social activities. She secures sufficient rest, grooms herself immaculately, and is emotionally and physically relaxed.

Sensory, motor, psychological, social, and cognitive components supporting Carolyn's occupational performance are accomplished and enhanced. Carolyn functions at a very high level of developmental competence.

Note. Adapted from an interview by Sandra Blanke, Department of Occupational Therapy, San Jose State University, 1987.

LATER ADULTHOOD

Occupational Performance

Later adulthood, ages 50 to 65, is a time of continued adaptation and often a time of consolidation. For men and women who have pursued careers, earlier plans and goals may come to fruition, or the individual may have to come to terms with his or her level of achievement.

Occupational and social roles in later adulthood include parent, grandparent, son, daughter, friend, colleague, and worker. The worker role may occur in a hierarchical pattern or a collegial one. The later-aged adult may also be a grandson, a granddaughter, a student, or a volunteer. At this stage the adult begins to experience role change and role loss.

Adaptive behavior involves continued growth toward one's potential. Adaptation is focused on coping with the changes that are occurring in relationships with friends and acquaintances as well as those occurring within oneself. Adjustment to physical and psychological deterioration, to the loss of friends and family, especially parents, and to one's own mortality is a key feature of this stage.

Self-care/self-maintenance activities mastered earlier are presumed to continue for independence of functioning. Independence in care of self, family (if applicable), and living quarters is expected. Financial independence and engagement in satisfying relationships and activities continue. Children may have achieved self-sufficient functioning just at the time when parents may be losing theirs.

Play/leisure activities may focus on interests to be developed now for later life. Hobbies, social games, travel, and sports may be pursuits of this stage.

In the work/education area, maintaining responsibility and commitment through employment, achievement, and successful fulfillment of obligations associated with one's job are characteristic. Homemaking and home-maintenance skills are still developing. The physical aspects of parenting may decrease, however they may be replaced with the physical aspects of caring for parents.

Relaxation as a part of the rest cycle and ensuring balance among self-care/self-maintenance, work/education, and play/leisure remain important for continued healthy development.

Occupational Performance Enablers

Signs of decline may begin to appear in tactile, visual, auditory, vestibular, gustatory, olfactory, proprioceptive, and kinesthetic functioning. Motor planning may also show evidence of deterioration, with a disparity between perceptual-cognitive planning and execution. Changes in form and space perception, equilibrium responses (balance), postural flexibility, and perception of body scheme occur as the adult ages.

Physical development may show decline to some extent. The coordination of extremities, as indicated in writing and walking, may show some alteration. Strength, endurance, and muscle tone change.

With regard to psychological/social development during this stage, the individual addresses the meaning of his or her life and accepts his or her life cycle as inevitable, even if some specific life events are not acceptable. Such acceptance is central to the achievement of inner peace. Egocentrism may begin to be evident as a function of aging.

In psychodynamic development, the individual copes with continued growth and cultivates an inner life. He or she is less defended against life, more open to the coming years.

Greater confidence in his or her ability to cope and survive may be apparent.

Social language development achieved earlier is used for communication. Language use is primarily verbal; however, nonverbal language is also employed.

In the sociocultural domain, affiliations with family, social organizations, interest groups, civic associations, work-related units, and other groups are important. The individual also cultivates solitary interests.

Moral development is reinforced by experience, wisdom, and/or religious beliefs. Cognitive development is at its peak. High-level integration, including conceptualization and memory, is well developed in the normal adult.

Occupational role performance in later adulthood is illustrated in Case Study 2-3.

Case Study 2-3

Roberta in Later Adulthood: Roberta, a 56-year-old widow, is the mother of three children. She describes her occupation as homemaker, having cared for a family and managed a household for 30 years. With the death of her husband and with her last child about to move away from home, Roberta is in a time of changing life roles. Her interests include international traveling and crafts.

Roberta fulfills the criteria of generativity in middle to older adulthood (Erikson, 1985) and is engaged in the developmental tasks of middle age (Havighurst, 1972). She is an active member of a women's philanthropical organization that sponsors young women through college and assists local community causes. The term ''sandwich'' generation (Sheehy, 1976), often assigned to midlife, is illustrated in Roberta's responsibility for her ailing father-in-law and her concern for her growing children. Roberta is in a time of transition, evaluating her past occupational roles and contemplating future ones. Among the possibilities are selling her house and traveling. She also may work outside her home, renew an interest in the sciences, and further develop an interest in crafts, hiking, and skiing. Experiencing the death of her husband has forced Roberta to consider her own mortality earlier in life than she might have otherwise.

Note. Adapted from an interview by Eileen Maddox, Department of Occupational Therapy, San Jose State University, 1985.

OLD AGE

Occupational Performance

Old age is described as 65 to 85 years. A wide range of adaptive responses are possible within this span of life. Significant life changes typically occur. Occupational and social roles may include parent, grandparent, son, daughter, grandson, granddaughter, friend, colleague, worker, volunteer, student, homemaker, and partner or spouse.

Adaptive behavior associated with these roles is focused on adjustment to: 1) changes in physical appearance; 2) decreasing physical strength and the possibility or the reality of declining health; 3) possible retirement and reduction in income; 4) the deaths of family members and friends, especially a mate; and 5) one's own impending death. A major choice is whether to adopt an activity orientation, opt for disengagement, or pursue a continuing-growth model for one's later years. The older person who chooses an activity orientation carries on much as he or she did in middle age, keeping up many activities and substituting others for those lost because of retirement or the death of friends or a mate. Widowhood demands changes in life roles and may offer greater freedom or restriction, depending on the individual. Disengagement is typified by gradually and selectively narrowing one's activities and commitments. According to disengagement theory, it is a normal pattern of aging and may begin to occur in the later years of this stage (Papalia & Olds, 1986). The continuing-growth model permits the older person to achieve new areas of competence in skills as he or she ages.

Independence in self-care/self-maintenance, care of the home, and management of finances may begin to change or decline. Some changes related to self-care may occur because of the death of a family member or a move from one location to another. Responsibility for aging parents may grow.

Play/leisure activities may increase as some people shift from significant time spent in work to significant time spent in leisure. Hobby interests may continue. Social activities may continue or decline. Travel may increase as more time becomes available. Participation in some sports may continue or resume.

Employment may demand less time or cease because of retirement, or it may continue, as with the self-employed. Responsibilities associated with employment may shift. Associations with fellow workers may decline or increase. Homemaking and home-maintenance responsibilities may shift. Child-care and parenting activities may decline; however, responsibility for elderly parents is likely to increase.

Balance among self-care/self-maintenance, work/ education, play/leisure, and rest/relaxation continues to be important. Patterns of rest vary greatly. Older people sleep fewer hours than younger people. Wakefulness at night may return. Daytime naps may be taken to compensate for loss of nighttime sleep.

Occupational Performance Enablers

Sensory development may decline gradually. Tactile, visual, auditory, vestibular, gustatory, olfactory, proprioceptive, and kinesthetic functioning may change noticeably. Motor planning, form and space perception, equilibrium responses, postural flexibility, and body scheme may begin to show signs of deterioration.

Both fine and gross motor coordination may show signs of change. Deterioration in strength, endurance, and muscle tone may occur and be seen in all parts of the body, with leg strength declining first.

Psychological/social development is focused on peer group and family relationships. Interaction with others contributes to the older person's sense of self. The ability to participate in a variety of groups continues. Egocentricity may return as the elderly adult begins to feel that he or she has lived long enough to have the privilege of speaking out without filtering his or her opinions and thoughts.

Psychodynamic development is characterized by mutually satisfying sexual relationships. Language is predominantly verbal. However, nonverbal behavior is also used for communication.

Sociocultural development centers on the family. An older person may be regarded as the wise member of the family or the peer group.

Cognitive development may continue or begin to decline. However, cognitive skills at this stage serve to balance physical decline. Years of experience and intellectual development often make it possible for the older person to solve problems mentally and to discover new ways of managing daily-life tasks that compensate for motor decline and sustain independent functioning.

Occupational role performance in old age is illustrated in Case Studies 2-4, 2-5, and 2-6.

Case Study 2-4

Ben in Old Age: Ben, now 69 years of age, retired five years ago following 43 years of employment. He is married, with two married children and three grandchildren. His period of development corresponds with the stage of ego integrity versus despair (Erikson, 1985). He expresses general satisfaction with his life, has a positive attitude toward his parents, and comfortably accepts the inevitability of death through the tenets of his religious faith.

Ben is coping with the gradual cessation of some leisure activities, imposed by health problems. Deterioration of physical coordination and strength due to slow-healing injuries and memory loss reflect occupational performance components requiring adjustment and adaptation.

Ben's retirement has been successful. His orientation to it illustrates disengagement (Papalia & Olds, 1986). He has

withdrawn from activities such as travel, golf, camping, and playing cards. However, he finds enjoyment and purpose in his everyday activities and in his family, church, and home responsibilities. His wife is a major source of companionship. This pattern is consistent with Ben's characterization of himself as a loner when he was younger.

Note. Adapted from an interview by Lisa Sarnicola, OTR, Department of Occupational Therapy, San Jose State University, 1984.

Case Study 2-5

Greta in Old Age: Greta, at 76, can be described as elegant. She exhibits physical changes of aging, such as wrinkles, skin discoloration, brittle nails, gray hair, some muscle atrophy, and a forward curvature of the spine. These characteristics are consistent with the description of the age in *The Mature Years* (Lewis, 1979).

Greta has achieved ego integrity (Erikson, 1985). She enjoys her life, expresses no regrets, and recognizes her worth to herself, others, and society. She receives considerable satisfaction from her occupational roles, which include sister, mother, grandmother, great grandmother, and widow. Greta delights in nurturing her family and sharing with them.

A common occurrence for women in Greta's age group was to move from the family home to the husband's home. This was the case with Greta. Although she does not regret the action and its aftermath, not until her husband's death did she face the need to become independent and more self-reliant and to discover competencies that were not required in her married state. Greta has made the needed adjustments to continue a successful life. She reports that loneliness is the worst part of widowhood.

Note. Adapted from an interview by Rebecca Gill, OTR, Department of Occupational Therapy, San Jose State University, 1984.

Case Study 2-6

Harold in Old Age: Harold is 78 years old. A widower for the past four years, he lives alone in a condominium in a quiet, middle-class neighborhood. He has successfully resolved three crises of old age: ego differentiation versus work-role preoccupation, body transcendence versus body preoccupation, and ego transcendence versus ego preoccupation (Peck, as cited in Papalia & Olds, 1986). He has also resolved the crisis of ego integrity versus despair (Erikson, 1985) and exhibits characteristics of maturity (Llorens, 1976).

Harold has coped well with forced retirement and has reorganized his life, separating his value as a person from his value as an employee. He believes that he has earned time to do what he chooses. Harold has also accepted and dealt with the effects of aging, now wearing strong eye-glasses and a hearing aid to compensate for visual and auditory deficits. He works at keeping fit by walking three miles per day. Harold realizes that he is nearing the end of his life and embraces death as a part of life. He considers his life well lived. He realizes that he has made mistakes, but he views them as a part of his growth and development as a person, and has no regrets.

While accepting and coping with the physical and neuro-physiological changes of aging and with the inevitability of death, Harold remains socioculturally dynamic. He takes an active role in the family and in community and civic affairs. His move from a larger home to a condominium was an adjustment to his declining physical condition and an opportunity to gain more time for intellectual development. For yard work and planting trees, he has substituted more reading and learning about new subjects. He continues to establish and maintain relationships with others in his age group through social functions.

Harold's childhood-activity history is closely related to his activity choices in adulthood. As a boy, he enjoyed telling and writing stories and poetry, pastimes in which he still engages. He also enjoyed problem solving, figuring things out for himself. He continues this activity in the form of working puzzles and assembling new appliances without reading the instruction manual. Harold lives a balanced life in old age.

Note. Adapted from an interview by Maryann Solberg, Department of Occupational Therapy, San Jose State University, 1986.

OLD-OLD AGE

Occupational Performance

The old-old are in the age group over 85 years. Their occupational and social roles may include parent, grandparent, friend, colleague, worker, volunteer, and student. Loss of roles is characteristic of the age, occurring for some in the worker role, as with a change in job status, and for others in the caregiver role, because of the death of parents and friends.

Adaptive behavior involves decision-making regarding continuing to grow and adapt or resigning oneself to declining sensory, motor, psychological, social, and cognitive skills. Continuation of growth requires adjustment to decreasing physical strength and possibly deteriorating health, changes in worker status and income, deaths of family and friends, reduced ability to meet social obligations, and one's own impending death.

Self-care skills mastered earlier may continue or decline. The old-old person may feed himself or herself independently with no or some spilling, or may lose the self-feeding ability altogether as a result of accident or injury. He or she may dress and wash independently or may gradually lose this skill. Manipulation of small buttons, zippers, and the like may become difficult. The person may lose interest in personal grooming and hygiene and may also become incontinent during the day or at night. The ability to care fully for financial responsibilities or to maintain a home independently may be lost as well. As skill levels decline, the loss of ability to perform competently may affect interest in life and motivation to assume role responsibility.

Play/leisure activities may be active or passive. They may include travel and participation in games, hobbies, or sports, as well as artistic and literary pursuits.

Work responsibilities related to home management and homemaking may continue or decline. Child-care and parenting activities are usually no longer required. Grandparenting, however, is often a joy of this age. Paid employment is usually not an activity. Exceptions may occur among the self-employed and the wealthy.

Rest requirements vary, with more rest being necessary for some. Patterns of sleep also vary, from a complete 8 to 10 hours of sleep at night only, to short spans of sleep at night with naps during the day. Some elders shift from being active predominantly during the day to being active at night and sleeping late in the morning. Balance between activity and rest/relaxation is important.

Occupational Performance Enablers

Sensory development may decline dramatically or gradually. Tactile, visual, auditory, vestibular, gustatory, olfactory, proprioceptive, and kinesthetic functioning may require technological enhancement to produce the responses required for adaptation. Motor planning, form and space perception, equilibrium responses, postural flexibility, and body scheme may show signs of deterioration. Habit and behavior patterns may assist compensation in areas of decline.

Motor coordination, both fine and gross, may decline. Strength, endurance, and muscle tone may show further deterioration.

Psychological/social development continues as a function of peer group and family affiliations. Interaction with others remains important in contributing to the sense of self. Participation in activities that have cultural meaning to the person is a factor in sustained growth.

Satisfying sexual needs as a function of psychodynamic development is a developmental task during this period, as it is in all other stages. Language is predominantly verbal, but nonverbal communication is still used.

Sociocultural development predominantly involves family and friends. It may also include caregivers other than family, as in the case of old-old people living in retirement communities or nursing homes. The wisdom of the old-old person may be highly or negatively regarded by the social community in which he or she resides. This will influence continued sociocultural growth.

Cognitive development may be maintained or decline. The intellectual development and the cumulative experience of aging may contribute to continued independence in function.

Case Studies 2-7 and 2-8 describe occupational performance in two persons in the old-old age group.

Case Study 2-7

Steve in Old-Old Age: Steve is 86 years of age, which places him in the developmental stage of old-old age. However, he continues to engage in self-care, leisure, and work activities, as he has for many years. Except for a slight decline in physical functioning and the loss of several friends, the events of this life stage, such as retirement, change in finances, new living arrangements, death of spouse, and major shifts in daily routine, have not occurred for Steve. He is an example of the activity theory of aging (Papalia & Olds, 1986). He works weekdays and some weekends as a piano tuner; is actively involved in building model trains, playing cards, and playing music; and takes pleasure in the company of friends and family. Although reminiscence is identified as a characteristic of the age, Steve does not reminisce as much as would be expected. He enjoys performing his occupational roles of worker, spouse, friend, and uncle.

There is a correlation between the types of play in which Steve engaged as a child and the types of work and leisure activities he has chosen as an adult. When he was a boy, Steve enjoyed music and took piano lessons; piano tuning has been his life work. He liked trains and playing cards as a child and as a young adult; these are his main hobbies in old-old age.

Note. Adapted from an interview by Karen Webenbauer, Department of Occupational Therapy, San Jose State University, 1987.

Case Study 2-8

Margaret in Old-Old Age: At 100, Margaret is healthy and alert, active and lively. She enjoys reminiscing and accepts her life, having no regrets. She demonstrates the activity orientation of aging (Papalia & Olds, 1986). She is particularly concerned that she maintain her intellectual skills and not "let her mind go." Therefore she practices learning and telling jokes, and she engages in intellectual games such as naming the states of the union and their capitals in alphabetical order. She refrains from sitting

around with "the old and boring people." Margaret lives in a retirement center and participates in as many activities as the center offers.

Margaret has some vision and hearing loss. Her occupational performance is not impaired, however, for she can carry out her remaining occupational roles. She has prepared for the possibility of blindness by teaching herself to perform activities without sight.

As a younger woman, Margaret was active in political movements, such as prohibition and women's rights. She was not encouraged to seek a career. However, following her husband's death, she launched a dress shop that became a successful business. There was no indication that this career choice was related to her activity interests as a child, which were associated with horseback riding. Survival may have been the motivating force.

Note. Adapted from an interview by Dena DeAngelis, OTR, Department of Occupational Therapy, San Jose State University, 1985.

FAMILY RELATIONSHIPS IN OCCUPATIONAL PERFORMANCE

Types of families have expanded in recent years. Family relationships, including those with either a natural or a created extended family, are important in developing competence in occupational performance and occupational performance components. This is particularly true in psychological, social, and cognitive functioning. Family configurations include the nuclear family, the single-parent family, the three-generation family, the middle-aged-couple or older-couple family, the institutional or foster family, the unmarried-parent or unmarried-couple family, the homosexual-couple family, and the communal family.

The nuclear family consists of husband, wife, and children living in a common household. In the traditional family, the husband has been the major source of income, and the wife has taken the role of home manager and child rearer. More families are evolving into units in which both husband and wife are workers outside the home and the husband shares the home-management and child-rearing responsibilities. The dyadic nuclear family consists of a husband and a wife who are childless, with one or both of them being gainfully employed.

The single-parent family comprises one parent and his or her preschool or school-age children. This family configuration can result from death, divorce, abandonment, separation, or nonmarriage. Single parenthood can affect the family's financial and social status and family members' prior or present relationships with the absent parent.

Three-generation families incorporate patterns in one

household that may include: (a) aged parents, grown children, and grandchildren; (b) middle-aged parents, grown children, and grandchildren; or (c) middle-aged adults, their aging parents, and their younger children. The values and the developmental crises of each generation must be considered and resolved in order for all family members to lead satisfactory lives.

The middle-aged or older couple also constitute a family unit. This family results when children have been launched in school, career, or marriage or when the couple have had no children. One or both members are employed or retired. This family typically enjoys the freedom to explore and continue to grow in much the same way as the dyadic nuclear family, but at a later point in life. However, the responsibility for grown children may reassert itself at any time within the couple's life span.

The institutional family and the foster family are constituted by society and used voluntarily or involuntarily. The institutional family is group oriented and cares for children in orphanages, residential schools, and correctional institutions. Foster families consist of one or more children and the foster parents to whom those children have been assigned for temporary care by a court or by an agency.

Several less traditional family units are emerging in society. These structures, which also influence children in their growth and development, include unmarried-parent or unmarried-couple families, homosexual-couple families, and communal families.

Unmarried couples with a child or children are families in which natural or adopted children are nurtured. Marriage may not be desired or possible. The unmarried couple may choose to live together for varying periods or as a permanent arrangement. The unmarried-couple family may experience developmental issues similar to those of the single-parent family that became so involuntarily.

The homosexual-couple family may comprise a male or a female couple and a child or children. The children may be formally or informally adopted, or in the case of a female couple, they may have been born naturally within the family.

Communal families, with monogamous couples and group marriages, feature sharing of facilities, resources, and experiences. Socialization of the children is considered to be a function of the group. Members of a communal family with monogamous couples share a household, but individual children are identified with their primary family unit. The communal family by group marriage maintains a household of adults and children who are known as one family in which all adults are married to one another and all are parents to the children.

Kinship networks or extended families, may be adjuncts to both traditional and less traditional family patterns. These networks provide a supportive, reciprocal system for the exchange of goods and services. The most effective ones typically consist of members in close geographical proximity. Emanating from natural or created family structures, such relationships can be very influential in the social and psychological development of the child (Kennedy, 1978).

RELATIVE NATURE OF DEVELOPMENTAL AGES AND STAGES

In seeking to understand human growth and development from the standpoint of stages, one must consider them as relative to circumstances in the lives of each individual rather than as absolute regarding a person's competence for adaptation. Occupational role behavior, performance, and performance components described for one age group or stage of development could occur or reach levels of competence in an earlier or later stage depending on circumstances, experience in basic component skills, and environmental resources. An example occurs in Case Study 2-3: Roberta is coping with being "sandwiched in" at age 56 in the stage of later adulthood. This phenomenon is described in the literature for the stage of middle adulthood, which encompasses ages 35-50. Another example is presented by widowhood, which generally occurs in later life, but can occur in any stage and at any age following marriage.

Role transitions in midlife and old age are also relative such that midlife and old age are not well demarcated in society and are subject to circumstance and experience. Rosow (1985) has examined various aspects of aging. The phenomenon of role loss in his description of role types is particularly cogent to this discussion: "The loss of roles excludes the aged from significant social participation and devalues them" (p. 71). Rejection, intolerance, deprivation of vital functions that support a sense of self-worth and self-esteem, assignment to marginal status, and alienation from the mainstream of society are some of the penalties in later life. Denial of rewards that were considered routine earlier in life too often occurs in the later part of the life span.

Old age is the first stage in the life cycle in which systematic loss of status is a factor to which an entire group is subject (Rosow, 1985). All previous periods, from childhood through earlier adulthood, are usually marked by steady social growth in self-care/self-maintenance, play/leisure, and work/education. Status acquisition in earlier stages of development "involves gains in competence, responsibility, authority, privilege, reward, and prestige" (p. 71). Status loss in old age represents a significant break in this pattern, beginning the reversal of the acquisitional trend.

Another major discontinuity from earlier patterns of growth and development is society's lack of social norms, expectations, and standards for role performance by the aged. This presents a bewildering situation in which people are left to fashion a life-style with ill-defined parameters. It may contribute to the lives of many elderly being "socially unstructured." Role definition or redefinition in the context of intrinsically motivated occupational performance can assist in the acquisition of acceptable new roles as a person ages. Social identity involves loss of social roles. Although role loss does not occur instantly, it occurs of necessity because one is constrained to give up some roles.

OVERCOMING DEVELOPMENTAL DEFICIENCIES

Role competence for adaptation at a given age and stage of growth and development requires assessment of occupational performance and performance components relative to environmental expectations, self-expectations, and normative behavioral and performance expectations in a sociocultural context. Appropriate intervention will take into account both remedial and compensatory strategies to overcome deficiencies and to move a person toward competence and mastery. Engaging an individual in activities, tasks, and interpersonal interactions that are consistent with intrinsic motivations and the extrinsic reward system, so that the individual can perform as competently as possible in his or her occupational roles, is a goal of occupational therapy.

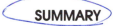

SUMMARY

The development of skills for independence in self-care/self-maintenance, play/leisure, work/education, and rest/relaxation is critical for the successful performance of occupational and social roles. The level of subskill development depends on the neurophysiological, physical, and psychological integrity of the human system as nurtured by social and cultural experiences.

Engagement in activities, tasks, and interpersonal interactions must be intrinsically motivated and extrinsically reinforced to facilitate mastery, achievement, competence, and generalization. Activities, tasks, and interpersonal interactions provide stimuli to the sensory systems, and they influence the processing and the integration of stimuli and the outcome of adaptation.

Study Questions

1. Differentiate between occupational performance and occupational performance components.

2. Describe levels of mastery for successful adaptation.

3. List the stages of development according to each developmental theorist.

4. Discuss the similarities and the differences among the developmental theorists.

5. Describe the developmental orientations of the occupational therapy theorists.

6. Name the occupational performance skill areas.

7. Name the occupational performance components.

8. What are the similarities and the differences among the occupational performance skills of humans across the life span?

9. Describe the adaptive behavior associated with life roles from infancy through old-old age.

10. What are extrinsically motivated activities?

11. What are intrinsically motivated activities?

12. List and discuss at least five family configurations that occur in Western society.

Recommended Readings

Clark, P.N., & Allen, A.S. (1985). *Occupational therapy for children.* St. Louis: C. V. Mosby.

Erikson, E. (1985). *Childhood and society.* New York: W.W. Norton.

Gilfoyle, E., Grady, A., & Moore, J. (1980). *Children adapt.* Thorofare, NJ: Charles B. Slack.

Havighurst, R.J. (1979). *Developmental tasks and education.* New York: David McKay.

Kennedy, C. (1978). *Human development: The adult years and aging.* New York: Macmillan.

Llorens, L.A. (1976). *Application of a developmental theory for health and rehabilitation.* Rockville, MD: American Occupational Therapy Association.

Papalia, D.E., & Olds, S.W. (1986). *Human development.* New York: McGraw-Hill.

Reilly, M. (1974). *Play as exploratory learning.* Beverly Hills, CA: Sage.

Rosow, I. (1985). Status and role change through the life

cycle. In R.H. Binstock & E. Shanas (Eds.), *Handbook of aging and the social sciences* (pp. 62-91). New York: Van Nostrand Reinhold.

Sheehy, G. (1976). *Passages*. New York: E.P. Dutton.

References

American Occupational Therapy Association. (1979). Policy: The philosophical base of occupational therapy. *American Journal of Occupational Therapy, 33*, 785.

American Occupational Therapy Association. (1989). Occupational therapy product output reporting system and uniform terminology for reporting occupational therapy services. In Reference manual of the official documents of the American Occupational Therapy Association (pp. VII.19-29). Rockville, MD: Author. (Original work published 1981).

Ayres, A.J. (1972). *Sensory integration and learning disorders*. Los Angeles: Western Psychological Services.

Ayres, A.J. (1979). *Sensory integration and the child*. Los Angeles: Western Psychological Services.

Clark, P.N., & Allen, A.S. (1985). *Occupational therapy for children*. St. Louis: C.V. Mosby.

Erikson, E. (1985). *Childhood and society*. New York: W.W. Norton.

Fidler, G.S., & Fidler, J.W. (1978). Doing and becoming: Purposeful action and self-actualization. *American Journal of Occupational Therapy, 32*, 305-310.

Gilfoyle, E., Grady, A., & Moore, J. (1980). *Children adapt*. Thorofare, NJ: Charles B. Slack.

Hall, G. (1979). *A primer of Freudian psychology*. New York: New American Library.

Havighurst, R.J. (1979). *Developmental tasks and education*. New York: David McKay.

Kennedy, C. (1978). *Human development: The adult years and aging*. New York: Macmillan.

Knoblock, H., & Pasamanick, B. (1974). *Gesell and Armatruda's developmental diagnosis*. New York: Harper & Row.

Lewis, S.C. (1979). *The mature years*. Thorofare, NJ: Charles B. Slack.

Llorens, L.A. (1970). *Facilitating growth and development: The promise of occupational therapy*. American Journal of Occupational Therapy, 24, 93-101.

Llorens, L.A. (1976). *Application of a developmental theory for health and rehabilitation*. Rockville, MD: American Occupational Therapy Association.

Llorens, L.A. (1984). Theoretical conceptualization of occupational therapy: 1960-1982. *Occupational Therapy in Mental Health, 4*(2),1-14.

Llorens, L.A., & Burris, B. (1981). Development of sensory integration in learning disabilities. In J. Gottlieb & S. S. Strichart (Eds.). *Development theory and research in learning disabilities* (pp. 57-79). Baltimore: University Park Press.

Maier, H.W. (1978). *Three theories of child development*. New York: Harper & Row.

Miller, R., Seig, K., Ludwig, F., Shortridge, S., & Van Deusen, J. (1988). *Six perspectives on theory for the practice of occupational therapy*. Rockville, MD: Aspen.

Mosey, A.C. (1968). *Occupational therapy: Theory and practice*. Medford, MA: Pothier Brothers.

Mosey, A.C. (1971). *Three frames of reference for mental health*. Thorofare, NJ: Charles B. Slack.

Papalia, D.E., & Olds, S.W. (1986). *Human development*. New York: McGraw-Hill.

Reilly, M. (1974). *Play as exploratory learning*. Beverly Hills, CA: Sage.

Rosow, I. (1985). Status and role change through the life cycle. In R.H. Binstock & E. Shanas (Eds.). *Handbook of aging and the social sciences* (pp. 62-91). New York: Van Nostrand Reinhold.

Sheehy, G. (1976). *Passages*. New York: E.P. Dutton.

CHAPTER CONTENT OUTLINE

KEY TERMS

Attention Strategies

Autonomic nervous system

Avoidant Strategies

Cognitive appraisal

Commitment

Coping

Emotion-focused coping

General adaptation syndrome

Primary appraisal

Problem-focused coping

Stress

Stressors

Sympathetic nervous system

Type A behavior

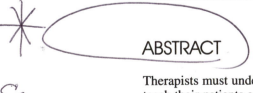

ABSTRACT

Therapists must understand the dynamics of coping and adaptation in order to
teach their patients and clients coping strategies that will help them successfully
deal with stressful situations and to identify those at risk. This chapter explores
the dynamics of coping; factors that influence coping, such as social support or
self-efficacy; current approaches to improving coping skills; and how coping
theory can be applied in practice to help individuals better contend with
stressful situations related to performance deficits.

Performance Deficits as Sources of Stress
Coping Theory and Occupational Therapy

Charles Christiansen

"Living organisms never submit passively to environmental forces; however primitive they may be, all of them attempt to respond adaptively to these forces, each in its own manner. The characteristics of this response express the individuality of the organism and determine whether it will experience health or disease in a given stituation."

—Dubos, 1965

OBJECTIVES

The information in this chapter is intended to help the reader—

1. distinguish between coping and adaptation.

2. identify several functions of coping.

3. list and classify various types of stressors.

4. explain what is meant by cognitive appraisal.

5. understand the personal and environmental factors that seem to influence coping efforts.

6. identify various types of coping strategies and determine which seem to be most effective on the basis of current research.

7. discuss various approaches designed to improve coping abilities.

8. understand how knowledge of coping theory can be applied to improve occupational therapy practice.

Occupational therapists typically experience an interesting phenomenon as part of their daily practice. They observe that patients or clients with similar deficits or the same disability frequently have remarkably different results. Some appear to respond quite well to treatment, adapt readily to changes in their life-style, and experience favorable outcomes. Others, however, have a more difficult time and seem to encounter many problems in adjusting to or resolving the stressful situations imposed by their conditions. Clearly, then, factors other than the nature or the severity of the condition, or even the type of intervention, account for these differences. It is likely that they can at least partially be explained by the manner in which people are able to deal with difficult situations.

The process through which people adjust to the stressful demands of their daily environments has been labeled **coping.** Occupational therapy can be viewed as a process that assists people in coping with problem situations and attaining satisfactory adjustment to living circumstances. By their very nature, performance deficits are associated with stressful situations, either through the challenges that they create or by virtue of the circumstances that imposed them. Despite this obvious relationship between performance deficits and stress, little has been written in the occupational therapy literature about how people adjust to stressful events, and little research has been done in the field to gain insight into coping behaviors.

In this chapter, the central role of performance in coping and adaptation is examined. For example, performance deficits can themselves represent or follow the harm, threat, or challenge situations that characterize stressful events. Moreover, the ability to successfully meet challenges or difficult situations requires a mustering of personal and environmental resources to deal effectively with them. Abilities, beliefs, and personality dispositions influence a person's perception of stressful events and thereby affect the manner in which one attempts to cope with stressful situations.

An assumption is made that performance deficits represent stressful events that require adaptive responses. On the other hand, task performance can be viewed as a means of coping with stressful circumstances, whether directed at the problem situation itself or used in other ways that help a person deal with emotional responses to such events.

Much of the recent research on coping and adaptation has been encouraged by a widespread interest in stress and its relationship to disease and medical treatment. However, because of the relationships between performance, stress, and coping, the factors that determine successful adjustment also have important implications for the work of occupational therapists. Thus, with increased understanding of the dynamics of coping and adaptation, therapists may be better able to teach coping strategies that can assist patients and clients in dealing successfully with the stressful situations that they are experiencing in their lives. Also, therapists may be able to identify people who are at risk for unsuccessful adaptation, either because their coping skills are limited or ineffective, or because their personal or environmental situations or resources have been shown to interfere with successful coping. Such people either require special approaches within the context of therapy or become candidates for specific coping intervention strategies.

ADAPTATION

Although the terms **coping** and adaptation are frequently used interchangeably, they are more appropriately viewed in a hierarchy, with adaptation as the more encompassing term. Successful coping leads to adaptation, but not all adaptive behaviors can be categorized as coping (Cohen & Lazarus, 1984). Coping always involves some type of stress. It thus requires effort over and above the routine or automatic actions that are adaptive, yet require little energy or conscious attention, such as looking before proceeding through an intersection or taking care with sharp objects. Although such actions can help to avoid crises (e.g., personal injury) and are important behaviors, they fall outside the meaning of coping in this chapter because of their routine nature.

Some scientists use *adaptation* in a biological sense, to identify a process that allows species to survive over time. However, the term is used throughout this chapter in its psychological sense. Thus, *adaptation* refers to the general category of processes that determine the satisfactoriness of fit between an individual and his/her environment. Successful adaptation equates with quality of life. To function effectively at the social level is to have adapted.

COPING

In order to achieve successful social adaptation, people must employ various strategies. They must achieve mastery over environmental challenges, they must have adequate defenses for responding to threat, and they must be able to adapt under particularly difficult conditions. Coping takes place when people adjust to the pressures of the environment by engaging in specific problem-solving efforts. Stated according to this framework, coping consists of the problem-solving efforts that a person makes when he or she views the demands of the environment as relevant to his or her welfare (that is, when the person confronts a situation of considerable jeopardy or promise) and when these demands tax the person's adaptive resources (Lazarus & Folkman, 1984).

Coping implies the use of personal resources and competencies to resolve stress and create new ways of dealing with problem situations. It has three components (White, 1974): First, a person must be able to gain and process new information that is needed for fully understanding the situation. Second, a person must be able to maintain control over his or her emotional state. This suggests, not the absence of emotion, but the ability to identify one's emotions correctly, express them appropriately, and control their expression. Mechanic (1974) refers to this as the ability to maintain a state of psychological equilibrium, noting that when people possess psychological equilibrium, they can direct their energies and skills toward meeting external as well as internal needs. He believes that successful coping also implies dealing with social and environmental demands and having the motivation to meet such demands. Finally, coping requires that a person have some freedom of response or realistic alternatives for dealing with the situation that he or she is experiencing.

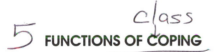

5 FUNCTIONS OF COPING

Coping skills may be required as a part of normal development, as suggested by Erikson's (1985) stage-related tasks. Alternatively, they may be required during stressful episodes that are situational and unanticipated, as may occur with illness or injury.

In a synthesis of the works of many writers who have explored the coping requirements imposed by illness, Cohen and Lazarus (1979) describe five main functions of coping: (a) to reduce harmful environmental conditions and enhance prospects of recovery, (b) to tolerate or adjust to negative events and realities, (c) to maintain a positive self-image, (d)

to maintain emotional equilibrium, and (e) to continue satisfying relationships with others. Each of the coping tasks just identified can be classified as either problem-focused or emotion-focused (Lazarus & Folkman, 1984b). **Problem-focused coping** is distinguished by efforts to manage the nature of the problem. **Emotion-focused** coping is characterized by attempts to regulate the emotions or the distress accompanying a stressful situation. More attention is given to these classifications later in the chapter. Many authors have noted that some problems (such as congenital conditions or terminal illnesses) may not be amenable to a person's efforts to change them. Under these circumstances, coping must of necessity be emotion-focused, directed at the feelings one has about the situation at hand.

STRESS

Stress is defined here as the body's generalized reaction to external threats. The physiologist Walter Cannon (1932) was the first scientist to use the term in a technical sense, suggesting that stress was a disturbance of homeostasis, or the regulatory balance of the body. Hans Selye (1936) further developed the concept, referring to stress as an orchestrated set of bodily defenses against any form of noxious stimulus. He used these physiological reactions to environmental demands to explain a phenomenon he called **general adaptation syndrome** (G.A.S.), consisting of an alarm reaction, a resistance stage, and an exhaustion stage. As research in this area continued, scientists began looking at the effect of stressors on hormonal secretions. This became a natural link to behavioral medicine and the idea that emotional responses to environmental stressors might partly explain subsequent impairments in health. More recently, a growing body of research has shown consistent relationships between psychosocial factors in the environment and health status.

The environmental conditions and the specific events that elicit stress reactions are frequently termed **stressors**. Coping can be viewed as the manner in which a person attempts to ward off or buffer the negative effects of stressors or stressful situations. There are clear responses to such situations at the physiological level; Elliott and Eisdorfer (1982) offer a comprehensive review. However, this chapter emphasizes the psychological processes and the behavioral responses that characterize a person's response to stressful conditions.

Types of Stressors

Stressors include specific events and environmental conditions. Although much attention has been focused on life events as stressors, environmental conditions that do not involve change can also produce psychological and physiological reactions. An example of an environmental condition that is not event related, but could evoke a stress reaction, is boredom. Also, when a person's expectations are not fulfilled, such as his or her not graduating on a planned date or not receiving an expected promotion, these conditions can be stressful.

Clearly, stressful events are not equivalent in their impact. They differ in the manner in which they are appraised and in the ability of the individual to cope with them. The timing, the duration, the frequency, the controllability, even the order of events, as well as their perceived and actual consequences, can affect their impact on a person's life.

Four types of stressors have been identified (Elliott & Eisdorfer, 1982, p. 150), distinguished mainly by their duration:

1. *Acute stressors*—time-limited events, such as experiencing a job interview or preparing for an important examination.
2. *Stressor sequences*—a series of events occurring over an extended period as a result of an initiating event, such as losing a job, which may trigger a family move, a reduced standard of living, and other events.
3. *Chronic intermittent stressors*—time-limited events that can recur daily, weekly, or monthly, such as visits from unwelcome relatives.
4. *Chronic permanent stressors*—circumstances that may be initiated by a discrete event, but always persist for an extended time, such as permanent disabilities, marital discord, or an unsatisfactory job situation.

Little is known about the relationship between the type of stressor and its effect on adaptational outcomes. Nor have scientists yet determined if different types of stressors require specific coping strategies. Because most research involving humans has concerned acute stressors, much less is known about the effects of chronic stressors or stressor sequences on adaptational consequences such as health and well-being.

Stress and Illness

A substantive body of literature has shown convincing relationships between stressful life events and both acute and chronic illnesses of physical and emotional varieties. For example, much attention has been paid to the impact of the high-stress, achievement-oriented life-style described as **Type A behavior** (Glass, 1977). People with this type of disposition show more reaction to stressors than people with more easygoing life-styles, who are classified as Type Bs. In fact, studies have shown that people with Type A

behavioral patterns are twice as likely to suffer heart attacks as those with Type B patterns. Research has also shown a relationship between stressful events and tension headaches (Holroyd, Appel, & Andrasik, 1983), ulcers (Smith, Colligan, Horning, & Hurrel, 1978), and high blood pressure (Talbott et al., 1985), as well as asthma, arthritis, and diabetes.

Although research into the physiological mechanisms underlying these relationships between stress and illness continues, the autonomic nervous system, the endocrine system, the immune system, and the brain appear to be involved in the triggering of physical and emotional responses to stressful situations. It is currently believed that stress affects the immune system by lowering its ability to resist infection (Jemmott et al., 1983).

Scientists have also studied stress as one of many factors involved in the development of psychological illness. Although the division between physical and psychological illness is becoming less distinct, some evidence has been found to link stressful events to depression, schizophrenia, and anxiety disorders. However, studies have not shown strong or consistent relationships between life stress and these emotional disorders. Moreover, the relationships have been moderated by social and cognitive variables, including the presence of family support and one's sense of vulnerability and personal control. In general, such findings underscore the complexity of the coping process and provide support for the transactional, process-oriented theory of coping mechanisms described in this chapter.

Measurement of Stressors

Much of current knowledge about the effects of stress is based on studies of life events and selected outcomes. As mentioned previously, a large amount of this effort has focused on the relationship between stress and health status. A study by Holmes and Rahe (1967) is frequently credited with stimulating great interest in this area of inquiry. Using the Social Readjustment Rating Scale, which contains 43 life events (listed in Table 3-1), these researchers found that the magnitude of life change experienced during a specified period could be used to predict the health status of a group of naval personnel serving aboard an aircraft carrier. As predicted, the people who experienced the greatest life stress as measured in life change units also reported significantly more health problems during an ensuing period.

This approach to measuring stress, using a scale of life events, formed the basis for a number of subsequent studies, most of which corroborated the relationship between life stress and health found by Holmes and Rahe. However, it soon became evident that the Social Readjustment Rating Scale was an imperfect measure of

Table 3-1
Social Readjustment Rating Scale

Rank	Life Event	Mean Value	Rank	Life Event	Mean Value
1	Death of spouse	100	23	Son or daughter leaving home	29
2	Divorce	73	24	Trouble with in-laws	29
3	Marital separation	65	25	Outstanding personal achievement	28
4	Jail term	63	26	Wife begin or stop work	26
5	Death of close family member	63	27	Begin or end school work	26
6	Personal injury or illness	53	28	Change in living conditions	25
7	Marriage	50	29	Revision of personal habits	24
8	Fired at work	47	30	Trouble with boss	23
9	Marital reconciliation	45	31	Change in work hours or conditions	20
10	Retirement	45	32	Change in residence	20
11	Change in health of family member	44	33	Change in schools	20
12	Pregnancy	40	34	Change in recreation	19
13	Sex difficulties	39	35	Change in church activities	19
14	Gain of new family member	39	36	Change in social activities	18
15	Business readjustment	39	37	Mortgage or loan less than $10,000	17
16	Change in financial state	38	38	Change in sleeping habits	16
17	Death of close friend	37	39	Change in number of family get-togethers	15
18	Change to different line of work	36	40	Change in eating habits	15
19	Change in number of arguments with spouse	35	41	Vacation	13
20	Mortgage over $10,000	31	42	Christmas	12
21	Foreclosure of mortgage or loan	30	43	Minor violations of the law	11
22	Change in responsibilities at work	29			

From Holmes, TH and Rahe, RH (1967). *The Social Readjustment Rating Scale. Journal of Psychosomatic Research, 11(2), 216. Oxford, England: Pergamon Press.*

stress. This was because the reliability of reporting life events was shown to have a limited duration (Jenkins, Hurst, & Rose, 1979) and because the assumption that both positive and negative experiences resulted in similar consequences (either psychological or physiological) was found to be incorrect (Rose, 1980; Vinokur & Selzer, 1975).

More recent attempts to measure stressful life events have attempted to eliminate these conceptual and psychometric problems. For example, the PERI Life Events Scale (Dohrenwend, Krasnoff, Askenasy, & Dohrenwend, 1978) is designed to consider the frequency as well as the intensity of a stressful experience. The Hassles and Uplifts Scales (Kanner, Coyne, Schaefer, & Lazarus, 1981) attempt to distinguish between negative and positive experiences and to focus on the day-to-day events that characterize living, rather than on the major acute stressors emphasized in the Social Readjustment Rating Scale. *Hassles* have been defined as "experiences and conditions of daily living that have been appraised as salient and harmful or threatening to the individual's well-being" (Lazarus, 1984, p. 376). On the other hand, *uplifts* are defined as "experiences and conditions of daily living that have been appraised as vital and positive or favorable to the endorser's well-being" (p. 376). Table 3-2 presents the 10 most frequent hassles and uplifts reported in Kanner *et al.*'s (1981) study. Research on hassles and uplifts using the Hassles and Uplifts Scales has shown them to be a better predictor of concurrent and subsequent psychological symptoms than a standard life-events scale (Kanner et al., 1981).

Studies continue in an effort to determine which approach to the measurement of stress will yield the most fruitful results in identifying people at risk for adverse adaptational outcomes. Zimmerman (1985) has published a useful review of the various scales being used to measure stressful life events.

Table 3-2
Ten Most Frequent Hassles and Uplifts
(N = 100)

Item	% of Times Checked
Hassles	
1. Concerns about weight	52.4
2. Health of a family member	48.1
3. Rising prices of common goods	43.7
4. Home maintenance	42.8
5. Too many things to do	38.6
6. Misplacing or losing things	38.1
7. Yard work or outside home maintenance	38.1
8. Property, investment or taxes	37.6
9. Crime	37.1
10. Physical appearance	35.9
Uplifts	
1. Relating well with your spouse or lover	76.3
2. Relating well with friends	74.4
3. Completing a task	73.3
4. Feeling healthy	72.7
5. Getting enough sleep	69.7
6. Eating out	68.4
7. Meeting your responsibilities	68.1
8. Visiting, phoning, or writing someone	67.7
9. Spending time with family	66.7
10. Home (inside) pleasing to you	65.5

Items are those most frequently checked over a period of 9 months. The "% of items checked" figures represent the mean percentage of people checking the item each month averaged over the nine monthly administrations.

From Kanner, AD, Coyne, JC, Shaefer, C and Lazarus, RS (1981). Comparison of two modes of stress measurement: Daily hassles and uplifts versus major life events. Journal of Behavioral Medicine, 4. New York, NY: Plenum Publishing Corporation.

THE COPING PROCESS

As might be expected, coping is a complex phenomenon. Table 3-3 depicts the various components that social scientists view as relevant to an understanding of coping. This transactional model shows that both the characteristics of a person's living environment and his or her personal disposition and intrapersonal resources affect the manner in which he or she perceives and appraises a particular stressful situation and responds to the situation on the basis of the appraisal. The term *transactional* is used purposely to emphasize that the process is extremely dynamic. That is, far from being a passive player who waits to fend off stressful situations when they occur, a person is capable of anticipating the possibility of a stressful environmental event and preventing its occurrence or at least buffering its effects.

An example offered by Moos (1984) helps to illustrate this point: A person with an attentive perceptual style (personal system) lives in a neighborhood with a high crime rate (environment). Perceiving the possibility of danger (cognitively appraising the situation), the person copes by placing safety locks on windows and doors and thus reduces the likelihood of experiencing a stressful event (being victimized by crime).

Coping Stages

Several writers have proposed that coping efforts occur in definable stages or sequences. For example, Shontz (1975) has posited a series of coping stages, including shock, detachment, encounter, retreat, and reality testing. In this formulation coping involves a continuous shifting between confrontation and avoidance or denial. Shontz asserts that the retreat phase prevents breakdown by permitting temporary withdrawal into safety. The process is viewed as a necessary stage preceding psychological growth.

In another stage model, Klinger (1975) has suggested that people initially respond to loss with increased effort and a higher level of concentration. This may be followed by frustration and anger if the efforts to overcome the stress are not successful. Ultimately, continued lack of success results in depression, which is characterized by pessimism and apathy. In Klinger's view, disengagement and depression are an adaptive way to cope.

Lazarus (1984), however, asserts that stage models of coping fail to consider the variability of individuals in terms of their situational contexts when confronted with stressful events. These situations are also influenced by the timing and the duration of stressful encounters, considered from the standpoint of a person's life history and experiences. Lazarus notes further that some shared cultural patterns may be exhibited in coping responses. However, it is more likely that responses are individually and situationally determined, and unlikely to reflect a dominant stage pattern of response.

In the following sections, current theory and findings regarding the individual and his or her appraisal of the nature of a stressful situation are examined. Attention is also focused on the role of the environment and the methods of coping that people use. This should help us gain a better understanding of the coping process and its implications for occupational therapy.

Personal Factors and Cognitive Appraisal

Although researchers agree that the factors of most concern in coping involve the individual, his or her environment, and the nature of the stressful situation, a key point of divergence seems to be related to **cognitive appraisal**, that part of the coping process during which a person evaluates a stressor and chooses a strategy for dealing with it. So-called structural approaches to studying coping tend to place less importance on cognitive appraisal, preferring to view personal, environmental, and situational factors as relatively equivalent structural elements. On the other hand, the transactional approach views the appraisal process as one of the principal determinants of coping behavior. For this reason it has special relevance for occupational therapy practice, a point that is discussed later in this chapter.

Lazarus and Folkman (1984a, 1984b) have been the principal proponents of the transactional model, schematically represented in Figure 3-1. As suggested earlier, this model views the coping process as heavily dependent on the personal resources of individuals and their appraisals of situations viewed as requiring a response. The premise is that people want to know what is happening to them and what it means for their well-being. Although these appraisals or individual attempts to understand the nature and the meaning of a particular stressful situation are strongly influenced by needs, motives, and other psychological characteristics, they are also based on accurate perceptions of the objective environment. Thus reactions to demanding and hostile environments are shaped interactively by personal factors and the objective nature of the environmental threat. It is also important to note that once a stressful situation is appraised, it is continually reappraised by the person in light of coping efforts and changes in the environment. Such reappraisal can be classified as ordinary or defensive in nature (which occurs if the event is perceived as a threat). Reappraisals may change the meaning of the event and thus lead to changes in one's coping strategies.

Lazarus (1984) defines stress as "an inharmonious fit between the person and the environment, or one in which the person's resources are taxed or exceeded, forcing the person to struggle, usually in complex ways, to cope" (p. 376). A person judges stressful events in two ways:

1. A *primary appraisal* in terms of the events' perceived significance for his or her well-being
2. A *secondary appraisal* in terms of his or her resources and options for coping.

A **primary appraisal** of an unusual or novel situation leads to its being interpreted as (a) irrelevant, (b) benign-positive, or (c) stressful. As might be expected, a situation viewed as irrelevant is not considered to have implications for a person's well-being and is ignored. An interpretation of the second type, benign-positive, signals that no coping action is necessary. A situation appraised as stressful is one in which the person has judged that environmental or internal demands will strain or exceed his or her adaptive resources. Such stress appraisals have been described by Lazarus as falling into three categories: (a) harm-loss, (b) threat, or (c) challenge.

Harm-Loss Appraisals. Harm-loss appraisals are judgments that damage has already occurred, whether through disease or injury, diminished self-esteem, or loss of a loved one. As might be expected, the most damaging events are those involving aspects of life with deep meaning or significance to the individual.

Threat Appraisals. When an event is appraised as holding the possibility of future harm, it is classified as a threat. A threat appraisal has great adaptational significance because people can prepare themselves for the event by planning and working through their coping responses. Common emotions accompanying threat are fear, worry, anxiety, and anger. These emotions may impede problem-focused coping efforts, however, so they increase the possibility of poor problem resolution. Coping, in fact, has been described as a means of mediating the emotional response to threat based on the individual's perceived significance of the event (Folkman & Lazarus, 1988a, 1988b).

Sometimes a situation evokes simultaneous appraisals of harm-loss and threat. An example is when a person suffers a serious disabling injury. The pain or the loss of function is an immediate concern, and there may be threatening implications for the future—such as whether or not the functional loss will permit a return to work. Events that result in loss frequently have negative implications for the future and are thus usually viewed as threatening.

Table 3-3
Important Dimensions of the Coping Process

Personal	Environmental
Personality dispositions	Types and nature of stressors
Perceptual styles	Social network
Cognition	Economic and educational resources
Historical and cultural factors	
Coping strategies	Situational ambiguity

and on

transactional model

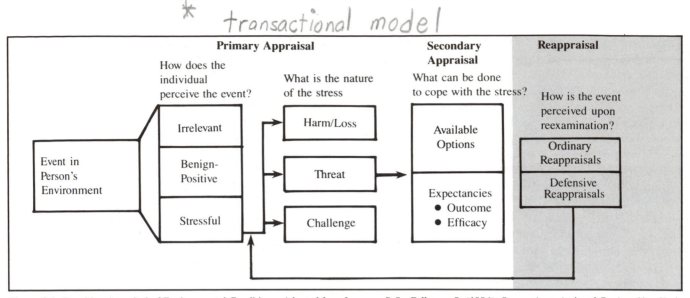

Figure 3-1. Cognitive Appraisal of Environmental Conditions. *Adapted from Lazarus, P.S., Folkman, S. (1984). Stress, Appraisal and Coping. New York: Springer Publishing Company.*

Challenge Appraisals. Situations viewed as challenging are events that hold the potential for mastery or gain, but also require the mobilization of coping resources. In general, they are accompanied by pleasurable emotions, such as hopefulness, eagerness, and confidence. Because they engender these positive emotions, challenge appraisals tend to facilitate effective problem-focused coping and to promote good morale.

Challenge and threat appraisals should not be viewed as mutually exclusive. A career opportunity can be appraised as a challenge in that it offers the potential for an increase in prestige, responsibility, and financial reward, but also a threat in that it poses the risks of increased demands and inadequate performance. Similarly, important examinations typically elicit simultaneous challenge and threat appraisals from students.

Factors Influencing Coping Success

Earlier it was noted that coping is influenced by situational factors, available resources, and characteristics of the individual. Because coping is a dynamic process, however, these factors interact to determine how a stressful situation is appraised. The appraisal then influences the type of coping activity used by the individual in responding to the situation. In the following sections, the environmental and personal factors known to be important to the coping process are examined.

Environmental Factors. The nature of a stressful situation itself influences the coping process through its effect on a person's appraisal of it. As situations are perceived more clearly, a person is better able to choose a coping response.

However, other elements in the environment, such as material or social resources, affect the person's choice of coping strategy and ability to cope. To fully understand how these factors, ambiguity and social support, interact to influence coping success, it is necessary to discuss them in more detail.

Ambiguity. An ambiguous situation is one that cannot be easily interpreted because its meaning is unclear. Ambiguity can play an important role during the cognitive appraisal of a stressful situation because it can raise anxiety and delay an appropriate coping response. A situation that nearly everyone has experienced illustrates the point: *At three o'clock in the morning, the sound of broken glass pierces an otherwise tranquil night. It appears to have come from the direction of the garage. Could it be an intruder? Or did a stray cat knock over an empty milk bottle?*

During the process of appraising a stressful situation, a person determines whether a condition of harm-loss, threat, or challenge exists. To the extent that the environment lacks clarity, the person will feel uncertain about the nature of the situation. This uncertainty, in turn, will delay or interfere with the important task of deciding on an appropriate course of action.

Unfortunately many stressful social situations are ambiguous and hence difficult to appraise. This lack of clarity and its consequent uncertainty may help to explain the popularity of various syndicated advice columns, such as "Dear Abby." There tend to be broad differences in the manner in which people react to various social contexts. For example, it is not unusual for one to conclude an interaction with another person and be puzzled by something he or she said or uncertain of what was meant by his or her nonverbal language.

Researchers have shown that conditions of uncertainty tend to increase the importance of personal factors, such as beliefs and personality traits, when a person selects a course of action, or a coping response. Thus a person with low self-esteem may interpret an ambiguous situation as an indication that he or she is inadequate in some way. In contrast, a person with high self-confidence and much more interpersonal experience might conclude only that the other person was preoccupied or having a bad day.

The ambiguous coping situation may be likened to a projective test, in which the experiences and the characteristics of the individual provide the basis for inferences about the meaning of the situation (Lazarus & Folkman, 1984b). As situational factors become clearer and more readily interpreted, personal factors are less likely to influence appraisal.

Social Support. Conventional wisdom has long held that in times of stress, it is helpful to have friends and family around to provide tangible assistance as well as emotional support. Does the empirical research on stress support these notions? To answer this question, various investigators have attempted to measure the presence of social support and its impact in buffering the effects of stressful life events. In general, these findings have consistently shown that such support can have a positive impact on coping outcomes. For example, people who have social supports may live longer than those who do not (Berkman & Syme, 1979), and social support shows a positive relationship to lowered incidence of physical illness (Cassell, 1976) and more positive mental health (Cobb, 1976). Further, diminished social resources have been associated with psychological distress and psychosomatic complaints (Dean & Lin, 1977; Theorell, 1976).

One difficulty associated with this research has been the definition and the measurement of social support. In addition to large numbers of family and friends being accessible to a person, the type of support available is likely to make a difference. Offering material assistance or emotional comfort are useful forms of social support. Providing information or conveying a sense of belonging can also be helpful. Someone who encourages expression of beliefs or feelings and acknowledges their appropriateness can be valuable (Silver & Wortman, 1980).

On the other hand, sometimes such support can be less than helpful because friends and family members can convey irritation and resentment when confronted with the frustration of chronic illnesses or stressful conditions that are not easily overcome (Suls, 1982). Also, the information provided by the members of one's social network may be inaccurate, thus thwarting rather than assisting the coping process. Moreover, the way in which the recipient views such support may be quite different from the way in which the giver intends it or the outsider perceives it.

Although one's spouse would be expected to be a source of social support, it is not unusual for marital relationships to increase rather than reduce stress. Furthermore, the availability of social support may not equate with its use by the person experiencing stressful life encounters. Some people may view support as an indication that they are unable to cope without assistance. As a consequence, social support serves only to threaten their self-esteem.

Lazarus and Folkman (1984b) have suggested an interesting and potentially confounding interaction between personal characteristics, coping styles, and social support: People who lack interpersonal competence may limit the social resources on which they can call during stressful situations. For example, a person with paranoid characteristics may alienate potential friends by misinterpreting their intentions, or a person with depressive characteristics may withdraw from social interaction and thereby diminish his or her chances to establish meaningful social contacts. Clearly too, the experience of prolonged illness or stressful episodes can itself diminish the opportunity for social interaction because of incapacitation or forced isolation. If poor adaptational outcomes are examined by researchers in such situations, diminished social support may be incorrectly viewed as a cause of inadequate coping rather than as an effect of the stressful conditions.

Similarly, some stressful episodes such as job loss, divorce, death of a loved one, or change of residence, are accompanied by social losses. Determining whether the observed outcomes are due to the stressors *per se* or the loss of social support that accompanies them is difficult.

The related personality characteristics of extraversion and need for affiliation may make some people more susceptible to the absence of social support during stressful episodes (Duckitt, 1984; Lefcourt, Martin, & Saleh, 1984). The importance of social support during stressful episodes appears to depend on the personality makeup of the individual.

People may learn to cultivate social relationships because they are aware of the importance of social interaction to their coping ability. In this sense, social support can be viewed as a type of coping mechanism rather than simply as an environmental resource.

One can conclude from the preceding discussion that the situation being experienced and the personality of the individual interact to determine the effect of social support on coping. Although social resources constitute an important factor in coping, social support is not always helpful, and the specific methods and circumstances governing the buffering effect of social resources are not yet understood.

Personal Factors. As noted earlier, during cognitive appraisal, personal characteristics interact with the dimensions of the situation to influence the manner in which an event is perceived and evaluated. These personal factors exert their influence by determining what is important to a person's well-being in a given situation, affecting his or her understanding of the event, and providing a basis for evaluating the success of coping efforts. Two important personal dimensions that influence appraisal are (a) **commitments,** or an individual's values, motives, and goals, which give meaning to life events; and (b) beliefs, or an individual's notions about reality. These are discussed in the following paragraphs, along with various other personality factors.

Commitments. Commitments are complex and tend to express themselves in patterns that may not be apparent solely on the basis of knowing a person's objective circumstances. For example, one person who loses an arm may be primarily concerned about the implications of the amputation for job performance, whereas another person may be more distressed about bodily disfigurement and the social stigma that accompanies it. These varying concerns reflect the different commitments held by each person that shape his or her appraisal and perception of the harm-loss event which has occurred.

Occupational therapists who have worked with people having amputated limbs are aware that these varying commitments also influence choice of coping strategy and appraisal of outcome. The person in the first of the preceding examples, fitted with a prosthesis that emphasizes function and permits a full resumption of previous vocational activities, will view the outcome as entirely satisfactory. The person in the second example, whose commitment is governed principally by appearance, may be equally satisfied with a cosmetically superior, but less functional, prosthesis.

Commitments influence appraisal by guiding people into (or away from) situations that can challenge, threaten, benefit, or harm them. Clearly people's choices of activities reflect what is most meaningful to them and most consistent with their needs and perceptions of self.

Commitments also influence appraisal through the manner in which they shape vigilance or cue sensitivity in various situations. Psychologists have shown that people tend to focus on different aspects of a situation, thus influencing their perceptions and appraisals of events. This was well illustrated in a study by King and Sorrentino (1983). The researchers carefully constructed 20 stimulus events depicting social situations that could be objectively described as cooperative or competitive in nature. Subjects were asked to compare all possible pairings of the events in terms of how they differed along 13 dimensions (friendly versus unfriendly, etc.). Data were analyzed to determine if the subjects had similar perceptions of the characteristics of

the situations. Although there was some evidence of general agreement regarding the characteristics, there was also wide variability among individual perceptions. This finding lends support to the suggestion that individual behavior varies within the same situation because of differences in how the situation is perceived. Perceptions, in turn, are influenced by personality characteristics and experiences that lend personal meaning to the situation.

A third and important way in which commitments influence cognitive appraisal is through their relationship to *psychological vulnerability*, or diminished ability to cope. When a person's coping resources are inadequate, he or she is said to be psychologically vulnerable to a potential threat. Such vulnerabilities may be based on various person-related factors.

In general, adequately functioning people who have resource deficits are psychologically vulnerable only if their deficits pertain to something that matters, something to which they have a high degree of commitment. Thus a sprained ankle can render a football player psychologically vulnerable if the threat to his popularity or to next year's salary is of importance to him (as it generally is). On the other hand, the same resource deficit (the inability to run fast and avoid obstacles) will not cause psychological vulnerability in a college professor, whose motivations and values are not as dependent on physical prowess. Psychological vulnerability, then, occurs when the nature of a deficit influences a person's ability to cope with a situation that has important meaning to him or her. As might be expected, the greater the strength of a commitment, the more vulnerable a person is to deficits in the area of that commitment.

Researchers have found that commitment patterns can result in unusual appraisals of potentially stressful situations. Although the potential for injury is usually regarded as a threat, an injury also represents an acceptable reason for avoiding responsibilities or otherwise aversive situations. A person whose commitment pattern is influenced by a need for social affiliation might appraise a broken leg from a ski trip as less of a loss than others would consider it to be, especially if it brings additional attention or sympathy. A psychological term for this phenomenon of advantage from adversity is *secondary gain*.

An interesting investigation by Kasl, Evans, and Niederman (1979) demonstrates the complex interactions of costs and benefits that characterize patterns of commitment. Studying West Point cadets, the researchers found that the incidence of infectious mononucleosis could be predicted by knowing the level of academic motivation, the family history of motivation, and the academic performance of the cadets. Cadets with poor academic performance and high academic motivation (commitment) were more likely to become infected, presumably because of the greater stress that they endured as a result of their commitments.

The more public a commitment is, the greater the perceived threat when the commitment is challenged. Once a commitment for a particular course of action is known to others, there are social pressures to maintain or honor it. To reverse a decision once made public carries with it certain social costs (referred to by sociologists as *loss of face*) that are typically steadfastly avoided in human social interaction. Accordingly, the more public a commitment is, that is, the more people who know about it, the greater is a person's perceived obligation to carry out the chosen course of action.

Knowledge of this aspect of commitment and its influence on behavior is sometimes used in training situations to "lock in" performance goals. This approach is analogous to *contracting* in behavior modification and has been used with success in various occupational therapy clinical situations.

The phrase *committed to action* seems quite appropriate here, suggesting that commitments can sustain efforts to ward off threatening situations even against formidable odds. Laboratory experiments have shown that commitment explains effort over and above the presence of external incentives. This motivating aspect of commitment might be evident in the frequency with which people with terminal illness live beyond their life expectancies. The particular commitments that sustain life in these situations may include a devotion to family or a desire to complete unfinished business. Nevertheless, patterns of commitment are clearly exhibited in a disposition sometimes referred to as a will to live. The opposite is also true: The absence of such a commitment pattern can quickly lead to death.

In summary, commitments are an important component in the understanding of stress and coping because they define areas of meaningfulness and thereby help people determine which situations are relevant to their well-being. Moreover, commitments influence the types of situations in which people find themselves, and shape their responsiveness to situational cues. Finally, commitments have a motivating quality that sustains coping efforts. By knowing a person's patterns of commitments, one can identify his or her areas of vulnerability. This may be particularly important for predicting the circumstances under which a person is likely to feel harmed, threatened, or challenged.

Beliefs. People have preexisting notions about reality that serve as perceptual sets or lenses through which they view events in their environment. During appraisal these beliefs help shape people's understanding of the meaning of events they experience.

Lazarus and Folkman (1984b) have identified two major categories of beliefs that are relevant to cognitive appraisal:

Rotter's locus of control

(a) beliefs about personal control and (b) beliefs about existential concerns. Beliefs about personal control influence whether people will have confidence in their ability to manage environmental demands or feel incapable and vulnerable in the face of threat. If they believe that they have some control over events, they will be more likely to perceive a stressful event as a challenge than to view it as a threat. If they feel vulnerable and at the mercy of fate or chance, the tendency will be to perceive nearly all stressful instances as threatening.

Beliefs about personal control can be general or apply only to specific types of situations. The best known theory of generalized control or expectancy was developed by Rotter (1966, 1975). In this concept a person with an *internal locus of control* believes that the outcome of events is contingent on his or her own behavior, and a person with an *external locus of control* believes that events are influenced by luck, chance, fate, or powerful others.

According to Rotter, generalized control expectancies have their greatest influence when situations are novel or ambiguous. Under these conditions, situational cues are minimal and the lack of clarity makes it difficult to ascribe meaning to events and thus appraise them as benign, threatening, or challenging. Consequently, beliefs about control exert more influence in appraising the meaning of the environmental situation. Thus a person with a disposition to view situations as controllable (an internal locus of control) is more likely to view a novel or ambiguous situation as challenging than to see it as threatening.

Generalized control expectancies have less influence when a situation can be clearly defined by the person experiencing it. Under such conditions the specific characteristics of an event have more influence in the appraisal process. Conversely, when a situation is more ambiguous, control expectancies exert a greater influence.

Dispositional optimism is a regulator of how well people respond to stress because it influences the strategies that they use in their coping efforts (Scheier & Carver, 1985). In general, optimists tend to do better than pessimists when confronted with stressful occurrences. They tend to engage in problem-focused coping, elaboration of coping, and seeking of social support. At the same time, they tend to avoid denial, disengagement, and emotion-focused coping strategies, which are viewed as less functional and adaptive.

Situation-specific feelings about one's ability to control events have been referred to as *self-efficacy*. Bandura's (1977) theory of self-efficacy distinguishes between *efficacy expectancy*, or a person's expectation that he or she will be able successfully to execute a course of action or strategy for dealing with an environmental demand, and *outcome expectancy*, or a person's belief that the behavior will lead to a desired outcome. Bandura places great importance on efficacy expectancies in shaping behavior because he believes that people tend to avoid threatening situations that exceed their coping skills. On the other hand, they engage confidently in situations that they judge themselves capable of handling.

These observations have important ramifications for coping behavior because efficacy expectancies not only influence the extent to which a person feels threatened in a given situation, but also affect the person's willingness to persist in the face of obstacles and aversive experiences. Bandura notes that efficacy expectancies, by themselves, are not sufficient to produce coping if a person has no stake in the outcome.

Despite the complex relationships existing between the personal factors of control beliefs and appraisals, certain conclusions can be reached about the effect of control beliefs on adaptational outcomes (Folkman, 1984). The degree of consistency between the perceived and the actual controllability of a stressful situation may be an index of the likelihood of a successful outcome. If a stressful encounter is realistically appraised as controllable, the factor that will most likely explain the outcome is whether the stressful event is appraised as a threat or as a challenge. Because of the more positive emotions elicited by challenge situations and their tendency to promote problem-focused coping strategies, this type of situation is more likely to result in satisfactory adaptation.

If a stressful situation is realistically viewed as uncontrollable, however, the outcome may be one of learned helplessness or depression. Alternatively, it may depend on reappraisals that can transform the meaning of the uncontrollable event with respect to its significance for well-being. According to a review of studies on coping with uncontrollable events, people who discover something positive in a negative situation show less distress than those who do not (Silver & Wortman, 1980). Also, the abandonment of old goals and the creation of new ones can serve to establish new definitions of the conditions and the outcomes that people can control. This can promote positive morale and preserve a person's general sense of control and self-esteem. An appropriate example is the gymnast with a spinal cord injury who realizes that she can do nothing to regain the use of her paralyzed legs, but establishes a new goal of learning how to get around in a wheelchair sufficiently well to be able to compete in wheelchair athletics.

The risk of maladaptive outcomes is greatest when the appraisal of control does not match reality (Folkman, 1984). An appraisal of an event as uncontrollable that is in fact controllable will likely result in the abandonment of necessary problem-focused coping, and harm or loss will be even more probable. In health care, such a situation might be represented by patients who fail to participate in

important treatment regimens because they believe the outcome to be beyond their control. For patients with high blood pressure, such a perception could have fatal results.

An interesting study by Ferington (1986) provides additional evidence of the importance of perceived and actual control. She found that depression, viewed as an index of coping effectiveness, was less likely to occur in people with spinal cord injury who perceived that options for control were available, regardless of their assessed preference for control. In another study of people with spinal cord injury, Frank et al. (1987) found that people with less perceived control over events tended to use wishful thinking and self-blame as ways of coping more often than those with more perceived control. Also, they reported higher levels of psychological distress and depression than people who demonstrated a greater belief in internal resources did.

Personality Factors. Researchers have been studying the relationship of personality factors to stressful encounters for a number of years. Because of the complexity of these issues, many methodological problems have plagued the investigations. Nevertheless, personality variables have been considered as a possible moderating factor in the relationship between stress and adaptational outcome, particularly as reflected in health and illness. Perhaps the most useful research in this area has shown a relationship between the personality disposition called Type A behavior, characterized by achievement orientation and drive, and increased risk of coronary heart disease (Glass, 1977).

A few studies have examined personality from the perspective of its potential for protecting or buffering a person against the effects of stressful encounters. For example, Hinkle (1974) found that in comparison with people who were more likely to become ill, people who remained healthy were emotionally insulated, showed a lack of concern for others, and were little involved in life affairs. More recently Kobasa (1979) has coined the term *hardiness* to refer to people who seem to have a resistance to illness despite their experiencing many stressful events. According to Kobasa (1982), the hardy personality is characterized by a strong sense of meaningfulness and commitment to self, an internal locus of control, and a tendency to view adaptational demands as challenging. Studying executives who had experienced high levels of stress, Kobasa found that those who experienced lower levels of illness despite their enduring relatively high amounts of life stress tended to exhibit a cluster of traits—commitment, control, and challenge—that Kobasa subsequently described as representing hardiness. Additional research has suggested that hardiness may work best when people are experiencing intensively stressful life events (Kobasa, Maddi, & Courington, 1981; Kobasa, Maddi, & Kahn, 1982).

In other research, the hardiness factor has received mixed support (Ganellen & Blaney, 1984; Holahan & Moos, 1985; Schmied & Lawler, 1986). This has led to speculation that these personality dimensions may act in different ways depending on the age, the sex, and the occupation of the person experiencing stress, or that they may act in combination with other factors, such as social support. Recent critiques of the hardiness hypothesis have suggested that future research concentrate on examining the individual traits that make up the constellation, especially commitment and control, rather than continuing to assume that hardiness is a unitary dimension (Funk & Houston, 1987; Hull, Van Treuren, & Virnelli, 1987).

Antonovsky (1979) has proposed that a sense of coherence is a common theme linking psychological, biological, and social resources to good health. People who view the world as manageable, comprehensible, and meaningful can be described as having a sense of coherence. In many ways, sense of coherence resembles Kobasa's hardiness constellation.

Holahan and Moos (1986) studied personality characteristics, coping styles, and social support in a large sample of families in the San Francisco Bay area. They found that both self-confidence and an easygoing disposition were related to reduced psychological consequences of life stress.

McRae and Costa (1986) have suggested a classification of personality traits into three broad domains: neuroticism, extraversion, and openness to experience. They argue that these domains encompass many established personality traits and could provide a basis for a more systematic examination of the links between coping and personality. In studies of several hundred community-dwelling adults, they found that types of coping (as listed in Table 3-4) were closely related to the personality dimensions of extraversion and neuroticism, and that more satisfactory coping outcomes were related to extraversion and problem-oriented styles of coping rather than to avoidance or denial.

Types of Coping

Several researchers have focused on the types of coping strategies employed by people when they are confronted with stressful situations. As explained earlier, the method of coping a person chooses is influenced by the way in which he or she appraises a situation and by the resources available to him or her, whether material or personal.

Different approaches exist for classifying coping efforts, depending on the method or the focus of the behavioral strategy used. In the method-of-coping classification (Moos, 1974), coping efforts are viewed as either cognitive, behavioral, or avoidant in nature. **Cognitive strategies** include attempts to manage the appraisal of the situation, as

Table 3-4
Rank Order of Mean Effectiveness Ratings for 27 Coping Mechanisms

	Effectiveness for		
	Problem Solving	Distress Reduction	Average Rank[*]
Hostile reaction	1	3	2.00
Rational action	25	21	23.00
Seeking help	26	25	25.50
Perseverance	19	14	16.50
Isolation of affect	6	7	6.50
Fatalism	13	8	10.50
Expression of feelings	23	22	22.50
Positive thinking	16	18	17.00
Distraction	9	13	11.00
Escapist fantasy	4	12	8.17
Intellectual denial	17	15	16.00
Self-blame	5	1	3.00
Social comparison	10	16	13.00
Sedation	14	17	15.50
Substitution	15	24	19.50
Restraint	22	19	20.50
Drawing strength from adversity	20	26	23.00
Avoidance	18	10	14.00
Withdrawal	11	6	8.50
Self-adaptation	24	20	22.00
Wishful thinking	3	4	3.50
Active forgetting	7	11	9.00
Humor	21	23	22.00
Passivity	8	5	6.50
Indecisiveness	2	2	2.00
Assessing blame	12	9	10.50
Faith	27	27	27.00

[*]Mechanisms ranked from least effective (1) to most effective (27).

From McRae, RR and Costa, PT, Jr. (1986). Personality, coping and coping effectiveness in an adult sample. Journal of Personality, 54(2). Durham, NC: Duke University Press.

through drawing on past experience or trying to see the positive aspects of the situation. **Behavioral strategies** include information-gathering or problem-related actions that are aimed directly at the source of the stress. **Avoidant strategies** attempt to reduce emotional attention through diversion or conscious efforts to circumvent or sidestep the source of stress.

This method-of-coping taxonomy has been applied to people adjusting to physical illness. Moos and Tsu (1977) believe that coping by people who are ill includes such strategies as (a) denying or minimizing the seriousness of a crisis, (b) seeking relevant information, (c) requesting reassurance and emotional support, (d) learning specific illness-related procedures, (e) setting concrete, limited goals, (f) rehearsing alternative outcomes, and (g) finding a general purpose or pattern of meaning in the course of events.

Ilfeld (1980) examined the interview responses of a large sample of adults living in Chicago to determine if patterns existed in styles of coping with stressful situations encountered in the marital role, on the job, in parenting, or in dealing with finances. From a total of 47 types of coping responses reported in the interviews, Ilfeld identified five principal styles or strategies: action coping (or problem resolution), rationalization/avoidance, acceptance, seeking outside help, and withdrawal/conflict. The first three cut across problems encountered in all four roles. The fourth emerged in regard to marital as well as parenting problems, and the fifth, characterized by cycles of appeasement and confrontation, was unique to marital problems.

Another approach to classifying coping is based on its focus—problems or emotions (Folkman & Lazarus, 1980). **Problem-focused coping** is characterized by attempts to do something constructive about the conditions that harm, threaten, or challenge. Behaviors in this category can include aggressive interpersonal efforts to alter a situation or deliberate, calm, rational problem-solving. **Emotion-focused coping** is distinguished by attempts to regulate or manage emotions and maintain emotional equilibrium, whether the focus of the regulation is behavior and expression, physiological disturbance, subjective distress, or all three. Included in this category are distancing, self-control, seeking of social support, acceptance of responsibility, escape/avoidance, and positive reappraisal.

The focus-of-coping classification has been designed to accommodate the fact that the same coping strategy can address both problem-focused and emotion-focused objectives, on separate occasions or simultaneously. The new mother who consults a book on child care, for example, is using information gathering as a coping strategy. She may find that her infant's skin rash is quite normal and derive emotional reassurance from the information. Alternatively she may determine that overdressing is causing the heat rash and take direct action to remedy the problem.

Both emotion-focused and problem-focused coping are frequently used in dealing with stressful encounters, and both are important (Folkman & Lazarus, 1980). For example, during a serious illness a patient must be alert to danger signals and active in preventing complications, at the same time maintaining his or her morale. Unfortunately, little is known about how various combinations of these two approaches affect adaptational outcomes.

Measurement of Coping

The classification schemes described in the preceding section have formed the basis for different approaches to measuring coping strategies. Some of the pioneering efforts in this area consisted of few items (Sidle, Moos, Adams, & Cady, 1969), were based on empirical analyses of interview data (Ilfeld, 1980), or attempted to measure global traits or styles (Gleser & Ilhilevich, 1969; Joffe & Naditch, 1977; Schutz, 1967). For a comprehensive review of various early approaches to measuring coping and adaptation, the reader is referred to Moos (1974).

More recent efforts to measure coping have reflected increased sophistication. The research relies less on asking people how they coped with stressful situations in terms of global behaviors and more on asking people to reconstruct recent experiences from the standpoint of how they thought, felt, and acted in response to those experiences (Folkman & Lazarus, 1980; Lazarus & Folkman, 1984b). This approach may provide greater insight into the complex and cognitively influenced issues surrounding coping.

The *Ways of Coping Checklist* used in this research can be self-administered, or data can be collected by a trained interviewer. The 67 items in the revised checklist call for subjects to indicate the degree to which they have used a particular coping behavior in response to a recently experienced stressful episode. Table 3-5 presents sample items. The coping responses can then be empirically classified according to function or type (problem focused, wishful thinking, mixed growth, minimization of threat, seeking social support, and self-blame). Although there are clear disadvantages to using self-report scales like the Ways of Coping Checklist, Lazarus and Folkman (1984b) argue that the advantages of the approach (such as being able to tap the important cognitive appraisal-oriented aspects of coping) outweigh the inferential and logistical disadvantages of other approaches. Further, they contend, as greater understanding of the processes underlying coping evolves, convergent approaches to measuring coping may be desirable. Such strategies might include the simultaneous use of self-report, behavioral observation, and physiological measures.

Relative Effectiveness of Different Coping Strategies

Several researchers have been interested in the relative effectiveness of different types of coping. In a statistical investigation of many studies (called a meta-analysis), Suls and Fletcher (1985) examined the relative benefits of avoidant versus attention strategies of coping. **Avoidant strategies** are types of coping in which a person focuses attention away from the source of stress or from his or her psychological and bodily reactions to it. Examples are

Table 3-5
Sample Items From the Ways of Coping Checklist (Revised)

Please read each item below and indicate, by circling the
appropriate category, to what extent you used it in the situation you have just described.

	Not Used	Used Somewhat	Used Quite a Bit	Used a Great Deal
1. Just concentrated on what I have to do next—the next step.	0	1	2	3
7. Tried to get the person responsible to change his or her mind.	0	1	2	3
13. Went on as if nothing had happened.	0	1	2	3
16. Slept more than usual.	0	1	2	3
21. Tried to forget the whole thing.	0	1	2	3
28. I let my feelings out somehow.	0	1	2	3
34. Took a big change or did something very risky.	0	1	2	3
45. Talked to someone about how I was feeling.	0	1	2	3
50. Refused to believe that it had happened.	0	1	2	3
56. I changed something about myself.	0	1	2	3

From Lazarus, RS and Folkman, S (1984). Stress, Appraisal and Coping. pp. 328-333. New York, NY: Springer Publishing Company. Reprinted with permission.

distraction, denial, and cognitive avoidance. **Attention strategies**, by contrast, are types in which a person focuses attention on the source of stress or on reactions to it. Examples are information gathering, problem-solving, and efforts to reduce anxiety or tension. Suls and Fletcher found that the effectiveness of avoidant strategies was associated with more positive adaptation in the early phases of stressful experience, whereas attention strategies were superior to avoidant ones for long-term outcomes.

Western cultures tend to equate successful coping with problem-solving or mastery over the environment (Lazarus & Folkman, 1984b). This view would necessarily give attention strategies preference over avoidance strategies. Although effectively overcoming a problem is clearly a desirable outcome, many stressful circumstances in life are not easily overcome. In these situations, coping strategies that serve to manage emotional responses or maintain self-esteem are not only helpful but essential. Thus they should be viewed as strategies of equal merit to active or problem-solving approaches.

Along these lines, health professionals in rehabilitation are frequently warned about the detrimental effects of denial following loss of function or during bereavement. Although denial has been defined in many ways, it most often refers to attempts to ignore reality. Clearly there are situations in which denial as a coping mechanism can yield unfavorable outcomes. However, a person's use of denial to cope with overwhelming situations in their early stages, to deal with harmful or threatening situations that he or she can do nothing constructive to overcome, or to manage his or her emotions while also employing active coping strategies, must be viewed as adaptive. The use of denial is maladaptive only when it interferes with the use of other strategies.

Weisman (1972) has made a distinction between denial of fact and denial of implication. A young man with a spinal cord injury, for example, may deny the permanent nature of his paralysis and as a result refuse others' attempts to help him learn new skills, hoping for a spontaneous recovery. This is denial of fact. Alternatively he may accept the reality of the situation, but deny any implication that it will interfere with his attainment of life goals. This is denial of implication. Denial of implication can be equated with positive thinking or hopefulness, which can be a valuable psychological resource. In the first instance denial as a coping strategy is maladaptive, whereas in the second instance it may clearly assist the young man in successfully adapting to a difficult life circumstance.

To complicate matters further, coping may lead to a positive adaptational outcome in one life domain while having negative implications in another. In the previously cited example of two persons coping with stress induced by the loss of an arm, they can reduce the stress caused by loss of independence by learning to use a prosthesis, but only at the potential cost of drawing attention to the disability and feeling stigmatized. In such a case, coping will simultaneously yield positive gains physically and negative gains socially. It is not unusual for domains to be affected differentially by a given coping strategy.

One can conclude from the foregoing that the success of a particular coping strategy will depend on the time at which the outcome is measured, the context of the situation in which coping occurs, and the domain that is affected. One should not universally expect positive adaptational outcomes as a direct result of any type of coping; rather, one should expect them as a result of specific types of coping by categories of people within certain contexts. This conclusion was underscored in a comprehensive study by Parkes (1986). She examined relationships between personality dimensions such as neuroticism and extraversion, and coping styles. She also considered environmental factors such as social support and work demands, as well as the type of stressful episode and its perceived importance to the individual. Parkes found that substantial proportions of the variation in coping styles in her sample were due to interactions between personal, environmental, and situational factors. Thus her study provided empirical support for the view of coping as a transactional process (Lazarus & Folkman, 1984b) and illustrated its complexity.

Improvement of Coping Abilities

Despite the complexities of the coping process and the sometimes contradictory evidence provided by many studies, it is possible to use existing knowledge to help people improve their coping skills. Approaches to improving coping skills vary according to the conceptual model of stress and coping endorsed by the practitioner. From the perspective of the person-environment transactional model described in this chapter, coping skills must be improved through strategies designed to strengthen problem-solving skills and the manner in which one reacts to and appraises a stressful situation.

As already explained, coping through environmental mastery or direct problem-solving involves active attempts by a person to prevent, circumvent, or overcome a problem situation. However, there are numerous situations for which satisfactory or practical solutions cannot be found. Moreover, it would be impossible to attempt to anticipate, much less prepare a person for, the infinite number of potential stressors encountered during life.

In a very real way, the process of social development

offers direct and vicarious experiences, as well as role models, for learning how to deal effectively with difficult situations. Society itself, through its culture and institutions, exerts a large influence in providing the skills and the solutions for environmental problems. Unfortunately these may be inadequate, and the experiences and the role models available to many people may not be sufficient to allow for the development of satisfactory coping skills.

Further, people's motivations are profoundly influenced by the incentive systems in society (Mechanic, 1974). Thus, behavioral patterns that are valued will tend to be those that are most learned and used, whether or not they prepare one for adequately dealing with environmental threats and challenges. To appreciate this, one need only observe the magnitude of the drug abuse problem in America, which must certainly be viewed as a maladaptive coping strategy that has been broadly embraced as the result of social incentives.

Moreover, although the human's biological tools for coping have evolved over millions of years, the demands of the environment have changed dramatically in a relatively short period, with the most extraordinary features of society having evolved within the past century. Today's increasingly sedentary life-style threatens people's physical well-being. Approaches to learning and tendencies of emotional response are probably influenced by the requirements of an earlier era. The result is that contemporary demands frequently exceed people's capacity to respond adequately to them. Stated in another way, although the number of stressful situations encountered by people in contemporary society is probably no greater than in earlier times, people may be less well equipped to deal with them because of their nature and complexity. Certainly, however, awareness of stress and its likely effects on health has prompted public as well as professional interest in how to cope with it.

For this reason a number of approaches have evolved with the purpose of assisting people in developing or acquiring effective coping strategies. These techniques are directed at helping people manage their appraisal or perception of a stressful event, manage their response to the event, or both. Examples of appraisal-oriented approaches are information acquisition and cognitive therapy. Response-oriented approaches include relaxation training, meditation training, biofeedback training, assertiveness training, social skills training, and modeling. Some approaches combine both appraisal- and response-oriented strategies. Stress inoculation training and problem-solving training are discussed as examples of combinations. Table 3-6 outlines the three types of strategies and the respective examples.

	Table 3-6	
	Intervention Strategies for Improving Coping	
Appraisal-Oriented Approaches	**Response-Oriented Approaches**	**Combination Approaches**
Acquisition of information	Progressive relaxation training	Stress inoculation training
Cognitive therapy	Meditation training	Problem-solving training
	Assertiveness training	
	Biofeedback training	
	Social skills training	
	Modeling	

Appraisal-Oriented Approaches.

Acquisition of Information. A major element in the coping process is acquiring information about the nature of the stressor. This information allows people to appraise whether they are confronting a harm, a threat, or a challenge. Because the absence of accurate information in such situations interferes with effective coping, it seems logical that providing information will facilitate the coping process.

This notion was tested by Janis (1958) in studies with patients about to undergo surgery. Those who were given specific information about what would happen to them before, during, and following surgery requested less medication for pain, were less demanding on staff, and were discharged earlier than a comparison group that received the usual information. The finding led to additional study of the usefulness of information in reducing stress among hospitalized patients.

Whereas the information provided to patients in this study concerned the actual procedures to be performed, more recent investigations have provided information on the sensations that are likely to be experienced during and following various procedures. In a review of this work, Kendall and Watson (1981) conclude that sensory information tends to be more valuable in facilitating coping.

There is some evidence that the coping styles of individuals may interact with information to produce different outcomes. In a study by DeLong (1971), people who actively acknowledged the negative aspects of a stressful situation (surgery) were more likely to benefit from the provision of specific information about what the procedure entailed. People who used avoidance as a coping strategy, however, tended to do less well if they were given information about the procedure.

More recently, Martelli, Auerbach, Alexander, and Mercuri (1987) found that intervention strategies that incorporated both problem-focused and emotion-focused coping styles were more successful in enhancing patients' adjustment to and satisfaction with surgery than either problem- or emotion-focused strategies exclusively. Better adjustment and satisfaction and lower self-reported pain from preprosthetic oral surgery were obtained when high information-preference subjects were given a problem-focused intervention and low information-preference subjects were given an emotion-focused intervention. This suggests the value of matching intervention approaches to patients' coping styles.

Cognitive Therapy. Ellis (1973) and Beck (1976) have been proponents of a type of intervention that is directed at the irrational beliefs and thought processes that lead to maladaptive behavior. The assumption underlying the approaches representing this type of intervention is that if people can be taught to view the world in a more accurate or logical way, the probability of constructive problem-solving will be enhanced.

These approaches rely on interaction between a therapist and a patient or a client in which an analysis of the thinking that has led up to inadequate coping behaviors takes place. As more logical ways of interpreting the environment are learned, exaggerated responses, overgeneralizations, and other products of emotionally influenced perception are reduced, and problem-solving is enhanced.

Stress inoculation therapy also uses a cognitive approach to restructure thinking or foster more accurate appraisals of stressful events. It is discussed in a later section because it also relies on behavioral skills that are response-oriented in nature.

Response-Oriented Approaches.

Several approaches to stress management involve training a person to respond in a nonstressful way to difficult situations through relaxation strategies, including progressive relaxation, meditation, and biofeedback. These techniques have been used with great effectiveness in reducing essential hypertension (viewed as a physiological indicator of stress) as well as headache, insomnia, and asthma (Agras, 1981; Seer, 1979). Moreover, research has shown that the effects of relaxation strategies can be maintained and generalized to settings outside the clinic (Blackwell, Bloomfield, & Gartside, 1976). As methods of coping, they can be classified as emotion focused because they seek to modify the individual's affective response to environmental stressors. Other response-oriented approaches are assertiveness training, social skills training, and modeling.

Progressive Relaxation Training. Two types of relaxation are commonly recognized and used by professionals for stress reduction: progressive and Bensonian. Jacobson (1938) is generally credited with introducing progressive relaxation as a means to reduce tension. In this technique, a patient or a client is trained to relax one muscle group at a time, progressing through the body until all muscle groups have become relaxed.

A rationale is provided for the procedure before it begins, usually in the form of an explanation that tension is the result of muscle activity. An environment that facilitates relaxation is necessary before the technique is started. This should include a comfortable chair and no potentially distracting lights or sounds.

Patients or clients are asked to breathe deeply and to exhale slowly. For purposes of demonstrating how a relaxed muscle should feel, they are next instructed to tense a particular muscle group (for example, the hand) and to maintain the tension for 10 to 15 seconds. Following this, they are told to release the tensed muscle group slowly, focusing on the soothing and relaxed feelings as the tension is released. They are then led through the same tensing-and-relaxation sequence with other muscle groups, including forehead, eyes, mouth, neck, shoulders, arms, back, stomach, thighs, calves, feet, and toes.

These breathing exercises may be repeated until the patient or the client achieves a deep feeling of relaxation. Emphasis is placed on attending to the feelings associated with the relaxed condition so as to minimize or diminish the external sources of anxiety and stress. Patients and clients can practice the techniques independently after learning them. Many commercial audiotapes are available that can be used as instructional aids for independent practice.

A variation of this technique, known as Bensonian relaxation (Benson, Beary, & Carol, 1974), is also used by some practitioners. Although also focusing on the reduction of muscle tension and the elimination of distracting stimuli, this technique adds the elements of repetitive sound and a passive attitude. The patient or the client usually sits in a comfortable position with eyes closed and muscles relaxed. Attention is focused on breathing deeply for about 20 seconds and silently repeating a sound (such as "one") with each breath. The repetition of sound is designed to prevent distracting thoughts and maintain muscle relaxation. No differences in outcome between progressive and Bensonian relaxation techniques have been described in the literature.

Meditation Training. Another approach to changing the response to stress is meditation. It involves a conscious attempt by the patient or the client to focus attention in a nonanalytic way on a single thought or image and to avoid contemplation or reflection that would be distracting. Although many people tend to associate this technique with particular religious orientations, it should not be equated with prayer in a clinical context. Instead, it should be considered a means of attending to the process of thinking. Meditation has been shown to be effective in reducing stress, anxiety, phobias, and hypertension. However, there is no evidence that the physiological changes are different from relaxation or other self-regulatory approaches to managing reactions to stress, such as biofeedback (Shapiro, 1985).

Biofeedback Training. During the late 1960s several researchers began to explore the possibility that people could consciously control biological processes such as heart rate, digestive secretion, and constriction of blood vessels, if they were given information or feedback about the status of these processes. The processes are normally involuntary, controlled by the **autonomic nervous system**. The efforts evolved from diverse areas of research in machine control, rehabilitation medicine, and psychology. Animal studies demonstrating that control of autonomic functions could be effected through reinforcement (Miller, 1969) were soon extended to human subjects by other researchers (Brown, 1970; Kamiya, 1969), who showed that humans were capable of learning to control their brain waves using electroencephalographic (EEG) feedback. This finding resulted in the commercial production of various biofeedback machines that measured muscle tension, skin temperature, blood pressure, heart rate, skin conduction, and other physiological processes for the purpose of training people to control them. Since that time, biofeedback has become a major treatment strategy for stress-related disorders (Blanchard et al., 1986).

Despite the broad array of systems that can be monitored, two major types of biofeedback predominate: electromyographic (EMG) and skin temperature. EMG biofeedback involves learning to affect muscle tension levels through the use of an EMG machine that measures the electrical discharge in muscle fibers. Measurement is generally accomplished by attaching electrodes to the skin surface over the muscles to be monitored. The level of muscle tension is reflected in a signal (visual, auditory, or both) that varies according to the degree of electrical activity present. An increasing signal is an indication of greater muscle activity or tension. For control of general tension, electrodes are frequently placed over the muscles of the forehead. This technique is also used in neuromotor rehabilitation (e.g., following a stroke), a procedure through which patients learn to increase rather than decrease muscle tension.

Biofeedback using skin temperature involves placing a temperature-sensitive resistor (known as a thermistor) on the skin's surface, generally on the fingers or the toes. The device indicates changes in skin temperature, which is influenced by stress. High levels of stress tend to constrict blood vessels, and this has the effect of cooling the temperature of the skin. Thus cooler temperatures on the surface of the skin may indicate stress or tension, although it should be emphasized that temperature biofeedback is not a direct indicator of tension or relaxation.

The goal of temperature biofeedback is to raise skin temperature by promoting dilation or relaxation of the peripheral blood vessels. This vasodilation, which warms the skin, accompanies relaxation.

Two other types of biofeedback are in less frequent clinical use. The first, EEG biofeedback, involves a measure of electrical activity of the brain. One type of electrical brain activity is reflected in alpha waves, which seem to be related to a state of relaxed wakefulness. A special type of EEG biofeedback, known as sensorimotor rhythm, is also in use clinically. It involves feedback from a limited range of frequencies, with the recordings emanating from the sensorimotor area of the cerebral cortex. This variation has shown promising results in reducing seizures (Green & Schellenberger, 1986), but requires a prolonged training period.

Although favorable outcomes in reducing tension headaches or blood pressure are assumed to come about through lowered muscle tension, some research has shown that people learning biofeedback have reduced their headache pain even while increasing the amount of muscle tension. A possible explanation for this phenomenon is that the person responds to what he or she appraises to be occurring. If this interpretation is accurate, it provides additional support for the importance of appraisal in the coping process (Andrasik & Holroyd, 1980).

Assertiveness Training. Assertiveness training is another approach to provide skills that can be useful in effective coping. Assertive behavior is defined as direct, honest, and appropriate expression of thoughts, feelings, desires, and needs (Lange & Jakubowski, 1976). The failure to assert oneself in situations may result in an increase in stress, anxiety, depression, or anger. Nonassertive behavior is thought to result from fear of rejection, the belief that one lacks the right to assert oneself or the conviction that assertion is dangerous. In many cases, nonassertive people are unable to distinguish between assertive and aggressive behavior and thus are incapable of asserting themselves in situations in which doing so would be appropriate.

Training to develop assertiveness skills typically begins with group discussions of the importance of positive beliefs and statements about oneself in shaping behaviors. Maladaptive beliefs and self-statements are elucidated, challenged, and replaced with more appropriate ones. Following this, skills training may begin. It consists of activities to help a patient or a client discriminate among the specific behaviors that reflect assertiveness or nonassertiveness. Such factors as eye contact, voice intonation, gestures, and body postures are modeled and discussed. Patients or clients then begin practicing asserting themselves in situations that they find difficult. Typically this occurs through observation of the trainer, followed by role playing. Feedback is given by the trainer and other group members, along with positive reinforcement for appropriate performance. Through successive approximations the patient or the client learns to implement the assertive behaviors appropriately and transfer them outside the training situation.

Social Skills Training. Social skill can be defined as the ability to act in a manner that facilitates social approval and avoids rejection, with its accompanying anxiety or punishment. The objective of social skills training is to teach a person more effective ways of interacting with others and with situations. Typically training occurs in group sessions, during which discussion centers on interpersonal behaviors and their effects on other people. Frequently, individual behavioral goals are defined, and group feedback is provided. Approaches to self-assessment and self-reinforcement may also be taught.

Modeling. As noted earlier, coping skills are learned during normal development through observing the performance of others. This type of social learning, called modeling, has been studied extensively by Bandura (1977) and has resulted in a method to assist children in coping with various types of medical procedures, including surgery. In this method, an actor with whom a child can easily identify is shown on film, first experiencing anxiety or fear and then successfully coping with the stressful situation. Studies (e.g., Melamed & Siegel, 1975) have shown that the timing of the intervention is important because anxiety increases immediately after viewing the film, then decreases with time. For this reason, sufficient time must be allowed following viewing to allow the modeling to affect the coping skills of the learner.

Combined Approaches.

Stress Inoculation Training. One of the more comprehensive approaches to developing coping skills is stress inoculation training, developed by Cameron and Meichenbaum (1982). It introduces a way of thinking about managing stressful episodes and a framework for considering the general factors that contribute to or interfere with effective coping. The developers identify four fundamental prerequisites for effective coping. First, a person must have a satisfactory (reasonably accurate) view of the world, himself or herself, and his or her activities. Second, a person must have an adequate repertoire of responses or skills for dealing with the continuing demands of life. Third, a person must use these responses or skills when they are needed. Finally, after dealing with a stressful episode, a person must be able to resume his or her usual pattern of activity without a long delay.

In recognition of these requirements, stress inoculation training involves three phases: conceptualization, skill acquisition, and rehearsal and application. The *conceptualization* phase is principally educational and involves problem-solving dialogue between the patient or the client and the provider. The aim is to identify problems that are causing stress and to examine maladaptive behavior patterns. Through more rational consideration the problems are redefined as manageable with appropriate coping skills. This phase of intervention addresses the appraisal component of the coping process.

In the second phase, *skill acquisition,* patients and clients learn to respond more effectively to stress-inducing situations. They acquire behavioral and cognitive skills. Examples of behavioral coping are assertiveness and relaxation. Cognitive strategies focus on the use of positive self-statements to facilitate appropriate coping behavior or reduce inhibitions that interfere with appropriate responses.

The third phase, *rehearsal and application*, is directed at practicing the skills learned in the previous phases. This permits the development of a sense of self-efficacy when the patient or the client observes that the learned coping skills can be effectively applied. This phase principally serves to establish lasting patterns of effective coping behavior.

These techniques were incorporated in a study of the relative effectiveness of various approaches to improving coping in hospitalized children (Zastowny, Kirschenbaum, & Meng, 1986). The researchers compared three groups that received various combinations of information, training in anxiety reduction, and training in active coping skills. As expected, the groups receiving information about the stressful situation plus either anxiety-reduction training or active-coping-skills training demonstrated fewer problem behaviors than the group receiving information only. A related

study (Peterson & Shigetomi, 1981) compared active-coping-skills training with modeling and information only. The results suggested that active-coping-skills training was more beneficial than modeling or information approaches, either singly or in combination.

Problem-Solving Training. Problem-solving is defined as a behavioral process that provides a variety of potential solutions (responses) to a problem situation. Effective problem-solving should increase the probability of a person's selecting the most effective solution from a potential array of solutions (Goldfried & Davison, 1976). Teaching problem-solving skills involves helping a person identify the most effective alternatives and select and implement one. The general model for this training includes five steps: (a) *problem orientation*, during which the patient or the client develops an attitude that an effective solution can be found and learns to inhibit acting on first impulse; (b) *problem definition and formulation,* during which the patient or the client is taught to define problem situations in detail to permit attending to relevant aspects of the situation; (c) *generation of solutions*, the core of problem-solving, which allows the uninhibited formulation of possible solutions to the problem; (d) *determination of a course of action to follow*, which involves rigorous examination of the expected consequences of each alternative through cost-benefit analyses; and (e) *verification of the effectiveness of the solution.*

COPING THEORY: IMPLICATIONS FOR OCCUPATIONAL THERAPY

Because coping is a process on which people call when environmental demands tax their adaptive resources, nearly every patient or client seen by an occupational therapist should be viewed as needing an ability to cope. Expressed in another way, by their very nature, performance deficits, or problems with living, require coping skills. Although the need for effective coping may be more readily apparent in people with severe physical disabilities who are involved in rehabilitation programs, even patients whose conditions hold prospects for complete recovery (e.g., patients with hand injuries) must contend with diminished function and emotional disruption during recuperation.

It is tempting to view the entire duration of treatment as a single stressful episode in the life of a patient or a client, but in fact, diminished functional performance typically leads to stressor sequences or a condition in which one is faced with a constant series of threatening or challenging situations. For example, people with permanent disability, in addition to having to deal with demanding physical challenges, must also contend with the stresses created by the prejudices of social stigma (Stensrud & Stensrud, 1981). Accordingly, from the standpoint of understanding how coping theory might lead to improved case management, therapists should be mindful that patients and clients are confronted with multiple stressful situations as a result of their conditions and that simultaneously their resources or abilities to cope have been diminished.

Coping and Activity Engagement

Although occupational therapists frequently emphasize the utility of activity in improving functional performance, they have also long recognized the importance of activity as a useful strategy for managing emotional distress. The use of activity in this regard was based originally on conventional wisdom that in times of stress or anxiety, it is helpful to engage in activity rather than remain passive. However, a number of studies have now been conducted to determine the role of activity in stressful situations and to ascertain whether objective evidence can be found for the value of activity in modifying or regulating stress responses.

In a review of several studies that examined activity versus passivity under stressful circumstances, Gal and Lazarus (1975) note quite contradictory findings. Some of the studies involved people under highly stressful combat conditions, whereas others were laboratory experiments in which humans or monkeys were subjected to stressful stimuli. When physiological indicators of stress for subjects in active and passive conditions were measured and compared, results did not consistently show that activity reduced the stress reactions during the stressful events.

Explaining that these measures might themselves be affected by bodily activity, the reviewers suggest that the duration of the responses is a better indicator of the subjects' emotional reactions to the stressful circumstances than is the magnitude. Furthermore, citing some evidence that activities directly related to the source of a threat may be more beneficial than indirectly related or unrelated activities, they suggest that a distinction be made between activity that is or is not functionally related to the threatening situation.

Gal and Lazarus speculate that activity affects stress reactions in three principal ways:

1. It may permit a person to experience feelings of mastery or control over a situation and thus reduce anxiety and feelings of helplessness. Even in instances in which activity does not provide actual control, the perception that it does is likely to be beneficial, especially for people whose psychological orientation is toward control of situations (i.e., people who have an internal locus of control).

2. Activity may serve as a means of diverting attention away from the source of stress. Neural studies have provided evidence that both cortical and peripheral evoked potentials can be reduced or eliminated when attention is diverted.

3. Activity may serve as a means of discharging energy. This mechanism is important from the standpoint of ''fight or flight'' reactions elicited under stressful or threatening conditions. The **sympathetic nervous system** is a part of the autonomic nervous system that mobilizes the body's resources during stressful situations. In animals, excitation in this system results in species-specific motor behavior to confront or avoid danger. In humans, however, cultural values and behavioral expectations often preclude these alternatives as means of dissipating the arousal caused by threatening or stressful situations. Activity, therefore, may very well serve the purpose of permitting a release of the tension accompanying physiological mobilization or arousal, thus providing an explanation for subjective feelings of reduced anxiety and well-being.

Although these speculations about the general role of activity in stress and coping are consistent with theories supporting the use of activity in occupational therapy practice, empirical evidence is inadequate to accept them as conclusive. Certainly, occupational therapists are in an excellent position to conduct research that will provide more solid substantiation for the general role of activity in coping. In a similar way, research on coping processes can be useful to occupational therapists in planning intervention and in understanding the behaviors and the emotions of their patients and clients.

The apparent benefits of activity in coping seem to provide general support for the value of occupational therapy in stressful situations, but a more comprehensive examination of the literature on coping is necessary to fully appreciate its implications for the field. Despite a considerable body of research, understanding of coping is far from complete. This is not surprising, given the many factors that have been shown to influence the manner and the success of coping efforts. Nevertheless, what is known can be useful to the occupational therapist both in understanding patients and clients and in planning successful intervention strategies.

Influences on Appraisal

Occupational therapists have traditionally emphasized the importance of a patient's or client's values and attitudes and their influence on motivation for treatment or engagement in tasks. From a coping perspective such consideration relates to the appraisal mechanism. People's view of diminished function as a condition of harm, threat, or challenge will affect their reaction to it. Also, certain personality attributes, such as sense of efficacy and locus of control, will influence their appraisal. As explained earlier, once appraised, stressful circumstances are constantly reappraised, so that the nature of the coping process employed may change, based on subsequent conditions. In the context of therapy, the occupational therapist can influence appraisal in various ways—for example, by demonstrating to patients or clients that they have control in circumstances in which they think they do not have it and by structuring interventions to yield successes that contribute to patients' and clients' sense of efficacy.

In short, how patients and clients frame or define problems will have an important influence on their efforts to engage in effective coping behaviors. This will, in turn, affect their motivation for therapy and their compliance with treatment approaches. As their perceptions of control and self-efficacy are enhanced, their coping will become more successful. Moreover, because threat appraisals are usually accompanied by negative emotions such as fear, anxiety, and anger, it is in the therapist's interest to help the patient or the client define the problem as a challenge rather than as a threat.

Another method of influencing appraisal to promote positive coping is careful establishment of well-articulated treatment goals. Setting clear treatment goals is more than a technique for documenting practice. It is a means of clearly defining the nature of a problem in a way that allows the patient or the client to appraise it properly and respond to the situation as a challenge rather than as a threat.

During goal setting, information that therapists provide to patients and clients about the nature of their deficits and the reasons behind various treatment approaches will be instrumental in reducing anxiety and fear and promoting successful coping. Information seeking is a coping strategy that helps a person reduce ambiguity and clearly define the nature of stressful circumstances.

In an earlier section, the importance of commitment, or that which has special meaning to the individual, was discussed. Therapists cannot depend only on the commitment that patients and clients bring to therapy at the outset of intervention. Commitment changes over time. At each step of the way, patients and clients must decide to do what therapists are asking in the treatment setting and decide to use what they learn in the environment outside the treatment setting. Such decisions reflect motivation (Lazarus & Folkman, 1984b).

To the extent that patients and clients view treatment goals as important, motivation will be greater. At the same time psychological vulnerability will be increased, so

structuring the treatment approach to provide early successes will be vital. Collaboration of patients and clients in establishing treatment goals helps to ensure commitment while increasing feelings of control, because choice implies a degree of control. When commitments to goals are expressed publicly, the degree of motivation is increased even more because failure to fulfill a publicly expressed commitment can result in loss of face. Astute therapists use their knowledge of this phenomenon to a patient's or client's advantage in planning and executing treatment regimens. Ferington (1986) advises caution here. Preferred scope of control may be an issue for patients and clients with low preferences for control. With them the need to exercise personal control might be limited to a few areas of personal concern, such as self-care activities. Ferington notes that if as White (1974) suggested, autonomy is the "freedom to think and act flexibly," then that freedom would necessarily include the option of choosing not to act.

Assessment and Augmentation of Environmental Resources

In addition to relying on the personal resources of efficacy and control, described in the previous section, coping depends on environmental resources. Material resources (such as money and a comfortable home setting) can be considered important assets in coping, but the most important environmental resource seems to be social support. Although therapists should be mindful of the potential negative effects of social support articulated earlier in this chapter, the benefits, such as information, emotional comfort, and a sense of belongingness, can be valuable. For the occupational therapist, this provides an additional reason for the effective use of self in the therapeutic process and suggests the importance of involving family members in treatment whenever possible. Certainly therapists should be aware of the social resources available to patients and clients, so that deficits in this area can be considered in treatment planning. For example, the therapist might arrange for group treatment sessions, so that some benefits of socialization might be realized. It has been observed that some conditions, such as depression or chronic illness, can result in social isolation or withdrawal. Under these circumstances social interaction in the treatment setting assumes even greater importance.

Support or self-help groups are also widely recognized as opportunities for receiving support and encouragement. Participation in such groups can yield benefits for both patients and clients and families, such as sharing common experiences, gaining information, and providing mutual help and support. Being of assistance to others can be a source of reassurance of one's own competence and usefulness, thus contributing to feelings of self-esteem and self-efficacy.

Patients and clients who lack interpersonal competence may be unable to cultivate social resources because of deficits in this area. Given the importance of social resources in coping, goals relating to interpersonal skills must be considered in treatment planning concurrently with interventions directed at cognitive or physical deficits. Of particular importance are skills related to impression management, that is, enhancing the interpersonal behaviors that facilitate positive social contacts. DeLoach and Greer (1981) have offered a number of suggestions for improving the social impression of people who are disabled or who simply lack adequate skills for eliciting favorable impressions in interpersonal contacts. Areas of importance include physical demeanor, physical distance, facial expression, and vocal behavior. Therapists should become familiar with the principles and the approaches necessary for improving the impression management of patients and clients with inadequate interpersonal skills.

These general principles derived from coping theory can improve the effectiveness of therapeutic intervention for nearly all types of patients and clients. Those with chronic and permanent conditions warrant special attention, however, because as noted earlier, their coping resources are challenged by an exceptional number of stressors over an extended period.

Coping and Chronic Conditions

Stressors commonly encountered during chronic illness or disability include medical crises, treatment regimens that require profound life-style changes, symptoms, family relationships, emotional upsets, and demands on time (Moos & Tsu, 1977; Strauss & Glaser, 1975). Simultaneously the person has fewer physical and emotional resources to bring to bear on these circumstances (Dimond, 1984). His or her ability to mobilize coping strategies that will yield a satisfactory adaptational outcome will depend on the type of onset and the expected course of the illness, the nature and the extent of limitation, and the type and the extent of changes in physical appearance and bodily functions.

To determine if there were basic differences in the types of coping strategies employed by people with varying kinds of chronic illness and if some strategies were more effective than others, Felton, Revenson, and Hinrichsen (1984) studied four groups of adults with either hypertension, diabetes mellitus, rheumatoid arthritis, or systemic blood cancer. Factor analysis of the specific coping strategies used by the participants in the study resulted in six major categories of coping:

1. Cognitive restructuring—efforts to find positive aspects of the illness experience and to regard the illness as an opportunity for inner growth
2. Emotional expression—becoming angry at other people or joking about the illness
3. Wish-fulfilling fantasy—indulgence in longing for the illness to be over
4. Self-blame—attempts to refocus attention in order to avoid accepting the illness as a chronic problem
5. Information-seeking—attempts to seek information and advice about the illness and its treatment
6. Threat minimization—conscious efforts to put distressing thoughts out of one's mind.

In the study, psychological adjustment was measured by acceptance of illness, self-esteem, and indications of positive and negative affect or mood. Despite wide variation in medical treatment demands, levels of disability, and immediacy of life threat, the coping strategies used by the illness groups were largely the same. That is, specific kinds of coping strategies were not related to the type of chronic illness. However, the use of cognitive strategies was associated with positive mood states, and the use of threat minimization was related to better adjustment as reflected in acceptance of illness. By contrast, the use of emotionally expressive, avoidant, and blaming coping strategies was associated with lower self-esteem and poorer adjustment.

These findings seem consistent with those obtained by other researchers. For example, among cancer patients, Worden and Sobel (1978) found inverse relationships between ego strength or self-esteem and hopelessness, frustration, and denial; and positive correlations between ego strength and successful problem-solving. Similarly Hyman (1975) found higher levels of self-esteem among people with various long-term conditions who had experienced rehabilitation success.

Collectively these findings underscore the importance of the patient's or client's view of self in predicting the success of rehabilitation efforts. Accordingly, in working with patients and clients with chronic problems or disabilities, a prominent goal must be the development of their self-image. Adams and Lindemann (1974) have asserted that one of the most important events in successful adaptation to chronic disability is acceptance by the individual that he or she is no longer sick, but "different." This suggests the significance of a clear appraisal of self-image. Rehabilitation professionals can help patients and clients develop realistic self-images through a concerted effort to reinforce the existence of altered life circumstances and to reaffirm new role expectations and responsibilities.

At the same time, preserving a sense of personal worth, keeping distress within manageable limits, maintaining or restoring relations with significant others, enhancing the prospects for recovery of bodily functions, and increasing the likelihood of working out a personally valued and socially acceptable life-style after maximum physical recovery has been attained, are important goals. These are vital component parts of the ultimate goal of altering the patient's or client's view of self in the future and establishing a modified ego ideal.

In light of the importance of coping to successful adaptation and overall well-being, therapists should consider the coping resources and skills of their patients and clients throughout therapeutic intervention. Performance deficits require the ability to cope in practical as well as emotional ways. Accordingly therapists may need to establish the development of coping skills as ancillary treatment goals with many patients and clients. Although occupational therapists may become directly involved in using some of the coping interventions described in this chapter, professionals in psychology, social work, nursing, and related disciplines might more appropriately conduct others. Through awareness of approaches to improving coping skills, the occupational therapist will be better able to refer patients and clients as necessary, so that they can attain and maintain the highest possible quality of life once they have overcome performance deficits.

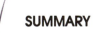

SUMMARY

Coping theory is concerned with the responses of people to stressful circumstances. The nature of a stressor, as perceived by the person experiencing it, interacts with personality dispositions and environmental factors to influence the specific coping efforts undertaken. Such efforts can be either problem or emotion focused. If they are effective, they lead to satisfactory adaptation.

Important personal elements that affect a person's appraisal of a stressful situation are self-esteem and self-efficacy, or the degree to which a person perceives that he or she can effectively implement specific coping strategies. These views of self are influenced strongly by successful experiences and feelings of control. A person's appraisal of a situation and ultimate choice of a coping strategy are also affected by the importance attached to succeeding (or the costs associated with not succeeding) in a particular stressful encounter.

Environmental resources are the material and the social resources necessary to deal effectively with stressful events. Studies have shown that social support is an important environmental resource that can have both positive and negative implications for coping. People whose interpersonal skills are poor or whose coping styles lead to social withdrawal may be reducing their ability to cope with stressful episodes.

Specific interventions to improve coping (or manage stress) include appraisal-oriented approaches, response-oriented approaches, and combinations of the two. Examples of appraisal-oriented strategies are information acquisition and cognitive therapy. Response-oriented strategies include training in relaxation, meditation, biofeedback, assertiveness, social skills, and modeling. Stress inoculation training and problem-solving training represent combination approaches.

With respect to occupational therapy practice, effective intervention requires an awareness of the coping needs and resources of all patients and clients. Although activity itself appears to yield useful benefits in emotion-focused coping, the therapist should plan intervention with an underlying aim of improving the patient's or client's coping efforts and resources, from appraisal to response. The importance of social skills to effective coping should not be overlooked.

Study Questions

1. Discuss the difference between coping and adaptation. According to Lazarus, which of the two always involves stress?

2. According to the model of coping developed by Lazarus and his colleagues, stressors can be appraised as falling into three general categories. List them.

3. Cite an example of an event that could be viewed as threatening and challenging at the same time.

4. Discuss the role of social support in coping. Cite an example of how social resources can have a detrimental effect on coping.

5. Distinguish between problem- and emotion-focused coping. Can the same behavior be classified as both? If so, cite an example.

6. What is the relationship, if any, between activity and coping? Does research support or refute the effectiveness of activity in managing emotional reactions to stressful circumstances?

7. Discuss the role of self-efficacy in coping. How can occupational therapists influence a person's sense of efficacy?

8. Ambiguity is an environmental characteristic that impedes coping. What kinds of life situations tend to exhibit environmental ambiguity? How do people tend to deal with ambiguous situations?

9. Cite several current approaches to improving coping skills. Which, if any, might be appropriate for use by an occupational therapist?

10. Why are performance deficits likely to be sources of stress? Cite examples of situations in your own life in which a physical or an emotional condition created additional stress for you or someone you knew. Describe the coping strategies that you or the other person used in dealing with the stress.

Recommended Readings

Coelho, G.V., Hamburg, D.A., & Adams, J.E. (Eds.). (1974). *Coping and adaptation*. New York: Basic Books.

Dubos, R. (1965). *Man adapting*. New Haven: Yale University Press.

Elliott, G.R., & Eisdorfer, C. (Eds.). (1982). *Stress and human health*. New York: Springer.

Hamburger, L.K., & Lohr, J.M. (1984). *Stress and stress management*. New York: Springer.

Lazarus, R.S., & Folkman, S. (1984). *Stress, appraisal and coping*. New York: Springer.

Mason, J.W. (1975). A historical view of the stress field. *Journal of Human Stress, 1*(2), 22-36.

Meichenbaum, D., & Jaremko, M.E. (Eds). (1983). *Stress reduction and prevention*. New York: Plenum Press.

Moos, R.H. (Ed.). (1977). *Coping with physical illness*. New York: Plenum Press.

Pelletier, K.R. (1977). *Mind as healer, mind as slayer*. New York: Delta.

Selye, H. (1974). *Stress without distress*. New York: J.B. Lippincott.

Selye, H. (1982). History and present status of the stress concept. In L. Goldberger & S. Breznitz (Eds.), *Handbook of stress: Theoretical and clinical aspects* (pp. 7-17). New York: Free Press.

References

Agras, W.S. (1981). Behavioral approaches to the treatment of essential hypertension. *International Journal of Obesity, 5* (Suppl. 1), 173-181.

Andrasik, F., & Holroyd, K.A. (1980). A test of specific and nonspecific effects in the biofeedback treatment of tension headache. *Journal of Consulting and Clinical Psychology, 48*, 575-586.

Andrew, J. (1970). Recovery from surgery, with and without preparatory instruction for three coping styles. *Journal of Personality and Social Psychology, 15*, 223-226.

Antonovsky, A. (1979). *Health, stress and coping*. San Francisco: Jossey-Bass.

Bandura, A. (1977). Self-efficacy: Toward a unifying theory of behavioral change. *Psychological Review, 84*, 191-215.

Beck, A.T. (1976). *Cognitive therapy and the emotional disorders*. New York: International Universities Press.

Berkman, L.F., & Syme, S.L. (1979). Social networks, host resistances, and mortality: A follow-up study of Alameda County residents. *American Journal of Epidemiology, 109*, 186-204.

Blackwell, B., Bloomfield, S., & Gartside, P. (1976). Transcendental meditation in hypertension: Individual response patterns. *Lancet, i*, 223-226.

Blanchard, E.B., Andrasik, F., Appelbaum, K.A., Evans, D.D., Myers, P., & Barron, K.D. (1986). Three studies of the psychological changes in chronic headache patients associated with biofeedback and relaxation therapies. *Psychosomatic Medicine, 48*, 73-83.

Brown, B. (1970). Recognition of aspects of consciousness through association with EEG alpha activity represented by a light signal. *Psychophysics, 6*, 442-446.

Cameron, R., & Meichenbaum, D. (1982). The nature of effective coping and the treatment of stress-related problems: A cognitive behavioral perspective. In L. Goldberger & S. Breznitz (Eds.), *Handbook of stress: Theoretical and clinical aspects* (pp. 695-710). New York: Free Press.

Cannon, W.B. (1932). *The wisdom of the body*. New York: W.W. Norton.

Cassel, J. (1976). The contribution of the social environment to host resistance. *American Journal of Epidemiology, 104*, 107-123.

Cobb, S. (1976). Social support as a moderator of life stress. *Psychosomatic Medicine, 38*, 300-314.

Cohen, F., & Lazarus, R.S. (1979). Coping with the stress of illness. In G.C. Stone, F. Cohen, N.E. Adler, et al. (Eds.), *Health psychology: A handbook* (pp. 217-254). San Francisco: Jossey-Bass.

Cohen, F., & Lazarus, R.S. (1984). Coping and adaptation in health and illness. In D. Mechanic (Ed.), *Handbook of health and health services* (pp. 608-635). New York: Free Press.

Dean, A., & Lin, N. (1977). The stress-buffering role of social support. *Journal of Nervous and Mental Disease, 169*, 403-417.

DeLoach, C., & Greer, B.G. (1981). *Adjustment to severe physical disability: A metamorphosis*. New York: McGraw-Hill.

DeLong, R.D. (1971). Individual differences in patterns of anxiety arousal, stress relevant information, and recovery from surgery (Doctoral dissertation, University of California, Los Angeles, 1970). *Dissertation Abstracts International, 32,* 554B.

Dimond, M. (1984). Social adaptation of the chronically ill. In D. Mechanic (Ed.), *Handbook of health and health services* (pp. 636-656). New York: Free Press.

Dohrenwend, B.S., Krasnoff, L., Askenasy, A.R., & Dohrenwend, B.P. (1978). Exemplification of a method for scaling life events: The PERI Life Events Scale. *Journal of Health and Social Behavior, 19,* 205-229.

Dubos, R. (1965). *Man adapting*. New Haven: Yale University Press.

Duckitt, J. (1984). Social support, personality, and the prediction of psychological distress. *Journal of Clinical Psychology, 40,* 1199-1205.

Elliott, G.R., & Eisdorfer, C. (Eds.). (1982). *Stress and human health*. New York: Springer.

Ellis, A. (1973). *Humanistic psychotherapy: The rational emotive approach*. New York: Julian Press.

Erikson, E. (1985). *Childhood and society*. New York: W. W. Norton.

Felton, B.J., Revenson, T.A., & Hinrichsen, G.A. (1984). Stress and coping in the explanation of psychological adjustment among chronically ill adults. *Social Science and Medicine, 18,* 889-898.

Ferington, F.W. (1986). Personal control and coping effectiveness in spinal cord injured persons. *Research in Nursing and Health, 9,* 257-265.

Folkman, S. (1984). Personal control and stress and coping processes: A theoretical analysis. *Journal of Personality and Social Psychology, 46,* 839-852.

Folkman, S., & Lazarus, R.S. (1980). An analysis of coping in a middle-aged community sample. *Journal of Health and Social Behavior, 21,* 219-239.

Folkman, S., & Lazarus, R.S. (1988a). Coping as a mediator of emotion. *Journal of Personality and Social Psychology, 54,* 466-475.

Folkman, S., & Lazarus, R.S. (1988b). The relationship between coping and emotion: *Implications for theory and research. Social Science and Medicine, 26,* 309-317.

Frank, R.G., Umlauf, R.L., Wonderlich, J.S., Askanazi, A.G.S., Buckelew, S.P., & Elliott, T.R. (1987). Differences in coping styles among persons with spinal cord injury: A cluster-analytic approach. *Journal of Consulting and Clinical Psychology, 55,* 727-731.

Funk, S.C., & Houston, B.K. (1987). A critical analysis of the hardiness scale's validity and utility. *Journal of Personality and Social Psychology, 53,* 572-578.

Gal, R., & Lazarus, R.S. (1975). The role of activity in anticipating and confronting stressful situations. *Journal of Human Stress, 1*(4), 4-20.

Ganellen, R.J., & Blaney, P.H. (1984). Hardiness and social support as moderators of the effects of life stress. *Journal of Personality and Social Psychology, 47,* 156-163.

Glass, D.C. (1977). *Behavior patterns, stress, and human disease*. Hillsdale, NJ: Lawrence Erlbaum Associates.

Gleser, G.C., & Ilhilevich, D. (1969). An objective instrument for measuring defense mechanisms. *Journal of Consulting and Clinical Psychology, 33,* 651-660.

Goldfried, M.R., & Davison, G C. (1976). *Clinical behavior therapy*. New York: Holt, Rinehart & Winston.

Green, J.A., & Schellenberger, R.D. (1986). Biofeedback research and the ghost in the box: A reply to Roberts. *American Psychologist, 41,* 1003-1005.

Hinkle, L.E. (1974). The effect of exposure to culture change, social change, and changes in interpersonal relationships on health. In B.S. Dohrenwend & B.P. Dohrenwend (Eds.), *Stressful life events: Their nature and effects* (pp. 9-44). New York: John Wiley & Sons.

Holahan, C.J., & Moos, R.H. (1985). Life stress and health: Personality, coping, and family support in stress resistance. *Journal of Personality and Social Psychology, 49,* 739-747.

Holahan, C.J., & Moos, R.H. (1986). Personality, coping, and family resources in stress resistance: A longitudinal analysis. *Journal of Personality and Social Psychology, 51,* 389-395.

Holmes, T.H., & Rahe, R.H. (1967). The social adjustment rating scale. *Journal of Psychosomatic Research, 11,* 213-218.

Holroyd, K.A., Appel, M.A., & Andraskik, F. (1983). A cognitive-behavioral approach to psychophysiological disorders. In D. Meichenbaum & M.E. Jaremko (Eds.), *Stress reduction and prevention* (pp. 219-260). New York: Plenum Press.

Hull, J.G., Van Treuren, R.R., & Virnelli, S. (1987). Hardiness and health: A critique and alternative approach. *Journal of Personality and Social Psychology, 53,* 518-530.

Hyman, M. (1975). Social psychological factors affecting disability among ambulatory patients. *Journal of Chronic Disease, 28,* 199-216.

Ilfeld, F.W. (1980). Coping styles of Chicago adults: Description. *Journal of Human Stress, 6*(2), 2-10.

Jacobson, E. (1938). *Progressive relaxation: A physiological and clinical investigation of muscle states and* their significance in psychology and medical practice (2nd ed.). Chicago: University of Chicago Press.

Janis, I.L. (1958). *Psychological stress*. New York: John Wiley & Sons.

Jemmott, J.B., Borysenko, J.Z., Borysenko, M., McClelland, D.C., Chapman, R., Meyer, D., & Benson, H. (1983). Academic stress, power motivation and decrease in secretion rate of salivary secretory immunoglobulin A. *Lancet, (i),* 1400-1402.

Jenkins, C.D., Hurst, M.W., & Rose, R.M. (1979). Life changes: Do people really remember? *Archives of General Psychiatry, 36,* 379-384.

Joffe, P.E., & Naditch, M.P. (1977). Paper-and-pencil measures of coping and defense processes. In N. Haan (Ed.), *Coping and defending: Processes of self-environment organization*. New York: Academic Press.

Kamiya, J. (1969). Operant control of the EEG alpha rhythm and some of its reported effects on consciousness. In C. Tart (Ed.), *Altered states of consciousness* (pp. 507-517). New York: John Wiley & Sons.

Kanner, A.D., Coyne, J.C., Schaefer, C., & Lazarus, R.S. (1981). Comparison of two modes of stress measurement: Daily hassles and uplifts versus major life events. *Journal of Behavioral Medicine, 4,* 1-39.

Kasl, S.V., Evans, A.S., & Niederman, J.C. (1979). Psychosocial risk factors in the development of infectious mononucleosis. *Psychosomatic Medicine, 41,* 445-466.

Kendall, P.C., & Watson, D. (1981). Psychological preparation for stressful medical procedures. In C.K. Prokop & L.A. Bradley (Eds.), *Medical psychology: Contributions to behavioral medicine* (pp. 167-213). New York: Academic Press.

King, G.A., & Sorrentino, R.M. (1983). Psychological dimensions of goal-oriented interpersonal situations. *Journal of Personality and Social Psychology, 44,* 140-162.

Klinger, E. (1975). Consequences of, commitment to, and disengagement from incentives. *Psychological Review, 82,* 1-25.

Kobasa, S.C. (1979). Stressful life events, personality, and health: An inquiry into hardiness. *Journal of Personality and Social Psychology, 37,* 1-11.

Kobasa, S.C. (1982). The hardy personality: Toward a social psychology of stress and health. In G.S. Sanders & J. Suls (Eds.), *Social psychology of health and illness* (pp. 3-32). Hillsdale, NJ: Lawrence Erlbaum Associates.

Kobasa, S., Maddi, S.R., & Courington, S. (1981). Personality and constitution as mediators in the stress-illness relationship. *Journal of Health and Social Behavior, 22,* 368-378.

Kobasa, S., Maddi, S.R., & Kahn, S. (1982). Hardiness

and health: A prospective study. *Journal of Personality and Social Psychology, 42,* 168-177.

Lange, A.J., & Jakubowski, P. (1976). *Responsible assertive behavior*. Champaign, IL: Research Press.

Lazarus, R.S. (1984). Puzzles in the study of daily hassles. *Journal of Behavioral Medicine, 7,* 375-389.

Lazarus, R.S., & Folkman, S. (1984a). Coping and adaptation. In W.D. Gentry (Ed.), *Handbook of behavioral medicine* (pp. 282-325). New York: Guilford Press.

Lazarus, R.S., & Folkman, S. (1984b). *Stress, appraisal and coping*. New York: Springer.

Lefcourt, H.M., Martin, R.A., & Saleh, W.E. (1984). Locus of control and social support: Interactive moderators of stress. *Journal of Personality and Social Psychology, 47,* 378-389.

Martelli, M.F., Auerbach, S.M., Alexander, J., & Mercuri, L.G. (1987). Stress management in the health care setting: Matching interventions with patient coping styles. *Journal of Consulting and Clinical Psychology, 55,* 201-207.

McRae, R.R., & Costa, P.T., Jr. (1986). Personality, coping, and coping effectiveness in an adult sample. *Journal of Personality, 54,* 385-395.

Mechanic, D. (1974). Social structure and personal adaptation: Some neglected dimensions. In G.V. Coelho, D.A. Hamburg, & J.E. Adams (Eds.), *Coping and adaptation* (pp. 32-44). New York: Basic Books.

Melamed, B.G., & Siegel, L.J. (1975). Reduction of anxiety in children facing hospitalization and surgery by use of filmed modeling. *Journal of Consulting and Clinical Psychology, 43,* 511-521.

Miller, N.E. (1969). Learning of visceral and glandular responses. *Science, 163,* 434-445.

Moos, R.H., & Tsu, V.D. (1977). The crisis of physical illness: An overview. In R. H. Moos (Ed.), *Coping with physical illness* (pp. 3-21). New York: Plenum Press.

Parkes, K.R. (1986). Coping in stressful episodes: The role of individual differences, environmental factors, and situational characteristics. *Journal of Personality and Social Psychology, 51,* 1277-1292.

Peterson, L., & Shigetomi, C. (1981). The use of coping techniques to minimize anxiety in hospitalized children. *Behavior Therapy, 12,* 1-14.

Rose, R.M. (1980). Endocrine response to stressful psychological events. *Psychiatric Clinics of North America, 3,* 1-15.

Rotter, J.B. (1966). Generalized expectancies for internal versus external control of reinforcement. *Psychological Monographs: General and Applied, 80* (Whole No. 609).

Rotter, J.B. (1975). Some problems and misconceptions related to the construct of internal versus external control of reinforcement. *Journal of Consulting and Clinical Psychology, 43,* 56-67.

Scheier, M.F., & Carver, C.S. (1985). Optimism, coping, and health: Assessment and implications of generalized outcome expectancies. *Health Psychology, 4,* 219-247.

Schmied, L.A., & Lawler, K.A. (1986). Hardiness, type A behavior, and the stress-illness relation in working women. *Journal of Personality and Social Psychology, 51,* 1218-1223.

Schroeder, D.H., & Costa, P.T. (1984). Influence of life event stress on physical illness: Substantive effects or methodological flaws? *Journal of Personality and Social Psychology, 46,* 853-863.

Schutz, W.C. (1967). *The FIRO Scales manual.* Palo Alto, CA: Consulting Psychologists Press.

Seer, P. (1979). Psychological control of essential hypertension: Review of the literature and methodological critique. *Psychological Bulletin, 86,* 1015-1043.

Selye, H. (1936). A syndrome produced by diverse noxious agents. *Nature, 138,* 2.

Shapiro, D.H. (1985). Meditation and behavioral medicine: Application of a self-regulation strategy to the clinical management of stress. In S.R. Burchfield (Ed.), *Stress: Psychological and physiological interactions* (pp. 307-328). Washington, DC: Hemisphere.

Shontz, F. (1975). *The psychological aspects of physical illness and disability.* New York: Macmillan.

Sidle, A., Moos, R., Adams, J., & Cady, P. (1969). Development of a coping scale. *Archives of General Psychiatry, 20,* 226-232.

Silver, R. L., & Wortman, C.B. (1980). Coping with undesirable life events. In J. Garber & M.E.P. Seligman (Eds.), *Human helplessness: Theory and applications* (pp. 279-340). New York: Academic Press.

Smith, T.W., Colligan, M., Horning, R.W., & Hurrel, J. (1978). *Occupational comparison of stress-related disease incidence.* Cincinnati, OH: National Institute for Occupational Safety and Health.

Stensrud, R., & Stensrud, K. (1981). Interpersonal stress as a consequence of being disabled. *Journal of Rehabilitation, 47,* 43-46.

Strauss, A., & Glaser, B. (1975). *Chronic illness and the quality of life.* St. Louis: C. V. Mosby.

Suls, J. (1982). Social support, interpersonal relations, and health: Benefits and liabilities. In G. Sanders & J. Suls (Eds.), *Social psychology of health and illness* (pp. 255-277). Hillsdale, NJ: Lawrence Erlbaum Associates.

Suls, J., & Fletcher, B. (1985). The relative efficacy of avoidant and nonavoidant coping strategies: A meta-analysis. *Health Psychology, 4,* 249-288.

Talbott, E., Helmkamp, J., Mathews, K., Kuller, L., Cottington, E., & Redmond, G. (1985). Occupational noise exposure, noise-induced hearing loss, and the epidemiology of high blood pressure. *American Journal of Epidemiology, 121,* 501-514.

Theorell, T. (1976). Selected illnesses and somatic factors in relation to two psycho-social stress indices: A prospective study of middle-aged construction building workers. *Journal of Psychosomatic Research, 21,* 499-509.

Vinokur, A., & Selzer, M.L. (1975). Desirable versus undesirable life events: Their relationship to stress and mental distress. *Journal of Personality and Social Psychology, 32,* 329-337.

Weisman, A.D. (1972). *On dying and denying: A psychiatric study of terminality.* New York: Behavioral Publications.

White, R.W. (1974). Strategies of adaptation: An attempt at systematic description. In G.V. Coelho, D.A. Hamburg, & J.E. Adams (Eds.), *Coping and adaptation* (pp. 47-68). New York: Basic Books.

Worden, J.W., & Sobel, H.J. (1978). Ego strength and psychosocial adaptation to cancer. *Psychosomatic Medicine, 40,* 585-592.

Zastowny, T.R., Kirschenbaum, D.S., & Meng, A.L. (1986). Coping skills training for children: Effects on distress before, during and after hospitalization for surgery. *Health Psychology, 5,* 231-247.

Zimmerman, M. (1985). Methodological issues in the assessment of life events: A review of issues and research. *Social Psychology Review, 3,* 339-370.

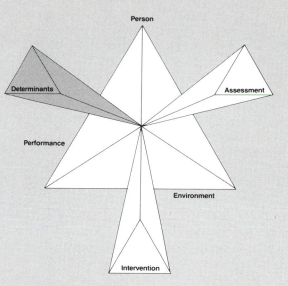

Section Two

Determinants of Occupational Performance

CHAPTER CONTENT OUTLINE

KEY TERMS

Assimilation

Bicultural

Culture

Cultural Filter

Disability behavior

Disease

Ethnicity

Explanatory models

Illness

Patterns of help-seeking

ABSTRACT

Culture has a great influence on human performance, and consideration of cultural bias and cultural variation is important in working with patients. This chapter emphasizes the need for therapists to assess the unique cultural identity of each person and its implications for human performance in order to implement appropriate intervention. Four important concepts borrowed from the social sciences are discussed: illness versus disease, culturally influenced explanatory models, the cultural notions of body structure, and culturally distinct patterns of help-seeking.

Cultural Influences on Performance

4

Laura H. Krefting
Douglas V. Krefting

"Healing is a powerful, culturally endorsed ritual. There is no doubt that if you trust the practitioner and if you share the same cultural myths, healing is better achieved."

—Hammerschlag, 1988

OBJECTIVES

The information in this chapter is intended to help the reader—

1. operationally define culture as it relates to occupational therapy practice.

2. provide a rationale for considering culture in assessment and intervention in occupational therapy.

3. identify five ways in which culture can affect the therapeutic relationship.

4. distinguish between culture and ethnicity.

5. distinguish between illness and disease.

6. define the concept of explanatory model and identify specific assessment questions that can be used to elicit patients' or clients' explanatory models.

7. identify the three major health care sectors and give three examples of practitioners in each one.

8. define the concept of the therapeutic management group and its relevance to occupational therapy practice.

INTRODUCTION

The concept of culture has been identified as important in the practice of occupational therapy, yet it is not clearly defined in the literature. Moreover, it is seldom considered in relation to how occupational therapists make decisions about assessment and intervention. Despite the growth of occupational therapy's body of knowledge and conceptual base, with regard to culture, therapists are still working on the level of personal experience and intuition rather than on the level of conceptually sound information that is supported by research.

The purpose of this chapter is to sensitize therapists to the need to consider variation in culture and its effects on practice. Using concepts borrowed from the social sciences, the chapter offers an operational definition of culture that relates to factors influencing human performance. This is accomplished by first discussing various definitions of culture and then comparing the definitions to ways in which the term has been used in the occupational therapy and health care literature. Examples of specific cultural influences on practice are used to enrich the operational definition. Finally, four concepts from clinical anthropology are presented to aid therapists in using the concept of culture in daily practice: those of illness and disease, explanatory models, cultural definitions of anatomy and physiology, and patterns of help-seeking.

DEFINITION OF CULTURE

In anthropology, entire books have been devoted to defining **culture,** suggesting the richness and the complexity of this central theoretical concept (for discussions, see Geertz, 1973; Keesing, 1981; Kroeber & Kluckholn, 1963). After decades of scholarly debate, anthropologists have not agreed on a single definition. However, certain commonalities among the definitions provide a basis for understanding the concept:

1. *Culture* is a system of learned patterns of behavior. The idea that it is learned rather than biologically inherited is important. Learning occurs through socialization; that is, culture is transmitted to the young of a group by other group members.

2. *Culture* is shared by members of a group rather than being the property of an individual.
3. *Culture* includes the concept of providing the individual and the group with effective mechanisms for interacting both with others and with the surrounding environment.

If one tries to identify the basic elements of culture, the list seems endless: morals, art, law, customs, speech patterns, interaction, economic and production patterns, goals, beliefs, and values are each constituents of culture. As explained by Tylor (1871/1958), one of the earliest anthropologists to address this question, **culture** can include anything acquired by humans as members of society.

The complexity and the plurality of the culture concept depend on one's theoretical orientation within anthropology (Litterst, 1985). Some anthropologists have narrowed the definition to look at culture as a mental or attitudinal construct, a shared understanding among a group. Others focus specifically on behavior or the artifacts of behavior. Anthropologists of this viewpoint, which is referred to as *material culture,* might study pottery shards, traditional ceremonial chants, or folk herbal cures. The debate between the two groups continues, but they agree that culture is a design or a model for behavior. That is, some kind of pattern or framework is expressed in the behavioral characteristics of each group of people. This framework guides behavior and provides meaning to life. Therapists need to understand the importance of the framework and recognize the power that it has in organizing people's lives.

The influence of culture on behavior is not always conscious; culture is taken for granted (Peacock, 1986). This observation seems to hold for occupational therapy practice. Although culture is acknowledged as an influence on human performance, therapists do not systematically assess it or use it in planning treatment. Hall (1959) calls it the "silent language" and describes cultural traditions and conventions as often subconscious. He argues that most people do not recognize the effect of culture on themselves, yet their behavior is rigidly influenced by it. For example, many North Americans are concerned about balancing work and leisure. In fact, expert leisure counselors deal with people who are considered *workaholics*. In other cultures, however, leisure is seen as a sign of laziness or incompetence, and productivity alone is valued. One of the purposes of this chapter is to bring the meaning of culture to the

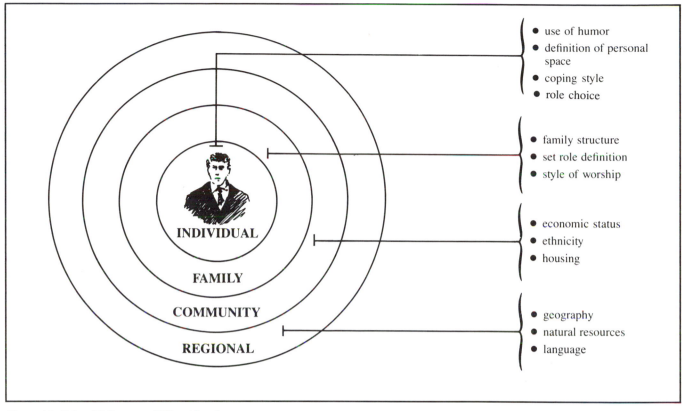

Figure 4-1. Cultural Influence at Different Levels.

consciousness of therapists, so that they can observe cultural influences on patients' and clients' behavior and on their own decision-making in the therapeutic setting.

Those who use culture in practical ways often adopt a multidimensional definition of it. Figure 4-1 shows examples of cultural influence at the levels of the individual, the family, the community, and the region. In the preceding definitions **culture** refers to visible, common patterns held by large groups; for example, states and nations. This dimension is represented in Figure 4-1 by the outer circle. It is most often apparent in cross-cultural studies—for example, a comparison of aging in the United States and Brazil. Language, types of industry, natural resources, and geographic diversity are pertinent factors. This level includes the popular definition of groups, such as the Moslem and Inuit cultures.

Within these cultures, however, there is variation. In considering culture at a community level, smaller more refined commonalities among people are apparent. For example, middle-class Caucasian suburbanites might be similar in type of housing, ethnicity, and economic background, particularly if they are compared with inner-city residents. People of lower socioeconomic class tend to behave more ethnically in health matters than people of the

same background who are of higher socioeconomic status (Clarke, 1983).

Even within these communities, cultures differ, as can be seen by comparing two neighboring families. Factors that might differ at the family level of culture include family structure, sex-role definition, and style of worship. For example, differences in behavior in reacting to disability may become apparent between the only child of a third-generation Bostonian family and the middle sibling of five in a single-parent family residing in the same neighborhood.

Finally, culture can be defined in terms of the individual. That is, each person can be considered to have an individual culture. Although culture is a shared phenomenon, sharing is seen in the context of transmission and socialization. Moreover, individuals learn culture from a number of different people and places, so each person's contact with and interpretation of culture is unique. For instance, siblings brought up in the same home culture might differ in definition of personal space, coping style, use of humor, and choice of role.

Generally an individual learns guidelines for behavior from being part of a particular family, a particular group of peers, a particular community, and a certain geographic region. These guidelines, which teach him or her how to view the world, form the basis of behavior. The same guidelines are transmitted to the succeeding generation. However, each person is also the integrated product of multiple levels of culture and can be considered to have a unique cultural identity. Thus culture cannot be seen as a monolithic force that operates on all members of society in a similar way (Brodsky, 1983). Each person has individual cultural factors that interact with genetic, biophysiological, and environmental factors to determine human performance.

This brief definition is intended to introduce therapists to the concept of culture and to illustrate the breadth of the idea. Although complex, the richness gives the concept relevance to the daily practice of occupational therapy. Against the background of this general definition of culture, some issues surrounding the misinterpretation of the concept are discussed in the next section.

Misinterpretation of the Concept of Culture

One of the most common misinterpretations of culture is to confuse it with **ethnicity.** Ethnicity is that part of identity derived from membership in a racial, religious, national, or linguistic group or subgroup, usually through birth (Hartog & Hartog, 1983). Ethnicity is an important component of culture, but the terms are not synonymous. For example, two people may come from the same barrio and share a strong Hispanic background, but differ in religion, education, family structure, and experience with the biomedical system. The importance of understanding culture as more than ethnicity can be seen in the possibility of greater contrasts between people of the same ethnic category but different educational and class levels, than between people of diverse ethnic backgrounds (Clarke, 1983). Consider the importance of cultural sensitivity in planning intervention for the following: the ``bag man'' who has just been admitted to the hospital for the 37th time in one year, the fundamental Christian who is refusing treatment, the recent Vietnamese refugee, or the first-generation Italian grandmother.

There are no specific rules for working with people of a particular culture. For example, the therapist will not find a definitive article on treating an elderly Lebanese person. This is a problem for medical or clinical anthropologists who are called in difficult situations to instruct the staff about ``how to manage the difficult patient from Transylvania, whose 17 family members will not leave the hospital room.'' It is important to understand the basic components of culture and necessary to assess the cultural identity of each person.

Another difficulty in understanding culture is in acknowledging commonalities within a group without inferring a consistency among people. That is, there are major differences between people of the same culture, for example, Irish Catholics or between Eastern European Jews. Varia-

tion within a cultural group highlights the multilevel understanding of culture. Sapir (1917) contends that the true importance of culture is at the individual level. This is the level at which the concept of culture can be most influential in occupational therapy.

In looking at heterogeneity within cultural groups, it is important to consider the assimilation of cultures. **Assimilation** refers to the process by which people of one culture lose their culturally unique characteristics and become more like those of the dominant culture. Assimilation is often used to describe how well immigrants have adapted to their new country. Some argue that the melting pot is a myth (e.g., Shawski, 1987), that there has been no significant assimilation of ethnic groups in middle-class-dominated American culture. Although a growing number of immigrant groups and subcultures make up North America, second- and third-generation immigrants may become similar at the community level. That is, they become more like each other than like the earlier generation of their own subgroup. Diversity within immigrant groups depends on such factors as length of residence in North America, residential area (i.e., ethnic neighborhood), language spoken at home, fluency in English, and contact with country of origin. Variety among groups, even recent immigrants, can be noted. Differing characteristics include membership in *cultural clubs* (such as Sons of Norway or the Laotian Students' Badminton Club), clothing style, language spoken at home, attendance at cultural festivals, and so on. This dilution of stronger cultural characteristics prevents anthropologists from making broad generalizations about how certain groups will behave.

Moreover, some people are **bicultural.** These individuals may adapt to the dominant culture at work, yet retain their own cultural values and customs at home (Blakeney, 1987). For example, a teenager who has recently arrived in North America from Ghana might resemble his peers during school hours, but after school and on weekends follow the customs and beliefs of another culture. This might include speaking another language, following particular dietary habits, and wearing special clothes. This biculturality can also be seen at the family level, in the contrast between a wife who stays at home with young children and thus retains more of the original cultural characteristics, and her husband, who works outside the home and thereby becomes more assimilated. Intergenerational comparisons illustrate this phenomenon too. For example, in groups in which knowledge has traditionally been passed orally, elders are the authority because they are the repositories of knowledge. When such groups immigrate to a new country or to a region with a different culture, the young may become powerful because through school attendance and peer contact, they may more quickly learn the knowledge that helps them adapt to new cultural rules. Often the young are the ones who learn how to complete Medicare forms and use credit cards.

THE CONCEPT OF CULTURE IN THE OCCUPATIONAL THERAPY LITERATURE

Using the preceding definition of culture as a framework, this section considers the variety of ways in which the term **culture** has been used to describe illness and disability. It focuses largely on the treatment of culture in the occupational therapy literature, but also refers to culture as used in the general medical literature that is relevant to the practice of occupational therapy.

A review of some of the key references in occupational therapy suggests that although culture is acknowledged on a theoretical and philosophical level, it is one of the least developed aspects of occupational therapy knowledge. For example, Reed and Sanderson (1980) include the sociocultural environment in their model of practice and describe culture as encompassing all human beings and organized patterns of living. They suggest that the environment can be influenced by cultural factors, which include institutions, mores and laws, architectural design, art and science, technical knowledge, history, and language. In another vein, they note that some occupational roles, such as in law and government service, are performed to meet the expectations of the sociocultural environment. Their definition supports the model of occupational performance; however, it does not go far enough in considering the practical aspects of assessing patients' and clients' cultural background.

Hopkins and Tiffany's (1983) treatment of culture makes the concept understandable in relation to practice. They explain that the perceptions of both the therapist and the patient or the client are filtered through a cultural screen. Also, they identify a number of cultural aspects to assessment, for example, time management, handling of anxiety, use of humor, and significance of food. Their treatment of the concept provides illustration; however, it does not provide a guide to treatment.

The concept of culture is also addressed in the model of human occupation. According to Barris, Kielhofner, Levine, and Neville (1985), culture is the environmental level that influences and organizes other levels of human environment—objects, tasks, social groups, and organizations—and is in turn constrained by them. Three dimensions of culture are particularly relevant to human performance: the nature of work and play, space/time, and transmission of knowledge and values.

Barris and coworkers' (1985) definition of culture has been examined by others in the field, for example, by Wieringa and McColl (1987), in their article about Canadian Natives. They state that the traditional models of care do not address cultural issues nor recognize cultural stereotyping. Using the model of human occupation as a framework, they discuss the Cree and Ojibway people in relation to role performance, role learning, work patterns, and interpersonal patterns.

Levine (1984) also addresses the concept of culture in the model of human occupation through an excellent case analysis. She notes that culture affects the delivery of home care through culturally sensitive selection of goals and treatment and through establishment of rapport. Such case histories are an important step in developing the concept of culture in that they act as a transition between conceptual models and practice.

The most common treatment of culture in the occupational therapy literature is to equate it with ethnicity or race. Examples are studies of maritime Canadians, Black Americans, or Vietnamese immigrants. In an occupational therapy study by Lindsay (1971), nationality and primary language spoken were examined among injured immigrant workers. Culture in this context was not rigorously defined; rather the author's general observations formed the basis for conclusions about the immigrant's culture.

This approach is common in the issue of *Occupational Therapy in Health Care* devoted to sociocultural implications. Here some writers attempt to provide background information on certain ''cultural groups.'' For example, McCormack (1987) discusses characteristic health beliefs and practices of Hispanics, Indo-Chinese, and Black Americans; and Blakeney (1987) uses Appalachian peoples as examples of the importance of addressing the values of a subculture. Such approaches represent a narrow definition of culture that neglects potential variation within groups (Litterst, 1985). The articles imply a homogeneity among group members, and the findings, if not carefully portrayed, can perpetuate stereotypes. Without a cultural assessment at the individual level, therapists can easily develop preconceived ideas about how groups of people will manage their illness or disability. The heterogeneity of disability behaviors is illustrated by Brodsky (1983), who, reflecting on her experience with over 2,000 disabled people, concludes that there are no cultural stereotypes and no disability behaviors specific to a single cultural group.

In a similar vein, articles describing disability or occupational therapy techniques in a particular country are fairly common. Here the term **culture** refers specifically to geographical location—for example, ''Rehabilitation in China'' (Bray & Chamings, 1983). Many of the materials produced by the World Federation of Occupational Therapists, Rehabilitation International, and the World Health Organization describe the cultures of different countries. This definition of culture, as represented in the circular model described earlier, is at the first and most general level.

An interesting variation on the term culture appears in an excellent article by Morse (1987) describing a program in which religion was the dominant cultural factor considered in treatment. Morse described a socialization and life-skills program for Jewish adults with developmental disabilities that made use of festivals, foods, and religious occasions, and staff that included a rabbinical student. Culturally sensitive individual therapy is not usually this straightforward, however.

Another means of using the concept of culture is seen in cross-cultural studies. Although cross-cultural studies comparing diseases and treatments are common in the general medical literature, few appear in relation to human occupation. Jamison (1985) considers cultural differences in styles of motivation, cognition, human relations, and social interaction as factors in working with disabled children. She specifically notes that culture is critical in the learning process, citing a number of references from the literature on cross-cultural education. Oddly, although she gives examples of the influence of culture on pediatric practice, she does not define culture. A cross-cultural approach is also evident in studies to validate instruments by establishing norms for different populations. Cultural norms have been developed for a number of assessments commonly used by therapists, including the *Miller Assessment for Preschoolers* (Miller, 1982) and the *Bay Area Functional Performance Evaluation* (Brockett, 1987).

An approach to culture that is frequently taken by anthropologists and sociologists is the study of disability as a subculture. Similar to more traditional anthropological studies that have investigated adolescents in Samoa (Mead, 1923) or untouchables in India (Freeman, 1979), this approach involves examination of a disability group with shared understandings. The few examples of this research in the occupational therapy literature include Kielhofner's (1981) work on persons with mental illness and Krefting's (1989) study on people with traumatic brain injury. A number of social scientists have explored disability groups as subcultures, and their writings are an important source of understanding for therapists. These include Becker's (1980) ethnography of deaf elderly persons, Estroff's (1981) excellent work on mentally ill people in the community, the Kauferts' (1984) work on long-term polio patients in Canada, and Locker's (1983) study of persons with rheumatoid arthritis.

In addition to addressing cultural influences on disability, another perspective is to consider the culture of disability and rehabilitation. In this sense rehabilitation professionals and their practices are examined as a subculture. Health care systems are cultural systems and thus are open to analysis by ethnographers just as other systems are. A study of the culture of occupational therapy would consider such phenomena as interactions between professionals, rehabilitation's place in the larger health care system, power structure, and so on. Gritzer and Arluke's (1985) historical study of physical and occupational therapy takes this perspective, although the authors do not identify it as such. More explicit studies representing the anthropology of disability include Gubrium and Buckholdt's (1982) exposé on the care of disabled persons in a rehabilitation ward and Roth and Eddy's (1967) study of a long-term care institution for the "unwanted." Such descriptions contribute a rich and all-encompassing picture of rehabilitation.

Another perspective on the culture of disability is the global view: the position of rehabilitation and disabled persons in the larger health care system. The relative status of rehabilitation as a subspecialty of medicine reflects the devaluing experienced by disabled and chronically ill people. The emphasis in Western society on values such as competence, independence, productivity, and mastery is mirrored in the health care system. This cultural perception can be noted from the level of the individual caregiver (e.g., the therapist who avoids long-term-care patients) to the national level (e.g., funding policies for service delivery and research that favor technological medicine). Aspects of the health care system that seem most valued in North America are those related to acute and emergency care and technological diagnostics, which in many ways are the antithesis of rehabilitation. Many patients and clients seen by therapists are never cured, nor is there a "quick fix" to their problems in human performance. Although they adapt to their disability or chronic illness, they are often viewed negatively as medical failures. In this sense, people who are chronically disabled or ill are constant reminders of the limits of therapeutic effectiveness within the health care system (Williams, 1987).

CLINICAL APPLICATION OF THE CONCEPT OF CULTURE

The previous sections have emphasized the definition of culture at the level of the individual. Translating this concept into occupational therapy practice means recognizing that each patient or client has a different cultural background and a unique definition of his or her illness or disability. Because each person's perspective on productivity, self-care, and leisure is influenced by culture, therapists must assess the cultural identity of the patient or the client and use this information to plan culturally sensitive interventions. The purpose of sensitizing therapists to cultural factors in human performance, then, is to improve practice. As Levine (1987) notes, culture can make therapy more meaningful to patients and clients and therefore influence outcome. She suggests that therapists search for activities that will stimulate and interest patients and clients as well as promote functional abilities and adaptive skills. Although these principles are basic to professional training, in many cases, assessment and intervention are made more difficult because of the complexities of a patient's or client's cultural background. Table 4-1 lists the cultural factors that can influence human performance.

The consequences of dismissing cultural factors in occupational therapy assessment and intervention are enormous. First, rapport will be difficult to establish, thereby decreasing the patient's or client's trust in the therapist. Poor rapport can develop into major communication problems such as the two parties holding different treatment goals and priorities. Different goals and priorities can in turn result in a patient's or client's noncompliance and dissatisfaction with treatment. Moreover, by ignoring cultural factors, therapists can come to feel helpless or develop a dislike of an individual or a group. Family members may be affected by cultural problems and become antagonists rather than facilitators of treatment. All of these consequences lead to less effective therapy and often a poor outcome. Below is a list of important factors influenced by culture that the therapist should consider in the occupational therapy assessment:

1. Use of time (reflecting *their* work ethic)
2. Balance of work and play
3. Sense of personal space
4. Values regarding finances
5. Role(s) assumed in the family
6. Knowledge of disability and sources of information
7. Beliefs about causality
8. View of the inner workings of the body
9. Sources of social support
10. Amount and level of assistance from others they will accept
11. Degree of importance attributed to physical appearance
12. Degree of importance attributed to independence/ autonomy
13. Sense of control over things that happen to them
14. Typical or preferred coping strategies
15. Style of expressing emotions

Case Study 4-1 illustrates the problems that can arise in therapy when cultural factors are ignored.

Table 4-1
Cultural Factors Influencing Performance

- Family structure
- Parental childrearing styles or practices
- Economic status and history
- Educational background
- Age
- Marital status and history
- Vocational status and history
- Religion or spiritual orientation
- Political orientation
- Immediate environment
- Beliefs (*about health, work, money, roles*)
- Customs
- Values
- Health-related experiences

Different cultural factors influence human performance and can affect the perception of occupational therapy.

Case Study 4-1

Cultural Differences Between Therapist and Patient: Frank was a 68-year-old man seen in the Occupational Therapy Department after a below-the-knee amputation. During the initial assessment Gordon, the therapist, noted that since Frank's retirement as the foreman of a construction crew, he had done very little. He had no hobbies, and he belonged to no special groups and clubs. Rather he seemed to enjoy watching television most of the day. Recognizing the importance of human occupation, especially in people recently retired, Gordon included the development of a hobby or a leisure interest in the treatment goals.

Over the two months in which Gordon worked with Frank, the two men developed no rapport at all. Whenever Gordon dealt directly with problems related to the amputation such as discussing bathroom adaptations, Frank listened in disinterested silence, and any mention of developing leisure skills caused Frank to become angry. Gordon tried to encourage Frank by describing his own grandfather's involvement in seniors' lawn bowling and volunteer work at the local school, but Frank quit coming to occupational therapy and never picked up the dressing aids that had been ordered for him.

At the discharge meeting Gordon described his lack of success in Frank's case. The head nurse noted that Frank was troubled about occupational therapy. He had complained, "Every time I went to occupational therapy, that young man was trying to get me to do some darn hobby or

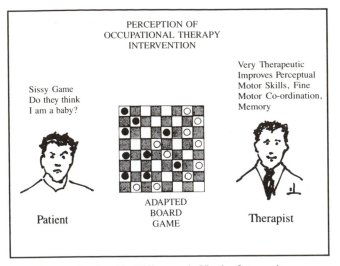

Figure 4-2. Patient/Provider Differences in Viewing Intervention.

join some sissy group with a bunch of old codgers. I've worked all my life, and now I can finally sleep in and watch TV—I deserve it."

It is clear that the therapist, Gordon, viewed productivity and healthy aging through a very different cultural filter than did Frank.

What makes culture even more important is the increasing number and variety of cultural groups in North America. Changing immigration laws and refugee policies and increased mobility within regions of North America have created a situation in which a therapist may work with people from nearly every cultural group in the world. Not only must therapists address the special characteristics of these cultural groups, but they may see new types of disabilities or ones that are no longer common in North America, such as post-typhoid paralysis, polio, and blindness due to vitamin A deficiency. New arrivals to a culture are also at risk for stress-related disorders or complications because of social, economic, and cultural dislocation (Clarke, 1983). This growing cultural diversity shows no sign of slowing down, so cultural factors will undoubtedly become more significant in occupational therapy practice.

Negotiation of Cultural Filters in Therapy

In moving the complex and rather abstract definition of culture into the realm of practice, it is helpful to see culture as a filter or a veil through which people perceive life's experiences. Each person has a unique filter. Even though people may participate in or observe an experience in the company of many others, they will not perceive it in exactly the same way because of their **cultural filters.**

Thus far in the chapter, the culture of the patient or the client has been the major focus, but in any therapeutic relationship the filters of the therapist must also be considered. That is, in treatment, both cultural backgrounds must be examined because they are the filters through which the two parties view the therapeutic endeavor. Some of the more obvious cultural filters are perceptions of illness and health in general and of the immediate illness in particular; perceptions of therapy; and beliefs about purposeful activity, productivity, and leisure. Table 4-1 also illustrates how different cultural filters can affect the perception of occupational therapy when a patient/client is asked to participate in a therapeutic game.

Addressing the therapist's cultural filter, Robinson (1987) notes that therapists are typically from white middle-class backgrounds and possess the inherent values, mores, and expectations of those backgrounds. Possible biases arising from such a cultural identity are a valuing of leisure activities, an attitude about the amount of responsibility that family versus institution should assume for disabled persons, and definitions of security and financial management. A therapist with this cultural identity might strive to return a person to work, whereas the person might prefer to stay on disability allowance. Shawski (1987) gives a very clear example of the cultural filter in noting, "I have caught myself saying that patients have sequencing problems if they brush their teeth differently than I (p. 47)." This illustrates ethnocentricity, in which unfamiliar cultures are judged or defined in terms of the therapist's own, with the view that the therapist's culture is superior.

What *is* important is that the two cultural filters be negotiated. Therapists must try to understand patients' or clients' backgrounds and identify how their personal values and biases may interfere with assessment and treatment. At the same time, therapists must recognize the nature of their own background and its influences on the therapeutic situation. In this way, both parties can arrive at a common understanding of the problem areas, their priority in treatment, and means of intervention.

THE INFLUENCE OF CULTURE ON THERAPY

The basic premise in this chapter is that illness and disability are shaped by sociocultural factors. This section addresses a number of disability-related factors that are influenced by culture, including disability behavior, definition of disability, communication between therapist and patient or client, and perceptions of therapy.

Disability Behavior

One of the central factors in occupational therapy practice is **disability behavior.** A concept borrowed from the social sciences, disability behavior is considered a special case of illness behavior. Illness behavior is defined as the ways in which people respond to bodily indications and conditions that they come to view as abnormal (Mechanic, 1986). Disability behavior describes the manner in which people monitor themselves, define and interpret symptoms, take remedial actions, and use sources of help. It encompasses behavior indicating the nature of a disability (e.g., wincing, being pushed in a wheelchair, and not attending to conversation) and behavior carried out in reaction to a disability (e.g., seeking help from a reflexologist and not attending therapy).

Cultural factors influence the perception, the classification, the labeling, the explanation, and the experienced meaning of disability symptoms. Even more important to disability behavior is how people monitor and respond to their symptoms over the course of a chronic illness and how this affects their behavior, the remedial actions they take, and their response to treatment. Disability behavior varies with all cultural factors, such as socioeconomic class, educational level, geographic location, and nature of the community.

One aspect of disability behavior is how individuals manage the signs and the symptoms of their disability or illness. Cultural variation in how illness and disability are experienced constitutes a large area of study in medical anthropology and sociology. The comparative work most cited in the literature is Zborowski's (1969) investigation of the influence of ethnicity on people's perceptions of and reactions to their symptoms. Zborowski noted different responses to pain in neurological patients of Irish, Italian, Jewish, and white Anglo-Saxon Protestant (WASP) backgrounds. In a similar study Zola (1966) examined Irish and Italian patients. Despite having an almost identical diagnosis, the Italian patients reported more symptoms and dysfunction than the Irish ones did.

People vary in their tolerance for discomfort, in knowledge about their illness or disability, and in the specific ways that their illness or disability affects role performance (Mechanic, 1978). For example, a therapist might mentally compare two individuals with similar backgrounds, diagnoses, and functional problems and try to explain how one could be such a complainer and the other such a model patient. An assessment of their cultural identity would have provided the answer. Culture, then, almost certainly influences the manner in which people learn to cope with difficult situations such as illness and disability.

Disability behavior is also influenced by a person's perception of the emotional impact of an illness or a disability and the amount of stigma involved. For example, people of Chinese background exhibit a well-documented tendency toward somatization of psychiatric disorders; that is, they convert mental experiences or states into bodily symptoms (Kleinman, 1986). This has been attributed to their believing that a greater stigma is attached to a mental illness than to a physical illness. Consequently, psychiatric illnesses often have psychosomatic manifestations.

Culture can also influence beliefs about the cause of disability and the actions taken in response to it. Studies of the Navajo, for instance, reveal that illness or disability is identified by the agent thought to cause it rather than by symptoms (Adair & Deuschle, 1970). Similarly, many people of the Moslem faith or from a predominantly Moslem country believe that disability is the will of God. They may not be motivated to seek treatment or to comply with plans made by health care professionals because doing so is viewed as transgressing God's will. This basic cultural orientation to nature and God influences whether an individual or a family actively intervenes in illness or disability or assumes a passively fatalistic approach. It may in part explain why congenitally disabled children in some developing countries are, by the clinical standards of North America, neglected. Case Study 4-2 describes such a situation in Indonesia.

Case Study 4-2

Behavior Influenced by Beliefs About Causes: Working in a community-based disability detection and prevention program in rural Asia, Brian, a rehabilitation professional, noted that some older children and young adults suffered from very severe cleft palate. Not only did this affect their ability to eat, but their physical appearance was visibly marred. At first he attributed the failure to correct the disability to the lack of services available to rural people in a developing country. However, the community-based program had been in operation in that area for over a decade, so most parents had had ample opportunity to bring their children in for referral. A local health volunteer explained that some parents did not want their children publicly identified as disabled. The people attributed cleft palate to negative actions by a mother during her pregnancy. If she was "rough" in behavior—for instance, if she swore or spit—she was punished for these actions by bearing a disabled child. Bringing the child to the attention of the community rehabilitation worker would be acknowledging her transgressions.

Definition of Disability

Another area influenced by culture is the way in which disability is defined. The identification of a specific disability is defined. The identification of a specific physical or mental impairment or health condition as a disability, varies from one culture to another as well as among social classes or ethnic groups within a single culture. Gliedman and Roth (1980) argue that some physical limitations in North America have been ''medicalized.'' For example, middle-class America views asthma, stuttering, and learning disabilities as handicaps, whereas other cultural groups view them as personal characteristics not directly related to health issues. The labeling of these as disabilities, then, is an interpretation that varies among cultural groups.

The definition of psychosocial disabilities is also affected by cultural factors. For example, whether anxiety or depression is regarded as an everyday experience or a psychiatric diagnosis found in the DSM III (*Diagnostic and Statistical Manual,* 3rd ed.) is culturally variable. This effect is often related to the social acceptability of symptoms within a cultural group.

Economic factors can also influence the definition of disability. Whether one is normal or abnormal, sick or well, is defined in some cultures by whether one can work and support oneself. Thus regardless of the severity of physical or mental limitations, if people are employed, they are not classified or treated as disabled.

Communication Between Therapist and Patient or Client

One of the major therapeutic factors influenced by culture is the communication between the therapist and the patient or the client. Although much of the literature on culture and communication in health care focuses on the physician-patient encounter (for example, Cassel, 1985; Garrity, 1981; Like & Zyzanski, 1987), the findings have clear implications for occupational therapists. One of the important factors in a cultural assessment is the language (both verbal and nonverbal) available to describe and express problems and distress. Far more important than the specific language or dialect spoken is the ability of patients and clients to communicate their distress. Some people do not have a sophisticated command of vocabulary to describe the problems that they are experiencing. For example, they may not be able to characterize muscles as ''stiff'' versus ''sore''; their muscles just ''hurt.'' The elderly often have difficulty articulating the problem, and when faced with questions from the therapist calling for a yes or no answer (e.g., ''Is the joint inflamed?''), they may answer arbitrarily or give the answer they believe the therapist wants to hear. Communicating about psychosocial problems is particularly difficult for some people. As noted previously, psychiatric problems may be highly stigmatized, and people may go to great lengths to avoid being considered psychiatrically disabled, for example, the phrase ''just a case of nerves'' has subsumed a variety of symptoms ranging from anxiety and depression to agitation and loss of contact with reality.

Communication involves more than the accurate translation of words. Language shapes thought (Ellmer & Olbrisch, 1983). Because various cultures with different languages perceive illness or disability in different ways, an understanding of their perspective is important. This directly influences information-gathering and establishment of rapport and may contribute to misdiagnosis and ineffective treatment. For instance, in some cultures lack of comprehension means losing face, so people would rather risk giving the wrong response than to admit that they do not understand the terms, such as *passing water* or *incontinence.* Therapists may find this kind of communication barrier common in working with older immigrants.

There are a number of other culturally based communication problems. The excessive use of complex medical terminology or unfamiliar labels may be a barrier to communication. A therapist noting ''dysfunction in the volitional subsystem or in the executive function of initiation'' may mystify parents who say that their brain-injured child ''just isn't motivated.'' There is also ample opportunity for miscommunication when people use the same word, but have different understandings of it. A person who has recently been diagnosed as having rheumatoid arthritis may view *rest* as something to do only when he or she is too sick to continue, but in the therapeutic sense *rest* may be a part of the treatment regime even when the person is feeling well.

In addition, it is critical for therapists to ensure that they understand a patient's or client's nonverbal communication. Areas that may be particularly important to the occupational therapist are how much personal space patients or clients are accustomed to, if and when a comforting touch is appropriate, and whether direct eye contact is important. Communication problems may also surround the use of humor and the amount of small talk that is necessary at the beginning of each therapy session. Members of many cultural groups need a prescribed period of social conversation before they embark on the real communication. An efficient, time-conscious therapist may miss such subtleties and jeopardize the therapeutic relationship.

Perceptions of Occupational Therapy

The cultural influence on occupational therapy can also be seen in a patient's or client's perceptions of health care providers. An example is people's responding more positively to someone wearing a white medical or lab coat than to someone not in clinical attire. Discrepancies between a patient's or client's expectation of the caregiver and the caregiver's actual performance may influence the degree to which the patient or the client continues to use services (Ellmer & Olbrisch, 1983). This is particularly important in occupational therapy where the word *occupation* is misleading to many people, who expect vocational specialists. People also favor treatments or labels that match their own views. Again, this may present a problem in occupational therapy practice because highly therapeutic activities often appear deceptively simple, especially in comparison with the high technology used in other health fields. Thus a person recovering from a stroke who has just completed a biofeedback muscle reeducation program may have difficulty accepting that sanding a cutting board works toward the same goals as biofeedback.

Another characteristic of the treatment situation that is influenced by culture is whether decisions are made individually or collectively. For example, many health care providers expect patients and clients to make autonomous, on-the-spot decisions (Mechanic, 1978). This creates conflict for members of some cultural groups because they are accustomed to the family making decisions about something as important as health care issues. Without an opportunity to consult with others, they may feel anxiety or be ill prepared to make a considered decision, particularly if it may affect other family members. The degree of family support itself is a cultural factor.

Folk Illnesses

A prominent subject in the medical anthropology literature is folk or cultural illnesses. These are defined as illnesses specific to a particular group, for which their culture includes an etiological explanation, a diagnosis, and intervention or prevention strategies. These unique symptoms and signs often have a symbolic, moral, or social meaning in the culture. Folk illnesses are considered to be culture-bound in that they are a unique disorder recognized mainly by members of a particular culture and generally have no counterpart. Several such illnesses have been identified by anthropologists and health care personnel. An example described by Good (1977) is *narahaitiye qalb*, or "heart distress." Found in Iran, this illness usually manifests itself in a pounding of the heart linked with anxiety and unhappiness. The symptoms appear after quarrels, childbirth, death, or the use of contraceptives. Like *narahaitiye qalb*, folk illnesses often link an individual illness with wider concerns such as the ill person's position or role in the family or community, or supernatural forces (Helman, 1984).

A folk illness found among Hispanic Americans is *susto*, or "magical fright." Clinically, *susto* includes depression, listlessness, restless sleep, and loss of appetite. The etiology is based on the idea that each person has one or more immaterial souls that may become detached from the body. This may be attributed to a sudden fright or the soul's being "stolen" by spirit guardians of the earth for deliberate or unintentional transgressions. The soul is held captive until the individual has atoned, often through employment of a *curandiero,* or folk healer. The folk healer coaxes the soul back into the body with various remedies. A number of epidemiological factors are associated with *susto,* including stressful social relationships and unmet social expectations (Rubel, 1977).

Although most folk illnesses are rare in North America, with increasing immigration, it is possible to encounter a folk illness in occupational therapy practice. Even if therapists do not have frequent contact with this type of illness, knowing about it is important to the understanding of culture because it is an obvious example of the transmission of culture. That is, a child learns to respond to and express certain symptoms in a culturally patterned manner. He or she learns to identify the folk illness in family and friends and then in himself or herself. Folk illnesses are also one of the most obvious and often one of the most sensational means of seeing the interaction between culture and disability and illness.

SOCIAL SCIENCE CONCEPTS USEFUL IN PRACTICE

This section addresses four social science concepts that can help the therapist assess and plan interventions around the unique culture of the patient or the client. These concepts were chosen because they illustrate ways in which individuals and cultural groups differ in matters pertinent to the practice of occupational therapy, and because they illustrate how occupational therapists can practically address the culture of the individual patient or client. The concepts are considered in terms of both treatment of individuals and, more broadly, occupational therapy service delivery.

Illness and Disease

One principle that highlights the importance of culture in working with people who have disabilities is the distinction between illness and disease (Kleinman, 1978). **Disease,** with its biological connotation, refers to abnormalities of structure and function in body organs and systems. It is a deviation from the norm of measurable biological variables and, as such, has been objectified and divorced from social and environmental contexts (Parry, 1984). Disease is what scientists study. **Illness** describes what people experience: devalued changes in being and in social function (Kleinman, 1978). Illness encompasses personal, interpersonal, and cultural reactions to sickness—how one is socialized to react to pain and how one expresses discomfort, for example. The experience of illness can also be based on social position, on previous illnesses, and on one's attitudes about certain labels or diagnoses. An important illustration of this is the practitioner's labeling an illness as psychological or psychosomatic when the patient believes the problem has an organic cause.

There is often a discrepancy between disease as conceptualized by practitioners and illness as experienced by patients and clients. Health professionals manage disease, whereas disabled people and concerned others manage illness. Disease focuses on the individual, whereas illness takes in the social relationship determinants. Disease-related problems identified by the therapist might be decreased range of motion in the shoulder girdle or inability to cross midline. Illness-related problems might include dependence on family and loneliness.

Another way of considering illness and disease is that there may be illness without disease. In this situation a person may feel that something is wrong physically, emotionally, and sometimes socially, but after examination by a health care professional is told that nothing is wrong, that there is *no* disease. A number of situations fall into this group: unpleasant emotions or physical symptoms for which no organic cause can be found, psychosomatic disorders (irritable bowel, hyperventilation syndrome), hypochondria, and some of the folk illnesses described in the preceding section (Helman, 1984).

Similarly there may be disease without illness. Physical abnormalities may be found on the chemical or cellular level, but the individuals experiencing the abnormalities (who do not consider themselves to be patients) may not feel ill. Common examples are hypertension, raised blood cholesterol, and some types of cancer. This situation often leads to noncompliance because the experience of the *patient* does not match the opinion of the clinician.

Health professionals have been systematically inattentive to the illness aspect of disability. This is in part responsible for noncompliance, patient and family dissatisfaction with health care, and inadequate clinical care (Kleinman, Eisenberg, & Good, 1978). Although occupational therapy philosophy is patient- or client-centered and holistic, the realities of practice often force therapists to deal with problems of disease. For example, in determining treatment priorities, therapists often address the more biomedically pressing issues even if patients or clients perceive another issue as more problematic. That is, what is important to the therapist may not concern the patient or the client. Case Studies 4-3 and 4-4 offer illustrations here.

Case Study 4-3

Different Definitions of Independence: Dennis suffered a spinal cord fracture in an ice hockey accident, which left him quadriplegic. After intensive rehabilitation he was discharged to his apartment with community rehabilitation support. Leslie, the occupational therapist, encouraged him to maintain the independent dressing and hygiene skills that he had mastered while in the hospital. However, after one month at home Dennis no longer seemed interested in independence in his morning routine and had a friend coming in every morning to help him. He also began talking about hiring an attendant to help him for four hours each morning on a permanent basis. On one home visit Leslie noticed that several hundred dollars worth of activities-of-daily-living aids were shoved in the back of a closet, apparently never used. Checking the kitchen on several occasions, she consistently found the refrigerator bare, with the exception of cold pizza and take-out Chinese food.

Leslie was concerned that Dennis was losing his independence, and she considered a readmission to the rehabilitation hospital to help him regain his skills. In reassessing him, however, she found that he could, in fact, still perform all the independent living skills; but he was choosing not to use them. As he explained, having help in the morning spared him two hours of time and energy, not to mention frustration. This freed him to look for work—a tough task. He said that he would feel more independent receiving a paycheck than showering by himself. Although his meals were not always nutritious, ordering in saved effort. Moreover, he was never a cook before his accident and had no interest in being one now.

The major goal of occupational therapy is to help patients and clients reach the highest level of independence possible. The culture of the individual influences this goal in terms of variations in people's definitions of independence. Therapists must be sensitive to the fact that the rehabilitation profession's definition of independence may not match that of the patient or the client or that of the independent living movement.

Case Study 4-4

The Human Side of Patienthood: As a result of a serious car accident, Marilyn sustained a severe closed head injury and multiple leg fractures, necessitating 12 months of inpatient occupational therapy and another six months of daily outpatient therapy. On the basis of a functional cognitive assessment, Marilyn's therapist recommended that she attend outpatient therapy for at least another three months. This recommendation was supported by the psychologist, who suggested that Marilyn's deficits could be addressed by a computerized cognitive retraining program. The two professionals agreed that Marilyn had excellent addressed by a computerized cognitive retraining program. The two professionals agreed that Marilyn had excellent potential, and they were looking forward to working with her in this next step of the therapy program.

On first hearing the plan, Marilyn's mother disagreed with it, insisting that Marilyn had had enough therapy. Not until the physician was called in to discuss her resistance did the mother reluctantly agree.

Over the next month, Marilyn missed seven sessions and was late almost every day. A conference was held to discuss Marilyn's and her mother's attitudes. The therapist discovered that they were both "sick to death" of going to the hospital, where they had spent almost every day of the past two years. Moreover, Marilyn was depressed by "all those stroke people who hang around occupational therapy" and had to be dragged to each therapy session by her mother. Most important, Marilyn's mother felt that it would be more beneficial for her daughter to be in a healthy environment with people her own age than in a place full of sick people. When these perceptions of illness were revealed, a plan was developed for Marilyn to attend a special school program and receive cognitive retraining in that setting.

Had the therapist been sensitive to, and based treatment decisions on, the illness experienced by Marilyn and her mother rather than on the disease data, therapy would have been more successful, and everyone involved would have been less frustrated and more satisfied with treatment.

Translating this point into occupational therapy practice means that therapists should be sensitive to patients' or clients' interpretation of their disability or illness and the implications for therapy. If patients or clients do not perceive the intervention strategy as helping their problems, motivation and compliance will decrease. The authors have sometimes been guilty of neglecting the illness aspect of dysfunction by focusing on exercise as a preventive and promotive occupation. Although research indicates that exercise is therapeutic for any number of disabilities, it may not have a place in the life of a person who values working 12 to 14 hours a day, nor will it be accepted as the treatment of choice.

In addition, patients and clients may be socialized to identify disease-related problems when interacting with health professionals and therefore may report disease symptoms, even though those symptoms may not be the more troublesome ones. For example, in a recent research project dealing with recovery after traumatic brain injury, when the occupational therapist presented herself as such, the disabled people and their families identified the critical problems as double vision, unstable walking, and swallowing difficulties. However, when the therapist represented herself as an anthropologist, they identified problems related to lack of finances, loneliness, and being labeled as retarded.

Probably the most common situation in which this disease-illness dichotomy appears is when the illness-oriented therapist works in a disease-oriented setting. An example is the conflict that was experienced by an occupational therapist working on a multidisciplinary kidney dialysis team in an acute care hospital. The therapist identified the need to provide leisure activity for a patient who was depressed and unmotivated by dialysis. This treatment plan was met with opposition from the other team members, who felt the therapist's job was only to supply a splint to protect the cannula. The illness aspect of supplying a leisure activity was viewed as "unmedical" and a waste of resources.

A broader illustration of therapists working in a disease-driven system can be noted in the fact that occupational therapy on a long-term or outpatient basis is not always funded, and follow-up visits are often considered a luxury. After the acute disease problems are addressed, the more complex and persistent illness problems are not considered sufficiently important to be covered by many medical plans. For a large number of people with disabilities, such as those with brain injuries and those with psychiatric disturbances, the greatest challenges and the greatest need for occupational therapy occur once the hospital doors close behind them.

Explanatory Models

Explanatory models are mental representations that people make about episodes of illness. Explanatory models address what illnesses are, what causes them, and what should be done about them. The models have both cognitive and affective components—knowledge, feelings, and attitudes (Galazka & Eckert, 1986; Helman, 1984). Explanatory models contain information about the etiology of an illness, its timing and mode of onset, its pathophysiological process, its natural history and severity (particularly the prognosis for it), and appropriate treatments and the rationale for them. Explanatory models also encompass ideas about the causes and the effects of illnesses—going outdoors with wet hair causes colds, for instance. Explanatory models of health contain ideas about what health is and what it is not. Each person's idea of what is normal or acceptable is an important part of an explanatory model of a disability. One person who must wear special orthoses and orthopedic shoes may consider himself or herself disabled because of these special adaptations, whereas another may not.

Explanatory models are developed in response to a particular illness episode and are different from general beliefs about illness. Each individual has a repertoire of

Table 4-2
Examples of Questions to Elicit Explanatory Models

What is your problem? What do you call it?

What do you think has caused your problem?

Why do you think this has happened?

Why has it happened to you in particular?

Why has it happened now? Why did it start when it did?

What has changed in your body or mind to cause this?

What do you think your illness does to you? How does it work?

What do you fear most about your illness?

In what ways has your life changed because of this illness?

How bad is your illness?

How long do you think it will last?

What would happen if nothing was done about it?

What should be done about it?

What will happen if this is done? How will your illness change?

What will change in your body or mind?

These questions can be used to discuss changes in the status of a disability or an illness or the development of a new disability or illness.

the "flu is going around," he may think the muscle pain that he previously attributed to arthritis is just the flu.

Explanatory models are partly conscious and partly outside an individual's awareness. They tend to be vague, contradictory, and as just described, dynamic. This elusive quality makes it critical for therapists to assess a patient's or client's explanatory model of an illness or disability episode. Some guiding questions for doing this are presented in Table 4-2. Often, explanatory models do not come to consciousness until an individual is specifically asked about them. Therefore, increasing a person's awareness of them is a therapeutic intervention in its own right.

What is important about explanatory models is that they form the basis of behavior in relation to the illness or the disability. They influence when a person seeks treatment, from whom, whether he or she complies, and whether he or she believes something is truly wrong.

Part of the assessment of explanatory models is determining if the patient or the client recognizes how a particular occupational therapy treatment will influence his or her disability. A clear rationale for each activity is also important—more so in occupational therapy because a ceramic project, adapted games, and kitchen activities do not appear to be treatment in the medical sense.

A common component of explanatory models in people with chronic illnesses is the relationship of stress to exacerbation of symptoms, such as flare-ups of rheumatoid arthritis or multiple sclerosis. Blumhagen's (1980) excellent study also illustrates the stress factor in explanatory models. He discovered that many of the patients explained their condition, which they called "hyper-tension," as arising from the tension or the stress of their daily lives.

Explanatory models are also held by health care professionals and family members. Although professionals' models are usually based on scientific models, they too are inconsistent and dynamic. Even in modern societies one finds an interesting blend of sophisticated scientific ideas and folk wisdom learned from friends or simply through intuition (Mechanic, 1978). If one asks a group of occupational therapists how to get rid of warts, their responses will be far from consistent, and many may be along the lines of "Kiss a frog." A more important inconsistency was revealed when I asked a group of occupational therapists why, and to what extent, purposeful occupation was therapeutic. The basic relationship between well-being and occupation was generally accepted, but the models explaining the relationship varied widely. Much of the current emphasis on research reflects an attempt to find a common explanation for why particular intervention strategies work.

health beliefs based on his or her own illness experiences as well as the illness experiences of others that he or she has observed. This is the background against which every episode is experienced.

Explanatory models are based on past experiences, on information from professionals (that is, the person's interpretation of that information), on media and literature (e.g., television programs with medical themes and *Reader's Digest* articles), and on information passed on by family and friends. Thus, they are strongly influenced by cultural factors.

Explanatory models are not always consistent and often contain contradictory information; for instance, it is important to rest an arthritic joint, but swimming and walking also help. Moreover, explanatory models are dynamic, changing with new information. Thus if a woman suspects that the cause of the pain in her ankle is a torn ligament, but she is sent to a rheumatologist, her explanatory model may quickly change to arthritis. Or if a man, in describing symptoms to his neighbor, is told that

An earlier section of this chapter describes the influence of culture on communication between professionals, patients or clients, and family. Incompatibility of explanatory models is one result of ignoring the cultural aspect of the patient or the client. Professionals and lay people differ greatly in their understandings of a particular illness episode, especially in etiology, labeling or diagnosis, and treatment. For example, most health care professionals focus on quantifiable data and do not take into consideration supernatural or interpersonal explanations of illness—that the illness is a lesson from God, for instance. Further, most people with a disease orientation do not consider the moral, social, or psychological contexts of the problems. Thus an essential part of therapy is to negotiate explanatory models to ensure that everyone on the team, including the patient or client and family, comes to a common understanding about the problem and its treatment. The necessity of this common understanding was made clear to me while working with a young man who was described by the family as neurotic, by the family physician as malingering, by the school teacher as lazy, and by the neuropsychologist as mildly brain injured.

Explanatory models can be incorporated directly into treatment. If the patient's or client's model is not consistent with the therapist's, intervention might employ components of the patient's or client's model in education programs. One way to do this is to use words or symbols that the person finds important. For example, if he or she says that ''hot blood'' underlies joint inflammation, therapists might use those words to describe inflammation and its treatment. Explanatory models about prognosis in disability and chronic illness are particularly important in therapy. Economic decisions are often affected by inaccurate models. If a family firmly believes that their paraplegic son will walk again, they will not consider environmental modifications of the home. The patient's understanding of prognosis is important regarding return to work. Some people with disabilities do not take the necessary steps to obtain the disability allowance that they require, because of their strong belief that they will soon be well. After two years of trying to return to competitive employment and failing, however, they will face difficulties in applying for disability allowance or financial compensation. At the other end of the spectrum, people who believe that their illness is so disabling that they will never return to work will only frustrate, and be frustrated by, the therapist's persistent attempts at vocational assessment.

Cultural Definitions of Anatomy and Physiology

People have many notions about their body. Most of the notions are acquired as part of growing up in a particular family and society, thus the influence of culture is obvious. These ideas, sometimes referred to as *ethnoanatomy* and *ethnophysiology*, are special, critical components of explanatory models. General explanatory models of a particular episode contain patients' or clients' appraisals of symptoms, assumptions about causes, and responses to professional advice. This is influenced by their theories of the body: ideal size, shape, and appearance (important in disfiguring disabilities such as burns), body structure, and body functions (Helman, 1984).

Of particular importance to the general practice of occupational therapy are the latter two ideas. Cultural notions about body structure have a commonality in that most people have very little concrete knowledge of anatomy. Bits of information are gleaned from advertisements for medicines in popular magazines, remarks from television shows or documentary programs featuring various illnesses or body systems, or the diagram on the running-shoe box. Many ideas are developed simply through speculation and theorizing, thus people may think the bladder and the gall bladder are connected functionally because their names are similar. Like explanatory models, these ideas are not static and often change with age and illness history. One person may claim to know the anatomy of the knee intimately after two ligament repairs. Another may describe intervertebral discs as 10 inches in diameter to correspond to the amount of pain experienced. As these examples suggest, the importance of ethnoanatomy is that it influences people's perceptions and presentations of problems.

In Helman's (1984) view, although beliefs about the body's structure can have clinical importance, beliefs about how it functions are probably more significant in their effect on people's behavior. He describes *ethnophysiology* as dealing with one or more aspects of the body, including inner workings; outside influences on inner workings, such as diet, exercise, and environment; and nature and disposal of the by-products of the body's functioning, for example, urine and menstrual blood.

There are a number of lay models of ethnophysiology. Two are pertinent to occupational therapy: (1) *the body as a machine*, and (2) *balance and imbalance*. The machine model is based on the idea that the body is like a battery-driven machine or an engine. A major implication is that fuel or energy is needed to drive it, for example, tonics or vitamins for *recharging* or special foods that are the right fuel. The machine model includes the notion that the body (like a bicycle or a car) consists of separate parts and that they may fail and need replacing. The notion has been reinforced by widespread use of medical transplants, such as organ transplants, implantation of pacemakers, and hip replacements. This is seen as substituting the new for the old. One of the negative aspects of the machine model is that people begin to view everything as replaceable (like the cornea or the femur head) and to believe that after surgery they will be "as good as new." The model has contributed to overuse and abuse of body parts that are nonreplaceable or at least not easily replaceable, such as the lungs, the liver, and joint surfaces.

The machine model is also reflected in ideas about aging. Many people subscribe to the wear-and-tear notion that body parts wear down just as washing-machine parts do, and that the pains accompanying aging are a result of this and are to be expected.

The *balance-and-imbalance model* of physiology suggests that the healthy working of the body depends on a harmonious balance between two or more elements or forces within it. The balance can be affected by internal conditions, such as one's emotional state or the number of hours of sleep the night before; by the external environment, such as diet and weather; and by supernatural causes, such as divine punishment for moral transgressions. One of the best examples is the hot-cold model of illness that is common in many Latin American and Asian cultures. In this model, health is controlled by the effects of heat or cold on the body. Heat and cold do not pertain to actual temperatures, but to the symbolic power in most substances, such as food, herbs, and cloth. Further, mental states and personal temperaments are grouped into hot and cold categories.

On the basis of this ethnophysiological model, patients or clients may ask for certain foods or treatments that they believe will help restore their balance. For instance, some Hispanics believe that cilantro will "cool" an infection, as will white foods such as yogurt. In addition, the color of pills and medicines is critical. If joints are hot and swollen, anti-inflammatories in cooling colors need to be prescribed.

Perceptions of anatomy and physiology do not always reflect scientific tenets and may in fact contradict biomedical knowledge. Such models are most common in disabilities that are not logical, for example, a foot that drops because of a burst vessel in the brain. An ethnophysiological model can actually be harmful to a patient or a client, as illustrated in Case Study 4-5. It is therefore important that therapists assess people's ideas about anatomy and physiology related to their illness and their notions about the effect of occupational therapy intervention.

Case Study 4-5

An Ethnophysiological Model of Muscle Activity: Jane, a 20-year-old woman, suffered multiple injuries in a sports accident. After several months of intensive rehabilitation,

she was discharged to her parents' home. Among her residual problems was an extremely spastic left arm. Her mother attended every therapy session while Jane was in the hospital and carried on therapy programs at home. Jane's father worked long hours during the day, but he visited her nearly every evening in the hospital. Once she was home, he helped with her evening exercise program to give Jane's mother time on her own.

In the first weeks after discharge, Jane seemed to be making slow but steady progress in all areas, except that the spasticity in her arm was increasing and she was very severely fatigued in the evenings. Jane's mother contacted the therapist at the rehabilitation hospital, who made a home visit when both parents were present. Asked about the nature of the evening exercise, Jane's father proudly described the "muscle building" program he had developed for Jane. He had reasoned that if muscles were not working, then they were not sufficiently built up, and that if weight lifters did repeated exercises with heavy weights to develop their muscles, Jane's arm muscle would benefit from the same sort of activity. He saw himself as Jane's coach and was encouraging her to work with homemade weights until she could no longer lift them.

Jane's father held a "jock" model of muscle activity, appropriate to normal and weak muscles, but not to those with spasticity. His ethnophysiological ideas were based on watching weight lifting on television and reading sports magazines. Although he was well intentioned, he was fostering disability behavior that was countertherapeutic.

Patterns of Help-Seeking

Patterns of help-seeking are the culturally distinct ways in which people go about finding help at particular times in an illness. **Help-seeking** refers to both how many alternatives are open to a person and how and why the person makes choices among various alternatives. Although many studies of help-seeking have been conducted, the majority focus on the professional health care network, such as physicians and public health clinics. However, people seek help for physical and psychological problems from a variety of other sources—families, friends, pharmacists, naturopaths, and so on.

To assess patterns of help-seeking accurately, therapists must be aware of the concept of pluralism in health care in general and in rehabilitation in particular. That is, many models of health care are open to patients and clients; therapists should not assume that theirs is the only alternative possible. One commonly accepted typology of health care alternatives describes three sectors of help: the biomedical, the popular, and the traditional (Kleinman, 1980). The biomedical system is the predominant one and the one within which most therapists work. It is defined by the well-organized, legally sanctioned healing professions. The biomedical system is physician-centered and specialty-

The biomedical system is physician-centered and specialty-oriented. Currently it is based on technological diagnosis rather than clinical evaluation.

The popular sector comprises alternatives that are not officially sanctioned (as those in the biomedical sector are), but do not directly contradict the predominant sector. Both professionals and lay people work in this sector. Although not directly contradictory of biomedical options, the options in the popular sector are materially or behaviorally divergent. Popular alternatives include self-treatment or self-medication, advice or treatment from a neighbor or a friend, self-help groups, and consultation with a nonmedical person who has special experience with a particular disorder or treatment. Helman (1984) identifies a number of sources of help in the popular sector, including paramedical personnel (e.g., medical receptionists and pharmacists) who are consulted informally and relatives or spouses of physicians. Their credentials are mainly based on experience rather than on specialist training. For example, the first author has never practiced as a therapist in the field of rheumatology, but because of her own personal experience with arthritis, she has been a popular health care resource for friends who suffer from joint pain.

Despite the variety of alternatives in the popular health care sector, it largely revolves around women, who are the customary caregivers in almost all societies, and the major focus of diagnosis and treatment is the family. One study found that 70 to 90 percent of health care took place within the popular sector, in both Western and non-Western countries (Kleinman, Eisenberg, & Good, 1978). The increasing visibility of this sector can be seen in a recent move by some American states to license pharmacists to both prescribe and dispense drugs (Selya, 1988).

An important characteristic of the popular health sector is that it is related to health maintenance, an activity as critical to people with disabilities or chronic illnesses as to healthy people. Each culture has guidelines for remaining healthy or minimizing the effects of a long-standing illness. These include beliefs about healthy eating, sleeping, and spirituality, among others. A belief implicit in occupational therapy is the importance of balancing work and leisure. This largely reflects a Western approach to health.

The third health care sector identified by Helman is of a traditional or folk nature that is usually seen as unorthodox and often in conflict with the principles of the biomedical sector. Examples include faith healing, herbalism, and reflexology. Folk practitioners often do not have a written medical tradition such as textbooks, nor is their knowledge systematized. Generally they have little formal training. Their skills are usually acquired through apprenticeship to an older folk healer. Many claim to have been born with a "healing power."

The folk sector is especially common in developing countries, where ill health is attributed to social causes (witchcraft, the evil eye, etc.) or supernatural forces (God, spirits, ghosts, etc.). Folk practitioners usually take a broad approach to illness and treat the person, the social environment, and the supernatural. The family is typically very involved in the diagnosis and the treatment of an ill person. In many of the healing rites, the reactions of the family as well as the ill person are considered. An interesting example of a folk-sector resource is *injectors*. These people usually have only the briefest experience with health care, perhaps as the driver for a local doctor, but possess extraordinary interpersonal and counseling skills. Their entire practice consists of *injecting* people with drugs (or in some cases colored water) to cure almost any illness.

The relationships between healers in the three sectors tend to be mistrusting (Helman, 1984). People in the biomedical sector see folk healers as quacks and view popular healers as "unqualified pseudoprofessionals who make people sicker rather than better."

In countries with few biomedical resources, governments are supporting popular and traditional methods. This support is evident in the World Health Organization campaign to enlist traditional birth attendants, herbalists, and the like in geographic areas where medical services are scarce. [The inequity in distribution of health care resources is evident when one compares ratios of physicians to people in developed and developing countries. For instance, in the United States in 1980 there were 595 people per physician, compared with 73,043 people per physician in Ethiopia (WHO, 1980).]

Complicating the picture even further is the fact that some practitioners do not fit neatly into the three-sector typology. For instance, acupuncture and chiropractic are becoming more acceptable and are often undertaken by practitioners who are also trained in the biomedical system.

A study by Lin, Tardiff, Donetz, and Goresky (1978) illustrates the importance of cultural background in patterns of help-seeking. These researchers focused on a sample of psychiatric patients with mixed cultural background in an urban North American setting. They noted that people of Chinese background tolerated even advanced psychotic symptoms in the home, and that when they sought help, it was for physical symptoms. Anglo-Saxon and European people revealed a different set of values. Although the families were involved in caring for the psychiatric patient, they contacted social, mental health, and health agencies early in the illness. A third pattern was noted among Native Americans, who showed neither the family solidarity of the Chinese nor the use of social and health services of the Anglo-Saxons and Europeans. Having no sociocultural support system, they appeared in treatment only in crisis and were passively passed among help-giving agencies.

The concept of help-seeking has a number of practical implications for occupational therapy assessment and intervention. First, the patient's or client's history of help-seeking (including perceived importance and success of each alternative) should be a part of any comprehensive assessment. Eliciting people's thoughts and feelings about the popular and traditional sectors is often difficult because they may be reluctant to disclose nonmedical or unsophisticated sources of help, despite using them. A way for therapists to facilitate this is to convey an accepting attitude about the range of alternatives, perhaps by introducing the topic with a comment about the number of people they see in therapy who use nonmedical options. Giving personal examples, such as experience with acupuncture and herbal remedies, can encourage people to reveal their patterns of help-seeking.

People are more likely to have used popular and traditional health alternatives if few biomedical services are available. This is especially relevant in the case of long-term or degenerative disabilities—chronic mental illness, dementia, amyotrophic lateral sclerosis, for example. Out of sheer desperation people will engage in folk and popular options, often more than one at a time. Unfortunately some of these people may become involved with charlatans who are more interested in making money than in the ill person's welfare.

When options from different sectors are used simultaneously or consecutively, considering help-seeking patterns is critical because the alternatives might conflict with the occupational therapy assessment and intervention. For example, if an herbalist advocates fasting for a condition that the occupational therapist is treating as a low-energy problem, the therapist's recommendation to eat healthy meals three times a day may create tension or anxiety for the patient or the client, or it may be disregarded. In some situations, occupational therapy can build on other sources of help to increase the therapeutic effect—for instance, by incorporating foods suggested by a naturopath into occupational therapy cooking sessions or by preceding occupational therapy treatment sessions with meditation or T'ai Chi exercises. Likely the most common overlap in patterns of help-seeking is between occupational therapy treatment and support provided by the family. An example is the therapist working on a self-feeding program for an older man while his family members feed him every evening and weekend.

In addition to looking at where patients and clients go for help, it is important to consider when they seek assistance. Because disability is often a lifelong proposition, people seek help for problems intermittently over many years.

Also, with degenerative illnesses new problems arise. An example is the timing of vocational services for people with brain injury. Because they experience a protracted and often unpredictable recovery, patients or clients may seek prevocational assessment or vocational services several years after the injury, long after their case is "closed." Getting back into the rehabilitation system when they are best prepared to make use of the resources can be difficult.

From a broader perspective, rehabilitation services are largely based on the acute care, institutional model, in which services are concentrated in the period immediately following the initial diagnosis. Often patients or clients find themselves on a "conveyor belt" of services, moving from acute care, to a rehabilitation hospital, to outpatient status. They may not consider what to do next because "that's the way all multiple sclerosis treatment programs go." There is rarely any mechanism to go backward on the conveyor belt—for example, to return to rehabilitation for intensive treatment after discharge. People are expected to follow the accepted pattern of use; if they do not, they are seen as noncompliant.

A concept closely linked to help-seeking behavior is the *therapeutic management group*. The therapeutic management group consists of individuals who take charge of decisions about an illness along with, or on behalf of, the sufferer (Helman, 1984). These decisions include diagnosis of illness, selection of helping alternatives, evaluation of whether the therapeutic alternative is working, and support of the ill person. Two aspects of the therapeutic management group are important. The first is the *identity of the people involved*. A therapeutic management group might include immediate family members such as parents, spouse, or children; a neighbor who has some health care background; an attorney (when disability payments are involved); and great Aunt Gertrude, the family matriarch. The occupational therapist's advice is considered by the members of the therapeutic management group, but the therapist is not part of the group, nor is his or her opinion necessarily the most powerful in the decision-making process. Therapeutic management groups illustrate the power structure in the social network of the patient or the client; that is, who is most powerful in terms of decision-making.

The second important aspect of the therapeutic management group is the *decision-making process*. This might include the style of decision-making (authoritarian vs. consensus), the number of people involved in the decision, the role of the patient or the client (whether he or she has much say), and the degree to which professionals are consulted.

Therapists often assume that unless the patient or the client is a child or is mentally incompetent, he or she makes all of the decisions. This is not always the case, and failures in therapy may result from dealing with the wrong player. An example of what can occur if the therapeutic management group is not identified and consulted, is ineffective discharge planning. The therapist and a female patient develop an ambitious program of outpatient therapy that requires transport to the hospital five days a week. The most powerful voice in the therapeutic management group, however, is the husband, who vetoes the idea because it will tie up the family car. Therefore, asking questions about who is involved in making health care decisions and how they are made is important. A good way to do this is to use a previous health care problem as an example and have the patient or the client talk about the decisions that were necessary. This aspect of the occupational therapy assessment fits well into the family section of an evaluation.

Although questions about health care decision-making should be included in all initial assessments, they are especially important when major health care decisions are being made, such as placement in a long-term care facility or high-risk surgery. They are most obviously important when mental competency is an issue, such as with Alzheimer's disease, psychosis, or severe brain damage.

Case Study 4-6

Cultural Differences in the Concept of Time: Karen, a new occupational therapy graduate, was one of two therapists in a small hospital located in an agricultural district. A number of Karen's patients were farmers, many of them Native Americans living on a reservation about 20 miles from town. Although Karen had always lived in a big city, she was enjoying small-town life, and her work was very satisfying, with the exception of case management. Somehow her patients never seemed to get to their appointments on time. It was not that they did not show up, but that they appeared whenever it was convenient for them. Not only were they late, but more often than not, they arrived with a relative or two who also had some sort of health problem with which Karen would be asked to help. This was a terrific frustration for Karen, who had been voted the most organized and efficient student in her year by her classmates. She had tried telephone reminders, written reminders, offered a wide choice of appointment times—but still few of them arrived when she expected them.

Finally, thinking she had nothing to lose, Karen began to confront her patients about their inability to attend on time. They explained they had to work when the weather was fair and came to town when it was foul or when they finished their work. As for the nonfarmers, they seemed concerned that she was frustrated, but came late for their next appointment anyway.

The term *Indian time* or *rubber time* is used in many areas of the world to describe being perpetually late. Although most North Americans view it negatively as disregard for custom, cultural differences in the concept of time are well documented. In this case, Karen was faced with a disjuncture between her own culturally defined ideas about promptness and her patients' sense of time.

SUMMARY

The purpose of this chapter is to sensitize therapists to the influence of culture on human performance. Although culture has been acknowledged as important in understanding human performance, the concept has not been developed to the point that it is meaningful in daily practice.

Culture is a system of learned patterns of behavior shared by members of a group that provides them with effective mechanisms for interaction. It can be represented as a series of concentric circles signaling different dimensions or levels: region, community, family, and individual. Therapists must use the definition at the individual level to assess the unique cultural identity of each patient or client.

Some of the ways in which culture can affect assessment and intervention are the shaping of disability behavior, definition of disability, communication between the therapist and the patient or the client, and the patient's or client's perception of therapy. By neglecting culture, the therapist diminishes the effectiveness of therapy. Inattention to the cultural identity of the patient or the client can result in lack of rapport and communication problems that can lead to noncompliance and dissatisfaction with occupational therapy and to frustration on the part of the therapist.

Of particular importance to the use of culture in practice is the idea that both the therapist and the patient or the client view the therapeutic endeavor through cultural filters. Therapists should be aware of their own cultural biases and also consider the cultural variation of their patients and clients. With this in mind, they must assess the unique cultural identity of each person and its implications for human performance, and then implement culturally appropriate intervention.

Four social science concepts give therapists specific tools with which to use culture in their daily practice. By assessing illness behavior and exploring explanatory models, particularly ethnoanatomy and ethnophysiology, therapists can make therapy illness-directed rather than disease-directed. The concept of patterns of help-seeking is also directed. The concept of patterns of help-seeking is also useful in providing culturally sensitive intervention.

Study Questions

1. Define the term culture and describe its elements in terms of the concentric-circles model.

2. Describe six ways in which the concept of culture has been used in occupational therapy.

3. What are the potential consequences of ignoring a patient's or client's cultural identity?

4. Describe four areas of practice that can be affected by culture and give an example of each.

5. Identify aspects of your cultural identity that could potentially bias your practice as an occupational therapist.

6. Distinguish between a disease and an illness and describe how a person can have a disease without having an illness, or an illness without having a disease.

7. Define the term explanatory model and describe its component parts.

8. Describe two models of ethnophysiology and give one instance of how they could affect the practice of occupational therapy.

9. Why are patterns of help-seeking important to occupational therapy? Distinguish between the three major health care alternatives.

10. How could the therapeutic management group influence occupational therapy practice?

Recommended Readings

Baer, H.A. (Ed.). (1987). *Encounters with biomedicine: Case studies in medical anthropology*. New York: Gordon and Breach.

Chrisman, N.J., & Maretzi, T.W. (Eds.). (1982). *Clinically applied anthropology: Anthropologists in health science settings*. Boston: R. Reidel.

Janes, C.R., Stall, R., & Gifford, S.M. (Eds.). (1986). *Anthropology and epidemiology: Interdisciplinary approaches to the study of health and disease*. Boston: D. Reidel.

Kleinman, A. (1980). *Patients and healers in the context of culture: An exploration of the borderland between anthropology, medicine, and psychiatry*. Berkeley: University of California Press.

Langness, L., & Levine, H L. (Eds.). (1986). *Culture and retardation*. Boston: D. Reidel.

Lock, M., & Gordon, D. (Eds). (1988). *Biomedicine examined*. Boston: Kluwer Academic Publishers.

Myerhoff, B. (1978). *Number our days*. New York: Simon & Schuster.

Schneider, J.W., & Conrad, P. (1983). *Having epilepsy: The experience and control of illness*. Philadelphia: Temple University Press.

References

Adair, J., & Deuschle, K. (1970). *The people's health: Medicine and anthropology in a Navajo community*. New York: Appleton-Century-Crofts.

Barris, R., Kielhofner, G., Levine, R., & Neville, A. (1985). Occupation as interaction with the environment. In G. Kielhofner (Ed.), *A model of human occupation: Theory and application* (pp. 42-62). Baltimore: Williams & Wilkins.

Becker, G. (1980). *Growing old in silence: Deaf people in old age*. Berkeley: University of California Press.

Blakeney, A.B. (1987). Appalachian values: Implications for occupational therapists. *Occupational Therapy in Health Care, 4*, 57-72.

Blumhagen, D. (1980). Hyper-tension: A folk illness with a medical name. *Culture, Medicine, and Psychiatry, 4*, 197-227.

Bray, G., & Chamings, P.A. (1983). Rehabilitation in China: Impressions and perspectives. *Journal of Rehabilitation, 49*, 56-60.

Brockett, M. (1987). Cultural variations in Bay Area Functional Performance Evaluation scores—Considerations for occupational therapy. *Canadian Journal of Occupational Therapy, 54*, 195-199.

Brodsky, C.M. (1983). Culture and disability behavior. *Western Journal of Medicine, 139*, 892-899.

Cassel, E.J. (1985). *Talking with patients, Vol. 1, The theory of doctor-patient communication*. Cambridge, MA: MIT Press.

Clarke, M.M. (1983). Cultural context of medical practice. *Western Journal of Medicine, 139*, 806-810.

Ellmer, R., & Olbrisch, M.E. (1983). The contribution of a cultural perspective in understanding and evaluating client satisfaction. *Evaluation and Program Planning, 6*, 275-281.

Estroff, S.E. (1981). *Making it crazy*. Berkeley: University of California Press.

Freeman, J.M. (1979). *Untouchable*. Palo Alto, CA: Stanford University Press.

Galazka, S.S., & Eckert, J.K. (1986). Clinically applied anthropology: Concepts for the family physician. *Journal of Family Practice, 22*, 159-165.

Garrity, T.F. (1981). Medical compliance and the clinician-patient relationship: A review. *Social Science and Medicine, 15E*, 215-222.

Geertz, C. (1973). *The interpretation of cultures*. New York: Basic Books.

Gliedman, J., & Roth, W. (1980). *The unexpected minority: Handicapped children in America*. New York: Harcourt Brace Jovanovich.

Good, B. (1977). The heart of what's the matter: The semantics of illness in Iran. *Culture, Medicine, and Psychiatry, 1*, 25-58.

Gritzer, G., & Arluke, A. (1985). *The making of rehabilitation: A political economy of medical specialization, 1890-1980*. Berkeley: University of California Press.

Gubrium, J.F., & Buckholdt, D.R. (1982). *Describing care: Images and practice in rehabilitation*. Cambridge, MA: Oelgeschlager, Gunn, & Hain.

Hall, E. (1959). The silent language. New York: Doubleday.

Hammerschlag, C.A. (1988). *The dancing healers: A doctor's journey of healing with Native Americans*. San Francisco: Harper & Row.

Hartog, J., & Hartog, E.E. (1983). Cultural aspects of health and illness behaviors in hospitals. *Western Journal of Medicine, 139*, 910-916.

Helman, C. (1984). *Culture, health and illness*. Bristol, England: John Wright and Sons.

Hopkins, H.L., & Tiffany, E.G. (1983). Occupational therapy—A problem-solving process. In H.L. Hopkins & H.D. Smith (Eds.), *Willard and Spackman's Occupational therapy* (6th ed.) (pp. 89-99). Philadelphia: J.B. Lippincott.

Jamison, M. (1985). The interaction of culture and learning: Implications for occupational therapy. *Canadian Journal of Occupational Therapy, 52*, 5-8.

Kaufert, P.L., & Kaufert, J.M. (1984). Methodological and conceptual issues in measuring the long-term impact of disability: The experience of poliomyelitis patients in Manitoba. *Social Science and Medicine, 19*, 609-618.

Keesing, R. (1981). Theories of cultures. In R. Casson (Ed.), *Language, culture, and cognition*. New York: Macmillan.

Kielhofner, G. (1981). An ethnographic study of deinstitutionalized adults: Their community setting and daily experiences. *Occupational Therapy Journal of Research, 1*, 125-142.

Kleinman, A. (1978). Lessons from a clinical approach to medical anthropological research. *Medical Anthropology Newsletter, 8*, 11-15.

Kleinman, A. (1980). *Patients and healers in the context of culture: An exploration of the borderland between anthropology, medicine, and psychiatry*. Berkeley: University of California Press.

Kleinman, A. (1986). *Social origins of distress and disease: Depression, neurasthenia, and pain in modern China*. New Haven, CT: Yale University Press.

Kleinman, A., Eisenberg, L., & Good, B. (1978). Culture, illness, and care: Clinical lessons from anthropologic and cross-cultural research. *Annals of Internal Medicine, 88*, 251-258.

Krefting, L. (1989). Community re-integration after head injury: The results of a disability ethnography. *Occupational Therapy Journal of Research, 9*, 67-83.

Kroeber, A.L., & Kluckholn, C. (1963). *Culture: A critical review*. New York: Vintage Books.

Levine, R.E. (1984). The cultural aspects of home care delivery. *American Journal of Occupational Therapy, 38*, 734-738.

Levine, R.E. (1987). Culture: A factor influencing the outcome of occupational therapy. *Occupational Therapy in Health Care, 4*, 3-16.

Like, R., & Zyzanski, S.J. (1987). Patient satisfaction with the clinical encounter: Social psychological determinants. *Social Science and Medicine, 24*, 351-357.

Lin, T., Tardiff, K., Donetx, G., & Gorsky, W. (1978). Ethnicity and patterns of help-seeking. *Culture, Medicine, and Psychiatry, 2*, 3-13.

Lindsay, J. (1971). The injured workman—Do cultural influences affect his rehabilitation? *Canadian Journal of Occupational Therapy, 38*, 15-19.

Litterst, T.A.E. (1985). A reappraisal of anthropological fieldwork methods and the concept of culture in occupational therapy research. *American Journal of Occupational Therapy, 39*, 602-604.

Locker, D. (1983). *Disability and disadvantage: The consequence of chronic illness*. London: Tavistock.

McCormack, G.L. (1987). Culture and communication in the treatment planning for occupational therapy with minority patients. *Occupational Therapy in Health Care, 4*, 17-36.

Mead, M. (1923). *Coming of age in Samoa*. New York: William Morrow.

Mechanic, D. (1978). *Medical sociology*. New York: Free Press.

Mechanic, D. (1986). The concept of illness behavior: Culture, situation, and personal predisposition. *Psychological Medicine, 16*, 1-7.

Miller, L.J. (1982). *Miller assessment for preschoolers.*

Littleton, CO: Foundation for Knowledge in Development.

Morse, A. (1987). A cultural intervention model for developmentally disabled adults: An expanded role for occupational therapy. *Occupational Therapy in Health Care, 4,* 103-113.

Parry, K.K. (1984). Concepts from medical anthropology for clinicians. *Physical Therapy, 64,* 929-933.

Peacock, J.L. (1986). *The anthropological lens: Harsh light, soft focus.* London: Cambridge University Press.

Reed, K., & Sanderson, S.R. (1980). *Concepts of occupational therapy.* Baltimore: Williams & Wilkins.

Robinson, L. (1987). Patient compliance in occupational therapy home health programs: Sociocultural considerations. *Occupational Therapy in Health Care, 4,* 127-137.

Roth, J.A., & Eddy, E.M. (1967). *Rehabilitation for the unwanted.* New York: Atherton Press.

Rubel, A. (1977). The epidemiology of folk illness: Susto in Hispanic America. In D. Landy (Ed.), *Culture, disease, and healing: Studies in medical anthropology* (pp. 119-128). New York: Macmillan.

Sapir, E. (1917). Do we need a super-organic? *American Anthropologist, 19,* 441-447.

Selya, R. M. (1988). Pharmacies as alternative sources of medical care: The case of Cincinnati. *Social Science and Medicine, 26,* 409-416.

Shawski, K. A. (1987). Ethnic/racial considerations in occupational therapy. *Occupational Therapy in Health Care, 4,* 37-49.

Tylor, E. (1958). *Primitive culture.* New York: Harper & Row (Original work published 1871).

Wieringa, N., & McColl, M. (1987). Implications of the model of human occupation for intervention with native Canadians. *Occupational Therapy in Health Care, 4,* 73-91.

Williams, G. (1987). Disablement and social context of daily activity. *International Disability Studies, 9,* 97-102.

World Health Organization. (1980). Health personnel and hospital establishments. In *World Health Statistics Annual.* Geneva: World Health Organization.

Zborowski, M. (1969). *People in pain.* San Francisco: Jossey-Bass.

Zola, I. K. (1966). Culture and symptoms: Analysis of patients presenting complaints. *American Sociology Review, 31,* 615-630.

CHAPTER CONTENT OUTLINE

KEY TERMS

Archetypal places

Behavior setting

Cognitive complexity

Cultural style

Environmental press

Mobility sphere

Proxemics

Resource environment

Schema theory

Stimulus-arousal properties

Symbolic associations

ABSTRACT

This chapter examines several components of the physical environment that influence performance, including the design of spaces (interiors and furnishings), design of tools and equipment, environmental protection and management of risk factors, behavior settings, and the interaction that must take place between the person and the environment in order for adaptation to occur. Several key studies of various methods and perspectives are presented to help examine the integrated human behavior patterns within the occupational settings that are of major concern to occupational therapists, including home environments, play environments, work environments, neighborhoods, and institutional environments.

The Physical Environment and Performance

5

Jean Cole Spencer

"With no particular knowledge of disabled people, the designer might conclude that accessible housing is housing (such persons) can get in and out of. If he turns to the design manuals that discuss accommodation of disabled people, he may also decide that it involves the dimensioning and arrangement of the house. This definition allows the disabled person to move in and around his dwelling, but it fails to convey a sense of what he does there. It lacks any feeling for the everyday life of disabled people, seeing them instead as abstractions or as extensions of the designer or people like him."

—Lifchez & Winslow, 1979

OBJECTIVES

The information in this chapter is intended to help the reader—

1. describe alternative ways of looking at physical environments that have emerged within various disciplines.

2. define key concepts from these disciplines that are useful to occupational therapists.

3. identify specific features of physical environments that influence intrinsic human performance factors.

4. describe studies of various kinds of occupational settings that illustrate application of the key concepts in practical daily situations.

5. describe alternative methods for conducting research on the effects of physical environments on human performance.

INTRODUCTION

This chapter examines physical environments to identify specific features that have been shown to affect various domains of human performance. Considering physical environments in isolation, apart from their close relationship to the social and cultural meanings that humans attach to physical objects and settings, is difficult. Often all of these features together shape individual behavior, social interaction, and complex activity patterns within a setting. For example, the physical arrangement of chairs in a waiting room can either facilitate or discourage social interaction among the room's occupants which in turn influences the activity patterns of any newcomers to the setting. In this chapter, the author discusses ideas from a variety of fields, including architecture, environmental design, ergonomics, anthropology, and psychology, that illustrate the diverse ways in which physical environments have been viewed and how these approaches can be used by occupational therapists in helping their patients and clients overcome performance deficits.

ALTERNATIVE PERSPECTIVES AND KEY CONCEPTS

Scholars from many fields have studied numerous aspects of physical environments. The fields can be broadly grouped into disciplines interested in design of spaces, design of interiors and furnishings, design of tools and equipment, environmental protection and risk management, and behavior settings. Table 5-1 lists the disciplines according to these aspects. This section highlights concepts in each of these areas that are useful to therapists. The next section examines ways in which therapists themselves have historically analyzed physical environments and points out areas in which therapists are beginning to recognize the great therapeutic potential of environmental management for improving patient and client performance.

Design of Spaces

Architecture and community planning are the disciplines most readily identified as addressing design of the built environment whether it is a single structure or an entire metropolitan area. One of the fundamental concepts within

the two disciplines is the notion that environments should be both functional for users and aesthetically attractive, although the relative weight given to functionality and asthetics has varied throughout the history of design disciplines. Several concepts from these fields seem particularly useful to occupational therapists.

Archetypal Places. One such concept is the notion of *archetypal places*, which was initially developed by Spivack (1973) and later adopted by Lifchez and Winslow (1979) for their book, *Design for Independent Living*. By the term **archetypal places**, Spivack means settings in the physical environment (rooms and furnishings) that focus and support fundamental human functions, including taking shelter, sleeping, mating, grooming, feeding, excreting, storing, establishing territory, playing, routing, meeting, competing, and working. "Such settings, taken together, in their smallest irreducible groups, are archetypal places" (Spivack, 1973, p. 46).

The concept of archetypal places implies an inherent connection between space and the activity patterns within it. The concept assumes that basic activity needs are primary, and spaces are analyzed in terms of how well they meet those needs. Some archetypal places such as facilities for grooming and feeding relate directly to physical performance components. Others focus on social and cultural aspects of behavior such as competition and establishment of territory. This contrast should alert therapists and others concerned with physical spaces to view them more than just in physical terms. To understand human behavior holistically, they must integrate the physical, social, and cultural aspects of functioning within an environmental context. Lifchez and Winslow (1979) emphasize the great importance of learning to understand physical spaces from the perspectives of occupants of various cultural backgrounds that may differ greatly from those of the architect or the therapist.

Proxemics. Another concept that supports the close interdependence of spatial and cultural aspects of physical settings is **proxemics**. Anthropologist Edward T. Hall (1966) initially formulated this concept by studying people's needs for space when they engage in various types of interactions. Hall found important differences among people of various cultures in what they considered to be appropriate and comfortable amounts of space and physical distances between people when they engage in a variety of interactions including intimate, close, social, and public interactions.

It is extremely important for therapists to be aware of potential differences among people in their perceived needs for amounts and types of space. In residential settings and in treatment environments, the need for privacy becomes a major issue for an optimal design of space for human functioning.

Resource Environment. A third important concept from space design is the notion of the *resource environment*. The term *resource* refers to both *instrumental facilities*, those that meet basic survival needs such as grocery stores, and *symbolic facilities*, those that meet more social or emotional needs such as parks and churches. Lawton (1977) used this concept to investigate how the spatial arrangement of resources in neighborhoods and communities and the distances that must be traveled to reach them, influenced the abilities of older people to lead self-supporting lifestyles. Clearly this issue of access to community resources is an important one to be considered by therapists in helping their patients and clients meet their responsibilities for self-care and home management in community settings.

Mobility Sphere. Directly related to the spatial arrangement of the resource environment is the concept of **mobility sphere**, the range of distance within which an individual can travel regularly (Cantor, 1979). A person's mobility sphere can be shaped by three components: 1) how far he/she can ambulate or travel by wheelchair or some other assistive device, 2) accessibility features of the neighborhood or the community, such as sidewalks, curb cuts, elevators, ramps, and accomodations for special equipment like wheelchairs or walkers, and 3) long-distance transportation options such as the availability of a personal car or van or public transportation (bus, subway, train, or airplane). Many studies (for example, DeJong, 1981) have shown that the availability of usable transportation is a major factor affecting the ability of disabled people to work, attend school, live independently, and participate in community life.

Unfortunately, in community planning efforts many of the provisions for circulation and routing of goods and people through space have been based on the assumption that everyone has roughly similar mobility options. This assumption has often excluded elderly or disabled people from much of the activity within the community (Bowe, 1980). Since health care trends demonstrate shifts away from institutional care settings toward community-based living, this concept of mobility sphere seems particularly important to therapists working with patients and clients in

Table 5-1
Alternative Perspectives on Physical Environments
Design of Spaces
Architecture
Community Planning
Design of Interiors and Furnishings
Interior Design
Industrial Psychology
Design of Tools and Equipment
Industrial Design
Ergonomics
Human Factors Engineering
Rehabilitation Engineering
Environmental Protection and Management
Public Health
Safety Engineering
Behavior Settings
Psychology
Anthropology
Sociology

these settings. Even though a person may appear to have a relatively rich resource environment with plenty of grocery stores, restaurants, and other necessary facilities within a half-mile radius, if the person's endurance allows him or her to walk only three blocks and no transportation is available, those resources may still be quite inaccessible. Therapists are thus challenged to consider not just the physical environments of the immediate dwelling or workplace but those of the whole neighborhood or the community within which patients and clients seek to function.

Design of Interiors and Furnishings

Disciplines such as interior design and industrial psychology have invested substantial effort to design building interiors and furnishings that encourage certain kinds of activities and that foster certain social-emotional atmospheres or moods among the inhabitants or workers. Professionals in these fields arrange and decorate interior spaces to maximize human functional performance and comfort. Psychologists have also attempted formal study of human responses to arrangement and decoration of interior spaces, such as studies on the effects of light and color on mood and emotions (Birren, 1969; Brunner, 1968; Pease, 1977), and a study on the ability of people to deal with complexity in one's surroundings (Claxton, 1980; Hunt, 1982; Lachman, Lachman, & Butterfield, 1979).

Cultural Style and Symbolic Associations. From these studies in design and their effects on work behavior, has emerged the term, **cultural style,** which is a collection of furnishings, objects, and decor that connote a certain life-style or behavior pattern. Although decor is not usually considered within the realm of therapy, a related tradition in psychiatric occupational therapy deals with **symbolic associations**. This notion suggests that individuals feel and act differently when certain objects are present within their environment because these objects represent something personal to them and their lifestyle. Symbolic associations can include both an object's broader, cultural connotations and its narrower, idiosyncratic associations for individuals or families. A classic contribution to the literature in this area is Searles' (1960) book, *The Nonhuman Environment,* which suggests that in residential settings, such as nursing homes or group homes where routine and uniformity contribute to a loss of individual identity, the individual's right to personalize his or her physical living space can be important in establishing a sense of individual identity. Sociologist Erving Goffman (1961) in his book, *Asylums*, describes the concept of "total institutions" where residents have lost their right to individualize their clothing and their living space with objects that symbolize their personal identity. The sociologist Lee Bowker (1982) in his research on humanization of residential settings, such as nursing homes, has also recognized the significance of the right of individuals to have a personalized space.

Stimulus-Arousal Properties. A second major concept that has been found important in studies of interior furnishings is their **stimulus-arousal properties**. The potential of various sensory stimuli to alert individuals is generally thought to be related to the intensity and pace of the stimuli. The novelty of the stimuli is also an important factor because repetition is thought to result in habituation or a decrease in alerting effects (Barris, Kielhofner, Levine, & Neville, 1985). Designers most frequently and consciously shape environments by varying the intensity and the pace of color, light, and sound. Therapists often use this stimulus-arousal concept when varying the intensity and the pace of vestibular and tactile stimuli to excite or inhibit alertness in patients and clients (Farber, 1982).

The stimulus-arousal properties of environments can substantially influence human functioning. The literature on the potentially deleterious effects of understimulation has been ably reviewed by Parent (1978), who points out

the important implications of the findings for therapists in settings such as intensive care units. At the other extreme, environments that overstimulate can overwhelm the brain's ability to sort, prioritize, and screen incoming stimuli (Ornstein, 1986). The hazards of overstimulating environments are well-known to therapists working with patients whose ability to screen stimuli has been impaired, including those with head injuries or strokes. Such patients are unable to maintain concentration in distracting settings.

Atmosphere. Closely related to the concept of how sensory stimuli affect people's capacity for concentration is the effect of sensory stimuli on the mood or the atmosphere of a setting. Both academic psychologists and human factors engineers have studied the psychology of color and light. Examples include Birren (1969), Brunner (1968), and Pease (1977).

Occupational therapists have used the relationship between color and mood in their clinical interpretation of projective tests in which patients and clients are asked to draw or paint how they feel. There are guidelines for therapists for interpreting the meaning of such tests, such as those developed by Azima and Goodman (Hemphill, 1982).

One very interesting finding in this area of how light and color effect mood is the research that has linked serious depression experienced by some people to the seasonal cycles. It appears that some people are more prone to experience depression in the winter months when daylight is much shorter than in the summer months (Rosenthal, Sack, Gillin, et al., 1984). This phenomenon, called seasonal affective disorder, is thought to be related to basic processes within the limbic system of the brain.

Cognitive Complexity. A final key concept that emerges from disciplines focused on the impact of environmental interiors and furnishings is the **cognitive complexity** of the setting. This concept has gained prominence through studies (Claxton, 1980; Hunt, 1982; Lachman et al.,1979) that focus on the variety, the familiarity, and the complexity of stimuli in settings and the potential for interactive feedback between setting elements and users. Yarrow, Rubenstein, and Pedersen (1975) studied the home environments of infants and demonstrated methods by which one can assess such variables as variety and complexity in the environment. The growing interest of clinicians in the cognitive rehabilitation of people with head injuries has given even more impetus to the study of these variables that define cognitive complexity in various environments (Rosenthal, 1984). For example, factors like the pace or the speed of activities can have a major impact on the level of cognitive complexity within an environment, particularly for those with impairments who experience slowed processing and response times, such as in head injury or stroke patients. Another example of the effects of cognitive complexity is the elderly person who might function quite competently driving in traffic in a small town but might be overwhelmed by the speed and the complexity of traffic on a large urban freeway.

Design of Tools and Equipment

Design of tools and equipment is a major area in which studies of various disciplines have been useful to therapists in analyzing physical environments. The disciplines of industrial design, ergonomics, and human factors engineering have tended to emphasize tools and equipment to increase productivity in the workplace. Studies have focused primarily on industrial production, ''high-tech'' fabrication facilities, and office environments, but through specialized fields such as rehabilitation engineering, this area of study has been expanded to include tools and equipment for people with disabilities.

Object Manipulation. One concern that has been central in this research is *object manipulation* and design of mechanisms that closely match the dexterity capabilities of human hands and upper extremities. This work has in some cases included research in special environments, such as in areas with high or low gravity forces. The applied fields of rehabilitation engineering and occupational therapy have invested substantial effort to design tools and equipment for people with hand or upper extremity impairments who have difficulty with grasp or stabilization.

In recent years, design of these tools and equipment has responded to the need for more gross motor skills and more stabilization of upper extremity function. This helped lay the groundwork for the current health care trends toward establishing *work hardening* treatment programs designed to maximize the individual's ability to return to work.

Performance Efficiency. A major approach that has evolved in the design of tools and equipment includes the study of *performance efficiency* or the goal of achieving maximum productivity in a given period. Such efforts began with early industrial time-and-motion studies intended to minimize unnecessary, wasted movement in using equipment. The field of ergonomics or human factors engineering has dramatically broadened this area to include many other factors that affect performance efficiency, such as response time and visual perception. Similar basic principles have traditionally been used by therapists under the rubric of energy conservation in working with patients and clients who have limited endurance and therefore must use their available energy to its best productive advantage.

Environmental Protection and Risk Management

Ever since the early years of the industrial revolution when environmental hazards were first recognized as contributors to illness, various disciplines have studied such hazards and ways to minimize their risks. The field of public health and community medicine began by focusing on the elimination of infectious diseases and later started to address factors such as air and water pollution as agents of disease in the environment.

The central concept in these efforts is the identification and *management of risk factors* believed to play a substantial role in causing disease. The same concept underlies the efforts of safety engineers and government regulatory agencies to prevent disaster and trauma, whether it is reducing amounts of dangerous chemicals in drinking water or assuring the safety of mass transportation services.

The basic concept of prevention through risk management has been adopted by occupational therapists in helping to assure the safety of clients who are at risk because of sensory loss or impairments in coordination and mobility. Environmental interventions such as installing safety features such as grab bars to prevent falls or improved lighting often help reduce the risk of injury in the homes of elderly persons.

Behavior Settings

Behavior settings is a term coined by psychologist Roger Barker (1963) that describes a physical location in which a customary pattern of behavior occurs without regard to the particular inhabitants of the setting. Barker was interested in culturally-patterned rules and expectations for behavior. Other social scientists, particularly anthropologists and sociologists, had studied this for many years, often in terms of cultural or social roles. Barker's contribution to this research area was his close linkage of behavior patterns to specific physical settings. Barker initiated studies in the field known today as ecological psychology, and established a most important concept for anyone interested in the physical environment and its effects on human behavior—the interrelation between physical, social, and cultural aspects of environments.

Cues. It is important to establish the concept of behavior settings here because of its value for therapists in considering physical surroundings. Therapists should be aware that physical objects, furnishings, and spaces have significance beyond their presence in treatment settings, residential institutions, and even in homes or the workplace. Physical objects serve as cues that can induce whole patterns of behavior and activity because they are familiar to and closely associated with certain expected behaviors of members of a particular culture. These cues of familiar objects or environment can help people get their bearings and adjust to new circumstances, such as disability, or new environments, such as hospitals or nursing homes. A phenomenon frequently noted clinically by therapists, although not well documented in the literature, is the attempt of disoriented stroke patients or clients to re-create a familiar environment by viewing people or objects in a new setting as if they were from their hometown or some other familiar cultural system. This seems to demonstrate the phenomenon of constructing the social and cultural aspects of behavior settings from the presence of a few physical cues.

Because occupational therapy clinics frequently use familiar and commonplace objects rather than elaborate special equipment, they seem particularly well suited to helping patients or clients adapt and draw on their past repertoires of behavior in new circumstances. Kielhofner (1983) has written about the potential of occupational therapy clinic environments to establish behavior settings that are familiar and therefore therapeutic for patients.

Environmental Press. The term **environmental press** was used originally by psychologist Henry Murray (1938) to characterize the congruence he observed between individuals and environments. *Press* refers to the tendency of environments to encourage or require certain types of behavior. In some instances, press may simply involve broad guidelines for appropriate or functional behavior. In other cases, it may include various sanctions enforced to produce the required behaviors, such that people who do not comply are eliminated from the setting. The notion of press is useful to therapists in helping patients and clients analyze the extent of compatibility between their personalities and the behavior patterns expected in a given setting.

Schema Theory. The field of cognitive anthropology has developed a useful concept to describe the basic activity patterns associated with a given setting. Called **schema theory**, this concept was also used by the psychologist Jean Piaget (1960) in developing his classic theory of human cognitive development. The notion of schema suggests that within a culture there are standard routine performances that occur in given situations in a typical sequence and with typical kinds of participants. Within the general framework or structure, the details of a given performance may vary, but the basic structure remains. For example, a host might set the table somewhat differently if six guests will be present at a meal instead of just three family members, but the basic pattern of setting the table will be consistent. The central point is that there are certain expectations for the organization of activity that will occur in physical settings.

OCCUPATIONAL THERAPY AND THE PHYSICAL ENVIRONMENT

In occupational therapy, the central concern is also activity and its deliberate use for therapeutic purposes. This is the profession's unique contribution to the collective body of knowledge of how people function. As we have seen in the disciplines and studies mentioned above, physical environments play a fundamental role in shaping and directing activity; and it is for this reason that physical environments are worthy of our special attention and understanding.

Mobility

Historically, occupational therapists have focused their attention on two major aspects of physical environments. One of these is the accessibility by wheelchair of spaces in the built environment, including homes, workplaces, and commercial structures. People with impairments in mobility often benefit from bathrooms and hallways wide enough for wheelchair turning and from elevators and ramped entrances rather than steps. Therapists have joined with other advocates, including organizations of disabled people and architects and designers, to develop and support standards like those of the American National Standards Institute (1980) pertaining to wheelchair accessibility. Such standards have been incorporated into regulations implementing federal legislation, for example, Section 504 of the Rehabilitation Act of 1973 and the Americans with Disabilities Act of 1990, which prohibit discrimination against people with disabilities. In many parts of the United States, these standards have also been incorporated into local building codes. Therapists frequently provide consultation to commercial builders and designers as well as to families who need to modify buildings, homes, or public spaces in order to apply general accessibility standards.

Activities of Daily Living

The aspect of physical environments traditionally addressed by therapists is support for patients and clients to function in *activities of daily living* (ADLs). Important settings for ADLs are kitchens and bathrooms, where people with disabilities perform the daily tasks of meal preparation, grooming, personal hygiene, bathing, and dressing. Therapy departments in almost all rehabilitation facilities have evaluation checklists that are used to assess the ability of patients and clients to manage tasks and ADLs in their own homes. As noted in the chapter on occupational performance assessment, some of these ADL instruments have gained general acceptance, such as the Klein-Bell Scale (Klein & Bell, 1982). ADL assessments also focus on people's ability to reach and manipulate the tools and the equipment they need for task performance. Therapists often provide a wide variety of specialized, adaptive equipment to help patients and clients manage tasks in spite of impairments of reach, stability, or grasp.

Negotiation of the Environment

Occupational therapists have concern with mobility and object manipulation to include attention to perceptual and cognitive skills, such as the client's orientation and memory. This has given rise to the development of consulting practices to address difficulties experienced by elderly people in various physical environments. Firms such as Geriatric Environmental Concepts, for example, employ occupational therapists who recommend that nursing homes or hospitals avoid the glare of waxed floors to improve the functioning of persons with problems in visual perception or suggest the use of simple and consistent signs using colors and pictorial symbols rather than lengthy wording to help persons with cognitive impairments find their way in institutional settings.

Symbolic and Cultural
Implications for Treatment

Therapists are giving consideration to the symbolic and cultural connotations of physical environments and the therapeutic application of such information in helping to evoke desired adaptive behavior and performance in patients and clients in home health care settings as well as in treatment environments (Kielhofner, 1983). Barris et al. (1985) have written creatively about environments at a theoretical level, and Barris, Kielhofner, and Watts (1983) have described the potential role of therapists as environmental managers in clinical practice. Various other therapists have explored these environmental issues at a more applied level with particular patient or client groups in specific community environments, including studies on relocation and stress in the elderly (Hasselus, 1978), on daily-life experiences of deinstitutionalized retarded people (Keilhofner, 1981), and on need-satisfaction of elderly people living in the community and in institutions (Tickle and Yerxa, 1981).

ADAPTIVE PROCESSES AND
PERSON-ENVIRONMENT INTERACTION

In the preceding sections, we examined key concepts from various disciplines that have studied physical environments. In this section, we will investigate the interactive processes by which humans function within physical environments. This involves examination of the effects of specific features of physical settings on the various human performance components outlined in other chapters.

Central to this discussion is the premise that effective human performance requires three fundamental adaptive processes:

(1) making sense of one's surroundings,
(2) understanding situational demands or options for performance
(3) executing appropriate performance output

In developing an integrated perspective on how environmental variables affect human functioning, it is important to remember the connection between physical environments and their social and cultural implications. Thus the discussion in this section frequently returns to Barker's (1963) notion of behavior settings, which focuses on the fundamental linkage between physical locations and the customary patterns of behavior that occur in them. Table 5-2 considers each of these adaptive processes, examining those environmental dimensions which interact with specific human performance components to allow a person to adapt to the environment.

Making Sense of One's Surroundings

Fundamental to effective functioning within any behavior setting is the ability to make sense of one's surroundings— to identify where one is and what is going on there. Several features of physical settings contribute to that environment's interpretability or coherence and help people assess where they are and what is happening.

At the level of physiological performance, the stimulus properties of a setting affect human arousal and attention. These are typically basic *exteroceptive stimuli* or input from the external environment such as light, color, noise, smell, and texture. (*Somatosensory stimuli* arise within the body and are detected through the proprioceptive, kinesthetic, and vestibular senses.) These stimuli may alert the individual and cause physiological arousal of the central and autonomic nervous systems, or the stimuli might be soothing and inhibit these systems. Unless a person can maintain arousal without becoming overstimulated, he/she will be unable to proceed to the more complex tasks of interpreting the significance of the stimuli. An optimal state of arousal requires not only the ability to detect incoming sensory signals, but the ability to screen out some stimuli to enable one to focus on the tasks at hand. This requires that one does not attend equally to all stimuli, but selectively focuses on what is judged relevant or important in the circumstances.

At a sensory performance level there are two fundamental processes: *discrimination* and *integration*. Being able to

Table 5-2
Adaptive Processes and Person-Environment Interaction

Adaptive Processes	Environmental Dimensions	Human Performance Enablers
Making sense of one's surroundings	Environmental interpretability and coherence Stimulus properties	Physiological systems Arousal Attention Inhibition
		Sensory systems Discrimination Integration
	Light, color, noise, texture, smell	
	Familiarity of cues	Perceptual systems Recognition Association
		Cognitive systems Memory
Understanding situational demands for performance	Environmental press Complexity, pace, variety, responsiveness	Cognitive systems Planning and sequencing
	Behavior settings (activity patterns and roles)	Hypothetical thinking
		Problem solving
Executing appropriate performance output	Environmental negotiability Accessibility Efficiency	Cognitive systems Executive functions
		Psychological systems Volition
		Neuromotor systems Mobility Object manipulation

detect and discriminate variations in the visual, auditory, and tactile properties of the physical environment is a crucial first step in making sense of one's surroundings. Blindness or deafness constitute extreme losses of visual or auditory discrimination, but more moderate losses frequently occur along with the normal aging process. Loss of touch discrimination is less frequently seen but can be equally disabling since it renders the individual unable to recognize and manipulate objects and tools. Loss of tactile sensation can greatly increase the risk of burns or other injuries since the individual is unable to discern painful sensations.

Not only must individuals be able to detect the sensory stimuli but they must be able to integrate or process the information for the brain to react appropriately. Measurement and analysis of sensory integration processes and remediation of sensory integration dysfunction have

become a major area of research in occupational therapy under the leadership of Ayres. One of the major contributions of Ayres' work has been confirmation of the notion that older and more basic sensory systems in the evolutionary sequence (vestibular, olfactory, and basic tactile processing) provide the groundwork on which later sensory systems depend (e.g., visual processing). Thus Ayres (1983) suggested that remediation of dysfunction in these more basic sensory systems can lead to more adaptive visual and auditory processing from the physical environment.

Finally, within the perceptual domain of human functioning are the complex brain functions called *recognition* and *association*. These crucial functions involve comparison of new incoming environmental stimuli with the stored memories of similar stimuli in the past. A striking example of the process of association is smelling a familiar odor like cinnamon that immediately conjures up childhood memories of having cinnamon rolls with milk or perhaps of baking apple pies. The capability of associating new stimuli with old memories is essential for humans to grow and develop in a cumulative fashion based on life experience. This association elicits information on several different levels. The first is the basic linguistic meaning of a given stimulus, in this case, that cinnamon is a spice. The second is the emotions one felt in the past in conjunction with the stimulus, in this case, pleasant memories of cinnamon rolls and apple pies. The third is the memory of how one properly uses this item in one's culture, in this case, that cinnamon is used in cooking certain types of foods such as fruits and pastries and is not used as seasoning for broccoli, or face powder, or bathtub scrubbing powder. These rather simple examples emphasize that perceptual association depends on familiarity with the cultural context of physical objects and spaces, and that being able to recall this context is essential to making sense of one's surroundings. As a child develops and learns, he/she gains a repertoire of familiar environments or settings and a knowledge of what should take place in those environments. Similarly children learn which causes generally lead to which effects.

Given the importance of one's memory in this process of successful association, it seems evident that people with memory impairment should be expected to have substantial difficulty interpreting physical settings. This difficulty may be a result of global impairment of all memory functions or it may be due to discrete and localized lesions in sensory association areas of the brain. The neurologist Oliver Sacks (1985) describes an individual with this sort of discrete impairment of sensory association in the book, *The Man Who Mistook His Wife for a Hat*.

Understanding Situational Demands for Performance

The second stage of adaptive human performance within an environment (see Table 5-2) involves understanding situational demands and options for performance. This means knowing what behavior is expected or appropriate within the setting—what one should say or do. Various features of physical settings influence the individual's ability to interpret environmental press and understand expectations for his or her performance. The field of information processing has emphasized the importance of features such as cognitive complexity (how many things are going on at once), pace (how quickly action proceeds), variety (how much change occurs in the setting), and responsiveness (whether events change in response to the behavior of the individual). People who have difficulty with cognitive processing often perform much better in a simple setting in which only one thing is happening and the pace is slow. People with more extensively developed processing abilities might find such an environment boring and lacking in features that evoke participation.

Analyzing the situation and planning what one will do or say in an environmental situation draws on a major group of cognitive skills such as memory, problem-solving, sequencing, and ability to think hypothetically. Certain task-specific cognitive skills such as reading and calculation may be required as well. Although these human cognitive processes often seem to center primarily on the hypothetical manipulation of social and cultural aspects of environments, anticipating how the physical environment will respond to one's actions is also very important. A person's past experiences of moving through space and manipulating objects help him/her judge how the environment will respond, whether a given behavior will achieve a certain outcome or whether the physical environment is unlikely to respond in ways intended by the individual. This involves the skill of *praxis*, or motor planning.

Executing Appropriate Performance Output

The final stage of person-environment interaction involves executing performance output. This phase has cognitive, psychological, and neuromuscular subsystems. Psychological factors play an important part in how actively engaged a person becomes in an environment and its behavior settings. Barris et al. (1985) have written about interests and values and their counterparts in intention within the volitional subsystem of the individual. This conceptualization asserts that human beings do not just respond in obligatory, instinctual ways to environmental stimuli and possibilities for action. Rather, free will and choice underlie human engagement in executing performance within the environment. These often are activated by the features of the setting itself including the atmosphere or the character of its space and furnishings, as well as by the array of available objects that suggest certain activity patterns.

Within the cognitive domain, execution requires a group of skills that are often termed *executive functions* (Rosenthal et al., 1984). These include initiation, monitoring of performance, and evaluation of results of behavior. Monitoring and evaluation bring the individual back to earlier stages in the adaptive process in which he/she reinterprets the setting and what is happening there, and reassesses options for future action in light of his/her own effects on the setting. The executive functions are generally regarded as higher-level cognitive skills localized in the frontal lobes of the brain. People with impairments in these functions may be unable to initiate a given action, even though they have just discussed verbally the behavior that they plan to perform. Also, people with frontal lobe impairments are commonly unable to monitor their performance. In rehabilitation of patients who have suffered head injury or stroke, one sign of progress is when they begin to recognize and later correct their own mistakes. These skills clearly require the ability to compare one's actual performance with some expected performance standard.

Finally, execution of performance output requires neuromotor abilities to move in space and to manipulate objects. These abilities of the individual are dramatically influenced by features of the physical environment, including what distances and routes must be traveled to execute an intended action and whether these are within the person's mobility sphere. They are also influenced by a person's coordination and strength which governs ones ability to manipulate objects and tools. In recent years, rehabilitation technology has dramatically altered the neuromotor capabilities of people with severe physical disabilities by giving them new tools for wheelchair mobility, object manipulation, environmental control, and speech. These technological developments are examined in another chapter.

HUMAN PERFORMANCE IN SETTINGS OF DAILY OCCUPATION

This section examines studies of integrated human behavior patterns within the five major kinds of occupational settings of concern to occupational therapists:
1) home environments where much of the occupational domain of self-maintenance takes place,
2) play environments,
3) work environments,
4) neighborhood and community environments where the remainder of self-maintenance occupations occurs, and
5) institutional environments which encompass the entire range of life activities for residents. Institutional settings are of special concern to therapists because many of their patients reside in institutions either temporarily or permanently.

The studies that are discussed were selected to represent a broad range of disciplines that have investigated person-environment interaction. They also focus on differing sets of variables within the physical environment and related behavior settings. These studies are not necessarily the most recent works in a given area. Rather they represent a range of methods and perspectives. Readers interested in more detailed information on the studies are urged to consult the primary sources that are cited in the references.

Home Environments

One useful approach to understanding person-environment interaction in home settings was developed in the School of Architecture at the University of California at Berkeley under the leadership of Raymond Lifchez (Lifchez & Winslow, 1979). The interest of Lifchez and his colleagues in this area emerged from their involvement with an activist community of physically disabled students at the university and architects who designed home environments for handicapped persons. The approach stressed the importance of extensive interaction between architects and users of space, so that architects came to understand what activities meant to clients and the mechanical steps clients use to perform activities. Lifchez and Winslow proposed to shape this interaction by use of design plans and models as projective stimuli to which clients responded and indicated how the space would work for their activities.

The content areas addressed in Lifchez and Winslow's (1979) analysis of home environments for physically disabled people are based on the concept of archetypal places, explained at the beginning of this chapter. Archetypal places are locations in which fundamental human activities occur such as taking shelter, sleeping, mating, grooming, feeding, excreting, storing, establishing territory, playing, routing, meeting, competing, and working (Spivack, 1973). Lifchez and Winslow's (1979) book, *Design for Independent Living*, provides a perceptive analysis of how the physical arrangement of home environments affects the concrete physical tasks such as grooming and feeding. It also examines implications for social activities such as establishing territory, meeting, or competing. In addition to discussing the obvious variables of mobility and object manipulation that are of concern to physically disabled people, Lifchez and Winslow make insightful comments about the socially and physically distancing effects of wheelchairs and other equipment used by disabled people and encourage home designs that minimize these effects.

Lifchez and Winslow's study illustrates a method frequently used in analyzing environments—intuitive judgment by experts with professional training (in this case architects). This method of study is subject to the criticism that it may lack reliability and validity; that is, that other experts with similar training may study this phenomenon and reach different conclusions. The claim of interpreter bias is a problem for architects, anthropologists, and health care providers who make clinical judgments based on their interpretation of the meaning of certain activities for other people. The great advantage of studies like the one conducted by Lifchez and Winslow is that it does include questions regarding meaning and values. Such qualitative variables are deliberately excluded from consideration in most approaches to quantitative research. If one believes that the domain of meaning has an impact on human functioning as did Lifchez and Winslow, then it is important to conduct research that takes into account such variables regardless of how difficult they may be to study.

Quite a different method was used by Yarrow, Rubenstein, and Pedersen (1975) of the National Institute of Child Health and Human Development to conduct an innovative study of the home environments of 41 black infants five to six months of age. Their purpose was to examine the effects of specific environmental variables on a child's functioning, including his or her cognitive and motivational development.

Carefully structured naturalistic observations were made using time-sampling methods of specific behaviors of the caregivers toward the infants and the complexity, the variety, and the responsiveness of the physical surroundings. The infants' functioning was assessed using the *Bayley Scales of Infant Development* and tests of problem-solving and exploratory behavior given in the infants' homes.

Relationships between infants' skills and motivation and environmental variables were analyzed using multivariate techniques that showed important differential effects between stimulation from caregivers and stimulation from the physical environment. The characteristics of objects available to infants were not related to either language or social development, but did relate to several aspects of cognitive and motivational development. The variety of objects was related to the largest number of infant development variables. Maternal affect seemed to encourage infants' stimulus-seeking behavior, thus mediating their environmental interactions. Caregivers smiling was correlated with only two aspects of stimulus-seeking behavior, whereas playing with the infant correlated with a number of variables, including social responsiveness, object permanence, and exploratory behaviors. This study substantiates the notion that effects of the physical environment are often mediated by social and cultural aspects of the behavior setting (in this case, the caregivers' behavior). The authors conclude that stimulation from caregivers and stimulation from the physical environment make both unique and important contributions to human development but have quite different effects.

Naturalistic observation is a research method that emanated from the Department of Psychology at the University of Kansas, where Roger Barker (1963) developed the notion of the behavior setting that has been prominent in this chapter. Today this notion is central to a whole field of study often called, *ecological psychology*, which looks at behavior as it naturally occurs in typical settings. Research conducted in these natural settings is without the artificial controls of an experimental laboratory in which variables are manipulated by researchers. In naturalistic observation, there are very specific and detailed rules for categorizing and coding behaviors to increase reliability and minimize the bias of different interpretations from observers. Precision is thus gained at the expense of ignoring a major domain of human functioning — that of meaning and values.

Play Environments

The work of Yarrow, Rubenstein, and Pedersen (1975) on home environments of infants focuses heavily on their play. Berg and Medrich (1980) also addressed the occupational domain of play in their study of the effects of four contrasting neighborhood environments on the *free play* (unsupervised) of children. They used a structured format to interview preadolescents and their parents. The four neighborhoods differed in terms of several variables, including terrain (hilly versus flat), separation of residential areas from commercial ones, population density, access to planned play areas, access to unmanaged space, vacant lots, role of streets and sidewalks, personal safety, traffic safety, and mobility options (walking, bicycles, public transportation, or cars driven by adults).

Interviews were conducted with a selected sample of parents and children in all four neighborhoods. Questions focused on children's actual activity and social interaction patterns and on opinions about neighborhood features such as availability of play spaces, resources, and friends. Substantial differences were noted among the children's behavior in various neighborhood environments, particularly in the following areas: the numbers and types of play activities; types of spaces used for play; proportion of time spent in solitary, dyadic, or group play; the range of social contact of the children; and the autonomy of the children in managing their leisure activities. From an occupational therapy perspective, many of these variables appear to have substantial consequences for a child's overall development. Thus settings for free play seem to be an important environmental concern for therapists.

The structured interview format used in this study is a much more efficient way to gather data on behavior than the labor-intensive naturalistic observation method used by Yarrow, Rubenstein, and Pedersen (1975). However, two possible drawbacks of this interview format are that it does not provide a precise level of detail in analyzing specific behaviors, and it presents a potential validity problem because people's responses to questions regarding their behavior may differ from their actual behavior.

Work Environments

Much of the research on person-environment interaction in work environments has been done in human factors engineering, ergonomics, and industrial design. Research in these disciplines usually involves experimental designs in which laboratory simulations of specific job tasks are carefully controlled. Through very precise manipulation of task demands, it is possible to measure the effects of specific task variables on human work performance.

A study by Cushman (1986) illustrates use of this experimental model to analyze reading ability under different environmental conditions. Reading is a perceptual-cognitive task commonly required in office settings. Asking subjects to read text continuously for 80 minutes, Cushman compared their reading performance using printed text versus performance using microfiche and video display terminals that had both negative images (light characters on dark ground) and positive images (dark characters on light ground). Work performance measures were reading speed, reading comprehension, and visual fatigue. Cushman found that visual fatigue was significantly greater when subjects read from negative microfiche projected on a metal screen or from video display terminals with positive images. However, when subjects read from microfiche projected on a high-reflectance matte screen or from a video display terminal with negative images, visual fatigue was no greater than with printed text. Reading speeds were slower for conditions with negative images, but reading comprehensions scores were similar for all conditions.

On the basis of these results, the choice of media for reading tasks in office environments appears to have significant impact on performance. In settings in which microfiche and video display technologies are used, it is important to provide tools that optimize performance, such as nonscintillating screens in glare-free environments for microfiche, video display terminals with a negative display mode, and lighting that can be adjusted for the special characteristics of a particular office setting.

A study by Braune and Wichens (1985) illustrates the use of experimental methodology to study the performance of pilots on simulated work tasks requiring perceptual-motor skills and information processing. The aircraft cockpit is a work environment that involves both perceptual and cognitive processing and neuromuscular output (to manipulate aircraft controls). Through elaborate statistical analysis of performance data on a battery of information-processing and motor coordination tasks, the authors identified a cluster of performance skills required in this

work environment that decline gradually over the age span of 20 to 60 years (primarily tasks requiring time-sharing or multiple-task attention). They conclude that pilots should periodically undergo individual testing on a battery similar to this one in order to calculate their functional age and govern the types of piloting tasks they are capable of performing adequately.

A study conducted by Armstrong, Radwin, Hansen and Kennedy (1986) also used experimental methods to analyze performance in a work setting. In hopes of discovering ways to minimize risk factors for repetitive trauma disorders in the upper extremities of the workers, they tried to estimate optimal work locations for specific tasks requiring reach, lifting, and hand-assembly performance. Their goal was to improve job analysis by estimating the optimal work locations using computer-based methods. This research is applicable to job environments that primarily require motor skills in hand-labor industries.

These three studies focused on aspects of work performance that are of great interest to occupational therapists, including sensory and perceptual processing, cognitive processing, and execution of motor output in response to repetitive environmental demands (like those in the hand-assembly industrial work) or unpredictable environmental demands (like those of aircraft control). The great advantage of the experimental research methods used in these studies is their precise control and measurement of both task and performance variables, which allow reasonable assumptions regarding cause and effect in analyzing human performance. The great disadvantage of experimental research is that it may give a somewhat inaccurate or unrealistic picture of what actually occurs in work settings. In actual work settings, there are always variables and tasks that can never be precisely controlled, and human performance is inevitably affected by people's values and meanings, which cannot be precisely measured.

Neighborhood Environments

Much self-maintenance activity for clients occurs at the neighborhood or community level, thus these environments should be the legitimate concerns of occupational therapy.

A study of 26 inner-city neighborhoods by Marjorie Cantor (1979) of the New York Department of Aging was conducted to assess the viability of inner-city areas as residential environments for the elderly. A survey research design was used to interview a random sample of 1,552 elderly persons of white, black, and Hispanic descent. The four central variables were (1) the extent of residents' life space, (2) their perceptions of their neighborhoods and of the availability of needed goods and services within these areas, (3) the social support systems they used, and (4) their views on the advantages and disadvantages of city life.

Residents' use of the physical environment and its resources was assessed by giving them a standard list of facilities commonly used in everyday life and asking them a series of questions regarding these facilities: which facilities they used, whether the facilities were inside or outside the neighborhood, how far from home were the facilities located, how often were the facilities used, and what usual mode of transportation was used to various facilities. Facilities included grocery stores, drugstores, clothing stores, doctors' offices or clinics, churches or synagogues, banks, restaurants or bars, parks, movies or theaters, clubs or organizations, and places of employment.

Most residents regarded their neighborhood as extending a radius of 10 city blocks or less from their homes, and the facilities that they most commonly used were six blocks or less from home. The most common mode of transportation was walking. Public transportation was used occasionally for longer trips. Although much of the life of these elderly people was conducted within their neighborhoods, 70 percent reported leaving the neighborhood occasionally, and over half reported going outside its boundaries at least once a week.

The study also investigated specific kinds of social support exchanged between elderly residents and their children, neighbors, and friends. The findings suggest that inner-city neighborhoods provide far more social support than is commonly believed and that elderly people are actively engaged in social-support networks. The types of social support frequently identified in the study often mediated the elderly person's need to use physical resources of the environment, neighbors who often did such as shopping for elderly residents. Such social exchanges decreased the amount of physical mobility required of the elderly. The balance may shift toward more dependency by elderly people on social support in neighborhoods where key resources are beyond their mobility spheres.

The survey methodology that Cantor used allowed her to draw conclusions about the entire elderly population of the inner city because of the large and carefully randomized sample of subjects who were actually interviewed. The great advantage of survey designs is that data can be efficiently gathered on large populations. Their major weakness is less rich information from each individual and potential for respondents to provide invalid information that cannot be confirmed.

Institutional Environments

The sociologist Lee Bowker (1982) and his associates at the University of Wisconsin in Milwaukee conducted a comprehensive study of four institutions for elderly people in order to identify features of these environments that support a humanistic philosophy of care in the major categories of physical setting, general administrative policies, programming, and social relationships. The study was conducted using qualitative ethnographic research methodology that emerged from the traditions of anthropology. Data were collected by participant observation and extensive interviewing of staff and residents at each facility. On the basis of over 300 hours of interviewing at each site, the project staff synthesized a typology of roles played by staff and residents. They also categorized recurrent themes related to the environment as described by staff and residents. Drawing on this interpretive analysis and using a method called grounded theory (Johnson, 1975), Bowker synthesized a total of 33 environmental variables identified by participants as humanistic. The nine physical environment variables identified as important features that foster humanization were: provision of space for personal possessions, use of color coding, provision of space for privacy (including opportunities for sexual expression), provision of space for social interaction, use of bulletin boards and other information-giving devices, use of both natural and artificial lighting, use of noninstitutional furniture, arrangement of furniture both in private rooms and public places, and use of living things to humanize physical structures.

The qualitative methodology employed in this study offers the advantage of allowing participants in a social or cultural system to define what is happening and what it means in their own terms and constructs. Interpretive categories are derived inductively from the detailed data, rather than being imposed by the researcher's frame of reference. The disadvantages of this methodology are its cost as a labor-intensive process and the potential for interpreter bias in defining themes or categories from the content of data. The methodology offers a richness of data that is particularly useful for generating hypotheses and new explanations of relationships among variables that have not previously been studied extensively. The method thus helps generate theory that can later be tested by more quantitative methods.

Case Study 5-1

Use of Environmental Assessment and Intervention to Improve Human Performance: Angela was a six-year-old girl with cerebral palsy that had resulted in a staggering gait, problems with arm and hand coordination, and slow but intelligible speech. On starting first grade in public school, she had difficulty making friends with other children and participating in classroom activities. She started crying frequently at home, did not want to return to school, and regressed in her abilities to walk, feed herself, and manage her toileting functions. Angela's mother took her to the local cerebral palsy center, where Angela had been seen for years. She hoped to find out why she was relating poorly to other children and was no longer using functional abilities that the entire family had worked hard with her to develop during her preschool years.

At the cerebral palsy center the occupational therapist performed an evaluation, which showed that in the special testing environment, Angela was able to walk, feed herself, and manipulate objects as well as she could previously. The therapist also conducted a naturalistic observation of Angela during her free play in the center's playground. The therapist observed that Angela played most energetically and interacted most positively with other children in two locations: the sandbox and a corner of the room where goods and play money were available for the children to establish a make-believe grocery store.

The therapist contacted an occupational therapist at Angela's school. Cooperatively they observed Angela's activities in the classroom and on the playground. They also conducted a resource survey of the classroom and the playground. The two therapists also documented the mobility sphere of Angela's classmates and the distances they regularly traveled between their classroom, lunchroom, playground, and assembly room. Conversations with Angela's teacher confirmed the therapists' hunches that Angela was having difficulty keeping up with the other children in verbal and written classroom tasks, in traveling long distances around the school, and in gross motor playground activities on the swings and merry-go-round.

The therapists recommended several environmental interventions to improve Angela's performance. An important recommendation involved advising Angela's teacher to add certain play objects to the classroom to foster representational play skills such as playing grocery store, gas station, or spaceship operation. These were learning and recreational activities that Angela could master and enjoy and ones which placed less emphasis on her verbal and written skills. The central focus of this intervention was to engage Angela and her peers in joint activities in which Angela could demonstrate her competencies.

The school therapist also developed a strategy for getting volunteers to add resources to the playground designed to stimulate constructional play. These included two sandboxes where playing allowed Angela to interact with friends in ways that did not make her feel conspicuous and awkward because of her staggering gait.

The third area in which recommendations were made centered on Angela's mobility sphere. Angela's family resisted the initial suggestion that she use a wheelchair for fast long-distance travel at school, so it was agreed that the family would get her a wagon to keep in the classroom. With this vehicle Angela could push herself long distances or be pulled by the other children, who themselves enjoyed using the wagon.

The school therapist, who was seeing Angela for individual therapy, followed her classroom, free play, and mobility activities. The changes that had been made in the physical environment did allow Angela to cultivate her competencies and establish informal peer interaction in settings that she could manage without feeling she was always behind the other children. In time, having success rather than failure experiences changed Angela's feelings about school. The regressive behavior and social withdrawal that had developed when she entered public school disappeared. Relatively simple environmental changes allowed Angela to successfully enter the mainstream of the public school system and to interact with her peers on the basis of her competencies rather than her disabilities.

SUMMARY

Many features of the physical environment shape the ability of inhabitants to make sense of their surroundings, analyze their performance options, and execute integrated patterns of occupational behavior appropriate to the setting and functional for their adaptive survival. A central premise of this chapter is that when functional occupational performance does not occur, the factors contributing to this outcome may lie in the individual or in the environment. More specifically, they may lie in the extent to which the individual's performance capabilities in many domains correspond optimally to the demands and the opportunities of the setting. By considering factors affecting performance in both individual and environmental domains, the occupational therapist has a broad array of intervention strategies available to change various factors and thereby modify the course of adaptive interaction between person and environment.

Study Questions

1. Choose a public behavior setting that is a part of your daily life and describe the customary patterns of behavior that occur there. Then describe a person who might have difficulty functioning in that setting.

2. On a map of the community in which you live, mark the territory that is part of your mobility sphere. Then describe a person who might have difficulty moving about within this territory.

3. Suppose that you have suddenly arrived in a city that you have never visited before. Describe features of the physical environment that you would use in the important adaptive tasks of making sense of your surroundings.

4. Describe a physical environment you know that would be considered to have a high level of cognitive complexity. What features of the setting contribute to this complexity?

5. Describe several research methods that have been used to analyze the impact of environments on human performance in daily occupational settings.

References

American National Standards Institute. (1980). *Specifications for making buildings and facilities accessible to and usable by the physically handicapped*. New York: Author.

Armstrong, T.J., Radwin, R.G., Hansen, D.J., & Kennedy, K.W. (1986). Repetitive trauma disorders: Job evaluation and design. *Human Factors, 28*, 325-336.

Ayres, A.J. (1983). *Sensory integration and learning disorders*. (2nd ed). Los Angeles: Western Psychological Services.

Barker, R. (1963). On the nature of environment. *Journal of Social Issues, 19*(4), 17-38.

Barris, R., Kielhofner, G., Levine, R., & Neville, A. (1985). Occupation as interaction with the environment. In G. Kielhofner (Ed.), *A model of human occupation: Theory and application* (pp. 42-62). Baltimore: Williams & Wilkins.

Barris, R., Kielhofner, G., & Watts, J. (1983). *Psychosocial occupational therapy: Practice in a pluralistic arena*. Laurel, MD: Ramsco.

Berg, J., & Medrich, E.A. (1980). Children in four neighborhoods: The physical environment and its effect on play and play patterns. *Environment and Behavior, 12*, 320-348.

Birren, F. (1969). *Light, color, and environment*. New York: Van Nostrand Reinhold.

Bowe, F. (1980). *Rehabilitating America: Toward independence for disabled and elderly people*. New York: Harper & Row.

Bowker, L.H. (1982). *Humanizing institutions for the aged*. Lexington, MA: D.C. Heath.

Braune, R., & Wichens, C.D. (1985). The functional age profile: An objective decision criterion for assessment of pilot performance capacities and capabilities. *Human Factors, 27*, 681-693.

Brunner, J. (1968). *Contemporary theory and research in visual perception*. New York: Holt, Rinehart & Winston.

Cantor, M.H. (1979). Life space and social support. In T.D. Byerts, S.C. Howell, & L.A. Pastalan (Eds.), *Environmental context of aging: Lifestyles, environmental quality, and living arrangements*. New York: Garland STPM Press.

Claxton, G.R. (Ed.). (1980). *Cognitive psychology: New directions*. London: Routledge and Kegan Paul.

Cushman, W.H. (1986). Reading from microfiche, a VDT, and the printed page: Subjective fatigue and performance. *Human Factors, 28*, 63-73.

DeJong, G. (1981). *Environmental accessibility and independent living outcomes*. East Lansing, MI: Michigan State University, University Center for International Rehabilitation.

Farber, S.D. (1982). *Neurorehabilitation: A multisensory approach*. Philadelphia: W.B. Saunders.

Goffman, E. (1961). *Asylums: Essays on the social situation of mental patients and other inmates*. Garden City, NY: Doubleday.

Hall, E.T. (1966). *The hidden dimension*. Garden City, NY: Doubleday.

Hasselkus, B. (1978). Relocation stress and the elderly. *American Journal of Occupational Therapy, 32*, 631-636.

Hemphill, B. (1982). *The evaluation process in psychiatric occupational therapy*. Thorofare, NJ: Slack.

Hunt, M. (1982). *The universe within*. New York: Simon & Schuster.

Johnson, J. (1975). *Doing field research*. New York: Free Press.

Kielhofner, G. (1981). An ethnographic study of deinstitutionalized adults: Their community settings and daily life experiences. *Occupational Therapy Journal of Research, 1*, 125-142.

Kielhofner, G. (Ed.). (1983). *Health through occupation: Theory and practice in occupational therapy*. Philadelphia: F. A. Davis.

Klein, R.M., & Bell, B.J. (1982). Self-care skills: Behavioral measurement with the Klein-Bell ADL scale. *Archives of Physical Medicine and Rehabilitation, 63*, 335-338.

Lachman, R., Lachman, J., & Butterfield, E.C. (1979). *Cognitive psychology and information processing*. Hillsdale, NJ: Lawrence Erlbaum Associates.

Lawton, M.P. (1977). The impact of environment on aging and behavior. In J.E. Britten & K.W. Schaie (Eds.), *Handbook of the psychology of aging*. New York: Van Nostrand Reinhold.

Lifchez, R., & Winslow, B. (1979). *Design for independent living: The environment and physically disabled people*. New York: Whitney Library of Design.

Murray, H. (1938). *Explorations in personality*. New York: Oxford University Press.

Ornstein, R. (1986). *The psychology of consciousness*. New York: Viking-Penguin.

Parent, L. (1978). Effects of a low-stimulus environment on behavior. *American Journal of Occupational Therapy, 32*, 19-25.

Pease, P. (1977). Clinical implications of color vision

research. *Journal of the American Optometric Association, 50,* 739.

Piaget, J. (1966). *The origins of intelligence in children.* New York: International Universities Press.

Rehabilitation Act of 1973. Public Law No. 93-112, 29 USC 701 (1982).

Rosenthal, M. (1984). Strategies for family intervention. In B. Edelstein & E. Couture (Eds.), *Behavioral approaches to the traumatically brain damaged.* New York: Plenum Press.

Rosenthal, N.E., Sack, D.A., Gillin, J.C., Lewy A.M., et al. (1984). Seasonal affective disorder: A description of the syndrome and preliminary findings with light therapy. *Archives of General Psychiatry, 41,* 72-80.

Sacks, O. (1985). *The man who mistook his wife for a hat.* New York: Summit Books, Simon & Shuster.

Searles, H. (1960). *The nonhuman environment.* New York: International Universities.

Spivack, M. (1973, October). Archetypal places. *Architectural Forum,* 140, 43-48.

Tickle, L., & Yerxa, E. (1981). Need satisfaction of older persons living in the community and in institutions, Part 1: The environment. *American Journal of Occupational Therapy, 35,* 644-649.

Yarrow, L.J., Rubenstein, J.L., & Pedersen, F.A. (1975). *Infant and environment: Early cognitive and motivational development.* Washington, DC: Hemisphere.

CHAPTER CONTENT OUTLINE

KEY TERMS

Arousal

Behavior setting

Environmental press

Group

Group roles

Institutionalization

Role

Social climate

Social support

Socialization

ABSTRACT

One's social environment is a very complex system of dimensions and components. It includes social groups and social systems, social networks and social support, and activity patterns, beliefs and expectations. The dynamics of the social environment and its influence on performance are explored through the person-environment interaction, the influence of family and home, the influence of play/leisure/recreation, the environment-person fit at work, and the social climate of educational settings, community settings, and institutional settings. The role of the occupational therapist as a teacher of social skills and as a social environmental manager is discussed along with recommendations for research.

Performance and the Social Environment

6

Harriett Davidson

"People need people in ways that health care professionals have only begun to examine."

—Blythe, 1983

OBJECTIVES

The information in this chapter is intended to help the reader—

1. describe dimensions of the social environment that potentially can impact a person's performance.

2. identify individual responses to the social environment that may enhance or limit performance.

3. examine social attitudes and social group behaviors that may limit or support the role performance of disabled individuals.

4. select social groups that appear particularly influential to the individual's development and performance.

5. suggest strategies for providing social support for particular behaviors or role performance.

6. suggest roles for the occupational therapist as a teacher of social skills and as a social environmental manager.

COMPONENTS OF THE SOCIAL ENVIRONMENT

A person's world, or environment, has been characterized in various ways. It is generally said to comprise physical, social, and temporal factors. Separating the three, either theoretically or practically, is difficult. Some theorists identify the environment as all the conditions surrounding and within the individual. Thus the individual is seen as the first-level environment, intimate relationships are seen as the second level, and community relationships as the third level (Llorens, 1984). The larger society is a distant fourth level. See Figure 6-1.

Barris, Kielhofner, Levine, and Neville (1985) describe layers of the environment as including objects, tasks, social groups and organizations, and culture. Some occupational therapists refer to objects in the individual's environment as human or nonhuman, thus apparently combining the physical, social, and cultural aspects of environment quite indivisibly. Spencer (1987) has proposed analyzing environments as (a) space and associated objects, (b) social systems and networks, and (c) culturally defined activity patterns, beliefs, and expectations.

The social environment can be represented at any moment in time, but the temporal dimensions of the environment indicate that it is dynamic and ever-changing as all the elements of family, social group, and organization interact (Anderson & Carter, 1974). In the process of living, people are performing various tasks and engaging in activity patterns and social interactions that are defined and given meaning by the various social roles that they play and by the culture in which the interactions take place. Social groups and networks are complex and unique in their configuration, and an individual moves in and out of them through time and space.

Knowledge about social environments has grown from the work of scholars in many disciplines, including the social and behavioral sciences and a variety of fields of clinical practice. Each discipline has contributed threads from which the whole cloth of current knowledge is woven. The concepts considered most useful to the knowledge and the practice of occupational therapy are presented in this chapter. These concepts relate to (a) social groups, (b) social systems, (c) social networks, and (d) socially defined activity patterns, beliefs, and expectations.

Social Groups and Social Systems

Psychologists have developed a tradition of small group work pioneered by Kurt Lewin in the 1930s and noted for such efforts as the National Training Laboratories that developed T-groups (sensitivity groups) in the 1950s and that continue to provide interaction/communication training. The **group** in this context is *"a plurality of individuals (three or more) who are in contact with one another, who take each other into account, and who are aware of some commonality"* (Olmsted, 1959, p. 21). Psychologists have tended to examine groups as small societies, using an experimental approach; they have tended *not* to consider the relationship between the groups they study and the society as a whole.

Social psychologists have attempted to consider both aspects. They incorporate the sociological approach that has historically examined the group as a cell in the social organism, or a building block in the larger society. Sociologists have studied groups as they occur in natural settings. They sometimes divide groups into primary groups

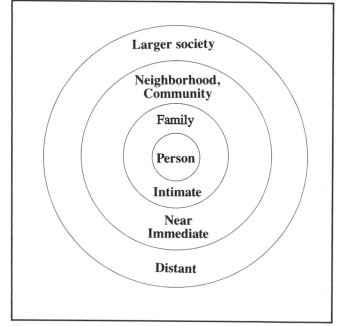

Figure 6-1. Levels of Social Environment.

that are small in which people have face-to-face interactions (e.g., the family), and secondary groups those that are larger in which people only have intermittent contact with each other (e.g., a large corporation). Anthropologists have contributed cross-cultural perspectives on how human groups form and how they function. Industrial psychologists have studied work groups in terms of motivation and productivity.

Clinical psychologists and psychiatrists have used group process and group dynamics as a treatment tool to effect change in the intra- and inter-personal functioning of their patients. The primary group has been the focus of their intensive study regarding the following: ways in which groups develop, the kinds of roles that people play in groups (including leadership roles), the ways in which group goals are set, how norms develop, how communication occurs, and how power is distributed within groups (Yalom, 1975; Zander, 1971).

Systems theorists have contributed a way of organizing knowledge about the complex nature of social environments into a hierarchy of systems and subsystems. The basic principles of systems theory were discussed in Chapter One.

Occupational therapists have historically addressed the needs of humans in treatment groups. They have elaborated on the study of how people learn and grow in *activity groups* and in *developmental groups*. An activity group can provide a behavior setting whose central focus is an activity in which humans routinely engage. Although the group is designed to be therapeutic and induce changes in the level of performance of the individuals, it replicates in many respects the natural social environment in which people perform their daily activity (Mosey, 1986; Ostrow & Kaplan, 1987). The activity group in psychiatric occupational therapy has gone through five eras:

1. the *project era* (1922-1936), in which the group was essentially a collective unit;
2. the *socialization era* (1937-1953), in which the group was seen as a socializing agent;
3. the *group dynamics or group process era* (1954-1961), in which group process was central to the treatment;
4. the *ego-building, psychodynamic era* (1962-1969), in which the intrapsychic part of the process was emphasized; and
5. the *adaptation era* (1970-present), in which the group is provided with structured, graded learning experiences that will lead to social adaptation through learning or practicing daily living and social skills (Howe & Schwartzberg, 1986).

Occupational therapists are beginning to document the relative efficacy of specific populations of activity groups as compared with verbal groups (De Carlo & Mann, 1985;

Mumford, 1974). One of the assumptions of occupational therapists is that the social learning that takes place in the clinic will generalize to situations in the community and will be relatively stable. However, such predictions will be valid to the extent that occupational therapists understand the variables of the environment into which patients and clients will move and the skills with which they are able to function adaptively in the environment.

The *developmental group* in occupational therapy is an application of knowledge from the fields of developmental psychology and sociology about the ways in which humans interact at different ages and stages in their lives. In this simulation of a real-world group, therapists design their roles as leader to emulate leaders that one might encounter in non-familial primary groups.

Social Networks and Social Support

Social networks are a way of conceptualizing dimensions of the social environment. Social groups and social networks are not the same. Social groups may include some paths of social networks, but the concept of social groups is not adequate for describing the linkages and the many paths that associations take (Bott, 1957)

A *network* is a "specific type of relation linking a defined set of persons, objects, or events" (Knoke & Kuklinski, 1982, p. 12). This total web of people with whom an individual is enmeshed, known as a network, is independent of a physical setting. In a social network, the people or social groups represented are sometimes called actors or nodes, and their relationships to one another can be depicted graphically either with lines connecting them or in a matrix to demonstrate the number of relations between any two actors or nodes. The people in these organizations or networks are selected for inclusion because of some attribute that they possess—for example, being a member of a family.

Network analysis allows the occupational therapist to analyze the individual patient or client in terms of personal interactions rather than in terms of other social units that might not be as descriptive. A network represents not just people but also their demographic characteristics, various relationships among people, the larger sociopolitical milieu, and time and space characteristics. Many types of units can be studied in network analysis including classrooms, street gangs, or even a leadership network in a community. Several dimensions are studied in analyzing networks and are used to describe them: range or the number of members, symmetry or the balance of power or profit, and intensity or the degree of commitment to a linkage.

Because one of the functions of a social network is to provide **social support,** the identification of such social support systems within social networks is an important function of health care professionals. All relationships in a network may not be supportive in nature. Some may be supportive or caring, some may be reciprocal, some may exercise power over others, and some may spread rumors, or have other unsupportive characteristics. (Wellman, 1980).

A *personal support network* is defined as a set of personal associations that provides the individual with support for his/her social identity and for emotional aid, material aid, and informational needs. Social support is widely viewed as important in the development and the maintenance of emotional and physical health and functional performance. Health care workers must work closely within that social support system of the client. In fact, health is defined within the social context, and that context often dictates how and when sick or disabled persons are allowed to return to healthy status. Therefore health professionals must share with the client's support systems some of the same expectations of what the patient or the client will be able to do and who will help him/her do it.

In many cultures, kinship networks are described as close, supportive, and plentiful, and can be available in case of illness or disability. Other networks are provided by tribal relationships or communities. In the United States, especially in urban areas, networks tend to be dispersed, with ties that may be neither close nor plentiful. The occupational therapist in this case must call on neighborhood, community, and friendship networks when mobilizing support.

The concept of social support has at least three components (Barrera, 1986):

1. *social embeddedness,* the connection that individuals have to significant others in the social environment (measured by marital status, participation in community organizations, presence of older siblings, contact with friends, etc.; that is, potential support resources)
2. *perceived social support,* or a cognitive appraisal of being connected to others (measured by perceived availability or adequacy)
3. *enacted support,* or actions that others perform when they actually render assistance to a focal person (measured by what people do when they provide support).

In other words, there is objective social relatedness, the client's perception of the relatedness, and the actual support received. For the health care professional, it is important to know the distinctions between these three components. The fact that an elderly person living at home has a daughter living within five miles may be important information for the therapist, but knowing that the daughter is disabled and cannot drive a car, or that the daughter works full time and

is a single parent, clearly alters the picture of that support system. In order to gain accurate information regarding a person's support systems, therapists certainly need to ask clients about their perceptions of their support system, rather than simply counting the number of available support people.

Social scientists have attempted to describe social support operationally. Although some theorists simply classify social support as expressive (emotional) or instrumental (doing things) (Pilisuk & Parks, 1986), Barrera (1986) specifies four factors in social support:

1. *directive guidance,* including giving of advice
2. *nondirective counseling,* including expressions of intimacy, availability, and esteem
3. *positive social interaction,* including joking, diversion, and discovery of interests
4. *tangible assistance,* including provision of shelter or money

There are potentially negative as well as positive aspects to social ties in supporting role performance. Very cohesive relationships can place undue pressure on individuals to conform or even generate collective rejection and scapegoating of individuals. If a person is rebellious or wants to change behavior, he/she may feel isolated and alone if the group is very unlike him/her (Moos, 1984). For example, a young woman planning to enter a university may feel alone if she comes from a close-knit family in which all the other females have not graduated from high school. The family may exert pressure on her to conform to old patterns of behavior in the family. During such a time when an individual is undergoing personal change, close support systems may support the status quo and make changes difficult.

A growing body of knowledge suggests a relationship between the adequacy of the social support system and the health or functional status of the individual (Brown & Harris, 1978). The dynamics have not been clearly established but studies indicate theory that support may provide a buffer effect rather than a direct effect for psychosocial or emotional health (Henderson, Byrne, Duncan-Jones et al., 1981; Vaux, Riedel, & Stewart, 1987). Some authors suggest that the individual's satisfaction with the social support, or their feeling of relatedness, is more important than the existence of the support (Huxley, Goldberg, Maguire, & Kincey, 1979).

Informal Networks. Support systems are often classified as formal or informal. Froland et al. (1981) refer to informal networks as either embedded or those that form naturally, or those that are created. The therapist can locate and use natural support systems that are already in place, but does not manipulate them. Froland et al. (1981) identify six kinds of informal helping networks:

1. family and friends
2. neighbors
3. natural helpers or people who naturally orient their lives toward helping others
4. role-related helpers, people who have a central position in the community
5. people with similar problems, such as members of self-help groups
6. volunteers, people who help informally in a formal organization.

Embedded networks have been found to develop over time even among groups of transients and among people living in single room occupancy hotels in large cities. Even in these seemingly disinfranchised groups, some individuals take over the caring and instrumental roles.

Created networks are designed usually by a formal agency to meet specific needs. They are often more specialized and depend on volunteers' willingness to help. These created networks may help people develop new roles, skills, and values, however, sometimes their services may not be as acceptable to the recipient. Some examples of informal, designed networks that have been developed in the community are:

1. volunteers who regularly visit elderly persons to just chat or do household chores and home repairs
2. Adopt-a-Grandparent program, which brings together adolescents and adults in their 70s or 80s, and for which the adolescents get school credit (Larronde, 1983)
3. programs to help elderly persons remain living independently at home when aided by volunteers who visit and provide transportation, food shopping, food preparation, sitting, cleaning, and home maintenance (Maguire, 1979)
4. an educational (social learning) program in which occupational therapists link long-term female psychiatric patients with members of a social service club for a series of work readiness seminars. In this program, the occupational therapist acts as the "culture broker" for the patient, interpreting the needs, appropriate behavioral expectations, and appropriate level of learning (Mauras-Corsini, Daniewicz, and Swan, 1985).

Caregiver is a label given to those who provide assistance to people with limitations in adaptive function. They can be found both in the informal network and in the formal one, but the majority of caregivers come from the family. Although they provide a rich natural resource, health care workers have begun to recognize the heavy burden and stress that they bear in many cases, especially in the care of patients with dementia.

The term *caregiver burden* has been given to that subjective feeling of being overwhelmed by the multiple tasks and the unremitting nature of the caregiving process. Research has shown the effects of caregiving on the emotional state, the social activity patterns, and the economic level of the caregiver. Some forms of social support can help ease caregiver burden, and much of this support is provided by family members and neighbors. Some communities are developing respite care programs to allow caregivers time to rest emotionally and physically. Respite care for caregivers need not negatively affect the care recipient's health to any great degree, although it may affect the caregiver-receiver relationship. But often this break is necessary to help caregivers continue their caregiving roles over long periods of time.

MacElveen (1978) has suggested that each individual has a "network style." He found that among home dialysis patients, some preferred to depend on themselves, others favored a kinship style of sharing with relatives, and others leaned toward sharing with friends. Some patients wanted to share with people who have common interests (associates), and others preferred a restricted style in which they shared with only a small number of people.

In the community there are certain people who, because of their job, have the opportunity to interact regularly with some needy populations. Postal carriers, cab drivers, and receptionists in doctors' offices have frequent contact with elderly and disabled persons and are in a good position to provide advice, support, and assistance. In some special projects, these individuals have been trained to watch for crises or conditions that need referrals (Hooyman, 1983). Thus the informal network can become more effective in providing support for those who need it.

Formal Networks. *Formalization* is the process of imposing standards to achieve control of the services provided by an agency or a group. Formal networks range from nationally organized voluntary groups to highly organized service agencies. It is best if a service agency can remain somewhat flexible and not too formalized in order to be responsive to the needs of individuals (Froland, et al., 1981)

A number of organized support groups are available to provide a variety of services to those learning to adjust to illnesses or disabilities. Several of these are described below:

- Reach-to-Recovery is a group sponsored by the American Cancer Society that provides a visitation program for women who have had mastectomies.
- The International Association of Laryngectomies is also sponsored by the American Cancer Society and provides visitation and educational programs to those who are undergoing laryngectomies.

- Mended Hearts is an organization founded in 1951 by four patients recovering from heart surgery and provides visitation to heart surgery patients before and after surgery, follow-up in local chapter meetings and educational programs.

Other groups are designed to provide support for family members:

- Make Today Count was founded in 1974 by a cancer patient, but now includes support groups for families of individuals with life-threatening diseases.
- The Alzheimer's Support Groups of the Alzheimer's Disease and Related Disorders Association are designed to help family and caretakers of people with Alzheimer's disease and related disorders.

Other groups are designed to support health and wellness practices and to help people adjust to new roles. For example, La Leche League International supports women who want to breastfeed their babies.

Although there are many support groups available, often patients or the clients do not know how to go about locating and using them. The occupational therapist may need to teach some patients and clients interpersonal skills or conduct role-playing or modeling to help them learn to listen, give and receive feedback, and express an opinion or feeling without offending others in order for them to take advantage of the services that are available (Blythe, 1983).

Formal and informal social support services may be complementary, but they do not substitute for each other; in fact, they appear to meet some different needs (Moscovice, Davidson, & McCaffrey, 1988). In some social groups the use of formal services is unacceptable, so they are not used, even though apparently available.

In summary, *social networks* are all the people who have relationships with a single individual, not all of whom know one another. They are embedded in total environments and sometimes provide social support and relatedness for an individual. In a complex society, informal networks cannot be expected to provide all of the physical and emotional support that a person needs, thus formal services develop. Health care workers assess these support networks, both formal and informal, in order to successfully provide services or emotional support that patients and clients might require.

Activity Patterns, Beliefs, and Expectations

Cultural expectations are shaped by beliefs, values, attitudes, and customs of the members of the social group with which the individual is associating. Not only do these expectations shape the development of task and role performance, but they demand that performance from those who enter the group.

Social systems make certain demands for task or role performance of the individuals interacting within that system. These expectations or demands are termed **environmental press** and are shaped by the beliefs, values, attitudes and customs of the social group. They require specific responses from the individual that encompass the range of skills including physiological, sensory, cognitive, neuromotor, and psychosocial. Barris et al. (1985) suggest that cultural expectations related to work and play and the use of time and space are particularly important to occupational therapists.

Socialization is the process of learning through responding to cultural and social expectations and explicit demands. Socialization should not be thought of as simply a child's automatic, unthinking internalization of cultural values, but as a dynamic process in which a person, throughout life, interacts with the social group and processes the values and behaviors of that group. The person may even alter those values and, in so doing, may change the social system (Brown, 1965).

The concept of **role** is borrowed from the theater. It implies the taking on of certain behaviors and even certain dialogues. Roles have certain prescribed actions and words and sometimes the behaviors are set down in print, as in a job description for a worker or a catalog for a college student. The individual has a certain leeway, and the role can be interpreted in many ways. Often roles must be learned and practiced, and during this initial stage the individual is self-conscious as in the case of a new college student, a new army recruit, or a new father (Brown, 1965). How well a person can perform a role depends at least in part on his/her innate abilities and the skills and the competencies that he/she has developed. It also depends on the ''goodness of fit'' between his/her competencies and the demands and the supports of the social environment.

Various environments may provide an excellent or a poor fit between an individual's competencies and the environmental press. A toddler just learning to eat with his/her fingers does not fit well in a formal restaurant setting. In contrast, a sophisticated middle-aged woman could be accepted and comfortable building a sand castle at the beach if she so chose. Thus, the more extensive repertoire of skills a person possesses, the more extensive is the range of environments in which the person can fit and perform life roles competently. Also, the more competent the individual, the greater the number and the kinds of settings in which he/she can perform (Lawton, 1982). The toddler is certainly limited in the number of environments in which he/she can function adequately because his/her repertoire of skills is very limited. This same messy eating with fingers that would draw very negative attention in a fancy restaurant would likely be accepted and maybe even encouraged by parents in the home environment or in a day care setting where children are being taught and encouraged to feed themselves. Hence, we see that the child has a much better fit with his home environment where there is support and acceptance.

Changing Roles of Sick and Disabled Persons. The social group has certain definitions and expectations for people who are sick and disabled. A person who is sick is exempted from regular performance expectations of the group and usually receives special treatment, concern, and support. Sometimes people with chronic or severe illnesses or disabilities get so accustomed to the role of being sick, they have difficulty returning to normal functioning (Kasl and Wells, 1985). Moos and Tsu (1977) have described the adjustment to severe illness in three stages: first, the individual denies the seriousness of the illness, then he/she seeks information about the condition and support from family and friends, and in the last stage, the person begins to learn specific behaviors necessary to play the *sick role*.

In some western cultures where independence and achievement are valued highly, the dependency associated with the sick role is viewed as undesirable and legitimate only when it is temporary. Society expects the sick person to recover as quickly as possible. There is a growing awareness that the traditional sick role does not contribute to the long-term maintenance of health and autonomy, and professionals encourage patients and clients to avoid the sick role and to take more responsibility for their health care. This new role of health manager encourages patients to become informed about health decisions and remain in control of the process (Burke, Miyake, Kielhofner and Barris, 1983).

The role of patient has changed over time in response to the dramatic changes taking place in the health care delivery system. Health care workers teach individuals the patient/client role depending on whether the program is oriented toward prevention, treatment, or rehabilitation (Brink, 1985). Expectations range from the traditional *patient role,* in which the individual is viewed as dependent and less able to engage actively in the job of getting healthy, to the *client role,* in which the person is expected to collaborate vigorously and actively in goal-setting and goal-achieving (Reilly, 1984). The manner in which health care professionals view those with serious illness or disability, the labels they attach to them, and expectations from them, can, in fact, influence their recovery or adjustment back into society.

As described in chapter one, the World Health Organization differentiates among the terms *impairment, disability and handicap. Impairment* is a deficit or abnormality at the anatomic, physiological, mental, or psychological level. A *disability* is a deficit in the performance area within physical and social environments. *Handicap* is a disadvantage resulting from an impairment or disability that interferes

with role performance and renders the person unable to live up to social norms. The distinctions are important since these labels have been known to influence how society views these people. A disability implies certain functional limitations, but a handicap implies a certain role set within a society (World Health Organization, 1980).

Burke et al. (1983) have suggested a new role for the person with a chronic disability—that of *health apprentice,* which has positive connotations of someone engaged in learning new role skills. The therapist's role in working with the health apprentice is that of teacher, collaborator, and advocate for full citizenship. In order to help maximize the client's competence, therapists should provide a treatment environment that is free of highly technical equipment and of professional attitudes that inspire a sense of helplessness.

Attitudes and Stigma. Relatively well-set feelings or dispositions toward people or situations are called *attitudes.* Attitudes toward people who are ill, disabled, or handicapped have been addressed in the literature regarding stigma. Illness or disability creates a "differentness" in terms of social identity. Differentness itself is neither good nor bad, but it does tend to set the different person apart from the group norm. This differentness may be of a physical nature (e.g., quadriplegia, hemiplegia, or obesity), of a character nature (e.g., mental disorder, homosexuality, or unemployment), or of a tribal nature (e.g., race, nation, or religion), and is referred to as a *stigma* by Goffman (1963).

Others tend to view these stigmatized people in stereotypical ways. Stereotyping in its worst form allows some to even view disabled or handicapped persons as being less human. Stereotyping is defined as a "hostile or negative attitude toward a distinguishable group based on generalizations derived from faulty or incomplete information" (Aaronson, 1984).

Erikson (1962) suggests that stigmatizing is a defense against people's anxiety about whether they have correctly classified circumstances or people and whether they have responded correctly to an unfamiliar situation. This defense mechanism of stigmatizing others makes people feel more normal when they negatively evaluate another person.

There is a variety of speculation about the origins of negative attitudes toward people with disabilities but Livneh (1984) listed four:

1. The culture places value on physical prowess and personal appearance.
2. A religious belief that views disability as punishment for sin.
3. Disabilities seem to make other people feel uncomfortable about their own body integrity or death.

4. The behaviors displayed by disabled persons invite prejudice.

Others have suggested other contributing factors such as economic and political competition (Aaronson, 1984), and whether one's disability is visible or invisible to society (Livneh, 1984).

It is possible for the stigmatized person to incorporate or reject societal demands or expected roles. Although the stigmatized one often takes on the social identity created for him, he may still feel that he is normal and able to function like everyone else. Hence he may experience self-hate and shame because society views him as not measuring up. Many professionals may be overzealous and wrongly interpret how a disabled person feels about himself/herself. They may " . . . *tell him what he should do and feel about what he is and isn't, and all this purportedly in his own interests*" (Goffman, 1963, pp. 124-125).

The choices and decisions are not always clear-cut or satisfying for these stigmatized individuals. They have the choice of joining the group of fellow sufferers who emphasize their differentness in an attempt to politicize their demands for acceptance, and in the process, they become even more set apart; or they may join the group which tries to integrate into society by teaching others how to behave around them and accept them which is, at best, only a conditional acceptance. Those whose differentness is "invisible" (one that cannot be detected by society), such as in the case of epilepsy or the early stages of AIDS, must decide whether to reveal or conceal their "secret." All of these dilemmas have no easy or totally satisfying solution. In fact, the only certain factor regarding relationships between able-bodied and disabled persons is that both groups make each other feel very uncomfortable (Archer, 1985). Many people have ambivalent, rather than negative views of disabled persons (Wright, 1988) and this confusion causes a tendency toward ignoring that population entirely. They are socially ill-defined and for all practical purposes "invisible" to the rest of society, suggest Murphy, Sheer, Murphy, and Mack (1988).

Degree of stigmatization of various groups often changes over time within a society. Depending on the attitudes and beliefs of a particular society, hierarchies of preference develop in which one type of disability may be viewed more or less favorably than others. Today's hierarchy indicates that the most preferred people are normal or gifted individuals and the least well-accepted include those with mental illness or mental retardation and those with disabilities that are believed to be self-imposed, such as alchoholism or obesity (review by Horne, 1985; Archer, 1985). Physical disabilities such as asthma, arthritis, and heart trouble are more easily tolerated and accepted.

Integration of Disabled Persons into Society. A number of social programs have been designed to integrate the disabled person into society and resulted in varying degrees of success. Three such programs are: (1) the *mainstreaming* of disabled children, (2) the *normalization movement,* and (3) the *independent living movement* (De Jong, 1981).

The *mainstreaming movement* (Gliedman & Roth, 1980) focused on the attitudes of schoolchildren, parents, teachers, and professionals in order to bring about change to integrate disabled children into the school mainstream. It was discovered that before mainstreaming could be successfully accomplished, parents, teachers and professionals needed to alter their expectations regarding the disabled children. Some had unrealistically high expectations and others had expectations that were too low. Both extremes had deleterious effects on the levels of performance of disabled children.

The *normalization movement* has also met with problems. Normalization has been defined as "utilization of means which are as culturally normative as possible, in order to establish and/or maintain personal behaviors and characteristics which are as culturally normative as possible" (Wolfensberger, 1972, p. 28). It became evident that effective normalization required an understanding of the normal social environment by those expected to integrate into it. Kielhofner and Takata's work (1980) suggested that just placing people with a disability into a "normal" situation does not necessarily integrate them. The authors concluded that people with retardation exist as a subordinate culture within a larger culture, and integration into that larger culture can occur only by understanding the retarded person's interpretation of the situation and by letting him/her participate in the decision-making processes of the social system.

The *independent living movement* has focused on self-help and self-organization of persons with disability to manage their own housing, transportation, and attendant care services in order to live independently in the community, or at the very least to have the freedom of choice in how they minimize reliance on others (De Jong, 1981).

The attitudes of professionals including occupational therapists should provide models for the social system. Some believe that occupational therapists have the opportunity to be powerful advocates for the disabled (Bruce & Christiansen, 1988). However, therapists' attitudes have been shown to be more negative than expected. Their attitudes vary widely according to age, gender, occupation, education, setting, and type of training received (Geskie & Salasek, 1988). One study found that occupational therapists reported favorable attitudes toward people with disabilities but still had difficulties wrestling with expectations on a case-by-case basis (Benham, 1988). Even when occupational therapists have favorable attitudes toward disabled persons, they can sometimes inadvertently foster prejudice by using words that connote confusion or prejudice, for example, carelessly interchanging the terms impairment, disability, and handicap (Bruce & Christiansen, 1988).

Acceptance appears to be promoted by regular interactions in which the individuals are relatively equal in social, educational, and vocational status and in which the differences can be directly confronted. Some researchers have studied the behavioral effects of increasing contact between the "different" person and the social group. One study showed that there were attitude changes toward racial minorities in the classroom when members of small groups had to depend upon one another for completion of assignments (Aaronson, 1984). This model has been suggested as a useful one for applying to situations with disabled persons. It appears that the most effective way to break down prejudice toward disabled persons and foster interaction is a combination of accurate factual information about the different groups and close association with them (with the consideration of a number of interpersonal or situational factors) (Horne, 1985).

From the studies, we can see that there are certain characteristics of the social environment that foster integration of different individuals:

1. a wide latitude of acceptance of differentness
2. an environment where the different individuals can participate in decision-making and are permitted to demonstrate skills and contribute to the social goals
3. an environment in which the different individuals are in close proximity and interact with others
4. the free acknowledgement of differences and adequate information about those differences.

Social Climates

The idea that a social environment has a "social climate", or a personality of its own, has been developed by Moos (1979). His approach was to use people's perceptions of the environment as a way to define the climate, which is seen as having an influence on the way people in those environments behave. Conversely, the environment is influenced by the people in that environment. Moos and his associates in the Social Ecology Laboratory have developed a number of inventories to assess social climates in such settings as the university, the correctional institution, etc. All these assessments use a common set of dimensions for examining the environments, including relationship dimensions, personal growth or goal orientation dimensions, and system maintenance and change dimensions. The measurement of perception of these common dimensions makes it possible to compare

environments and also to compare people's behaviors in different environments. Evidence from research shows that when people perceive positive qualities in the relationships, they express more satisfaction and show more engagement in a variety of activities in different settings.

A related perspective for describing social expectations is that of the behavior setting described by Barker (1965). The **behavior setting** is a physical environment where a combination of stable patterns of activities take place, for example, the classroom is a behavior setting where similar kinds of behavior are expected and occur. The size of the setting has certain implications for the expectations and demands made on the individual by the setting. For example, in a small workplace where there are fewer personnel, people tend to be more highly involved in activity and more different kinds of actions. It is entirely possible in a small high school that one individual might be the editor of the school paper, a cheerleader, and the president of three clubs. This perspective is more fully described in the chapter on physical environments.

DIMENSIONS OF SOCIAL ENVIRONMENTS

The occupational therapist is accustomed to teaching function and to designing clinical environments that support role and skill performance. A newer role is the appraisal of community and special environments to which patients and clients may return or enter. Therapists must assess environments, and if they are found to be unfavorable, they must assist clients in the adaptation process and work to redesign them or find new environments for the patient. In order to do this, the therapist must identify variables of the social environment that might potentially influence performance. Social groups, social systems, and networks may be examined in terms of their structural and functional dimensions, their relational dimensions, and their temporal dimensions. The following case study illustrates the variables in the environment that can influence performance.

Case Study 6-1

Rodolfo: Rodolfo is a 13-year-old Mexican-American boy who was hospitalized with complaints of headaches and nervousness for the past year and recently hearing voices telling him to run out in front of a moving car. He was diagnosed as having a complex partial seizure disorder, severe stress related to having two disabled parents (about whose health he worries), and poor school performance. He has a history of numerous accidents since babyhood.

Rodolfo's ability to play family roles is complicated by his seizure behavior, in which he has aggressive episodes and later does not remember the incident. The mother, age 52, is unemployed and suffers from hypertension, chest pains and arthritis. The father, age 50, is unemployed (he reports having incurred two on-the-job accidents) and complains of having a nervous condition as well as physical difficulties. Both parents speak Spanish primarily and rely on a daughter to translate into English. The family moved from California to Texas recently, reportedly for better job opportunities. Also living at home is an older brother who is not employed and who drinks alcohol excessively and an older sister who is employed in a hospital.

Analysis of Rodolfo's parents as models reveals they did not model competence in work or family settings or in their relations with the community. Their status was that of unemployed individuals living on disability payments. They had little energy to give to nurturing behaviors and tended to reward or excuse Rodolfo's illness behaviors. The older brother modeled similar behaviors. The values of the models were dissimilar to the mainstream culture, except for the older sister.

In the neighborhood, Rodolfo tended to be a loner and did not belong to a social group. At school, he played with younger or older kids, usually in a follower role. With his peers he was often aggressive. He did not compete well academically and was held back from grade promotion on two occasions. Thus, he experienced few if any, feelings of competency. He reported having some work experience soliciting for the local newspaper. He expressed interest primarily in sports activities.

In looking at social groups that would support Rodolfo's performance, the occupational therapist identified the older sister who helped him sometime with his schoolwork. She provided a model for school performance, as she had completed high school and had obtained a job, although Rodolfo tended to see the female and the male roles as sharply delineated. The large classroom school setting had not provided the task expectations and the environmental cues that he needed for optimum performance. His parents were not firm about insisting that he turn off the television and study.

Dilantin improved his seizure status, although it was believed he still experienced seizures in the form of aggression. He was placed in small classroom groups in which he first tended to doze off in class but later began to incorporate the classroom values of involvement in learning. Because the learning was individualized, he was able to exhibit accomplishment, he began to do his homework, to be more involved and even exhibit a sense of humor on occasion, although he still exhibited cognitive limitations. In occupational therapy, he initially interacted socially only with staff, but with cueing for task behavior, he was soon able to concentrate and remain task-focused within a small group in the clinic.

There was a community youth center in Rodolfo's neighborhood which provided a variety of activities for Mexican-American youth. Rodolfo knew about the center but had never voluntarily attended. The occupational therapist arranged for some of the participants at the center to invite Rodolfo and he began attending. Although not the star athlete, he is now taking part in games there.

The work setting has the potential to provide Rodolfo with a value system and approval for performance. His current job is a solitary one, but he is considering possible options. He has moved from dreaming of being an astronaut to considering blue-collar kind of work, but is still not ready to select the specific kind of job. He is incorporating the limitations imposed by his seizure condition, and the information about his competencies given by the participants at the youth center is helping him evaluate his own skills.

Structural and Functional Dimensions

Social groups and organizations may be studied in terms of size, density, function, permeability of boundaries, and structural complexity (Barris, Kielhofner, Levine, & Neville, 1985). *Size* relates to the number of people who are involved in the group. Groups that are smaller tend to have less role specialization of members and to have more expectation for independent responsibility of members. For example, students going to a small high school may be expected to be involved in more activities and to hold more offices. Both large and small groups can arouse different emotions or feelings in different individuals. For example, students in a small class may feel tense because they know they will be expected to participate in the class discussion. Such people may prefer a large class where they can sit on the last row and stay uninvolved. Other individuals may feel tense being in a large class in which they are uncertain of the expectations and how they will be able to compete and distinguish themselves. This latter set of individuals would feel more comfortable in a small class. *Density* or concentration is created by the number of people in an environment. Crowding is relative to the demands of the settings for tasks or functions and to individuals' perception of what is expected in that setting. For example, a dance floor may not be considered crowded when people are in close proximity to one another, yet in another setting, such as an occupational therapy clinic where therapists are trying to treat patients, the same closeness would be considered crowding.

Permeability of boundaries refers to the difficulty getting into the group and susceptibility of the group to outside influences. The more requirements there are for entrance into the group and the more specialized the skills of those entering, the more commitment to the values of the group is required. For example, it is relatively difficult to gain entry into a medical school and to pass the board examinations. Those who accomplish this are highly committed to the values of medicine and support each other's practice.

A group's *function* is its central purpose and relates to its reason for being. Function will determine some of the group's structural characteristics. Performance demands are related to the function of the group. Social and cultural values and role norms also shape the performance demands. Work groups tend to be more structured and to press for more specific behaviors with certain procedures and standards. They may also demand internalization of certain values. Play groups tend to be less structured and demanding.

Structural complexity refers to the type of relationships or networks found among members and is somewhat related to the size of the group or organization. As an organization gets larger, it tends to develop hierarchies, and roles tend to become specialized. A small country store may have one owner and salesperson who deals with a variety of merchandise. In contrast, Macy's Department Store is much larger geographically and includes several executives, managers for several departments, many salespeople, and stockboys, each of whom has a specialized position. Both for the worker and for the consumer, this environment is more complex to negotiate physically, socially, and cognitively.

Relational Dimensions

Relational dimensions are determined by role norms, by the context of the setting, and to some degree by the individual characteristics of the person. Relations are defined by content and form. *Content* refers to the characteristics of the association such as helping, supporting, supervising, or kinship. *Form* refers to the particular properties of the connections between or among the individuals (Wellman, 1981), such as availability, strength, and symmetry.

Availability refers to physical presence as well as emotional accessibility between or among people. If a person is in close physical proximity but emotionally inaccessible, the relationship would not be said to be available. Relationships may be available densely or sparsely, in clusters or in various structures (Wellman, 1981).

Strength is the intensity of the relationship. For example, a relationship with a daughter may provide more support for an elderly woman than a relationship with a husband because the daughter may be able to take the woman grocery shopping or to the doctor.

Symmetry refers to whether the relationship is reciprocal or as strong in one direction as in the other. Is the exchange of resources equal? Does the daughter in the above example rely on the mother for the same degree of support as the mother gets from the daughter?

Temporal Dimensions or Change Processes

Social systems are dynamic and change over time. Moos (1974) has identified three temporal dimensions: system

organization/system maintenance, participant influence, and system change.

System organization/system maintenance refers to the rules or values that organize the behaviors of the members and serve to support the ability of the group to remain stable. Values govern the rules and the structure of the organization. The rules of a college course establish that members must enter at registration time, attend routinely, and stay throughout the semester if they are to complete it successfully. Therefore one would expect group membership to remain stable throughout the semester even though individuals within the group will experience change in level of knowledge.

Participant influence is determined by the function, size, permeability, and structural complexity of the group. Some groups are relatively responsive to attempts of members to change the system, others are not. For example, a person is much more likely to influence the local parent-teacher organization than the state legislature in California.

The *degree of system change* that is possible is determined by organization and participant influence. The change can be at the person level, at the level of the immediate setting, or between or among settings (*mesosystem*). Changes at the mesosystem level require an understanding of the social regularities or patterns of social relations, connections, or linkages. Change at this level takes place through public policy. A parent may convince her disabled child that she is capable of functioning in the public school system (person level). The parent may persuade the superintendent of the local school to let her child enter the school (immediate setting level), but it takes Public Law 94-142 to persuade the United States public educational system that all disabled children should enter public schools (mesosystem level).

Person-Environment Interaction. People move into and out of social settings throughout a lifetime. These social settings are determined by availability, choice, and the ability of the individual to interact adaptively within the setting and have a reasonable number of needs met. The assumption is made that the adaptational processes are characterized by several factors:

1. the individual's ability to identify roles, activities, and tasks that are possible in a selected environment
2. the ability to perform selected roles, activities, and tasks with the social constraints and supports of that environment
3. the ability to effect change in selected environments

Identifying Possible Roles, Tasks, and Activities

In the social group into which an individual is born, certain patterns of activity are characteristic. The child's initial task is to understand what others are doing and what others expect of him/her. A person's interaction with the social system is governed by the following: the stimulus properties of the human models available in the environment; the individual's sensory reception, perception, discrimination, and integration; and the selective attention given to these models. Through reasoning and awareness of self and environment, individuals are able to understand what they might be capable of doing.

The neuromotor skills necessary to respond include skills to move in space and skills to identify and explore the objects and people that are found in the environment. For the infant, the mother or caretaker provides these objects and conveys, through words and actions, the social values and expectations related to them. In this exploration, the infant needs social interactional skill to communicate about these expectations, such as when an infant learns to reciprocate and respond with a social smile. Whether the individual develops or uses certain neuromotor skills depends to some degree on whether the use of such skills is sanctioned. For example, society's current emphasis on physical fitness and exercise for both women and men is vastly different from that of the nineteenth century when women were encouraged to be delicate and frail.

Physiologic responses of autonomic nervous system arousal will influence the degree of excitement with which an individual greets an environment. If the people and the expectations are matched with the individual's needs and abilities, the individual's cardiovascular, psychoneuroendocrine, and hormone levels will respond and the person will tend to identify the activity as pleasing. If demands exceed the ability to respond, the person will interpret the environment as stressful or aversive, and avoidance or maladaptive responses may result. The presence of social support can modify the effects of stressful demands or expectations. An individual who has had no role models and has not developed social expectations, may respond to situations with apathy or with asocial behavior. The absence of role models in the early years can create profound deficits in function.

Motivation, volition and problem-solving are involved in choosing a setting or in choosing models. It has been shown that people prefer and choose to interact with: (1) those with whom they have a greater opportunity to interact, (2) those who have desirable values and norms, (3) those most like themselves in values, attitudes, and social background, (4) those perceived as viewing them favorably, (5) those who view them as they view themselves, and (6) those in whose company they can meet their own needs (Secord, Bachman, & Slavitt, 1976).

Performing Roles, Tasks, and Activities

The structure of the social system and the explicit nature of the role expectations influence the way in which the individual actually performs the activities and tasks related to roles. Some of these expectations and rules are quite explicit and inflexible, as in some work settings. Some have boundaries that are quite broad and open to individual interpretation, as in some leisure or play settings.

Choice, or volition, is involved to some degree as to where the individual chooses to work and play and live, although disabled people with a lower level of adaptation have fewer choices. A combination of psychological and cognitive factors will determine how the individual interprets the demands of the environment. One person will interpret a work situation, for example, as stressful and aversive, whereas another will see it as challenging. A social environment that is moderately high in support, that allows for clarity of communication and some role flexibility, will tend to support work role performance.

Demands from the neuromotor systems or cognitive systems vary according to the type of role or task. For example, some types of work do not provide opportunities for maintaining skills, and in those cases, the individual may look for ways to develop those skills in other roles. Business executives who have little requirement for neuromotor behavior in their jobs may choose to work out in a gym or play tennis in order to prevent those neuromotor skills from declining.

Effecting Change in Environments

Changing social environments require many special skills: being able to establish goals, to plan, and to develop and execute behavioral programs. Volition and the social skill to effect this change are also necessary. Once the change has been made, evaluation of the change requires sensory reception, perception, integration, and interpretation of results. Lastly, one must make use of cognitive skills and abstract reasoning to assess the effects of change.

FAMILY AND HOME INFLUENCE ON HUMAN PERFORMANCE THROUGHOUT THE LIFE STAGES

The factors that influence human behavior have been the subject of endless studies by psychologists, psychiatrists, anthropologists, sociologists, social workers, physicians, nurses, and other health professionals. Although it would be impossible to discuss all the factors that have been studied, some of the most important ones will be presented.

The nuclear family is still considered to be a most

powerful social influence on the behavior of a person. However, certain conditions may compromise the integrity of the family unit or dilute its influence. The contemporary family in our socially mobile society is often a one-parent family or one in which both parents are employed and the child care responsibility is shared with nonfamily caregivers. Families are smaller and today's mother may be inexperienced in child care or limited in her knowledge of human development. In addition, many traditional parenting tasks have been taken over by professionals, so children receive little socialization toward parenting as a primary role.

Statistics show an alarming number of adolescent mothers who are unmarried in the United States. For those mothers and their children, there is not a primary nuclear family to render support. It has been shown that children of unmarried mothers tend to have increased rates of school dropout, out-of-wedlock births, separation, divorce, and welfare use (independent of economic status effects).

Prenatal, Perinatal, and Postnatal Influences

Scientific technology and medicine today have greatly increased the survival rate of premature babies, but their survival does not guarantee a healthy, thriving child. In fact, many premature infants have physical problems. The infant may be ill or developmentally immature and may not be able to interact as the family expects or to tolerate a great deal of social stimulation by the family. A number of studies demonstrate that when the low birth weight child is at risk, the home environment and related socioeconomic status influence positive outcomes (Escalona, 1984).

The social environment of the fetus can influence competency. There is some evidence that psychological stress of the pregnant mother is related to the physical development of the fetus, although these studies have often been flawed (Newman & Newman, 1978). Anxiety in the pregnant mother has been associated with a number of maternal complications such as hyperemesis gravidum (pernicious, excessive vomiting in pregnancy), difficult and prolonged labor, habitual abortion, and fetal complications (Burstein, Kinch & Stern, 1974; MacDonald & Christakos, 1963). Women with little social support (both emotional and tangible) and high life stress have been found to have a significantly higher rate of complications than those with high support (Norbeck & Tilden, 1983; Tilden, 1983). Both parents are vulnerable to stress during the prenatal period. Studies have linked the amount of social support with positive attachment to the fetus and newborn and to more positive outcomes in the child's language and cognition.

It has also been shown that how the society perceives the pregnant woman, whether she is perceived as adequate or vulnerable and whether she is treated with solicitude or shame, will make a difference in her activity level and maternal care during pregnancy and in the birth process. Other factors that have been shown to affect the nature of the bonding process between mother and child include whether the mother is anesthetized, whether the birth takes place in a hospital or at home, and whether there are perinatal complications.

The expectant mother readies herself to bond with the infant during the nine months of gestation, and the perinatal and immediate postnatal period are considered critical for that process. If that readiness period is shortened because of premature birth, the social climate is one of crisis rather than readiness. Birth order creates its own social climate for the infant because first-time mothers are more awkward and anxious than experienced mothers.

The Early Years

The family is the primary agent for early support and for training or developing competencies. Opportunities for intimacy and emotional response are available in the ideal family relationship (Olmsted, 1959). The importance of the reciprocal nature of the relationship between mother and infant has recently received attention (Brazelton, Koslowski, & Main, 1974). For example, the child's crying elicits a response from the mother. Once the child's crying predictably elicits the mother's response, the child is freed to try other kinds of communication behaviors and thus can modify the level of demands. This can lay the groundwork for the child's feelings of competency (Bell & Ainsworth, 1972). Yarrow, Rubenstein, and Pederson (1975) identified several social aspects of maternal care and demonstrated the relationship between maternal behaviors, particularly playing with the infant, and the child's development.

Infants' responsiveness to the human environment varies according to sex, temperament, consolability, activity level, and state of health. The readiness of the infant for stimulus/interaction is one determinant of the infant's response. Brazelton and Als (1979) analyzed early interactions of infants. They found the newborn infant to be visually alert during daylight about 3 percent of the time. For the caregiver to provide stimulation/interaction at those times fosters adaptation. Meaningful stimuli, human and non-human, presented at a distance and a rate the child can accommodate, are necessary for adaptive response. Babies as young as two weeks old will look longer at a mother's face than at a stranger's, and will look distressed if the face is presented out of context. If the stimuli (human or non-human interaction) are presented too soon or with too great an intensity, irritability or depression of infant function may occur (White & Held, 1967).

Cultural values will guide the responses of the parent, the amount and kinds of stimulation, and what behaviors of the child will be accepted or rejected. The parents' own knowledge and skills also influence these behaviors. Poor parenting skills or physical or emotional disability can distort the parent-child relationship and reduce the infant's ability to respond and cope. In the process of defining their own roles, parents will define the child's role (Newman & Newman, 1978).

Each culture has its ideals by which children are shaped, socialized, and rewarded, and these tend to be interpreted by the family. A number of studies have suggested ethnic differences in infants' response styles to interactions. Kagan, Kearsley, and Zelana (1978) found that at three-and-one-half months of age, Caucasian and Chinese infants had similar smiling and vocalization responses but by eight months, differences were emerging. For example, they found a more variable heart rate in Caucasians under various stimulus conditions.

Childhood

Role of Fathers. In a 1974 study, Bronfenbrenner found that fathers had only 2.7 interactions per day with their infant one-year-olds, and these lasted an average of 37 seconds. Although there is a tendency for fathers to take a more active role in parenting today, this is not universally true. If one parent is absent in the family, it is most likely to be the father. Fathers and mothers may provide different functions in the child's development. It has been suggested that mothers tend to provide more linguistic support to the child, whereas fathers make more demands for role performance. If the father is not present and there is no other father figure to provide this role, the child may suffer performance deficits.

Fathers may also have an indirect effect on the child's developing competencies. Some suggest the secondary effects of the father's emotional and economic support of the wife allow her to provide more emotional support to the child (Lewis & Weinraub, 1976). Because many mothers work today, fathers may no longer assume this role and may seek new instrumental roles in the family (Mosey, 1986).

Learning to Walk: A Father's Influence on a Child with Cerebral Palsy

The wonderful rapport between us — father and daughter — greatly eased the monstrous task of learning to walk. Dad made it seem natural, washing away bitterness with love. It was a challenge we both worked at. There were no threats, no rigid schedules. I wasn't told I had to learn to walk: I wanted to. And Dad was always there ready to help.

Sometimes in teaching me to balance, Dad would plant my feet firmly on his wide, muscular hand and lift me into the air, letting go just briefly. His other hand was always there, ready to catch me if I would fall. As a child these moments with Dad were exciting.

But then it was time to take that first step — alone, without clinging to his comforting hand. Dad would stand against the living room wall and teach me to come into his outstretched arms.

Bitterly I would sob, "I can't."

"Come, Dad would urge, "I know you can."

I wanted to — desperately — but I couldn't. My feet were frozen to the spot with fear — a fear I still could taste as I sat in Dr. Retman's office, listening to Dad say, "Actually walking took a long time in coming."

From Heymanns, B (1977). Bittersweet triumph. Garden City, NY: Doubleday and Company, Inc. (p. 27)

Family Size and Birth Order. The size of the family may influence performance skills. Large families tend to foster a sense of privacy and independence in which children develop competencies (Haviland & Scarborough, 1981). Birth order can also make a difference: firstborns have been shown to be more likely to achieve success and show academic excellence, although there is no difference in intelligence (Newman & Newman, 1978).

Working Mothers and Day Care. The increase of women in the workforce has created a group of children without parental influence for long periods of time. A large number of school-age children, called "latchkey" children, return home from school to households with no adults present. There is concern among professionals over the possible effects of working mothers and the absence of adults in the home. Gaps in nurturance and guidance have not been adequately identified, but it is thought that if proper resources are made available, children can find alternative sources of support (Hoffman, 1974).

As the number of mothers in the work force increases, more children are spending their time in informal and formal child-care agencies. Such day care may be in the child's home, in another home of a relative or nonrelative, in unregulated family day care, or in licensed day care. Day care may act as a support network for both parent and child, providing instrumental support, emotional support, and information and referral services (Long, 1983). There has been a great deal of concern about the detrimental effects of day care, but most studies have failed to show such effects.

Although almost all studies agree that the attachment formed with the mother is the strongest and most influential for the infant, there is evidence that nonparental influences (siblings, peers, and adult caretakers) provide important social systems (Rutter, 1981). An emerging role for parents today is that of a coordinator of their children's socializing and early education experiences, including day care, special classes, and summer camps. (Long, 1983).

Families without Support Systems. The absence of social support or the lack of ability of parents to engage the support are frequently noted in families where child abuse has taken place. It has been shown that social isolation of the parents correlates with child maltreatment (Garbarino, Stocking, & associates, 1980). The social isolation may be the result of long-standing personality problems or it may be situational. Such programs as Parents Anonymous, a self-help group, are designed to foster social support for abusing and neglectful parents. How successful they are depends on the parents' ability to use the social relationships to relieve stress and begin to change their behavior.

Network Support for Families with Young Children. Some neighborhoods have a network of natural helpers that make it easier to locate day care services and to find answers to questions about parenting. When the family is not intact or when special problems occur, the need for a supportive social network increases. The network can help the parents in their role learning and maturation as parents, can help broaden the repertoire of parenting behaviors, and can link the parents to the outside world in new ways. The effects of personal networks on a child's development can be summed up as follows:

> "Network influence is both direct and indirect. It includes the sanctioning of parental behavior and the provision of material and emotional support for both parent and child. Network members also serve as models for parent and child, they stimulate the child directly and they involve the child more generally in network activities. These processes interact with the developmental age of the child to stimulate the basic trust, empathy and mastery of the reciprocal exchange skills essential to network building." (Cochran & Brassard, 1979, pp. 606-607).

Recent trends in supportive services include employee-sponsored child care (which has been met with indifference by many employees), comprehensive child care programs such as Head Start and Home Start, and resource and referral centers which provide education, advocacy, and political action groups, as well as networking and linking functions (Long, 1983).

Adolescence

Although adolescents are still members of the family, they must separate from the family to achieve adult status. Because of the importance of the peer group, adolescents can be described as moving into a miniculture of their own. This may be less true in rural communities in which adolescents grow up as part of the community as a whole rather than segregating into a peer group.

The peer group is a kind of social network that is considered developmentally important to the child and adolescent; and the occupational therapist is concerned with the nature and quality of these groups. Perceived emotional support of friends and number of reciprocal best friend relationships is an important contributor to measure of social and perceived self-competence measures in early adolescence (Cauce, 1986). Living in close proximity to one another appears to be the most important factor in selecting the peer group (Hollingshead, 1949).

Studies have been conducted on the kinds of groups developed by adolescents to meet their needs for developing autonomy, self-identify, and value clarification. Two examples of these groups are cliques and gangs. Cliques are small groups that tend to be mutually exclusive and marked by certain rules and visible characteristics, such as a high school group that socialize together, dress alike, and perhaps even talk alike. Those not conforming are excluded. Isolated and impulsive adolescents tend to be excluded from cliques (Dunphy, 1963).

Yablonsky (1970) identified three main types of adolescent gangs:

1. *social gangs,* in which long-lasting relationships center around the interests of group members such as team sports. Conformity to group goals is required and determines who joins.
2. *delinquent gangs,* in which the group rules violate the rules of the larger society and members are often rewarded with material goods or power. Conformity is required.
3. *violent gangs,* which are made up of members with unstable personalities who are not accepted by other groups. Proximity and conformity determine membership.

Although the peer group is a dominant social influence upon performance for adolescents, the family remains an important element in the social environment. Two important dimensions of parenting styles have been identified as (1) degree of warmth or rejection and (2) degree of control or permissiveness. Extremely controlling parents tend to have children with dependency on authority and lower self-esteem. Delinquents describe their parents as hostile and either authoritarian or permissive or swinging from one to the other (Haviland & Scarborough, 1981).

Adolescents of single-parent families have usually gone through the stress of their parents' divorce. Adolescents are more likely than younger children to have extra-family supports such as friends and schoolmates, and so may recover from the stress sooner. This may act to make them closer to friends and more distant from the family over the long term. Following the loss of a parent, adolescents are more likely to be given more responsibility for younger siblings and for their own life. With good support from friends and continuity of life situations, this situation can result in increased sense of competency for the adolescent. Without supports, the sense of competency may diminish (Haviland & Scarborough, 1981).

Early Adulthood

Marriage and childrearing are often a tasks of early adulthood. There is substantial evidence that marriage has a profound positive influence on health and thus on role performance. A number of health risks are associated with living alone. Men living alone whether single, separated, widowed, or divorced experience higher mortality rates; this occurs to a lesser degree in women (see Berkman, 1985, for a review of the literature).

It is during early adulthood that many people begin to have and raise children, which can greatly change the social support system and social network of the family (Boyce, 1985). Families with children tend to develop networks of others with children. Having children may result in more extensive interactions with kin but fewer with nonfamilial people (Hammer, Gurwirth, & Phillips, 1982). Spousal support appears the most potent social support for the mother, at least in terms of psychological well-being (D'Arcy & Siddique, 1984).

Societal values have changed to accept and even somewhat support the single lifestyle for carrying on roles of intimacy, work, and play without participating in marriage and childrearing roles. It is also possible and completely acceptable for a woman to go through medical school working long shifts required of internship, and still rear a family and maintain a home.

Middle Adulthood

Primary roles during middle adulthood involve work and homemaking. For the person with a family, work and family life are inextricably linked at this stage of life. Many studies have shown a relationship between health indicators and social support and work roles. There is evidence of a "spillover effect" of bringing work stresses into family life, such that men and women may experience fatigue, low motivation, and physiological responses that interfere with family role function. In a study of women married to Type A, top-level administrators, the wives reported negative effects on family roles; they experienced negative impact on family life, lower emotional support from a social network, and feelings of depression and isolation (Burke, Weir, & DuWors, 1979). It seems that wives may see their role as a

supporter of their husbands and expect to derive satisfaction from performing that role and are often disappointed as the husband distances himself from family life while trying to build up his career (Kasl & Wells, 1985). When both spouses work there may be different dynamics at work. For example, working wives feel that equity (reciprocity) in their marriage is more important than intimacy. Their levels of dissatisfaction, even depression, tend to be influenced by their husbands' not appreciating them or disagreeing about helping with the housework (Vanfossen, 1981).

During the middle adulthood years, people may experience other stressful situations such as their children leaving home, the stabilization of their careers, the added financial responsibility of children in college, and their parents who might need dependent care. So, particularly for women, the "freedom" they looked forward to during these years may not occur. Some women may even experience the added stress and isolation caused by the premature death of a spouse. All of these events require support systems to carry the families through these crises.

The Later Years

Performance in the later years can be influenced by physical and mental impairments, by a decrease in social support from spouses and social networks, and by an unpreparedness for the role and performance demands of old age. Elderly persons in learning and defining their roles often have limited access to their social networks because of chronic disabling conditions, economic limitations, and deaths of many members of their social network. How well one negotiates successful retirement from work and continues to function productively depend upon the timing or when it occurs, the stage of the retirement process (Minkler, 1985), and the kind of work done (Haynes, McMichael, & Tyroler, 1977; Martin & Doran, 1966; Stokes & Maddox, 1967). The person is less likely to be healthy and productive if valued social contacts are lost. Sometimes social resources may buffer the possible negative effects of retirement (Minkler, 1985).

Because most older Americans live in their own homes, they are often able to retain their social network as they get older. A relatively small number of older people move to age-segregated housing that limits their interaction with people of other age ranges. The effects of this move cause a decline in some relationships and improvement in others, although most of those who choose this arrangement report being satisfied (Perlmutter & Hall, 1985). A small proportion of the elderly live in institutional settings, primarily nursing homes, which may severely separate them from relationships. The feelings of separation and isolation that accompany a move into a nursing home can often cause a decline or even death. In essence, the elderly person's total social network decreases, often resulting in depression and decrease in function because of a chronic state of coping with the unremitting sense of loss of spouse and friends.

Loss of a family member is a major stressful and traumatic life event. It has been shown that the surviving spouse is considered at increased risk for morbidity and mortality (Minkler, 1985), particularly during the first six months after the death (Parkes, Benjamin, & Fitzgerald, 1969), and this is particularly true among men (Helsing, Comstock, and Szklo, 1981). Married men who lose a spouse appear to be at greater risk than married women, particularly older women, who are not found to have the same severe response. Neugarten (1979) suggests that older women may cope better because perhaps they anticipate and expect this event in their later years and are thus more prepared for it.

In addition to diminishment of social networks, older people have less varied sources of contact to call upon for help (Pilisuk & Parks, 1986). Kulys and Tobin (1980) found that most elderly named close relatives when asked who would be responsible for them in a crisis. Some of the respondents were unsure of whether or not they could really count on this person, because in some cases this relative was not nearby or emotionally close. When those relatives named were told of this choice, some were found to be surprised or annoyed by the choice (Kulys & Tobin, 1980). There are few available well-controlled studies to demonstrate that social support from health care providers during this period can make a difference in the mortality/morbidity level, but those available appear to demonstrate a positive outcome (Raphael, 1977).

Older people are often not prepared for their roles of old person, retiree, and widow or widower. The aging person may find himself in a devalued position that has ambiguous norms and expectations (Rosow, 1974). In later years, the older person loses many of his/her former roles such as spouse, or parent (if isolated from their children), or bread winner, and there may not be other roles to replace them (Rosow, 1974). Blau (1954) points out that widows tend to be excluded from their groups of married friends and cannot find viable substitutes for the relationships until their social groups become composed of a large portion of widows. Their status is often diminished, and there are no formal or respected contexts in which to learn or adjust to their new roles. This all contributes to a sense of worthlessness, isolation and even depression.

Case Study 6-2

91-year-old Lydia: Lydia is a 91-year-old female, widowed and living alone on a farm in a sparsely populated rural community approximately three miles from the nearest town, which has a population of about 8,000 residents. She entered the hospital with a diagnosis of acute myocardial infarction, had an uneventful recovery, and within five days of admission was evaluated for her ability to return to her home alone. Daily living skills evaluation revealed that she could manage her personal hygiene, dressing, and grooming with the exception of pulling dresses over her head and putting on support hose. However, because of limitations of strength and endurance, and need for bed rest and graded activities, she was unable to manage homemaking tasks and occupational tasks of managing the farm chores. The decision about whether she needed nursing home care or whether she could stay at home was dependent upon information about her social resources, since her finances were limited and she was dependent upon Medicare assistance for her medical bills.

The Kinship Network Analysis revealed a good number of potential resources for assistance among relatives; however, none of them lived in the home. Two daughters lived about 50 miles away, were working mothers, but were available on weekends. One son, about 150 miles away, was retired and thus able to leave his family for periods of time. Another son, 500 miles away, was willing and able to contribute financially. A nephew and his wife living six miles away agreed to call periodically and drop by to help with non-routine tasks. Thus, a plan was developed for having family members alternate spending time with Lydia. At that time, reevaluation revealed that Lydia was able to manage daily tasks, including returning to driving, but the family was not comfortable with her being alone at night. Funds from the son enabled the family to hire a retired but active woman to stay at the farm at night.

The other social systems in which Lydia was embedded were evaluated in relation to support for motivation, health behaviors, and community activity. Several groups were a part of this network including her church, United Methodist Women's group, American Association of Retired Persons, and the quilters' group at the community center program for senior citizens. Members of the church's Sunday School class, a close-knit group that provided not only spiritual support but also a great deal of reality orientation during their Sunday School classes, and instituted a telephone network to see that everyone was doing well and was well informed about everyone else.

The AARP was used by the respondent as the basis for information. Lectures were provided on social policy and health-related issues. The recreational opportunities provided by the AARP were largely ignored. The members of the quilting group provided recreation and social support. They visited, laughed, shared, and criticized each other freely if needed (that is, offered advice about behavior). They had into center funds. They also provided each other with a great deal of medical information. Some was related to folk remedies, but most of it was related to the latest medical treatments available. This exchange provided valuable health information. Shopping around for health care in her community required skill. There was only one hospital which was threatening to close. A visit to a specialty clinic might require taking the van to a town over 50 miles away and sitting long hours in a clinic to get the kind of special care they felt appropriate.

Lydia identified a strong value for being cognitively able and independent. Though sources for financial support were limited in the strict monetary sense, she received and gave things of value frequently. For example, almost every visitor to her home brought something, whether it was a plant, some food, or a garden tool. And most went away with flowers, eggs, homemade bread, or garden produce. She was very careful to exchange fairly. The trade may also be made for practical assistance and food or flowers.

Identification of social resources confirmed that, with minor adjustments, Lydia was able to remain in her home and be a valuable and valued member of the community.

Note: From Wolfensberger, W. (1973). A selective overview of the works of Jean Vanier and the movement of L'Arche.

Special Influences on the Family

Pets. Although animals have been viewed as important to humans throughout history, it has been only recently that behavioral scientists and health care workers have taken an interest in the potential value of their relationships to people. Pets may provide the following functions: (1) companionship, (2) something to keep one busy, (3) something to care for, (4) something to touch and fondle, (5) a focus of attention, (6) exercise, and (7) safety (Katcher & Friedmann, 1980). The findings of a survey conducted in 11 states in the United States showed that 87 percent of the respondents considered their pets to be members of the family, while a lesser percent stated that they thought of their pets as people (Cain, 1979). There is a heightened interest in considering pets as a part of the social environment and investigating their effect on the health and functional behavior of their owners.

Not all people view pets as desirable. Pets might be avoided because of cultural values, health reasons, because they get under foot and may cause falls and injuries, or because of the inability to meet the demands they make for care and attention.

Families with Physically Disabled Children. Families of physically disabled children have unique problems in rearing their children and most are totally unprepared for this special role. Many of the special problems stem from parents' ignorance of the nature or the capacities inherent in the disability and a tendency for parents to overprotect and perform functions for the child that he/she is able to accomplish on his/her own (Lindemann, 1981). For exam-

ple, if it takes an hour for a disabled child to dress himself/herself, parents may dress the child to save time. Such tendencies to do things for the child, may make it difficult for the child to develop accurate self-knowledge and to perform to capability. Over the longterm, the child may feel comfortable with this overprotection and begin to play the role of "special" or "pitiful" child. Overprotection of the disabled can be a problem at any age and can result in a lack of environmental challenge and blandness; some authors have proposed that risk and novelty be programmed into the lives of disabled persons.

Therapists often call upon parents to provide therapy and other related support for their disabled child. This new role as therapist can often alter the relationship between parent and child. When asking parents to take on a new role such as performing therapeutic exercises with the child, therapists need to be sensitive to what is occurring and try to reinforce comfortable and positive interactions. Tyler, Kogan, and Turner (1974) studied the responses of mothers to training designed to implement therapy with their children and found that mothers were apparently uncomfortable with the role of therapist, and they showed more control and negative responses when giving therapy than when in free play with the child. They also found a longitudinal decrease in expression of moderate warmth both among therapists and mothers. Tyler and Kogan (1977) found that it was possible to alter the negative affective interaction of the mother and child by providing immediate feedback to decrease negative behavior. They concluded that mothers could manage therapeutic tasks in moderation if given training and support. There is no doubt that there is added stress and responsibility in raising and caring for children with disabilities that requires special training and support from health professionals and the community.

Families of the chronically ill and disabled child usually adapt more effectively if they have social networks available to them. The network members can perform a variety of needed tasks such as taking the child to the doctor, administering medicines, and offering emotional support (Hansen & Rosenthal, 1987).

Special Problems of those with Psychosocial Dysfunction. The social networks of people with major psychiatric illnesses have been described as different from those with the less severe emotional problems of a normal population. It is difficult for people with psychotic conditions to engage in reciprocal relationships. They tend to have a small primary network, with less interpersonal intimacy, greater asymmetry in helping exchanges, and less stability, and minimal friendship ties (Gottlieb, 1985; Pattison, Llasman, & Hurd, 1979; Pilisuk & Parks, 1986). Network ties may be described as often ambivalent at best rather than supportive.

Because of the chronic nature of psychiatric illness and the subsequent demands on the helping network, these patients create a feeling of burden in the helping network (Froland, et al., 1979).

Families of those with psychosocial dysfunction have in the past sometimes been implicated as contributing to the dysfunction. Research findings have been questionable regarding this because of inadequate controls and researchers' bias, and the difficulty of measuring degree of support and perception of people with mental and emotional conditions who often cannot perceive others as being supportive.

Intense emotional relationships appear to be poorly tolerated by people with schizophrenic disorders. This has been demonstrated in family relationships (Caton, 1984) and in community treatment settings (Linn, et al., 1979), where more positive social functioning was seen when patients were involved in the more object-focused activity of occupational therapy than when they participated in intensive group therapy.

People with less serious psychiatric problems are described as having a somewhat larger network than the seriously ill, but the network often involves distant people or having ties that may be negative (Henderson et al., 1978). Depressed patients were found to lack confiding relationships, experience loneliness, and engage in both fewer leisure activities and activities involving others, when compared to nonpsychiatric controls (Eisemann, 1985). Some researchers have found evidence that relationships can protect against depression when people experience severe life events (Brown, 1978).

It is well accepted that there is a correlation between social support and recovery from illness, both physical and psychological. Different kinds of support appear differentially helpful. For example, support and information from the doctor may influence psychological adjustment to breast cancer, but not physical recovery (Wortman & Conway, 1985).

The fact that a person has relationships does not always assure positive effects on recovery. Sometimes friends and family may find aspects of an illness or disability so distressing, that they may tend to avoid the sick or disabled person. Quite understandably, this avoidance might be interpreted as rejection by the one who is ill or disabled. Peters-Golden (1982) found that approximately 75 percent of respondents said that people treated them differently after learning they had cancer.

The Therapist's Role

Because psychiatric patients do not have reliable social support systems on which to call for help, health care professionals tend to create networks for them. This can sometimes be a self-defeating activity as it has been shown that better effects are achieved when therapists foster natural, embedded networks of their clients even when these networks seem fragile (D'Augelli, 1983).

In learning to play supportive roles for the ill, therapists should study natural helping behaviors that people use when helping others. It is also useful to ask the patient what they think might be a helpful approach. Because patients often do not know when and how to ask for help, patients with poor prognoses may receive little support from health care workers when they need it the most. Therapists can identify strategies that seem to elicit support and then educate patients about how to use such strategies. Therapists may need to help patients practice such skills as sociability, assertiveness, comfort with intimacy, and the ability to empathize with others. This ability to empathize can help patients understand their family members' discomfort about their illness or disability. They may also need to explore their values and beliefs about appropriate times to ask for help (Wortman & Conway, 1985).

PLAY/LEISURE/RECREATION: INFLUENCE ON PERFORMANCE

Play is often said to be a child's work and although expected to elicit pleasure and laughter, it is often taken very seriously by the child. The importance given to play by occupational therapists is illustrated in this statement:

> "Children who do not play come to adulthood ill prepared. They lack task and interpersonal skills, have no sense of their place in the world, feel unable to effect change on their environment, do not know what to expect, or what is expected. They are basically naive, and often angry." (Mosey, 1986, p. 84).

Play is considered essential for later activity, task, and role performance. A play environment is initially mediated by a parenting adult. Later on, the play environment is self-selected and offers the opportunity for peer socialization and time away from adults. Objects, task activities, and people in the play environment provide opportunities for exploration and sensory, motor, psychosocial, and cognitive growth.

Play in the Home and Family

The home setting is traditionally where early play takes place. The child is more or less free to explore and play. The home environment must be safe and invite exploration. The objects in the environment should have just the right amount of both novelty and familiarity. The humans in the environment act as mediators of the play objects, project a certain playfulness and pleasure in the play, and act as models for play behavior. The mother is usually considered the most central figure in family modeling, although the father's role is also important. If a mother is unable to care for herself or experience pleasure in her roles, she is an unsatisfactory model for her children in terms of social competence. If this mother is labeled "mentally ill," a status not valued by society, the psychological outcome for her children would likely be social incompetence. In cases like these where unsatisfactory role models exist, the child then will need some alternative or additional model to develop task and interpersonal skills.

In addition to analyzing these parental models, the therapist should analyze the family organization in terms of status, value, and psychological outcome. It has been shown that many chronically disabled clients share common characteristics with the victims of poverty and can be described in terms of the same cultural values (Reilly, 1974).

Playgrounds

Much of the older child's play takes place outside the home. The playground, planned or natural, is ideally perceived as an environment in which the child can make choices and express himself freely. In other words, the child is relatively free from parental influence and more likely to be influenced by peers. However, in reality, the child in a given neighborhood may have the task of adopting or adapting to whatever is available whether it is the street or alley or a vacant lot (Berg & Medrich, 1980). In this case the neighborhood becomes the playground and may be analyzed as such. Peers are likely to be those living nearby. If a child's playground should be one in which he is freed from management by adults, the disabled child who cannot move or act to manipulate the environment or take part freely in usual play activities is doubly disadvantaged. Disabled children are severely limited in playground activities by their physical disabilities and the physical and social barriers of the play environment (Takata, 1971). Thus the disabled child experiences deficits in play and in play environments. Differences have been reported in the developmental age levels of play between handicapped and non-handicapped children (Behnke & Menarcheck-Fetkovich, 1984; Munoz, 1986). Gralewicz (1973) found that handicapped children spent significantly less time in play and spent less time with adults and with other children than did the nonhandicapped. For disabled children, the time that might be used for play was needed for treatment instead.

The therapist's task of creating the "just-right" environment for the disabled child requires skill, energy, and creativity. The autobiography of Cristy Brown who was born with cerebral palsy (Brown, 1971) is a compelling account of the impact of parental belief, support, instrumental behaviors, and a strong play network in producing competent behaviors regardless of severe barriers.

The Hospital and Play Behavior

The hospital environment has been examined in terms of its influence on play behaviors. In the hospital, the normal rhythms of activity are all centered around routine medical care and not play activity. The parents are inhibited by the fact that this is not their territory, and the children are not able to cultivate their private play spaces. They tend to see themselves as being unable to control the environment (Kielhofner, et al., 1983).

If successful play is the foundation of adaptive function, then occupational therapists offer an important role in designing play spaces in hospitals and in designing remedial play programs. There seems to be disagreement regarding how much structure and initiative in the play situation should be provided by the therapist or caretaker of the child with developmental delays (see Munoz, 1986, for a review of the evidence). It appears that the severity of the disability, particularly in the cognitive realm, interferes with spontaneous play and increases the importance of the therapist as mediator of the social environment. However, there may be an equal danger of overstructuring the activity and preventing the emergence of spontaneous play.

Michelman (1974) has developed a play agenda for "the deficit child" in which she specifies environmental elements that will (a) evoke interaction with the environment, (b) foster mastery of symbols, and (c) develop risk-taking, problem-solving, and decision-making. She describes the therapist as mediating between the child and the environment by arranging objects, spaces, and tasks that are matched to the child's capabilities and which will arouse curiosity, require a gradation of play experiences for growth, and offer opportunities for experiencing feelings of efficacy. The social environment that she describes consists of adults that model the excitement of exploration and older children who can model behavior. Social activity should alternate with solitary activity, and the children in the group should allow for interaction, cooperation, and competition.

In summary, since ordinary play settings may not be accesible to the child with disability, parents and therapists must design environments that encourage success and include adults who are resource people and role models, and peers who offer developmental age-appropriate interaction and feedback.

Leisure Activity Settings

Throughout the lifetime, a person needs a time away from work and responsibilities, a time to restore oneself and find meaning in life. The term *leisure* is commonly used for this activity. Leisure is characterized by relative choice and is usually shared by people of like interests. The activity may be something one likes to do alone or with other people. The leisure environment may be solitary or crowded with people. The social mood is usually one of playfulness and one that is relatively free from standards and rules (although religious and sports occasions may involve a great many rules specific to those groups).

These settings are those away from work and away from the management of the home or personal living situation; they include recreational, religious, and esthetic activities (Shera & Johnson, 1984). Mosey (1986) reminds us that leisure should be seen as a time to seek meaning in life and to be free to be self-determined. Leisure pursuits are influenced by age, gender, occupation, marital status, and education. They may be solitary or social activities.

Choice of groups in which one engages in leisure activities is based on a compromise between mutuality and equal status and on a need for interaction and activities that are inherently rewarding. Membership in the leisure activity group may require people to interact with others with whom they might have little in common except for interest in the activity itself (Secord, Backman, & Slavitt, 1976). For example, one might go on bird-watching expeditions with others with whom he/she would not otherwise normally associate.

Solitary activities are not necessarily lonely activities. The element of choice appears to be critical in differentiating between the two. Often people who work in high-contact, stressful jobs select silence and solitude for their leisure activity. Reading and engaging in hobbies may or may not be shared with another. However, when the activity is solitary because the individual lacks mobility or the social skills to engage in social activity, a problem is identified. People living in institutions often do not have the luxury of a solitary activity because they lack private space.

PERFORMANCE IN THE WORKPLACE

"Work is an instrumental activity in which one struggles with the environment for compelling material reasons: physical survival, social survival, and rewarding social status. It is any formal activity that involves or prepares one to earn a living, i.e., education or remunerative employment. It is limited by time, place, and structural organization " (Mosey, 1986, p. 71).

In a complex society, work is organized in such a way that the needs of the ongoing social group are met. Different social groups have different values, regulations, and laws related to who works and how work is done, and these may

come in conflict with the person's needs. For example, although a 70-year-old person may still be productive and motivated to work, he/she may be legally required to retire.

Early work settings tended to combine work and play in a rhythm quite different from many modern workplaces. The industrial era ushered in a demand for ways to make workers more productive. The studies known as the Hawthorne or Western Electric studies conducted in the early 1900's were the outgrowth of just that demand. The researchers discovered some important things about how work groups function in the work settings. They found that people in continuous contact with each other can form strong, cohesive groups with norms for behavior and with patterned ways of working together. They discovered that some group norms contribute to productive behavior and some do not. For example, groups may set rates for quality of work that restrict as well as enhance productivity. Olmsted (1959) found that workers assume individual roles within the group and subgroups form that may compete with each other.

In a complex society, work settings are many and varied. Many work settings are organizations that are social units or human groups, deliberately constructed to seek specific goals (Parsons, 1964). These organizational goals are primary and the function of management is to see that people's capabilities and needs fit well with the organization's goals. The work environment demands certain standards of performance.

Demands of Work Settings

Work requires varied degrees of skill in physical, cognitive, and psychosocial areas. Work environments demand both general work skills, such as getting to work on time and getting along with fellow workers, and specific job-related skills. The *general work skills* are usually acquired through general socialization processes, and *specific work skills* are usually acquired by specific training or education. In addition to performing job tasks, a particular type of work may require specific other behaviors, such as one might be expected to dress in a certain style or engage in certain social behaviors both inside and outside the work setting.

Environment-Person Fit at Work

Development of the worker role is seen as a lifetime process in several stages. The child learns about self, tries out behaviors, and develops interests and identity in what has been termed, *the fantasy stage.* The adolescent, in *the tentative stage,* may try worker roles, analyze the fit between personal competencies and the demands in various settings, and thus gradually narrow the choices. In *the realistic stage,* the choices are actually made.

It is no longer assumed that the individual will work in one setting for a lifetime. Often the individual pauses to reassess during adulthood and may change worksettings or occupations (Ginsberg, 1957). Thus an occupational career is a developmental and a lifelong process. When there is a *good fit* between the demands of the work setting and the individual, the person is likely to be satisfied in terms of economic needs, needs of self-esteem, and mastery needs. Stress occurs when there is a *poor fit* between the individual and the worker role or the work setting. A job is stressful when it does not provide rewards and supports to meet a person's motives and when a person's ability falls below the job demands required to receive the rewards and supports. The way the individual appraises (cognitively and emotionally) the situation, determines the level of stress perceived.

Stress and Job Performance

Four working conditions that might produce stresses are identified by Levi, Frankenhaeuser, and Gardell (1986):

1. *quantitative overload*: too much to do, time pressure, or repetitive work flow, in combination with one-sided job demands on attention, such as mass production technology or routine office work;
2. *qualitative underload*: too narrow, one-sided job content, a lack of stimulus variation, no demands on the individual's creativity or problem-solving skills, or low opportunities to have social interaction;
3. *lack of control*, specifically in relation to work methods or work pace;
4. *lack of social support* at home, in the community, or from fellow workers.

In examining the environmental press and arousal and choice of work settings, some authors have characterized work by the amount of decision-making and the work demands of the job. Some jobs make high demands but have a large margin for decision-making and are therefore considered stimulating, such as managers or journalists. Other jobs make few demands but have a reduced margin for decision-making and provide relatively little stimulation, such as a night watchman. Stress is perceived when work makes excessive demands and allows little control.

Certain job characteristics or working conditions, are by their nature, high in such stresses. For example, assembly line work appears to be related to feelings of lack of control, monotony, social isolation, lack of freedom, and time pressure. Observers of assembly line work have described resulting discontent, stress, and alienation among the workers. Jobs that are highly automated and demand strict attention to detail and where errors can produce dire consequences are particularly stressful as in the case of air traffic controllers.

The social structure of the work setting can also contribute to stress. If workers are paid collectively by the number of objects produced, there tends to be social pressure from their fellow employees. If workers are paid only by what they individually produce, there may be a reluctance to help each other. This is evidenced by the fact that fewer injuries were reported in industries such as mining and logging when management changed from the piecework system of reward to fixed salaries (Levi et al., 1986).

The human factors aspects of a job are often the most stressful. For example, working as a nurse with terminally ill and dying patients is generally considered to be a stressful occupation. Yet one study gave some surprising results when 327 health care workers were asked what caused their stress. They reported the stress of working with sick patients to account for only 15 percent of the stress, 36 percent of the stressors was attributed to the organization of the workplace and communication problems, and the largest stressor reported was "team communications problems" (Vachon, 1987).

Social support may act as a buffer against the stressors of the job and may also represent a coping strategy when mobilized by the individual. However, social relationships may themselves be stressors and interfere with job performance. An example of family interference is the working mother whose performance suffers because she loses sleep while staying awake with a sick child. However, not everyone needs the same amount of social support to counter job stress. Brown (1978) found that those who did not seek help could be divided into two categories, self-reliant respondents who had well-integrated networks but did not choose to use them, and reluctant non-seekers who showed the least effective coping repertoires and lowest self-esteem.

People can cope with the stress by talking with others in the workplace. Caplan (1971) studied NASA administrators, scientists, and engineers and found that they were less likely to experience work-related stress if they perceived high levels of interpersonal supportive relationships. However, he concluded that not all types of support are equally effective and not all types of stress and health are equally affected. Generally, work-related stressors are best buffered by supervisors' and coworkers' social support, although there are some effects of stress such as boredom that are not buffered by support. It has been found that supervisors are the most powerful source of support especially for those at lower levels. Spouses can be important sources of support, but Caplan found friends and other relatives to be less important as social supports.

Wells (1987) suggests the following social strategies to manage the stresses of technical environments (*techno-stress*):

1. Promote interaction among workers and involve the

workers in developing the strategies, whether they are creating work groups or coordinating rest breaks

2. Increase job decision latitude, for example, let three workers cooperate to decide the best approach to their task.

3. Train supervisors to provide support to the workers they supervise (workers feel less stress if supervisors are supportive).

4. Make work hours flexible, so that employees can benefit from support from home.

5. Promote the health and well-being of workers.

Other Influences on Work Performance

Choice seems to be an important motivational factor in the performance level of an occupation. Mullen (1986) found that women who have choices about whether to work or be homemakers tend to have better health than those who must assume the work role in order to survive (e.g., single mothers).

Another positive influence on work performance is whether the work fosters self-esteem. When the work is considered dirty, disagreeable or dangerous, or unlawful, this may reduce self-esteem. If the person has poor work performance and cannot do the job, again he/she may experience low self-esteem. When the social group does not value the work, the individual tends not to find it valuable or meaningful.

Because of the standards and demands for performance, many disabled people do not work and do not expect to work. Some disabled people may not be able to work because of impairments in mobility or manual dexterity. Others may not have developed general work skills, or they may be handicapped by the attitudes or reactions of potential employers or fellow workers (Mosey, 1986).

PERFORMANCE IN THE INSTITUTIONAL SETTING

Occupational therapists have long sought to introduce normal patterns of activity into institutions and have studied institutions from two primary perspectives: the influence of institutionalization on posture and sensorimotor behaviors and the impact of **institutionalization** on certain vulnerabilities of the individual.

Institutionality is a multidimensional construct. Goffman (1961), in his book *Asylums*, defines the *total institution* as "a place of residence and work where a large number of like-situated individuals, cut off from the wider society for an appreciable period of time, together lead an enclosed, formally administered round of life" (p. xiii). The total nature of the institution is characterized by a barrier to

social intercourse with the outside world and a barrier to departure. The key fact of total institutions is that they are set up to handle large groups of people by a "bureaucratic organization" of people. Social distance is great between staff and inmates, and work and play for the inmates has a different meaning from that of the outside world.

Many people living in institutions suffer from institutional neurosis. Institutional neurosis is characterized as a disease involving apathy, lack of initiative, loss of interest (especially in things of an impersonal nature), submissiveness, apparent inability to make plans for the future, lack of individuality, and sometimes a characteristic posture and gait (Barton, 1976; Beck & Callahan,1980; Wing & Brown, 1970). This is can be attributed to a combination of the illness or disability itself and the effects of inadequate environmental stimulation.

Institutional life can be made more appealing if opportunities for fellowship exist. In addressing this need, Wolfensberger (1973) has written:

> For retarded adults who are unlikely to marry, I now see more fully the need to create occasions and settings which bring joy and create a spirit of communal life and fellowship. Much as in the armed forces, monasteries, vessels at sea, and similar celibate settings, only deeply-felt fellowship and the love of comrades can compensate most adults, including retarded ones, for that which they ordinarily seek in an spouse and children.

Nursing Homes

The typical nursing home resident is white, female, widowed, and alone. Residents in nursing homes generally suffer from multiple chronic conditions and functional impairments. However, for every elderly person who is institutionalized, there are at least two other people living in the community who have about the same degree of functional impairment. Only a small percentage will leave the nursing home to return to their homes, and in many cases, little effort is made to encourage a return to independent living.

The nursing home has been the target of much criticism. Certain social conditions of the nursing home have been identified as increasing the risk of loss of performance capacity or opportunity. It has been suggested that nursing home care is directed toward the least competent person (Posner, 1974), and that competent behavior may be considered inappropriate by the cultural expectations of the nursing home. The resident has a different lifestyle imposed, one that fosters a passivity and one that does not threaten the routine of the nursing home. When investigators observed more than 1000 residents in 44 nursing homes over a two-day period for social contacts, nearly three-fourths of the residents were observed to have no contact with any staff member. And for more than one-half of the observation period, the residents were not engaged in a meaningful activity (Gottesman & Boureston, 1974). Jones and van Amelsvoort Jones (1986) studied communication patterns between nursing staff and elderly persons in an extended intermediate care facility and found that at peak interaction time, the nursing staff spoke an average of seven words per hour with residents, and most of the communication consisted of commands.

Relocation from one's home or normal living situation is viewed as a stressful life event with severe responses in many people. Many earlier researchers have identified increased mortality and morbidity factors related to relocation to a nursing home, but do not agree on its cause (Blenkner, 1967). More recent studies have failed to replicate early findings, perhaps because more attention is paid to careful pre-location planning (Minkler, 1985). Other studies have indicated factors that appear to influence the health and function of those entering nursing homes including: (1) the person's participation in the decision of whether to enter the nursing home, (2) the ability to plan and participate in the transition process (Jasnau, 1967; Novick, 1967), (3) the degree of social support (Minkler, 1985), (4) the extent to which the event is predictable, and (5) the extent to which the individual has control (Schultz & Brenner, 1977).

An involuntary move into a nursing home is much more traumatic than a voluntary one. Involuntary moves are often precipitated by the loss of spouse or other social supports, an illness, or loss or diminishment of physical function. The loss of control associated with an involuntary move leads to a realization that one's life is controlled by outside forces, an expectation for future loss of control, and a belief that one's actions cannot influence the outcome of events. This feeling of "learned helplessness" is said to result in such symptoms as passivity, frustration, depression, and anxiety (Seligman, 1975). It involves the person's motivation, cognition, and behavior, and is manifested in ways similar to that of a reactive depression. This "helpless" individual no longer participates in activities that were previously perceived as pleasant, and is thus further removed from social situations in which support can be received. The performance of daily living activities, both productive and leisure activities, is absent or reduced. The complications of inactivity ensue and morbidity is increased.

Returning some sense of control to the individual seems to lessen helplessness (Seligman, 1975). Some studies have demonstrated differences in function when residents were given opportunities to exercise control (Langer & Rodin, 1976; Mercer & Kane, 1979). Langer and Rodin provided an experimental group of nursing home residents with the opportunity to choose and care for a plant after hearing a discussion on the responsibilities and opportunities for decision-making. The control group members were given plants for which the staff had the responsibility to care. Eighteen months later members of the group who cared for their own plants were reported to be more active and alert, while 71 percent of the control group were rated as more debilitated.

Langer (1975) has described the "illusion of control" or the possibility of limited decision-making, in which the individual perceives that he is exercising control in a specific situation. The exercise of this limited control can help maintain or even develop a sense of competency in which the individual's performance is optimized. Averell (1973) has described three types of control that a resident might exercise: *behavioral, cognitive,* and *decisional.* An example of behavioral control might be a patient doing range of motion exercises for himself/herself rather than allowing the therapist to conduct passive exercises. Cognitive control is represented by the patient's access to information with which he can then control events, for example, the therapist gives information about what happens to the musculoskeletal system and how to prevent deformities. Decisional control is using the opportunity to choose from among several options, such as deciding whether to do exercises in a group setting or whether or not to participate in a sport.

It is important to differentiate between choice and control. It is assumed that people scan the environment and identify the range of choices available to them. The opportunity for choices increases motivation, which in turn improves performance on a task. However, the exercise of the choice alone is not sufficient to increase a sense of control.

Nelson and Ferberow (1980) have suggested that if nursing home residents lack a sense of control, they may attempt to reestablish control by some acts of non-compliance, such as refusing to get out of bed, smoking, or violating a diabetic diet. This may be a way of indirect suicide. In this case, the sense of control is maintained at a great cost to the individual, and it is indeed self-destructive. A goal for therapists or other health professionals should be to help replace these destructive behaviors with more healthy behavior that provides the same sense of control. For example, allowing patients to plan their own menu might be a decisional control option that could promote adherence to diet.

By Goffman's definition of *total institutions,* work and play take on different meanings in a nursing home. But when work and play behavior link them to the community, they share the same definition as in the community. In a study by Hatter and Nelson (1987), significantly more of the residents participated when asked to make Christmas cookies for children at a preschool than when invited simply to make cookies to eat.

The physical and organizational environment can influence social climate in nursing homes (Moos, 1984). Settings with more physical amenities, better social-recreational aids, more available personal space, and more options for personal choices were likely to foster more cohesive and independent performance of the residents.

Institutions for Mentally Retarded Persons

The social climate of an institution for mentally retarded persons can likewise support either competent or incompetent performance. Kielhofner and Takata (1980) ethnographically analyzed the perception of the mentally retarded person's relationship with the institutional environment. They concluded that the social world of institutionalized mentally retarded persons is composed of a limited number of staff, usually a social worker, maybe workers at an activity center and fellow residents. The "normals" are seen as being powerful, and rewarding inactivity and incompetence by "helping" residents but not reinforcing autonomy. So helplessness is perceived as a purposeful strategy on the part of the residents. Because privacy is nonexistent, hoarding becomes a reaction. Ways in which therapists can help increase competent performance in institutionalized people are by: 1) evaluating the individual's strengths in ways of managing the environment adaptively, 2) establishing a horizontal rather than vertical or helper relationship, and 3) requiring that clients be involved in their own decision-making and development of competencies.

Performance in Prisons

A number of studies have explored the idea that the social climate of the prison makes demands for odd and specific kinds of responses. For example, in order to avoid confrontation with prison guards, new prisoners quickly learn to show an apathetic and blank face (called dogfacing). The prisoners quickly learn to behave like prisoners in order to survive.

Haney, Banks, and Zimbardo (1973) and Haney and Zimbardo (1977) described an interesting study in which they had students play roles of prisoner or guard. It was found that once involved in the role, the guards often found themselves becoming brutal and the prisoners passive as each role demanded. Although these studies were criticized for methodological problems, they are frequently cited as evidence that the social context supports such behaviors and that public policy authorizes such situations, and creates routines where such abusive behavior can occur, and where dehumanization can take place (Rodin, 1985). Thus, prisons may reinforce the excluded status of criminals, and the structure and the values may support abuse and recidivism.

So we see that institutions are places in which roles and temporal dimensions are constricted. In institutions, the natural rhythms of life are distorted and people often feel disoriented and devalued. Therapists and other health care professionals can help create an environment that fosters physical comfort, involvement in decision-making, activity patterns congruent to residents' interests and life tasks, their integration into the community, and increased performance of activities, tasks and roles.

PERFORMANCE IN TREATMENT SETTINGS

The psychologist, Rudolf Moos, and his associates at Stanford University Social Ecology Laboratory have done a great deal of work in studying the social environment of various treatment settings. They began by studying psychiatric treatment settings, both hospital-based and community-based. In general, they found that the programs that tend to lead to improvement in self-care and community skills are the ones that emphasize practical, task-oriented learning, encourage independence, and support personal responsibility. If programs are poorly organized, have unclear goals, or poor staff and peer support, there is a higher dropout rate from treatment.

Different kinds of patients react differently to specific aspects of the environment depending on their level of emotional disturbance. More disturbed patients need a more tolerant, relatively structured setting that does not require too much interpersonal stimulation (Cronkite, Moos, & Finney, 1983).

Kaplan (1988) has applied the principles of structure and support with a group of psychiatric patients with a minimal level of functioning. She used a directive approach and structured the environment to assure maximum participation of all members. She reported that it was successful in helping the patients reorganize and prepare for a more verbal and mature level of function.

Schooler and Spohn (1982) provide a thought-provoking analysis of a "resocialization" program that they instituted over 20 years ago. With a group of patients diagnosed with schizophrenia, they attempted to provide an experimental "socioenvironmental" ward to counteract the social disengagement commonly seen in these patients. Patients were provided with group leaders who were trained to lead feeling-oriented group discussions twice a day and to attempt to foster the group's feeling of social unity. Baseline measurements were made and again taken two years after the program began. Results showed the experimental group showed a higher level of interaction but also poorer performance on psychological tests. Reseachers observed the effects of environmental design and used the information to modify treatment approaches and to better understand the patients' needs.

Twenty years later they concluded that their social environmental design was contraindicated. Their conclusions and current theory suggest that schizophrenics use social withdrawal as a protection against the cognitive-perceptual overload and emotional arousal produced by the social contact. One patient's reaction revealed that before the experimental environment he had likened his self-isolation to a glass shell from which he could see out but not hear activities around him. When staff and other patients forced interaction, he felt as if they were trying to shatter his shell which frightened him. This study serves to warn therapists to constantly assess the effects of the social environment and modify them as needed.

Hospital Environment. By definition, people in hospitals are sick and the sick role implies a moratorium on all demands for competent performance of life roles. Gray (1972) challenged occupational therapists to reexamine this definition and the treatment environment of a hospital setting. If hospitalization is prolonged, the patient may lose his/her work-play skills even when there are no disabling sequelae. Expectations and demands of hospitals do not reinforce normal values or practices of work and play and temporal adaptation. Gray even suggests that many health care workers do not model good work-play values or even physical fitness. This situation may be worsened by the fact that in the patient's absence, the family constellation may have shifted, and others may have taken on his/her roles and responsibilities. Even though the trends are toward much shorter hospital stays, these problems of the hospital environment still exist.

Several investigators have studied the stress of hospitalization itself (Volicer, 1974; Volicer, 1978; Williams, 1974; Wilson-Barnett, 1976; Wu, 1973). Wu suggested that hospitalization may influence behavior more than the illness itself. Volicer (1974) developed the *Hospital Stress Rating Scale* to measure the stress experienced by hospital patients. From a sample of 216 patients in cancer, surgical, and medical wards, he found that the most stressful agent was the threat to the patient's body and/or life, but identified other highly stressful factors such as the hospital environment, separation from the family, and financial considerations. He also found that high scores on the Hospital Stress Rating Scale correlated with increased patient reports of pain, lower physical status during hospitalization, and less improvement after discharge (Volicer, 1978).

The Occupational Therapy Clinic. The occupational therapy clinic has been described as providing a specific culture in which activity, interaction, growth, and role definition are fostered (Pierce & Dickerson, 1962; Schmalz, 1969). Reilly (1966) described a model occupational therapy program as a ''total culture which acknowledges competency, arouses curiosity, feeds in universal knowledge, deepens appreciations, and demands behavior across the full spectrum of a human's abilities. . . . It presses for the exercising of life skills in a balanced pattern of daily living'' (pp. 63-64).

Barris and co-workers (1985) lend specificity to these guidelines by articulating principles for creating treatment environments. These include:

1. Treatment environments should be optimally arousing to the patients/clients (e.g., removing distractions or providing complex tasks for those in need of stimulation).
2. The environment should support the client's sense of internal control (e.g., provide options for client decisions or include enough support that confused clients can predict certain events).
3. The environment should be continuous with the client's cultural background and interests (have familiar activities, expectations, and roles).
4. A variety of settings should be available for the patients to practice their competencies in the treatment setting and in the community.

Mosey (1981) states that three of occupational therapy's legitimate tools are use of the human and nonhuman environments, the use of activity groups, and the therapeutic use of self. This implies the strength of the human environment to effect change and to promote competent performance.

In summary, a hospital, clinic, or other treatment setting has a social environment that can be defined and consciously altered. The environment should be congruent with a patient's lifestyle and beliefs. It should provide for enough arousal for patients to engage in their own health process but not so much as to inhibit it. The individual should be actively involved in decisions. Competent behavior matched with his abilities should be required, and activity patterns should be familiar and valued.

PERFORMANCE IN EDUCATIONAL SETTINGS

The school is considered by some to be an important socializing agent for the individual and under optimal circumstances can support competent performance of the child. Student morale, interest in the subject matter, and sense of academic self-efficacy are fostered by positive relationships with teachers and peers and a focus on student participation in a well-organized classroom.

Fraser and Fisher (1983) found that students placed in classes with their preferred environments (supportive, competitive, clear structure, and innovative) developed more positive attitudes toward the subject being taught. Classes that set specific academic goals and remain task-oriented combined with clear structure and supportive relationships, result in student gains on standard achievement tests. They also found if achievement was stressed without warmth, even though substantial achievement may be gained, students' interest and creativity may be lacking. Another study shows absenteeism increases if support and student involvement are lacking even when there is competition in the classroom with teacher control (Moos, 1979).

As might be expected, problem students have more difficulty adapting to variations in classroom environments than do non-problem students (Wright & Cowen, 1982). The size of the school has been related to the level that students participate in activities, with those students in smaller schools having greater school extracurricular participation (Berk & Goebel, 1987).

In summary, in order for a school to assist an individual in developing performance skills, it must offer a social environment in which competencies are acknowledged and a variety of learning methods are available. If the social values of an individual are not reflected in the school, and the system does not acknowledge the student's "differentness," then the system may simply reinforce his/her belief that he/she does not "fit in" as a student.

PERFORMANCE IN THE COMMUNITY

A community is a social group that shares one or more of the following: a specific location, government, heritage, common characteristics, or common interests. Communities are held together primarily by feelings and sentiments. Communities may be of place, nonplace or mind, or kinship (Tonnes, 1957). Communities are considered to be entities and may even be described as the client or recipient of services (Anderson & McFarlane, 1988). Much of the individual's interaction with the social environment takes place within the community.

The community is the term most commonly used to describe the setting into which health care workers hope to integrate their clients. Community connotes a social group that is immediate and important to the individual where there are shared resources, interests, and goals. Transitional programs attempt to help the client integrate back into the community.

Neighborhoods are considered a subset of communities. A neighborhood may be a small geographical area in which people know each other and exchange favors, or it may be a larger area that one would describe when asked "where do you live?" (Froland et al., 1981). Neighborhood cultural values determine the role of a "good neighbor." Cantor (1979), Spencer (1987), and others have proposed that the neighborhood is a useful unit for assessing and managing social environments, particularly for those clients with limited mobility or adaptive capacity. For such populations, neighborhoods may be a rich source of social support. Neighborhoods may be analyzed in many ways. For occupational therapists, it may be useful to analyze them in terms of mobility spheres, physical and social resources, and activity patterns (Spencer & Davidson, 1988).

Neighborhoods provide a primary setting in which children spend unstructured time. They can experiment, explore, discover places where children can gather without adult surveillance, and overcome physical obstacles. Through daily living arrangements they can form habits that carry over into adult life. For adults, the neighborhood provides the social structure that supports daily living patterns.

THE OCCUPATIONAL THERAPIST AS ENVIRONMENTAL DESIGNER AND ADVISER

Exploring Change

Competence has been described as being able to interact effectively with the environment while maintaining individuality and growth (White, 1960). This means the opportunity to explore the environment, engage in activity, and manipulate the environment. Kielhofner and Miyake (1983) have identified ability as only one of four dimensions of human competence; the other three are avoiding circumstances in which limitations would hinder the person, finding resources to aid performance in areas in which success is possible, and finding a reference group that respects the person's level of capacity. In other words, competence is described in terms of *person-environment fit*. By careful assessment and deliberate manipulation of the person-environment fit, the therapist can help a client realize his or her potential.

In attempting to improve the performance capabilities of the individual client or groups of clients, the therapist functions in four major ways:

1. *The occupational therapist is concerned with improving the social skills of the client so that the client can better engage in social exchanges in a variety of settings.*

2. *The therapist improves the ''fit'' between the expected environment and the client.* This might involve relaxing the social expectations in the environment, adding supportive people to the environment, or exchanging one environment for another that is more friendly or in which there is better fit between demands and needs, for example, moving a client to another community in which supportive relatives live. Increasing individual performance components increases the likelihood that the individual will be able to move flexibly between and among various environments. Thus the therapist does not introduce environmental adaptations as an alternative to effecting individual change, but rather as a means of increasing individual performance.

3. *The therapist in the clinic becomes a part of the social environment of the patient/client and assumes a variety of roles as indicated by the patient's needs.*

In addition to the classic therapeutic role, the occupational therapist assumes the roles of teacher, supervisor, coach, player, craftsman, and so forth (Barris, Kielhofner, & Watts, 1983). The therapist uses groups to influence performance in the clinics. He/she modulates the number and kind of people who serve as part of the group and the kind of activity in which the group engages. In the social milieu of the clinic, the therapist guides the client through progressively more complex social environments, by means of such techniques as moving from parallel toward a mature group (see Mosey, 1986). The following description illustrates the varity of roles the therapist may be called upon to play.

The Many Roles of a Therapist

I spent the afternoon working with a resident who is presently not living in the (L'Arche) community. My role in the beginning was that of evaluator: seeing how much skill he had nailing wood, positioning pieces to be nailed, placing the nail, keeping the nail perpendicular. Later I took the role of instructor: teaching how to use a nail punch and determining the correct department. Later I became work organizer: anticipating how to organize the material so he did not run out of work. Later I became inspector: checking the work that was completed. The resident skill level improved so readily that he needed infrequent supervision. Later I became a co-worker and role model: working parallel to the resident. Finally I became supporter: encouraging and praising the resident's accomplishments.

Note: From Wintz, GS (1988). Specialty fieldwork in a psychosocial environment: An exploratry study of the therapeutic community--A L'Arche approach. Unpublished professional paper. Houston, TX: Texas Woman's University.

One of the primary tasks of the therapist is to help the client use the social resources available to him/her. There is a growing body of evidence to support the efficacy of using social skills training with some psychosocially dysfunctional populations, such as those with schizophrenia. There is also evidence for support of assertion-training (a subset of social skills training) for those who are non-assertive, such as individuals with depression (see Ostrow & Kaplan, 1987, for a complete review of these studies). The social environment in the clinic is designed so that all interpersonal encounters can have therapeutic value, and the physical and task environment communicates an expectation of socially competent behavior (Barris et al., 1983).

Sharrott (1983) has suggested the following social sequence for addressing the client's needs:

1. Deal with the patient's here-and-now bodily conditions.
2. Encourage clinical interpersonal relationships to progress from staff relations (predictable performances according to role) to ''we-relations'' in which people relate as individuals.
3. Address the family relationships which often must be redefined during the illness or disability.
4. Explore the community relations in which clients can try out the new definitions and skills that have been developed in therapy. The social environment should provide the patient with opportunities to test and legitimatize his old perceptions, beliefs and values, as well as his new ones.
5. The therapist acts as teacher and advisor to the client who wants to assume control of their interaction with environments and as a change agent in communities.

The client at this stage should be able to adapt to a variety of environments but is also involved with community education, advocacy, and legislative affairs that might help people with performance deficits to better use their capabilities.

Limitations of the Approach

Occupational therapists using this approach must understand social systems and must be involved in community planning. In this capacity, the occupational therapist may sometimes appear to overlap functions with other professionals such as social workers and community planners. The occupational therapist's holistic viewpoint, while focusing on the performance aspects of the client's life, can make him or her both well-suited and unique.

Recommendations for Research

Research in the area of social environments is beset by all the problems most feared by traditional scientists who are committed to the experimental design. The laboratory conditions that these methods require essentially distort the phenomena being examined, and the method of choice for research of this kind appears to be careful and systematic observation in naturalistic settings. Whereas some aspects of the social environment have been examined in great detail (e.g., the relationship between social support and health), others offer little information on which to base predictions of outcomes. Occupational therapists, because of their knowledge about human activity and because of their understanding of the needs of special populations, are uniquely suited for research with those populations (i.e.: the high-risk neonate, persons with developmental delay, and cognitively disabled persons). Models of community planning and alternate social environments for these people need research to support public policy decisions.

A first step is refinement of assessment instruments and strategies which can generate some sound theoretical models of practice. The clinician needs to consider carefully what aspects of human groups are most cogent for study and decide on priorities of investigation so as to provide innovative and efficacious services.

Knowledge of how to understand and use the social environment therapeutically is in its early stages. Research in this area is a challenge therapists should not refuse.

SUMMARY

As individuals go about their daily activities, they do so within a social environment that greatly influences both what they do and how they do it. Because of the many ways that the social environment can affect performance, it is important for occupational therapists to understand types of social influence and their characteristics. Fortunately, the knowledge provided by many disciplines helps us to better understand the social groups, networks and other components which provide the structure, support, role expectations and demands, and other characteristics which collectively shape the degree of fit between the person and the environment. When performance is adversely affected as a consequence of dimensions within the social environment, intervention may be necessary. Occupational therapists may often be in a position to use their understanding of the social environment to serve as agents of change; potentially assuming multiple roles in this process.

Study Questions

1. Analyze the social environment of your classroom and consider these questions:

- How does the size of your class influence your role specialization?
- How difficult was it to get into your class and what is required for you to remain a member of the class? Is this related to your commitment to staying in the class?
- What is the central function of your class? How does this relate to what you do every day in class and to the rules, standards, and values that guide the activities?
- How complex is the structure of the class? How difficult is it to determine how to get things done within the class?
- What kinds of relationships exist within the class? Are feelings shared as well as tasks? Do members cooperate in learning or are relationships competitive? What is the relative status of students and professor?
- How do these elements change over the course of the semester? How much can the class influence the change?
- What are the effects of all these factors upon your performance in this class?

2. Compare and contrast the ideal social environment that you would provide for the young child at home and the elderly person in the nursing home. What elements would be very similar? What would be very different?

3. The severely mentally ill person has few people in his social network and has difficulty relating to people in close, high-emotion situations. If you want to improve the person-environment fit, what kind of social environment would you choose for this individual?

4. What social behaviors of a coworker would provide social support for a worker in a high stress (high demand-low control) work setting? What kind of organizational systems characteristics would provide support?

5. Exchange is an important aspect of social relationships, that is, what the person gives as well as what the person gets. Consider some of the possible "commodities" the following person might give in a social exchange with you:

- An 89-year-old woman, once a pilot in the 1930's, who is now nearly blind, walks with a walker, and requires assistance with grocery shopping, laundry, and housecleaning.
- A 63-year-old accountant who has recently had to take a medical retirement because of a stroke. He has always worked hard, was a good father to his children, but never traveled to all the places he wanted to go.

- A 29-year-old man, hospitalized with a complication of human immunodeficiency virus (HIV) or Acquired Immune Deficiency Syndrome (AIDS), who has been a fashion designer and has enjoyed a homosexual lifestyle for years.

6. What are the characteristics of a "total institution" (e.g., a prison)? What effects do the social relationships in this kind of setting have upon human performance?

7. Some groups of disabled persons have developed strong advocacy positions and have achieved a great deal, both in terms of recognition as valuable persons (not stereotypes) and in terms of removing the stigma of their disability; others have not made such gains. What are some of the factors that have contributed to the attitudinal changes in the current society?

8. Based on what you know about the roles of occupational therapist and social worker, how might the interventions of the two disciplines differ in the way they view a client's neighborhood? How might they complement each other's work?

References

Aaronson, E. (1984). *The social animal* (4th ed.). New York: W.H. Freeman.

Anderson, E.T., & McFarlane, J.M. (1988). *Community as client*. Philadelphia: J.B. Lippincott.

Anderson, R.E., & Carter, I.E. (1974). *Human behavior in the social environment*. Chicago: Aldine.

Archer, D. (1985). Social deviance. In G. Lindzey & E. Aronson (Eds.), *The handbook of social psychology, Vol. 2* (3rd ed., pp. 743-804). New York: Random House.

Averell, J. (1973). Personal control over aversive stimuli and its relationship to stress. *Psychological Bulletin, 80*, 286-303.

Barker, R.G. (1965). Explorations in ecological psychology. *American Psychologist, 20*, 1-14.

Barrera, M.E. (1986). Distinctions between social support concepts: Measures and models. *American Journal of Community Psychology, 14*, 413-445.

Barris, R., Kielhofner, G., Levine, R.E., & Neville, A.M. (1985). Occupation as interaction with the environment. In G. Kielhofner (Ed.), *A model of human occupation: Theory and application* (pp. 42-62). Baltimore: Williams & Wilkins.

Barris, R., Kielhofner, G., & Watts, J. (1983). *Psychosocial occupational therapy: Practice in a pluralistic arena*. Laurel, MD: RAMSCO.

Barton, P. (1976). *Institutional neurosis* (3rd ed.). Bristol, England: John Wright & Sons.

Beck, M.A., & Callahan, D.K. (1980). Impact of institutionalization on the posture of chronic schizophrenic patients. *American Journal of Occupational Therapy, 74*, 332-335.

Behnke, C., & Menarcheck-Fetkovich, M. (1984). Examining reliability and validity of the play history. *American Journal of Occupational Therapy, 38*, 94-100.

Bell, S.M., & Ainsworth, M.D.S. (1972). Infant crying and maternal responsiveness. *Child Development, 43*, 1171-1190.

Benham, P.K. (1988). Attitudes of occupational therapy personnel toward persons with disabilities. *American Journal of Occupational Therapy, 42*, 305-311.

Berg, J., & Medrich, E.A. (1980). Children in four neighborhoods: The physical environment and its effect on play patterns. *Environment and Behavior, 12*, 320-328.

Berk, L.E., & Goebel, B.L. (1987). High school size and extracurricular participation: A study of a small college environment. *Environment and Behavior, 19*, 53-76.

Berkman, L.F. (1985). The relationship of social networks and social support to morbidity and mortality. In S. Cohen & S.L. Syme (Eds.), *Social support and health* (pp. 241-262). Orlando, FL: Academic Press.

Blau, Z. (1954). Structural constraints on friendship in old age. *American Sociological Review, 59*, 379-383.

Blenkner, M. (1967). Environmental change and the aging individual. *Gerontologist, 7*, 101-105.

Blythe, B.J. (1983). Social support networks in health care and health promotion. In J.K. Whittaker & J. Garbarino (Eds.), *Social support networks: Informal helping in the human services* (pp. 107-133). New York: Aldine.

Bott, E. (1957). *Family and social network*. London: Tavistock.

Boyce, W.T. (1985). Social support, family relations, and children. In S. Cohen & S.L. Syme (Eds.), *Social support and health* (pp.151-173). Orlando, FL: Academic Press.

Brazelton, T.B., & Als, H. (1979). Four early stages in the development of mother-infant interaction. *Psychoanalytic Study of the Child, 34*, 349-369.

Brazelton, T.B., Koslowski, B., & Main, M. (1974). The origins of reciprocity: The early mother-infant interaction. In M. Lewis & L.A. Rosenblum (Eds.), *The effect of the infant on its caregiver* (pp. 49-76). New York: Wiley Interscience.

Brink, P.J. (1985). On the patient role [editorial]. *Western Journal of Nursing Research, 7*, 397-399.

Bronfenbrenner, U. (1974). The origins of alienation. *Scientific American, 231*, 53-61.

Brown, C. (1971). *The story of Cristy Brown*. New York: Pocket Books.

Brown, G.W., & Harris, T. (1978). *Social origins of depression*. New York: Free Press.

Brown, R. (1965). *Social psychology*. New York: Free Press.

Brown, R.B. (1978). Social and psychological correlates of help-seeking behavior among urban adults. *American Journal of Community Psychology, 6*, 425-439.

Bruce, M.A., & Christiansen, C.H. (1988). Advocacy in word as well as in deed. *American Journal of Occupational Therapy, 42*, 189-191.

Burke, J.P., Miyake, S., Kielhofner, G., & Barris, R. (1983). The demystification of health care and demise of the sick role: Implications for occupational therapy. In G. Kielhofner (Ed.), *Health through occupation* (pp. 197-210). Philadelphia: F.A. Davis.

Burke, R.J., Weir, R., & Duwors, R.E. (1979). Type A behavior of administrators and wives' reports of marital satisfaction and well-being. *Journal of Applied Psychology, 64*, 57-65.

Cain, A. (1979). A study of pets in the family system. *Human Behavior, 8*, 24.

Cantor, J.H. (1979). Life space and social support. In T.D. Byerts, S.C. Howell, & L.A. Pastalan (Eds.), *Environmental context of aging: Lifestyles, environmental quality, and living arrangements* (pp. 33-61). New York: Garland STPM Press.

Caplan, R.D. (1971). Organizational stress and individual strain: A social-psychological study of risk factors in coronary heart disease among administrators, engineers, and scientists. Unpublished doctoral dissertation, University of Michigan, 1971.

Caton, C.L. (1984). *Management of chronic schizophrenia*. New York: Oxford University Press.

Cauce, A.M. (1986). Social networks and social competence: Exploring the effects of early adolescent friendships. *American Journal of Community Psychology, 14*, 607-628.

Cochran, M.M., & Brassard, J.A. (1979). Child development and personal social networks. *Child Development, 50*, 601-616.

Cronkite, R., Moos, R., & Finney, J., (1983). The context of adaptation: An integrative prespective on community and treatment environments. In W.A. O'Connor & Lubin (Eds.) *Ecological models in clinical and community health*. New York: Wiley.

D'Arcy, C., & Siddique, C. M. (1984). Social support and mental health among mothers of preschool and school age children. *Social Psychiatry, 19*, 155-162.

D'Augelli, A. (1983). Social support networks in mental health. In J.K. Whittaker & J. Garbarino (Eds.), *Social support networks: Informal helping in the human services* (pp. 74-106). New York: Aldine Publishing Company.

DeCarlo, J.J., & Mann, W.C. (1985). The effectiveness of verbal versus activity groups in improving self-perceptions of interpersonal communication skills. *American Journal of Occupational Therapy, 39*, 20.

DeJong, G. (1981). *Environmental accessibility and independent living outcomes*. East Lansing, MI: Michigan State University, University Center for International Rehabilitation.

Dunphy, D.C. (1963). The social structure of urban adolescent peer group. *Sociometry, 26*, 230-246.

Eisemann, M. (1985). Depressed patients and non-psychiatric controls: Discriminant analysis on social environment variables. *Acta Psychiatrica Scandinavia, 71*, 495-498.

Erikson, K. (1962). Notes on the sociology of deviance. *Social Problems, 9*, 307-314.

Escalona, S.K. (1984). Social and other environmental influences on the cognitive and personality development of low birthweight infants. *American Journal of Mental Deficiency, 88*, 508-512.

Fraser, B., & Fisher, D. (1983). Use of actual and preferred environment scales in person-environment fit research. *Journal of Educational Psychology, 75*, 303-313.

Froland, C., Pancoast, D., Chapman, N., & Kimboko, P. (1979, September). Professional partnerships with informal helpers: Emerging forms. Presented at the Annual Convention of the American Psychological Association. New York, NY.

Froland, C., Pancoast, D., Chapman, N., & Kimboko, P. (1981). *Helping networks and human services*. Beverly Hills: Sage Publications.

Garbarino, J., Stocking, S., & Associates. (1980). *Protecting children from abuse and neglect: Developing and maintaining effective support systems for families*. San Francisco: Jossey-Bass.

Geskie, M.A., & Salasek, J.L. (1988). Attitudes of health care personnel towards persons with disabilities. In H.E. Yuker (Ed.), *Attitudes toward persons with disabilities* (pp. 187-200). New York: Springer Publishing Company.

Ginsberg, E. (1957). *Occupational choice: An approach to a general theory*. New York: Columbia University Press.

Gliedman, J., & Roth, W. (1980). *The unexpected minority: Handicapped children in America*. New York: Harcourt Brace Jovanovich.

Goffman, E. (1961). *Asylums: Essays on the social situation of mental patients and other inmates*. New York: Doubleday.

Goffman, E. (1963). *Stigma: Notes on the management of spoiled identity*. Englewood Cliffs, NJ: Prentice-Hall.

Gottesman, L.E., & Boureston, M.C. (1974). Why nursing homes do what they do. *Gerontologist, 14*, 501-506.

Gottlieb, B.H. (1985). Social support and community mental health. In S. Cohen, & S.L. Syme, (Eds.), *Social support and health* (pp. 303-323). Orlando: Academic Press, Inc.

Gralewicz, A. (1973). Play deprivation in multihandicapped children. *American Journal of Occupational Therapy, 27,* 70-72.

Gray, M. (1972). Effects of hospitalization on work-play behavior. *American Journal of Occupational Therapy, 26,* 180-185.

Hammer, M., Gutwirth, L., & Phillips, S.L. (1982). Parenthood and social networks: A preliminary view. *Social Science and Medicine, 16,* 2091-2100.

Haney, C., Banks, W.C., & Zimbardo, P.G. (1973). Interpersonal dynamics in a simulated prison. *International Journal of Criminology and Penology, I,* 69-79.

Haney, C., & Zimbardo, P.G. (1977). The socialization into criminality: On becoming a prisoner and a guard. In J.L. Tapp & F.J. Levine (Eds.), *Law, justice, and the individual in society: Psychological and legal issues.* New York: Holt, Rinehart, and Winston.

Hansen, J.C., & Rosenthal, D.R. (1987). *Family stress.* Rockville, MD: Aspen Publishing Company.

Hatter, J.K., & Nelson, D.L. (1987). Altruism and task participation in the elderly. *American Journal of Occupational Therapy, 41,* 379-381.

Haviland, J.M., & Scarborough, H.S. (1981). *Adolescent development in contemporary society.* New York: D. Van Nostrand Company.

Haynes, S., McMichael, A., & Tyroler, H. (1977). The relationship of normal involuntary retirement to early mortality among U.S. rubber workers. *Social Science and Medicine, 11,* 105-114.

Helsing, K., Comstock, G.W., & Szklo, M. (1981). Mortality after bereavement. *American Journal of Epidemiology, 114* (1), 41-52.

Henderson, S., Byrne, D., Duncan-Jones, P., Adcock, S., Scott, R., & Steele, G. (1978). Social bonds in the epidemiology of neurosis: A preliminary communication. *British Journal of Psychiatry, 132,* 462-466.

Heymanns, B. (1977). *Bittersweet triumph.* Garden City, NY: Doubleday & Company, Inc.

Hoffman, L.W. (1974). Effects on the child (pp. 32-62). In L.W. Hoffman & F. Nye (Eds.) *Working mothers.* San Francisco: Jossey Bass.

Hollingshead, A.B. (1949). *Elmtown's youth.* New York: John Wiley & Sons.

Hooyman, N. (1983). Social support networks in services to the elderly. In J.K. Whittaker & J. Garbarino (Eds.), *Social support networks: Informal helping in the human services* (pp. 134-166). New York: Aldine Publishing Company.

Horne, M.D. (1985). *Attitudes toward handicapped students: Professional, peer, and parent reactions.* Hillsdale, New Jersey: Lawrence Erlbaum Associates, Publishers.

Howe, M.C., & Schwartzberg, S.L. (1986). *A functional approach to group work in occupational therapy.* Philadelphia: J.B. Lippincott.

Huxley, P.J., Goldberg, D.P., Maguire, G.P., & Kincey, V.A. (1979). The prediction of the course of minor psychiatric disorders. *British Journal of Psychiatry, 135,* 535-543.

Jasnau, K.F. (1967). Individualized versus mass transfer of non-psychotic geriatric patients from mental hospitals to nursing homes. *Journal of the American Geriatrics Society, 15,* 280-284.

Jones, D.C., & van Amelsvoort Jones, G.M.M. (1986). Communication patterns between nursing staff and the ethnic elderly in a long term care setting. *Journal of Advanced Nursing, 11,* 265-272.

Kagan, J., Kearsley, R.B., & Zelazo, P.R. (1978). *Infancy: Its place in human development.* Cambridge: Harvard University Press.

Kaplan, K.L. (1988). *Directive group therapy.* Thorofare, NJ: Slack.

Kasl, S.V., & Wells, J.A. (1985). Work and the family: Social support and health in the middle years. In S. Cohen, & Y.S.L. Syme (Eds.), *Social support and health* (pp. 175-198). New York: Academic Press.

Katcher, A.H., & Friedmann, E. (1980). Potential health value of pet ownership. *The Compendium on Continuing Education, 2,* 117-122.

Kazak, A.E., & Wilcox, B.L. (1984). The structure and function of social support networks in families with handicapped children. *American Journal of Community Psychology, 12,* 1984

Kielhofner, G., Barris, R., Bauer, D., Shoestock, B., & Walker, L. (1983). A comparison of play behavior in nonhospitalized and hospitalized children. *American Journal of Occupational Therapy, 37,* 305-312.

Kielhofner, G., & Miyake, S. (1983). In G. Kielhofner (Ed.), *Health through occupation* (pp. 257-266). Philadelphia: F.A. Davis Company.

Kielhofner, G., & Takata, N. (1980). A study of mentally retarded persons: Applied research in occupational therapy. *American Journal of Occupational Therapy, 34,* 252-258.

Knoke, D., & Kuklinski, J.H. (1982). *Network analysis.* Beverly Hills, CA: Sage Publications.

Kulys, R., & Tobin, S.S. (1980). Older people and their "responsible others." *Social Work, 25,* 138-145.

Langer, E. (1975). The illusion of control. *Journal of Personal and Social Psychology, 32,* 311-328.

Langer, E. & Rodin, J. (1976). The effects of choice and enhanced personal responsibility for the aged: A field experiment in an institutional setting. *Journal of Personality and Social Psychology, 34*, 191-198.

Larronde, S.A. (1983). Adopt-A-Grandparent. *Modern Maturity, 26*, 50-51.

Lawton, M.P. (1982). Competence, environmental press, and the adaptation of older people. In M.P. Lawton, P.G. Windley, & T.O. Byerts (Eds.), *Aging and the environment: Theoretical approaches*. New York: Springer.

Levi, L., Frankenhaeuser, M., & Gardell, B. (1986). The characteristics of the workplace and the nature of its social demands. In S.G. Wolf, & A.J. Firestone (Eds.), *Occupational stress* (pp. 54-67). Littleton, MA: PSG Publishing Company.

Lewis, M., & Weinraub, M. (1976). The father's role in the child's social network. In M.E. Lamb (Ed.), *The role of the father in child development*. New York: Wiley.

Lindemann, J.E. (1981). *Psychological and behavioral aspects of physical disability*. New York: Plenum Press.

Linn, M.W., Caffey, E.M., Klett, C.J., Hogarty, G.E., & Lamb, H.R. (1979). Day treatment and psychotropic change in the aftercare of schizophrenic patients. *Archives of General Psychiatry, 36*, 1055-1066.

Livneh, H. (1984). On the origins of negative attitudes toward people with disabilities. In R.P. Marinelli & A.E. Dell Orto (Eds.), *The psychological and social impact of physical disability*. New York: Springer Publishing Company.

Llorens, L.A. (1984). Changing balance: Environment and individual. *American Journal of Occupational Therapy, 38*, 29-34.

Long, F. (1983). Social support networks in day care and early childhood development. In J.K. Whittaker & J. Garbarino & Associates (Eds.), *Social support networks: Informal helping in the human services* (pp. 189-217). New York: Aldine Publishing Company.

MacDonald, R., & Christakos, A. (1963). Relationship of emotional adjustment during pregnancy to obstetric complications. *American Journal of Obstetrics and Gynecology, 86*, 589-601.

MacElveen, P.M. (1978). Social networks. In D.C. Longo & R.A. Williams (Eds.), *Clinical practice in psychosocial nursing: Assessment and intervention*. New York: Appleton-Century-Crofts.

Maguire, G.A. (1979). Volunteer program to assist the elderly to remain in home settings. *American Journal of Occupational Therapy, 33*, 98-101.

Martin, J., & Doran, A. (1966). Evidence concerning the relationship between health and retirement. *Sociological Review, 14*, 239.

Mauras-Corsino, E., Daniewicz, C.V., & Swan, L.C. (1985). The use of community networks for chronic psychiatric patients. *American Journal of Occupational Therapy, 39*, 374-378.

Mercer, S.O., & Kane, R.A. (1979). Helplessness and hopelessness among the institutionalized aged: An experiment. *Health and Social Work, 4*, 91-113.

Michaelman, S.S. (1974). Play and the deficit child. In M. Reilly, (Ed.), *Play as exploratory learning*. Beverly Hills, CA: Sage Publications.

Minkler, M. (1985). Social support and health of the elderly. In S. Cohen & L.L. Syme (Eds.), *Social support and health* (pp. 199-216), Orlando: Academic Press, Inc.

Moos, R.H. (1974). *Evaluating treatment environments: A social ecological approach*. New York: John Wiley and Sons.

Moos, R. (1979). *Evaluating educational environments: Procedures, methods, findings, and policy implications*. San Francisco: Jossey-Bass, 1979.

Moos, R.H. (1984). Context and coping: Toward a unifying conceptual framework. *American Journal of Community Psychiatry, 12*, 5-36.

Moos, R.H., & Tsu, V.D. (1977). The crisis of physical illness: An overview. In R.H. Moos (Ed.), *Coping with physical illness* (pp. 12-15). New York: Plenum Press.

Moscovice, I., Davidson, G., & McCaffrey, D. (1988). Substitution of formal and informal care for the community-based elderly. *Medical Care, 26*, 971-981.

Mosey, A. (1981). *Occupational therapy: Configuration of a profession*. New York: Raven Press.

Mosey, A. (1986) *Psychosocial components of occupational therapy*. New York: Raven Press.

Mumford, M.S. (1974). A comparison of interpersonal skills in verbal and activity groups. *American Journal of Occupational Therapy, 28*, 281-283.

Munoz, J.P. (1986) In *American Occupational Therapy Association. Play: A skill for life*. Rockville, MD: author.

Murphy, F.R., Scheer, J., Murphy, Y., & Mack, R. (1988). Physical desirability and social liminality: A study in the rituals of adversity. *Social Science and Medicine, 26*, 235-242.

Nelson, F.L., & Farberow, N.L. (1980). Indirect self-destructive behavior in the elderly nursing home patient. *Journal of Gerontology, 35*, 949-957.

Neugarten, B. (1979). Time, age, and the life cycle. *The American Journal of Psychiatry, 136*, 887-894.

Newman, B.M., & Newman, P.R. (1978) *Infancy and childhood*. New York: John Wiley & Sons.

Norbeck, J.S., & Tilden, V.P. (1983). Life stress, social support, and emotional disequilibrium in complications of pregnancy: A prospective multivariate study. *Journal of Health and Social Behavior, 24*, 30-46.

Novick, J.B. (1967). Easing the stress of moving day. *Hospitals, 41*, 64-74.

Olmsted, M.S. (1959). *The small group*. New York: Random House.

Ostrow, P.C., & Kaplan, K.L. (Eds.). (1987). *Occupational therapy in mental health: A guide to outcomes research*. Rockville, MD: American Occupational Therapy Association.

Parkes, C.M., Benjamin, B., & Fitzgerald, R.G. (1969). Broken hearts: A statistical study of increased mortality among widowers. *British Medical Journal, 1*, 740-743.

Parsons, T. (1964). *Social structure and personality*. London: Collier-Macmillan Ltd.

Pattison, E.M., Llasmas, R., & Hurd, G. (1979). Social network: Mediation of anxiety. *Psychiatric Annals, 9*, 56-67.

Perlmutter, M., & Hall, E. (1985). *Adult development and aging*. New York: John Wiley & Sons.

Peters-Golden, H. (1982). Breast cancer: Varied perceptions of social support in the illness experience. *Social Science and Medicine, 16*, 483-491.

Pierce, C.M. & Dickerson, R. (1962). The occupational therapy shop as a culture. *American Journal of Occupational Therapy, 16*, 231-235.

Pilisuk, M., & Parks, S.H. (1986). *The healing web: Social networks and human survival*. Hanover: University Press of New England.

Posner, J. (1974). Notes on the negative implications of being competent in a home for the aged. *International Journal of Aging and Human Development, 5*, 357-364.

Raphael, B. (1977). Preventive intervention with the recently bereaved. *Archives of General Psychiatry, 34*, 1450-1454.

Reilly, M. (1966). A psychiatric occupational therapy program as a teaching model. *American Journal of Occupational Therapy, 20*, 61-67.

Reilly, M. (Ed.). (1974). *Play as exploratory learning*. Beverly Hills: Sage Publications.

Reilly, M. (1984). The importance of the client versus patient issue for occupational therapy. *American Journal of Occupational Therapy, 38*, 404-406.

Rodin, J. (1985). The application of social psychology. In G. Lindzey & E. Aranson (Eds.), *The handbook of social psychology. Vol II.* (pp. 805-881). New York: Random House.

Rosow, I. (1974). *Socialization into old age*. Berkeley: University of California Press.

Rutter, M. (1981). Attachment and the development of social relationships. In M. Rutter (Ed.), *Scientific foundations of development psychiatry*. Baltimore: University Park Press.

Schmalz, H.A. (1969). Occupational therapy as a socialization process. Unpublished master's thesis, University of Southern California, Los Angeles.

Schooler, C., & Spohn, H.E. (1982). Social dysfunction and treatment failure in schizophrenia. *Schizophrenia Bulletin, 8*, 85-98.

Schultz, R., & Brenner, G. (1977). Relocation of the aged: A review and theoretical analysis. *Journal of Gerontology, 32*, 323-333.

Secord, P.F., Backman, C.W., & Slavitt, D.R. (1976). *Understanding social life*. New York: McGraw-Hill Book Company.

Seligman, M.E.P. (1975). *Helplessness: On depression, development and death*. San Francisco: W.H. Freeman and Company.

Sharrott, G.W. (1983). Occupational therapy's role in the client's creation and affirmation of meaning. In G. Kielhofner (Ed.), *Health through occupation* (pp. 213-235). Philadelphia: F.A. Davis Company.

Shera, W., & Johnson, F.A. (1984). Leisure and changing values. In R.C. Nann, D.S. Butt, & L. Ladrido-Ignacio (Eds.), *Mental health, cultural values, and social development* (pp. 162-163). Dordrecht, Holland: D. Reidel Publishing Company.

Spencer, J.C. (1987). Environmental assessment strategies. *Topics in Geriatric Rehabilitation, 3*, (1), 35-41.

Spencer, J.C., & Davidson, H.A. (1988, April). Use of neighborhood environments by elderly persons. Paper presented at the American Occupational Therapy Association Conference, Phoenix.

Stokes, R.G., & Maddox, G.L. (1967). Some social factors on retirement. *Journal of Gerontology, 22*, 329-333.

Takata, N. (1971). The play milieu: A preliminary appraisal. *American Journal of Occupational Therapy, 25*, 281-284.

Tilden, V.P. (1983). The relation of life stress and social support to emotional disequilibrium during pregnancy. *Research in Nursing and Health, 6*, 167-174.

Tonnes, F. (1957). *Community and society*. Trans. Charles P. Loomis. Michigan State University Press.

Tyler, B., & Kogan, K.L. (1977). Reduction of stress between mothers and their handicapped children. *American Journal of Occupational Therapy, 31*, 151-155.

Tyler, N.B., Kogan, K.L., & Turner, P. (1974). Interpersonal components of therapy with young cerebral palsied. *American Journal of Occupational Therapy, 28*, 395-400.

Vachon, M.L. (1987). *Occupational stress in the care of the critically ill, the dying, and the bereaved*. Washington: Hemisphere Publishing Corporation.

Vanfossen, B.E. (1981). Sex differences in the mental

health effects of spouse support and equity. *Journal of Health and Social Behavior, 22*, 130-143.

Vaux, A., Riedel, S., & Stewart, D. (1987). Modes of social support: The social support behaviors scale. *American Journal of Community Psychology, 15*, 209-237.

Vollicer, B.J. (1974). Patients' perceptions of stressful events associated with hospitalization. *Nursing Research, 23*, 235-238.

Vollicer, B.J. (1978). Hospital stress and patient reports of pain and physical status. *Journal of Human Stress, 4* (2), 28-37.

Wellman, B. (1978). Applying network analysis to the study of support. In B.H. Gottlieb (Ed.), *Social networks and social support* (pp. 171-200). Beverly Hills: Sage Publications.

Wells, J.A. (1987). Social support strategies for technostress management. In A.S. Sethi, D.H.J. Caro, & R.S. Schuler (Eds.), *Strategic management of technostress in an information society* (pp. 116-138). Lewiston, NY: C.J. Hogrete, Inc.

White, B.L. & Held, R. (1967). Plasticity of sensorimotor development in the human infant. In J. Hellmuth (Ed.), *Exceptional infant* (Vol 1). New York: Brunner/Mazel Publishing Company.

White, R. (1960). Competence and the psychosexual stages of development. Nebraska Symposium on Motivation, pp 1-12.

Williams, F. (1974). The crisis of hospitalization. *Nursing Clinics of North America, 9* (1), 37-45.

Wilson-Barnett, J. (1976). Patients' emotional reactions to hospitalization: An exploratory study. *Journal of Advanced Nursing, 1*, 351-358.

Wing, J.I., & Brown, G.W. (1970). *Institutionalization and schizophrenia*. Cambridge: Cambridge University Press.

Wintz, G. S. (1988). Specialty fieldwork in a psychosocial environment: An exploratory study of the therapeutic community—A L'Arche approach. Unpublished professional paper, Texas Woman's University, Houston, TX.

Wolfensberger, W. (1972). *Normalization: The principle of normalization in human services*. Toronto: National Institute on Mental Retardation.

Wolfensberger, W. (1973). A selective overview of the works of Jean Vanier and the movement of L'Arche.

World Health Organization. (1980). *International classification of impairments, disabilities, and handicaps: A manual of classification relating to consequences of disease*. Geneva: World Health Organization.

Wortman, C.B., & Conway, T.L. (1985). Social support and recovery from illness. In S. Cohen & Y.S.L. Syme (Eds.), *Social support and health* (pp. 281-302). Orlando: Academic Press, Inc.

Wright, B.A. (1988). The fundamental negative bias. In H.E. Yuker (Ed.), *Attitudes toward persons with disabilities*, (pp.-3-21). New York: Springer Publishing Company.

Wright, S., & Cowen, E. (1982). Student perception of school environment and its relationship to mood, achievement, popularity, and adjustment. *American Journal of Community Psychology, 10*, 687-703.

Wu, R. (1973). *Behavior and illness*. Englewood Cliffs, NJ: Prentice-Hall.

Yablonsky, L. (1970). *The violent gang* (rev. ed). Baltimore: Penguin.

Yalom, I.D. (1975). *Theory and practice of group psychotherapy*. New York: Basic Books.

Yarrow, L. J., Rubenstein, J. L., & Pederson, F. A. (1975). *Infant and environment: Early cognitive and motivational development*. New York: Wiley and Sons.

Zander, A. (1971). *Motives and goals in groups*. New York: Academic Press.

CHAPTER CONTENT OUTLINE

KEY TERMS

Cost containment

Equality of access

Health policy

National health insurance

Re-privatization

Public good

Special interest groups

Third party payment

ABSTRACT

Current public health care policy in the United States has developed around economic, political, sociological, and scientific influences that have shaped society since the American Revolution. These influences are examined in chronological sequence in relation to the evolution of health care policy in the United States and their impact on the shape of the health care system in general and occupational therapy in particular. There has been considerable focus on the impact of the Medicare/Medicaid legislation of 1965 and the subsequent Amendments which designated how and where public funds were to be allocated for health care for poor and elderly persons. The chapter concludes with a view toward the future and a challenge to occupational therapists to become involved in public policy making in order to ensure funding for occupational therapy services and enhance the quality of services provided.

Public Policy and Its Influence on Performance

Mary Sladky Struthers
Barbara Boyt Schell

"One cannot be in the practice of any of the health professions today without being keenly aware of the many forces shaping one's future roles and responsibilities."

—West, 1967

OBJECTIVES

The information in this chapter is intended to help the reader—

1. examine how occupational therapy services are provided within the context of a complex health care system.

2. identify key components of a health care system.

3. explain the historical context in which the U.S. health care system developed.

4. identify the impact of U.S. health policy on the development of the occupational therapy profession.

5. define the concepts of equality of access and cost containment and explain how these concepts currently shape health care policy.

6. identify the ways in which health policy affects performance of occupational therapy patients and clients.

7. identify ways in which individual occupational therapists and the profession can influence health policy.

INTRODUCTION

Occupational therapists in the United States and the individuals they serve are affected by policies that have evolved and shaped the American health care system. Occupational therapy exists as a provider of service in a vast health care system that is characterized by numerous special interest groups, all competing for the health care dollar. Although the industry evolved in the U.S. as primarily a private enterprise, since approximately 1912, the federal government has assumed an increasingly significant role in the economic aspects of health care. The major driving force toward more federal involvement was the concept of **equality of access**. Americans had come to believe that health was a basic human right. However, by 1987, this belief, coupled with a predominantly market-driven system, produced health care costs projected at more than $500 billion (Statistical Abstract of the United States, 1987). Consider this cost figure in growth terms. In 1950, the yearly national health expenditures were $12.7 billion or about one billion dollars per month. By 1985, this figure grew to $425 billion per year or about one billion dollars per day (Schramm, 1987). In a world of finite resources, this escalating cost of health care has forced policymakers to shift focus away from equality of access to cost control.

In this chapter, we will discuss policy from several perspectives. First, public and health policy will be defined along with the major issues surrounding these definitions. Second, a review of the health care system as it has developed in the United States will provide a foundation for understanding health policy, and models of health systems will be presented as conceptual aids. We will trace the evolution of health systems through the legislative process, using Medicare as an example, and will examine the impact of health policy on occupational therapy as a profession. Through a series of case studies, we will look at how several selected health care policies specifically influence the performance of individuals and groups within the United States. Finally, we will take a look at what the future holds for occupational therapy, focusing on the emerging political and ethical issues that are the subject of current debate and certain to shape policy decisions of the future.

POLICY

Policy consists of the recognized principles which govern and produce a course(s) of action. Taken in a broad context, policy also means the art and science of applying governing principles (Crichton, 1981). Public policy exists to direct governmental resources toward the solution of problems which are felt to be in the public interest to solve. **Health policy** is therefore concerned with the principles and interventions by a people with regard to the health of its individual and collective members. The outcome is the organization of systems for the provision of health services. Figure 7-1 shows an overview of how a nation might consider the concept of health. Elements of the physical and social environments combine with biological status to determine the well being of individuals. Health is determined by such factors as education, nutrition, home environment, natural environment, work environment, and genetic makeup. Indeed, this leads us to one of the central problems in the formation and evaluation of health policy. No one definition of health exists. Is health merely the absence of disease and disability as the medical model typifies? Not according to the World Health Organization (WHO), which defines health as a "state of well-being" (de Kervasdoue, Kimberly, & Rodwin, 1984). This broad definition of health from the WHO and the broad spectrum of determinants of health seen in Figure 7-1 reveal the far-reaching possibilities for government intervention in the health of a population. If one were to make comparisons among nations, it would be clear that nations have organized their health delivery systems according to very different views of what constitutes health (Roemer, 1985). Thus, health policy is not only the rationale for governmental intervention in health affairs but also the methods utilized to achieve those goals. Health policy is influenced by tacit assumptions embedded in the religious, political, ethical, moral, and economic history of a people. An understanding of basic concepts underlying our own democratic government will uncover some of the dynamics underlying our current system, or non-system of national health policy. Americans have traditionally believed that the management of public affairs begins at home with the family, the church, and city hall (Bellah et al., 1985). Common opinion holds that those who succeed do so

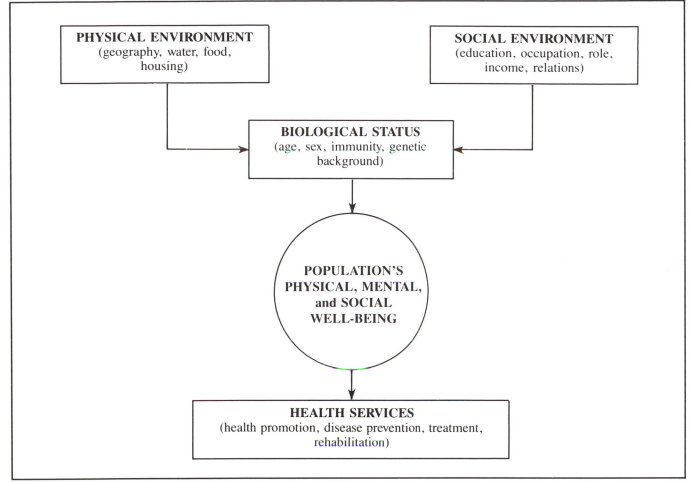

Figure 7-1. Determinants of Health. *From Roemer, M.I. (1985). National Strategies for Health Care Organization: A World Overview. Ann Arbor, MI: Health Administration Press.*

through strength of character and those who do not succeed have wrought their own hardship. The economy is dominated by a market-based strategy where government and private economies are viewed as separate and distinct (Wilhite, 1958). Additionally, from the time of the Continental Congress, the distribution of power between the federal, state, and local governments in the U.S. favored the local community. The American approach to social order and issues has always rested more on states' rights, secularism, and more recently on regionalism, than on any concept of national order. The federal government traditionally has exercised power over those activities which could not be handled on a local level. These have historically been military protection, international trade, and interstate commerce. Federal involvement in social programs has been justified by these narrow traditions. To understand the impact of these traditions on U.S. health policy, we must look to the evolution of its health care system.

EVOLUTION OF THE HEALTH CARE SYSTEM IN THE UNITED STATES

Early Beginnings

Federal involvement with the nation's health began as far back as 1798. Under the Act For the Relief of Sick and Disabled Seamen, the Fifth Congress and President John Adams provided health services to seamen. Funding for the program was provided by the seamen themselves through a wage deduction of twenty cents per month. The wage deduction and the program in general were to be administered on a local level by marine hospital directors who were appointed by the President (Mullan, 1989). However, the policy rationale was related to the federal objectives of maintaining the armed forces in a state of readiness and protecting the economically important shipping industry (Stevens & Stevens, 1974).

The American general hospital has its origins in sixteenth

century England. Local officials who were beset by the problems of the orphans, homeless, insane, and chronically and acutely ill poor people, created the almshouse/workhouse funded through public monies. Aid was refused to the poor in their homes for fear of the spread of pauperism (Dowling, 1982). At the same time in England, the voluntary hospital developed. Funded through private charity, these hospitals were governed by boards of prominent people.

As the British colonies evolved in North America, the underlying social, political, and economic values from 17th and 18th century England constituted the basis for health care development on the new continent. The almshouse evolved as a means of handling local dependent and indigent people. Populations in the almshouse were a mix of orphans, prostitutes, alcoholics, medical/surgical patients, vagrants, homeless childbearing women, handicapped persons, chronically ill, and criminals. Those who were well enough provided care for the other residents. Poor urban workers who became ill were sent to the almshouse for ''care.''

For the upper and middle classes, health care was primarily the responsibility of the family. Illnesses were treated and babies were born in the home. Medical insurance did not exist; middle class and wealthy persons paid privately for physician, midwife, and dental services.

By 1800, there were only two voluntary hospitals in America, Philadelphia's Pennsylvania Hospital and the New York Hospital. The hospitals were governed differently than the almshouse. Privately funded, these institutions selectively admitted acutely ill patients and attracted resources and medical staff through social connections. These institutions were developed and run under the social attitudes of hierarchy and the responsibility of wealth. The hospital in early America was defined by need and dependency, not the existence of sophisticated medical or technological resources (Rosenberg, 1987).

Without great changes in medical technology or therapeutics, the function and form of the American hospital remained unchanged until the later half of the 1800's. In addition to the increased need for medical care and surgical procedures brought by the Civil War, the late 1800's brought the startling expansion of the American city. Growth occurred from rural migration as well as unprecedented immigration from abroad.[1]

As cities grew, poverty intensified. The overcrowding, coupled with poor nutrition, and lack of sanitation and clean water systems, created many health related problems. As cholera and yellow fever epidemics wiped out high percentages of these poor city dwellers, local policy began to form. Because these epidemics transcended social boundaries, the upper class had to realize that disease was not related to the moral inferiority of the poor. Public sentiment began to change regarding the purpose of hospital care. Almshouse populations were sorted out and separate units of care were established for differing patient needs.[2]

Some city or municipal hospitals, still charged with the care of indigent persons, evolved from the almshouse but with slightly altered perspectives on care and governance. Voluntary and religious hospitals also grew in number.[3]

The Emergence of a Federal Role

Between 1870 and 1917, the American hospital evolved into the orderly, professionally run, physician-dominated, technologically-oriented system of today (Stevens, 1989). After 1900, both the American Medical Association and the American Hospital Association were formed. Since that time, these two special interest groups have played key roles in the evolution of the American health care system. Both have had a strong influence on the type of care produced, the settings in which care takes place, and the payment mechanisms designed to cover the cost of care.[4]

From the early 1900's on, the impact of new technology on the health care system was profound. The advent of anesthesia played a major role in the shift from home based health care to a system where institutional based care became the rule. Sterile conditions were needed to ensure safe surgery. Additionally, more highly trained personnel were needed to staff these hospitals. The formal profession of nursing evolved within this context. Technological advances in combination with the changing nature and content of medical education collided with the social and economic elements, yielding a contrived, yet disorderly evolution of system of care.[5]

1. For detailed discussion of urban growth during the 1800's, read *The Private City: Philadelphia In Three Periods of Its Growth* (1968), by Sam Bass Warner, Philadelphia: University of Pennsylvania Press and America Becomes Urban: The Development of U.S. Cities and Towns 1780-1980. (1988) by Eric H. Monkkonen, Berkeley, CA: University of California Press.

2. Frequently, the separation of patient groups was based upon social notions of illness. Insanity was viewed as a moral disturbance rather than an illness. This illness was segregated from others through the establishment of not only separate wards, but separate hospitals. Occupational therapy got its start in these institutions: its roots are in the moral era of treatment. For a more thorough discussion, refer to Reed and Sanderson, Concepts in Occupational Therapy.

3. *In The Care of Strangers: The Rise of America's Hospital System,* Charles Rosenberg portrays the professional and social transformation of the American hospital from 1800 through 1920.

4. For a complete discussion of the elements impacting on the development of the hospital and its relationship to American societal values, see Rosemary Stevens, *In Sickness and in Wealth: American Hospitals in the Twentieth Century,* New York: Basic Books.

Sentiment toward regional cooperation and disease control also grew from this time period. The policy rationale for expanding beyond local control was economic in nature, justified by the potential harm to interstate commerce and concern for the protection of the growing national and international economy (Duffy, 1985).

New federal initiatives in health policy were facilitated by the changing sentiment regarding individual and collective welfare, the rising economic influence of health professionals and institutions, and the increase in health technology. The first laws relating to food and drugs were passed. In 1912, the federal government recognized the special interests of children with the establishment of the Children's Bureau under the U.S. Department of Labor. The formation of the Children's Bureau reflects an important transformation in thinking. Federal policy began to form around certain segments of the population which were recognized as at risk and for which strong public support existed.[6]

1930 to 1965: Securing the Federal Role

The depression of the 1930's brought great hardship to large segments of the American population. The high percentage of unemployed strained the already sagging local economies. In answer to these problems, the federal government intervened to provide social insurance for unemployment, worker's compensation, retirement income for the country's workers, and public assistance through the states for individuals unable to work. The Social Security Act of 1935 was the landmark legislation of the era. It greatly expanded the federal role in health care and supported the notion that health care was a right of all citizens. This unprecedented role of the federal government in the state and local economies set the tone for public policy for the next 30 years.

Public reaction to the depression also served to stimulate private initiatives in health resources. Hospital economies were heavily affected by the depression. In an attempt to increase revenues, the American Hospital Association introduced a **third party payment** mechanism in the form of 39 pre-paid health insurance plans sold to employee groups. These plans eventually evolved into the Blue Cross plans. The American Medical Association initiated a similar mechanism seeking reimbursement for physicians' services in the hospital environment, and the Blue Shield plans were born.

By 1930, the role of research in disease control was recognized. With the promise of more advanced medical technologies, sentiment grew for establishing a federal research policy. In 1930, the Randall Act created the first National Institute of Health (NIH). This legislation initiated the federal role as one of the major funding sources for health research. By 1950, seven national institutes existed, and today there are thirteen. Federal funding for the NIH exceeded $16.5 billion in 1989 (Mullan, 1989).

World War II brought more major changes in federal involvement. The Emergency Maternal and Infant Care Program provided for the health needs of wives and children of servicemen. In 1943, a program of rehabilitation for veterans was funded through the Veterans Administration. Also in 1943, states were provided with money to develop civilian rehabilitation programs.[7]

Although mechanisms were in place to pay for patient services, voluntary hospitals were still suffering from a lack of endowment dollars to pay for capital improvements. It was widely believed that rural populations suffered from a lack of inpatient hospital beds. The Hospital Survey and Construction Act (Hill-Burton) was passed in 1946 to set up a system of matching grants to pay for hospital construction. The bill was originally designed to increase access to health care and, due to pressure from special interest groups, was amended to establish funding for nursing homes, rehabilitation centers, ambulatory care centers, and other capital projects.

Social welfare sentiment following the depression and the harsh realities of World War II set in place public attitudes regarding access to and the quantity of health care services which exist today. The government undertook legislative action to support these public concerns. However, indirectly the government supported the private enterprise of medicine. There was also the influence of certain special interest groups during this period. Both the American Medical Association and the American Hospital Association used the legislative process very effectively to protect the interests of their respective members. These two groups had major influence in the ''art and science'' of policy implementation through the control of finance and delivery system strategies. At the same time, the government failed to develop mechanisms to ensure quality or to assess or challenge resource consumption. Hospitals and physicians

---

5. For thoughts on the role of science and technology, see Renee Fox, *"Medicine, Science and Technology"* in *Applications of Social Science to Clinical Medicine and Health Policy,* edited by Linda Aiken and David Mechanic, 1987. New Brunswick, NJ: Rutgers University Press.

6. This support of special groups led to the development of the categorical grant as a funding mechanism. The grant remained a key funding strategy throgh the 1960's.

7. This legislation created the link between rehabilitation and medicine, thus moving the primary control of rehabilitation away from the educational system. See Gritzer and Arluke.

gained firm control of both the costs and nature of services provided (Starr, 1982).

1965 to 1982: The Rising Costs of Health Care

Federal involvement as a major financier of health care took another giant step in 1965 with the passage of the Medicare (Title XVIII) and Medicaid (Title XIX) amendments to the Social Security Act. With the Medicare legislation, the government recognized the increasing need for health care in the aging population. These expanded federal dollars went toward the payment of medical bills to social security beneficiaries. To implement the program, the federal government contracted with private insurance carriers to serve as intermediaries, the majority of which were the Blue Cross organizations. In contrast, Medicaid was a federal grant program which allocated money to the states to support health care for the poor. The federal government allowed states a great deal of autonomy in determining eligibility and the types of services for which funds would be provided.

As the "Great Society" expanded, so did the public's notion of equality. The increased need for health services in various sectors of the population necessitated more trained health care workers. As a result, the federal government expanded its role in financing the education of health professionals. The 1963 Health Professions Education Assistance Act provided both scholarships and loans as well as construction funds for schools. This legislation was followed in 1964 by the Nurse Training Act, in 1965 by the Health Professions Assistance Amendments, in 1966 by the Allied Health Professions Personnel Training Act, and in 1968 by the Health Manpower Training Act. Various training legislation continued through the 1970's.

The health industry was now growing rapidly. Not surprisingly, national attention began to focus on strategies to manage the rising cost of health care. The focus of public sentiment shifted from the previously held view of unquestioned autonomy of physician and hospital practice. Hospital planning councils and federal planning programs attempted to streamline the system with emphasis on coordinating services and reducing unnecessary duplication and costs. States adopted certificate of need statutes which required that need be established before additional hospitals were built. Professional Standards Review Organizations were mandated by federal legislation and required that patient records be reviewed for appropriateness of services provided. The nascent concept of managed care began with the introduction of the Health Maintenance Organizations (HMO's). The HMO began as an attempt to coordinate service delivery and control costs. The health care system began to focus on the quality and appropriateness of care.

1982 to the Present: The Shift to Cost Containment

By 1982, hospital costs accounted for 43 percent of the yearly $49.2 billion expended for Medicare (Health Care Financing Administration Fact Sheet, 1983). As the costs continued to escalate, the integrity of the Social Security System came into question. After a number of unsuccessful administrative attempts to initiate reform, a Republican-dominated Congress supported the Reagan administration in signing into law the greatest revamping of payment mechanisms since the 1965 Medicare legislation—the Tax Equity and Fiscal Responsibility Act of 1982 (TEFRA) (P.L. 97-248) and the Social Security Amendments of 1983 (P.L. 98-21). These laws were designed to focus primarily on hospital care.

The TEFRA legislation reversed the incentives for the hospital industry by changing payment from a retrospective to a prospective payment system. Hospitals were reimbursed according to a pre-specified amount for particular illnesses/injuries, rather than the old system of reimbursing for the actual costs incurred during the time of care. Illnesses were grouped into 467 categories for payment and these groups were termed *Diagnosis Related Groups* or DRG's. Since the hospitals were reimbursed according to these pre-determined amounts for each illness/injury, if the cost of a patient's care exceeded this amount, the hospital had to absorb these costs and hence lost revenue. Thus additional services provided to a health consumer resulted in expense to the hospital rather than revenue.

Hospital administrations responded to this **cost containment** challenge in two important ways: (1) by shortening lengths of stay in the hospital because unnecessary time spent in the hospital became an expense to the hospital rather than the payor; and (2) by encouraging physicians to reconsider their practice patterns of ordering tests and ancillary services since such services also became expenses to the hospital under the new prospective payment system.[8]

The era of cost control was firmly established. Private insurers were forced to adopt prospective pricing systems or bear the burden of shifting hospital costs. Both Health Maintenance Organizations and Preferred Provider Organizations (PPO's) became familiar alternatives to the traditional health insurance programs.[9]

---

8. Occupational therapy was one of the ancillary services which converted from revenue to expense during this era.

U.S. HEALTH CARE POLICY COMPARED TO OTHER NATIONS

Since 1883, nearly half of the nations in the world have adopted some form of national health service or insurance mechanism. The initial concept of **national health insurance** developed in Europe and the United States simultaneously in response to increased urbanization and industrialization and the demise of extended families to care for the ill (Litman & Robins, 1984). But as many European countries developed national health systems, the United States developed a system that serviced only select programs and populations and fostered the preservation of the private health care delivery mechanisms. Today, the United States is the only western nation without a comprehensive national health insurance system that covers the entire population (Mechanic, 1989).

Our current health policy has developed around the economic, political, sociological and scientific influences which have shaped our society since the American Revolution. These include the influence of a market economy, the importance of **special interest groups** to American life, and the individualism of the population which is manifest in orientation to local control rather than national systems of control. As a result, American public policy implementation can best be characterized by the term ''disjointed incrementalism'' (Kissick, 1988).

THE HEALTH SYSTEM

The outcome of health policy is the organization of systems for the provision of health services. Two models are presented here to describe both health systems development and the component parts of a health system. Health care practitioners can utilize these models to develop an understanding of the systems in which they deliver services and how these systems affect the performance and outcome of the American health care consumer.

Health Systems Development

The terms, *health system, health services system, health care system*, and *health services* are used interchangeably in the literature. DeMiguel (1975) has defined health system as ''the set of relationships among institutions, social groups, and individuals that is directed toward maintaining and improving the health status of certain human populations.'' DeMiguel's model for health systems (which has been adapted from work by Weinerman) presents the health system not only as a structure, but also a process (Figure 7-2). Historical experience, cultural values, and societal resources combine to form social policy and define national priorities. These result in the application of knowledge, arrangement of services, and the allocation of resources that comprise the health care system. From this system, outcomes are produced. Outcomes are related to the health status of a population and can be measured in various ways. Examples of outcome measures are the quantity of services by cost, the quality of improved health status, and the accessibility of services. These outcomes flow back into the system, and create feedback as input for system change and adaptation.

Health System Components

The health system is very complex. It has multiple functions, such as patient care, education of health professionals, and health education of the public. In National Strategies for Health Care Organization (1985), Roemer describes the essential components of a health service system (Figure 7-3). He sees the essential components of the health care system as follows:

Production of Resources. Resources include health manpower, facilities, commodities, and knowledge. These resources provide support for the existence of the system. *Health manpower* is human resources of skilled individuals, such as physicians, nurses, pharmacists, technologists, and occupational therapists. *Health facilities* are those sites in which care is delivered, such as hospitals, ambulatory care centers, emergency care centers, laboratories, private clinics, nursing homes, and rehabilitation centers. *Health commodities* are products necessary for health care such as drugs, prosthetic devices, bandages, laboratory chemicals, and technological equipment. *Knowledge* is produced from experimental research and observation and is passed on through education. Knowledge results in improved technologies and affects all the other resource areas.

Organization of Resources. Resources must be pulled together in an organization to develop or deliver health services. These functional groupings constitute programs that may be sponsored by government, voluntary non-profit organizations, or profit-oriented companies and corporations.

---

9. These are types of managed care systems. Physicians and other health providers contract to provide services under pre-arranged payment agreements. Primary physicians act as case managers by reviewing and pre-approving all expenditures for individual subscriber care. Financial incentives are provided to the primary physicians that encourage a reduction of the number of specialty consultations, tests, and ancillary services.

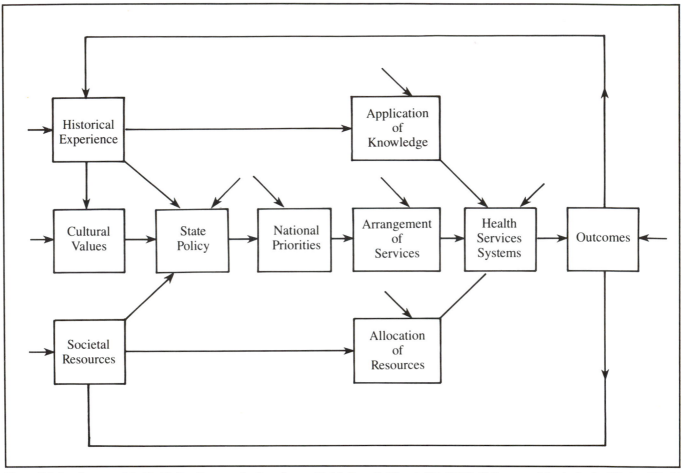

Figure 7-2. Development of the Health Care System—An Open System Model. *From DeMiguel, J.M. (1975). "A Framework for the Study of National Health Systems," Inquiry Supplement 12(14). Adapted from Weinerman, E.R. (1971). "Research on Comparative Health Service Systems." Medical Care, 9, 272-290.*

Economic Support. Programs are organized and developed with money. The funding of health care comes from individuals through direct payment, employers, voluntary health insurance, social insurance, charity, and government taxation.

Management. Management plays a supporting role in the organization of programs. This includes planning, administration, regulation, and evaluation. Today's management efforts in health care are being directed by the interests of payers towards issues of evaluation of effectiveness and regulation of care.

Delivery of Services. The outcome of all the above components is the delivery of services to people. Basic services are termed preventive, therapeutic, and rehabilitative. These services can be delivered in primary care settings, such as general hospitals or doctors' offices. They

may also be delivered in more specialized secondary facilities and tertiary care (comprehensive diagnostic facilities) or special programs. The variations in facilities, personnel, and technology among delivery settings are considerable and are important in accurately evaluating the outcomes as related to the resources consumed.

ADVOCACY IN HEALTH POLICY

From these models it becomes clear that government can directly influence the development and organization of programs, and therefore the delivery of services, through both regulatory controls and economic incentives. Health professionals must look beyond daily patient care responsibilities to the larger systems which affect their work. Changes in any one of the components of the health

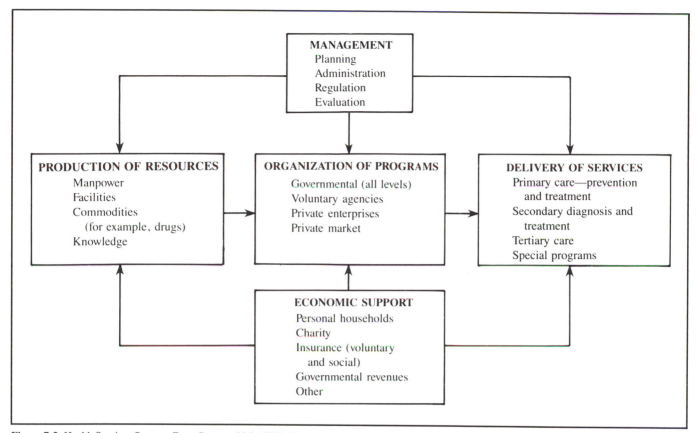

Figure 7-3. Health Services System. *From Roemer, M.I. (1985). National Strategies for Health Care Organization: A World Overview. Ann Arbor, MI: Health Administration Press.*

delivery system could create either a positive or negative impact on a health consumer's ability to obtain services. Improving the performance potential of individuals in our society necessitates an understanding of the rationale for policy decisions and the art and science of policy implementation.

Policy Implementation: The Medicare Example

The concept of equality of access guided political and social opinion from the Depression until the 1970's when the current economic/cost containment rationale took precedence. The political climate of 1964 supported the rationale of social equity. A growing concern existed over the rising cost of health care for the aged and public support for some type of national health insurance for this population was high. The concept of national health insurance had long been debated, but the powerful interest groups of the American Hospital Association and American Medical Association had opposed any such legislation. Physicians feared a less than favorable reimbursement package under such a plan. The hospitals, with newly

financed facilities and capital projects, were also concerned with altering payment mechanisms.

Strong public support coupled with a Congress controlled by a Democratic majority provided the leverage for the passage of health insurance for the aged. Representative Wilbur Mills was the powerful chairman of the House Ways and Means Committee. Under his sponsorship, the Medicare legislation was passed. It was a three-part implementation package which had more to do with special interests and compromise than the original policy objective of health insurance for the aged. *Medicare Part A* was a compulsory hospital insurance program for the elderly. *Medicare Part B* was a government subsidized voluntary insurance to cover outpatient hospital costs and physician fees, both inpatient and outpatient. The third part, *Medicaid*, provided federal grants-in-aid to the states to subsidize health care for the poor. Medicare A was proposed by the Democrats, Part B by the Republicans, and Medicaid was an expansion of the 1970 Kerr-Mills legislation proposed by Representative Wilbur Mills. Although frequently viewed as one program, this three-part legislation encompassed very diverse policy goals (Morris, 1985).

Congress now had the task of developing implementation strategies which would satisfy the powerful special interest groups. Medicare Part A resulted in *cost plus reimbursement* contracts for hospitals, whereby hospitals were allowed to charge the government the cost plus overhead for such items as capital costs and medical education. Part B developed a new payment mechanism for physicians' services. Service to Medicare beneficiaries provided a new source of income to physicians.[10] Medicaid implementation was to take place on a state level. This resulted in extremely varied strategies which depended upon the individual state's health policy objectives.

Thus, out of a policy desire to provide national health insurance to the aged, the federal government also authorized state funding for the poor. Implementation strategies were designed to enhance growth in the private sectors of the health industry. Hospitals and physicians who had once feared such a national plan, grew wealthy under the Medicare reimbursement system. Individual health providers controlled the amount of services provided to beneficiaries and the cost of those services. The federal government

implemented no mechanisms to control either the cost or the quality of services.

Legislation and the Growth of Occupational Therapy

Hospital-based occupational therapy also grew under the Medicare legislation as hospitals were driven to maximize services under Part A to generate income. According to Scott (1985), Medicare is the largest single payor of occupational therapy services. She estimated that in 1985, 20 percent of all occupational therapists and assistants were serving Medicare beneficiaries.

In contrast, occupational therapy growth did not occur in outpatient facilities or private practice because occupational therapy was not included in Part B coverage. Because of a lack of political support, the American Occupational Therapy Association (AOTA) could not mobilize efforts to ensure coverage of occupational therapy in the 1965 legislation (Gritzer & Arluke, 1985).[11] Recognition of this problem led AOTA leadership to develop a framework for political action.[12]

Political activities in the 70s and 80s on the part of AOTA have resulted in the further expansion of occupational therapy as a service provider. The Education for All Handicapped Children Act of 1975 (P.L. 94-142) and Amendments of 1986 (P.L. 99-457) provide funding for the education of handicapped children. Occupational therapy is covered as a related service. The 1986 Social Security Amendments included coverage for occupational therapy in outpatient settings, skilled nursing facilities, and in private clinics. Table 7-1 shows current Medicare coverage for occupational therapy services. State initiatives have taken place also. Over 90% of the states now have occupational therapy practice acts.

Public policy, as enacted through legislation and regulation has shaped a good deal of occupational therapy practice. As with other health care services in the United States, occupational therapy operates in a marketplace in which services correspond to payment mechanisms. Compare the primary employment settings for occupational therapists from 1973 to 1986 (Table 7-2) with the summary of payment sources for therapy services (Table 7-3). During

---

10. Other professional services with strong political action initiatives were also funded under Part B. These groups include Speech Pathologists and Physical Therapists.

11. For a discussion of occupational therapy's market mistakes, see Gritzer and Arluke, *The Making of Rehabilitation: A Political Economy of Medical Specialization,* pp. 135-145.

12. AOTA developed a Government and Legal Affairs Division which was later renamed the Legislative and Political Affairs Division. Additionally, the AOTA authorized the formation of the American Occupational Therapy Political Action Committee (AOTPAC) that supports legislative campaigns of politicians supportive of the objectives of the AOTA and the special interest groups served by the profession.

Table 7-1
July 1, 1987 Coverage for Occupational Therapy Services Under Medicare Parts A and B

Setting	Part A	Part B
Comprehensive Outpatient Rehabilitation Facility (CORF)		
Health Maintenance Organization/ Competitive Medical Plan (HMO/CMP)	Covered if HMO/CMP serves Medicare beneficiaries.	Covered if HMO/CMP serves Medicare beneficiaries.
Home Health Care	Covered. Need for occupational therapy alone does not qualify patient for benefits, but occupational therapy may continue after qualifying services end.	Covered. Need for occupational therapy alone does not qualify patient for benefits, but occupational therapy may continue after qualifying services end.
Hospice	Covered.	
Hospital Inpatient	Provided at the hospital's option under Prospective Payment System (*Exempt* psychiatric and rehabilitation hospitals and units *must provide* occupational therapy).	
Hospital Outpatient		Covered if rendered by hospital personnel under supervision of physician.
Other Outpatient: a) Physician's Office/Physician Directed Clinic		a) Covered if rendered as ("incident to physician's services.")
b) Rehabilitation Agencies		b) Covered.
c) Home Health Agencies		c) Covered when beneficiary is not under a home health plan of treatment.
Skilled Nursing Facility	Covered.	Covered.
Independent Practice		Covered under independent provider number. Subject to $500 limit per beneficiary.

Adapted from Occupational Therapy Medicare Handbook. (1987). Rockville, MD: American Occupational Therapy Association, Inc.

that time, the primary settings for employment correspond to those environments covered by public funding—general hospitals, rehabilitation hospitals, and the public school system. Thus we see that public policy directed toward specific segments of the population creates private incentives for growth in the health care sector. This was no exception for occupational therapy.

THE IMPACT OF POLICY ON INDIVIDUAL PERFORMANCE

So far in this chapter, we have focused on developing an understanding of public policy, the health care system, and their relationship to occupational therapy. How does all this influence performance? Public policy and the health care system determine the context and parameters of many of the services that occupational therapy patients receive. As people try to fulfill their roles in society, the social, political, and economic realities continue to govern their ability to engage productively in the occupational areas of work, home management, self-care, and leisure. When performance is disrupted, the mix and availability of timely services can make a significant difference in an individual's ability to overcome problems and return to productive life.

The major pieces of legislation that have influenced occupational therapy patients and clients are summarized in Table 7-4. The best way to explain how these laws can

Table 7-2
Primary Employment Setting by Year

Setting	OTRs 1973 %	1977 %	1982 %	1986 %	COTAs 1973 %	1977 %	1982 %	1986 %
College, 2 yr.	1.4	1.2	0.8	0.7	0.8	0.9	0.6	0.8
College/Univ., 4 yr.	5.6	4.9	4.1	3.1	0.7	0.6	0.9	0.3
Comm. Mental Health Ctr.	4.2	4.3	2.4	1.6	4.0	3.5	3.1	3.8
Correctional Institution	0.2	0.2	0.1	0.1	0.3	0.2	0.1	0.2
Day Care Ctr./Program	1.4	1.1	1.0	1.1	1.2	2.4	2.0	4.3
Halfway House	—	—	—	0.0	—	—	—	0.1
HMO (incl. PPO/IPA)	0.3	0.2	0.2	0.3	0.7	0.3	0.3	0.2
Home Health Agency	0.9	2.2	3.8	4.6	0.2	0.4	0.8	1.2
Hospice	—	—	0.0	0.1	—	—	0.0	0.0
Gen. Hospital-Rehab.	—	—	—	4.2	—	—	—	4.5
Gen. Hospital-all other	20.5	19.8	25.3	22.0	15.1	12.7	17.8	14.1
Pediatric Hospital	2.9	20	1.6	1.7	1.5	1.2	0.8	0.4
Psychiatric Hospital	13.8	11.2	7.4	6.9	22.6	14.3	9.7	8.4
Outpatient Clinic (free stdg.)	—	—	2.5	2.4	—	—	1.7	0.9
Physician's Office	—	—	—	1.1	—	—	—	0.2
Private Industry	—	—	0.7	0.5	—	—	1.0	0.5
Private Practice	1.3	2.1	3.5	6.0	0.3	0.4	1.2	1.9
Public Health Agency	1.6	1.5	0.8	0.9	0.5	0.5	0.3	0.4
Rehab. Hospital/Center	13.4	10.9	8.9	10.5	9.5	11.0	8.4	8.4
Research Facility	0.3	0.3	0.4	0.2	0.2	0.3	0.1	0.0
Residential Care Fac. incl. Group Home, Ind. Liv. Ctr.	—	4.4	4.2	3.3	—	8.5	7.6	7.5
Retirement or Senior Ctr.	—	—	—	0.2	—	—	—	1.1
School System (includes private school)	11.0	14.0	18.3	17.0	3.6	6.2	11.3	14.4
Sheltered Workshop	0.7	0.7	0.7	0.4	1.4	0.9	1.9	1.6
Skilled Nursing Home/Int. Care Facility	6.2	7.9	6.0	5.8	22.8	26.1	22.5	20.1
Vocational or Prevoc. Prog.	—	—	—	0.7	—	—	—	1.6
Voluntary Agency (e.g., Easter Seal/U.C.P.)	—	1.7	1.7	1.4	—	0.4	1.2	1.2
Other	14.2	9.4	5.4	3.2	14.7	9.3	6.7	2.2
Total	99.9%	100.0%	99.8%	100.0%	100.1%	100.1%	100.0%	100.0%

Note: Missing data are due to changing employment categories on the various administrations of the surveys. Recoding of additional settings in the "other" category into existing alternatives may explain the decline in the "other" category. For this reason, small differences in the percentages over time should be interpreted with care.

specifically influence patients' or clients' performance is to examine individual case studies. The following case studies demonstrate the impact of policy on individual human performance.

Case Study 7-1

Medicare-Skilled Nursing Facility: Mrs. Moss was an elderly widow who lived by herself in her own home until she suffered a stroke. She did not have any close relatives living nearby. Among other problems, the stroke left her with severe swallowing problems that made it impossible for her to gain adequate oral nutrition. She was receiving supplemental feedings through a nasogastric tube. The medical team recommended that a gastrostomy tube be implanted since she had not made rapid progress in regaining swallowing skills. The gastrostomy would allow liquid feedings to pass directly to her stomach, so that the nasal tube could be removed. The occupational therapist wanted to see the tube removed, as it was

---

Table 7-3
Payment Sources for Occupational Therapy in the United States

PROGRAM	SERVICES COVERED
Medicare	Pays for services in hospitals, outpatient facilities, home care, hospices, physician offices, and in independent practice. Restrictions apply in all these settings.
Medicaid	Service is eligible but each state varies.
CHAMPUS	Civilian Health and Medical Program of the Uniformed Services is an insurance program for retired members of the armed forces and their dependents. It pays for occupational therapy provided in inpatient and outpatient settings. It has a special rehabilitation benefit.
Education for All Handicapped Children Act	Services provided when identified as a necessary related service for a child to benefit from special education and must be incorporated in the Individualized Education Plan (IEP) for the child. Occupational therapy has also been designated as a primary intervention service in the Early Intervention Program mandated in the 1986 amendment to this act.
Workmen's Compensation	(state level, employer-supported program) Services frequently paid for as part of the health benefit package provided to workers injured on the job.
Vocational Rehabilitation	(state-level programs) Services and adaptive devices frequently paid for as part of a plan to help disabled individuals to become employed or to live independently. Services may be provided as rehabilitation engineering or technology services.
Private Insurance Plans	Coverage varies greatly. They frequently provide some level of occupational therapy coverage for inpatient medical care, and may cover part or all of outpatient services.
Pre-paid Health Plans	Health Maintenance Organizations (HMO's) and Social/Health Maintenance Organizations may cover when services are considered part of a managed plan of care. This is particularly true when these plans seek to provide care to Medicare recipients, as all covered services must be available.
Self-Pay	(Individual Payment) Individuals receiving services may pay part or all of the fees associated with occupational therapy services.
Consultation Services	Some industries and businesses also pay for services as a direct or consultation service to provide preventive and restorative services to employees. Consultation services may be employed to assist in the design and distribution of products to meet the needs of the disabled and to provide education about and to those with special needs.

From Current coverage for occupational therapy services under Medicare parts a and b. In Scott, S (Ed.) Payment for occupational therapy services: Federal, Medicare. pp. 1-4. Copyright 1988 by The American Occupational Therapy Association. Reprinted with permission.

irritating Mrs. Moss's throat and most likely interfering with some of her swallowing abilities and delaying her recovery.

As she had slowed in her progress at the rehabilitation facility, a decision was made to discharge Mrs. Moss to a nursing home where she could continue to receive skilled care and therapy services available to support her continued recovery. To qualify for the Medicare coverage of a nursing home stay, one must require skilled nursing care. While management of a nasogastric tube requires skilled nursing care, a gastrostomy does not. Even though the insertion of the gastrostomy would have allowed Mrs. Moss to return to her home, the team knew Mrs. Moss could not manage at home without home care services. The occupational therapist wanted Mrs. Moss to return to her own home but realized that Mrs. Moss did not have sufficient self-care and homemaking skills to manage independently at this time. Under Medicare, Mrs. Moss with a gastrostomy would only have been eligible for minimal home care services twice a week.

In this case, although Medicare had provided financial aid to support Mrs. Moss through the acute and subacute stages of recovery, the restrictions regarding her extended care served as a disincentive for the rehabilitation team and Mrs. Moss to focus their efforts on regaining her independence. Such efforts might have been directed toward her learning to swallow and providing alternate nutrition systems. But Medicare focuses only on meeting medical care needs and sometimes restrictions actually encourage patients to remain in a sick role in order to continue to receive care under those restrictions. The end result many times is reduced performance for the patient.

Table 7-4
U.S. Legislation Affecting Occupational Therapy Clients

Social Security Act of 1935 (PL74-241) and Amendments
The social security system provides financial support for disabled workers, as well as retirement income to the elderly. Extensive medical benefits are also provided to the elderly through this system.

Disability Insurance Benefit Program, 1956
Provides cash benefits to disabled persons who have qualifying work experience.

Title 19 (PL 89-97) Medicare Program, 1965
Provides coverage for medical care to the elderly. Occupational therapy is a covered service within limits.

Title 18 (PL 89-97) Medicaid Program, 1965
Provides grants to states for medical assistance to the poor. Occupational may be a covered service, at the state's discretion.

Medicare Amendments (PL 92-603), 1971
Placed limits on the amount of reimbursement hospitals could receive for routine costs.

Supplemental Security Income Program, 1974
Provides cash benefits to needy disabled who do not have qualifying work experience. Served to supplement state welfare programs.

Housing and Community Development Act, 1974
Encouraged building and provision of housing to the disabled by providing federal dollars to private builders.

Tax Equity and Fiscal Responsibility Act (PL 97-248), 1982
Extended limits on reimbursement to hospitals to include ancillary services, including occupational therapy.

Omnibus Social Security Act (PL 98-210), 1983
Replaced the cost based payment system with a prospective payment system, using diagnostic related groupings as the determinant of payment.

Social Security Amendments (PL 96-265), 1980
Removes certain disincentives to work by allowing disabled people to deduct independent-living expenses in computing income benefits.

Deficit Reduction Legislation Acts (PL 98-369), 1984, (PL 99-272), 1985, (PL 99-509), 1986
Modified Medicare laws, including amendment which extended occupational therapy coverage in Part B.

Older Americans Act (PL 89-73), 1965 and Amendments
Established an Administration on Aging with objectives to expand state and local networks to assist the aged and provide resources to health care professionals working with the aged. Established nationwide network of area agencies on aging. Provided oversight for prevention of discrimination to aged.

Architectural Barriers Act (PL 90-480), 1968
Requires federally funded buildings and rented sites to be accessible.

Urban Mass Transportation Act (PL 91-453), 1970
Requires eligible recipients to plan and design accessible mass transportation facilities and services.

Federal Aid Highway Act (PL 91-453), 1970
Requires transportation facilities receiving federal assistance through this act be accessible. Allows funding to be used for constructing accessible crosswalks.

Rehabilitation Act (PL 93-112), 1973 & Amendments (PL 93-516), 1974
Established Rehabilitation Services Administration and provided for vocational rehabilitation of the handicapped, with emphasis on the severely disabled. Provided for grants to improve independent living potential for individuals for whom vocational goals were not feasible. Established Architectural Transportation Barriers Compliance Board to oversee compliance with federal access legislation. Prohibited employment discrimination against qualified handicapped people in programs that are federally funded. Prohibited public service programs funded by Federal dollars from denying service to individuals solely based on disability.

Department of Transportation Appropriations Act (PL 93-391), 1975
Requires purchase of mass transit equipment or facility construction to be accessible to elderly and handicapped.

Developmental Disabilities Assistance and Bill of Rights Act (PL 94-103), 1975
Establishes protection and advocacy systems for developmentally disabled people.

Education of All Handicapped Children Act (PL 94-142), 1975 and Amendments (PL 99-457), 1986
Provides for a free appropriate education for handicapped children in the least restrictive environment. Provides funding for related services, including occupational therapy, as required to assist handicapped children to benefit from special education. Amendments added funding to meet the needs of preschoolers and mandated a program of early intervention to infants and toddlers with handicaps.

National Housing Act Amendments (PL 94-173), 1975
Established the Office of Independent Living for disabled people in U.S. Department of Housing and Urban Development. Included removal of barriers in federally supported housing.

Rehabilitation Comprehensive Services and Developmental Disabilities Amendments (PL 95-602), 1978
Established independent living as a priority for state vocational rehabilitation programs, including federal funding for independent living centers.

Americans with Disabilities Act, (PL 101-366) 1990
Requires businesses to make provisions for disabled workers and to ensure accessibility in all businesses with more than 15 workers.

Information was obtained from Litman's *Health Politics and Policy,* Appendix 2, "Chronology and Capsule Highlights of Government in Health in the United States (9), and DeJong & Lifchez's article in the *Scientific American* entitled "Physical Disability and Public Policy (14). Additional sources of information were from the American Occupational Therapy Association.

Case Study 7-2

Social Security Disability Income: George was a 19-year-old who was employed as a laborer before receiving a spinal cord injury as the result of a diving accident. His injury left him a paraplegic, but he retained full use of his arms and hands. He received vocational rehabilitation services from his state vocational rehabilitation agency, which sent him to school to be a small engine repair mechanic. Vocational rehabilitation laws served as an incentive to George, as they paid for the full cost of his retraining. However, George was unable to find full-time work, as many engine repair jobs require repairs at levels that George could not reach from his wheelchair.

Because of his condition, George was able to qualify for Social Security Disability Income (SSDI), which provided him with money on which to live. However, in order to receive this income subsidy, George had to be declared totally and permanently disabled and unable to work. Even parttime work would cause him to lose his disabled status and the disability income.

In this situation, public policies had served as an incentive for work performance through support of training in alternate job skills but yet, in the end, the restrictions served as a disincentive for George to return to work . This can occur both when full-time employment opportunities are limited or when the disabled worker does not have sufficient endurance for full-time work.

Case Study 7-3

Medicare—Home Health Care: Mary was an 82-year-old woman who lived in a large home in a rural area with her 92-year-old husband. Before she suffered a stroke, she was very active as a homemaker and in church activities. She also did a great deal of needlework, especially crocheting. She actively participated in several service and religious organizations. She had several grown children who lived in the community, and who were available to help with grocery shopping and similar chores.

The stroke left Mary with residual weakness in her right arm and leg. She was able to ambulate with a cane; however, she required some minimal assistance with dressing, toileting, and bathing activities because she was unable to adjust her clothing adequately. She was unable to carry objects when ambulating because of the weakness in her arm and the need to use her upper extremity to maintain balance. She also had a mild speech deficit, but was easily understood and processed information accurately.

After her discharge, Mary received occupational therapy and speech therapy in the home. Occupational therapy services were directed toward increasing coordinated function of her right arm and increasing independence in the home environment. Although Mary made some progress, it was clear to the therapist that she was more motivated to return to her community activities than to household chores. The therapist would have preferred to involve Mary in more community outings to increase her confidence level in outdoor mobility and her functional communication. However, one of the qualifying indicators for eligibility for home care services is that the person must be confined to home due to a functional limitation that restricts his/her ability to leave the home.

Again we see that the same policy that provides important services necessary to increase performance, also limits performance. In this case, Mary was inadvertently discouraged from pursuing her social activities outside her home because of such restrictions.

Case Study 7-4

Education of All Handicapped Children Act (PL 94-142): Johnny was an eleven-year-old boy who was having difficulty keeping up with his peers in school, most noticeably in handwriting activities. He had a diagnosis of mild cerebral palsy, and was therefore eligible to receive special services to enhance his potential for learning. He was referred by the school to occupational therapy for services to improve his handwriting. Before this referral, Johnny had never received therapy services of any kind, as he lived in a rural area that was generally underserved by health and rehabilitation personnel.

After an evaluation, the occupational therapist determined that Johnny's performance could be improved through the use of specific positioning techniques, implementation of appropriate work heights, and introduction of graded grasp and release activities to improve hand function. While providing consultation to the teacher and education to Johnny's parents, it became evident that these same strategies would also improve a number of Johnny's self-care skills, such as self-feeding, managing clothing fastenings, and toileting activities.

Johnny's performance was certainly enhanced by these services. Due to a public policy that affirms the right of all children to have access to an appropriate public education, he was provided with services that enhanced not only his educational opportunities, but all aspects of his performance.

Case Study 7-5

Worker's Compensation: Harry worked as an employee of a manufacturing firm. His responsibilities included loading trucks, driving them to delivery points within the city, and unloading the truck at the delivery site. During one of his trips Harry was injured when the tire blew out on his truck, resulting in a collision with a telephone pole. Harry sustained a serious whiplash, fractured his right wrist, and severely traumatized his lower back. Because this occurred during the course of his work duties, he was eligible for both medical and income benefits under his state's workmen's compensation law. This covered all medical expenses necessary to restore his ability to return to work and two-thirds of his normal wage in income support. (Note: Because worker's compensation is administered at the state level, the level of payment may vary.)

After an inpatient hospitalization and outpatient physical and occupational therapy, the medical team found Harry able to return to work with a restriction not to lift anything over 50 pounds. Harry's employer was required by law to either continue paying the income benefit or place him in another job that was within his physical capabilities at comparable wages. Harry's employer was concerned about Harry's usefulness as an employee now that he no longer had sufficient strength to load and unload the truck, even though he could still drive. Harry recognized his employer's hesitation and was reluctant to return to work for fear of either re-injuring himself or being fired. He knew if he accepted work, he would no longer be considered disabled and would lose the benefits of workers' compensation.

In this case, although the state law provided support to ensure that Harry received adequate medical attention, the workers' compensation created a disincentive for him to return to work. This negatively effected his overall performance and inhibited the opportunity for him to realize his fullest performance potential.

THE FUTURE

This overview of health policy would not be complete without a discussion of the future. As health care personnel tackle policy issues, inherent in their assessment is an understanding that professionals have the ethical responsibility to police their own practice for the protection of the consumer. In the past, consumer protection has too frequently been overshadowed by concerns for economic gain and concern for particular practice arenas. The implications of this ethical dilemma cannot be ignored today. We are beginning to see the meshing of the ethical concerns with the economic concerns as American health care consumers demand appropriate outcomes for their investment of time and money. It is clear that this demand for health professionals to take responsibility for the outcome and quality of services they provide will become even stronger as the American public continues to spend increasing amounts of personal funds for health care.

Our health industry is pluralistic in nature and will continue as such. However, society must make choices regarding the nature and quantity of services provided and paid for through public monies. Will we continue to pay the price for lengthy hospital stays in intensive care units for a severely debilitated elderly person with a terminal disease? Or would the public be better served by using the costs of those hospitalizations to provide prenatal care to a number of low income mothers who would not otherwise receive proper prenatal care? This is a purposefully provocative question, but a realistic one—there are no simple answers. How does a society make such difficult choices when it comes to health care and quality of life? How does a nation without a defined health care rationale for its people begin to address these questions? As a nation, we have no assurance that even if we did have carefully defined priorities, we could overcome the economic, political, social, and technological imperatives which we have already discussed.

The American health care system is rooted in a social system which is class based. As health care providers, it is important to understand the two-tiered systems of care which exist in this country. Without this understanding and acceptance, we will be unable to conceive of a more equitable system for all people.

There is no question that science and technological advancement have benefited world health. Infants born in 1980 can be expected to live 27 more years than infants born in 1900 (DeJong & Lifchez, 1983). However, not all the results have been positive. One by-product of the analytic scientific concept of cause-and-effect has been medical specialization which nurtures a health system that views the patient in terms of a sick or malfunctioning body part that needs to be corrected or healed. The outcome of such attitudes and practice is rarely the overall good health of the patient and attainment of optimal functional performance. The goal of all health care should be a productive, meaningful life for the patient.

As science, technology and medicine advance the boundaries of life, health professionals will be treating new varieties of severely and chronically disabled consumers. Treating the premature infant of 24 weeks gestation or the 85-year-old jogger with a sports injury will provide challenges to even the most innovative practitioner to assist these individuals to develop or regain meaningful life roles. As more people continue to live into their 80's or 90's, the elderly population will become the dominant age group.

The current economic crisis in health care will persist. The debate will continue regarding the role of the federal government in the health and well-being of the American people. Historically, the government intervened in questions of equity or fairness of distribution, access or availability (particularly for the disadvantaged) and market imperfections such as the uneven distribution in rural areas. These questions will be readdressed as the cost containment era progresses. A substantial portion of the current rationale for policy is to create opportunity for the **re-privatization** of the health industry. In the coming years, both the site of health care delivery and the nature of services provided will change as private market forces take advantage of new opportunity. Professionals will move beyond the confines of clinic practice into other areas such as private industry, corporate program development, wellness programs, and health education programs. (See Chapter 27)

It is important that health practitioners understand not only the great health policy debate, but become active in the process. As policy continues to focus on outcome measurements, more and more references exist in the literature to functional outcome and human performance. The suggestion was made early in the debate that perhaps quality health care can only be measured when the individual has been returned to productive, meaningful life roles (Zubkoff & Blumstein, 1978). Occupational therapists refer to this as human occupation and have been claiming it as a specialty since the early 1900's (Kielhofner, 1983). From the economic perspective, the combination of these two factors creates "opportunity." The political and social climates of the coming decades could lend credibility to this notion. Chapter 28, Professional issues in a changing environment, addresses what occupation therapists can do to make a difference in the policies of the future.

SUMMARY

This chapter has attempted to provide an overview of public policy from the perspective of its influence on health care services; and therefore, on the availability and nature of services to address human performance deficits in the United States. It has been shown that public policy develops around economic, political, sociological and scientific interests. As the federal government in the U.S. has become more involved in funding health services, there has been an understandable interest in controlling costs. This, in turn, has engendered legislation designed to shape the health care sytem through influence on resources (which include personnel, facilities, commodities and knowledge) and their organization, on the management of those resources, and on the delivery of services.

It has been shown that the implementation of Medicare and Medicaid as well as subsequent legislation, has a direct effect on occupational therapy. It was shown that the nature of services provided by therapists have been influenced by specific payment mechanisms provided for in this legislation. The prospective payment system, implemented subsequent to the passage of the Tax Equity and Fiscal Responsibility Act (TEFRA) of 1983, was presented as a notable example of this influence. It was also emphasized that when mechanisms are not in place to provide payment for specialized services, such as occupational therapy, patients and clients may not attain a level of independent function consistent with their personal satisfaction and the public good.

Study Questions

1. The definition of health is crucial to the development of health policy. How do you define health?

2. What do you think is the federal government's responsibility for health care of its citizens? What is the basis for your beliefs?

3. Managed care has emerged as a major cost containment strategy within health care during the last decade. What services do occupational therapists offer that managed care systems would likely see as important cost effective measures?

4. There is some debate that physical rehabilitation is not really a medical service because the goal is not to cure, but rather a social service that focuses on returning people to productive personal and community life. If this definition is adopted as the basis for policy decisions, what are the implications for the occupational therapy profession and the individuals who need rehabilitation?

5. Think of patients and clients you have seen on recent fieldwork experiences and choose a group of specific interest to you. Name at least four specific methods you would use to examine how health policy issues influence their performance.

6. Americans believe citizens have a right to health care. As you were growing up, how did you come to realize your rights to health care? Give examples of how these beliefs have been implemented in daily life.

7. How do you see current regulations affecting your access to health care? What would you like to see changed?

Acknowledgment

The order in which the authors' names appear for this chapter is by agreement and may not reflect relative contribution.

References

Anderson, O. (1985). *Health services in the United States, a great enterprise since 1875.* Ann Arbor, MI: Health Services Administration Press.

Bair, J. & Gray, M. (Eds.) (1985). *The occupational therapy manager*. Rockville, MD: The American Occupational Therapy Association. Rockville, MD: The American Occupational Therapy Association, Inc.

Bellah, R., Madsen, R., Sullivan, W., Swidler, A., & Tipton, S. (1985). *Habits of the heart: Individualism and commitment in American life*. Berkeley, CA. University of California Press.

Crichton, A. (1981). *Health policy making: Fundamental issues to the United States, Canada, Great Britain, Australia*. (p. 23). Ann Arbor, MI: Health Administration Press.

DeJong, G. & Lifchez, R. (1983). Physical disability and public policy. *Scientific American, 6*, 42.

DeMiguel, J. (1975). A framework for the study of national health systems. *Inquiry*, Supplement to XII, 10-19.

de Kervasdoue, J., Kimberly, J., & Rodwin, V. (1984). *The end of an illusion: The future of health policy in western industrialized nations*. Berkeley, CA: University of California Press.

Dowling, H. (1982). *City hospitals*. Cambridge, MA: Harvard University Press.

Duffy, J. (1985). Social impact of disease in the late 19th century. In Leavitt, J. & Numbers, R. (Eds.). *Sickness and health in America: Readings in the history of medicine and public health*. (pp. 414-421). Madison, WI: University of Wisconsin.

Fox, R. (1987). Medicine, science, and technology. In Aiken, L. & Mechanic, D. (Eds.). *Applications of social science to clinical medicine and health policy*. New Brunswick, NJ: Rutgers University Press.

Gritzer, G. & Arluke, A. (1985). *The making of rehabilitation: a political economy of medical specialization, 1890-1980*. Berkeley, CA, University of California Press.

Kielhofner, G. (Ed.) (1983). *Health through occupation: theory and practice in occupational therapy*. Philadelphia, PA: F.A. Davis Company.

Kissick, W. (1988). Medicine Management: Two cultures in search of excellence. *Business and Health*, 1988, 52.

Litman, T. & Robins, L. (1984). *Health politics and policy*. New York, NY: John Wiley & Sons.

Mechanic, D. (1989). *Painful choices: Research and essays on health care*. New Brunswick, N.J.: Transaction Publishers.

Morris, J. (1985). *Searching for a cure: National health policy considered*. Washington, DC: Berkeley Morgan.

Mullan, F. (1989). *Plagues and politics*. New York: Basic Books.

Occupational Therapy News (1987). Rockville, MD: The American Occupational Therapy Association. Vol. 41, No. 9, p. 12.

Reed, K. & Sanderson, S. (1980). *Concepts of occupational therapy*. Baltimore, MD: Williams & Wilkins.

Rodwin, V. (1984). *The health planning predicament: France, Quebec, England and the United States*. (p. 41). Berkeley, CA: University of California Press.

Roemer, M. (1985). *National strategies for health care organizations—A world view*. Ann Arbor, MI: Health Administration Press.

Rosenberg, C. (1987). *The care of strangers: The rise of America's hospital system*. New York, NY: Basic Books.

Schramm, C.J. (Ed.). (1987). *Health care and its costs*. New York: W.W. Morton and Company.

Scott, S. (1985). Payment for occupational therapy services. In Bair, J. & Gray, M. (Eds.) *The occupational therapy manager*. Rockville, MD: The American Occupational Therapy Association, Inc.

Smith, H. R. & Fottler, M. (1985). *Prospective payment: Managing for operation effectiveness*. Rockville, MD: Aspen Systems Corporation.

Starr, P. (1982). *The social transformation of American medicine*. New York, NY: Basic Books, Inc.

Stevens, R. (1989). *In sickness and in wealth: American hospitals in the twentieth century*. New York, NY: Basic Books.

Stevens, R. & Stevens, R. (1974). *Welfare medicine in America: A case study of Medicaid*. New York, NY: The Free Press.

U.S. Department of Commerce (1987). Statistical abstract of the United States. National Health Care Expenses, Table 125. Washington, D.C.

U.S. Department of Health and Human Services (1983). *Health care financing administration fact sheet*. Baltimore, MD.

West, W.L. (1967). The 1967 Eleanor Clark Slagle Lecture: Professional responsibility in times of change. *The American Journal of Occupational Therapy*, Vol. XXII, No. 1.

Wilhite, V. (1958). *Founders of American economic thought and policy*. New York: NY: Bookman Associates.

Zubkoff, M. & Blumstein, J.F. (1978). The medical marketplace: Health policy formulation in consideration of economic structure. *National Commission on the Cost of Medical Care*. Vol II. Monroe, Wisconsin: American Medical Association.

CHAPTER CONTENT OUTLINE

Introduction

What is Physical Fitness?

Components of Physical Fitness

Responses and Adaptations

Reasons for Diminished Fitness

Other Factors Affecting Performance

Enhancing Performance Through Improved Physical Fitness

Summary

KEY TERMS

Aerobic power

Alarm reaction

Disuse atrophy

Dynamic flexibility

Dynamic strength

Ergometry

Exhaustion

Goniometer

Mechanical efficiency

Oxygen consumption

Principle of overload

Resistance development

Static flexibility

Static strength

ABSTRACT

The physiologic factors affecting performance are considered within the framework of the five components of health-related physical fitness. Cardiorespiratory function, muscle strength, muscle endurance, flexibility and body composition are each examined in light of their responses and adaptations to exercise and specific mechanisms of change. In addition, the parts these factors play in supporting human activity are examined. The chapter concludes with an overall prescription for enhancing performance through improved physical fitness.

Physiological Dimensions of Performance

8

Marian A. Minor

"Exercise ferments the humors, casts them into their proper channels, throws off redundancies, and helps nature in those secret distributions, without which the body cannot subsist in its vigor, nor the soul act with cheerfulness."
—Joseph Addison, 1711

OBJECTIVES

The information in this chapter is intended to help the reader—

1. identify the five components of health-related physical fitness.

2. understand the clinical implications of varying levels of physical fitness in the measurement of performance.

3. describe the difference between exercise response and adaptation to repeated bouts of service.

4. understand principles for improving the five components of fitness.

5. relate the effects of inactivity, aging and fatigue to performance.

p. 213 (Summary) chart!

INTRODUCTION

It is not the purpose of this chapter to present a crash course in exercise physiology. Detailed discussions of glycolytic pathways, the Krebs cycle, electron transport system, and the wonders of cyclic adenosine triphosphate will be left to the exercise physiology texts. If you are intrigued by the physiologic underpinnings of human performance, you will be able to explore the field in greater depth at your leisure. If you decide that this domain is not your favorite, then hopefully this chapter will afford you a basic appreciation of the part physiologic factors play in supporting human activity.

The physiologic factors will be discussed within the framework of the five components of physical fitness: *cardiorespiratory function, muscle strength, muscle endurance, flexibility,* and *body composition*. Each factor is discussed in light of response and adaptation to exercise and the mechanisms of change. We focus on the continual interplay between the physiologic factors that influence activity and the effect of activity and inactivity on the physiologic responses. By the time you have finished this chapter, you will appreciate the extent to which certain aspects of human physiology can both limit and enhance performance.

✳ WHAT IS PHYSICAL FITNESS? ✳

To perform activities and to accomplish tasks, a person must be able to move body parts, manipulate objects, and move the body through space. The physical ability to perform these activities in a meaningful way is dependent on a person's state of physical fitness.

What is physical fitness? Physical fitness is often defined in terms of particular sports interests or physical goals. To some people, being able to jog three miles is being physically fit, and to others physical fitness means a regimen of weight training. Quite commonly people equate flexibility with fitness or view being thin as being fit. According to exercise scientists and physical educators, physical fitness is a multifactorial concept that includes several components: 1) cardiorespiratory function, 2) muscle strength, 3) muscle endurance, 4) flexibility, and 5) body composition. The definition offered by David Lamb

(1984) is particularly appropriate to our discussion. Lamb defines physical fitness as *"the capacity to meet successfully the present and potential physical challenges of life."* Physical fitness is a result of heredity, activity levels, and the presence of pathology on these five areas. With no inherited or pathological limitations, and regular activity performed at training levels, one can enhance physical fitness to achieve excellent ratings in these categories.

On the other hand, fitness can be limited by inheritance, acquired pathology, or by prolonged periods of inactivity or immobilization. Physical and mental limitations do not exclude people from the possibility of being physically fit. There is good news and bad news about one's ability to control their own fitness. The bad news is that there are factors, such as heredity, that are beyond one's control. For example, if one's ambition is to be an elite marathon runner but one did not inherit the potential for a high maximal **oxygen consumption** and a high percentage of slow-twitch muscle fibers in calf and thigh muscles, then those goals may be unattainable. Being a marathon runner would likely be out of the question for a person who inherited rheumatoid arthritis and the resulting bouts of systemic inflammation, fatigue, and pain requiring periods of prolonged rest and severely restricted activity. In cases like these, performance goals may need to be reevaluated and new, more realistic goals established.

However, the good news is that every person can achieve the goal of maximal personal fitness to support individual performance, and physical fitness does respond positively to appropriate physical activity. After an acute illness when the medical need for immobilization is past, a gradual return to adequate levels of physical activity will produce measurable improvements in both fitness and performance measures. The consequences of disease and trauma can produce very real physical handicaps. Too often the ensuing consequences of inactivity also produce limitations. Insufficient activity after a disease or injury can often produce chronic limitations in performance. In a program of rehabilitation, it is important to consider physical fitness as the foundation on which functional capacity and skill learning are built. Improvement of physical fitness enables people to extend their capacities to successfully accomplish desired activities and maximize performance.

Physical Fitness as an Organizational Concept

An understanding of health-related physical fitness as a

multifactorial concept can be applied as an organizational tool in the study of human performance. The five physical fitness factors of cardiorespiratory function, muscular strength, muscle endurance, flexibility, and body composition encompass the physiologic bases of human performance.

The five components have been defined quantitatively and can be measured to reveal differences over time and between individuals. The concept and the measurement tools are applicable to a wide range of ages, abilities, and fitness levels. As we discuss physical fitness, it is essential to remember that the components, although specific, are interdependent. Not only is the overall assessment of physical fitness dependent on the various components, but also the actual and measured level of one component is often dependent on function in another component. For example, poor muscular endurance will not only lessen aerobic capacity, it may hinder attempts to accurately measure the cardiorespiratory component. Body composition, which is the proportion of lean body weight to fat weight, will affect assessment of cardiorespiratory fitness in terms of oxygen consumption. Although we consider the components of physical fitness as discrete areas for purposes of discussion and measurement, the components are interrelated so that a change in one component is often associated with predictable changes in other components. The components of fitness are also capable of adapting to exercise demands (training) or lack of adequate demands (inactivity).

There are three major reasons to use physical fitness as an organizing concept to study human performance.

1. The components of physical fitness and the human performance paradigm share a common outcome measure: the capacity to perform work. The foundation of the human performance paradigm rests on the capacity of the individual to accomplish activities and to sustain effort to complete tasks. In the vocabulary of physical fitness, this concept is termed *physical working capacity (PWC)* or *physical performance capacity*. The definition of physical working capacity is sometimes expressed in the precise terms of the exercise scientist to describe the results of laboratory assessment of **aerobic power.** The object is to determine performance levels. Performance capacity can be expressed either in terms of the aerobic power or maximal oxygen consumption of which the individual is capable, or in terms of the amount of work that the individual can perform.

2. In the context of occupation, work capacity is defined as the ability to accomplish production goals without undue fatigue and with safety for self and coworkers. The energy expenditure or percentage of maximal

power that can be sustained over an eight-hour period is the measure used to describe the level of fitness or work capacity. In addition to the shared outcome measures of the human performance paradigm and physical fitness, there is a wealth of objective, and valid measurement tools that require little or no conversion from their originally intended use as physical fitness measures to be directly applicable in describing physical performance. When choosing from the wide variety of measurement instruments available, it is extremely important to choose the instrument that specifically measures the component of interest, has been validated for your particular application, and that requires a minimal degree of motor skill on the part of the subject.

3. These five physiologic components have the capacity to respond to and adapt to demands, both acute and chronic, imposed by changes in physical activity. It is this ability of the body to respond and adapt that influences, and is influenced by, activity and performance.

COMPONENTS OF PHYSICAL FITNESS

Cardiorespiratory Function

Cardiorespiratory fitness is dependent on the respiratory (lungs) and cardiovascular (heart, blood vessels, and blood components) systems and specific cellular components that help the body use oxygen during exercise (Pollock, Wilmore, & Fox, 1984). The respiratory and cardiovascular systems comprise the oxygen transport system which delivers oxygen to the working muscles and removes chemical waste products. Cellular metabolism within the muscle and liver cells functions to replenish energy supplies required by the working muscles.

Cardiorespiratory fitness can be defined as the ability to take in, transport, and use oxygen. The cardiorespiratory functioning of our bodies is continuous, recognized externally by the signs of a pulse and breathing. When these signs are severely altered or absent, death is imminent.

Our cardiorespiratory functioning is amazingly sensitive and responsive to our needs, even to our anticipation of need. For example, consider pulse, rate of breathing, and blood pressure, all of which are indicators of cardiorespiratory work. At rest in the supine position, one might have a pulse of 60 beats per minute, respiration rate of 12 breaths per minute, and a blood pressure of 100/60 mm Hg. Sitting up puts a slightly greater load on the cardiorespiratory system by using greater muscle activity to support the head and trunk and to overcome the force of gravity on venous return of blood from the abdomen and lower extremities. In the seated position, pulse might increase to 65 beats per minute, breathing rate to 14 breaths per minute, and blood pressure to 110/60 mm Hg. As one stands up, there is even more increased demand to supply oxygen to a greater number of recruited muscle fibers and to counteract a greater effect of gravity on venous return. Now one might have a pulse of 70 beats per minute, breathing rate of 16, and a blood pressure of 120/80 mm Hg. The gradual increase in these vital signs indicates the increasing amount of work being performed by one's cardiorespiratory system.

Stepping on a motor-driven treadmill, climbing onto a bicycle ergometer, or engaging in a progressive lifting task where one experiences a gradual increase in workloads will result in pronounced increases in heart rate, breathing, and blood pressure as the work becomes harder and longer until one reaches maximal capacity. At this point, a person's ability to respond reaches a plateau, and increasing workloads will not elicit increased responses. If demand continues at this intensity, one will soon reach the point of exhaustion and will have to stop or collapse.

Pulmonary Factors. Pulmonary factors such as lung volume, vital capacity, breathing rate, and pulmonary ventilation do not limit physical activity unless the person has significant respiratory disease or is at a high altitude. Even during intense exercise, ventilation is only about 60 to 85 percent of a healthy person's maximum capacity for breathing. Under most conditions the arterial blood leaving the heart is 97 percent saturated with oxygen. Therefore, in the absence of respiratory disease, most of the limitation to endurance performance depends not on our ability to inspire and diffuse oxygen into the blood, but on the ability of the heart and circulatory system to deliver oxygen, and cellular mechanisms to use the oxygen for energy production. Respiratory impairment can limit cardiorespiratory fitness both directly and indirectly. Cardiorespiratory fitness is affected directly by inadequate pulmonary ventilation in which the amount of oxygen in the blood does not meet the increased cellular needs of exercising muscles. Respiratory impairment indirectly affects cardiorespiratory fitness by the increased energy required to breathe. In respiratory disease, breathing itself may become exhaustive work and the oxygen supply may be greatly reduced to the nonrespiratory muscles, resulting in diminished performance (McArdle, Katch, & Katch, 1986). Studies investigating the effect of endurance or aerobic exercise training on people with chronic obstructive pulmonary disease (COPD) show that endurance can be improved by participation in an endurance training exercise program. However, studies to date have shown no significant improvement in pulmonary

function to explain this increase in endurance performance (Atkins, Kaplan, Timms, et al., 1984).

Cardiovascular Factors. The cardiovascular system is made up of the following components:

1) the heart, which provides the force for blood flow and maintains circulation;
2) the arterial system, which conducts oxygen-rich blood to tissues, regulates blood flow, and maintains pressure through the vascular circuit;
3) the capillaries, which provide the medium for exchange between the blood and tissues; and
4) the veins, which return blood to the heart and serve as an active blood reservoir.

The amount of blood that the heart pumps in a minute is the *cardiac output* and is measured in milliliters per minute (ml/min). Cardiac output is the primary indicator of the ability of the heart to meet the demands of physical activity. Cardiac output is a product of the *heart rate* (beats per minute) and *stroke volume* (milliliters of blood ejected with each stroke).

The heart responds to a demand for increased blood flow with greater cardiac output by increasing both heart rate and stroke volume. The aerobically trained and conditioned heart muscle will produce a greater cardiac output at the same heart rate as an untrained heart by virtue of a greater stroke volume. This means that the conditioned heart can produce greater cardiac output at a lower heart rate than the untrained heart. Less work, by virtue of a lower heart rate, results in lowered oxygen demand by the heart muscle itself and longer periods of relaxation (*diastole*) in which the ventricles can fill. Longer filling time favors increased stroke volume.

Stroke volume will change with body position and is greatest in the prone or supine position. In this position, it changes very little with increasing physical exertion, but in the upright position, the return flow of blood to the heart is resisted by the force of gravity and stroke volume decreases. Increasing exertion in the upright position will eventually result in stroke volume that approaches that of the horizontal position.

Negative Effects on Cardiovascular Function. The presence of coronary disease and/or deconditioning affect the ability of a person to be physically active because of compromised blood flow, and therefore limited oxygen supply to the heart muscle. This reduces cardiac output, and therefore limits blood flow and oxygen to the working skeletal muscle. Insufficient blood flow to support the needs of the contracting heart muscle may result in *exertional angina*, experienced as severe chest pain.

Insufficient activity for prolonged periods causes a

deconditioning effect on cardiac function and can result in higher resting heart rates, less capacity to increase stroke volume (as part of increased cardiac output), decreased maximal cardiac output, and decreased heart muscle mass and contractility. Prolonged periods of inactivity affect the heart through all of the cardiac regulatory channels: neural, hormonal, and intrinsic. *Atherosclerosis* further diminishes the functional capacity of the vascular system to transport blood.

The terms cardiovascular and cardiorespiratory are often used interchangeably. Strictly speaking, the term cardiovascular excludes the pulmonary function and the components of cellular metabolism but the term cardiorespiratory encompasses all of them. The two terms are considered synonymous in popular usage.

Another term that often appears in the vocabulary of physical fitness is aerobic. We hear of aerobic fitness, aerobic training, and aerobic endurance. Aerobic means "with oxygen." Aerobic fitness can also refer to the cardiovascular fitness component, but really describes the processes involved rather than the structures involved. Regardless of whether or not one considers the capacity of working muscle to use oxygen in the replenishment of energy supplies (*aerobic metabolism*) as part of the cardiovascular component or the muscle endurance component, it is an important factor in physical fitness.

Cardiorespiratory Response to Sudden Increases of Activity. The magnitude of cardiorespiratory response to a period of exercise is closely related to the intensity and duration of the exercise. Just before beginning exercise there is an anticipatory rise in both heart rate and respiration. As exercise progresses, heart rate, cardiac output, and respiration rise until they reach a plateau. If the exercise intensity is light to moderate, this plateau occurs when ventilation and heart rate are sufficient to meet the needs produced by the exertion. If the exercise is strenuous, the plateau is at the point of exhaustion when the individual reaches a maximal capacity and no further increase is physically possible. The greatest increases in stroke volume occur in the transition from rest to moderate exercise. For a physically trained person, stroke volume can increase 50 to 60 percent above resting values, and cardiac output can increase five to eight times over what it is at rest. In the untrained person, the major increase in cardiac output is produced by an increase in heart rate, with little increase in stroke volume, and therefore maximal cardiac output is limited.

Even at rest, the trained person will have greater stroke volume than the untrained person. Because resting cardiac output is relatively unchanged by training, the consequence is that the trained heart can beat more slowly to sustain the resting cardiac output. After the exercise bout is over, cardiorespiratory signs gradually return to pre-exercise levels. It is felt that training results in a more rapid return to resting levels; however, the reasons for this do not all lie within the cardiorespiratory system itself.

Cardiorespiratory Fitness. Although definitions for cardiorespiratory fitness can be quite specific and therefore quite varied, there is general agreement in exercise literature that cardiorespiratory fitness is the ability of the individual to perform large muscle or whole body activities continuously at a submaximal level of intensity for a sustained period of time. Cardiorespiratory fitness is assessed by how well one responds to prolonged and increasing work loads. It is dependent on the individual's capacity to take in, transport, and utilize oxygen. The level of cardiorespiratory fitness is assessed by monitoring heart rate, blood pressure, and cardiac function, and sometimes by direct measurement of oxygen consumption while the person is performing known and progressively strenuous workloads. The most common methods of measuring this work (**ergometry**) used in cardiorespiratory fitness testing are the motor-driven treadmill and bicycle ergometer. Other methods that also allow monitoring of both response and workload are step tests and arm crank ergometry.

Oxygen consumption is the difference between the rate at which inspired oxygen enters the lungs and the rate at which expired oxygen leaves the lungs. The most common measurement used to indicate cardiorespiratory fitness is maximal oxygen consumption (VO_2max). VO_2max is the greatest amount of oxygen that the individual can use in a given amount of time. The better the cardiorespiratory fitness, the higher the maximal oxygen consumption. VO_2max can be expressed in absolute terms of milliliters of oxygen per minute (ml/min), or in relative terms of milliliters of oxygen consumed per kilogram of body weight per minute (ml/kg/min). By relating oxygen consumption to body size, we are able to compare fitness levels of individuals of different sizes.

In general, men tend to have higher VO_2max than women, even after correcting for body weight. However, when oxygen consumption per kilogram of lean body mass is calculated, the sex differences become much smaller. Oxygen consumption can be measured directly in an appropriately equipped exercise laboratory or can be estimated from measures of heart rate at known submaximal workloads. Other terms synonymous with maximal oxygen consumption are maximal oxygen uptake, maximal oxygen intake, and maximal aerobic power. Although VO_2max is considered to be the gold standard in assessment of cardiorespiratory fitness, there are other indices that are also used.

Measuring Energy Expenditure: MET

MET (metabolic equivalent) is an expression of energy cost relative to the resting energy expenditure. Resting energy expenditure, considered to be approximately the same for all persons, is set at 3.5 ml of oxygen consumption per kilogram of body weight per minute. Therefore, one MET is oxygen consumption at rest and is considered to be 3.5 ml/kg/min. An energy expenditure of 5 METs is equal to oxygen consumption of 17.5 ml/kg/min ($5 \times 3.5 = 17.5$). The rate of energy expenditure or oxygen consumption for an activity that requires 5 METs is 5 times that required to support the energy needs of the person at rest.

Individual differences in resting oxygen consumption and in energy expenditure for actual performance, limits the usefulness of METs as a method for comparing actual energy expenditure between individuals. METs are primarily useful as a technique for assessing the relative rates of energy expenditure between activities. Therefore, METs can be a general guide to exercise intensity and energy expenditure. The greater the METs, the more intense the activity and greater the energy expenditure required to support the activity. Excitement, anxiety, obesity, and poor economy of effort may produce excessive metabolic increases so that METs expended during the performance of an activity may be greater than expected.

Initial fitness levels and health status determine the intensity and duration of the work that a person is asked to perform in the cardiorespiratory assessment. For example, a conditioned long-distance runner who wants to assess the effects of a three-month intensive training program might start with treadmill running at a speed of five miles per hour and increase the slope and speed every one or two minutes until exhaustion. A 75-year-old man who had a myocardial infarction four weeks prior and is now ready to be discharged to home would be assessed by the cardiac rehabilitation team using a low-level exercise test that could start at two miles per hour with no slope and gradually increase slope by 3.5 percent every two minutes with no increase in speed. Both procedures are assessing cardiorespiratory function.

Principles of Exercise to Improve Cardiorespiratory Fitness. The following six principles should be used to guide activity programs aimed at improving cardiorespiratory fitness:

1. The physical activity should require rhythmic, dynamic contractions of large muscle groups.
2. The intensity, duration, and frequency of the activity program should be based on current cardiovascular status and should be gradually progressive.
3. The activity should impose a demand on the cardiovascular system above accustomed levels. For a person who is markedly under-conditioned, any regular program of activity that moderately elevates heart rate and breathing above resting levels for at least five to ten minutes will lead to some aerobic endurance benefits. For a person who already has good cardiovascular endurance, the exercise must be more intense to provide the overload stimulus necessary to produce improvement. Activity so intense that it interferes with the ability to carry on a normal conversation is unnecessarily intense, increasing the risk of injury without concomitant training benefit.
4. The activity should be begun gradually with adequate warm-up to prepare the heart for an increased workload.
5. An exercise heart rate range should be individually established based on age, medical status, and current activity level. A heart rate beyond which a given individual should not exceed should be set and steadfastly observed.
6. Activities that require excessive upper-extremity exercise, particularly with arms elevated above chest height, or intense, sustained isometric contractions tend to elevate blood pressures but produce no training effects for improved cardiovascular (aerobic) endurance. Heavy resistance weight training programs or aerobic routines that rely on arm movements above the head are not appropriate methods to improve cardiovascular endurance. If elevated blood pressure is a risk factor, such activities can be dangerous.

Clinical Implications of Cardiorespiratory Fitness. It is appropriate to emphasize the importance of at least a two-minute warm-up preceding any strenuous activity. The objective of this warm-up is to gradually increase the blood flow to the heart muscle so that there will be sufficient oxygen available to support the demands made on the heart by the strenuous activity. Studies have shown that undertaking strenuous exercise without prior warm-up can result in abnormal heart function. These abnormalities were nearly all abolished when a two-minute warm-up was added (Lamb 1984).

Consideration of all of the above principles can help to build a therapeutic intervention with attention to an aerobic endurance component. To design and implement a true cardiovascular conditioning program requires that the therapist be involved in a comprehensive evaluation of the client's medical history and cardiac risk status in cooperation with a physician and exercise specialist. This evaluation usually includes an exercise stress test with electrocardiogram. It serves as the basis for writing an individualized exercise prescription containing detailed guidelines for exercise intensity, duration, and frequency, and monitoring the client's progress.

[handwritten: Exercise Program 3-4× wk for 30-40 min./session]

Most experts agree that the best exercise program with the least risk for improving cardiovascular function of a sedentary adult should include exercise performed at a frequency of three to four days a week, progressing to a duration of 30 to 40 minutes each session, and performed at an intensity that elevates the heart rate to 60 percent to 80 percent of maximal heart rate. The exercise prescription should include instructions for warm-up and cool-down activities as well as the aerobic conditioning segment. It should also detail the method of self-monitoring by the client and the level of supervision required, if any, by trained staff.

Increasing numbers of therapists are becoming involved in hospital- and community-based cardiac rehabilitation programs and are learning the specifics of exercise testing, prescription, and monitoring. General fitness programs for the healthy public should also be based on the principles of the exercise prescription. A diversity of assessment methods may be used to field test cardiovascular fitness in this population before participation in an exercise program, such as heart rate and distance covered in a 6 or 12 minute walk/jog or heart rate and time to walk a mile.

Muscle Strength

Muscle strength is the amount of force that can be exerted by one or a group of muscles in a single voluntary contraction. Strength can be developed and measured in several ways. In general, we speak of either **static strength**, developed in an isometric contraction or **dynamic strength**, developed in an isotonic or isokinetic contraction. In terms of functional performance, there is relatively little association between static and dynamic strength. Training to improve static strength will not show comparable gains in dynamic strength of the same muscle.

[handwritten: MET (Measuring Energy Expenditure)]

Table 8-1
Metabolic Equivalents for Work and Leisure Activities*

WORK/SELF MAINTENANCE		PLAY/LEISURE		WORK/SELF MAINTENANCE		PLAY/LEISURE
1½ METs	Desk work	Walking (1 mph) standing, playing cards, driving car, sewing, knitting	6-7 METs	Shoveling (10 lbs)		Walking (5 mph) bicycling (11 mph) tennis singles square dancing (folk) water skiing
2-3 METs	Auto repair Radio, TV repair Janitorial work Bartending	Walking (2 mph) billiards, bowling golf (power cart) fishing (on bank) playing piano shuffleboard level bicycling (5 mph)	7-8 METs	Carrying (80 lbs) Digging ditches Heavy carpentry		Jogging (5 mph) bicycling (12 mph) basketball (social) touch football downhill skiing ice hockey
3-4 METs	Bricklaying Machine assembly Wheelbarrow (100 lbs) Cleaning windows Lawn mowing (power)	Walking (3 mph) horseshoe pitching golf (pulling bag cart) bicycling (6 mph) archery fly fishing (standing)	8-9 METs	Shoveling (14 lbs)		Running (5½ mph) bicycling (13 mph) handball (social) jump rope (60-80 skips/min) fencing
4-5 METs	Painting Light carpentry Paper-hanging raking leaves bicycling (8 mph) Hoeing	Walking (3½ mph) table tennis golf (carry bag) tennis (doubles) ballroom dancing	10 METs	Shoveling (16 lbs)		Running (6 mph)
5-6 METs	Digging garden Light shoveling	Walking (4 mph) bicycling (10 mph) skating (recreational) badminton fishing (in waders)	13½ METs	Climbing stairs with 25 pound load		Handball (competitive) jump rope (120/min) skiing, cross country (at >5 mph)

* 1 MET = 3.5 ml O_2/kg/min = 1.25 kcal/min for 70 kg person

[handwritten notes at top of page:]
Isometric (p.853) contraction in which there is no joint movement & minimal change in muscle length (ie pinch, lock jaw, carrying a heavy package)

STATIC vs DYNAMIC = Isotonic / Isokinetic

Isometric strength is also specific to the joint angle at which the strength training was done.

The force exerted in a voluntary contraction depends on a number of factors: 1) recruitment of muscle fibers and their contractile state, 2) mechanical advantage of the lever system, 3) neuromuscular mechanisms, and 4) motivation. For the most part, muscle size and strength are closely associated. The larger (cross-sectional area) muscle is generally the stronger one, but not necessarily the most successful in performance when factors of speed, power, coordination, or endurance are required. The growth in the cross-sectional area of a muscle is due primarily to an increase in muscle fiber size (*hypertrophy*), rather than an increase in the actual number of fibers (*hyperplasia*). Current research indicates that the larger, fast-twitch muscle fibers that have a greater capacity to develop tension show a more pronounced hypertrophy in response to strength training than do the slow-twitch fibers. Adaptations in slow-twitch fibers occur primarily in response to muscle endurance training. These adaptations are concerned with changes in enzymatic content of the slow-twitch fibers rather than increased fiber size.

Isometric Strength. In isometric activities, there is little or no joint motion as the muscle exerts the necessary force to accomplish the task, such as when sustaining a pinch, carrying a heavy package in your arms, or clenching your jaw. There are also isometric phases of most muscular activity. Isometric strength can be expressed in terms of muscle tension as a percentage of the maximum voluntary contraction (MVC) exerted under static conditions. At 15 to 20 percent MVC the contraction can be maintained for a considerable period of time. Tensions above that level are fatiguing and maximum contraction can be maintained for only a few seconds to a few minutes. Maintaining a high intensity isometric contraction for more than a few seconds becomes an anaerobic activity. Because the blood vessels supplying oxygen to the working muscle are occluded by intense contraction, aerobic metabolism becomes impossible.

Dynamic strength measurements are more related to performance in sport and work than are isometric measurements. Isometric strength, however, is important in considerations of posture and balance.

Isotonic Strength. Isotonic strength is defined as the maximum weight that can be lifted at one time. Isotonic contractions may result from force generated as the muscle shortens (concentric) or from force exerted as the muscle lengthens (eccentric). Measurement of the concentric contraction is really a measure of strength at the hardest part of the lift, and this may be at the beginning or the end of the

range, depending on the muscle lever system and the length-tension ratio. Activities of daily life are accomplished by varying combinations of isometric and isotonic work. *ADL*

Response Mechanisms. Muscle strength is influenced primarily by changes in the amount of contractile proteins (actin and myosin) in fast-twitch fibers. It is the increase in the amount of protein filaments and cross bridges that produces increased muscle cross-sectional areas (hypertrophy) and stronger muscles.

Muscle Protein (Actin & Myosin)

Clinical Implications of Muscle Strength. Good nutrition with adequate caloric intake and an adequate protein composition is essential for an effective muscle-strengthening program. The body will preferentially use dietary protein for maintenance and repair requirements. Only after these requirements are met will synthesis of contractile proteins be allowed. This nutritional situation needs particular attention for some older, chronically-ill or institutionalized clients who tend to have low protein intake. The most effective strengthening program will strengthen the muscle(s) in the same manner that the strength will be used. The most efficacious strengthening programs are based on functional requirements for type of contraction, speed of contraction, and joint angle.

Principles of Exercise to Improve Muscle Strength. There are principles that apply to strength training in general and more specific techniques that apply to a particular type of strengthening. They are derived from research based on testing the theories of overload and specificity of training. For the most part, this research has been done on healthy, generally young, subjects with unimpaired musculoskeletal systems. It is believed that adherence to these principles will produce maximal strength gains in normal, healthy people. Application of these principles in the rehabilitation setting requires consideration of many additional factors including muscular and neural pathology.

Principles underlying muscle strength training include the following:

1. Greatest strength gains are achieved by performing a regular program of overload at maximal or near-maximal resistance. The load must be progressively increased to keep pace with strength gains and to continue to provide an overload stimulus. High-resistance, low-repetition exercise regimes are considered to be the most effective for producing strength gains.
2. Apply the overload to the specific muscle groups or movements that are to be strengthened.

3. To avoid early-onset fatigue in small muscle groups, start exercising large muscle groups before smaller ones.

4. Maximum strength gains are made when the muscle is overloaded at the same length (static) or at the same velocity (dynamic) in training as in testing or actual performance.

5. The rate of strength gain is greatest when the muscle is weakest in relation to maximal potential strength.

6. Allow adequate recovery between individual exercise sessions and between exercise bouts. Fatigued muscles are not able to respond and adapt to overload stress as well as muscles that have recovered from previous exercise. Frequency of strength training is often prescribed for every other day rather than daily to allow the muscle time to recover. Many exercise physiologists feel that training adaptations actually occur during the recovery period as the muscle fibers are repairing the microinjuries caused by the resistance overload.

Suggested Techniques for Static Strengthening (Lamb, 1984). *Isometric & Negatives*

1. Isometric exercise should be practiced at several different joint angles because the training effect tends to occur mostly at the angle selected for training.

2. Each training contraction should be a ''maximal'' voluntary contraction.

3. Optimal training effect is achieved by holding each contraction for two to five seconds. Holding the contraction longer than this increases the possibility of experiencing pain and stiffness after the exercise and produces no additional training.

4. The ''maximal'' isometric contraction should be repeated one to five times during each exercise session with two to three minutes rest between each contraction. Isometric strength training produces the most rapid results with daily exercise sessions, if there is no undue soreness.

5. Strength gains of isometric training can be maintained with one exercise training session per week.

6. Isometric contractions produce an extreme rise in both diastolic and systolic blood pressure if held for more than one or two seconds and should be avoided by people with cardiovascular disease.

Suggested Techniques For Dynamic Strengthening (Lamb, 1984).

1. During each exercise session, three or four sets of each exercise should be performed with the heaviest weight that can be correctly lifted one to six times during each set. The amount of weight is called a *repetition maximum* ~~1 to 6~~ (R.M.). The amount of weight decreases progressively from one R.M. to six R.M.'s. Research suggests that a few repetitions (no more than six) with near maximal resistance produce the greatest strength gains. For a person who is just beginning a weight training program, it is safest to begin lifting weight at 12 R.M. and gradually increase the amount to a range of one to six R.M.

2. During the exercise session allow five to ten minutes for recovery between sets of the same exercise. Frequency of training sessions should be at least three and no more than four times a week.

3. Strengthening of muscles responsible for a complex movement should be accomplished with exercises designed to incorporate or imitate that movement. Strengthening contractions should be done through the full range of motion.

4. Isotonic strength gains can be maintained with two exercise sessions per week. Isokinetic strengthening techniques rely on specialized equipment that is capable of producing variable resistance throughout the range of motion. Isokinetic training assures a constant activation of muscle fibers throughout the range of motion by matching resistance to available muscular force. There is a variety of isokinetic equipment with different methods of producing the isokinetic effect. The isokinetic training program will be determined by the equipment being used, training goals, and the abilities and needs of the trainee. The general principles of strengthening apply to isokinetic training. Special attention should be paid to the velocity of training contractions. For improvement of strength in a complex movement, the velocity of training contractions should be as close as possible to the velocity of contractions used in the functional, unloaded motion.

Muscle Endurance

Given the strength needed to perform an activity, additional improvement in performance depends on muscle endurance. Endurance means the ability to persist. Muscular endurance is defined and measured as the repetition of submaximal contractions (isotonic) or submaximal holding time (isometric). The use of the term muscular endurance should not be confused with cardiovascular endurance. It is possible to develop considerable endurance in a small muscle, such as a finger flexor, without having any noticeable effect on cardiovascular endurance (Sharkey, 1984). The oxygen required for a small muscle mass to sustain activity over an extended period of time can be satisfied without noticeably stressing the cardiovascular system much above resting levels. Thus most people can type, do needlework, or play the guitar without raising their respiration, heart rate, blood pressure, or oxygen consumption above their usual sedentary levels. The active muscles have the endurance to persist to accomplish the activities without imposing a stress on cardiovascular performance. When there is a greater demand for larger muscle mass to perform an activity, for example, the repetitive contraction of the quadriceps required to pedal a bicycle, the magnitude of the oxygen requirement to sustain muscular activity increases dramatically. Also this more strenuous activity involving large muscles requires the work of the cardiorespiratory system to activate and sustain increased circulation to the active muscles. When the size of the active muscle mass produces an increased demand for oxygen to sustain activity, and/or when the intensity of the muscular work produces an increased oxygen demand, then cardiorespiratory endurance and muscular endurance become interrelated. For example, a total-body activity of relatively low level of intensity, such as walking at a natural pace, will require certain levels of both cardiorespiratory and muscular endurance to sustain the activity for more than a few minutes. If the intensity increases from walking to jogging, increased demands are made on both the active muscles, to sustain the rhythmic activity, and the cardiorespiratory system, to maintain the increased circulation. The muscle mass/exercise intensity relationship is demonstrated well by the differences in energy expenditure between bicycle and arm ergometry. The smaller muscle mass of the upper extremities engaged in arm ergometry requires less oxygen per unit of time than a comparable effort on the bicycle ergometer powered by the considerably greater muscle mass of the lower extremities.

Response Mechanisms. Muscular endurance is influenced primarily by slow-twitch (oxidative) muscle fibers, and their mitochondrial material and oxidative enzymes. An increase in mitochondrial material and associated oxidative enzymes is related to improved muscular endurance for dynamic work.

Clinical Implications of Muscle Endurance. Specific muscular endurance may be improved by low-intensity, repetitive exercise localized to a specific muscle group or groups. Consequently, it is possible to increase muscular endurance for low-intensity activities such as walking, eating, and a variety of seated and bed activities while imposing little stress on the cardiorespiratory system.

Principles of Exercise to Improve Muscle Endurance. Whereas muscle strength is measured as the maximum amount of force that a muscle can exert in a single contrac-

tion, muscle endurance depends on the capacity of a muscle to repeatedly perform submaximal contractions. Muscular endurance is measured by the number of repetitions that can be performed or the period for which activity can be sustained. Cardiovascular endurance is improved by whole-body activities that stress the oxygen delivery system, but muscle endurance is only improved by local, muscular activity that stresses the capacity of the muscle to use oxygen and produce energy. When a person jogs or cycles to improve cardiovascular endurance, muscle endurance of the active lower-extremity muscles will probably improve as well. However, there will not be an improvement in muscle endurance in the upper extremities without specific activities included to produce local, adaptive changes.

Muscular endurance is related to muscular strength. Adequate strength must precede endurance training and adequate strength improves endurance. Endurance increases when a muscle group is able to work at a smaller percentage of maximal capacity. This occurs when either the muscle becomes stronger or the amount of force required to perform the motion decreases. If a person's muscular strength is deficient it may require a near maximal effort for that person to lift hand to mouth. Such a person would not be able to repeat this motion in a given amount of time as often as a person who performs this motion with normal strength and minimum effort.

If muscular strength is constant, endurance decreases as the intensity of effort required to produce the movement increases. For example, level running at six miles an hour can be sustained for a much longer time than level running at ten miles an hour or running up a grade. Thus, when we talk about muscle endurance we must also consider the muscular strength and intensity of effort relevant to the activity being performed.

The following is a summary of principles related to improving muscle endurance:

1. The overload (resistance) principle applies to training for muscle endurance as well as to strength training. Although more repetitions are required in endurance training, some overload is necessary for improvement to occur.
2. Appropriate overload for endurance training will generally produce improvements in both muscle strength and endurance.
3. Overload should be gauged so that the individual can perform at least 20 full-range repetitions of the motion and/or be able to sustain the activity for at least 30 seconds. If adding external resistance is not possible, overload can be achieved by gradual increases in the speed of the motion. If both strength and endurance are low, initial training may need to progress only by increasing the number of repetitions.

4. Constant attention to balancing resistance and repetitions in the exercise program is the key to achieving optimal improvement. Although ''low resistance, high repetition'' is the popular slogan for endurance training, too little resistance produces limited improvement.

5. In the absence of limiting factors, endurance training should occur three to five times per week and include two to three sets of 20 repetitions each while maintaining appropriate overload. Most of the literature from exercise physiology deals with muscular training in terms of weight loads. However, the same principles can be applied to training programs that use activities of daily living, work-related tasks, or recreational activities. In the rehabilitation setting it is possible to use these principles by adjusting the number of repetitions, speed of performance, frequency and duration of training sessions, and/or the application of external resistance.

Evaluation of Muscle Strength and Endurance. In clinical practice a test of muscle strength is often used in an evaluation of functional level. Because function depends to a great extent on the ability to sustain activity for a desired period of time, it would add much to the usefulness of the evaluation if an assessment of muscle endurance was included at a level of effort comparable to that required for the performance of the functions in question. Adequate dynamic strength of the deltoid, shoulder external rotators, and scapular stabilizers is required to move the upper extremity into a position necessary to brush teeth or comb hair. Adequate static strength is necessary to maintain the position momentarily. Endurance, both dynamic and static, must also be adequate for the task to be accomplished.

Flexibility

In keeping with our organizational framework, we will examine flexibility as one of the components of health-related physical fitness. In this context, we will not consider limitations in flexibility due to disease or trauma. In the therapeutic setting, many of the limitations in range of motion stem from pathological changes, and treatment requires specific knowledge of etiology, prognosis, and therapeutics. But for the purposes of our discussion here, we will confine our discussion of flexibility to the realm of general fitness, exploring ideas that may sometimes be overlooked in the therapeutic intervention.

Flexibility is the component of physical fitness that describes the range of motion of a joint or sequence of joints. Flexibility is determined by the following factors: 1) the elasticity of soft tissues surrounding the joint (skin, muscle, and periarticular connective tissue); 2) conditions within the joint that may restrict motion, such as bony deformity, malalignment, or inflammation; and 3) excessive body fat or muscle mass that can be an external obstruction limiting range of motion. The presence of pain, both acute and chronic, can also restrict flexibility. Even in the absence of disease-related restrictions of flexibility, range of motion varies with age, occupation, sex, and activity levels. It is difficult to establish norms.

Tables of normal range of motion are widely used in clinical assessment even though there is disparity among published normal values. The following are values that are widely accepted (Luttgens and Wells, 1982).

Normal Flexibility Values

hip flexion = 100 to 120 degrees
knee flexion = 120 to 145 degrees
shoulder flexion = 130 to 180 degrees

These normative tables seldom describe how the measurement was made, from what population the values were taken, nor the standard deviations for the mean values. Without this information normative data should only be applied in the broadest of terms. The current use of radiologic and electronic technology may be helpful in gaining a clearer picture of ideal values and adequate ranges of joint motion.

Static Flexibility and Dynamic Flexibility. There are two important concepts relating to joint motion within the domain of flexibility; one is **static flexibility** and the other is **dynamic flexibility**. Static or extent flexibility refers to the actual range of motion that a joint will allow. This is commonly referred to as joint range of motion. Clinically, we measure static flexibility with a **goniometer** and describe the magnitude of the motion in degrees. Measurement of static flexibility may be achieved by either active or passive motion of the body segments surrounding the joint. Dynamic flexibility refers to the ease of movement rather than the amount of movement produced by joint motion. Dynamic flexibility can be defined and measured as the amount of resistance of a joint to movement or the ability of a joint to make rapid and repeated flexing movements (Winnick & Short, 1985). Although dynamic flexibility is not commonly measured in a clinical setting, the ease or ''looseness'' of movement can be an important evaluation to make in assessing the functional consequences of impaired flexibility. In research settings, dynamic flexibility has been measured with *arthrography* (Byers, 1985) to determine the amount of resistance to passive motion of a joint. Another method is to simply count the number of repetitions of active joint motion that can be accomplished within a given time period. Both of these methods are subject to error introduced by active resistance to motion or by limitations in muscle strength and endurance.

Active, static stretching (preferred

Assessing Flexibility. What is adequate flexibility? Our definition of physical fitness as the capacity to successfully meet the present and potential physical challenges of life provides us with a framework for defining adequate flexibility. Assessing flexibility strictly in terms of the client's present needs is rather straightforward. For example, one might need to determine how much shoulder flexion is required to reach an upper cabinet or how much knee and hip flexion is necessary to descend stairs. Or one might need to determine how much cervical rotation is needed to provide a safe field of vision for a person driving in reverse or merging into freeway traffic.

It is evident that flexibility required to perform most tasks of daily living does not make use of the full potential range available. Flexibility assessment should not be limited to merely meeting clients' present requirements but should consider meeting potential physical challenges if the joint must move beyond its present range. Injuries occur when motion is forced beyond the existing range, so adequate flexibility must include range above that normally required. Currently, to evaluate flexibility deficits and to determine reasonable expectations of flexibility, we must continue to rely on judicious interpretation of the existing normative tables and on the tried and true assessment of bilateral range of motion.

The rehabilitation process usually contains specific objectives and therapeutic exercise regimens designed to improve or maintain range of motion in the presence of disease or trauma. The goal of flexibility is achieved by applying various techniques, some of which may be specifically addressed to the underlying causes of the flexibility deficit, such as upper motor neuron lesion spasticity, the rigidity of Parkinson's disease, paralysis from peripheral nerve damage, or decreased flexibility associated with rheumatological conditions. Therapeutic stretching techniques, based on Golgi body tendon functioning and reciprocal innervation, are typically employed when the restricted motion is associated with neuromuscular and contractile elements of the muscle.

In this discussion of flexibility, we will focus on the principles of achieving adequate flexibility of muscle and periarticular connective tissue in relation to the extensibility inherent in these structures, rather than therapeutic exercise regimens for specific diseases. In order to increase static or extent flexibility, exercise techniques are based on gradually producing minor distensions in connective tissue. The summation of these minor changes can produce major changes in overall extensibility of the periarticular structures and can result in gains in range of motion.

Passive Stretching versus Active Stretching. The techniques employed to increase flexibility are classified in two ways, either by the source of the force producing the movement or stretch, or by the characteristic of the applied stretch which is either constant or rebounding. *Passive stretching* is that which is applied externally by either another person or gravity and *active stretching* is when the movement occurs from one's own internal muscular force. *Static stretching* is holding the lengthened or stretched position without movement, while *ballistic stretching* is bouncing or repeated rhythmic movements intended to produce a rebound stretch at the outer limits of the range.

Current thought in both medical and sports literature appears to favor active, static stretching techniques. This active, static stretching has been found to be more beneficial because of less risk of overstretching and injury, less post-exercise soreness, less energy consumed, and less opposing muscle activity to impede optimal stretching (Luttgens & Wells, 1982).

Active, static stretching includes active movement to the outer limit of the current range, active effort to stretch slightly past this point, and holding the lengthened position from 6 to twelve seconds. The exercise should be repeated several times a day. The decision as to how far to stretch beyond current range must be an individual one. Some maintain that the stretch should not exceed 10 percent of the normal range. Others assert to stretch just to the point of increased tension. Stretching that produces increased pain is probably counterproductive in most cases.

Flexibility can be overdone. Flexibility is excessive when it overcomes the natural supportive function of the periarticular connective tissue and surrounding muscle. Excessive flexibility (*hypermobility*) results in joint instability and increased risk of strain and injury. The protective supporting role of periarticular connective tissue and muscle is particularly important for weight-bearing joints that are subjected to repeated stress in the course of normal daily activities.

Response Mechanisms. The property of extensibility lies in the structure of dense, ordinary, periarticular connective tissue that includes ligaments, tendons, synovial membrane, fasciae, and fibrous joint capsules. Extensibility or the ability of tissue to stretch is based upon the two main components, fibroblast cells and the extracellular matrix made of collagen and elastin fibers and the ground substance. Extensibility of connective tissue depends partially on adequate hydration because water makes up 60 to 70 percent of total connective tissue content. Maintenance of a critical distance between the fibers that assures free gliding of fibers and possibly preventing excessive cross-linking between fibers; and normal fibril orientation during fiber synthesis. These mechanisms are absolutely dependent on the movement of the connective tissue to maintain or increase extensibility (Donatelli & Owens-Burkhart, 1981).

Extensibility or ability of tissue to stretch

Clinical Implications of Flexibility. In both the clinic and the gym, range of motion or flexibility exercises are typically performed before more vigorous exercises aimed at improving muscular or cardiorespiratory fitness. The rationale for this is to provide a cardiorespiratory and muscular warm-up period. As we mentioned previously, preparing the heart for an increased workload is necessary for safety. Warmed-up muscles and connective tissue are more extensible and less susceptible to strain and injury. Therefore, the traditional stretching and mild active exercise routine designed to ease one into more vigorous exercise has become standard practice.

There is now evidence to support the benefits of an exercise regimen that includes active, static stretching both before and after the more vigorous portion of the routine. Active static stretching performed after vigorous exercise on the muscle groups involved in the aerobic or strengthening routines seems to measurably decrease postexercise muscle soreness. For most people, decreased discomfort tends to favor a return to more exercise. If increased flexibility is one of the primary objectives of a rehabilitation program, when designing interventions therapists should remember extensibility is greater when the tissues are warm. By performing flexibility exercises (active or passive) after a period of more vigorous, heat-producing activity, we can maximize joint range and minimize discomfort.

Principles for Improving Flexibility. Some guidelines for improving flexibility are as follows:

1. Static stretching is preferable to ballistic stretching, because static stretching reduces the risk of injury from overstretching, requires less energy, and tends to relieve rather than cause muscle soreness.
2. Increased flexibility is produced by overstretching, yet overstretching should not exceed normal muscle length by more than 10 percent.
3. Static stretch should be held from six to twelve seconds.
4. More repetitions are required to increase flexibility than to maintain it.
5. Flexibility exercises should be performed both before and after endurance and/or strengthening activities.
6. Stretching exercises performed actively make best use of neurophysiologic mechanisms favoring increased flexibility.

Body Composition

Body composition as a component of physical fitness refers to the fat and nonfat elements of the body or to the relative leanness/fatness of the individual. The frequently used height and weight tables can give us some idea of what total body weight should be for people of the same sex,

similar age and frame size. These tables tell us who is overweight or underweight with respect to the general population. However, these tables are not good measures for judging whether the individual has appropriate body fat. For example, consider two men who are both 48 years old and six feet tall. Harry weighs 210 pounds and has spent 25 years as a lumberjack. John weighs 185 pounds and is a computer programmer and enjoys reading, bridge, and cooking as leisure activities. According to the height and weight chart posted at the doctor's office, Harry (the lumberjack) is 25 pounds too heavy and should lose weight. John's weight, on the other hand, appears to be just right at 185 pounds. However, if we measured percentage of body fat for these two men, even though Harry weighs more, he has only 12 percent body fat. This is well below the recommended 15 percent for males. Whereas, John who weighs less, measures at 20 percent body fat, which is considered at the borderline obesity level for men.

Which of these two men is more fat? Harry's extra weight is lean tissue, primarily muscle built up in the course of his habitual and demanding daily exercise; hence he should not be considered as overly fat. In contrast, John who is well within the desired range for body weight, is over the recommended level for body fat. His sedentary lifestyle is probably primarily responsible for this excess body fat; however, other factors such as inherited body type, a preceding illness, or prolonged period of inactivity could be involved.

It is generally accepted that body composition in terms of percent body fat and percent lean weight is a more valid indicator of fitness than total body weight. The total amount of body fat exists as either essential fat or storage fat. Essential fat is needed for normal physiologic functioning and is the fat stored in bone marrow, throughout the nervous system, and in all organs of the body. Without a certain amount of essential fat, body function would deteriorate. In women, essential fat also includes sex-characteristic fat deposits in the breasts, uterus, hips, and thighs.

Storage fat is the fat deposited in the adipose tissue throughout the body and serves as an energy reserve, insulator from cold, and protector of vital organs from physical trauma. Major storage fat deposits are located beneath the skin (subcutaneous fat) and around major organs such as the heart and kidneys. It is storage fat that is most subject to change with alterations in diet and exercise. Approximately 50 percent of body fat is subcutaneous storage fat. Both men and women have a similar recommended percent of storage fat, 12 percent for women and 15 percent for men. There is a much greater difference between the sexes with regard to essential fat which is approximately 3 percent for men and 12 percent for women. To define obesity in terms of body fat, for men the standard

Recommended Total Body Fat Ranges for Adults			
	Athlete	Nonathlete	(Obesity)
Men	4–12%	15–22%	>22%
Women	13–18%	22–32%	>32%

is 20 percent and for women it is 30 percent. For young adults, the desired body fat percent is considered to be 13 to 15 percent for males and 25 percent for females.

Although body composition tables show an increasing percentage of body fat with advancing age, there is no particular reason to believe that this increased percent of body fat is an inevitable consequence of aging. Most exercise physiologists feel that the tendency of people to reduce physical activity with aging is responsible for greater body fat in relation to lean body weight in the older population, and that this trend is neither necessary nor desirable.

The health risk consequences of obesity are well known. But we are finding that being too lean may also have health risks. People with body fat measurements below the essential fat percentages of 3 percent for males and 12 percent for females often exhibit health problems.

In women, adipose tissue is used for estrogen storage. Young women with extremely low body fat, such as those who have undergone strenuous physical training or severe dieting, sometimes experience amenorrhea and osteoporosis. This may be associated with insufficient essential body fat to support the normal physiologic functioning of the menstrual cycle or bone remodeling.

Because it is not possible to directly measure body fat in a living body, we rely on indirect measures and estimates of body fat and lean body weight. The two methods used most often are *hydrostatic weighing* (underwater) and the *skinfold measurement* technique. Hydrostatic weighing, used most often for research purposes, is based on determining body density with underwater weighing and then using existing formulae to convert body density to percent body fat. Hydrostatic weighing requires a laboratory setup and considerable time and motivation from each person to be tested. The skinfold technique, a practical method for body composition screening, can be applied in a wide variety of settings and requires little more than passive cooperation on the part of the subject. By using special calipers, skinfold thickness is measured at specific body sites. The thicker the skinfold, the more subcutaneous fat. Because subcutaneous fat is 50 percent of human body fat, thickness of skinfolds is a valid indicator of total body fat. Both methods require a trained examiner and accurate instruments to produce reliable results.

Response Mechanisms. Body fat (adipose tissue) is composed of many cells containing triglyceride fat molecules. Up to about 16 years of age, a person's total body fat increases by both greater filling of fat cells already present (*hypertrophy*) and by an actual increase in the number of fat cells (*hyperplasia*). After adolescence, fat increases by cell hypertrophy. Fat cell number does not decrease with weight loss, but the size of the cells can be dramatically reduced by diet and exercise. Excessive fat storage occurs when the energy consumed in the diet is greater than the energy expended in daily activities. Obesity is defined as body fat in excess of 20 percent for men and 30 percent for women. By this definition, a person can be obese even when the height and weight charts do not indicate it.

To lose weight, it is necessary to create a negative energy balance between consumption and expenditure. This can be done by restricting food intake, increasing energy expenditure, or by a combination of both. Traditionally we thought that dietary restriction was the most effective way to lose weight. However, current research is showing that for most people a combination of moderate calorie restriction and an increase in mild to moderate aerobic exercise produces the most desirable results. It has been shown repeatedly that the major difference between obese individuals and their non-obese counterparts is the amount of physical activity. In most cases, the non-obese individuals consume at least the same amount of calories as the obese people. These findings have held true for babies, young children, and adults. The benefits of regular exercise for weight control go beyond just the direct burning of calories. Regular exercise has been shown to result in appetite suppression and, in some cases, an actual reduction in food intake by the exercisers.

Weight loss accomplished through exercise is almost entirely due to fat loss with a maintenance or gain in lean tissue. Weight loss through dietary restriction alone produces weight loss that includes a large loss of water and some lean tissue, especially early in the program.

Although the energy used in a single episode of exercise may be relatively small, energy expended through regular exercise has a cumulative effect. For example, 45 minutes of brisk walking can use about 350 kilocalories of energy. Although one session will not materially reduce fat, ten sessions of 350 kilocalories each will result in the loss of approximately one pound of fat with no change in diet. It also appears that weight loss and maintenance is most successful over the long term when regular physical activity becomes a part of the lifestyle. Current recommendations for weight loss generally suggest that half the caloric deficit be achieved through dietary restriction and the other half achieved with increased activity levels.

Clinical Implications: Body Composition. Implications for performance of daily personal, vocational, and leisure activities in relation to body composition are seen at both ends of the spectrum. Having too much fat tissue in relation to lean body weight or too little fat in relation to lean body weight have deleterious consequences. It is important to remember that neither of these two conditions is always apparent from physical appearance even though the condition might be severe enough to result in measurable performance deficits.

Obviously, the most frequently occurring condition is too much body fat. In the rehabilitation setting, we may see people within normal weight ranges, or even underweight, who have a disproportionately high percent body fat in relation to lean tissue. The balance between percent fat and lean tissue is influenced not only by excessive fat storage but also by loss of lean tissue, the primary component of which is skeletal muscle. Lack of muscular activity leads to loss of muscle mass. As little as one to two months of inactivity can result in muscles that have atrophied to one-half normal size. If food consumption is maintained at a level to prevent weight loss, this loss of muscle mass may not be readily apparent. However, the loss will eventually be evident in deficits in muscular strength and endurance and decreased aerobic capacity. If the inactivity is not prolonged, a return to adequate regular exercise can result in a restoration in lean tissue mass, as well as a decrease in fat.

People who have not exercised vigorously for months or even years can increase their lean tissue (muscle) weight through regular, moderate exercise such as brisk walking, bicycling, or water activities. People who are already reasonably fit will not be able to increase muscle mass through the same moderate intensity exercises. People who possess muscle mass adequate to meet current performance demands will need to perform heavy resistance exercise to increase muscle growth.

Although assessment of body composition will probably not become standard clinical practice in most occupational therapy settings, it is important to understand that it is the lean weight/fat weight ratio, not total body weight or appearance, that influences physical fitness and function.

Table 8-2
Physical Fitness Assessment

COMPONENT & DEFINITION	PRIMARY STRUCTURES INVOLVED	ASSESSED BY
Cardiorespiratory Function (ability to take in, transport and use oxygen)	heart vascular system lungs blood components cellular respiration	• oxygen uptake • cardiac output • heart rate • blood pressure
Muscle Strength (l x) (maximum amount of force that can be exerted in one contraction)	Type II muscle fibers myoneural mechanisms muscle energy stores anaerobic enzymes	• isometric strength by make/break test • isotonic strength by 1 repetition maximum
Muscle Endurance (maintenance of activity at submaximal exertion)	Type I muscle fibers systemic energy stores mitochondria oxidative enzymes	• isometric endurance by holding time • isotonic endurance by number of repetitions to fatigue
Flexibility (range and ease of joint movement)	joint structures periarticular tissues	• static/flexibility using goniometry • dynamic flexibility by resistance testing
Body Composition (proportion of fat to lean body mass)	lean body mass body fat (storage & essential fat)	• percentage of body fat using underwater weight or skin fold measurement

Principles for Improving Body Composition. A healthy proportion of lean body weight to body fat is part of good physical fitness. Achieving and maintaining this balance is important because obesity is a risk factor in many diseases and an adequate lean body mass of muscle and bone is essential to support functional activity. In the past, obesity has primarily been treated with dietary restriction to reduce the caloric input. Nutrition experts tell us that there is more to successful obesity treatment than mere calorie reduction, and exercise physiologists tell us that physical activity plays an important role in reducing the percent of body fat in several ways. The following principles summarize important relationships between exercise and body composition:

1. Participation in regular exercise can lead to a reduction in appetite. Several studies have shown that subjects who were physically active actually ate less than sedentary controls.
2. Moderate to vigorous exercise not only increases metabolic rate during the exercise itself, but also tends to elevate the metabolic rate for up to 24 hours following the exercise. An increased metabolic rate results in greater caloric expenditure.
3. Weight loss accomplished through exercise is almost entirely due to fat loss with a maintenance or gain in lean tissue/muscle (Lamb, 1984).
4. Moderately intense exercise such as brisk walking, when sustained for more than 45 minutes, tends to stimulate the metabolism of stored fat (glycogen sparing) for energy to support the activity.
5. An exercise program to increase muscle mass (a muscle strengthening program) is also an effective component in a weight-gain regime. By combining increased calorie consumption with physical activity to increase lean body mass, the most healthful weight gains can be made.

RESPONSES AND ADAPTATIONS

Physiological Stressors

Physiological systems respond to stimulation. Sometimes the stimulus is called a stress. Repeated or continuous stress on a physiologic system frequently leads to adaptations in how the system functions. Within our context of physical fitness, we will consider physical activity as the stimulus or stress on the various components, affecting both immediate responses and long-term adaptations. Physical activity can be an appropriate and positive stressor. This means that the physiologic components respond to the stimulus of physical activity and that physiologic adaptations can occur from repeated activity demands causing increased functional capacity.

Not all stressors are appropriate or positive. Cigarette smoking is a negative physiologic stressor that produces acute responses and long-term adaptations in the respiratory system. However, these changes have a negative effect on pulmonary function. Bed rest is another physiologic stressor that produces changes throughout the body, but many of the adaptations that occur with the stress of continued inactivity produce diminished functional capacity.

The Body's Response to Physical Activity

Physiologic reaction to physical activity can be divided into two categories: response and adaptation. Response is the immediate reaction to activity. Response involves the sudden, temporary changes that occur with a single bout of activity and disappear shortly after the activity is over. Increased heart rate and respiration are examples of response to a brisk 10-minute walk.

Adaptation is a more or less persistent change in structure or function following repeated bouts of activity (Lamb, 1984). It is adaptation that enables the body to eventually respond more easily to subsequent episodes of the same activity. The following are examples of likely adaptation: 1) the muscle hypertrophy and increased strength following an eight-week program of progressive resistance exercise; 2) an increased maximal oxygen consumption after 10 weeks of a walk/jog program; or 3) a change in body composition from 30 percent to 25 percent fat after a six-month combined program of a diet of 1200 calories per day and moderate exercise five days per week.

In rehabilitation and training for improved physical fitness, we are generally interested in producing adaptations by imposing appropriate and positive stressors on the physiologic systems. Although adaptation for improved function is the goal, we regulate activity (training) stress by monitoring the immediate response to the activity. Careful monitoring of the responses to each episode of activity is necessary to make adjustments in the activity to ensure maximum safety and effectiveness.

Response to a single bout of exercise is also the method of evaluating progress toward adaptation. For example, if the goal of your program is to increase the client's endurance for performing activities of daily living, the therapist might begin by developing a schedule for increasing ambulatory time periods in the course of preparing a meal. The goal is for the client to be able to sustain ambulation and meal preparation tasks without assistance or rest periods. The repeated bouts of activity will eventually produce adaptations in strength and endurance to help reach the goal of sustained performance. Monitoring response to the individual bouts of ambulatory activity will allow the therapist and the client to keep the activity within safe limits, to adjust the level of activity stress if need be, and to verify that adaptations are occurring. This can be done by measuring heart rate, respiration, and blood pressure, and by keeping track of self-perceived exertion, fatigue, and pain.

For activity to produce adaptation, it must in some way impose an increased load or stress on the system sufficient to produce change but not so great as to cause injury. Monitoring immediate response to activity will allow you to regulate the activity to stay within safe but effective limits. If the client, after being on his feet and working for five minutes, has a heart rate of 180 beats per minute (bpm), blood pressure of 90/50 mm Hg, respiration of 24, and feels that he is working as hard as he can, then you know that the activity session is too strenuous and needs to be shortened or made less intense. On the other hand, if after 10 minutes of ambulatory activity, there is essentially no change in these measures above resting levels, you will know that there is insufficient stress to produce change. In this case, you should increase the effort required and thereby continue to progress toward the goal of increased endurance.

Because nearly all the adaptations brought on by exercise training tend to reduce the relative stressfulness of exercise, the response to the training periods will become less pronounced as adaptation begins to occur. Heart rate and respiration will decrease for the same amount of work, blood pressure will stabilize, perceived exertion will lessen, and fatigue will be delayed or reduced. Therefore, the positive changes in observable responses over time can be a method of evaluation for positive feedback and reinforcement for the client and the therapist during the course of the program.

Now that we have reviewed the concept of physical activity as an appropriate positive stress for improving physical fitness and the difference between response and adaptation, we can proceed to a discussion of how specific changes in the various components of physical fitness can and do occur. The stress-response-adaptation phenomenon has been described by Dr. Hans Selye as the general adaptation syndrome (Brooks & Fahey, 1984). He defines the three stages of general adaptation syndrome as **alarm reaction, resistance development,** and **exhaustion,** and explains how these stages relate to each other.

Alarm reaction or response is the immediate reaction to imposed stress. If the stress is at a low enough level, the body may be able to adjust to the stressor by its current response mechanisms and maintain homeostasis without further changes. A healthy, normally active person re-

sponds easily to the physiologic stress of moving from lying down to standing up. We can see that there is a response by the slight increase in heart rate. However, this stress level can be handled by the body through existing response mechanisms. Yet the body has only limited capabilities to adjust to stress through its immediate response mechanisms. If the stress imposed is greater than the response mechanisms can handle, then adaptation must occur so that the body can handle the stress and regain homeostasis. This is the stage that Selye calls **resistance development**. It is during the resistance stage that the body improves its capacity to eventually handle the stressor more easily and that changes in the physiologic components of physical fitness occur. If the stress imposed is too great it becomes intolerable and the third stage occurs, **exhaustion** or *distress*. The stresses that result in physiologic exhaustion can be either acute or chronic. Acute exhaustion could come from an activity that required lifting too much weight or performing too many repetitions. Chronic physiologic exhaustion can be the result of such different stressors as unrelieved anxiety, sleep disorders, or physical overtraining (Brooks & Fahey, 1984). Anyone involved in prescribing or employing physical activity to promote health and function must know how to achieve and maintain balance in the stress-response-adaptation phenomenon and understand the application of two of the major principles: the overload principle and the principle of specificity. *(work hardening)*

The Overload Principle

Application of the appropriate positive stress is sometimes referred to as overloading the system. The **principle of overload** states that repeatedly imposing a stress above that normally experienced will cause adaptations to occur in the physiological systems experiencing the overload. The only mechanism by which adaptive changes for improved function can occur is through the application of this overload principle. If there is no overload, there is no adaptation for improvement. Overload is a positive stressor that can be quantified according to intensity, duration, and frequency of the activity being performed. The appropriate overload for an individual is achieved through varying the intensity, duration, and frequency of the activity program. The combination of intensity, frequency, and duration that constitutes an appropriate overload is dependent on the individual, the activity, the time, and the place. A woman who normally runs three miles daily in 30 minutes will need to run more miles or at a faster pace to achieve overload. A sedentary woman recovering from an acute flare of rheumatoid arthritis in which she was in bed for two weeks, may very well be at appropriate overload with an activity

Resistance

Alarm   Exhaustion

Sedentary (used often to imply no movement)

Table 8-3
Muscular Adaptations

STIMULUS	PRIMARY ADAPTATIONS	FUNCTIONAL IMPACT
Endurance exercise Repeated contractions (of low to moderate intensity)	Mitochondrial materials increase Increased oxidative enzymes Anaerobic pathways relatively unchanged	Increased endurance Increased glycogen sparing Decreased lactate production Insignificant hypertrophy
Strength training (heavy resistance with overload)	Fiber hypertrophy	Increased strength and power Little change in endurance
Immobilization	Muscle atrophy Decrease in oxidative enzymes	Decreased strength Decreased endurance Decreased coordination

---

program of five minutes of ambulation, three times daily. A man who walks a 15-minute mile every day in Atlantic City may find that in Denver he can only do a half-mile or has to slow down to a 20-minute mile to avoid becoming short of breath. For this man, the altitude in Denver has the effect of increasing the intensity of his exercise effort and producing an overload.

Application of overload is required for improved fitness and people at all levels of function and fitness can be afforded the opportunity to engage in appropriate activities to improve fitness and function with knowledgeable individual assessment and activity prescription. Although any of the three exercise variables (intensity, duration, or frequency) can be adjusted to produce the desired overload, research shows that *intensity* is the most potent factor for producing adaptations. By correctly applying the principle of overload, we are able to prescribe and monitor activity programs that will result in improved fitness for even the most de-conditioned or disabled individual.

The Principle of Specificity

The principle of specificity as it applies to achieving improvements in physical fitness and performance refers primarily to the specificity of training or the specific adaptation that occurs in response to the overload applied. We know from experience that stressing or training one body part or system does little to effect changes anywhere

else. It is obvious that progressive resistance exercises for the triceps would not produce change in knee extension strength nor would passive flexibility exercises for the low back improve abdominal wall strength.

Identifying specificity of training is not so obvious for increased muscle strength and/or endurance. In this instance, the specificity applies to the type of contraction (isometric or isotonic) and the joint angle or speed of shortening of the contraction. For example, it is well known that isometric strength training for the biceps done at 90 degrees of elbow flexion will not greatly improve strength or endurance measured during either dynamic elbow flexion or isometric contraction at 20 degrees.

Attention to the specificity of training for muscular fitness is crucial in the rehabilitation setting where improved function often depends on maximization of limited resources. The activity of eating involves a combination of isometric and isotonic strength of the shoulder girdle and upper extremity in order to grip a utensil and produce the necessary movement. Endurance is also needed for the movement to be repeated over the course of a meal. If the individual can accomplish the movement, then using the actual movement as the training exercise is usually the most effective path to improved function. However, if the individual is not able to accomplish the movement, it is necessary to identify the limiting factors—whether it is a deficiency in strength, endurance or a combination of both—and in which muscle groups the deficiency lies.

The principle of specificity tells us that the most effective training routine is the one that most closely parallels the requirements of the performance desired. By knowing the muscular requirements of the activity and the muscular resources at hand, you can apply the principle of specificity of training to develop an effective training program. Using activities of daily living in training to improve performance in those activities is the most efficient and effective method. For example, when the goal of training is for the person to be able to rise from a sitting position in a chair, the more quickly strengthening exercises for quadriceps and hip extensors can be sequenced to match the movement patterns of rising from a chair, the faster this functional performance will improve.

Physiology versus Performance

Physiologic adaptations and changes in observable performance are closely related but do not necessarily tell the same story. Although pure physiologic adaptations in cardiorespiratory function, muscular fitness, or flexibility are governed by the principles of overload and specificity, the variables affecting changes in performance are more diverse.

For example, a study is conducted with two young

[handwritten: Why a person of same physiological factors may vary in work done:]

women, Helen and Anne, who can be tested in all the components of fitness. Tests show that they have the same measurements for maximal oxygen consumption, muscular strength and endurance, flexibility, and percentage of body fat. They are the same age, height, and weight, and both have trained equally diligently for cross-country running. During the season, Anne usually wins or places among the first three finishers, whereas Helen is usually one of the last runners to finish or drops out.

What is responsible for such differences in the performances of two people who appear to be so similar and capable of equal effort and outcomes? There is, of course, no one answer that applies in all cases. Possible explanations for differences in performance can vary from motivation, self-efficacy, pain threshold, and fear of injury, to differences in economy of effort, glycogen and lactic acid metabolism, or muscle fiber composition. Although we understand a great deal about the physiologic adaptations and training needed to improve fitness and human performance, in many respects the variables of individual human performance remain an enigma.

It is impossible in real life to have two people exactly the same; however, we often see people who appear to be very similar physiologically who exhibit differences in observed performance. We even see changes in the same person's performance from one day to the next. Clinicians and trainers often think that if they could just uncover this secret of performance, they would have the key to success and be able to help people achieve their maximal performance. But there are undoubtedly many keys for unlocking this mystery of human performance, and they include not just physiological factors but psychological and social factors as well.

A methodical approach to this question of performance can yield valuable information and all possibilities should be examined. However, in this chapter we are exploring only one facet, the physiologic bases of performance using the organizational framework of physical fitness. This approach is relatively new to the rehabilitation process. Too often in the past, therapists have focused on the clinical diagnosis of pathology as the primary explanation for performance levels, and if a disease state does not provide the answers, then psychosocial variables such as motivation, depression, or helplessness are considered. Rarely have therapists looked at the underlying foundation on which performance capacity rests in either their assessments or prognoses.

The recent national attention given to physical fitness and exercise as basic lifestyle considerations underlines the importance of evaluating physical fitness as part of the clinical assessment. Looking at the example of Anne and Helen who were physiologically equal but whose

performances varied, it was important to first measure fitness levels to discover that they were physiologically equal rather than just assuming equal fitness because the women appeared so much alike in age, height, weight, and involvement in the same training program. As we have discussed, differences that cannot be observed without proper testing such as maximal oxygen consumption, percentage body fat, or muscular fitness, could certainly be the reasons for their performance differences. Therapists all too often tend to overlook a thorough fitness examination and instead focus on age, sex and disease-related factors as the basis for performance deficits. A comprehensive evaluation of performance must include information on physical fitness. Deficits in fitness must be addressed in the therapeutic intervention to achieve the best results.

REASONS FOR DIMINISHED FITNESS

Inactivity and Immobilization

[handwritten: • Deconditioning • Hypokinesia]

The human body requires the stresses imposed by an upright posture and regular physical activity to maintain homeostasis and the healthy functioning of all physiologic systems. Prolonged periods of inactivity produce an imbalance in the normal relationship between rest and physical activity which causes a negative stress on every system in the body. Prolonged periods of inactivity can be institutionally imposed or self-imposed, such as bed rest prescribed for the treatment of an acute illness or injury, neuromuscular inactivity due to paralysis, or just a sedentary existence. Depending on the degree and duration of the inactivity, adaptations occur as the body responds to this situation (see Table 8-3). The result of these adaptations is a deterioration in all aspects of physical fitness, commonly known as deconditioning. Extreme forms of this deconditioning are known as hypokinetic degenerative disease, the immobilization syndrome, or hypokinesia.

It is now well accepted that prolonged inactivity alone can produce illness. Observation of the effects of weightlessness during space flight has stimulated research into the effects of inactivity and loss of postural stimuli on healthy subjects during bed rest and immobilization (Sandler and Vernikos, 1986). These studies allow us to separate the effects of inactivity from the effects of an existing illness. Although bedrest is necessary and prescribed for some medical conditions, over extended periods, it can sometimes lead to a worsening of one's condition.

When a client is being evaluated and a therapeutic intervention planned, therapists should consider both the level of the person's regular physical activity before the onset of disease or injury and the degree and duration of inactivity after it. Applying the principle of overload to the stress of inactivity demonstrates that the more intense, frequent, and prolonged the inactivity, the greater is the amount of adaptation to that stress in terms of deconditioning. For example, if two men both 75 years old come to the clinic for evaluation and rehabilitation following a right hemisphere cerebrovascular accident, evaluation of their physical fitness could provide insights into the differences in their performance levels. Even with a similar neurologic impairment, they may be quite dissimilar in their ability to perform activities of daily living. Evaluating each man regarding his prior activity habits and his activity history since the cerebrovascular accident will reveal a great deal about the physiologic status that each man brings to the rehabilitation setting.

Cardiorespiratory Deconditioning. Prolonged inactivity results in adaptations by the cardiorespiratory system that compromise its ability to adequately respond to changes in activity level and changes in body position. Prolonged, insufficient activity results in increased basal heart rate, loss of blood volume, decrease in heart volume, decrease in stroke volume and cardiac output, decreased coronary blood flow, reduced orthostatic tolerance, and reduced aerobic capacity or maximal oxygen consumption.

Clinical manifestations of cardiorespiratory deconditioning are: 1) reduced exercise tolerance which is demonstrated by increased heart rate and respiration at low work loads, 2) early onset of fatigue, 3) possibly exertional dyspnea, and 4) perception of doing heavy or maximal work at low to moderate workloads.

If the person has been at rest in the horizontal position, he/she may experience a marked rise in heart rate and drop in blood pressure upon standing up (*orthostatic hypotension*). Standing upright may also produce syncope and fainting if the hypotension is severe or if the person is particularly sensitive to the low pressure. Diminished cardiorespiratory fitness makes a person less capable of adjusting to the increased physiologic demands of strenuous exercise, particularly exercise of sudden onset. As we have seen, strenuous exercise for one person may not be strenuous exercise for another. For a person who is severely deconditioned, it is possible that arising from bed and walking 50 feet could be strenuous exercise.

Muscular Deconditioning. Lack of muscle use leads to loss of muscle mass, commonly called **disuse atrophy**. It may take only four to eight weeks of disuse for muscle to atrophy to one-half normal size. If activity is resumed within that time, full function usually returns. However after four months of inactivity, a significant number of

muscle fibers deteriorate, and full recovery is unlikely. In the case of loss of nerve supply (denervation), muscle fibers will eventually be replaced by fat and connective tissue, and after two years this process is essentially complete.

During bedrest or immobilization, muscles necessary for upright posture (anitgravity muscles) and muscles necessary for locomotion are the most affected and undergo proportional decreases in strength and in actual muscle mass. Muscle tissue responds to activity stress. Under normal conditions, the demands of muscle-loading and movement produce a balance between the synthesis and degradation of contractile proteins so that muscle mass is maintained or increased. With insufficient loading or movement, such as during bedrest or immobilization, there is greater degradation than synthesis. Products of muscle breakdown appear in the blood and urine indicating that muscle atrophy is underway.

Innervation is an important factor in the balance between synthesis and degradation of contractile proteins as observed by decrease in muscle protein content that occurs when the nerve supply to a muscle is interrupted. Loss of contractile proteins causes a decrease in cross-sectional muscle mass which is directly proportional to loss of muscle strength. Decreased muscle endurance and maximal oxygen consumption are also a consequence of muscle atrophy due primarily to the selective nature of fiber deterioration that occurs in disuse atrophy.

Muscle disuse is typically associated with significant atrophy of the slow-twitch (Type I) muscle fibers and a decrease in the oxidative enzymes needed for energy production during endurance activities. In a study of morphological changes in muscle immobilized by casting, it was found that after one month in a cast, the proportion of Type I fibers decreased from 80 percent to 57 percent. Retraining after cast removal resulted in a return to pre-cast values (Sandler & Vernikos, 1986). Because Type I fibers provide the oxidative energy systems needed to support sustained activity, a reduction in the proportion and number of these fibers decreases the aerobic capacity for muscular work. A reduction in the aerobic energy systems diminishes the body's potential for maximal oxygen consumption. Thus, the decreased maximal oxygen consumption of inactivity that was mentioned as a cardiorespiratory adaptation is not only a consequence of the diminished capacity of the heart to deliver oxygen to working muscles, but also a result of diminished capacity of the muscles to use oxygen.

Adaptations in muscle tissue are responsive to the type and duration of the inactivity. A completely denervated muscle may lose 90 to 95 percent of its normal bulk. In the case of immobilization by splinting, the degree of muscle atrophy is only 30 to 35 percent. Loss in strength is progressive over time. Some studies have shown a 20 percent loss of residual strength for each week of inactivity. Although muscle can adapt to increases in activity imposed by a retraining program, the rate of recovery is much slower than the rate of loss. Valbona (1982) says that the expectation from a vigorous restrengthening program is probably no more than a 10 percent increase of initial strength per week.

Diminished Flexibility. Flexibility of connective tissue decreases rapidly with inactivity. In muscles and around joints where flexibility is required for normal motion, there is a loose meshwork of areolar connective tissue that allows a considerable and easy range of motion. When a body part is immobilized or the normal range of motion is restricted, the mere continuation of normal metabolic activity of connective tissue leads to diminished flexibility. When undisturbed by motion, the connective tissue network will shorten to the length to which the tissue is regularly asked to stretch. The old adage of "if you don't use it, you lose it" seems to apply here.

Normal connective tissue adapts to the stress of imposed motion, reorganizing the meshwork to allow more or less flexibility as required. Significant shortening in the connective tissue meshwork can occur within one week of restricted motion. If motion is restricted due to imposed immobilization or because of edema, trauma, or impaired circulation, the body will not only reorganize the connective tissue meshwork to a shorter length, but will also produce a dense connective tissue at the involved site. This dense connective tissue replaces the normal loose, areolar connective tissue and this dense fibrosis may start in as few as three days (Kottke, 1966).

Increased Percentage of Body Fat. The effect of inactivity on body composition is significant and goes beyond mere energy expenditure. We are all aware of the balance between energy expenditure and weight control that demonstrates that weight is gained when more calories are consumed than are expended in physical activity, and weight is lost when more energy is expended than is consumed. However, if we want to change body composition and decrease the percent of body fat, we can do this most effectively with an increase in physical activity.

Conversely and unfortunately, insufficient physical activity will result in an increase in percentage of body fat. Without physical activity, the percentage of body fat will increase even if there is no overall weight gain. Even when calories are reduced to produce weight loss, the decrease in percentage of body fat will occur more rapidly when accompanied by increased physical activity.

Physical activity helps to maintain appropriate body composition in more ways than just burning excess calories

that would otherwise be stored in adipose tissue. Other advantages of physical activity are: 1) Moderate intensity activity will tend to mobilize stored fat deposits and encourage the burning of fat as a source of energy. Exercise must be performed in at least 30 minute regimens on a regular basis for this to take place. 2) Physical activity also raises the metabolic rate during the exercise and for some time following it, so that energy expenditure can be increased even at rest. 3) Increased physical activity can cause actual increases in muscle mass (hypertrophy) for people who have been primarily sedentary. Engaging in quite moderate exercise such as walking, jogging, or bicycling will cause muscle tissue to adapt to the increased stress with actual increases in muscle mass. As pointed out before, this kind of activity will not increase muscle mass in those who are already engaged in regular vigorous physical exercise, since they must engage in muscle-building exercise to increase muscle mass.

Inactivity results in an increased proportion of body fat to lean body weight not only because excess calories are stored as adipose tissue but also because of the adaptive decrease in muscle mass, or disuse atrophy. As you remember, adequate levels of fat are about 15 percent for men and 25 percent for women. Aside from the well-known, health risk factors associated with adult obesity such as coronary heart disease, hypertension, and Type II diabetes, high body fat percentage more directly affects performance. The trade-off in body composition between fat and lean body weight occurs between secondary fat deposits (a storage compartment) and muscle mass (an active work-producing compartment). These are the two largest body compartments, and they are closely related metabolically. Therefore, an increase in percentage body fat compromises adequate muscle mass that is necessary for the strength and endurance to support functional performance.

Inactivity and immobilization affect all systems in the body. In this chapter, we have specifically addressed only those decrements related to physical fitness, but prolonged inactivity can lead to a myriad of other physical and mental conditions. Table 8-4 lists several clinical manifestations of prolonged immobilization. In fact, prolonged inactivity affects every organ in the body, disturbs hormonal and metabolic functions, and contributes to bone mineral loss and osteoporosis. The adaptations to prolonged inactivity may at times cause a greater degree of disability than the original incident that caused the person to become inactive.

Aging

There is no question that physiologic capacity and performance are to some extent age-dependent. Physiologic capacity tends to increase rapidly through childhood, peaking in the late teens to early thirties, and then gradually declines with increasing age. Results from research on aging point to more differences than similarities in both the processes of aging and the consequences for performance. The changes that we associate with aging occur at different rates in different people, and even at different rates within the same person. We have found that there are large differences between chronological age and biological age even within age groups. We have also found that changes long associated with aging appear to be not so much age-dependent as they are activity-dependent.

We will not attempt to address all the social, cultural and medical variables that could affect this process of aging, but rather we will present a representative clinical picture of the older client, knowing that this picture is greatly influenced by individual social, cultural and medical variables.

Gerontologists agree that the most universal change with age is a decreasing ability to respond to physical or emotional stress and return to prestress levels in a reasonable time (Weg, 1983). This is a diminished homeostatic capacity that may only become manifest when the current stressor is greater than that normally encountered. In general, resting values are less indicative of aging changes than response and recovery values.

Table 8-4
Clinical Manifestations of Prolonged Immobilization

Muscular
Decreased Strength
Decreased Endurance
Muscle Atrophy
Impaired Task Precision
and
Poor Coordination

Skeletal
Osteoporosis
Joint Fibrosis and Ankylosis

Cardiorespiratory
Increased Heart Rate
Decreased Cardiac Output/Reserve
Orthostatic Hypotension
Phlebothrombosis
Decreased Vital Capacity
Decreased Maximal Voluntary Ventilation
Impairment of Coughing Mechanism

Psychological
Depression
Apathy
Intellectual Dulling

Cardiorespiratory Changes with Aging. A decrease in maximal heart rate occurs with age and is not related to sex or to cardiorespiratory fitness. Age-predicted maximal heart rate can be estimated by the following formula:

$$220 - age = maximal\ heart\ rate\ (+\ 10\ beats\ per\ minute).$$

The clinical application of decreasing maximal heart rate with age will become apparent when we discuss exercise prescription. Conversely, the resting heart rate appears to be more sensitive to level of fitness than to age, and improved fitness is often reflected in a lower resting heart rate.

Other cardiorespiratory changes are a decrease in cardiac output because of decreased maximal heart rate and diminished stroke volume, decreased maximal oxygen consumption because of lowered efficiency of the heart in pumping blood, and a decreased muscle mass. There seems to be little change in the ability of the oxidative energy systems to use oxygen. With advancing age there can be a reduction in respiratory efficiency, and pulmonary function may become a limiting factor in maximal oxygen consumption.

Age-related changes in cardiorespiratory fitness are often compounded by the deleterious effects of inactivity and atherosclerosis. In the absence of coronary and peripheral vascular disease, people in their 80's have been shown to be able to engage in progressive cardiorespiratory training programs and exercise vigorously enough to produce physiologic adaptations and improved aerobic capacity (Smith & Gilligan, 1983).

Any training program for older clients should be based on individualized prescription, be well supervised, be gradually progressive, include a thorough warm-up period, and be initiated only after a thorough medical assessment.

Muscle Changes with Aging. Muscle mass and measured muscle strength, both static and dynamic, diminish progressively with age. However, it appears that the effect of inactivity plays a large role in explaining this decline. Exercise programs can result in improvements in strength, oxidative capacity, and some muscle hypertrophy.

A research finding of particular clinical interest is the discrepancy between performance of a brief arm-cranking test and measured muscle strength in 80-year-old subjects. When compared with middle-aged values, these subjects showed a 45 percent reduction in the work performed by arm cranking, but only a 28 percent decline in strength (Shephard, 1978). There are many possible reasons for this discrepancy. It may be inadequate speed of contraction needed to generate enough power to perform the task or poor coordination resulting from fatigue, lack of practice at the motor skill, inefficient muscle fiber recruitment, or any number of other reasons. From these results, we can see that a manual muscle test indicating "good strength" in a muscle group indicates little about the ability to generate adequate muscular power to perform a given task at a functional level.

With aging, lack of sheer muscle strength is generally not the primary limiting factor in performance capability for activities of daily living. Muscle biopsy studies of age-related changes in muscle fiber composition show that the greatest deterioration is in the fast-twitch (Type II) fibers that are responsible for high-intensity/velocity contractions. The primary metabolic systems of these muscle fibers are anaerobic, providing energy for muscle work that can generate great power but cannot be sustained for more than a matter of seconds.

Slow-twitch fibers (Type I) show less deterioration with aging. Type I fibers are the site of aerobic muscle metabolism and are responsible for supporting low to moderate muscular work for long periods of time. Marathon runners and postal delivery people are relying on their Type I fibers.

It is still unclear how much of this selective fiber deterioration is explained by aging itself and how much is due to disuse. Because activity patterns tend to become less physically demanding with aging, it is possible that the change of muscle fiber composition is an adaptive response to lower level stress demands of activities that are low to moderate in intensity and are typically required by a retirement lifestyle. In general, older muscle tissue shows a slow decline in strength, tone, speed, and endurance. However, appropriate exercise regimens can result in physiologic adaptations and improved performance at any age (Weg, 1983). In fact, studies of people who have maintained vigorous exercise programs into their 80's show that physical activity is effective in delaying and reducing changes in muscle strength and endurance.

Changes in Flexibility. Problems with decreased flexibility and the risk of connective tissue injury increase with advancing age. Here again, both biological aging and insufficient activity contribute to these problems. Studies done on connective tissue at the cellular level indicate that the aging process does result in loss of elastic tissue and alterations in the structure of the collagen molecule, reducing flexibility in muscle, tendon, ligament, and joint capsule. Age-related changes in the structure of articular cartilage appear to make it less resilient and more susceptible to injury. Loss of resiliency, thinning, and degenerative changes have been noted in articular cartilage as early as the second decade of life (Shephard, 1978).

Changes in molecular structure and vascularization of connective tissue increase the risk of injury to muscle, tendon, and articular structures and decrease the ability of these tissues to repair themselves. During the aging process, there appears to be a progressive decrease in capillaries and an increase in tendon calcification. These changes, associated with the increased likelihood of tendon ruptures, are also known to accompany reduced physical activity.

For all of these reasons, the clinical approach to the older or deconditioned person in respect to flexibility should be one of caution. Gradual progression of exercise activities that include adequate warm-up and gentle, active static stretching, both before and after the conditioning period, will help reduce the incidence of sprain and strain injuries. The common features of the aging joint are too often loss of both mobility and stability. Appropriate physical activity can have a preventive and a rehabilitative role in maintenance of good flexibility.

Changes in Body Composition in Aging. In industrialized societies where there are adequate food supplies and socioeconomic pressure for retirement, population studies show that increasing age is associated with increased percentage body fat. Reported percentages for body fat average around 28 percent for elderly men and 38 percent for elderly women, in contrast to 15 percent and 25 percent, respectively, for young men and women. Although there is a normal degree of muscle wasting that begins between the fifth and seventh decades of life, the increase in percentage body fat is felt to be a consequence of inactivity rather than a natural phenomenon of aging. Studies of master-class male athletes in their 70s, 80s, and 90s have shown no more than 14 percent body fat (Shephard, 1978).

An increase in percentage body fat with age is not always accompanied by an increase in body weight. In fact, body weight tends to climb from the mid-20s to mid-40s, and then begins a gradual decline while percentage body fat is increasing. This increase in body fat can be masking a gradual decrease in lean body tissue, primarily of skeletal muscle and bone (Shephard, 1978). Decreased muscle mass, due to a reduced synthesis of muscle proteins, results in decreases in muscle strength, power, and endurance, and lessened maxVO$_2$.

Osteoporosis or loss of bone mass is a major problem of aging, particularly in women, and is associated with age and/or inactivity. It is the loss of bone density and strength that occurs when more bone is resorbed than is formed in the remodeling process. If severe, osteoporosis can result in compression fracture of vertebrae and fractures in long bones. Osteoporosis is often a contributing factor to hip fractures in the elderly. Postmenopausal women are particularly at risk for severe osteoporosis. Other risk factors include: sedentary lifestyle, insufficient calcium intake, smoking, alcohol consumption, a slight build, and northern European lineage. Therapeutic recommendations for the prevention and treatment of osteoporosis include supple-

---

Table 8-5
Clinical Indications of Fatigue

Muscular
Decreased strength
Decreased contraction time
Increased recovery time
Tremors with contraction
Increased muscle lengthening time

General
Decreased coordination
Decreased smoothness/rhythm of performance
Appearance of compensatory/extraneous movements
General slowing down
Loss of concentration
Loss of interest
Increased frustration

---

mentary dietary calcium; moderate-intensity weight-bearing exercise such as walking; reduction of lifestyle risk factors; and often estrogen replacement therapy for postmenopausal women.

When planning programs for a person who is known or suspected to be at risk for osteoporosis, attention must be paid to avoiding situations that produce increased pressure on the vertebrae. Spontaneous compression fracture is most common in the thoracic vertebrae. Fracture resulting from increased loading is most common in lumbar vertebrae. Therefore, in the treatment setting avoid those postures that cause increased stress in the thoracic and lumbar regions such as extreme trunk flexion, slouched sitting posture, sudden forceful movements of the spinal column, and lifting heavy weights. It is also extremely important to observe all safety precautions to prevent falls.

When advanced age is a factor in a client's situation, it is important to look beyond a normal body weight for measures of individual muscular and skeletal fitness. Trying to assess a client's habitual activity level through self-report can be risky. It has been noted that older people and obese people tend to overestimate their physical activity both in terms of time spent in activity and in terms of the intensity of the activity itself. Most studies indicate that the general trend with age is toward less physical activity.

It is often not easy to make the distinction between age-related and activity-related changes in an elderly client. As the field of gerontology grows there will be larger, longitudinal studies producing information that will help us better understand aging and activity as they relate to performance. But for the present, we must use the knowledge we have to address both age-related and activity-related changes of these clients in clinical practice.

Disease

Illness and injury are, by definition, conditions that interfere with our ability to perform. Whether the condition is acute or chronic, traumatic or insidious in origin, physiologic changes are produced that alter our capacity for performance. Rehabilitation deals with reversing or minimizing the effects of the pathology to maximize functional performance. The growth of specialization in rehabilitation reflects the diversity of needs and specificity of therapeutic approaches.

This discussion of disease, in relation to the physiologic bases of performance, will not attempt to present pathophysiology or therapeutic interventions. Rather, it suggests a clinical perspective with which to view alterations in performance that are accompanied by illness and/or injury. This perspective includes assessment of physical fitness in addition to the traditional evaluation measures that often are disease-specific or function-specific. This assessment of physical fitness gives crucial information to our evaluation. Whatever the cause of the performance deficit, addressing fitness through the five component areas helps us differentiate between the disease-specific effects and the health-related fitness effects on performance and define and locate the areas of ability and disability. This information will be useful for effective treatment planning.

When planning a treatment program it is important to know if the performance decrements are a direct consequence of the pathology or if they are confounded by other causes. A clinical approach that includes attention to physical fitness as a factor affecting performance is also a positive and optimistic approach. We know that the components of fitness are amenable to improvement with appropriate training at any age, any stage of deconditioning, and in the presence of disease.

It is rare that performance cannot be improved by appropriate training to improve some parameter of fitness. For example, cardiorespiratory conditioning programs are used for both primary prevention and rehabilitation of coronary heart disease. It has also been successfully used to improve performance in rehabilitation programs for people with such varied diagnoses as COPD, chronic pain syndrome, and clinical depression. Even individuals with paraplegia due to spinal cord injury can improve cardiorespiratory fitness and maintain healthy cardiac status through conditioning programs using upper extremity aerobic exercise such as arm cranks and self-propelled wheelchair exercise regimes.

Physical fitness and disease are not opposite ends of the health spectrum. They are both factors in the multifactorial paradigm of human performance. There are two important facts to remember for the therapist planning rehabilitation programs: 1. The presence of illness or injury does not exclude the possibility of fitness or of improving fitness with appropriate conditioning. 2. The absence of sufficient physical activity on a regular basis leads to declining fitness and can lead even to disease or injury.

OTHER FACTORS AFFECTING PERFORMANCE

Aging, inactivity, and disease can have a direct effect on the components of fitness and thereby have the potential to influence observable performance. Fatigue and poor economy of effort are more likely to be signs of diminished fitness which appear during performance.

Fatigue

The exercise physiologist defines fatigue as the inability to maintain a given exercise intensity. The clinician is familiar with fatigue as a symptom reported by the client. The concept of fatigue includes both physiologic and psychosocial variables and implies a decrement in performance. In determining level of performance and perception of fatigue, the psychosocial variables of motivation, fear, pain tolerance, and general mental state may be just as important as the physiologic variables, especially in low-intensity, sustained-duration activities encountered in vocational and leisure pursuits.

The physiology of fatigue is a complex phenomenon. There is active research and controversy regarding the anatomical site(s) and mechanisms of fatigue that implicate the central nervous system, peripheral nerves, myoneural junction, and the muscles as possible sources of fatigue. There is debate about whether fatigue is due to accumulation or depletion of specific metabolites or is a general homeostatic response. What is clear is that there is no one site or mechanism that explains fatigue in all cases (Lamb, 1984). For example, fatigue occurring when a person attempts to maintain a tight grip for 20 seconds is due primarily to anaerobic mechanisms supporting contraction in the finger flexors and intrinsics of the hand; however, the possibility of changes at the neuromuscular junction cannot be disregarded. Fatigue occurring when a person begins a gait-retraining program could be due to inadequate oxygen transport or utilization by the active muscles or a variety of neural and/or muscular causes.

Fatigue is activity-specific for the intensity and duration of the activity and for the body parts involved in the activity. The physiologic status of the individual is a major determining factor in onset of fatigue. Fatigue is also influenced by environmental stressors such as heat, altitude, and humidity. The more complex and sustained the activity, the more difficult it is to determine specific causes of fatigue.

Fatigue is not always a negative factor. For physiologic adaptations to take place some physiologic fatigue must occur. Activity that is strenuous enough to result in a sense of general tiredness or some fatigue is associated with improved sleep behaviors and improved sense of well-being and relaxation. There is an important distinction between exercise-induced fatigue and exhaustion. Exercise to the point of exhaustion is appropriate only in the most controlled laboratory testing procedures with on-site medical supervision. The purpose of such exercise regimens is diagnostic or scientific enquiry, not training. It is the therapist's or trainer's responsibility to monitor physical activity to provide the sufficient overload that will allow adaptation without producing exhaustion.

It is necessary to be able to identify the onset of fatigue and understand its implications in the clinical setting. Clinical observation and client self-report should both be used to monitor fatigue. Table 8-5 lists the signs and symptoms of fatigue. Client self-report can be an important tool for monitoring fatigue from day to day, for assessing improvement over time, and for helping the client develop skills to monitor his or her own exertion and fatigue level outside the clinic.

Clinical observation to determine onset of fatigue can be systematic and is based on our knowledge of a number of performance-related principles. The inability to maintain or repeat the production of a given force by muscular contraction, another definition of fatigue, describes the first observation of fatigue. The clinical onset of muscular fatigue will be evidenced by changes in muscular performance such as decreased strength, decreased time of contraction and/or increased time of recovery, increased time for muscle lengthening following contraction, tremors with contraction, and substitution and compensatory movements. If the fatigue is related to insufficient coronary circulation and/or insufficient oxygen delivery (*hypoxia*), the clinical signs may be shortness of breath, increased heart rate and respiration with no increase in workload, sweating, or general sense of tiredness, especially in the exercising muscles. General performance may slow down and attention may wander. Symptoms such as chest pressure or pain, nausea, and numbness in upper extremities should be considered as a coronary event and emergency procedures should be followed. Only in the presence of heart disease will normal daily exercise requirements be limited by actual fatigue of the heart muscle or by the inability of the heart to provide adequate cardiac output.

Fatigue is associated with muscular incoordination. Thus, an easily observable clinical sign of fatigue is a change in the smoothness, the rhythm, or the coordinated

FATIGUE

effort with which a task is performed. The key to this observation is the word "change." Poor coordination and extraneous movement are often normally seen in the early stages of motor skill learning, so in that case these symptoms would not be indicative of fatigue. The incoordination and extraneous movements must be a deviation from an established rhythm or pattern to be considered a sign of fatigue. Some people actually develop recognizable fatigue patterns that appear as they tire at a particular task. Normally the change in movement pattern that accompanies the onset of fatigue requires even more effort and speeds the fatigue process.

The standing fatigue posture that relies on ligamentous structures and balanced body segments requires less muscular effort to maintain than does the normal upright stance; however, ambulation with this posture is more energy consuming than ambulation with good posture because of the extra work required of hip and knee musculature. The incoordination may appear as a general loss of rhythmic motion, or more specifically, as difficulty in performing movements that require rapid contraction and relaxation of antagonistic muscle groups or that require sequenced movement of body parts.

Loss of concentration is also often a sign of early fatigue. If activity continues past the point of appropriate overload, and fatigue becomes pronounced, harm can result.

Pronounced fatigue brings with it an increased susceptibility to injury as muscular control and protective tension are lost. Sprains and strains become more likely, and the ability of the muscle to respond to loading and to dissipate shock is reduced. Post-exercise muscle soreness increases with undue fatigue. This has been viewed as a possible reason for the poor exercise compliance rates associated with exercise regimes that are severely fatiguing to individuals.

Continuing exercise past the point of fatigue is counterproductive for both motor skill acquisition and physiologic muscle fiber adaptation. Practice for motor learning is most effective when neuromuscular capacity to sense and respond to both internal and external stimuli is not diminished by fatigue, and when motivation and concentration on the task at hand are high. Muscle fiber adaptation to physiologic overload appears to occur during periods of rest when the muscle fibers are being repaired from the microinjuries incurred during vigorous exercise. This process occurs during both endurance training and strength training. However, it is felt that the injury-repair process is particularly crucial to muscle-strengthening programs involving the fast-twitch muscle fibers that respond to overload with hypertrophy. Weight-lifting programs are recommended only three times a week in order to allow the repair and adaptation process to occur.

Exercise activity can be adjusted to prevent undue fatigue by changing any of the three exercise parameters: intensity, duration, and/or frequency. The adjustments to make can be based on the type of fatigue that occurs. Intensity and duration of the exercise are the most commonly manipulated variables; however, the frequency of the activity can be of vital concern. Frequent, intense training can lead to a state known as overtraining. Overtraining, recognized as a serious concern by coaches and athletic trainers, is characterized by deterioration in performance and general conditioning and a loss of interest or motivation. Overtraining is most likely a combination of prolonged physical and psychological fatigue. It is probably an all-too-common and unrecognized impediment to continued progress in intensive rehabilitation programs. By recognizing overtraining as a potential difficulty and by manipulating activity type, intensity, duration, and frequency; the therapist will be able to engage the client in safe and effective rehabilitation.

Fatigue can also be symptomatic of the disease itself. Many of the systemic, rheumatologic disorders such as rheumatoid arthritis, systemic lupus erythematosus, and polymyalgia rheumatica include marked fatigue as a clinical sign of heightened disease activity. In these cases, effective disease control is generally accompanied by diminished fatigue.

In the case of multiple sclerosis, undue fatigue can have prolonged effects on performance. Traditionally, medical recommendations have been to avoid strenuous activity. However, too little physical activity and poor fitness can add to the debilitating effects of this disease. It may be that one of the difficulties people with multiple sclerosis have in determining appropriate levels of activity is the inability to recognize signs of muscular fatigue as early as a person without nervous system pathology. It is possible that the person with multiple sclerosis may be recognizing exhaustion rather than fatigue. Exercise programs for the person with multiple sclerosis must be carefully monitored and systematically progressed to provide the opportunities for enhanced fitness without exacerbating the signs and symptoms of the disease.

Activity programs that provide conditioning stimuli and result in improved physical fitness are improving the body's capacity to respond to the activity stress. In other words, improving fitness is actually making the activities less stressful. The changes in performance that can be observed include: less effort required to accomplish the task, less marked response to the stressor, and a lengthened amount of time before the onset of fatigue.

Economy of Effort

The cost of production is a central concern in fields as diverse as economics, automotive engineering, and exercise physiology. The amount of input (dollars, gasoline, or calories) required to produce a given product (profit, miles traveled, or useful work) is expressed proportionally (percentage of profit, miles per gallon, or calories per hour). In the field of human performance, this ratio of energy input to work output can be expressed in both mathematical and clinical terms. **Mechanical efficiency** is calculated as a percentage of the actual mechanical work accomplished divided by the input of energy. The term work is used in the physical science concept of force acting through a vertical distance and applies only to external work performed. The mechanical efficiency of the locomotor activities of walking, running, or cycling is between 20 and 30 percent.

The primary factor that affects efficiency is the energy required to overcome internal and external friction. In terms of the efficiency equation, this is wasted energy because it does not produce measurable work. Mechanical efficiency varies between individuals, activities, and speed of performance. To a point, mechanical efficiency can be improved with training (McArdle, Katch, & Katch, 1986). Economy of effort is used in a clinical sense to describe differences in energy requirements between individuals and individual performances over time. It is the more clinically useful concept, requiring only a gauge of the energy input or effort required to produce a given performance. Economy of effort is commonly based on the amount of oxygen consumed while performing a particular activity. Because heart rate during submaximal exercise is proportional to oxygen consumption, the more easily monitored heart rate during performance can be used to evaluate economy of effort for an individual over time. To compare individuals, it is necessary to evaluate effort as a percentage of predicted maximal heart rate achieved. The less energy expended to produce a given amount of work, the greater the economy of effort.

Whether you consider mechanical efficiency or economy of effort, the bottom line is to produce the most work for the least cost. This efficiency of performance is most relevant to activities that require effort lasting more than a few minutes. Sustained performance relies on aerobic endurance that is affected by oxidative capacity, availability of energy stores, and the energy needed to perform the activity.

We can improve endurance performance, that is, lengthen the performance time, by improving oxidative capacity, increasing energy stores, or reducing the energy required to perform the activity. By reducing the energy requirement, there will be less stress on oxidative capacity, less depletion of energy stores, and the activity will be able to proceed for a longer time. Reducing the energy requirement is synonymous with improving the economy of effort. When the ability to sustain performance is a goal, any

adjustment that improves economy of effort directly translates into improved performance. Economy of effort relates to endurance performance, just as writing checks relates to your bank balance at the end of the month; the more you use early in the month, the less you have to get you through to the end of the month. If you withdraw too much too early, your ability to sustain activity at the desired level may be seriously diminished. Economy of effort can be affected by a number of factors. Those most relevant to rehabilitation and training are fatigue, skill, speed of performance, and biomechanical factors such as weight and posture.

Fatigue interferes with economy of effort. As muscular fatigue occurs, more and more motor units are recruited to produce or maintain tension. More active motor units require greater energy consumption. Consequently, for the same work output, greater input is being required and efficiency is reduced. In the more general sense, as fatigue sets in, established skill levels may be reduced as rhythmical and sequenced movement patterns are disrupted. Extraneous and inefficient motions appear. Fatigue is often accompanied by loss of attention and motivation, both important factors in efficient performance.

Motor Skill Proficiency and Economy of Effort. As skill or proficiency in performing an activity increases, the economy of effort improves. Early motor learning or relearning is characterized by unnecessary muscular tension and extraneous, poorly coordinated movements. As skill improves with effective practice and training, observers can see the performance become smoother, less effortful, and more productive. The performer notes improvement as motions become more automatic, more comfortable, and less tiring. As skill improves, less energy is being used to accomplish the task and economy of effort improves as well. Thus the task can be accomplished more satisfactorily and for longer periods of time. This relationship between motor skill proficiency and economy of effort is one of the most important aspects of the principle of specificity of training. It is only by practicing the activity itself that motor skill learning and increased efficiency can occur.

Speed of Performance and Economy of Effort. Speed of performance also affects mechanical efficiency and economy of effort. In a pure muscular contraction, increasing velocity of the contraction is associated with decreased tension production and reduced efficiency. In complex motor patterns required for ambulation and self-care, the association between speed and efficiency is not so clear cut. For any complex motor pattern, there appears to be a range of speed in which optimal efficiency occurs. Performance that is either much slower or faster than the optimal range results in poor economy of effort.

Submaximal exercise

A great deal of research has been done regarding mechanical efficiency of running and walking speeds, and we can use this as an example to illustrate this concept of speed and efficiency. Gait analysis studies tell us that the most efficient walking speed for the nondisabled adult is approximately 2.4 miles per hour (4 kilometers per hour). Efficiency of walking is similar for healthy adults, and varies with speed and incline. Walking slower than 2 miles per hour requires more energy and is less efficient than walking at slightly faster speeds. When walking increases to speeds greater than about 5 miles per hour, it becomes more efficient to run than to walk. The techniques of racewalking are aimed at reducing energy costs as much as possible while adhering to the requirements of maintaining a walking rather than a running pattern. For people who need to maximize endurance performance (marathon runners, production workers, freight loaders, and therapists), it is important to develop movement patterns and rhythms that expend less energy because the less energy required to perform, the longer the performance can be maintained.

For people who are interested in producing an energy deficit or training overload, economy of effort may not be the goal. For example, to develop a greater caloric deficit in an exercise program the individual may choose to walk at 5 miles per hour rather than to jog. In this way he or she will be using more energy per distance covered. Walking or running on sand or with additional weight on the feet or ankles increases the workload.

Although these actions reduce mechanical efficiency, they can be used to produce an overload for strength or endurance training. Taking advantage of mechanical inefficiency to produce a training effect can benefit people who have an extremely low exercise tolerance. In a study of the energy cost of extremely slow walking in cardiac patients, Franklin and colleagues showed that walking speeds between .8 and 2 miles per hour imposed similar metabolic and cardiac demands, approximated 7 ml/kg/min oxygen consumption, and could be useful in exercise training for select individuals with coronary heart disease (Franklin et al., 1983). The clinical implication of these findings is that even extremely slow walking can be a conditioning activity.

Psychosocial Factors that Affect Performance

There are many factors that affect performance other than the physiologic variables that we have discussed. These other factors include motivation, fear, pain, self-efficacy, and sociocultural norms, and are discussed in depth elsewhere in this text. These factors can affect an individual's observed performance during functional assessment in the clinical setting. They can influence actual individual daily activity levels that in turn affect physical fitness. We must always remember that human performance is the product of physiologic and psychosocial variables that together influence individuals. Observable performance should never be assumed to be a clear indication of physiologic capacity.

ENHANCING PERFORMANCE THROUGH IMPROVED PHYSICAL FITNESS

This section discusses training principles that have been developed for improving the five components of health-related physical fitness: cardiovascular function, muscle strength, muscle endurance, flexibility, and body composition. These principles provide a scientific rationale for implementing programs that provide appropriate and positive physiologic stress to promote some aspect of physical fitness. A knowledge of these principles also helps the therapist interpret changes in performance that occur during the course of rehabilitation. For the most part, these research- based principles have been developed through the study of athletes and healthy, normal populations. To apply these principles properly in the clinical setting, the therapist must include them in a comprehensive knowledge base of clinical assessment and therapeutic intervention.

Exercise Prescription for Physical Fitness

An exercise program for physical fitness is prescribed using the same strategies as all individualized health-related recommendations including: 1) a thorough assessment of the individual, 2) mutual goal-setting, 3) intervention strategies, 4) implementation, and 5) monitoring for harm and benefit. The specifics of the physical fitness prescription address the five components of physical fitness described in this chapter, and a comprehensive prescription will be based on assessment and intervention in all five areas, if needed. Table 8-2 outlines the assessment of the physical fitness components.

For the asymptomatic adult, the core of the exercise program is cardiovascular conditioning. This is the period of aerobic exercise that should provide appropriate overload to produce improvement in both cardiovascular and muscle endurance. Exercises for improvement of flexibility are included in the pre- and post-aerobic periods commonly called the warm-up and cool-down. Muscle strengthening is accomplished with a weight-training program that can be performed on the same or alternate days as the aerobic endurance exercise. Herbert A. de Vries (1980) defined the essential components of a scientific prescription of exercise:

    1. Determine the objectives of the exercise program. This requires assessment of the individual in the five

components of health-related fitness and mutual goal-setting.

2. Choose the exercise modality appropriate to achieving the goals. The exercise programs for improving upper-extremity strength, increasing low-back flexibility, or improving cardiovascular endurance will be different and specific.

3. Develop the exercise program with specific recommendations for exercise intensity, duration of the exercise at each session, and frequency of the sessions. The intensity recommendations should be stated as ranges with established upper level values that the client should not exceed and lower level, "insufficient load" values.

4. Determine realistic expectations for rate of change and amount of improvement to be achieved. Change is a function of various factors in each individual including initial fitness levels, intensity of the training, type of training, age, general health and psychosocial dimensions.

The American College of Sports Medicine (ACSM) has developed thorough guidelines for clinical exercise testing (ACSM, 1986). These should be understood and followed before prescribing any exercise program that requires unaccustomed activity levels. In the medical environment where much rehabilitation occurs, many of the ACSM requirements will be met by virtue of developing a diagnosis and/or treatment plan. For those in the community who want to begin a physical fitness exercise program, ACSM guidelines frequently require a medical history and exercise stress test including physician review of the electrocardiograms.

Benefits of Physical Fitness and Regular Physical Activity

There are both physiological and psychological benefits of being physically fit and participating in the regular physical activity required to stay fit. The physiological benefits, particularly in the area of cardiovascular health, are well documented. Although we cannot say that cardiovascular fitness will prevent coronary heart disease, atherosclerosis, or hypertension, we do know that populations that are physically active have less incidence of the symptoms and early deaths associated with heart disease. Current research in the area of cardiac rehabilitation certainly places aerobic exercise programs firmly into the therapeutic program.

The contribution of regular exercise, particularly weight-bearing activities, to healthy bone formation was emphasized by NASA studies on the effects of space flight and weightlessness on bone remodeling. Now we include daily weight-bearing exercise routines in management of osteoporosis.

Regular, moderate physical activity and endurance training are becoming part of management of both Type I and Type II diabetes, chronic obstructive pulmonary disease, obesity, anorexia nervosa, chronic pain syndrome, Parkinson's disease, multiple sclerosis, and arthritis.

In addition to these well-documented physiological benefits of regular exercise and fitness, we are now becoming more aware of the psychological benefits of exercise and fitness programs. Light- to moderate-intensity exercise in the form of walking, when measured by electromyography, has been shown to reduce muscle tension more than muscle-relaxant medication (deVries, 1986). Walk/jog and running programs are common in the treatment of depression and anxiety states and appear to be associated with measurable benefits in a number of studies. There are several theories concerning the mechanisms that are involved. Some believe that depression is a movement disorder, and a direct intervention is improving movement through exercise. Others believe that the effect is gained through the exercise-induced release of neurotransmitters such as norepinephrine, dopamine, and serotonin. Still another theory is the increase in cerebral blood flow that occurs with exercise. Improvements in self-esteem and self-concept with participation in exercise programs have been noted as well, although these have not been consistent findings.

The sense of well-being that many exercisers describe is a phenomenon still under study. The release of endorphins by the brain appears to be stimulated by physical exercise. Endorphins are natural morphine-like substances believed to be partly responsible for a range of psychological states associated with vigorous exercise including general feelings of well-being or "runner's high," exercise euphoria, and exercise addiction.

SUMMARY

This chapter has examined physiological factors which influence human performance from the standpoint of physical fitness. Cardiorespiratory function, considered in terms of the efficiency with which the oxygen demands of working muscles are met, can limit the frequency, intensity and duration of activity engagement. Isometric and isotonic muscle strength are also necessary for daily activities, respectively serving postural and stability requirements and providing forces needed in joint motion. Flexibility at joints is an additional factor which influences activity and task performance, while muscle endurance is necessary to sustain effort. In addition to the factors which are directly related to movement; body composition, considered as the proportion of fat and lean elements of the body, affects fitness through several mechanisms. These include modifying energy requirements and determining the amount of muscle tissue available to perform activity.

Certain conditions and circumstances diminish fitness, including immobilization and inactivity. These conditions can work in conjunction with the physiological changes accompanying aging and disease to more greatly limit performance. The general principles of exercise and fitness should be considered in planning intervention programs. An understanding of fatigue, including how it can be recognized and avoided through economy of effort, is also important to therapists. Finally, while physiological factors and their effect on fitness and the ability to perform daily occupations have been highlighted in this chapter, their influence on performance must be viewed in the context of other factors, such as psychosocial variables. This is in keeping with the general systems perspective of this book.

Study Questions

1. Describe the five components of health-related physical fitness. How is physical fitness applicable to clinical assessment?

2. Why is cardiorespiratory fitness important? What are the effects of prolonged inactivity on cardiorespiratory fitness?

3. Discuss the aging versus inactivity question in relation to muscle strength and muscle endurance.

4. Can human performance be accurately predicted by objective measurements of physiologic performance? Why or why not?

5. Describe some of the manifestations of prolonged bed rest.

6. What is meant by the principle of overload?

7. Describe some of the clinical manifestations of fatigue.

References

American College of Sports Medicine. (1986). *Guideline for exercise testing and prescription*. 3rd edition. Philadelphia: Lea and Febiger.

Andersen, K.L., Rutenfranz, J., Masironi, R., et al. (1978). *Habitual physical activity and health*. Copenhagen: World Health Organization.

Atkins, C.J., Kaplan, R.M., Timms, R.M., et al. (1984). Behavioral exercise programs in the management of chronic obstructive pulmonary disease. *Journal of Consulting and Clinical Psychology, 52*, 591-603.

Brooks, G.A., & Fahey, T.D. (1984). *Exercise physiology: Human bioenergetics and its applications*. New York: John Wiley and Sons.

Byers, P.H. (1985). Effect of exercise on morning stiffness and mobility in patients with rheumatoid arthritis. *Research in Nursing and Health, 8*, 275-281.

deVries, H.A. (1980). *Physiology of exercise for physical education and athletics*. 3rd edition. Dubuque, Iowa: William C. Brown.

deVries, H.A. (1981). Tranquilizer effect of exercise: A critical review. *The Physician and Sports Medicine, 9*(11), 47-55.

Donatelli, R., & Owens-Burkhart, H. (1981). Effects of immobilization on the extensibility of periarticular connective tissue. *Journal of Sport and Physical Training, 3*, 67-72.

Franklin, B.A., Pamatmat, A., Johnson, S., et al. (1983). Metabolic cost of extremely slow walking in cardiac patients: Implications for exercise testing and training. *Archives of Physical Medicine and Rehabilitation, 64*, 564-565.

Kottke, F.J. (1966). The effects of limitation of activity upon the human body. *Journal of the American Medical Association, 196*, 117-122.

Lamb, D.R. (1984). *Physiology of exercise responses and adaptations*. New York: MacMillan Publishing Company.

Lawrence, R.M. (1983). Psychological aspects of exercise. In A.A. Bove & D.T. Lowenthal (eds.), *Exercise medicine, physiological principles and clinical applications*. New York: Academic Press.

Luttgens, K., & Wells, K.F. (1982). *Kinesiology: Scientific basis of human motion*. 7th edition. New York: CBS College Publishing.

McArdle, W.D., Katch, F.I., & Katch, V.L. (1986). *Exercise physiology, energy, nutrition and human performance*. 2nd edition. Philadelphia: Lea and Febiger.

Noble, B.J., Borg, G.A.V., Jacobs, I., et al. (1983). A category-ratio perceived exertion scale: Relationship to blood and muscle lactates and heart rate. *Medical Science and Sports Exercise, 15*, 523-528.

Pollock, M.L., Wilmore, J.H., & Fox, S.M. (1984). *Exercise in health and disease: evaluation and prescription for prevention and rehabilitation*. Philadelphia, PA: W.B. Saunders.

Sandler, H., & Vernikos, J. (eds.) (1986). *Inactivity: Physiological effects*. Orlando, FL: Academic Press.

Sharkey, B.J. (1984). *Physiology of fitness*. 2nd edition. Champaign, IL: Human Kinetics Publishers, Inc.

Shephard, R.J. (1978). *Physical activity and aging*. Great Britain: Crooms Helm Ltd., Publishers.

Smith, E.L., & Gilligan, C. (1983). Physical activity prescription for the older adult. *Physical Sports Medicine, 11,* 91-101.

Valbona, C. (1982). Bodily responses to immobilization. In *Krusen's handbook of physical medicine and rehabilitation.* 3rd edition. Philadelphia, PA: W.B. Saunders.

Weg, R.B. (1983). Changing physiology of aging. In D.S. Woodruff & J.E. Birren (eds.), *Aging, scientific perspectives and social issues.* 2nd edition. Monterey, CA: Brooks/Cole Publishing Company.

Winnick, J.P., & Short, F.X. (1985). *Physical fitness testing of the disabled.* Champaign, IL: Human Kinetics Publishers, Inc.

CHAPTER CONTENT OUTLINE

Sensation Effects Performance

Development and Functions of
Sensory Systems

Evolution of Sensory Systems

The Sensory Systems

Role of Arousal and Attention in
Sensory Processing

Summary

KEY TERMS

Autogenic facilitation

Autogenic inhibition

Balance of power

Centrifugal control

**Compensatory action of the
nervous system**

Convergence

Corporal potentiality

Divergence

Multidimensional map

Plasticity

Release phenomenon

Sensory registration

Suppression

Threshold

Tonotopic

Topographic

ABSTRACT

Sensation is a critical factor in the performance of human activities and tasks
necessary in daily life. Motor systems rely heavily on information from sensory
systems to help individuals effectively respond to the environment. This chapter
investigates the development and functions of each of the sensory systems
(gustatory, olfactory, somatosensory, vestibular, auditory, visual,
proprioceptive) and the role of arousal and attention in sensory processing.

Sensory Dimensions of Performance

9

Winnie Dunn

"How do you know anything about your world? . . . The answer is through your senses. In fact, without your senses of vision, hearing, touch, taste, and smell, your brain — the organ that is responsible for your conscious experience — would be an eternal prisoner in the solitary confinement of your skull. . . . In fact, the minds of all living, thinking organisms are prisoners that must rely on information smuggled into them by the senses. Your world is what your senses tell you it is. The limitations of your senses set the boundaries of your conscious existence. Because our knowledge of the world depends on our senses, it is important to know how our senses function. Such faith in our senses is built into the very fabric of our lives . . . "

—Coren, Porac, & Ward, 1984

OBJECTIVES

The information in this chapter is intended to help the reader—

1. appreciate the importance of sensation in the performance of life tasks.

2. identify basic neurological mechanisms which support sensory processing, such as centrifugal control, balance of cellular actions, intersensory integration, plasticity and compensatory actions.

3. understand the critical relationship between sensory processing and motor performance.

4. review the development and specific functions of gustatory, olfactory somatosensory, vestibular, auditory, visual, and proprioceptive sensory systems.

5. identify similarities in function among sensory systems as well as unique characteristics of specific systems.

6. understand the role of arousal and attention in sensory processing.

7. explain why the loss of even one sensory system can affect individual performance.

8. understand the concepts of arousal/alerting and discrimination/mapping.

SENSATION EFFECTS PERFORMANCE

The purpose of this chapter is to explore the functions of the sensory systems as intrinsic components necessary for adequate performance of activities and tasks in our lives. Sensation is the conduit through which environmental information reaches the central nervous system (CNS) giving us data to form accurate and reliable maps of ourselves and our environment. We rely on these maps to remind us how task performance has occurred in the past and to develop skills to adapt performance to future demands.

Sensation is a critical prerequisite to normal human performance. As the quotation introducing this chapter suggests, sensation provides the mechanism for introducing the organism to its environment. Each sensation provides a unique point of view about the environment for the brain's benefit. Some of the sensory mechanisms are focused on providing information about the internal environment of the body. Other senses focus their attention on external environmental variables. Still other sensory mechanisms seem to be responsible for developing and maintaining appropriate interaction between the map of the environment and the map the individual has constructed of self.

This dynamic interaction of the various sensory systems forms a complete picture of self and environment which enables people to remain correctly oriented and to respond to task demands in an appropriate way (Bischof, 1974). From a neurological point of view, disorientation seems to be the result of poor interaction of the sensory inputs which results in the brain being unable to tell whether the body or the environment is the source of the stimulation (Bischof, 1974). Although sensations may seem more simple and discrete early in the developmental process, "It is important to recognize that in the course of everyday life motions to which the (organism) is exposed are complex . . . " (Benson, 1974, p. 283). Pure sensation from one sensory system is not likely to occur during normal human activity. As the various sensory systems gather information simultaneously, a multidimensional view of the body in the environment evolves. Bischof (1974) states that this accumulation of life experience reduces the individual's chances for making errors in decisions about perceptual events because equivalent messages can be compared before decisions are made about appropriate responses to stimuli. If only one sensation was available to an individual, their perception of the environment would be unidimensional and would lack the depth and dimension necessary for normal task performance.

For example, if the visual system was the only available sensation, it would be like living on the page of a *Better Homes and Gardens* magazine. Although there would be a rich visual environment with colors and contrast, the environment would provide a flat, unidimensional view of objects within the picture. Without other sensations at work, we would not be able to perceive textures such as a soft couch or the warmth of a glowing fire that might be in the picture. In essence, we would lack a full understanding of the environment. We understand the depth and texture of objects in the visual environment through other sensory experiences. As is seen in clinical practice, the lack of accuracy from one sensory system can seriously distort the individual's ability to perform life tasks efficiently. These individuals are responding to the environment with distorted information that is causing their performance to appear strange or different when compared to a standard of performance which responds to accurate information.

In practice, therapists often rely on observation of motor performance to monitor both present and changing status as the therapeutic process proceeds. Although there are discrete motor dysfunctions, many outward signs of motor inefficiency are related to dysfunction or difficulty with the receipt and processing of sensory information. "All parts of the motor system receive sensory messages directly or indirectly so that their neurons respond to vestibular, somatosensory, visual, or auditory stimuli similar to the neurons in sensory areas" (Kornhuber, 1974, p. 582). As will be discussed, the motor systems are heavily reliant on information from their sensory partners in order to produce effective responses to the environment. Further, as we will see, the motor systems are intimately connected neurologically with the sensory systems, forming a sensory-perceptual-motor relationship (Gilfoyle, Grady, & Moore, 1981; Guedry, 1974).

Actually, there are only three mechanisms through which the central nervous system can manifest itself: 1) the autonomic nervous system (ANS), 2) the motor output systems, and 3) the emotional/affective circuits which most frequently are manifested through autonomic and motor behaviors. Each of these output mechanisms relies heavily on sensory input from the internal or external environments to determine appropriate action. The dilemma in clinical practice is that without the use of invasive procedures to quantitatively record from electrodes at sensory neurons, clinicians must rely on observable behaviors to assist them in determining the effectiveness of therapeutic intervention. The error that is frequently made is to conclude that the problem always lies in the output system that produces the observable performance. Clinicians must become astute observers so they can clearly distinguish the differences between motor output difficulties and sensory processing difficulties in the same behaviors. Often these differences are subtle.

Not only motor performance, but perceptual, cognitive, and language functions are judged by observing outward behavior. Judgments must be made not only about the output itself but also about the input and internal mechanisms that are enabling that performance to occur (Hermelin & O'Connor, 1970). Several authors hypothesize that some psychiatric, social, and behavioral problems can be linked to a failure to accurately process incoming sensory information (Ayres, 1985; deQuiros & Schrager, 1978; Hermelin & O'Connor, 1970).

Research Models

Studies on sensory deprivation, sensory enrichment, and the sensory environment of high-risk infants have provided models from which one can hypothesize about the strong effects of sensation on performance and behavior. For example, men and women placed in environments that are devoid of sensation tend to hallucinate or attempt to recapture the sensation (Cotman & McGaugh, 1980; *Mind and Behavior*, 1980). In studies done on infant monkeys, deprivation of mother's touch has led to significant changes in the anatomical, physiological, and the behavioral systems (Coren, Porac, & Ward, 1984). Rosenzweig, Bennett, and Diamond (1972) conducted the classic animal studies on sensory enrichment. Rats in enriched, stimulating environments not only demonstrated more complex outward behaviors, they also developed more complex brain structures, as seen in postmortem examinations. Another study showed that although specific species of birds are disposed genetically to certain song patterns, the birds must be exposed to them in order to correctly develop the capability to sing (Cotman & McGaugh, 1980).

Studies of high-risk infants demonstrate that they survive and thrive better when provided with a controlled sensory environment than when they are completely isolated from sensory experiences. It appears that during periods of early development, the central nervous system is vulnerable and cannot adapt to random bombardment of stimuli. Therefore caregivers must provide the appropriate amount and type of

sensory experience to maximize positive response and outcome from the infants (Oehler, 1985).

A full-term newborn's first actions in the environment are responses to sensory stimulation. Many of the early reflexes are the result of touch and motion (Barnes, Crutchfield, & Heriza, 1984). These reflexes enable the organism to begin to respond to the environment in appropriate ways. As the individual grows and develops higher order control over motor interactions with the environment, sensations also become more complex because a wider array of experiences become available to the individual. The sensory systems must continually adapt to this changing environment to keep the brain apprised of the organism's status within its environment.

Clinical Implications

As individuals grow to adulthood, adult behavior is based on the ability to monitor the sensory experiences that constantly are occurring and decide which are the most important to respond to at any given moment. Judgments are made about the adequacy of our behavior based on our ability to appropriately choose the sensations to which we must attend and respond. People are judged abnormal or inefficient within their environment based upon any one of the following criteria: 1) if they do not choose the appropriate stimuli to respond to, 2) if they cannot attend to the stimuli long enough to make an appropriate response, or 3) if their neurological mechanisms do not enable them to receive or interpret the available information in a way that will produce an appropriate response. The challenge to the occupational therapist is to identify the subtle signs that will lead to diminished performance so that both direct intervention techniques and adaptations to life environments can maximize independence. The more frequently an individual has access to accurate and reliable sensory information, the more likely it is that the individual will develop functional occupational roles.

DEVELOPMENT AND FUNCTIONS OF SENSORY SYSTEMS

Before beginning a discussion of specific sensory systems and how they function, it is important for the reader to understand basic neurological principles that support the normal processing of sensation. These principles are important for occupational therapists to understand because they subserve all the functions of the central nervous system. By knowing these principles the occupational therapist can organize activities that are compatible with the way that the central nervous system functions, thus maximizing their effects on the client's performance outcomes. If unaware of these principles of central nervous system actions, the occupational therapist can develop activities that appear appropriate on the surface, but that do not maximize the responsiveness of the central nervous system itself.

Centrifugal Control

The first and most basic principle of central nervous system activity is the principle of **centrifugal control**, which is the brain's ability to regulate its own input. This principle is critical because it demonstrates the power of the central nervous system to ensure that the information received is the most valuable for its own function. Four types of centrifugal control will be discussed here: **suppression**, the **balance of power**, **divergence**, and **convergence** (Noback & Demarest, 1987).

Suppression. Suppression is the ability of the central nervous system to screen out certain stimuli so that others may be attended to more carefully. Normally we are constantly bombarded with an array of sensory stimuli. Through suppression the brain determines which stimuli warrant a response and which stimuli can be ignored safely. A common behavioral problem that appears with poor suppression is distractibility. People have a difficult time engaging in purposeful behavior because they are constantly distracted by other stimuli available in the environment. Another type of problem with suppression is an inability to screen out the appropriate stimuli for behavioral demands. If the wrong stimuli are screened out or if they are screened out in a rigid, ritualistic pattern, rather than in response to environmental demands, inappropriate or even dangerous situations can occur.

Balance of Power. The balance of power in the central nervous system refers to the complementary functions of the various parts of the brain. For example, certain parts of the brain are in charge of responding to arousal stimuli and increasing the activity level of the brain, whereas other parts of the brain are responsible for providing inhibitory control over those arousal centers. Some parts of the brain are responsible for initiating movement and other parts are responsible for stopping or controlling the amount of movement that occurs. In a normally functioning nervous system, there is a balance of power for all functions. This balance of power enables the central nervous system to finely tune responses and to produce the amount of response that will meet the environmental demand without being either overly responsive or unresponsive.

When the balance of power is upset in the central nervous system it is described as a **release phenomenon**. For example, frequently when there is brain damage in higher cortical centers, we see a release of the arousal mechanisms, resulting in hyperactivity or distractibility. These behaviors are not the result of dysfunction in the reticular activating system per se, but rather represent an unleashing of the arousal and activating mechanisms from the control usually provided by modulating centers. The reticular cells can continue activity without the inhibitory counterpart to balance this activity and keep it within the normal range. The release phenomenon can occur in any part of the central nervous system and can occur in relation to any function. Many of the abnormal behaviors observed and documented by occupational therapists can be attributed to a release phenomenon, or poor maintenance of the balance of power in the central nervous system.

Divergence. Divergence is the ability of the brain to send information it receives from one source to many parts of the central nervous system simultaneously. For example, if the brain receives a stimulus signalling potential harm, it would be important for that information to get to many areas simultaneously so that a "fight or flight response" could be generated. Divergence would also be important in the motor system to ensure that an entire muscle is engaged in action when a movement is required, rather than a small number of muscle fibers.

Convergence. Convergence is another mechanism of centrifugal control. Convergent neurons are those that require input from a variety of sources before a response will be generated. For example, a specific neuron may activate only if it receives three or more types of input. Convergent neurons enable the central nervous system to temper responsiveness to specific stimuli. The following is an oversimplified example to illustrate the importance of convergent cells:

> You are standing and hear a very loud and angry voice in back of you yell your name. With this sound, the auditory system might send a signal to prepare you for a "fight or flight response." Then you feel someone place a hand on your shoulder from behind and the somatosensory system also signals potential harm. Finally, when you turn and see that the individual is a friend who was teasing you with the gruff voice, the visual system provides more information to help you conclude that this is not a dangerous situation.

Because the three stimuli did not match in the above situation, convergent cells would not activate and, therefore, would enable the person to keep behavior within normal limits. Convergent cells can prevent a person from reacting inappropriately to partial stimuli available in the environment. Without this convergent neuronal network, the individual would respond to every stimulus. A person who is overly responsive to stimuli in the environment may have poor integration of the convergent neuronal network.

Balance of Excitation and Inhibition

Another basic principle of nervous system action is the balance of excitation and inhibition in the central nervous system. *Excitation* is the depolarization of neurons that moves them closer to the activation **threshold**, whereas *inhibition* is the hyperpolarization of neurons that makes it more difficult for the neurons to activate. We will consider a variety of types of excitation and inhibition.

Excitation. Excitation can occur in both temporal and spatial patterns. Temporal patterns are those that occur over time. Temporal summation would occur when a neuron is repeatedly stimulated, enabling the neuron to either be slowly depolarized or to continue sending a message over and over again such as is required to maintain muscle tone for postural control. Spatial neuron patterns are those that occur simultaneously over many areas of the brain at the same time. The repeated use of the neuron (temporal) is not as important as the use of many neurons at the same time (spatial) to engage the central nervous system components. Spatial summation is necessary to notice a sound, recognize it as a baby's cry, decide the baby is hungry, and proceed to fill that need.

Inhibition. Inhibition is the ability of the central nervous system to decrease its responsiveness to specific stimuli at any given moment. Although neuroscientists frequently discuss descending inhibition (higher centers having an effect on lower centers), the sensory systems are rich with interneuron networks within the sensory receptor areas that can inhibit neighboring cells; this is called *lateral inhibition*. This inhibitory field serves to make the target stimulus clearer and stronger. Lateral inhibition is very important for the accurate receipt and organization of sensory input.

Excitation and inhibition also encompass two other characteristics, those of feed-forward and feedback mechanisms.

Feedback and Feed-Forward Mechanisms. Feedback is the ability of the central nervous system to send information back to itself as a check and balance. Feedback allows an individual to judge whether actions already initiated need to be modified and to store the outcomes in memory for future reference. Noback & Demarest (1981) describe two general types of feedback: local feedback and reflected feedback. *Local feedback* inhibition occurs when small interneurons within a neighboring circuit form connections that stop a stimulus that has been occurring in a large neuron. This mechanism helps keep activity from continuing beyond its

useful period. For example, a local feedback circuit can stop the ongoing firing of a motor neuron by sending an inhibitory signal to the motor nerve, thus allowing a person to relax the muscle and stop the movement. But this inhibition occurs only if the local circuit neuron information is stronger than other messages on that large motor neuron. *Reflected feedback* occurs when higher centers of the central nervous system send descending fibers to influence the sensory or motor neurons. These higher centers can send excitatory or inhibitory messages making it either easier or more difficult to activate the neurons.

Feed-forward circuits exert influence in a forward direction coinciding with the information flow of the neurons. This most frequently occurs in ascending sensory systems to either alert higher centers about incoming information or inhibit some areas in order to strengthen the focus of more important parts of the environmental stimuli. Feed-forward inhibition is critical for task performance, because people always are confronted with more stimuli than are needed to complete the task successfully.

Intersensory Integration. Intersensory integration is a critical feature of the action of the central nervous system. There are interneurons in the spinal cord that participate in primitive intersensory integration, but the brain stem is a primary site for this activity. Several nuclei in the brain stem receive input from several sensory sources. This allows organization and integration of information at this low level of the central nervous system. For example, the vestibular nuclei receive input not only from the vestibular organ, but also from the visual system and proprioceptors. Intersensory integration allows the individual to develop a **multidimensional map** of self and environment and a map of how self and environment interact appropriately.

Plasticity

Plasticity is the ability of the central nervous system to adapt structurally or functionally in response to environmental demands. In the past, it was thought that plasticity was the most evident during the prenatal stage and during childhood, but now researchers are studying the effects of plasticity in other realms, for example the possibilities of axon regrowth in the central nervous system. Other investigations are directed at various types of internal and external environmental alterations that support or inhibit the manifestation of plasticity (Lund, 1978). It is likely that such findings will have a large impact on rehabilitation practices. For example, when individuals participate in treatment that requires more functional patterns of movement, they receive organized patterns of sensory feedback as well. It may be hypothesized that this sensory feedback alters the internal environment, creating opportunities for axon reorganization, altered synaptic activity, or dendritic branching, just as an enriched environment supports these actions during the developmental process. This theory might also support early initiation of activities in order to "force" the system to adapt and accomodate (Bach-y-Rita, 1980; Moore, 1980).

Compensatory Action of the Nervous System

The parts of the central nervous system are interdependent. This concept is described by Josephine Moore (1980). When damage occurs to one or more portions of the system, the interdependency relationships are disrupted; the resulting observable behaviors and performance are hypothesized to be compensating for the loss of information from one of its members. This compensatory model suggests, for example, that the basal ganglia do not function on their own to initiate action, but the basal ganglia network along with other parts of the central nervous system may be what enables initiation of action to occur. When the basal ganglia data are not available to the system because of damage, the network is disrupted, making it difficult for initiation of action to occur. What we observe is the result of an incomplete and compensating nervous system.

Knowledge of the basic principles of the central nervous system function will enable an occupational therapist to establish baseline parameters and develop both treatment activities and environmental alterations that will maximize the individual's ability to respond to intervention. These basic principles form the foundation for further understanding of the sensory systems.

EVOLUTION OF SENSORY SYSTEMS

Studies report on the development of myelin in various central nervous systems and the relationship between these events and behavioral observations. Because the presence of myelin on a nerve cell significantly increases its efficiency, knowing when it is established in each system is helpful for accurate interpretation of performance. Researchers record the time when the myelin pattern observed in the developing organism matches adult patterns of myelination. Yakovlev and LeCours (1967) and Langworthy (1933) provide a wealth of information relating myelin patterns to emerging behaviors and structural development.

Figure 9-1 illustrates the onset and course of myelination of various sensory and motor systems (Moore, 1980; Moore, 1987). From this figure, one can see that there are many interrelationships among systems during the formation of myelin. Myelinated systems are often preferred modes of input, perhaps because this information travels more efficiently to its destinations. Clinicians who work with people during the early stages of development can profit from the association between myelination and performance capabilities. For example, the myelin of the trigeminal nerve, which is responsible for sensation of the face and head, is laid down very early in development, thus making sensory experiences to the face very powerful. This might provide one explanation why infants put most objects toward the face or in the mouth during early periods of development.

Gottlieb (1983) notes that information regarding the onset and course of sensory system development is very significant to program development. He comments that this knowledge "supports the concept of cross-modal competence" (p. 20). Because tactile sensitivity develops early while the visual system develops late, Gottlieb hypothesizes that tactile experiences can influence the way the visual system will respond as it develops. The later-developing systems may rely on the maps that have been laid down by the earlier-developing systems for orientation and reference. Because meaning already has been established in the early-developing systems, this meaning can perhaps set the parameters for the interpretation of information from the later-developing systems. Evidence of these hypotheses can be seen in the actions of both children and adults. When presented with a new experience or task, adults frequently rely on more established memories for interpretation, and children continue to use movement and touch to explore objects long after they have developed efficient use of the visual and auditory systems. People often describe new events in terms of how they feel, smell, or taste. So we see that although the images in the mind are often thought of as visual, they frequently are made up of other sensory components.

Those who work with children can take advantage of this knowledge to establish an approach that acknowledges the role of myelinated neurons in efficient processing of sensory input and motor output. As Gottlieb (1983) suggests, use of tactile experiences can lay the groundwork for the pattern of visual and auditory responsivity later on. When planning intervention strategies for adults, therapists must consider the prior sensory relationships that are likely to already have been established. For example, if the therapist knows some details about the routines and interests of the client, the therapist may gain access to multidimensional sensory and motor memories by stimulating intact mechanisms within familiar routines and environmental conditions. Perhaps this is one reason why some individuals recover function more successfully in their own homes.

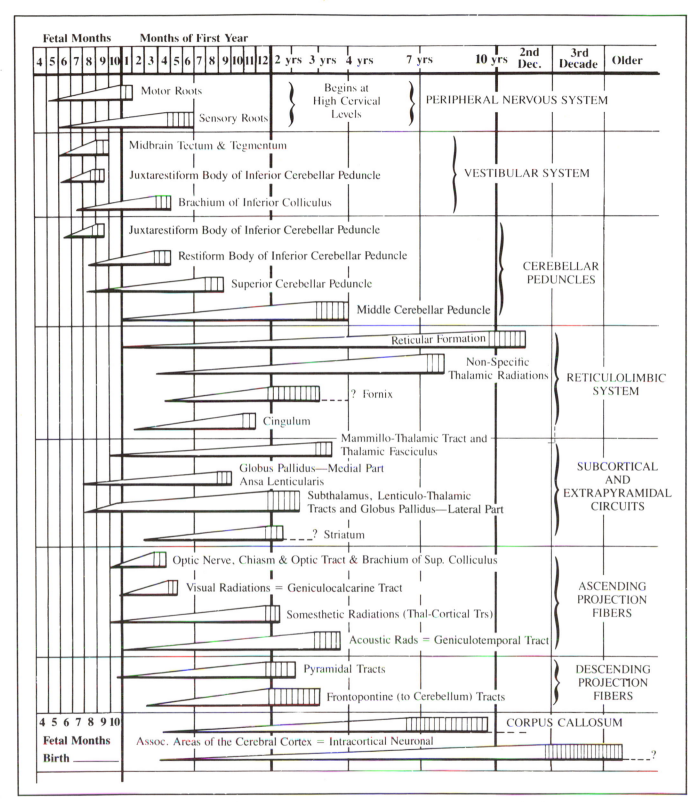

Figure 9-1. Myelogenesis of the Nervous System. *Adapted from Yakoylev, PA and LeCours, AR. "The Myelogenetic cycles of regional maturation of the brain." In Minkowski, A (1967). Regional development of the brain in early life. pp. 3-30. Oxford, England: Blackwell Scientific Publications, Ltd. Reprinted with permission of Josephine Moore, PhD, OTR, who designed this adaptation of this chart.*

SIMILARITIES AMONG SENSORY SYSTEMS

Although each sensory system is unique, there are some basic similarities in the way all sensory systems develop and function:

1. Each sensory system is responsible for bringing information from the environment to the nervous system for processing.
2. Each sensory system processes its own special brand of information at a variety of central nervous system levels, including the receptor site, spinal cord, brain stem, thalamus (except for olfactory), and higher cortical centers.
3. The sensation from each sensory system is complex and multidimensional.
4. Each sensory system processes information for two primary purposes: a) identifying stimuli in the environment, making the central nervous system aware of these stimuli, determining which require attention and which are potentially harmful (arousal or alerting mechanisms) and b) gathering information to construct maps of self and environment to be used by the central nervous system for organization and planning (discrimination or mapping).

In the normally functioning organism, the arousal/alerting and discrimination/mapping components complement each other to form a balance of power. This allows the individual to interact with the environment and gather information for discrimination and mapping under most conditions, while always having the capability to notice potentially harmful stimuli. This balance of power is a delicate one, requiring constant assessment of environmental stimuli so that all potentially important stimuli are noticed without interfering with ongoing purposeful activity. The components of arousal and mapping will be discussed with each sensory system.

THE SENSORY SYSTEMS

This section will introduce the specific actions of all of the primary sensory systems. The olfactory (smell) system and gustatory (taste) system are primitive, chemically-based sensory systems signaling the central nervous system about odors and taste. The somatosensory, proprioceptive, and vestibular systems enable an individual to develop an accurate map of self and how one interacts with the environment. Finally, the visual and auditory systems are responsible for mapping environmental variables so that interaction with the environment can be accurate and reliable.

The Gustatory System

The gustatory system is responsible for our sense of taste. Early in evolution, the differentiation between the gustatory and olfactory systems was minor because primitive organisms lived in the sea. When early organisms moved to the land to live, these two systems differentiated to serve the organism in very different ways. The gustatory system became the final checking system for food that was to enter the body, whereas the olfactory system became the chemical sense that could determine the location or direction of stimuli (e.g., food or predators) from a distance. The olfactory system became important for mapping the environment for survival (Coren, Porac, & Ward, 1984). From a neuroanatomical standpoint, senses of smell and taste travel by very different routes to inform the cerebral cortex about environmental events.

The taste of items that we place in our mouths is determined by their solubility, intensity, and amount. Authors generally agree that there are four basic taste qualities that can be labelled with language: sweet, salty, sour, and bitter (Coren, Porac, & Ward, 1984). They are discriminated both by the types of molecules found and by the way they are broken down by the chemicals within the system. The taste buds are the receptor organs for the gustatory system. There are as many as 10,000 taste buds available to young people; this amount decreases during the aging process.

Gustatory information travels from the sensory receptors in the tongue to portions of the brain stem where the information is relayed to the thalamus. The thalamus is responsible for sending the information to the appropriate location on the somatosensory cortex, which maps the mouth and tongue. Additionally, gustatory information reaches both the hypothalamus and the cortical taste area in the inferior frontal gyrus. The hypothalamus connections are important because of their believed contributions to feeding behaviors which drive the organism to ingest food (Bellingham, Wayner, & Barone, 1979). The cortical taste area is closely related to the sensory homunculus in the parietal lobe and enables us not only to have an accurate map of the tongue in the mouth but also to allow conscious sensation of taste (Heimer, 1983). Because taste is part of the cranial nerve network, its functions are jeopardized by brain stem trauma.

The characteristic taste patterns of the tongue have been mapped by many authors. Although the separation of function is important from a neuroscience standpoint, from a functional standpoint the overall appeal of food is the major consideration. An individual's responses to taste are very unique and seem to rely not only on experiential information but also on the genetic make-up of the individual. Some researchers have reported groups of people as being immune to tastes for certain substances. One of these substances is caffeine. Studies have shown that there are those who taste caffeine and those who do not (Blakeslee & Salmon, 1935; Coren, Porac, & Ward, 1984; Hall, Bartoshuk, Cain, & Stevens, 1975). From testing various substances, researchers hypothesize that there is a genetic mechanism that either allows or does not allow responsiveness to specific chemical changes that the substances produce.

Because of the deterioration process with aging, elderly persons often complain about blandness of food. Helpern and Meiselman (1980) found that salting food is in part a person's attempt to reach their specific threshold for taste. Recovery from stimulation in the gustatory system occurs within ten seconds after the stimulus, so a slower eating process or a process of mixing bites of salty food with bites of unsalty food is likely to produce less continuous seasoning of food during the meal.

Olfactory Sense

The olfactory system responds to odors in the environment. The process of smell is a complicated one, beginning with the intake of substances by the olfactory epithelium in the top portion of the nasal cavity. There are some unique features of the olfactory pathways that point out important functional differences from other sensory mechanisms. The first difference is seen in the two-neuron circuit that transmits information from the olfactory receptor sites into the central nervous system; other sensory systems require three neurons to reach central connections. Second, the internal cells of the olfactory system project directly to portions of higher centers and bypass the thalamus, unlike all other sensory systems.

The olfactory system is a very sensitive system, even more sensitive than its chemical counterpart, the gustatory system. However, unlike the taste system, researchers have been unable to discover basic categories of smell. It appears that the system is so complex and capable of responding to so many types of odors, that classification becomes extremely difficult.

Humans tend to underrate the role and effects of the olfactory system on performance and functioning in daily life. With specific connections to the limbic system, the olfactory system has the potential to establish memories and associations of our roles as children and adults. Olfactory stimulation can trigger memories of events that have occurred in recent or distant past. These memories are very specific to each individual's life experience and so may not be comparable between individuals. Because of the direct connections with arousal networks, the olfactory input also can increase our level of responsiveness quickly. Use of strong odors to arouse

people in semi-comatose states points out the powerful role of olfactory input.

Clinicians must remain aware of this sensory system in the planning and provision of services. Because individuals emit specific odors themselves, persons may recognize their therapist not only from visual, auditory, and somatosensory cues, but also from olfactory cues. This may be one factor that contributes to disorientation and agitation when substitutions occur. Additionally, therapists must be very careful about the additions of odors such as shampoos, perfumes, and laundry detergents. Although these factors go unnoticed by the normally functioning nervous system, a vulnerable system may react in unpredictable ways. Competent therapists consider all possibilities when unusual behaviors present themselves; observable behavior provides a window to central nervous system activity.

Olfactory input is also important in the environments where persons are served. The sterile environment of the hospital provides a type of olfactory sensory deprivation (Moore, 1980). In the familiar home environment, the olfactory system can contribute to orientation by noticing familiar odors.

Often clients who have difficulty with the olfactory system begin to complain about the taste of foods. Even though the smell of foods does not contribute directly to their taste, people seem to associate the smell of food with the taste. Because both taste and smell relate to individuals' food preferences, therapists should be cautious regarding interpretations of food complaints.

Somatosensory System

The somatosensory system responds to stimuli from the surface of the skin and neighboring tissues. Because of the unique placement of these receptors, one can characterize this system as being responsible for telling where the body ends and where the world begins. Somatosensory receptors continue to be the object of much research. The map of one's body is comprised of many types of stimuli. Receptor thresholds are partially determined by the structure of the receptor end organ itself and partially by its placement within the skin layers. The Pacinian corpuscle, for example, has been studied the most frequently. It is a capsular structure in which the nerve ending is surrounded by several layers of connective tissue. This receptor is very deep in the skin layers. Because of the placement and structure, it seems to be a rapidly adapting receptor that responds to pressure on the skin.

The combined input from various somatosensory receptors forms a multidimensional picture of skin stimulation. Receptive fields also contribute to multidimensional maps; a receptive field is the location on the surface of the skin that is innervated by one neuron.

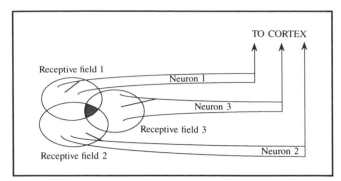

Figure 9-2a. Three overlapping receptor fields send information to the cortex. This shared information helps localize the touch sensation.

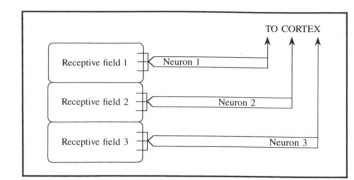

Figure 9-2b. Three receptive fields that do not overlap. Separate pieces of information make it difficult to determine exactly where the touch occurred.

Accurate somatosensory perception requires not only that the receptive fields function accurately, but that they function in concert with each other. If one were to isolate a somatosensory neuron, one could identify the skin surface (receptive field) that this neuron serves. The receptive fields overlap a great deal on the head, hands, and arms (Figure 9-2a), whereas on the back the receptive fields overlap very little (Figure 9-2b). This is functionally significant because human beings identify the exact location of the touch experience on body surfaces that have overlapping receptive fields, but can only identify the general area being touched when the receptive fields are discrete. When a specific place is touched on the forearm, hand, or face, the various neurons from several receptive fields that share that location report information to the brain simultaneously. Multiple input from various sources enables the brain to narrow the possible locations until it can identify the one spot on the surface of the skin that is shared by all of the activated neurons.

When the receptors send information to the central nervous system, the neurons travel into the spinal cord to ascend to higher centers (See Figure 9-3). In certain ascending pathways of the somatosensory system, synapses occur immediately upon entrance to the spinal cord, while others travel to the brain stem before their first synapse occurs (See Figure 9-4). Traditionally, the posterior columns have been characterized as the pathways for touch-pressure and proprioception, whereas the lateral spinothalamic pathways have been considered responsible for light touch, pain, and temperature reception. Recent evidence suggests that a broader view of somatosensory processing is required to interpret clinical observations accurately. It is common when studying brain systems, to attempt to explain the very complex actions of the central nervous system in an oversimplified way. As research techniques and technology become more sophisticated, scientists and practitioners gain knowledge and achieve a

better understanding of the complexity of the central nervous system.

Heimer (1983) reports that the ascending sensory pathways can be divided into three categories.

1. The first category is the *anterolateral system*. This is located in the anterior (front) and side portions of the spinal cord and appears to be responsible for processing of pain and temperature information. This includes the spinothalamic tract, which is traditionally named as the pain and temperature pathway, and the spinoreticular and spinotectal tracts. Because they are very closely related anatomically, damage to one often involves damage to the others as well.

   The anterolateral pathways synapse at the spinal cord level that corresponds to the receptor input location, the second neuron crosses over to travel in the anterior or lateral aspect of the spinal cord to the thalamus, and then to the sensorimotor cortex. Collateral fibers synapse with the reticular cells in the brain stem en route to the thalamus. The spinoreticular tract also synapses in the reticular cells of the brain stem. Reticular connections are important when examining the characteristics of arousal.

2. The second category includes pathways for touch-pressure, vibration, and proprioception. Although the *dorsal columns* have been seen classically as the pathways that carry out these functions, recent studies have shown that the *dorsolateral fasciculus* (which lies just laterally to the dorsal columns and the posterior horn of the gray matter) also carries this information, especially from the lower extremities. Researchers have also shown weak processing of touch-pressure input via anterolateral pathways.

   The dorsal column fibers take a somewhat different route to the thalamus and cortex. The neuron at the receptor site travels into the spinal cord and directly up through the posterior columns to the medulla (the lowest portion of the brain stem). At this point, a synapse occurs and the new fibers cross to the other side of the brain stem and travel to specific parts of the thalamus (ventrobasal complex of thalamus). This set of neurons synapses in the thalamus and then the next neuron carries information on to the sensorimotor cortex, specifically the postcentral gyrus of the parietal lobe. The postcentral gyrus contains the map of an individual's body from a sensory point of view. It is frequently referred to as the sensory homunculus.

The fibers that travel in the dorsolateral fasciculus synapse at the cervical level and the spinal cord. The new neuron crosses to the other side of the spinal cord and travels with the spinothalamic tract to the thalamus and on to the cortex. It is likely that the source of some of the earlier confusion about the function of the ascending pathways is due to the mixed anatomical and functional relationship of the dorsolateral fasciculus with the dorsal columns and the anterolateral system.

3. The third functional category reported by Heimer

(1983) includes the *unconscious proprioceptive pathways*. The spinocerebellar tracts serve the very specific function of providing the cerebellum with direct accurate sensory information before it is processed at higher levels of the brain. These pathways travel directly from the receptor side through the spinal cord and into the cerebellum. Pathways such as these allow the cerebellum to orchestrate motor activity through access to the sensation that stimulates a response. The higher motor centers also send processed information to the cerebellum, and so a comparison takes place between the original stimulus and this processed information in order to plan the motor event correctly. One can experience the action of the unconscious proprioceptive pathways when attempting to correct one's own movements. The cerebellum compares the plan and the sensation to determine

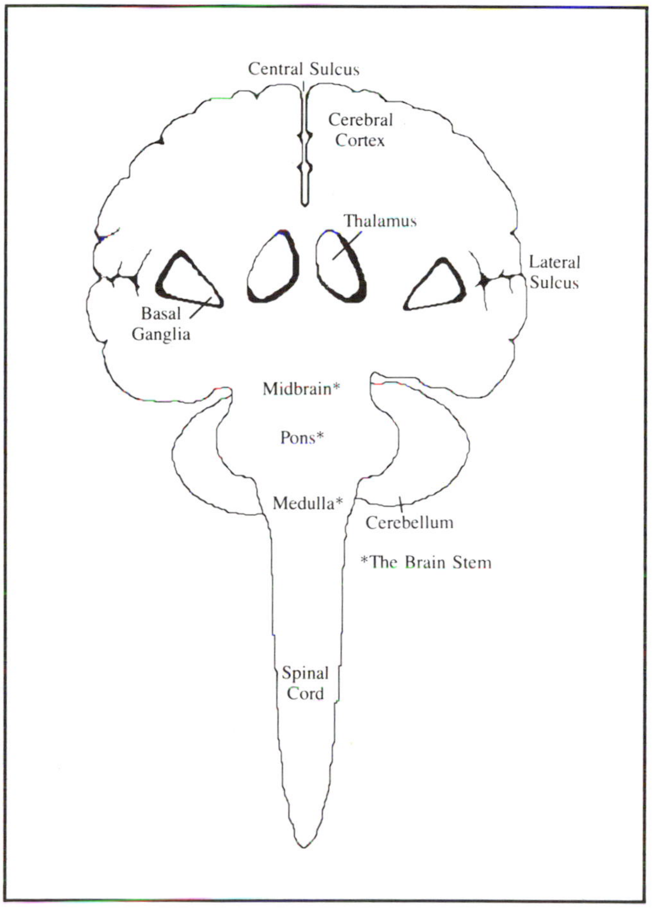

Figure 9-3. Schematic diagram of the major structures of the central nervous system.

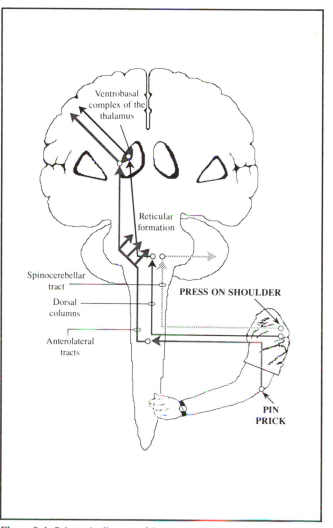

Figure 9-4. Schematic diagram of the somatosensory pathways.

whether an alteration must occur. It is this process that allows one to avoid knocking a glass over by picking it up correctly.

It is important to acknowledge the functional significance of the anatomical relationships among these pathways. Some somatosensory sensations are ipsilateral to the pathways that carry the input while others are contralateral to their corresponding pathways in the spinal cord. When there is damage in the spinal cord, pain and temperature loss is contralateral to the lesion while touch-pressure loss is ipsilateral to the lesion site. However, once nerve fibers reach the brain stem level all the sensory fibers have crossed, leading to all sensory losses being contralateral to the lesion site.

Concepts of Pain.

Gate control theory of pain. In 1965 Melzack and Wall proposed a new theory of the mechanisms of pain, entitled "The Gate Control Theory of Pain." According to this theory, information is processed at the spinal cord level by a variety of types of neurons. Smaller neurons (classified as C fibers) appear responsible for the transmission of the pain stimulus, while the more powerful neurons (classified as A fibers) transmit other information about the touch experience. Melzack and Wall hypothesized that interneurons within the gray matter of the spinal cord (called substantia gelatinosa) modulate the types of sensations that reach the cortical level. When the large fiber (A) is stimulated, it sends information to higher centers for discrimination and mapping, and simultaneously activates the interneurons which stop the pain message. The small pain fiber (C) sends the pain stimulus and simultaneously blocks the interneurons, which allows the pain message to continue. Melzack and Wall suggested that this spinal cord action "opens the gate," as it allows the transmission of the pain message (See Figure 9-5a).

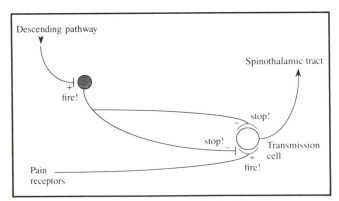

Figure 9-5a. The Gate Control Theory of Pain. Pain receptor neurons facilitate the transmission of pain. Large fibers can be stimulated to fire, leading to inhibition of the pain message being transmitted (close the gate).

In 1968 Melzack and Casey reported that pain could be divided into two operational components: the *sensory-discriminative* and the *affective-motivational* aspects of pain. The sensory-discriminative component localizes and identifies the stimulus (e.g., one's pain threshold or assessment of the intensity of the pain). The affective-motivational characteristics are more generalized, such as unpleasant feelings or the desire to escape the pain. People with frontal lobe lesions lose this affective-motivational component of pain, and although these individuals can identify the location of pain, and talk about its characteristics, they do not appear worried or concerned about their pain (Fields, 1987).

As with all theories which break new ground in our comprehension of complex functions, many researchers since this time have found alternate explanations for the transmission or inhibition of pain in the central nervous system (Fields, 1987). However, it is important to remember from a scholarly point of view, that theorists such as Melzack and Wall have played a very important role in the study of pain. By making these hypotheses, Melzack and Wall set the stage for others to investigate pain mechanisms. For example, the Gate Control Theory of Pain has enabled many researchers to develop devices (such as TENS units) for the inhibition of the pain stimulus at local levels.

Presently, researchers believe that in addition to spinal cord mechanisms, there are additional pain-control mechanisms from higher centers of the brain. Researchers found that electrical stimulation of the midbrain decreased pain responses in lab animals (Perl, 1984). This process is called stimulus-produced analgesia (Fields, 1987). It appears that the periaqueductal gray of the midbrain can be stimulated from spinal cord output to produce biochemicals that induce an analgesic effect on spinal cord neurons. Cortical contributions to this process have not yet been clarified (Fields, 1987). Figure 9-5b is a diagram of these descending influences. Opium derivatives are thought to be the strongest analgesic agents, with Beta-endorphins, dynorphins, and enkephalins being the most likely neurotransmitters to serve this function (Fields, 1987). As research continues in the area of pain, theories about the internal mechanisms will be refined; therapists will need to keep apprised of this information in order to make appropriate adaptations in devices and techniques used in pain treatment. Therapeutic techniques and devices that correspond to central nervous system mechanisms will be more successful. In fact, therapeutic trials are a major source of information for the development and modification of theoretical constructs.

Vestibular System

Structure and Function. The vestibular system makes a unique contribution to the multidimensional maps that enable individuals to interact with the environment effectively. The other sensory systems primarily provide information about self or environment. By providing constant and ongoing information about how the body interacts in the environment, the vestibular system enables the individual to remain oriented in space and time.

> "In the final analysis, one may have a well-developed sensory map of the external world and a well-developed motor map of movement from one place to another, but if one does not know where they are with respect to that map, they are virtually incapable of using that spatial mapping information. And the vestibular system appears to be the system that gives information about the individual's location in the overall spatial map." (Cool, 1987, p. 3)

The vestibular organ is comprised of five components: three semicircular canals and two chambers; collectively they respond to type, direction, angle, and speed of movement, and head position. Information from these receptor sites combine within the central nervous system to determine the exact orientation of the head. Receptors in the three semicircular canals are most sensitive to angular movements, whereas the receptors of the chambers are responsible for linear movement (Heimer, 1983; Kornhuber, 1974; Goldberg & Fernandez, 1984). Gravity provides a major source of information for the vestibular receptors.

There are three *semicircular canals* in each inner ear. The three semicircular canals are oriented at right angles to each other just like the three surfaces that meet in the corner of a room. If one would place one semicircular canal on each wall and the floor of the corner this would provide a good visual image of how the semicircular canals are related to each other anatomically. The structure of both sets of semicircular canals allows the brain to determine all head positions and movements. Corresponding canals on the right and left side respond in a complementary way so that the brain can determine which direction the head is moving. When the head moves in one direction, the canals on one side will produce an excitatory response while the corresponding canal on the other side will be inhibited. This causes a differential effect in central connections between the two sides and allows the brain to interpret the direction of head movement.

In order to fire the vestibular nerve, there must be a change in head position, rate (acceleration or deceleration), or direction the head is moving. When a person is engaged in a continuous angular movement (such as spinning at a constant speed and direction), the vestibular nerve does not fire. The two chambers are called the *utricle* and the *saccule*. The chambers respond to linear movement, especially along and against the force of gravity. Jumping up and down, running, and riding a wheeled toy provide linear stimulation.

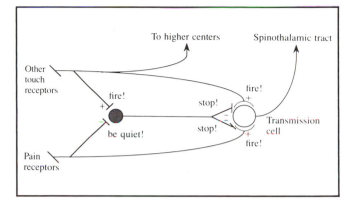

Figure 9-5b. Newer research indicates that higher brain centers can send inhibitory impulses downward to produce an analgesic effect.

Direct input from the vestibular organ travels to the vestibular nuclei (at the pontomedullary junction of the brain stem) and to a specialized portion of the cerebellum dedicated to vestibular processing (the flocculonodular lobe). The vestibulocerebellar connections are critical for postural control. Both the vestibular nuclei and the cerebellum receive vestibular, proprioceptive, somatosensory, and visual input. This multisensory information is organized to produce basic background movements necessary for postural control.

Postural Control Network. The postural control network is comprised of three primary descending motor pathways that work together to create background movements which enable an individual to engage in other activities. The *lateral vestibulospinal tract* is the larger of the tracts; it facilitates the extensor muscles, especially in the upper trunk and neck (Heimer, 1983; Noback and Demarest, 1981). The *medial vestibulospinal tract* is a smaller tract that facilitates flexor tone while inhibiting extensor tone. The third pathway establishes the balance of power within the system; the *reticulospinal tract*, provides additional support for excitation of flexion and inhibition of extension. These pathways work together to modulate body posture (see Figure 9-6). The vestibulocerebellar connections are well-documented pathways which also have an important role in the maintenance of posture and orientation. As stated above, the cerebellar connections with the vestibular nuclei provide the inhibitory control necessary for maintenance of posture.

Postural control is a basic, primary functional behavior. Even in controlled studies where the vestibular organ has been removed, there is a serious initial change in postural stability but within a short period of time compensatory action reinstates some of the functions that have been lost (Darian-Smith, 1984). It is believed that other reflexive and

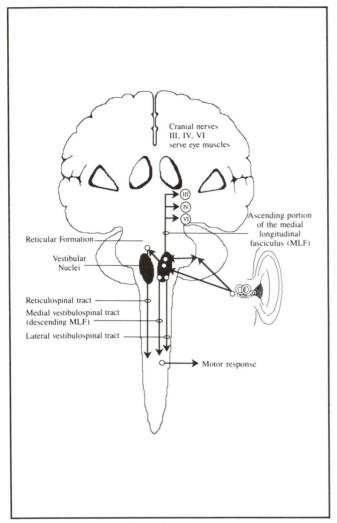

Cranial nerves
III, IV, VI
serve eye muscles

Ascending portion
of the medial
longitudinal
fasciculus (MLF)

Reticular Formation

Vestibular
Nuclei

Reticulospinal tract

Medial vestibulospinal tract
(descending MLF)

Lateral vestibulospinal tract

Motor response

Figure 9-6. Postural control network.

The vestibular system acts as the silent partner during task performance, actively contributing postural control while the person's attention is focused on something else (Kornhuber, 1974). When an individual is carrying out a task, attention must be focused intently on the cognitive and perceptual components of that task. As other systems are providing information to the brain about the task, the vestibular system must automatically maintain the body's dynamic orientation in space to support task performance. If one were to have attention directed away from cognitive tasks every time vestibular stimulation were provided, human beings would be unable to engage in purposeful activity. deQuiros and Schrager (1978) use the term **corporal potentiality** to describe the ability to screen out vestibular and postural information at conscious levels in order to enable the cortex to engage in higher cognitive tasks. When individuals must expend a lot of energy processing vestibular information for postural control, cognitive processing may be disrupted.

Vestibulo-ocular Pathways. The vestibulo-ocular pathways enable the individual to coordinate head and eye movements. The medial longitudinal fasciculus (MLF) travels within the brain stem connecting the vestibular nuclei with the cranial nerve nuclei that serve the eye muscles (specifically cranial nerves III, IV, and VI, the oculomotor, trochlear, and abducens nerves, respectively). This ability to distinguish the source of the movement is necessary to maintain orientation in space. When there is a conflict between expected and obtained sensory information from eyes, eye muscles, and/or vestibular organ, connections with the autonomic nervous system generate a reaction (e.g., nausea, sweating); these reactions are usually classified as "motion sickness." Kornhuber (1974) relates motion sickness to limbic system connections, including the hypothalamus which drives the autonomic nervous system. He states that the limbic system establishes the relationships among patterns of stimuli and particular autonomic reactions. The individual's control of motion and spatial orientation is threatened when the various sensory inputs simultaneously demand mutually incompatible postural adjustments.

Connections and Higher Cortical Connections. Physiological studies have demonstrated that certain brain centers produce short latency (quick) responses after vestibular stimulation. For example, through the collateral connections with the reticular cells, it is thought that vestibular information reaches higher centers of the brain for arousal and alerting responses. Reticular cells connect with the limbic system and would thus be associated with emotional feelings related to the movement experience.

There is some evidence to show connections to the

sensory systems which contribute to postural control as well take over the orientation functions. Dependence on visual and proprioceptive input seems to occur when vestibular input is no longer available. The interrelationships among the sensory systems form the core of the multidimensional maps that allow appropriate interaction of self in the environment. As Jongkees (1974) states,

"The vestibular organ is only one of the organs that inform us about our position in space. It cooperates with visual and kinesthetic sensations from muscles, joints, etc. As long as the information from these various sources is the same, we are well-informed about our position and our movements and everything is balanced. But as soon as they do not agree our balance is lost and we are subject to the frightening sensation of having lost contact with the world around us (p. 414)."

thalamus which is the major integrating structure for the cortex. Simple animal experiments show that various portions of the thalamus may respond to vestibular stimulation including the ventral posterior-inferior nucleus (a sensory relay area) of the thalamus, the ventral lateral nucleus (although its primary role is motor relay) and the medial geniculate body (an auditory relay area)(Abraham, Copack, & Gilman, 1977; Buttner & Henn, 1976; Deecke, Schwartz, & Fredrickson, 1974; Liedgren & Rubin, 1976; Magnin & Fuchs, 1977; Wepsic, 1966). Several authors have postulated that collateral vestibular fibers enter the lateral geniculate body (a visual relay area) to signal the visual system to prepare for potential head movement, so that visual images can coincide with head and eye movement and the individual can maintain orientation in space and time (Kornhuber, 1974). None of these authors cite specific locations as solely vestibular relays, but conclude that vestibular information is integrated with other types of information at the brain stem and higher levels (Darian-Smith, 1984). This hypothesized pervasive influence is compatible with clinical observations of disorientation when a child or adult has vestibular dysfunction.

Connections to cortical regions are also being studied (Darian-Smith, 1984). Two regions in the parietal lobe have been sited as the most likely locations for vestibular processing: the inferior temporal lobe and a portion of the primary sensory areas of the parietal lobe. Darian-Smith (1984) hypothesizes that the first region is related to one's perception of the body in space, while the second area seems to relate vestibular input to the motor output that is generated by the motor cortex.

Muscular Afferents (Proprioception)

Muscular afferents, usually discussed as part of the motor system, are receptors housed within the muscle belly, tendons, and joints to provide ongoing information to the central nervous system about the integrity of the muscle. Most people are familiar with these receptors as the *muscle spindles* and *Golgi tendon organ* (GTO). These receptors provide an excellent example of the intimate relationship between sensory and motor functioning within the neuromusculoskeletal system.

The muscle spindle is a small muscle fiber surrounded by connective tissue that is housed within the fleshy part of the muscle belly. These encapsulated fibers are dispersed throughout the muscle belly so that they may respond to any changes in muscle integrity. The muscle spindles are responsive to the length and changes in length of the muscle.

The muscle spindles contribute to a function called **autogenic facilitation,** which is the ability to stimulate one's own muscle to contract. For example, when the muscle belly is stretched, the muscle spindle fibers are also stretched and send an impulse into the spinal cord. The spinal cord interneurons and the motor neurons can then fire to facilitate contraction of the actual muscle belly fibers themselves. When the muscle belly contracts, the spindle is no longer stretched and the action can stop (Crutchfield & Barnes, 1984). The muscle spindle may play an important role in initial learning or relearning of motor movements by supporting the tension of those muscles as the individual experiments with the movements (Crutchfield & Barnes, 1984). Although spinal cord action is the focus when studying the muscle afferents, this information is also traveling to the cortex via ascending sensory pathways and interacting with descending motor influences. When the descending influences are altered because of trauma or disease, the balance of power is upset at the spinal cord level leading to a release phenomenon. The inhibitory control from higher centers is lost, "releasing" the muscle spindle from this modulating influence. When the muscle spindle acts continuously without inhibitory modulation, autogenic facilitation predominates the muscle action, producing spasticity (Crutchfield & Barnes, 1984).

The Golgi tendon organ is located within the tendons at the end of each muscle belly. The GTO is interwoven within this collagenous fiber so that when changes in tendon tension occur, the GTO can notice and respond to these changes. This can occur both when muscle contraction pulls on the nonelastic tendon or during the extreme ranges of passive stretching. The GTO functions through a process known as **autogenic inhibition**. Autogenic inhibition is the process of inhibiting the muscle which generated the stimulus while providing an excitatory impulse to the antagonist muscle. This process prevents the individual from over-using or damaging the muscle and the corresponding joints.

Through this mechanism, the GTO seems to contribute to cramp relief. During muscle cramping, the muscle is shortened and contains a high degree of tension. When the individual stretches the cramped muscle, the tendon stretches, firing the GTO. When the GTO impulse reaches the spinal cord, an inhibitory impulse is produced (autogenic inhibition) allowing the muscle with the cramp to relax (Crutchfield & Barnes, 1984).

Because the GTO inhibits its own muscle and excites the antagonist, the two sets of GTO's in complementary muscles maintain a balance of power across joints. The stability that is produced across a joint by complementary muscle action is called co-contraction. Weight-bearing positions rely on co-contraction, as do goal-directed movements which are supported by a stable joint or body area. Stability can be provided both proximally and distally. Movement of extremities is supported by trunk stability (e.g., reaching for a glass on the counter), while movement in the trunk can be supported through stability in the extremities (e.g., when an individual is on hands and knees, the elbows, wrists and knees provide stability, enabling mobilization of the hips and shoulders for swaying back and forth).

By understanding the concepts of autogenic facilitation of the muscle spindle and autogenic inhibition of the GTO, the therapist can better control the sensory and motor environment when planning intervention. For example, a quick stretch activates muscle spindles (changes in muscle length) engaging autogenic facilitation of the stretched muscle, whereas a maintained stretch past the tension state of the muscle is more likely to fire the GTO producing autogenic inhibition, relaxing the muscle being stretched.

The Visual System

The visual system is one of the most advanced sensory systems in the human organism. Although cell clusters form early in fetal life, this system becomes most functional in the postnatal period. Vision is the most prominent sensation; there are more fibers in the optic nerve than in all the sensory tracts in the entire length of the spinal cord (Kandel & Schwartz, 1985). Because of its anatomical organization from the front to the back of the cortex, it also provides an excellent vehicle for localization of central nervous system problems.

Retina. The retina is the receptor mechanism of the visual system. The retinal cells have been studied extensively because they are an extension of the central nervous system. When the central nervous system environment has been altered in a way that might affect the nerve cells or supporting structures, these changes can be observed in the retina. The retinal cells operate to maximize the reception of both light and color. Additionally, the complex interneuron network is set up to facilitate the transmission of the clearest visual image through lateral inhibition of neighboring cells. Specific retinal cells activate a specific optic nerve cell; this pattern of organization continues to the occipital lobe. This **topographic** or retinotopic organization allows the cortex to construct an accurate and reliable map of the visual environment.

Visual Pathways. The pathways for visual input travel from the front of the cortex (behind the eyeball) to the back (occipital lobe); the other sensory systems ascend from the receptor site to the cortex. This makes the visual system quite vulnerable to all types of cortical damage, but also provides a consistent source of diagnostic data for localizing the injury site. As with other sensory systems the visual

system has two subsystems that enable both alerting and mapping to take place efficiently.

The first visual system is referred to as the geniculocalcarine or geniculostriate system (Noback & Demarest, 1981). Figure 9-7 provides a diagram of the visual pathways. The nerve cells exit the eyeball, having obtained input from the retina and course backward toward the occipital lobe. The first segment, the *optic nerve*, covers the region from the eyeball to the converging point for all the optic nerve cells, called the *optic chiasm*. Complete severing of the optic nerve results in total blindness of the eye served. At the optic chiasm, central vision is carried through nerve cells that do not cross. These cells remain in the lateral aspects of the convergence point. Peripheral vision is carried through nerve cells that cross over at the optic chiasm, therefore if the crossed fibers are damaged, the individual loses peripheral vision; this is commonly known as *tunnel vision*.

After passing through the optic chiasm region, the fiber pathway is known as the *optic tract*; these fibers travel to the lateral geniculate body (a nucleus of the thalamus). The optic tract carries all information from the contralateral visual field. Just after exiting the lateral geniculate body, the fibers travel forward and out before coursing backward; this curved portion of the optic radiations is called Meyer's loop. This curve is necessary so that the fibers can travel around the lateral ventricles. This new bundle of fibers is called the optic radiations. As with the optic tract, the optic radiations carry information about the contralateral visual field. The optic radiations travel back to the occipital lobe, specifically, the calcarine sulcus (area 17), hence the name geniculocalcarine pathways.

The geniculocalcarine system seems to provide answers to the question "What is it?" by gathering information about the characteristics of the objects in the environment. The maps that are formed in the primary and association visual areas allow the individual to determine the identity and function of objects.

The second visual system is called the *tectal system*. The tectal system seems to answer the question "Where is it?", by identifying presence and location of stimuli for the individual (orienting). The fibers that serve this function pass through the optic nerve, chiasm and tract, but synapse in the tectal region of the midbrain (Schiller, 1984). (Remember that the midbrain is the highest portion of the brain stem and the tectum is made up of the superior and inferior colliculi.) Although the superior colliculus is considered a primary relay station for visual input through tectal system connections, it is also a relay station for somatosensory and auditory input (Kandel & Schwartz, 1985), allowing a coordination of these inputs for proper orientation to the arousing stimulus. An individual with cortical brain damage may alert to visual stimuli because the tectum is operating at the brain stem level, but will be unable to follow through with a goal-directed behavior related to the stimulus because the pathways that lead to the cortex are disrupted.

Visual System Functions and Therapeutic Interventions. The visual system is designed to recognize contrasts (Kandel & Schwartz, 1985). When the visual environment is diffuse or homogeneous, the cells of the visual system have difficulty responding. They search for the highest contrast possible, attempting to make this area distinct. The eyes continuously change position with very tiny movements to activate new retinal cells. In this way, the brain gets ongoing information about the object and can keep the image clear. Busy visual environments can be difficult for the visual system to handle. With too many competing images, the visual system cannot isolate significant high-contrast locations to generate the nerve impulses. For example, think of how difficult it is to find something in the "junk drawer" in the kitchen. This is because there are many overlapping objects of varying shapes, sizes, and colors; the competition is so great that clarity is frequently lost.

Altering the sensory environment to increase the chances for success in task performance enables the individual to actively engage the environment. This in turn increases accurate and reliable sensory feedback that can be stored and used for future tasks. Therapists can improve orientation in a visually disoriented individual by providing a high-contrast visual environment. For example, one could place dark handles on white cabinets in the kitchen, or place a very dark cloth or board on the counter top to help distinguish light-colored food items when preparing food. Contrast between the bed covering and the night stand in the bedroom would facilitate getting on the bed. Therapists can advise clients of ways to minimize problems with visual competition by organizing cabinets, shelves, and drawers into sections for predetermined items or placing tool outlines (shadows) on walls or racks to show which utensils or tools belong in each location. This not only provides a high contrast foreground-background for the items, but also minimizes stacking or cluttering of objects on top of each other.

The most common visual field defects that therapists encounter are tunnel vision (loss of peripheral vision) and *homonymous hemianopsia* (loss of one side of the visual field). Figure 9-8 demonstrates where these problems occur in the pathways. Because visual field loss is often permanent, it can have a significant impact on task performance. Consider the risks that are present when peripheral vision is not available to an individual. Many stimuli to which people attend are first noticed in the peripheral field, and much of one's body orientation relies on peripheral field input. Therapeutic intervention must incorporate patterns of movement that compensate for the loss of peripheral vision. For example, one can set up activities that require the individual to move the head from side to side, minimizing the effects of peripheral loss, and facilitating routine use of head movement to obtain visual input from a wider area (e.g., placing important stimuli to the side). Automatic use of head-turning and body-repositioning will contribute greatly to independence.

Homonymous hemianopsia is the loss of one side of the visual field. This can impair a person's independence because the individual can miss important cues from nearly half of the visual environment. Individuals with a homonymous hemianopsia frequently complain that objects are missing, when in fact they may be present but outside of the remaining visual field. Therapeutic intervention for these individuals must incorporate new head-positioning to maximize use of intact visual fields and minimize the effects of the lost visual field. This can be achieved by turning the head toward the lost visual field which places the retained visual field in front of the individual and moves the lost field over the shoulder. This new position facilitates more awareness of the immediate visual environment. The therapist must design methods that make this postural change an automatic one. For example, one can place items that are most important to the individual in the lost visual field to increase head-turning to look for them, or play a card game and place the deck in a position to facilitate head-turning. Auditory cues such as "look to the left, Mr. Jones" can be helpful initially, but there is a danger that the individual will become dependent on cues from others and never internalize this adaptation for independent task performance. Family education is also important to balance emerging adaptive behavior with safety.

Auditory System

Structure and Function. The auditory system is also one of the newer sensory mechanisms in the central nervous system. The auditory system processes sound primarily for communication, but also as a means of environmental orientation. Direction, distance, and quality of sound all contribute to the ability to orient within our environment from an auditory perspective (Kiang, 1984). Although other professionals specialize in working with problems of the auditory system, occupational therapists must also be aware of the basic mechanisms within the auditory system so that therapeutic approaches and environmental adaptations can accommodate difficulties that might arise from dysfunction in this system.

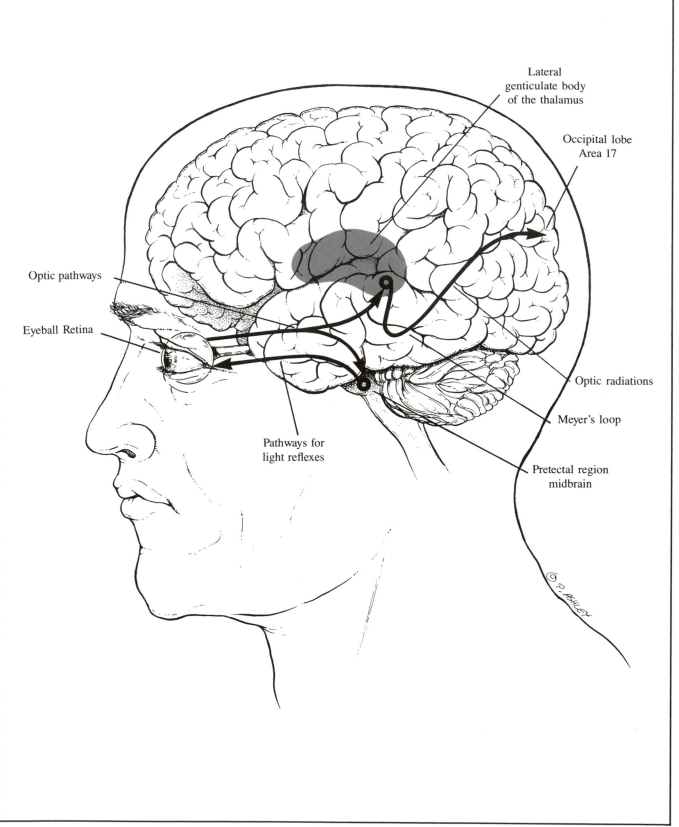

Figure 9-7. Schematic diagram of primary visual pathways.

The auditory receptor is divided into three sections: the outer, middle, and inner ear. Through these three components, airwaves are transformed into pressure waves within a fluid system. The pressure waves displace hair cells located in the inner ear and this action fires the nerve cells. The outer ear consists of the auricle (the part of the ear visible to us), the ear canal, and the ear drum or the *tympanic membrane*. The outer ear is vulnerable to obstructions in the canal or perforations of the eardrum, both of which diminish hearing on that side.

The middle ear is a chamber that contains three small bones (*malleus, incus,* and *stapes*) and two small muscles (*tensor tympani* and *stapedius*). When the ear drum vibrates, the small bones vibrate, which then emits pressure on the surface of the inner ear (*cochlea*). The Eustachian tube connects this self-contained chamber with the throat to provide a passageway to equalize pressure in the middle ear. The Eustachian tube is frequently the site of infection because bacteria or viruses can easily get trapped within its small diameter. This blocks the passageway into the middle ear making the pressure increase. Ear infections such as these occur frequently with young children, partly because their Eustachian tubes are less angled, allowing for less efficient drainage. This is a major reason why many children have plastic tubes placed in their ears during early childhood. The tube is inserted through the ear drum and provides an alternate means for pressure maintenance in the middle ear.

The cochlea is shaped like a snail with several chambers inside. The movement of the fluid within these chambers allows displacement of the hair cells. When the hair cells are displaced, the auditory nerves fire. Specific hair cells are responsible for specific sounds, and fire specific nerve cells. This process is known as **tonotopic** organization and is the mechanism by which the central nervous system can identify the sounds heard.

The central connections of the auditory system are unique in comparison to other sensory systems. Figure 9-9 illustrates the auditory pathways. The ascending pathways of the auditory system are bilateral in nature; this is significant because loss of the input on one side will not completely stop the information processing to both sides of the brain. In terms of functional performance, the individual experiences inability to localize sounds from the environment with loss of hearing to one ear or auditory nerve. Under normal conditions, the brain is able to compare the loudness of the sounds from the two ears to determine from which direction the sound is coming. When one ear has lost its ability to transmit information, the brain no longer can locate the direction, hence the person can hear the sound clearly, but has more difficulty finding it. Clinically, these individuals respond to sounds by changing posture or looking around to search for the origin of the sound.

These bilateral connections in the ascending auditory system extend throughout the brain stem. The inferior colliculus is a major relay point for auditory fibers (remember it is in the midbrain and is part of the tectum as described in the visual section). The inferior colliculus functions to alert the individual to auditory stimuli in the environment. From the brain stem, information travels to the medial geniculate body (in the thalamus) and the temporal lobe.

The auditory system also has a feedback mechanism that performs an important function. This feedback system follows a similar course as the ascending pathways but in a more unilateral pattern. This fiber pathway inhibits hair cells carrying extraneous or unimportant background noise from the environment, thus allowing the individual to attend to important sounds. This process is called auditory figure-ground perception. This is the mechanism which allows students to filter out such noises as rustling paper and shuffling feet in the classroom so they can hear the teacher's voice more clearly.

Although other professions may test the auditory system in more detail and may work on specific auditory compo-

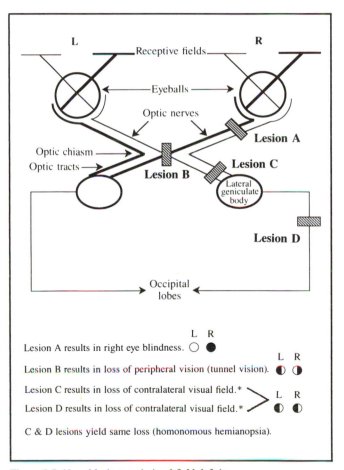

Figure 9-8. Neural lesions and visual field deficits.

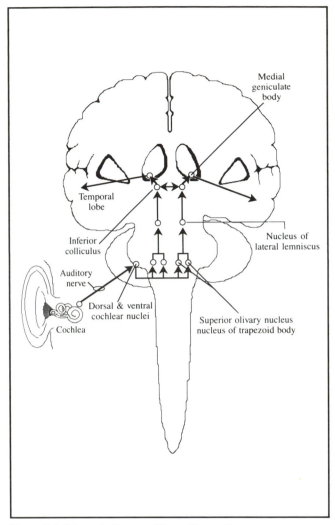

Figure 9-9. Schematic diagram of the auditory pathways.

nents in their intervention plans, the occupational therapist is responsible for the effects of auditory deficits on task performance. Therapists must decide whether treatment should be set up in a quiet isolated place to avoid noisy environments and decrease the amount of effort required by the auditory system or in a more natural environment in which the individual must develop inhibitory skills. Both choices are therapeutically sound, but must be actively chosen as part of the treatment goals. For example, the therapist may choose to work in quiet environments early in the treatment process so that other areas of concern such as postural control can be addressed without competition. The therapist might choose a simpler postural task while working in a more competing auditory environment to help the individual learn to screen out the extraneous noises that will always be part of the natural environment. A portable tape

recorder and earphones are helpful to introduce controlled auditory stimuli, which can later be incorporated into other activities. The therapist can control the type of sound (e.g., clinic noise, classroom noise, neighborhood noise, music, talking) and the volume on the tape so that as the client adjusts to one condition, it can be altered slightly. Therapists monitor performance in relation to task difficulty and the amount of environmental competition for attention, as this is another subtle variable that certainly can affect task performance.

ROLE OF AROUSAL AND ATTENTION IN SENSORY PROCESSING

Sensory processing is a critical prerequisite to task performance, but sensory processing cannot occur until the individual notices the stimulus. DeMoja, Reitano and Caracciolo (1985) describe the relationship between arousal and performance as a complex matrix affected by three variables: the structure of the individual's personality, the difficulty of the task, and the structure of the situation in which the task is to be performed. Vinogradova (1970) describes several events which must occur in order for the central nervous system to register a stimulus. First, the appropriate receptors must recognize that a change has occurred in the environment. Second, the central nervous system must determine whether such a stimulus has occurred before. Third the central nervous system must decide whether or not to act on the stimulus.

It appears that under normal conditions the central nervous system investigates stimuli that are not familiar and inhibits conscious awareness of familiar stimuli (McGuinness & Pribram, 1980). As with other actions of the central nervous system, a balance of power exists within the arousal network so that an individual can screen out extraneous input when engaged in a task, but simultaneously has the potential to alert to important or dangerous stimuli if they occur. It has been hypothesized that the balance of power is maintained for **sensory registration** by the interaction of three mechanisms: *arousal, activation,* and *effort* (McGuinness & Pribram, 1980).

Arousal is a neurological mechanism by which the central nervous system notices environmental stimuli. Arousal can occur with any change in the environment, including changes in parts of stimuli. At a very basic level, one network of the central nervous system is identifying any changes in the environment, while other mechanisms assist to determine the significance of these events. It is thought that the *amygdala,* a structure of the limbic system, has a primary role in arousal (Heimer, 1983; Pribram & McGuinness, 1975). The amygdala receives sensory input directly from the olfactory system, and indirectly from other senses via the reticular formation.

Activation is a longer-lasting response (several seconds) that seems to allow the individual to figure out a plan of action in response to the stimulus. There seems to be a large degree of cortical inhibition during activation, which screens out extraneous stimuli to allow the central nervous system to assess the situation. The central nervous system must: 1) search through information from past experience to determine whether the present stimulus is familiar and 2) appraise present body status in case action is required to respond to the stimulus.

Let's examine a common life task as an example of how arousal and activation function within normal performance. Imagine yourself sitting on your own comfortable couch watching a murder mystery on television. The mystery has been building to an exciting climax and the murderer is about to be revealed. Just at this moment, something flashes by the window in your living room. What are the first things that happen? Initially, there is a quick shift of attention to notice the stimulus (arousal), and then there are a few seconds in which you assess the situation (activation). You are likely to miss the identification of the murderer on television while your central nervous system determines the familiarity and relevance of the stimulus.

Effort is the voluntary phase of the sensory registration process (McGuinness & Pribram, 1980; Pribram & McGuinness, 1975). This is the component that allows the individual to carry out the chosen plan of action. Purposeful, goal-directed activity in response to a sensory event injects meaning into those experiences and also simultaneously provides additional sensory feedback. Meaningful interaction with the environment is necessary to establish accurate, reliable maps that become part of one's memory stores and therefore the source of comparison for future sensory events (Pribram & McGuinness, 1975).

Dysfunctional Performance Related to Sensory Registration

Each of the components of sensory registration is necessary for normal task performance. Abnormal behavior is a likely outcome when the balance of power is upset within the system. One might consider four basic categories of dysfunctional performance due to problems with this sensory registration mechanism (Jarrard, 1980; Ogulnick, 1981; Pribram & McGuinness, 1975):

1. resistance to identifying new stimuli

2. overresponsivity to new stimuli
3. errors in attending decisions
4. difficulty in the use of one's maps

Resistance to Identifying New Stimuli. If the central nervous system receives a stimulus and improperly determines that the stimulus is insignificant, no behavioral response is generated. One might use words such as lethargic or unresponsive to describe behaviors. Following this line of thinking into treatment planning, the occupational therapist would want to provide intervention that would increase the opportunities for an arousal response to occur. Optimum treatment planning in these cases is facilitated by knowledge of how the central nervous system seems to process arousal input.

To increase the opportunities for arousal to occur, the therapist must know which types of sensation are more likely to be processed by reticular cells and are therefore more likely to generate an arousal response in the amygdala. By reviewing information previously presented, one can conclude that the alerting portions of each system are more likely to generate activity in this arousal network. Various arousal inputs include light touch, variable and angular movement, sudden and high-intensity visual and auditory stimuli, and quick changes in body position. When incorporated into purposeful activity, these are appropriate treatment approaches to generate increased arousal.

Overresponsivity to Environmental Stimuli. The second type of problem that might occur is overresponsivity to environmental stimuli. In this case, the central nervous system is incorrectly determining that each new stimulus is novel and should therefore be noticed. One might use words such as distractible, overly active, or poor impulse control to describe this behavior pattern. Because individuals with this problem are frequently disrupted from tasks to notice a new stimulus, they do not have the opportunity to develop accurate, reliable maps about task performance. As a result, a circular problem emerges: without maps, stimuli continue to be perceived as new; when stimuli are perceived as new, arousal is likely to occur; arousal to all stimuli impedes purposeful task completion, which then reduces the ability to form maps; and the cycle continues.

It is important for the therapist to understand central nervous system processing when choosing an appropriate intervention strategy for the individual. It is possible to design strategies to increase activation and effort to allow task completion to occur. The discriminative components of each sensory system appear most capable of facilitating goal-directed activity, and in turn producing accurate, reliable, sensory feedback. Therapists focus on activities that incorporate discriminative sensations, such as proprioception, touch-pressure, and linear and positioning movements. For example, when an individual reaches for a glass to take a drink, attention is directed toward the actions of reaching, grasping, and bringing the glass toward the mouth, but it is also one's position, movement, and visual receptors that provide feedback to keep the central nervous system on the task and develop sensory maps for future use. Therefore, the sensation produced from purposeful activity provides a three-fold benefit for overly-responsive individuals: it assists with on-task behavior, it provides feedback that allow adjustments to be made if necessary, and it contributes to maps that can be referred to later. The therapist must create a therapeutic environment which provides reasonable opportunities for the individual—tasks which can be completed and yet provide an adequate challenge.

Errors in Attending Decisions.   The third type of problem involves errors made in attending decisions. Not only is accurate sensory interpretation important for perceptual and cognitive processes, it helps individuals attend to the appropriate stimuli and screen out other sensory stimuli at any given moment, and then to shift attention as tasks demand. Problems with selecting the proper stimulus and shifting attention appropriately are frequently seen in those with head trauma. These individuals can focus attention, but seem to focus either on inappropriate stimuli in the environment or on one stimulus for an inappropriate length of time. These inappropriate choices frequently lead to frustrating or dangerous situations. For example, while driving, the individual may attend only to the forward movement of the car, missing the stimuli from the side or rear views; such situations place the driver in a vulnerable situation. According to McGuinness and Pribram (1980), this process is further complicated when the individual has perceptual and motor problems.

Intervention for this type of problem is quite challenging. DeMoja, Reitano, and Caracciolo (1985) and Shek and Spinks (1985) suggest that an individual who is already aroused by any sensory system is more capable of carrying on perceptual tasks, and is less likely to be distracted. Furthermore, all types of stimulus changes increase both recognition and recall skills (Ben-Shakhar, 1980; Bernstein, 1981; Shek & Spinks, 1985). Thus, it may be helpful to practice stimulus selection and attentional shift across sensory systems. To return to the driving example, the therapist might ask the individual to maintain visual attention to the front, while reporting noticed auditory cues to the side. In this way, an arousal state is initiated and maintained, increasing the overall potential of the system in several areas.

Difficulty Using Sensory Memory Maps.   The fourth type of problem involves incorrect use of one's multidimensional maps. As a stimulus becomes available in one's environment, the central nervous system determines whether the stimulus is familiar by comparing it to past experiences. Two important components of this process are the creation and refinement of maps and the efficient storage and retrieval of maps. The *hippocampus*, a structure of the limbic system, mediates these actions (Jarrard, 1980; Ogulnick, 1981; Pribram & McGuinness, 1975; Delacour, 1980; Gerbrandt & Fowler, 1980); the association cortex houses the complex memories.

When an individual has difficulty creating maps, there does not seem to be a background of stored information, and so behavior is very simplistic. It is difficult for this individual to create appropriate responses to stimuli, because internal resources are limited. When given a toy or other object, such an individual might engage in very simplistic repetitive use of the item as if no other ideas are present (Ayres, 1985). Although lack of experiences can be related to lack of establishment of memories, a poorly functioning input system can also prohibit development of memory stores.

Difficulties also arise when the storage and retrieval mechanism is dysfunctional; the individual is unable to retrieve the memories of past sensory experiences. The individual has developed memories, but has difficulty accessing them in response to specific demands. Behavior may be frustrating to others because these individuals often exhibit behaviors in a free choice situation but cannot perform the same behavior on command. Others begin to believe that the individual "just isn't trying." Different central nervous system mechanisms generate free-choice and directed performance. Consider what has happened to you when you make the comment, "I wish you hadn't asked me to remember that name; I knew it before you asked me." You are describing the difference between generating information from within the cortex and engaging the retrieval mechanisms of the hippocampus.

The hippocampus seems to be responsible for the filing system for memories, making the retrieval of information efficient. Imagine how difficult it would be to retrieve information if one had to search through all possible memories for every situation. This would either considerably slow down responsiveness to demands (e.g., The therapist asks the individual what he had for breakfast and he does not respond. As they continue with the next activity, the individual suddenly bursts out "bran muffin and coffee") or lead to inappropriate responses through random use of the next available response (e.g., The therapist asks the child what she planted in the yard and the child says, "We are going to ride horses in Girl Scouts").

Intervention strategies focus on methods for developing efficient use of maps. In the first situation (lack of stored information), the therapist must use very simple activities that the individual can successfully complete, so that maps can form from the sensory feedback. Pouring liquids is an example of a simple task which can be completed successfully and produces good sensory feedback. The therapist can initially control amounts and container size to minimize opportunities to fail, and can then slowly introduce other variables. This activity produces sensation for several systems: proprioception, somatosensory, visual, and auditory.

Team collaboration is critical to successful intervention when retrieval problems exist. Because these individuals demonstrate poor access to their maps, the team must establish an efficient storage and retrieval mechanism for the individual. For example, all of those assisting the individual might agree on using the same command such as "come, sit down," so the individual will get many opportunities to match the command with the expected behavior, which can then become an easily retrieved response.

It is extremely important to pre-empt failure with this individual, because incorrect completion of a task allows incorrect maps to form and increases frustration. The therapist must anticipate outcomes and set up situations that maximize successful performance. Instead of posing an open-ended question such as "Where is the pan?", the therapist might ask "Is it on top or underneath?" If the child plays on the scooter board and wants to knock down the tower of blocks, the therapist might initially guide the scooter toward the tower with a rope, keeping the child moving in the right direction. Once the individual gains access to that response, external cues can be diminished.

Sensory registration is an important precursor to all human performance. To be able to respond to the environment appropriately, one must first notice what is occurring in the environment. The occupational therapist must recognize the behaviors associated with these problems in order to plan intervention strategies that are well suited to the individual's needs.

SUMMARY

Because it provides the maps of self and environment necessary for our actions in daily life, sensation is essential to human performance. Sensory processing, which is provided through the gustatory, olfactory, somatosensory, vestibular, proprioceptive, visual, and auditory systems, is dependent on basic neurological mechanisms. These include centrifugal control, balance of excitation and inhibition, plasticity, and compensatory action. In turn sensory processing is affected by arousal and attention, both of which can be influenced by environmental factors. Knowledge of the principles underlying the development and function of sensory systems is critical to understanding dysfunctional performance. For this reason, it is important for therapists to acquire a thorough understanding of these principles, as well as the structures and mechanisms which support sensation.

Study Questions

1. Explain how loss of one mode of sensory input can affect an individual's performance.

2. Describe one unique characteristic of each sensory system discussed in this chapter.

3. Why is centrifugal control a critical feature of sensory processing?

4. Describe the input pathways for each sensory system.

5. Explain the functional significance of sensory registration.

6. Explain why both arousal/alerting and discrimination/ mapping are necessary for normal performance.

Recommended Readings

Aitkin, L.M., Irvine, D.R.F., & Webster, W.R. (1984). In I. Darian-Smith (Ed.). *Handbook of physiology, Section 1: The nervous system; Volume II: Sensory processes, Part 2* (pp.675-738). Bethesda: American Physiological Society.

Ayres, A.J. (1980). *Sensory integration and the child.* Los Angeles: Western Psychological Services.

Ayres, A.J., & Tickle, L.S. (1980). Hyperresponsivity to touch and vestibular sitmuli as a predictor of positive response to sensory integration procedures by autistic children. *American Journal of Occupational Therapy, 34*(6), 375-381.

Bishop, P.O. (1984). Processing of visual information within the retinostriate system. In I. Darian-Smith (Ed.). *Handbook of physiology, Section 1: The nervous system; Volume II: Sensory processes, Part 2* (pp.341-424). Bethesda: American Physiological Society.

Damasio, A.R. (1978). A neurological model for childhood autism. *Archives of Neurology, 35,* 777-786.

De Armond, S.J., Fusco, M.M., & Dewey, M.M. (1976). *Structure of the human brain.* New York: Oxford University Press.

Faingold, C.L., & Hoffmann, W.E. (1981). Effects of bemegride on the sensory responses of neurons in the hippocampus and brain stem reticular formation. *Electroencephalography and Clinical Neurophysiology, 52,* 316-327.

Gold, M.S., & Gold, J.R. (1975). Autism and attention: Theoretical considerations and a pilot study using set reaction time. *Child Psychiatry and Human Development, 6*(2), 68-80.

Grossberg, S. (1982). Processing of expected and unexpected events during conditioning and attention: A psychophysiological theory. *Psychological Review, 89*(5), 529-572.

Guyton, A.C. (1972). *Structure and function of the nervous system.* Philadelphia: W. B. Saunders.

Held, R., Leibowitz, H.W., & Teuber, H-L. (Eds.). (1978). *Handbook of sensory physiology, Volume VIII: Perception.* New York: Springer-Verlag.

Jacobson, M. (Ed.). (1978). *Handbook of sensory physiology, Volume IX: Development of sensory systems.* New York: Springer-Verlag.

Johnson, L.L., & Moberg, G.P. (1980). Adrenocortical response to novelty stress in rats with dentate gyrus lesions. *Neuroendocrinology, 30,* 187-192.

Kroese, B.S., & Siddle, D.A.T. (1983). Effects of an attention-demanding task on amplitude and habituation of the electrodermal orienting response. *Psychophysiology, 20*(2), 128-135.

Leaton, R.N. (1981). Habituation of startle response, lick suppression, and exploratory behavior in rats with hippocampal lesions. *Journal of Corroborative and Physiological Psychology, 95*(5), 813-826.

Liebman, M. (1983). *Neuroanatomy made easy and understandable.* Rockville, MD: Aspen.

Matson, D.L. (1980). The sternomastoid differential orienting response: Why we face the speaker. *The Journal of Auditory Research, 20,* 217-226.

Matzke, H.A., & Foltz, F.M. (1979). *Synopsis of neuroanatomy.* New York: Oxford University Press.

Micco, D.J., Jr., & McEwen, B.S. (1980). Glucocorticoids, the hippocampus, and behavior: Interactive relation between task activation and steroid hormone binding specificity. *Journal of Corroborative and Physiological Psychology, 94*(4), 624-633.

Midgley, G.C., & Tees, R.C. (1981). Orienting behavior by rats with visual cortical and subcortical lesions. *Experimental Brain Research, 41,* 316-328.

Mitchell, D.E., & Timney, B. (1984). Postnatal development of function in the mammalian visual system. In I. Darian-Smith (Ed.). *Handbook of physiology, Section 1: The nervous system, Volume II: Sensory processes, Part 2* (pp.507-556). Bethesda: American Physiological Society.

Oetter, P. (1986). A sensory integrative approach to the treatment of attention deficit disorders. *Sensory International Special Interest Section Newsletter, 9*(2), 1-3.

Passingham, R.E. (1985). Premotor cortex: Sensory cues and movement. *Behavioral Brain Research, 18,* 175-185.

Pelland, M. (1986). Unilateral neglect: Visual field defect, oculomotor dysfunction, or body scheme disorder? *Sensory International Special Interest Section Newsletter, 9*(4), 1-5.

Post, R.B., & Leibowitz, H.W. (1986). Two modes of processing visual information: Implications for assessing visual impairment. *American Journal of Optometry and Physiological Optics, 63*(2), 94-96.

Reeves, G.D. (1985). Influence of somatic activity on body scheme. *Sensory International Special Interest Section Newsletter, 8*(2), 1-2.

Royeen, C.B. (1985). Domain specifications of the construct tactile defensiveness. *American Journal of Occupational Therapy, 39*(9), 596-599.

Saccuzzo, D.P., & Braff, D.L. (1981). Early information processing deficit in schizophrenia. *Archives of General Psychiatry, 38,* 175-179.

Schmidt, R.F. (Ed.). (1978). *Fundamentals of neurophysiology.* New York: Springer-Verlag.

Sharpless, S., & Jasper, H. (1956). Habituation of the arousal reaction. *Brain, 79,* 655-681.

Shepherd, G.M. (1979). *The synaptic organization of the brain.* New York: Oxford University Press.

Stanton, T.L., Beckman, A.L., & Winokur, A. (1981). Thyrotropin-releasing hormone effects in the central nervous system: Dependence on arousal state. *Science, 214,* 678-681.

Treisman, A.M. (1969). Strategies and models of selective

attention. *Psychological Review, 76,* 282-299.

Tsal, Y. (1983). Movements of attention across the visual field. *Journal of Experimental Psychology: Human Perception and Performance, 9*(4), 523-530.

Turkewiwtz, G., & Kenny, P.A. (1985). The role of developmental limitations of sensory input on sensory/perceptual organization. *Journal of Developmental and Behavioral Pediatrics, 6*(5), 302-306.

Vanderwolf, C.H. (1981). Reticulo-cortical activity and behavior: A critique of the arousal theory and a new synthesis. *The Behavioral and Brain Sciences, 4,* 459-514.

Vinogradova, O.S., Brazhnik, E.S., Karanov, A.M., & Zhadina, S.D. (1980). Neuronal activity of the septum following various types of deafferentation. *Brain Research, 187,* 353-368.

Watson, C. (1977). *Basic human neuroanatomy.* Boston: Little, Brown.

Young, L.R. (1984). Perception of the body in space: Mechanisms. In I. Darian-Smith (Ed.). *Handbook of physiology, Section 1: The nervous system, Volume II: Sensory processes, Part 2* (pp.1023-1066). Bethesda: American Physiological Society.

References

Abraham, L., Copack, P.B., & Gilman, S. (1977). Brain stem pathways for vestibular projections to cerebral cortex in the cat. *Experimental Neurology, 55,* 436-448.

Ayres, A.J. (1985). *Developmental dyspraxia and adult onset apraxia.* Torrance, CA: Sensory Integration International.

Bach-y-Rita, P. (Ed.). (1980). *Recovery of function: Theoretical considerations for brain injury rehabilitation.* Baltimore: University Park Press.

Barnes, M.R., Crutchfield, C.A. & Heriza, C. (1984). *The neurophysiological basis of patient treatment: Volume I, Reflex development.* Atlanta: Stokesville Publishing Co.

Bellingham, W.P., Wayner, M.J., & Barone, F.C. (1979). Schedule-induced eating in water-deprived rats. *Physiology and Behavior, 23,* 1105-1107.

Ben-Shakhar, G. (1980). Habituation of the orienting response to complex sequences of stimuli. *Psychophysiology, 17,* 524-534.

Benson, A.J. (1974). Modification of the response to angular accelerations by linear accelerations. In H.H. Kornhuber (Ed.). *Handbook of sensory physiology, Volume V1/2, Vestibular system Part 2: Psychophysics, applied aspects and general interpretations.* New York: Springer-Verlag.

Bernstein, A.S. (1981). The orienting response and stimulus significance. Further comments. *Biological Psychology, 12,* 171-185.

Bischof, N. (1974). Optic-vestibular orientation to the vertical. In H.H. Kornhuber (Ed.). *Handbook of sensory physiology, Volume V1/2, Vestibular system, Part 2: Psychophysics, applied aspects and general interpretations.* New York: Springer-Verlag.

Blakeslee, A.F., & Salmon, T.H. (1935). Genetics of sensory thresholds: Individual taste reactions for different substances. *Proceedings of the National Academy of Sciences of the U.S.A., 21,* 84-90.

Buttner V., & Henn, V. (1976). Thalamic unit activity in the alert monkey during natural vestibular stimulation. *Brain Research, 103,* 127-132.

Cool, S.J. (1987). A view for the "outside": sensory integration and developmental neurobiology. *Sensory Integration Newsletter, 10*(2), 2-3.

Coren, S., Porac, C., & Ward, L.M. (1984). *Sensation and perception.* Orlando: Academic Press.

Cotman, C.W., & McGaugh, J.L. (1980). *Behavioral neuroscience: An introduction.* New York: Academic Press.

Crutchfield, C.A., & Barnes, M.R. (1984). *The neurophysiologic basis of patient treatment: Volume III, Peripheral components of motor control.* Atlanta: Stokesville Publishing Co.

Darian-Smith, I. (1984). The sense of touch: Performance and peripheral neural processes. In I. Darian-Smith (Ed.). *Handbook of physiology, Section 1: The nervous system, Volume II: Sensory processes, part 2* (pp. 739-788). Bethesda: American Physiological Society.

Deecke, L.D., Schwartz, W.F., & Fredrickson, J.M. (1974). Nucleus ventroposterior inferior (VPI) as the vestibular thalamic relay in the rhesus monkey. *Experimental Brain Research, 20,* 88-100.

Delacour, J. (1980). Conditioned modifications of arousal and unit activity in the rat hippocampus. *Experimental Brain Research, 38,* 95-101.

DeMoja, C.A., Reitano, M., & Caracciolo, E. (1985). General arousal and performance. *Perceptual and Motor Skills, 61,* 747-753.

deQuiros, J.B., & Schrager, O.L. (1978). *Neuropsychological fundamentals in learning disabilities.* San Rafael, CA: Academic Therapy Publications.

Fields, H.L. (1987). *Pain.* New York: McGraw Hill.

Gerbrandt, L.K., & Fowler, J.R. (1980). Arousal-related sustained potentials in neocortex and hippocampus of rats. *Progress in Brain Research, 54,* 109-116.

Gilfoyle, E.M., Grady, A.P., & Moore, J.C. (1981).

Children adapt. Thorofare, NJ: Slack Inc.

Goldberg, J.M., & Fernandez, C. (1984). The vestibular system. In I. Darian-Smith (Ed.). *Handbook of physiology, Section 1: The nervous system, Volume II: Sensory processes, Part 2* (pp. 977-1022). Bethesda: American Physiological Society.

Gottlieb, G. (1983). Psychobiological approach to developmental disabilities. In *Handbook of child psychiatry: Volume II, Infancy and developmental psychobiology*. New York: Wiley.

Guedry, F.E. (1974). Psychophysics of vestibular sensation. In H.H. Kornhuber (Ed.). *Handbook of sensory physiology, Volume VI/2, Vestibular system Part 2: Psychophysics, applied aspects and general interpretations* (pp. 3-154). New York, Springer-Verlag.

Hall, M.J., Bartoshuk, L.M., Cain, W.S., & Stevens, J.C. (1975). PTC taste blindness and the taste of caffeine. *Nature (London), 253*, 442-443.

Halpern, B.P. & Meiselman, H.L. (1980). Taste psychophysics based on a simulation of human drinking. *Chemical Sense, 5*, 279-294.

Heimer, L. (1983). *The human brain and spinal cord*. New York: Springer-Verlag.

Hermelin, B., & O'Connor, N. (1970). *Psychological experiments with autistic children*. New York: Pergamon Press.

Jarrard, L.E. (1980). Selective hippocampal lesions and behavior. *Physiological Psychology, 8*(2), 198-206.

Jongkees, L.B.W. (1974). Pathology of vestibular sensation. In H.H. Kornhuber (Ed.). *Handbook of sensory physiology, Volume VI/2, Vestibular system Part 2: Psychophysics, applied aspects and general interpretations* (pp. 413-450). New York: Springer-Verlag.

Kandel, E.R., & Schwartz, J.H. (1985). *Principles of neural science*. New York: Elsevier.

Kiang, N.Y.S. (1984). Peripheral neural processing of auditory information. In I. Darian-Smith (Ed.). *Handbook of physiology, Section 1: The nervous system, Volume II: Sensory processes, Part 2* (pp. 639-674). Bethesda: American Physiological Society.

Kornhuber, H.H. (1974). The vestibular system and the general motor system. In H.H. Kornhuber (Ed.). *Handbook of sensory physiology, Volume VI/2, Vestibular system Part 2: Psychophysics, applied aspects, and general interpretations* (pp. 581-620). New York: Springer-Verlag.

Kornhuber, H.H. (Ed.). (1975). *The somatosensory system*. Stuttgart: Georg Thieme Publishers.

Langworthy, O.R. (1933). Development of behavior patterns and myelinization of the nervous system in the human fetus and infant. *Contributions to Embryology, 24*, 1-57.

Liedgren, S.R., & Rubin, A.M. (1976). Vestibulo-thalamic projections studied with antidromic techniques in the cat. *Acta Oto-Laryngology, 82*, 379-387.

Lund, R.D. (1978). *Development and plasticity of the brain: An introduction*. New York: Oxford University Press.

Magnin, M., & Fuchs, A.F. (1977). Discharge properties of neurons in the monkey thalamus tested with angular acceleration, eye movement, and visual stimuli. *Experimental Brain Research, 28*, 293-299.

McGuinness, D., & Pribram, K. (1980). The Neuropsychology of attention: Emotional and motivational controls. In W. Hiack (Ed.). *The brain and psychology* (pp. 95-139). Orlando: Academic Press.

Melzack, R., & Wall, P.D. (1965). Pain mechanisms: A new theory. *Science, 150*, 971-978.

Melzack, R. & Casey, K.L. (1968). Sensory, motivational, and central control determinants of pain. In D. Kenshalo (Ed.). *The Skin* (pp. 423-439). Springfield: Charles C.. Thomas.

Mind and behavior: readings from Scientific American. (no author or editor) Intros by R.L. Atkinson & R.C. Atkinson. (1980) San Francisco: W. H. Freeman Co.

Moore, J. (1980). Neuroanatomical considerations relating to recovery of function following brain lesions. In P. Bach-y-Rita (Ed.). *Recovery of function: Theoretical considerations for brain injury rehabilitation* (pp. 9-90). Baltimore: University Park Press.

Moore, J. (1987, October). Myelogenesis of the nervous system from the proceedings of the 10th Adaptation Symposium. Denver, CO.

Noback, C.R. & Demarest, R.J. (1981). *The human nervous system*. New York: McGraw-Hill.

Oehler, J.M. (1985, December). Examining the issue of tactile stimulation for preterm infants. *Neonatal Network*, 25-33.

Ogulnick, M.L. (1981). A hippocampal model of extraversion based on arousal, activation, and chunking: Tests of the chunking hypothesis. *Dissertation Abstracts International, 41*(9), 3585-B.

Perl, E.R. (1984). Pain and nociception. In I. Darian-Smith (Ed.). *Handbook of physiology, Section 1: The nervous system, Volume II: Sensory processes, Part 2* (pp. 915-976). Bethesda: American Physiology Association.

Pribram, K.H., & McGuinness, D. (1975). Arousal, activation. and effort in the control of attention. *Psychological Review, 82*(2), 116-149.

Rosenzweig, M.R., Bennett, E.L., & Diamond, M.C. (1972). Brain changes in response to experience. *Science, III*, 117-124.

Schiller, P.H. (1984). The superior colliculus and visual function. In I. Darian-Smith, *Handbook of physiology,*

Section 1: The nervous system, Volume II: Sensory processes, Part 2 (pp. 457-506). Bethesda: American Physiology Society.

Shek, D.T.L., & Spinks, J.A. (1985). Effect of the orienting response on sensory discriminability. *Perceptual and Motor Skills, 61*, 987-1003.

Vinogradova, O.S. (1970). Registration of information and the limbic system. In G. Horn & R.A. Hinde (Eds.). *Short-term changes in neural activity and behavior* (pp. 95-139). Cambridge: Cambridge University Press.

Wepsic, J.G. (1966). Multimodal sensory activation of cells in the maguocellular medial geniculate nucleus. *Experimental Neurology, 15*, 299-319.

Yakovlev, P.A., & Le Cours, A.R. (1967). The myelogenetic cycles of regional maturation of the brain. (pp. 3-70). In A. Minkowski (Ed.). *Regional development of the brain in early life*. Oxford: Blackwell Scientific Publications.

CHAPTER CONTENT OUTLINE

KEY TERMS

Center of gravity

Coordination

Endurance

Habituate

Lower motor neuron

Motor unit

Prime mover

Reflex

Stabilizer

Synergist

Tone (tonus)

Upper motor neuron

ABSTRACT

This chapter defines neuromotor performance and identifies the current views
regarding the structures of the nervous system that are involved in the
production, regulation and execution of movement. The components and
properties of both the musculoskeletal system and the nervous system that relate
to movement and action are explained. The interrelationship of the nervous and
motor systems, and the major motor learning theories are also presented. The
chapter reviews therapeutic techniques and emphasizes the need for further
research to help provide a better understanding of the neuromotor factors that
underlie human performance.

Neuromotor Dimensions of Performance

Shereen D. Farber

"Motion signals life as surely as an untimely twitch betrays a cornered opossum to a foraging fox."

—R.D. Selim, 1982

OBJECTIVES

The information in this chapter is intended to help the reader—

1. define the term "neuromotor performance."

2. identify components and properties of muscle that are necessary for understanding movement and action.

3. identify important components and properties of the nervous system that relate to movement and action.

4. examine the relationship between sensory and motor systems.

5. review major motor learning theories.

6. summarize the factors which influence the quality and quantity of neuromotor performance.

7. review the principles underlying effective therapy for neuromotor dysfunction.

8. identify useful avenues for future research to help us better understand the neuromotor factors underlying human performance.

DEFINITION OF NEUROMOTOR PERFORMANCE

For the purposes of this text, *neuromotor performance* is defined as a complex functional behavior resulting from the activation of central and peripheral nervous system motor structures, executed by the musculoskeletal system, and influenced by a myriad of inputs from the subject's internal and external environment. Normal neuromotor performance is flexible and allows the individual to use multiple action plans. The systems and structures responsible for movement within an individual are constantly evolving throughout the developmental process (Mulder & Hulstyn, 1984).

Movement produced by an organism is a sign and symbol of life, and in fact, neuromotor performance is one of the major determinants of survival. Without movement capabilities, persons may not be able to care for themselves, express emotion, fulfill ambition, or escape from danger. Although technical advancements have made it possible for people to live with severe movement dysfunction, in these cases, continuous support is required.

NERVOUS SYSTEM AND MUSCULOSKELETAL STRUCTURES INVOLVED IN NEUROMOTOR PERFORMANCE

Cortical Structures

Association Cortex. The association areas of the cortex serve a more complex function than perception of sensation (Brown, 1980). These cortices also determine the need for participation in motor acts. Association cortices interpret the various sensory messages by determining the type, location, and intensity of the stimuli in order to make appropriate judgments. Primary cortical regions project to related association cortices, and connections are known to occur among the association cortices within a hemisphere and between hemispheres (Brown, 1980; Jensen, 1980; Matzke & Foltz, 1983; Shepherd, 1979). (Figure 10-1). Action of these cortices allows us to develop cross-modal activity. For example, if a person smells smoke, he/she can visualize flames and direct the motor system to activate an escape.

Motor Cortices. Several cortical areas are related to motor function including: (1) the primary motor area (Brodmann's area 4), (2) a secondary motor area that incorporates a supplementary motor area (Brodmann's area 6), (3) the frontal eye field (Brodmann's area 8, lower portion), (4) Broca's speech area, and (5) the prefrontal cortex. (See Figure 10-2, a & b.)

The primary motor area is located in the precentral gyrus, along the anterior wall of the central sulcus and in the anterior part of the paracentral lobule; it is said to be responsible for execution of motor activity (Barr & Kiernan, 1988). Somatotopic representation in the primary motor area mirrors that of the post-central gyrus (Matzke & Foltz, 1983). See Figure 10-3. Besides a somatotopic organization, this cortex is also arranged in columns which allows the precentral gyrus to amplify incoming sensory stimuli and inhibit extraneous sensory input (Lohr & Wisniewski, 1987). Input to the primary motor area (area 4) is primarily from area 6, the post-central gyrus (areas 3, 1 and 2), and the ventrolateral and ventroanterior nuclei of the thalamus. Major output from this area is projected into the corticospinal tract, which is one of the primary neural structures influencing fine voluntary movement (Lohr and Wisniewski, 1987). When area 4 is stimulated, contralateral muscular contraction is usually elicited with neural codes being generated for force, rate, and direction of movement. It does not directly control coordinated purposeful action.

The premotor area (area 6) is located directly anterior to area 4, and major input to area 6 is from the ventroanterior and ventrolateral thalamic nuclei and the prefrontal cortex. The major function of the premotor area is to supervise the output of area 4 and to learn new motor programs or modify older motor programs, based on new information or requirements. Area 6 communicates with area 4 and contributes to the corticospinal tract. In contrast to area 4, area 6 does control complex motor tasks, especially those related to the visual system (Porter, 1983). The supplementary motor region is located, in part, within area 6. Electrical stimulation of the supplementary motor region can produce activation of muscles bilaterally (Barr & Kiernan, 1988; Porter, 1983).

The frontal eye field is located in area 8 of the cortex. Its main function is to coordinate conjugate eye movements. When a lesion occurs in this region, the subject's eyes deviate to the side of the lesion (Barr & Kiernan, 1988).

Broca's speech area (area 44) is another cortical region with associated motor function and is located in the frontal cortex directly above the lateral sulcus. The function of this region is to control the expression of speech (Noback & Demarest, 1981). If an individual has pathology in this region in the dominant hemisphere, he or she will have expressive aphasia, the inability to formulate and produce speech. The prefrontal cortex (areas 9, 10, 11, and 12) influences the expression of behavior related to emotion.

Sensory Cortices. The primary sensory cortex (somesthetic) is in the post-central gyrus (areas 3, 1, and 2 in Figure 10-2a) This cortical region is somatotopically organized with the representation for the head situated near the lateral sulcus (Figure 10-3a), and the foot located on the medial aspect of the strip (Figure 10-3b). Cortical areas representing the face, mouth, and hand are disproportionately large suggesting the importance of these body parts to survival. This also gives us a valuable clue regarding which areas of a patient's body we should stimulate if we want to influence a large area of cortex. The post-central gyrus receives input from the ventroposterolateral nucleus of the thalamus. The primary sensory cortex contributes to the corticospinal tract and interacts with motor cortices, hence

the name sensorimotor strip. Lesions in this region will produce decreased discriminative touch contralaterally and such lesions can disrupt movement of body parts (Barr & Kiernan, 1988).

There is a small secondary somesthetic area located near the lateral sulcus near the post-central gyrus. This region has bilateral body part representation with predominate contralateral patterns. Projections to this region are from the intralaminar nuclei and posterior nuclei of the thalamus. It is said that the secondary somesthetic region is involved in less discriminative sensation (Barr & Kiernan, 1988). (See Figure 10-2a.)

Primary cortical areas exist for each type of sensory modality, such as area 17 for vision. Each primary area projects to nearby association cortices, for example, area 17 projects to areas 18 and 19. A general integration occurs among the association areas for each sensation within each hemisphere and between hemispheres. Several non-cortical structures, such as the cerebellum, the superior colliculus, the vestibular nuclei, the hippocampus, and the corpus striatum, are known to receive multisensory (and motor) input. The specific relationship of each of these brain regions to sensory integration and motor behavior is under investigation. It is interesting to note that sensory integration occurs in many

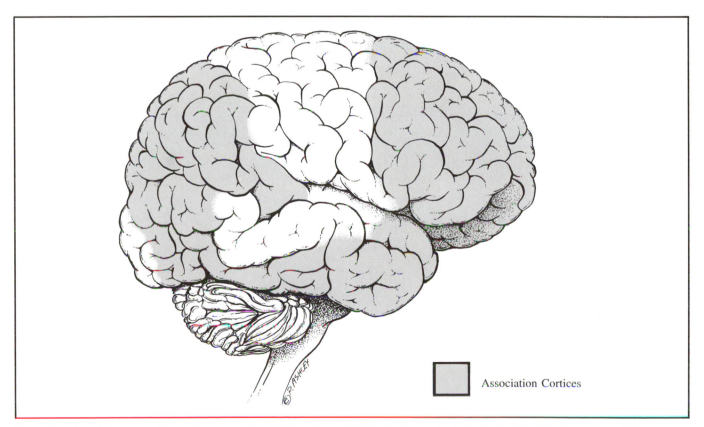

☐ Association Cortices

Figure 10-1. Association areas of the cerebral cortex. *Modified from Nolte, J. (1981). The Human Brain. St. Louis, MO: C.V. Mosby Co. p. 269.*

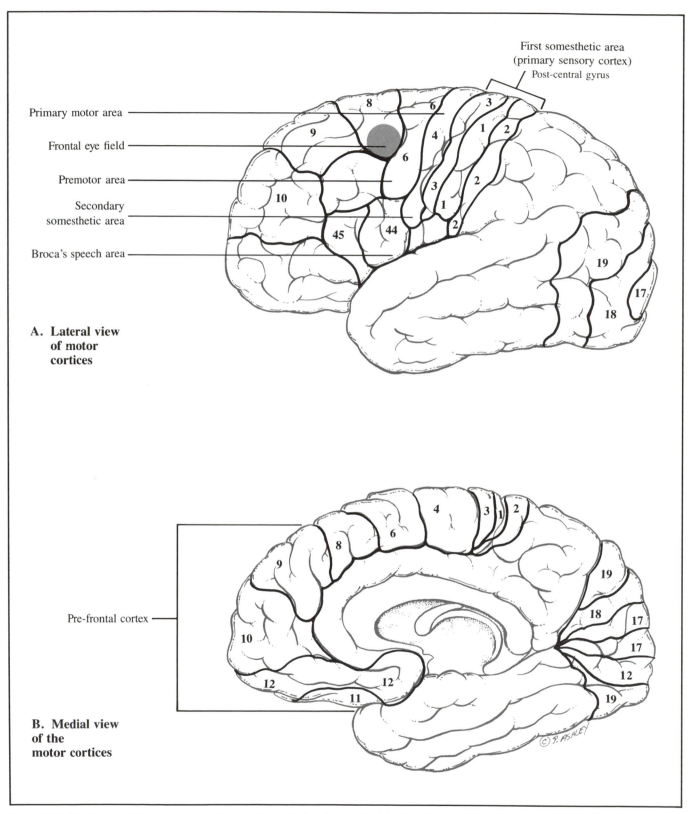

First somesthetic area
(primary sensory cortex)
Post-central gyrus

Primary motor area

Frontal eye field

Premotor area

Secondary
somesthetic area

Broca's speech area

**A. Lateral view
of motor
cortices**

Pre-frontal cortex

**B. Medial view
of the
motor cortices**

© P. ASHLEY

Figure 10-2a&b. Motor and Sensory Cortices. Brodmann's map (selected areas). *Modified from Noback, CR and Demarest, RJ (1981). The Human Nervous System. New York, NY: McGraw Hill, p. 486.*

locations within the nervous system. Each location may subserve a different aspect of sensory integration function or may serve as a backup center for the other.

Limbic Cortex. The limbic system oversees emotional tone and expression related to survival of both the individual and the species. The limbic system consists of cingulate gyrus, parahippocampal gyrus, hippocampal and dentate gyrus, and a number of structures that are functionally related including the hypothalamus, certain thalamic nuclei, specific regions of the brain stem tegmentum, epithalamus, orbital gyri, preoptic area, and the septal nuclei (Matzke & Foltz, 1983). The hippocampal component is known to contribute to memory function (Barr & Kieman, 1988). Without the limbic system the drive to move might not exist; and it has a profound effect on our emotional well-being. (See Figure 10-4.)

Motor Tracts Descending from the Cortex. The function of the *corticospinal tract* is to control fine, skilled movement, primarily in the contralateral upper extremity (Iv-

ersen, 1981; Matzke & Foltz, 1983). This tract is a major descending tract emanating from areas 3, 1, 2, 4, and 6 of the cortex. This tract sends collaterals to various structures as it courses downward. Approximately 80% of the fibers cross in the pyramids of the brain stem. Some of the fibers break up on the pontine nuclei and then enter the cerebellum to communicate intended action. The remaining fibers continue downward to the spinal cord with 10% of them ending directly on lower motor neurons and 90% ending on interneurons.

The corticonuclear tract is another group of fibers descending from the neocortex. The purpose of these tracts is to regulate the activity of cranial nerve nuclei.

Upper Motor Neurons. Motor structures known as **upper motor neurons** (UMN) are found throughout the central nervous system. In the telencephalon, the motor cortices and basal ganglia contain upper motor neurons. The thalamus and subthalamus house the upper motor neurons of the diencephalon. Many upper motor neurons reside in the brain stem including the red nuclei, motor nuclei of the

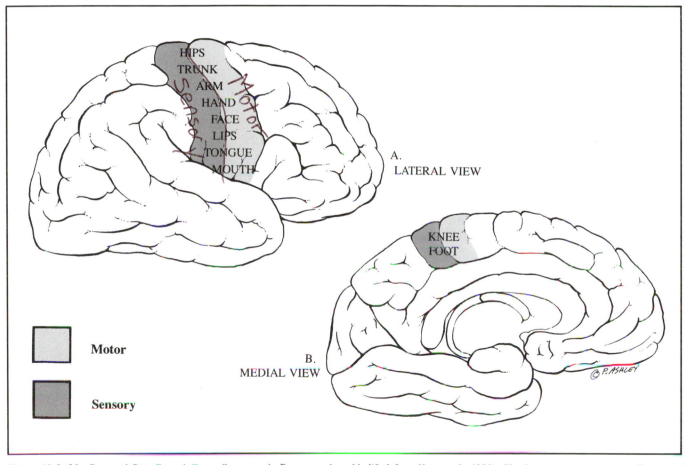

Figure 10-3a&b. Pre- and Post-Central Gyrus Somatotopic Representation. *Modified from Hermer, L (1983). The human nervous system—Functional neuroanatomy and dissection guide. New York, NY: Springer Verlag, p. 351.*

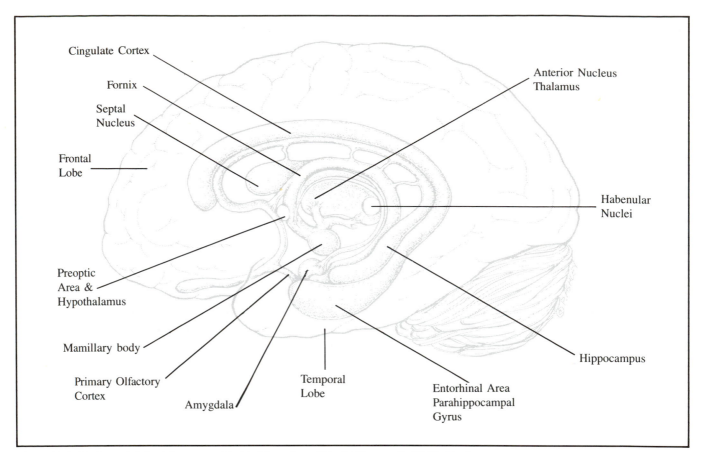

Figure 10-4. Limbic and Related Structures. *Modified from Barr, MA, & Kiernan, JA (1983). The human nervous system: An anatomical viewpoint. Philadelphia, PA: J.B. Lippincott, p. 270.*

reticular formation, amd the medial and lateral vestibular nuclei. Upper motor neurons give rise to descending tracts that control **lower motor neurons**. Interconnections among the upper motor neurons provide one basis for motor coordination (Figure 10-5).

Subcortical Structures

Basal Ganglia. Basal ganglia are upper motor neurons that are said to influence proximal musculature, stereotyped movements, auxiliary movements such as arm swings during gait, postural and tonal adjustments, initiation of movement, selection of appropriate subroutines, and the movement response to the environment (Brooks, 1986; Brown, 1980; Matzke & Foltz, 1983; Noback & Demarest, 1981). The main components of the basal ganglia consist of the caudate nucleus, the putamen, and the globus pallidum. The subthalamic nuclei and substantia nigra are closely associated. The basal ganglia surround the thalamus in the diencephalon with the internal capsule separating the thalamus and basal ganglia. The caudate receives input from all lobes of the cortex and in turn sends axons to the putamen.

The globus pallidus serves as the major output pathway for the basal ganglia and projects axons to the thalamus and the subthalamic nucleus. The substantia nigra has reciprocal connections with the caudate and putamen (Evarts & Wise, 1984; Farber, 1982; Iversen, 1981; Matzke & Folz, 1983). (See Figure 10-6.)

Cerebellum. The cerebellum receives sensory input from sensory modalities of sensory receptors and in turn communicates with specific upper motor neurons in order to coordinate muscular action. It also receives input from descending motor systems, so that it is informed about impending motor activity. Although the basal ganglia are said to influence initiation of motion, the cerebellum modifies action once it has commenced. Other functional roles of the cerebellum include error correction, **coordination** among groups of muscles (synergies), equilibrium responses, and tonal adjustments. The synaptic interaction among the cells of the cerebellar cortex have been studied by motor experts and are considered to be vital to motor learning (Brooks, 1986; Brown, 1980; Matzke & Foltz, 1983; Shepherd, 1979).

Thalamus. The thalamus is the largest component of the diencephalon and is composed of a variety of nuclei (sensory, motor, and autonomic) that serve as a sorting station for both ascending and descending information. It maintains specific connections with various regions of the cortex and interacts with a medley of subcortical structures.

Red Nucleus. The red nucleus is an upper motor neuron located at the junction of the diencephalon and midbrain, and may serve as a motor integration center (Shepherd, 1979). In addition, the red nucleus contains cells that are known to activate co-contraction patterns of wrist musculature in primates (DeLuca & Mambrito, 1987). This wrist co-contraction may serve to stablize the wrist so that skill can occur in the hand. Although all the connections to the red nucleus are unknown according to Barr and Kiernan (1988), input to the red nucleus arises primarily from the cerebellum, with minor components from the cerebral cortex and globus pallidus. Red nucleus outputs cross the midline and coalesce to become the rubrospinal tract, a tract that influences extensors (flexor bias tract) and contributes to fine flexor control in the upper extremity. Additional output from this nucleus synapses on the facial nucleus and the inferior olivary nucleus, a structure that sends axons to the cerebellum (Barr & Kiernan, l988; Brown, 1980).

Reticular Formation. The reticular formation, located chiefly in the tegmentum of the brain stem, consists of diffusely organized nuclei and tracts. All ascending and descending tracts send collaterals to the reticular formation thus influencing both sensory and motor activity. The complex functions attributed to the reticular formation are beyond the scope of this discussion; however, damage to the reticular formation can produce coma. The pontine reticular formation gives rise to a motor tract that is an extensor bias tract (*pontine reticulospinal tract*), while the medullary reticular formation produces a flexor bias tract (*medullary reticulospinal tract*) (Barr & Kiernan, l988; Matzke & Foltz, 1983).

Vestibular Nuclei. The secondary sensory nuclei for the vestibular system are located in the brain stem. Two of these nuclei, the medial and lateral vestibular nuclei, are also upper motor neurons and give rise to descending motor tracts. The lateral vestibular nucleus gives rise to the *lateral vestibulospinal tract*, which is an extensor-bias tract that stimulates midline body extensors and is important in the maintenance of balance and posture.

The medial vestibular nucleus gives rise to the *medial vestibulospinal tract,* which projects to the cervical and thoracic spinal cord levels and descends to the muscles of the neck in order to control head movements for appropriate

equilibrium responses (Barr & Kiernan, 1988; Noback & Demarest, 1981). The vestibular nuclei also give rise to ascending projections that travel in the medial longitudinal fasciculus and synapse on cranial nerve nuclei III, IV, and VI. The function of these projections is to enhance the coordination between head and eye movements. Connections between the vestibular nuclei and the reticular formation, cerebellum, and cortex may also impact on motor function.

Lower Motor Neurons of the Brain Stem. Lower motor neurons associated with the brain stem belong to the cranial nerve nuclear group, and control head and neck muscular activity. Table 10-1 shows a list of the neurons included in this group and the functions for which they are responsible (Matzke & Foltz, 1983).

Spinal Cord and Peripheral Structures

Lower Motor Neurons. One simplistic way to view communication among the components of the motor system is to say that upper motor neurons "talk" to lower motor

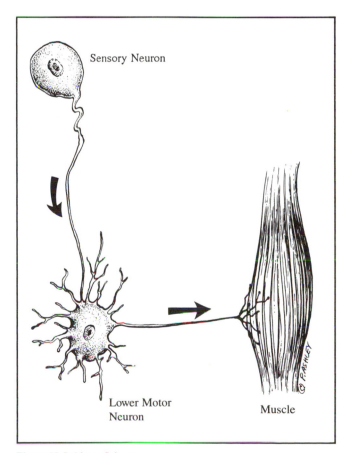

Figure 10-5. Motor Schema.

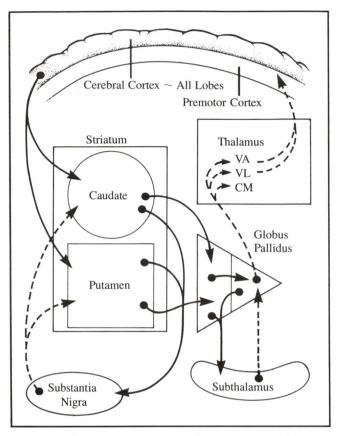

Figure 10-6. Schematic View of the Basal Ganglia and Related Structures. VA = Ventral Anterior; NVL = Ventral Lateral Nuc.; CM = Centromedian Nuc.

neurons, who then "talk" to muscles (Figure 10-5). Many descending tracts, interneurons, and sensory neurons synapse on each motor neuron. One source estimates that there are approximately 15,000 synapses on an average lower motor neuron (Selim, 1982). Two main varieties of lower motor neurons of the spinal cord, the *alpha motor neurons* and *gamma motor neurons*, exist in the ventral horn of the spinal cord. The alpha motor neuron innervates extrafusal (voluntary) muscle fibers and is the larger of the two types. Gamma motor neurons supply the intrafusal fibers found in muscle spindles.

Motor Unit. A **motor unit** is comprised of one alpha motor neuron and the muscle fibers that it supplies. Muscles with a fine degree of control have motor units consisting of only a few muscle fibers, while muscles with gross motor control like those of the back have numerous muscle fibers per alpha motor neuron. For example, extraocular muscles have motor units with three muscle fibers per neuron (Selim, 1982).

Types of Muscles. One element of the movement activation system is voluntary (*striated*) muscle. This muscle is

comprised of contractile protein. Some of the methods for classifying muscle are listed below:

Agonist muscles (**prime movers**)—A prime mover has the principle responsibility for a given action. In addition to the primary action, many muscles demonstrate secondary functions that are weaker movement patterns. For example, the anterior tibialis muscle is the prime mover for dorsiflexion with a secondary function of inversion.

Antagonist muscles—Antagonist muscls work in opposition to prime movers. Selim (1982) states that there is a fluid collaboration between the prime movers and the antagonists based on Sherrington's principle of reciprocal innervation. Sherrington noted that when a prime mover contracts or shortens, the antagonist muscle receives an inhibitory message causing the antagonist to lengthen. Lesions in the central nervous system may disrupt the smooth coordination between agonist and antagonist muscles.

Synergist muscles—Synergist muscles function by inhibiting extraneous action from muscles that interfere with the prime movers.

Stabilizer muscles—Stabilizers hold one attachment of a prime mover or may hold a bone or body part steady, thus providing a firm foundation for movement. Often muscle pairs, agonists and antagonists, coactivate around a joint to achieve stability. De Luca and Mambrito (1987) found that coactivation patterns are engaged under the following conditions: when an individual demonstrates uncertainty in a motor task or when a compensatory force correction is required. This degree of coactivation around a joint decreases as skill increases.

White muscle and dark muscle—White muscle is characterized by fast-twitch fibers and decreased **endurance**. White muscle also shows decreased myoglobin, increased glycolytic enzymes, and increased adenosine triphosphate (ATP) activity in the myofibrils (Hay & Reid, 1982). In contrast, dark muscle is characterized by slow-twitch fibers and increased endurance. Dark muscle also shows increased myoglobin, decreased glycolytic enzymes, and decreased ATP in the myofibrils. All human muscle is a mixture of light and dark fibers although one variety usually predominates in a given muscle. The gastrocnemius muscle is an example of a muscle consisting primarily of fast-twitch (white muscle) fibers.

Many variables interact to effect the composition of a muscle. For example, training can affect muscle composition. For example, the leg muscles of sprinters (who rely on quick muscle movement for short periods of time) that show a higher percentage of white muscle in comparison to the same muscles of marathon runners (who rely on endurance over long periods of running) that show a higher percentage of dark muscle (Hay and Reid, 1982). Age is another influencing factor and, as an individual ages, the percentage of white muscle fibers decreases in specific muscles (Bass, Gutmann, & Hanzlikova, 1972; Larsson, 1978).

Types of Muscle Contraction. Muscle contraction is traditionally defined as an increase in tension or a shortening in muscle fibers. This definition does not allow for all varieties of contractions such as when fibers actually lengthen.

Isometric contractions or *hold contractions* occur when the ends of a muscle are maintained in a fixed position or stabilized with an increased tension evenly distributed throughout the muscle. Isometric contractions are preferred for use in exercise programs for people having painful inflamed joints (Sandler & Vernikos, 1986). During isometric contractions, the muscle experiences increased blood flow, and systemic blood pressure tends to rise (Lamb, 1984). This response should be considered when developing treatment programs for hypertensive individuals.

An *isotonic contraction* occurs when a muscle shortens against a constant load. An individual can produce a maximum force in this type of contraction.

Concentric contraction involves muscular shortening during the contraction process as the muscle overcomes resistance, whereas *eccentric contraction* involves the lengthening of muscle fibers. It is shown that during eccentric contractions, there is less electromyographic activity, less oxygen uptake by the muscle, fewer motor units are activated, and less recruitment is measured. Gravity can participate in eccentric contractions, but the individual must produce a controlled lengthening for a smooth contraction to occur (Hay & Reid, 1982). Although eccentric contractions seem to be easier to perform than concentric contractions, repetitive exercise using eccentric muscular contractions may produce muscle soreness. Because of the greater force produced by eccentric contractions, fibers may sustain microinjury resulting in muscular pain (Lamb, 1984).

Muscle fatigue is defined as a decreased ability to maintain a contraction at a given force (Lamb, 1984). Many factors contribute to or cause muscular fatigue including central nervous system disease, muscle disease, decreased physical conditioning, decreased energy substrates, poor blood supply, metabolic disturbances, and peripheral nerve pathology or problems at the neuromuscular junction (Lamb, 1984). Fatigue is a common problem seen in patients with neuromotor pathology. Occupational therapists must monitor the amount of activity a patient is asked to perform to prevent fatigue while at the same time building the patient's endurance.

Bone-muscle Relationships. Without the bony component of the musculoskeletal system, muscle action could not occur. Muscles and bones interact in order to produce movement at joints. The type of movement depends on which muscles and joints are activated, specific patterns of muscle-to-bone attachments, and the type of resistance to movement.

Bone-muscle relationships have been classified into a lever system with three distinct types. In any lever, the *fulcrum* is the point on which the lever turns. The *load arm* is the space between the fulcrum and the load, whereas the *power arm* is the region between the fulcrum and the muscle (Figure 10-7). In general, the power arm is usually shorter than the load arm (Selim, 1982).

Class 1 lever—the fulcrum is located between the load and the resistance, thus producing efficient, fast movement but with diminished force (see Figure 10-8a). An example of this type of arrangement in the body is when a child throws a rock across a room. The arm acts as a Class 1 lever with the elbow serving as the fulcrum. Force acts upon the resistance through the fulcrum.

Class 2 lever—the resistance is located between the fulcrum and the load thus promoting power instead of speed (see Figure 10-8b). An example of this movement is a short woman standing on the balls of her feet trying to achieve more height to reach an object on a high shelf. Her toes act as the fulcrum, her body weight is the resistance, and her calf muscles are the muscular force.

Class 3 lever—the force is located between the fulcrum and resistance (see Figure 10-8c). With this muscle-to-bone arrangement, it is necessary for the individual to produce rapid movement in order to generate force. Force increases as speed increases (Selim, 1982). An illustration of this lever arrangement in the body can be seen when a teenager lifts a free-weight in a biceps curl. The biceps exert an upward force pulling the forearm toward the shoulder. The weight acts as the resistance.

Table 10-1
Lower Motor Neuron Functions

Neuron	Function
Nuclei III, IV and VI	Extraocular movements
Nuclei V	Mastication
Nuclei VII	Facial expression
Nuclei IX	Innervation of stylopharyngeus muscle
Nuclei X	Supply axons to muscles of pharynx, larynx, esophagus
Nuclei XI	Nerve supply of sternocleidomastoid and trapezius
Nuclei XII	Innervation of muscles of tongue

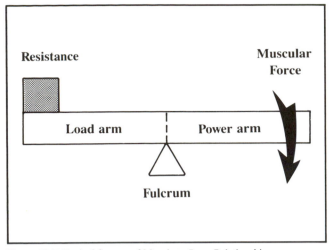

Figure 10-7. Typical System of Muscle to Bone Relationship.

Sensory Receptors

Sensory receptors are classified into types by function and location (See Table 10-2).

There are also special sensory receptors for each sense. Sensory input is transduced by receptors and reported to the central nervous system. For example, mechanical pressure delivered at a pressure receptor is transformed into electrochemical impulses that are meaningful to the central nervous system. This sensory information can then influence motor function.

The *muscle spindle*, an encapsulated sensory receptor, is included here as an example of the interaction between sensory input and motor performance. Muscle spindles are attached in a parallel arrangement to the myofibrils within the belly of voluntary muscle. When a muscle is stretched, the nerve endings of the muscle spindles report muscle fiber length and tension data to alpha motor neurons. At the time these messages enter the spinal cord, collaterals ascend to the cerebellum and other higher centers. The gamma motor neurons innervate the intrafusal fibers (those muscle fibers inside the capsule) and are stimulated by higher centers shortly after alpha motor neurons fire (alpha-gamma coactivation). Gamma motor neuron stimulation is said to bias the muscle spindle fibers and prevent collapse of the intrafusal muscle fibers so that they can remain sensitive to stretch.

It has been suggested that the sympathetic division of the autonomic nervous system innervates the nucler bag fibers of the muscle spindle. Thus if the individual is distressed, the muscle spindles may be overly taut so that slight stretches will result in contraction and perhaps hypertonia or excessive resistance (Boyd & Gladden, 1985; Swash & Fox, 1985).

The participation of the muscle spindle in the stretch reflex is one way in which muscle **tone** is modulated. According to Selim (1982), a stretch reflex occurs within 1/20,000 of one second as impulses travel from the muscle spindle to the alpha motor neuron at the rate of 200 miles per hour.

MOTOR LEARNING THEORIES

Closed Loop Theory

The closed loop theory was first described by Adams (1971; 1976) with self-regulation as a major theoretical feature (Figure 10-9). Muscular activity serves as feedback to the nervous system where an error-detection and error-correction system exists. New movements are made possible as the central nervous system uses feedback to compare novel movement requirements with existing memory and perceptual traces, thus allowing appropriate modification to be generated (Mulder & Hulstyn, 1984).

Open Loop Theory

Lashley (1917) proposed the open loop theory in which he suggested that motor programs were stored in a sequence of commands structured before a movement event occurred without input from peripheral feedback. This theory has been criticized because the research done to validate the theory employed lower level vertebrates known to possess innate motor programs. In studies with higher level mammals, methodological problems existed including incomplete eradication of sensory input. Thus the theory has not been adequately tested. Keele and Summers (1976) hypothesize that gross rhythmic activities may not require peripheral feedback but that sensory input is necessary for expression of fine manipulative skills.

Schema Theory

The schema theory was presented by Schmidt (1975; 1976a). Schmidt believes that schema or motor plans are constructed via experience and are modified after each trial. In order to achieve a novel movement, Schmidt postulates that the individual enters an existing schema with information regarding the desired outcome and the initial conditions, and this allows schemas to be appropriately modified.

Environmental/Ecological Theory

Those who support the environmental or ecological theory stress the importance of assessing the total, meaningful, goal-directed activity. This theory includes consideration of both the environment and the total performance (Stadler, Schwab, and Wehner, 1978) and is in contrast to the work of the motor learning theorists who analyze subsets of simple movement in laboratory or

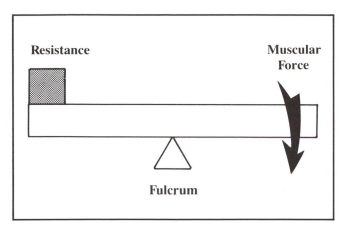

Figure 10-8a. Class 1 Lever.

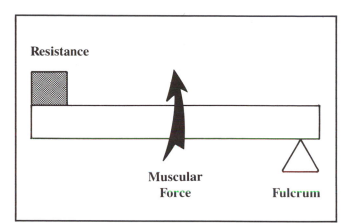

Figure 10-8c. Class 3 Lever.

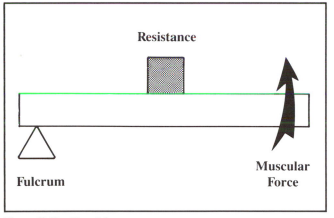

Figure 10-8b. Class 2 Lever.

simulated situations (Mulder and Hulstyn, 1984).

Reed (1982) describes the physiology of activity where the organism is in constant non-equilibrium with its environment, thus necessitating adaptation. *Adaptation* is the ability to make flexible changes in motor behavior that enhance survival. The process of adaptation occurs over a period of time.

Heterarchical Theory

First described by Turvey (1977), heterarchical theory suggests that control of motor function is not unidirectional as in a hierarchy. Instead, there are relatively autonomous structures at *all* levels in the nervous system that interact to distribute control to achieve a desired outcome. Turvey recognizes the influence of the Russian scientists, such as Luria and Bernstein, in the development of a heterarchical theory of motor control. At present, many neuroscientists and motor learning specialists subscribe to this theory including Newell (1981), Greene (1982), and Mulder and Hulstyn (1984). Heterarchical organizations provide for

more flexibility than hierarchies. Action plans are formulated at the executive levels of the heterarchy, whereas pattern movements may exist autonomously in lower regions of the system. Kugler and associates (1980) described a low-level pattern where muscle groups are linked together functionally into collectives.

Another aspect of the heterarchical theory is the concept of tuning. Environmental conditions or some aspect of the subject's nervous system can influence without actually producing the outcome. For example, if the sympathetic nervous system is overstimulated, the muscle spindles may be excessively taut so that when a slight stretch occurs, the resultant muscle tone is exaggerated. This is similar to tuning a stringed musical instrument that will not produce sound unless directly plucked or bowed but will enhance the musical product after tuning (Turvey, 1977).

Posture and Movement Theory

This theory views control of posture and movement as organized into three different levels (Brooks, 1986). The highest level consists of the association cortex with major input from the limbic cortex. The drive to move is coordinated with relevant perceptions and motor plans. According to Brooks, the limbic system input is critical in assisting the association cortex in translating needs into goals. Plans and strategy are synthesized by the highest level, assisted by interconnections with the caudate nucleus to accomplish goal-directed behavior.

In the middle level, strategy is converted into motor tactics. This level contains the sensorimotor cortex, cerebellum, the putamen loop of the basal ganglia, and brainstem structures.

The lower level or spinal processing level executes movement and posture. The spinal cord can function autonomously via **reflex** and automatic movements but is influenced by higher centers. There are multiple

Table 10-2
Functions of Sensory Receptors

Type of Receptor	Function
Exteroceptors	Provide information from the external environment
Proprioceptors	Report sensory data regarding the position of the body in space and the relationship of the body parts to each other
Interoceptor	Located in hollow viscera and send messages to the nervous system regarding the status of the particular organ
Chemoreceptors	Report chemical levels
Baroreceptors	Report pressure and stretch

interconnections among the components of the motor system, and no one of these components works without influencing the other.

Spatial Temporal Theory

Gilfoyle, Grady & Moore (1978) have incorporated many of the components of motor learning into a theory of spatiotemporal adaptation of individuals in their environment. They describe four aspects of a process of interaction including: assimilation, accommodation, association, and differentiation. *Assimilation* involves obtaining sensory information from either internal or external sources. *Accommodation* describes the subject's motor adjustments in order to receive sensory input. *Association* explains the integrational process between sensory input and motor response in addition to comparisons between past and present movement patterns. *Differentiation* requires identification of specific behavioral elements that must be produced for appropriate modification of the motor response. Gilfoyle and Grady believe that the final process is adaptation. The theory of spatiotemporal adaptation shares many common features with other motor learning theories but embodies appropriate occupational therapy intervention.

SENSORY SYSTEM AND MOTOR PERFORMANCE

Denis (1985) describes sensation as an aspect of human behavior turned inward, whereas motor activity represents human performance turned outward; sensation is private whereas motor activity is public. In this section, we will explore the relationship of sensation to motor performance.

Development of the Sensory Systems

The various sensory systems develop at different rates. Light-moving touch applied to the perioral region of a 7-1/2-week-old fetus produces an avoidance response (Hooker, 1977). This behavior represents one of the first sensorimotor reflex arcs to be demonstrated in development. Previously, therapists oversimplified the developmental process of sensory systems due to our interpretation of the neuroscience literature, the lack of operational definitions in the area of sensory system development, and the lack of state-of-the-art developmental research (Ayres, 1972; Farber, 1982). For example, it was believed that the vestibular system was one of the early-developing sensory systems with differentiation during the first trimester of pregnancy, and visual and auditory systems were attributed to later stages of development (Arey, 1974; Lowrey, 1973). While it is true that the visual system continues to develop for years after birth, we now know that, in fact, many components of the system are in place early in development and begin interacting with the vestibular system shortly after birth.

Therapists presume that stimuli representing early developing sensory systems should be introduced during the initial stages of neurorehabilitative or sensory integrative therapy. This hypothesis is based on the knowledge that early developing systems interact with the functional development of later developing systems. For example, if the vestibular system is dysfunctional, input to the cranial nerve nuclei that control eye movements will be compromised (Farber, 1982). As a result, eye tracking may not be of optimum quality. Such hypotheses need to be tested in controlled therapeutic intervention studies. It is important for therapists to carefully collect data regarding the interdependence of the development of the various sensory systems as they relate to human performance.

Receptors

Sensory receptors are the first structures to greet incoming information, then they translate this incoming information into a form that is meaningful to the central nervous system. In general, afferent messages will not synapse until they reach the central nervous system, thus assuring faithful reporting of information gathered from the environment. The threshold for a given receptor varies with age, sex, autonomic status, location of the receptor, and many other factors. If synapses occurred on peripheral nervous system structures like dorsal root ganglion cells, messages might be modified before reaching the nervous system. When sensation is continuous and repetitive,

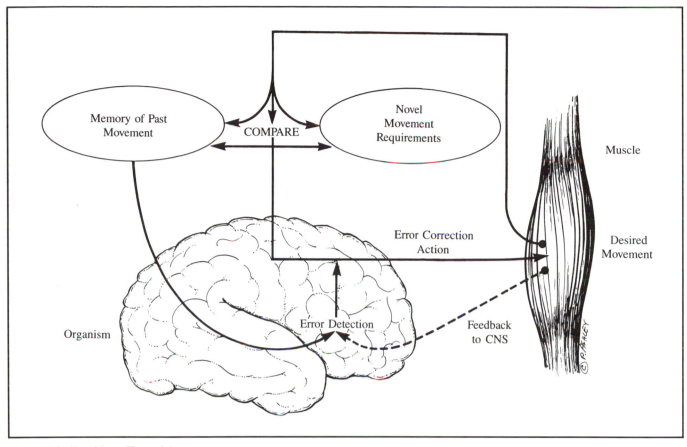

Figure 10-9. Closed Loop Theory Schema.

sensory receptors adapt (**habituate**) and may ignore input unless it is vital to survival.

Sensory Integration

Sensory integration occurs when a structure receives two or more types of neural communication (sensory, motor, or autonomic) and fuses that input into functional adaptive responses. Many different sensory integration centers exist within the central nervous system, each subserving different general functions. The manner in which the various centers relate to each other is still the subject of many investigations.

Types of Sensory Stimulation

Natural Versus Artificial Stimulation. The lack of apparent agreement in the use of natural versus artificial sensory stimuli underscores the need for improvement in operational definitions used in health professions. The following demonstrates how differently some authors define these terms. Some authors recommend that sensory stimuli be as natural or appropriate to the life experience of the subject as

is possible in order to produce adaptive responses (Farber, 1982). For example, weight-bearing through the arms and shoulders is a significant part of the sensory experience of an infant who is 6 to 8 months old. Thus, joint approximation designed to promote weight-bearing through the upper extremities is considered a desirable and natural stimulus for development or redevelopment of proximal stability at the shoulders.

In contrast, Mulder and Hulstyn (1984) prefer the use of *artificial stimuli* because they view natural stimuli as (1) qualitative (providing motivational or reinforcement information), (2) subjective (depending on the therapist's alertness), (3) superficial (allowing for only the most overt behavioral response to be monitored), and (4) slow in delivery (supplying feedback after the response has already occurred). These authors favor artificial stimuli such as biofeedback or electrical stimulation for muscle re-education because these stimuli are (1) quantitative (providing actual numbers for measurement because of monitoring devices), (2) objective (not requiring the therapist's attention during the stimulation), (3) accurate (providing information even at the level of the neuromuscular junction instead of just at the superficial overt behavioral level) and (4) immediate (with sensory feedback present even during the response). These authors believe that using artificially stimulated biofeedback for re-educating muscles is beneficial because the therapist can monitor individual motor units and provide quick auditory feedback to the patient.

Single Sensory Versus Multisensory Stimulation

Complex multisensory stimuli may not be appropriate for people having central nervous system lesions or immature nervous systems. Any stimulus that combines elements of more than one sensory modality is considered multisensory (Farber, 1982). In a classic study, Ritvo (1969) compared *postrotatory nystagmus* in age-matched normal children to autistic children. Postrotatory nystagmus is the rhythmical oscillation of the eyeballs occuring after a rotational vestibular stimulation. When the children received rotatory vestibular stimulation in a lighted room, the autistic children demonstrated significantly reduced postrotatory nystagmus compared to the normal controls. When rotatory input was delivered in a dark room with the children having their eyes open, no significant differences were observed between the groups. Ritvo concluded that the autistic children were unable to process the multisensory input. Whether application of multisensory versus single sensory input might reduce the quality of other motor responses in patients with distinct disease entities remains to be explored.

Guided Practice

Guided practice occurs when the performer is directed, cortically or subcortically, to activate a movement or movement components guided by feedback provided by a support person (therapist or coach). The support person must have excellent timing, anticipating when movement components are to be initiated.

Newell (1978) reports that once the additional feedback is withdrawn, the quality of the performance decays. In order to prevent the deterioration of action, the feedback must be applied in an intermittent manner. Schmidt (1976b) claims that sensory feedback from reflexes can be used to rapidly modify a motor act (50-80 msec) as long as central processing is not required to alter the action plan. If adjustments are required by central structures, sensory feedback will require longer time periods to effect change (120-200 msec) (Schmidt 1982). MacKenzie and Marteniuk (1987) suggest that visual feedback used to correct motor accuracy takes approximately 150 msec. They conclude that an integrated store of sensorimotor information is at the base of all coordinated movements. This store defines the relationships among body parts and of the body to the environment, so that movement goals can be achieved.

Effects of Decreased Sensation

Many researchers have asked the question, ''Will motor quality decrease if sensory feedback is eradicated?'' Scientists have investigated the consequences of destroying various sensory structures including the sensorimotor cortex, tracts, and afferent nerves. Research has shown that the body compensates for partial sensory losses with only a slight decrease in quality of motor activity. However, a total decrease in sensory input will result in motor deficit (Asanuma, 1986). Studies of total sensory deprivation are rare because of the difficulties in producing permanent dysfunction in certain sensory pathways that provide sensory input vital to survival (i.e., pain).

COMPONENTS OF NEUROMOTOR PERFORMANCE

Action Versus Movement

Proponents of the environmental theory stress the importance of examining action versus movement. Mulder and Hulstyn (1984) identify action as having an action plan, an intent to move, and specific goals that will shape the sequence and organization of voluntary movement components. Any given action is the sum of individual movements. Brooks (1986) describes movement as a process of trunk or limb repositioning that occurs between postures. Lohr and Wisniewski (1987) concur and extend the definition to specify change in position resulting from the action of striated muscles. There are simple movements that are learned early and more complex multijoint movements acquired later in development that require more coordination. For example, initially a neonate moves its limbs in phasic random bursts. With learning, the infant progresses to controlling specific body parts during an activity. This control requires coordination among many muscles, joints and all compoents of human performance.

Reciprocal Movements

One of the earliest forms of movement observed in humans is random *reciprocal movements*. As described earlier in this chapter, reciprocal movement occurs between agonist and antagonist muscle pairs. With developmental modification, reciprocal movement patterns are incorporated into higher level actions, including the swing phase of gait and rapid reaching movements. With these developmental refinements, we are able to replace random expression with precision in the performance of reciprocal movements. Sherrington did the classic experimental work in reciprocal movement (see under Antagonist Muscle discussion). As early as 1925, Tilney and Pike identified the cerebellum as critical to switching from a reciprocal pattern to one of coactivated muscular action. More recent studies support this contention (Terzuolo, Soechting, and Viviani, 1973).

One clinical example of reciprocal behavior is the sucking response of infants. Initially, sucking is a reflex that is vital to survival. As the baby learns to coordinate lips, tongue, head, throat, hands, and other elements in order to drink from a cup, sucking is replaced as a primary method of liquid intake. Sucking gradually becomes a voluntary motor act and the sucking reflex is integrated.

Posture and Postural Set

Brooks (1986) says that *posture* is the static position assumed by any body part or by the body in general that requires muscular effort. Subjects must make postural adjustments as they move body parts or change activity levels. Multiple structures and pathways contribute to postural skill because its maintenance is vital to survival (Brooks, 1986). Brown and Frank (1987) state that successful execution of voluntary movement demands a precise interaction between anticipatory postural adjustments and primary movement. Many authors believe that there are separate control centers for posture and for movement, with postural control occurring at lower levels of the motor system (Brown & Frank, 1987; Cordo & Nashner, 1982; and Nashner & McCollum, 1985). Therefore, one might speculate that a patient with damage in the postural control areas such as the vestibular system, might have difficulty with anticipating and producing tonal change necessary for precise movement.

Good body alignment occurs when the **center of gravity** of each body segment is located over the supporting base of the body (Selim, 1982). This ideal alignment, known by the lay public as ''good posture,'' provides maximum support for each part along with minimum strain (Brooks, 1986).

Postural set refers to a subcortical process in which the subject predetermines the tension and length of muscles to be used in a given activity. Brooks (1986) calls this ''bracing.'' Brown and Frank (1987) refer to it as ''preparatory set'' and manipulate the preparatory set of their subjects by informing them of the type movement to anticipate before the movement is activated.

Reflexive and Stereotypic Movement

A *reflex* is an involuntary motor response that remains relatively consistent for a given stimulus (Selim, 1982). For example, if one pricks the bottom of a patient's foot, the patient should withdraw that foot in a reflex pattern. This response is known as the flexor withdrawal reflex and occurs at the spinal cord level. Recent studies show that reflexes are not hard-wired, but demonstrate contextual and adaptive modification (MacKenzie & Marteniuk, 1987). Reflexes can be modified by many factors, including maturation, stress, alcohol, decreased sleep, drugs, intention, and biomechanical positioning.

Use of the Jendrassik maneuver demonstrates how reflexes may be modified (Figure 10-10). This is accomplished by first testing a subject's muscle stretch reflexes at base line, before any type of manipulation or intervention occurs. Then the subject is asked to perform the Jendrassik maneuver by interlocking hands and then pulling each hand in opposite directions. The maneuver will amplify the muscle stretch reflexes by a process known as *central facilitation*, which is the activation of higher centers that in turn send descending input to the lower motor neurons (Barrows, 1980).

Each level of the central nervous system has characteristic reflex patterns that change with maturity and disease. Spinal cord reflexes tend to be *phasic* (quick movement bursts), like the flexor withdrawal reflex. Brainstem postural reflexes tend to be characteristically *static* (tonic, holding responses) such as asymmetrical tonic neck reflex, symmetrical tonic neck reflex, and the tonic labyrinthine reflex. Midbrain reflexes are integrated in the brainstem tectum and are characterized as righting responses (designed to keep the head and body parts in alignment as the body moves through space), whereas cortical responses are said to be equilibrium responses (Crutchfield, Barnes, & Heriza, 1978; Fiorentino, 1973).

We know that many primitive reflexes and responses seen at low levels of the central nervous system are integrated by higher levels of the nervous system. They may also be biomechanically inhibited. For example, the spontaneous walking reflex seen in neonates seems to disappear. However, when an adult is supported in a pool of water, the spontaneous walking returns. It would appear that body weight inhibits this walking reflex seen in infancy. Yet, when an adult is supported by the buoyancy of water which removes the element of body weight, then the walking reflex is again seen. This can be an effective therapeutic measure to help adults reinitiate a walking pattern.

Stereotypic motor acts include repetitive movements like rocking, hand waving, and head banging. Normal children exhibit stereotypic motor behavior, but this behavior is exaggerated in developmentally disabled children (MacLean & Baumeister, 1982; Thelen, 1979, 1980). The manifestation of stereotypic behavior increases during the normal developmental process without preventing normal movement. This usually occurs at various stages when a child progresses from one developmental posture to another (Thelen, 1979). Stereotyped movement becomes abnormal when the intensity, frequency, amplitude, and duration interfere with functional movement. Stereotypic movement

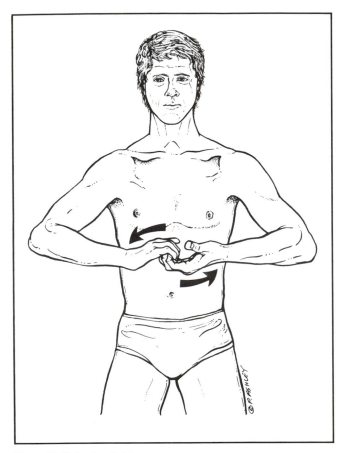

Figure 10-10. Jendrassik Maneuver.

range of motion and produce various soft tissue changes that further limit movement. In addition, the sympathetic nervous system is more active with increasing age. Consequently, muscle tone and resistance to passive movement may increase with age.

Co-contraction

Joints are mobilized by muscle groups that generate forces in opposite directions (DeLuca & Mambrito, 1987). Two variables are at work around joints: stiffness and torque (the force that causes a structure to twist around its axis). When there is high torque and low stiffness, the muscles around a joint will work individually. When the torque is reduced to zero and the stiffness is high, coactivation results (DeLuca & Mambrito, 1987). Proximal co-contracted joints serve as stable bases from which limbs can operate. Patients who lack proximal stability often use distal fixation as a method to achieve stability and stiffness. Unfortunately, distal fixation is not an adaptive compensation for deceased proximal stability because it can disrupt dexterity and prevent fine coordination. For example, learning diabled children often are hypotonic and lack midline postural extensor tone and proximal stability. Their posture can be poor both in sitting and in standing. Imagine such a child attempting to sit in a chair that provides poor support and at a desk that is the improper height to promote trunk stability. Imagine further this same child trying to write in cursive lettering. In addition to the perceptual difficulties such children may experience, the neuromotor problems are immense.

Weight Shift

The ability to shift weight involves both reciprocal innervation and co-contraction in a continuum. One can consider weight shifting in a dynamic locomotor pattern as a dynamic process of loading and unloading the respective extremities. As the stance extremity moves towards co-contraction with an increase in stiffness and decrease in torque, the unloaded extremity experiences increasing torque as it is unloaded and swings free. People who lack the ability to shift weight move forward through space with great difficulty.

Trunk and Limb Rotation

Human movement employs rotatory components in both the limbs and in the trunk. Defense pattern movements of ancient martial arts such as Tae Kwon Do are diagonal movements and said to be the most natural human movements and the easiest to perform. *Proprioceptive neuromuscular facilitation* (PNF), a treatment system for those with central nervous system pathology, also employs diagonal patterns (Knott & Voss, 1968). During diagonal

may occur to promote development and establish neural pathways (MacLean & Baumeister, 1982). This would imply that the behavior is adaptive at certain points in development.

Tone

Muscle tone is defined as resistance to stretch and is generated by lower motor neuron activity, viscoelastic properties of muscles and joints, and sensory feedback (Brooks, 1986). Tone is modified throughout the developmental continuum. Premature infants are frequently hypotonic whereas normal full-term neonates demonstrate physiological flexion. Babies soon start to develop extensor tone. With increasing maturity and integration of postural reflexes, normal children demonstrate a continuum of tonal balance throughout their bodies. At the other end of the developmental chronology, older people frequently do not demonstrate as much phasic motor activity compared to younger people because of many factors including changes in muscle fiber composition, sensory receptor activity, and central nervous system modifications. Inactivity can reduce movements, maximum muscular stretch is evoked (Brooks, 1986). When a therapist treats an individual with hypertonia throughout the trunk and limbs, rotation of the trunk and of the individual limbs is often employed to reduce tone so that normal movement can occur.

Coordination

One of the main functions of the cerebellum is coordination among the muscle groups involved in an activity. Humans rarely use a muscle in isolation. Most often, muscles are functionally grouped during activity. For example, as a man attempts to scratch the back of his neck, he must activate all of the following muscles: the abductors, external rotators, scapular protractors, supinators, and elbow, wrist, and finger flexors. Gross coordination develops in cephalocaudal and mediolateral directions. Fine motor coordination will be discussed in the next section.

Dexterity and Skill

Motor skill is defined as a relationship between those action plans stored in the central nervous system and the ability to translate them into visible motor behavior (MacKenzie & Marteniuk, 1987). Because there is constant change in the environment and in every movement, the skillful performer must be able to adapt a specific action to the environmental conditions. For example, a therapist working with a patient with neuromotor damage will make modifications on any given day in the amount of resistance applied, the location of hand placement, and the velocity of movement.

Skill enhances economy of movement and energy expenditure to render predictable high quality performance (Newell, 1981). Thus, we see that not just any "practice makes perfect" but rather "*perfect practice* makes perfect." People who practice using incorrect form will not necessarily obtain skill. Feedback from an objective observer is often helpful depending on how quickly and constructively it is delivered. Performers who have knowledge of results of their own action can determine if the skill was successfully learned. This knowledge is a critical factor in skill-building (Salmoni, Schmidt & Walter, 1984). As an individual improves within a given skill, fewer corrections are required so that the movement is smoother (Brooks, 1986).

Dexterity is frequently used synonymously with skill. The dexterous individual usually demonstrates precise movements in the distal segments of the upper extremities. Persons with bilateral upper extremity amputation often develop dexterity in their feet, substituting use of feet for hand function.

The new therapist who is learning to improve handling skills when treating a patient with neuromotor involvement might consider videotaping the treatment sessions. This allows the therapist to observe his/her own skills. This can be very helpful in making changes or alterations in handling procedures.

Strength

Strength is the force generated by a specific muscle. One method of building muscular strength is to contract against ever-increasing resistance. For example, as a toddler starts to build strength in arms and trunk, he/she is able to lift heavier toys and then carry them around. In treatment, gradual increases in the resistance are recommended to avoid muscular tears and joint injury. Good body alignment is also critical when contracting against resistance as certain joints are excessively vulnerable to damage. An example of this is when an individual lifts a heavy weight over the head without adequately aligning the trunk. Lifting the weight can shift the person's center of gravity and jeopardize trunk balance. If the person places too much torque on the sacroiliac joint or the lumbar spine, low back damage may result.

Endurance

Endurance is the ability to sustain a given activity over time. To increase endurance, one must increase the number of repetitions of a given exercise or activity. Without sufficient endurance, motor expression is compromised. Therapists should plan for the systematic increase of patient endurance during treatment sessions as well as in client's lifestyle. Because lifestyles become more sedentary as people get older, therapists must take into consideration this general decrease in endurance with age.

Velocity

Each human exhibits unique velocity patterns for specific motor activities. When first building skill, people may move at a slower rate and rhythm, but usually they increase the velocity as the movement becomes automatic. Therapists must consider this concept when treating people with impaired neuromotor performance. It is critical to help the individual to move at different rates and rhythms. Some people can perform an activity with high level of skill at a slow velocity, but when velocity increases the skill level decreases.

Range

Every joint has a range of motion that is determined by the conformation of the joint and the extensibility of the musculotendenous structures around the joint (Hay and Reid, 1982). There is an optimum range of motion or degree of flexibility available at each joint in order to achieve balance between mobility and stability. Too much range in a joint (hypermobility) that supports the body weight can result in instability. Decreased range of motion in a joint (hypomobility) that is actively participating in a phasic burst of movement can yield damage to the muscles and tendons around that joint. When individuals activate movement in their own joints, they may not utilize all available range at a given joint. Most human movement does not encompass the total continuum of range possible for each joint. In contrast, when passive range of motion is facilitated in a patient by a therapist, the scope of movement at any given joint may exceed that which the patient actively achieves in daily activities. Thus, therapists must exercise caution when passively ranging a patient in order to avoid damaging a joint.

Center of Gravity

The *center of gravity* is an imaginary point where the body weight is equally distributed. It can be located anywhere in or near the body depending on the position of the body in space and the alignment of the body parts. Individuals must continuously shift their center of gravity as they move through space. When the center of gravity is misplaced, because of muscular imbalance and poor body alignment, decreased balance and uneven gravitation pressure will result (Selim, 1982).

The following is an exercise that demonstrates this concept of center of gravity. Ask a friend to sit in a chair with feet directly below the knees with the hips in 90 degrees of flexion and trunk located squarely over the pelvis. While the subject is in this position, notice the alignment of the head. The ear lobe should be aligned over the apex of the shoulder when viewed from the side. Now ask your friend to move the pelvis out to the edge of the chair and tilt the pelvis posteriorly so that the person is now sitting on the sacrum. This movement will automatically protract the chin, and the head will move forward. This inappropriate alignment will produce strain around the superior angle of the scapulae and make upper extremity movements more difficult. The poor body alignment changes the location of the center of gravity so that the arms now feel heavy to the subject. Many patients sit with a posterior pelvic tilt and forward head alignment. By changing the patient's posture in the sitting position, one can promote a more physiologic location of the center of gravity that can result in better use of the upper extremities.

FACTORS AFFECTING NEUROMOTOR PERFORMANCE

Other Biophysical Forces

In addition to the physical factors such as strength, endurance, tone, and coordination which are described above, there are other physical forces that are relevant to neuromotor performance. These forces of gravity, friction, and fluid resistance are commonly studied in physics but do, in fact, act upon on the movement components mentioned above. Further review of these biophysical properties and laws is beyond the scope of this chapter.

Chronological and Developmental Age

At various ages, a given motor act is performed differently depending on the size of the lever arms or limbs, balance, coordination, cognition, and purpose. For example, we notice that a one-year-old toddler will walk with a wide base of support accompanied by increased ankle and knee flexion and decreased reciprocal swing. This is a different pattern than that exhibited by a two-year-old (Sutherland, 1984). O'Donovan (1985) illustrates the importance of developmental changes by reporting that muscle fibers increase in number during the neonatal period, whereas lower motor neurons decrease to the correct proportion so that motor units can be formed for control. Some of the characteristics of action or movement patterns observed in toddlers reappear in the geriatric population because of modifications in activity levels, disuse atrophy, decreased endurance, decreased white muscle fiber, and center of gravity alterations.

In general, the changes in action observed during the developmental continuum occur in an orderly manner. Females reach a performance plateau in some measures of motor performance at 13 years of age, whereas males may continue to improve if the skills require power, muscular endurance, and strength (Branta, Haubenstricker and Seefeldt, 1984). Generalizations regarding performance and age are difficult because task proficiency seems to vary with the specific task requirements.

Sex and Race

Many studies examining sexual and racial effects on neuromotor performance cannot factor out the additional influencing variables such as culture, socioeconomic class, nutrition, and specific tasks to be measured. Interracial marriage further obscures the differences that were said to exist between members of the alternate races (Selim, 1982).

Blacks seem to outnumber Caucasians in certain areas of professional sports, however, it is not clear whether this is because of increased ability due to genetic physiological influences or cultural influences, or to some combination of both factors. It has been shown that Blacks excel at running, jumping, speed, and agility (Selim, 1982). Anatomical differences do exist between Caucasians and Blacks in relation to limb size, hip size, and location of fat deposits; exactly how these differences contribute to neuromotor performance is still under investigation.

Sexual differences are more obvious than racial variations since we know that girls reach puberty approximately two years before boys. After puberty, fat deposits increase and bone growth decreases in females, while males demonstrate increased muscle bulk. This increased muscle bulk in males is a result of the positive effect of the male hormone testosterone on muscle development. Although men have more muscle than women, it is not necessarily of a better quality than that of women (Selim, 1982).

Anatomical and functional differences have been shown to exist between men and women. Women possess wider hips, increased percentage of their total body weight as fat, lower centers of gravity, better balance, increased flexibility, enhanced buoyancy, and amplified endurance. Men pump more blood per stroke, demonstrate slower heart rates, and sustain increased blood viscosity (Selim, 1982). Eaton and Enns (1986) report that males are more active than females although age is a critical variable.

Training

The effect of training on neuromotor performance has been analyzed by many researchers. Training stimuli of short duration may produce temporary changes in behavior that revert to baseline once the stimuli are removed. It takes repetition over time to produce persistent changes in structure or function or adaptive behavior (Lamb, 1984). Adaptive behavioral changes resulting from training help reduce the shifts that occur within the body's homeostasis. For example, with specific training for a given exercise, one becomes more efficient in the execution of this activity and can reduce the change in body temperature, heart rate, and exertion, and thus increase endurance (Lamb, 1984).

Training has also been shown to change the characteristics and fiber composition of muscle. For example, training for long distance running will produce a higher percentage of dark muscle compared to white. Weight-lifting will not change the type of fiber in the muscle but will increase the size of the fast-twitch fibers. Contractile speed and metabolic rate of muscle fiber can also be modified by training (Lamb, 1984). One study showed training enhanced performance on specific skills when age and sex were controlled (Clifton, 1978).

In addition, some have found a link between knowing what is expected in a movement pattern (such as during training) and refining the movement. Newell (1978) believes that perception and action are dynamically linked, so that "knowing" facilitates "doing," which in turn enriches "knowing."

Motivation

We have all heard stories of women who have found their children trapped under heavy objects and performed feats of strength to lift the objects and save their children. This classic example illustrates the influence of motivation on motor performance. Such exaggerated acts of strength are not unusual in cases of emergency when motivational levels are high. Likewise, when motivation is low, the quality of the motor performance is not likely to reflect a true indication of the individual's skill or potential. Mental states such as depression can also reduce one's motivation to move. In many cases, this starts a vicious cycle whereby the inactivity exacerbates the depression.

Health status

Many diseases can impact on an individual's ability to move efficiently. Hyperthyroidism (producing excess thyroid hormone) will result in an overabundance of dark, slow-twitch fibers which can compromise fast, phasic movement. In contrast, hypothyroidism reduces the amount of slow-twitch muscle available, so that static holding patterns may be attenuated (O'Donovan, 1985).

Meniere's Disease is another example of a disease that can compromise neuromotor performance. In this condition, the endolymph of the inner ear is not properly absorbed, creating possible aberrant stimulation of the vestibular receptors resulting in vertigo (dizziness) with movement of the head. During these vertiginous episodes, one feels as if the room is spinning. This sensation may be accompanied by autonomic features such as nausea and sweating. Such attacks of vertigo could have serious consequences for a construction worker who is required to stand on narrow steel girders of high-rise structures. Maintaining balance could be impossible, and this might necessitate modification in job responsibilities for the construction worker. We have only mentioned a few examples, since there are many diseases that compromise neuromotor performance (both temporarily and permanently).

Drugs, Diet, Caffeine

Drugs have various effects on neuromotor performance depending on the class of drug and the amount ingested. Antianxiety drugs were tested on a group of college-age women who demonstrated either high or low levels of trait anxiety, neuroticism, or extroversion. A mirrored drawing test was used to assess dexterity. During pre-drug testing, those with high anxiety/neuroticism demonstrated decreased performance when compared to low-anxiety subjects. Administration of the antianxiety drugs reduced the performance decrement between the two groups, but it also decreased the speed of performance in the low-anxiety group. This demonstrates that the personality traits of individuals and the degree to which a specific test will induce anxiety should be seriously considered before using antianxiety drugs (Nakano et al., 1978).

Wait and associates (1982) examined the effects of alcohol ingestion on perceptual motor coordination using controls for sex and amount of alcohol intake. They found subjects who consumed alcohol demonstrated impaired performance on a mirror-tracing task, but that alcohol intake did not produce a significant difference in performance in a dart-throwing task. This study highlights the need to avoid simple generalizations regarding any drug or chemical agent and potential effects on neuromotor performance. Each agent may affect different parts of the central nervous system and peripheral nervous system, thereby having specific behavioral effects.

Drinking 2-1/2 cups of coffee (caffeine) 1-1/2 hours before an activity will increase the utilization of fatty acid instead of glycogen. Burning fat yields a slow-energy release. Caffeine may also increase nervousness (Selim, 1982).

Anabolic steroids are becoming increasingly popular among young athletes as they are known to amplify muscular bulk and strength. The side-effects of using steroids are so dangerous that a massive campaign has been waged to prevent steroid use. The effects of steroids include muscular hypertrophy with augmented strength, liver disease, enhanced aggression, and decreased sperm production (Selim, 1982).

The study of dietary effect on motor performance is still in its infancy. Thus far, diets have been studied in relationship to energy release. Simple carbohydrates are said to release energy rapidly and comprise approximately 60 percent of our average diets (Lamb, 1984). Complex carbohydrates are metabolized more slowly compared to simple carbohydrates. Fat, which makes up 30 percent of our diets, burns slowly, and thus releases energy at a slow rate. Protein comprises only 10 percent of our diet and is not useful for energy production; however, the psychological influence of eating a big steak before an athletic event may be of significance but has yet to be fully evaluated (Lamb, 1984).

Environment

The controversy over whether human behavior is a product of environment or genetic predisposition has been ongoing for many years. We can prove that certain factors within the environment can modify both structure and function. For example, in a study of histology technicians who were exposed to formaldehyde, deficits were measured in equilibrium, dexterity, and memory. The exposure time correlated with the degree of severity of the deficit (Kilburn, Warshaw, & Thornton, 1987). There are positive environmental influences as well; a family that enthusiastically supports (both emotionally and financially) a child's athletic interest may indeed contribute to enhancing the child's performance.

Culture

Members of each culture may exhibit a unique movement repertoire sometimes exhibited in the form of characteristic dances or games (Selim, 1982). In primitive cultures, dance plays a primary role in communication, religious expression, and various other celebrations. A therapist who is treating a patient from a different culture must work closely with the patient and family members to determine whether additional therapy is necessary in order to regain certain abilities that will allow the patient to participate in vital cultural activities.

Inactivity and Disuse Atrophy

Immobilization and inactivity changes every system of the body. One obvious change is a reduction in muscle fiber diameter with disuse (Selim, 1982). After only one to two months of disuse, atrophy will reduce a muscle to one-half of its normal size. At this point, if activity is reinstated, a complete recovery of muscle fiber diameter is possible. If inactivity persists beyond two months, some atrophy will remain (Sandler & Vernikos, 1986). Antigravity muscles are most involved following bedrest, according to Sandler and Vernikos (1986). Inactivity alters sensory perception, functional maintenance of muscle and coordination, and ultimately produces a decrease in motor ability and task precision. (Sandler & Vernikos, 1986).

Cognition

Awareness of the environment is thought to motivate people to move within it. Mental retardation has been associated with a delay in walking, but this is not a universal finding among all mentally retarded people. Subgroups of mentally retarded have been shown to walk independently at the appropriate age at all levels of cognition. Hreidarsson, Shapiro and Capute (1983) suggest that cognition is not the sole determinant for achievement of independent walking. Although it is probable that if the subject sees no reason to ambulate and explore, he or she will not.

IMPLICATIONS FOR OCCUPATIONAL THERAPY

Suggested Therapeutic Techniques

As we attempt to refine our therapeutic practice based on concepts of motor learning and neuromotor performance, it is clear that therapy must do more than just rebuild or restore individual components of motion. Our therapeutic intervention must rebuild action and facilitate purpose (Mulder & Hulstyn, 1984). This concept is compatible with current theories of occupational therapy. For example, in the case of a patient who has suffered a stroke and has limited use of the upper extremities, increasing upper extremity movement alone may not improve the patient's performance. The therapist must help this person learn the action plans necessary to accomplish activities relevant to his/her various occupations.

Use of sensory stimulation is often employed by therapists and must be capable of inducing adaptive responses over time to be considered most beneficial. Weaning patients from sensory input is also important so that the patient does not become totally dependent on that extrasensory input. This may necessitate teaching the patient methods of self-stimulation when appropriate, such as sitting in a rocking chair in order to promote even, repetitive input for reducing muscle tone and stress.

Therapists attempting to rebuild a subject's strength must overload the weak muscles, taking care not to produce muscular fatigue. It is important to avoid using exercise for general strengthening or for other motor goals without addressing the specific purposes. Therapists should attempt to address each client's functional strength in specific activities. For example, if one considers a patient with a spinal cord lesion at the T10 level, appropriate occupational therapy would include activities designed to increase the patient's ability to transfer, push up in the chair, and perform necessary homemaking and self-care activities. It would be helpful for this patient to lift weights to strengthen upper extremities and trunk, however this is generally performed in physical therapy. It is crucial that occupational therapists determine the strength requiremeaants for all necessary occupatioabnal activities and assist the patient in developing endurance in those activities.

When people reside in rehabilitation centers, they receive daily therapy and maintain a certain level of conditioning. After discharge many patients undergo deconditioning. Consequently, the home therapy program must be able to interest and motivate the patient to maintain skill levels. Therapeutic intervention must address all the variables that can interfere with function. This is a challenge to occupational therapists to be creative in their therapeutic regimens while still focusing on the client's problems.

Research

The studies of motor learning theories and activity (Gliner, 1985) as used in occupational therapy should be of major interest to therapists. Basic to professional practice is the need to learn and analyze the effects of detailed activity and patients' performance in order to match the most appropriate activity to the specific problem manifested by a patient. It is then essential that occupational therapists further establish the value of using occupation for rehabilitation. There are several important areas that need further study: sensory feedback, including the most effective type to use at each stage of development; methods of delivering sensory stimulation; and the effectiveness of specific sensory modalities in treating people with certain disease entities.

SUMMARY

Human movement is a complex functional behavior dependent upon the motor structures of the peripheral nervous system, execution by the musculoskeletal system, and input from the environment. If therapists are to provide effective assessment and intervention, they must have a thorough understanding of the structures and functions of these components and their interrelationships. Additionally, they must be conversant with current theories of motor learning and the specific muscle components and movements necessary for action. When actions are viewed in the context of meaningful task performance, intervention is more likely to be effective and of optimal benefit to the client.

Study Questions

1. Compare and contrast the way the basal ganglia relates to movement control and the methods used by the cerebellum.

2. Identify two motor tracts that facilitate extensor tone.

3. Use of eccentric contractions in therapy has advantages and disadvantages. Identify them.

4. Define transduction.

5. How does the autonomic nervous system influence sensory receptors?

6. How does guided practice improve motor performance?

7. How does reciprocal movement modify with the individual's development.

8. Is stereotyped movement normal or abnormal? Support your answer.

9. In what way can hypermobility produce joint damage?

Recommended Readings

Boyd, I.A. & Gladden, M.H. (1985). *The muscle spindle.* New York: Stockton Press

Brooks, V.B. (1986). *The neural bases of motor control.* New York: Oxford University Press.

Carpenter, M.B., & Sutin, J. (1983). *Human neuroanatomy.* (8th Ed). Baltimore: Williams and Wilkins.

DeArmond, S.J., Fusco, M.M., & Dewey, M.M. (1984). *Structure of the human brain.* New York: Oxford University Press.

Farber, S.D., (1982). *Neurorehabilitation: A multisensory approach.* Philadelphia: W.B. Saunders Co.

Kandel, E.R., & Schwartz, J.H. (1985). *Principles of neural science..* (2nd Ed). New York: Elsevier.

Peterson, B.W., & Richmond, F.J. (1988). *Control of head movement.* New York: Oxford University Press.

Sutherland, D.H. (1984). *Gait disorders in childhood and adolescence.* Baltimore: Williams and Wilkins.

References

Adams, J.A. (1971). A closed loop theory of motor learning. *Journal of Motor Behavior, 3,* 111-150.

Adams, J.A. (1976). Issues for a closed loop theory of motor learning. In G.E. Stelmach (Ed.). *Motor control: Issues and trends.* New York: Academic Press.

Arey, L.B. (1974). *Developmental anatomy. 7th ed.* Philadelphia: W.B. Saunders.

Asanuma, H. (1986). Recovery of motor skill following deprivation of direct sensory input to the motor cortex in the monkey. In D.L. Akron & C.D. Woody (Eds.). *Neural mechanisms of conditioning (pp. 187-196).* New York: Plenum Press.

Ayres, A.J. (1972) *Sensory integration and learning disorders.* Los Angeles: Western Psychological Services.

Barr, M.L., & Kiernan, J.A. (1988). *The human nervous system: An anatomical viewpoint. 5th ed.* Philadelphia: J.B. Lippincott.

Barrows, H.S. (1980). *Guide to neurological assessment.* Philadelphia: J.B. Lippincott.

Bass, A., Gutmann, E., & Hanzlikova, V. (1975). Biochemical and histochemical changes in energy-supply-enzyme pattern of muscles of the rat during old age. *Gerontologia, 21,* 31-45.

Boyd, I.A., & Gladden M.H. (1985). *The muscle spindle.* New York: Stockton Press.

Branta, C., Haubenstricker, J., & Seefeldt, V. (1984). Age changes in motor skills during childhood and adolescence. *Exercise and Sports Sciences Review, 12,* 467-520.

Brodal, A. (1981). *Neurological anatomy in relation to clinical medicine. 3rd edition.* New York: Oxford University Press.

Brooks, V.B. (1986). *The neural bases of motor control.* New York: Oxford University Press.

Brown, D.R. (1980). *Neurosciences for allied health therapies.* St. Louis: C.V. Mosby.

Brown, J.E., & Frank, J.S. (1987). Influence of event anticipation on postural actions accompanying voluntary movement. *Experimental Brain Research, 67,* 645-650.

Clifton, M.A. (1978). Effects of special instruction and practice by preschool-age children on performance of object projection and stability tests. *Perceptual and Motor Skills, 47,* 1135-1140.

Cordo, P.J., & Nashner, L.M. (1982). Properties of postural adjustments associated with rapid arm movements. *Journal of Neurophysiology, 47,* 287-302.

Crutchfield, C., Barnes, M., & Heriza, C. (1978). *Neurological basis of patient treatment. Vol. 2.* Reflex testing. Morgantown, WV: Stokesville Publishing Co.

DeLuca, C.J., & Mambrito, B. (1987). Voluntary control of motor units in human antagonist muscles: coactivation and reciprocal activation. *Journal of Neurophysiology, 58,* 525-542.

Denis, M. (1985). Visual imagery and the use of mental practice in the development of motor skills. *Canadian Journal of Applied Sport Science, 10,* 4S-16S.

Eaton, W.O., & Enns, L.R. (1986). Sex differences in human motor activity level. *Psychological Bulletin, 100,* 19-28.

Evarts, E.V., & Wise, S.P. (1984). Basal ganglia output and motor control. *Ciba Foundation Symposia, 107,* 83-102.

Farber, S.D. (1982). *Neurorehabilitation: A multisensory approach.* Philadelphia: W.B. Saunders Co.

Fiorentino, M. (1973). *Reflex testing: methods for evaluating central nervous system development. 2nd ed.* Springfield, IL: Charles C. Thomas.

Gallistel, C.R. (1980). *The organization of action: A new synthesis.* Hillsdale, NJ: Lawrence Erlbaum Associates.

Gilfoyle, E.M., Grady, A.P., & Moore, J.C. (1978). *Children adapt.* Thorofare, NJ: Charles B. Slack.

Gliner, J.A. (1985). Purposeful activity in motor learning: An event approach to motor skill aquisition. *American Journal of Occupational Therapy, 39,* 28-34.

Greene, P.H. (1982). Why is it easy to control your arms? *Journal Motor Behavior, 14,* 260-286.

Gutmann, E., & Hanzlikova, V. (1972). *Age changes in the neuromuscular system.* Bristol: Scientechnica Publ. Ltd.

Hay, J.G., & Reid, J.G. (1982). *The anatomical bases of*

human motion. Englewood Cliffs, NJ: Prentice-Hall, Inc.

Hooker, D. (1977). Evidence of prenatal function of the central nervous system in man. In Payton, et al. (Eds.). *Scientific bases for neurophysiologic approaches to therapeutic exercise*. Philadelphia: F.A. Davis Co.

Hreidarsson, S.J., Shapiro, B.K., & Capute, A.J. (1983). Age of walking in the cognitively impaired. *Clinical Pediatrics, 22*, 248-250.

Iversen, S.D. (1981). Motor control. *British Medical Bulletin, 37,* 147-152.

Jensen, D. (1980). *The human nervous system*. New York: Appleton-Century-Crofts.

Kandel, E.R., & Schwartz, J.H. (1985). *Principles of neural science. 2nd ed*. New York, Amsterdam: Elsevier.

Keele, S.W., & Summers, J.J. (1976). The structure of motor programs. In G.E. Stelmach (Ed.). *Motor control: Issues and trends*. New York: Academic Press.

Kilburn, K.H., Warshaw, R., & Thornton, J.C. (1987). Formaldehyde impairs memory, equilibrium, and dexterity in histology technicians: Effects which persist for days after exposure. *Archives of Environmental Health, 42*, 117-120.

Knott, M., & Voss, D. (1968). *Proprioceptive neuromuscular facilitation. 2 ed*. New York: Harper and Row.

Kugler, P.N., Kelso, J.A., & Turvey, M.T. (1980). On the concept of coordinative structures as dissipative structures: I. Theoretical line. In G.E. Stelmach & J. Requin (Eds.). *Tutorials in motor behavior*. Amsterdam: North Publ. Co.

Lacquaniti, F., & Soechting, J.F. (1982). Coordination of arm and wrist motion during a reaching task. *Journal of Neuroscience, 4*, 399-408.

Lamb, D.R. (1984). *Physiology of exercise: Response and adaptation. 2nd ed*. New York: MacMillan Pub. Co.

Larsson, L. (1978). Morphological and functional characteristics of the aging skeletal muscle in man, a cross-sectional study. *Acta Physiologica Scandinavia, (Suppl) 457*, 1-36.

Lashley, K.S. (1917). The accuracy of movement in the absence of excitation from the moving organ. *American Journal of Physiology, 43*, 169-194.

Lohr, J.B. & Wisniewski, A.A. (1987). *Movement disorders: A neuropsychiatric approach*. New York: Guildford Press.

Lowrey, G.H. (1973). *Growth and development of children. 6th ed*. Chicago: Year Book Medical Publishers, Inc.

MacKenzie, C.L., & Marteniuk, R.G. (1987). Motor skill: Feedback, knowledge, and structural issues. *Canadian Journal of Psychology, 39*, 313-337.

MacLean, W.E., & Baumeister, A.A. (1982). Effects of vestibular stimulation on motor development and stereo-typed behavior of developmentally-delayed children. *Journal of Abnormal Child Psychology, 10*, 229-245.

Matzke, H.A., & Foltz, F.M. (1983). *Synopsis of neuroanatomy. 4th ed*. New York: Oxford University Press.

Mulder, T., & Hulstyn, W. (1984). Sensory feedback therapy and theoretical knowledge of motor control and learning. *American Journal of Physical Medicine, 63*, 226-244.

Nakano, S., Ogawa, N., Kawazu, Y., & Osato, E. (1978). Effects of antianxiety drug and personality on stress-inducing psychomotor performance test. *Journal of Clinical Pharmacology, 18*, 125-130.

Nashner, L.M., & McCollum, G. (1985). The organization of human postural movements: A formal basis and experimental synthesis. *Behavior and Brain Science, 8*, 135-172.

Newell, K.M. (1978). Some issues on action plans. In G.E. Stelmach (Ed.). *Information processing in motor control and learning*. New York: Academic Press.

Newell, K.M. (1981). Skill learning. In D. Holding (Ed.). Human skills. London: John Wiley and Sons.

Newell, K.M., Morris, L.R., & Scully, D.M. (1981). Augmented information and the acquisition of skill in physical activity. *Exercise and Sport Science Review, 13*, 235-261.

Noback, C.R., & Demarest, R.J. (1981). *The human nervous system: Basic principles of neurobiology. 3rd ed*. New York: McGraw-Hill.

O'Donovan, M.J. (1985). Developmental regulation of motor function: An uncharted sea. *Medicine and Science in Sports and Exercise, 17*, 35-43.

Porter, R. (1983). Functional organization of the motor cortex. In J.E. Desmedt (Ed.). *Motor control mechanisms in health and disease. (pp. 301-320)*. New York: Raven Press.

Reed, E.S. (1982). An outline of a theory of action systems. *Journal of Motor Behavior, 14*, 98-134.

Ritvo, E.R., et al. (1969). Decreased postrotatory nystagmus in early infantile autism. *Neurology, 19*, 653-658.

Salmoni, A.W., Schmidt, R.A., & Walter, C.B. (1984). Knowledge of results and motor learning: A review and critical reappraisal. *Psychological Bulletin, 95*, 355-386.

Sandler, H., & Vernikos, J. (1986). *Inactivity: Physiological effects*. Orlando, San Diego: Academic Press Inc. (Harcourt Brace Jovanovich).

Scelsi, R., Marchetti, C., & Poggi, P. (1980). Ultrastructural aspects of m. vastus lateralis in sedentary old people (age 65-89 years). *Acta Neuropathologie (Berl), 51*, 99-105.

Schmidt, R.A. (1975). A schema theory of discrete motor skill learning. *Psychological Review, 82*, 225-261.

Schmidt, R.A. (1976a). The schema as a solution to some persistent problems in motor learning theory. In G.E. Stelmach, *(Ed.). Motor control: Issues and trends*. New York: Academic Press.

Schmidt, R.A. (1976b). Control processes in motor skills. *Exercise and Sport Sciences Reviews, 4*, 229-261.

Schmidt, R.A. (1982). *Motor control and learning: A behavioral emphasis*. Champaign, IL: Human Kinetics Publ.

Selim, R.D. (Ed.). (1982). *Muscles: The magic of motion*. New York: Torstar Books.

Shepherd, G.M. (1979). *The synaptic organization of the brain. 2nd ed.*, New York: Oxford University Press.

Stadler, M., Schwab, B.P., & Wehner, T. (1978). The regulation sensorimotorische lernprozesse durch biosignale externe bioregulation. *Zeitschrift fur Psychologie, 186*, 341-381.

Sutherland, D.H. (1984). *Gait disorders in childhood and adolescence*. Baltimore: Williams and Wilkins.

Swash, M., & Fox, K.P. (1985). Adrenergic innervation of baboon and human muscle spindles. In I.A. Boyd & M.H. Gladden, *(Ed.). The muscle spindle*. New York: Stockton Press.

Terzuolo, C.A., Soechting, J.F., & Viviani, P. (1973). Studies on the control of some simple motor tasks. II. On the cerebellar control of movements in relation to the formulation of intentional commands. *Brain Research, 58*, 217-222.

Thelen, E. (1979). Rhythmical stereotypes in normal human infants. *Animal Behavior, 27*, 699-715.

Thelen, E. (1980). Determinants of amounts of stereotyped behavior in normal human infants. *Ethology and Sociobiology, 1*, 141-150.

Tilney, F., & Pike, F.H. (1925). Muscular coordination experimentally studied in its relation to the cerebellum. *Archives of Neurology and Psychiatry 1*, 289-334.

Traub, M.M., Rothwell, J.C., & Marsden, C.D. (1980). A grab reflex in the human hand. *Brain, 103*, 869-884.

Turvey, M.T. (1977). Preliminaries to a theory of action with reference to vision. In R. Shaw & J. Bransford (Eds.). *Perceiving, acting, and knowing*. Hillsdale, NJ: Lawrence Earlbaum Associates.

Wait, J.S., Welch, R.B., Thurgate, J.K., & Hineman, J. (1982). Drinking history and sex of subject in the effects of alcohol on perception and perceptual-motor coordination. *International Journal of Addiction, 17*, 445-462.

Walton, J., & Tindall, B. (1983). *Introduction to clinical neuroscience*. London: William Clowes Limited.

OUTLINE

KEY TERMS

Aphasia

Automatic processes

Bottom-up processing

Effortful processes

Encoding

Episodic memory

Levels of processing

Long-term memory

Memory processes

Memory structure

Procedural memory

Semantic memory

Sensory memory

Short-term memory

Top-down processing

ABSTRACT

Occupational therapists must understand the cognitive components that underlie performance and performance-based deficits. This chapter explores the fundamental components of cognition: attention, memory structures and processes, language acquisition and comprehension, and problem-solving; and the performance deficits related to each. The chapter includes a brief discussion of neural substrates and demonstrates how the study of cognition can be incorporated into occupational therapy practice.

Cognitive Dimensions of Performance

Janet Duchek

"The human mind is a particularly interesting device that displays remarkable adaptiveness and intelligence. We are often unaware of the extraordinary aspects of human cognition. Just as we can easily overlook the enormous accumulation of technology that permits a sports event on television to be broadcast live from Europe, so we can forget how sophisticated our mental processes must be to enable us to understand and enjoy that sportscast. One would like to understand the mechanisms that make such intellectual sophistication possible."

—Anderson, 1985

OBJECTIVES

The information in this chapter is intended to help the reader—

1. appreciate the value of the information processing approach to the study of cognition.

2. understand how cognitive dimensions influence the performance of life tasks.

3. identify fundamental components of cognition and deficits related to each.

4. describe stages of language acquisition and the processes of speech interpretation.

5. distinguish between episodic and semantic information and declarative and procedural memory.

6. identify the stages involved in everyday problem solving.

7. describe how the study of cognition can be incorporated into the practice of occupational therapy.

INTRODUCTION

What is cognition? In the broadest definition, it refers to the acquisition and use of knowledge or the process of thinking. Given such a definition, it is obvious that cognition is a basic fundamental property of humankind. In fact, Descartes found proof for his existence through his ability to think, saying, "I think, therefore I am." Although people have been writing about cognition for centuries, it is only recently that cognition has been studied scientifically. The field of cognitive psychology is devoted to the scientific study of human cognition. In Ulric Neisser's 1967 seminal work, *Cognitive Psychology*, he defined the study of cognition as " . . . all processes by which the sensory input is transformed, reduced, elaborated, stored, recovered, and used." Thus, cognition encompasses many different, yet related mental skills from the simplest of transforming and recognizing the pattern "t" as a letter to solving simultaneous equations.

The relationship between cognition and performance is both necessary and complex. Nearly all aspects of performance are guided by cognition. In order to understand some deficit in performance, one must have a clear understanding of the cognitive components underlying it. Suppose an individual is experiencing difficulty in dressing. In addition to the motor components, there are many cognitive skills involved in dressing oneself. For example, it could be that the individual has an attentional deficit and has difficulty in sustaining attention over an extended period of time in order to finish dressing. A memory deficit may be involved such that the individual is unable to remember the therapist's request to get dressed. The individual may be experiencing some language difficulty and thus not fully comprehend the therapist's request. Finally, the inability to dress may reflect higher integrative problem-solving processes involved in formulating or initiating a plan of action. Any or all of these cognitive mechanisms may influence the client's ability to dress. Thus, it is important to have a clear understanding of these cognitive components and their interaction in order to remediate the performance deficit.

INFORMATION PROCESSING APPROACH

Information processing refers to a general approach taken in the study of cognition. The approach grew out of the late 1950's with the advent of the computer as an information processor. The computer with both its hardware and software has provided a powerful model for human cognition.

According to an information processing approach, people process information in much the same way a computer processes information. Referring back to the definition of cognition, one can see that the acquisition and use of information involves a number of complex steps, and an information processing approach attempts to identify each step and understand what happens at each step. It is assumed that cognition or the way people process information can be broken down into a series of stages that can be studied. Of course, the processing of information begins with some sensory input from the environment. This sensory input is then transformed through a series of stages in the cognitive system. An information processing analysis involves tracing the flow of the input and mental processes associated with a given cognitive task. Models of human information processing and systems are often presented in the form of a flow chart. This will be seen clearly in the discussion of memory structure. Implicit in the information processing approach are the following assumptions (Best, 1989).

1. Cognitive processes can be broken down into separate stages.
2. Many times these stages occur in a serial order.
3. These processes or stages are subject to experimental analysis.

ATTENTION

Attention is basic to the initial stage of information processing. Attention needs to be directed to the sensory input before interpretation can take place. It is difficult to find a precise definition of attention. Although we have all used the expression "pay attention" and know how to react to it, it is still difficult to define exactly what takes place when one is "paying attention." Suppose you are sitting in a classroom taking an exam. You are intently thinking about a particular question, when suddenly someone drops a book on the floor. You jump a little and turn around to see who dropped the book and then return to the exam question. Then, someone next to you asks you for another pen. You first finish answering the question and then hand him a pen.

This scenario illustrates several aspects of attention. Attention seems to involve an ability to focus mental effort, an ability to sustain this focus, and shift this focus back and forth when necessary. In order to more precisely understand our ability to "pay attention", we will discuss three senses of attention as defined by Posner and Boies (1971): *alertness, selection,* and *allocation.* These three components of attention are not necessarily mutually exclusive, but all represent different aspects of our attentional system.

Alertness

One primary component of attention is the *alertness* or preparedness of the individual. Alertness refers to both the physical and mental level of arousal that is necessary to respond. Furthermore, arousal can be tonic or phasic (Posner & Rafal, 1987). *Tonic arousal* refers to a general level of wakefulness from one time of the day to another. In general, people are more alert at the beginning of the day than at the end of the day after a large dinner. Tonic arousal depends upon physiological indices such as body temperature and diurnal patterns and undergoes a slow modulation over time. *Phasic arousal* refers to a specific level of alertness due to some kind of warning signal. Immediately following a warning signal, the individual experiences a heightened readiness to respond. For example, the sprinter is at a high level of arousal and readiness to respond at the sound of the starter gun. Unlike the slow changes in tonic arousal, phasic arousal can be changed instantaneously and depends upon the functioning of the ascending reticular formation (Posner & Rafal, 1987).

Thus, in our example of the student taking the exam, one's level of tonic arousal would be affected by when the exam was taken, either in the morning or in the afternoon after eating a heavy lunch. Phasic arousal would be activated when the instructor warns, "Only five minutes to finish up."

Selection of Attention

A second component of attention involves the ability to selectively attend to certain information at the exclusion of other information. At any given moment, we are bombarded with sensory stimulation. As you are reading this book, you are hopefully unaware of the many sources of sensory input impinging upon you, such as the sound of the florescent lights humming, someone coughing, a television in the other room, or a dog barking outside. If we were aware of all these sources of stimulation, it would be impossible to perform or complete any given activity. Thus, a crucial function of our attentional system involves the selection of attention.

Many studies have been conducted to understand which sensory inputs are selected for attention and when this selection takes place in the attentional system. Selective listening studies have been used to predict success in a flight training program in the Israeli Air Force (Gopher & Kahneman, 1971) and to predict the accident rate of bus drivers (Kahneman, Ben-Ishai, & Lotan, 1973) in which listeners had to switch attention between different messages presented to each ear.

Not only are we able to selectively focus our mental effort on certain information in the environment, but we are also able to mentally shift this focus of attention. This selectivity and shifting of attention can be seen at party where one is able to selectively "tune-in to" or attend to a particular conversation amidst a variety of other conversations with little difficulty (*selectivity*) and then quickly shift the focus of attention (*shifting*) to another conversation across the room when some highly relevant stimulus is presented (i.e., someone mentions your name). You can then briefly tune-in on that conversation to hear what someone else is saying about you, while still politely smiling at the hostess to whom you are supposedly listening. Thus, we can control both the selection or focusing of mental effort and the shifting of that mental effort to another source of stimulation.

Allocation of Attention

Attentional capacity refers to a limited pool of cognitive resources available for allocation (Kahneman, 1973). A certain amount of this attentional capacity is allocated for use for any given cognitive task. A difficult cognitive task will utilize more capacity than a simple cognitive task. For example, more attention will be allocated when driving in rush hour traffic in downtown Boston than when driving across the Kansas plains. Because driving on the Kansas plains requires less attention, there will be enough capacity "left over" from this attentional reservoir to carry on an in-depth conversation with your friend as you drive. In contrast, driving in traffic in Boston uses up most of one's attentional reservoir and not much is left over to carry on a conversation at the same time.

Reconsider the example of the party where one was seemingly listening to one person while straining to hear a conversation across the room. It is very difficult, if not impossible, to focus one's attention on two conversations at one time; hence, the smile pasted on the face of the listener who cannot really attend to the conversation of the hostess. Thus we see that attention is not only selective and shiftable, but is limited.

Cognitive psychologists often experimentally look at attention capacity usage through a secondary task technique. In this technique, individuals are given two

Table 11-1
Characteristics of Memory Structures

	Sensory	Short-term Memory	Long-term Memory
Information Code	sensory	acoustic	semantic
Capacity	large	small & limited	large & unlimited
Duration	visual (250 msec)	up to 30 seconds	permanent

Adapted from Craik, FIM and Lockhart, RS (1972). Levels of processing: A framework for memory research. Journal of Verbal Learning and Verbal Behavior, 11, 671-684.

cognitive tasks to perform. For example, reading a passage may be the primary task and responding to an auditory signal may be the secondary task. The time taken to respond to the auditory signal is an indication of the amount of attentional capacity used to read the passage. If the passage is easy to read, then a person should be quick to respond to the auditory signal, since there is additional capacity left over. If the passage is difficult to read, then the person should be slow to respond to the auditory signal since there is little capacity remaining.

Automaticity

When a task becomes very well-practiced or *automatized*, it requires less attentional capacity from the reservoir. In the example above, if a child were given the same easy reading passage as the adults, the child's response time to the auditory signal would most likely be slower. This is because a child must allocate more attentional capacity for reading an easy passage because a child has very little practice in reading compared to the adult. Reading is a task which combines many component skills and is cognitively demanding for the young child. According to LaBerge and Samuels (1974), elementary component skills must become automatic so that attention can be allocated to the more complex component skills. For example, the child must first have extensive practice recognizing the features of letters so this skill becomes automatic, then he/she can focus attention on converting letters into sounds, and eventually focus attention on extracting meaning from the word. While the adult reader has acquired automaticity in all of these processes, the same processes drain the attentional reservoir of the child. But through practice, capacity-demanding tasks can become automatic (i.e., learning to ride a bike, play tennis), thus freeing attentional capacity for the processing of other information.

Attentional Deficits

Attentional deficits are commonly seen in brain-injured patients. Ben-Yishay, Rattok and Diller (1979) list the following attentional deficits of the brain-injured patient: (1) insufficient alertness, (2) inability to selectively attend to relevant stimulation and filter out irrelevant stimulation, (3) inability to sustain attention over a period of time, and (4) response perseveration due to an inability to shift attention. Any of these attentional deficits may impair learning and daily functioning in the brain-injured patient. Ben-Yishay has developed a remedial program to both assess and rehabilitate attentional functioning in individuals who have suffered severe head trauma (Ben-Yishay, Rattok, & Diller, 1979; Ben-Yishay, Piasetsky, & Rattok, 1987). This Orientation Remedial Module (ORM) attempts to improve phasic arousal by training individuals to respond to a warning signal while performing a series of five tasks which progressively increase in attentional demands. The selectivity of attention is improved by training individuals to react to selective environmental cues and screen out distractor cues. Focusing and sustaining attention is improved by training individuals to estimate time and respond to complex rhythm patterns. Training on the ORM tasks in 40 brain-injured patients resulted in improved attentional performance on these tasks with improved carryover to some psychometric tasks (Ben-Yishay, Piasetsky, & Rattok, 1987).

There is also evidence that learning disabled children do not perform as well as normal children in selective listening tasks (Cherry & Kruger, 1983). They have more difficulty in selectively attending to a relevant auditory stimulus and filtering out an irrelevant auditory stimulus. More recently some theorists argue that children with an underlying attentional problem referred to as *attentional deficit disorder* (ADD) can be distinguished from children with other learning disabilities (Kuehne, Kehle, & McMahon, 1987). Thus, a clear understanding of the specific type of attentional deficit can then lead to an appropriate remedial program.

MEMORY

Trying to remember the twelve cranial nerves for a physiology exam, forgetting the phone number you just looked up, understanding the meaning of dyspraxia, and knowing how to play the piano, all involve some aspect of memory. In an attempt to organize the wealth of information about memory, we will separately discuss memory structure and memory processes. **Memory structure** refers to the unvarying physical or structural components of memory and **memory processes** refer to the strategies for dealing with information which are under the individual's control.

Memory Structure

One popular information processing model of human memory proposes that our memory is made up of three basic structures: **sensory memory, short-term memory,** and **long-term memory** (Atkinson & Shiffrin, 1968). These storage components have different functions and operating characteristics, yet all three act together.

Sensory Memory. When a sensory input from the environment first enters the system it is presumably held in a sensory register. The information is held in a raw uninterpreted sensory form for a very brief period of time. Visual information is briefly stored in a register much like a photograph, whereas auditory information is stored much like an echo. Thus, the information is said to be modality specific. It is presumed that there is a sensory register for each sensory modality, but most research has been conducted on the visual and auditory sensory stores.

The purpose of the sensory store is to briefly extend the sensory input beyond the actual physical stimulus so that pattern recognition can occur. Presumably, while the information resides in the sensory store, it is pre-categorical in nature (Crowder & Morton, 1969) and subject to very rapid decay. It has been estimated that information is held in visual sensory memory for approximately 250 milliseconds, about one-quarter of a second (Sperling, 1960) and in auditory sensory memory for approximately 2 to 3 seconds (Darwin, Turvey, & Crowder, 1972; Balota & Duchek, 1986; Cowan, 1984). Information that does not decay is then transferred to another store for further analysis, that of short-term memory.

Short-Term Memory. *Short-term memory* (STM) differs from sensory memory in many respects. (See Table 11-1.) First, information transferred to STM is coded differently than in sensory memory. In STM, information is most often coded acoustically or verbally (Conrad, 1964; Hintzman, 1967) in contrast to sensory memory where information is still in sensory form.

Second, unlike sensory memory, STM has a limited capacity. Evidence indicates that STM is limited to approximately seven items (Miller, 1956). If you try to recall a string of letters or digits, you would have little or no difficulty recalling seven items, however, as soon as you begin to increase the list to nine, for most people, the task becomes much more difficult. It is no surprise that phone numbers and postal zip codes do not exceed seven digits.

Short-term memory capacity can be increased by grouping the information into more meaningful units (*chunking*). For example, you would have difficulty trying to remember the letter sequence, "NBCFBITWACIAIBM", however, recall would be much easier if the letters were grouped into smaller units, such as "NBC FBI TWA CIA IBM." One can only hold about seven chunks of information in STM. The importance of chunking was illustrated by the work of de Groot (1966) who indicated that a major difference between the master chess players and novices lies in their ability to group information into larger chunks (de Groot, 1966).

Third, information can reside in STM for a longer period of time than in sensory memory. Information can last up to 30 seconds in STM if not rehearsed and longer if rehearsed (Table 11-1). Rehearsal serves to refresh or regenerate the information. However, if the rehearsal is interrupted, the information can quickly be lost from STM. An example of this would be if you locate a plumber's phone number out of the phone book and walk over to the phone to dial it. As you walk to the phone you repeat the number over and over (*rehearsal*). As you begin to dial, your child runs in and tells you that she spilled a jar of water colors on the carpet. The interfering message not only raises your blood pressure, but erases the plumber's phone number from your STM.

The function of STM is very important. It is often referred to as "working memory" (Baddeley & Hitch, 1974) and is likened to our consciousness. It is closely tied with the other memory stores in that STM takes information from the other stores (i.e., sensory and long-term memory) and elaborates or transforms that information. For example, while reading this sentence, your working memory is combining the sensory information from the page (i.e., the letters) with your knowledge in long-term memory (i.e., the meanings of the words and their relationships in the context of the sentence). Furthermore, because STM is limited in capacity, this limits our ability to simultaneously perform other cognitive tasks. Thus, STM is closely tied to attentional processes as well.

Long-Term Memory. Given the limited duration and capacity of STM, it is obvious that there must be a more permanent memory store for all the information we have. This more permanent memory store is *long-term memory* (LTM). Information is transferred from STM to LTM where it is presumably stored more permanently. In fact, some memory theorists argue that information is never lost from LTM, but it may be inaccessible. Hence, the reason that you can't remember the name of your first grade teacher is not because that information is lost but rather because you cannot retrieve the information from LTM. If you were given two names from which to choose, it is likely you would choose the correct name.

Table 11-2
Differences Between Episodic and Semantic Information

Episodic	Semantic
Memory for personal events	Memory for general knowledge
Autobiographical reference	No autobiographical reference
Temporal tag	No temporal tag
Retrieval guided by context	Retrieval guided by meaning, associations, or rules

It has also been suggested that LTM has no capacity. See Table 11-1. There is always room for new information to be stored in LTM. Because of the enormous amount of information stored in LTM, it must be coded or organized in such a way that it is relatively easy to access. Otherwise, we would have to search the entire contents of our LTM every time we tried to remember something. Some researchers suggest that information is most likely coded semantically or according to meaning so that we only must search a limited area of our LTM. Other theoretical frameworks have been proposed to help define the nature of LTM.

Episodic vs. Semantic Memory. Tulving (1972) distinguishes between **episodic memory** or memory of personal episodes or events that have some temporal reference and **semantic memory** or memory of general knowledge. An example of the difference between these two types of memory can be illustrated in trying to answer two questions: *What did you have for breakfast yesterday?* and *Is a whale a mammal?* Both of these questions require a search of your LTM, but they seem to tap different types of stored information. To answer the first question, one must recall a personal event that happened yesterday, but to answer the second question, one must recall the defining characteristics of a mammal and decide whether a whale fits those characteristics.

Although both episodic and semantic memories represent information that is stored in long-term memory, the type of information differs in several dimensions. (See Table 11-2.) First, episodic memories have some personal or autobiographical reference, such as remembering what you had for breakfast, your first date, your favorite high school teacher, or the title of the last book you read. Semantic memories do not have any personal or autobiographical reference, such as knowing that a whale is a mammal, knowing that white wine should be chilled before serving, or the meaning of the word "facade." This information is not stored in memory as a

personal event but instead is stored as general knowledge without any autobiographical reference.

Episodic memories are different from semantic memories because they are stored with some temporal reference. Episodic memories are stored along with a time-tag for the occurrence of the event. Although the knowledge stored in semantic memory was acquired at a particular point in time, that time-tag is not stored along with the knowledge, perhaps because of the passage of time since the original knowledge was obtained.

Retrieval characteristics differ in episodic and semantic memory. Retrieval from episodic memory is guided primarily by the temporal tags stored with the relevant information. For example, when asked to learn a list of words, one must search LTM for those words. Those words are already stored in LTM along with many other words, thus one must search one's memory to find some time-tag or context-tag associated with the words in order to remember them. In contrast, semantic memory is organized as a complex network and retrieval can be guided by several dimensions such as meaning, associations, or rules.

Although there has been some debate as to whether episodic and semantic memory are indeed separate memory systems or represent different types of information in the same system (Anderson & Ross, 1980; Duchek & Neely, 1989; Hermann & Harwood, 1980; Neely & Durgunoglu, 1985; Shoben, Wescourt, & Smith, 1978), it is clear that both types of memories often interact. When one is asked to learn a list of words, one is not "learning" those words for the first time; they are already a part of semantic memory. One might even use the associations among those words as an aid to remembering them. But the actual memory experiment itself and having to recall those specific words in the context of the experiment is a personal event that could become part of one's episodic memory. In a later section, we shall see that the distinction between episodic and semantic information has proven useful in understanding different memory deficits.

Declarative vs. Procedural Memory. Another useful distinction for stored memories is the distinction between declarative and procedural knowledge. *Declarative knowledge* represents our knowledge for factual information. This type of knowledge is represented as a series of related statements and can be easily described verbally, such as the process of photosynthesis. Our declarative knowledge seems to be well organized in memory and can be reorganized if new information is added to the existing knowledge structure. The phrase "knowing that" is often used to describe declarative knowledge. (See Table 11-3.)

Procedural knowledge represents our knowledge for the necessary procedures to perform some activity. This type of knowledge is not represented as a series of statements, but rather as a set of procedures. Procedural knowledge does not lend itself to verbal description, as in the example of riding a bike. It is very difficult to describe to someone how to ride a bike; it is easier to simply demonstrate it. We are unsure of the way procedural knowledge is organized and reorganized in memory. The phrase ''knowing how'' is often used to describe procedural knowledge.

There does seem to be some interaction between declarative and procedural knowledge. In other words, procedural knowledge may first start as declarative knowledge. It has been suggested that there are three stages in the acquisition of a procedural skill (Anderson, 1983, 1985; Fitts & Posner, 1967):

1. *the cognitive stage* in which the learner gains declarative knowledge about the skill. The learner may memorize a series of statements and actually rehearse these statements while trying to perform the skill. For example, you may buy a book about tennis and verbally rehearse the steps involved in serving the ball.

2. *the associative stage* in which the learner starts to work out the skill and recognize and correct errors in performance. At this stage the declarative information is gradually transformed into procedures, and both forms of knowledge may coexist at this stage. This is when you begin to work on correcting the height of the ball toss and perfecting your swing.

3. *the autonomous stage* in which the knowledge is totally procedural in nature and the skill has become continuous and automated through practice. At this stage, the declarative knowledge is lost. For example, after much practice, your tennis serve has become a skillful, smooth and fluid motion.

As we shall see, the distinction between declarative and procedural knowledge has proven very useful in our understanding of memory deficits, such as amnesia.

Memory Processes

Memory processes refer to those cognitive processes that are typically under our control when dealing with information. Although the structural models have furthered our knowledge of memory, there has also been much interest in memory processes. An alternative to the structural or ''box model'' of memory are models which describe memory as a function of the types of processes used in dealing with information. We shall limit our discussion to the processes of encoding and retrieval and the distinction between automatic and effortful processing.

Levels of Processing and Encoding.

Encoding refers to those processes or strategies used to initially store information in memory. When we encode

information, we impose some type of organization on the information before it is stored so that later retrieval is made easier.

According to the **levels of processing** approach (Craik & Lockhart, 1972), the durability of the memory trace is a function of the level to which the information was encoded or processed. One can process on a superficial, perceptual level for a particular stimulus or process on a deeper, more meaningful level. For example, when studying for an exam you can merely skim the reading material and lecture notes without taking much time to really process the material. On the other hand, you can carefully go over the material taking time to think about the meaning of what you are reading and integrating the material with what you have already learned. Your memory for the material will depend upon how ''deeply'' you processed the material.

Encoding can occur along a continuum from shallow to deep, in which shallow processing emphasizes perceptual, acoustic, or nonsemantic analyses; and deep processing emphasizes more elaborate, meaningful, or semantic analyses. (See Table 11-4.) Indeed, semantic processing leads to better memory performance than nonsemantic processing (Craik & Tulving, 1975).

Mnemonic Strategies and Encoding. The use of *mnemonic strategies* to aid memory dates back to the Greeks. Any mnemonic technique involves imposing some type of organization on the to-be-remembered material at encoding. Today there are books written on techniques to improve one's memory, and some people claim to know methods to greatly improve one's memory capabilities. Strategies may include the use of verbal or visual aids. Verbal mediators consist of turning the item to be remembered into a meaningful sentence or story, such as remembering the musical notes on the treble clef by the phrase ''Every Good Boy Does Fine'' (E, G, B, D, and F). The use of visual imagery seems to be a common memory aid. Two popular

Table 11-3 Differences Between Declarative and Procedural Memory	
Declarative	**Procedural**
Knowing that	Knowing how
Represented as factual statements	Represented as a set of procedures
Verbally described	Not easily described verbally
Well-organized in memory	Unsure of organization

Table 11-4
Levels of Processing

Level of Processing	Type of Processing	Memory Trace
Shallow	Nonsemantic	Weak
Deep	Semantic	Durable

mnemonics involve visual imagery: keyword technique and method of loci.

The *keyword technique* involves two stages: (1) forming an association between the to-be-remembered item and a keyword and (2) forming a visual image of the keyword. For example, in order to remember a person's name, one might associate the name with a face. A colleague of mine reported using this technique to remember my last name of Duchek (pronounced dew-chek). He associated the keyword "dew" and formed a mental image of me *check*ing the dew on my lawn in the early morning, hence making a "dew check." Although this takes some effort on the learner's part and seems a bit peculiar, it does seem to aid memory for names (Morris, Jones, & Hampson, 1978) and has also proven useful in learning a foreign language (Atkinson & Raugh, 1975).

The *method of loci* is a mnemonic technique that also utilizes visual imagery and is useful when trying to remember a list of items. It involves imagining a familiar path with a number of familiar spatial locations and associating the to-be-remembered items with each location. When attempting to retrieve information, one merely has to take a walk down the path to remember the items. For example, in order to remember to pick up items at the grocery store including cheese, milk, spaghetti, tomatoes, butter, and apples, I might associate these items located along a path from the front door of the building to my office. I might imagine some cheese on the steps of the building, milk spilled on the front door, the receptionist with spaghetti on her head, tomatoes in the faculty mailboxes, butter on the doorknob of my office, and an apple from an admiring student on my desk. To remember these items when I get to the food store, I just mentally walk through that familiar path and remember the visual images of the grocery items.

It can be seen that these mnemonic strategies involve *chunking* information into larger units in STM and using existing information in LTM to encode the information in a more meaningful way. Then of course, it might just be easier to simply write a grocery list!

Encoding Specificity. Although we are discussing encoding and retrieval as separate memory processes, it is virtually impossible to separate the effects of encoding from retrieval. *Retrieval* is the act or process of accessing information that has already been stored in memory. The ease of retrieval depends on how effectively the information was encoded initially. Thus, the two processes are intimately related. The interaction between encoding and retrieval is referred to as the *encoding specificity principle* (Tulving & Thomson, 1973). According to this encoding specificity principle, the extent to which information will be retrieved depends upon the compatibility between the encoding and retrieval contexts. A retrieval cue will be more effective if it more closely reinstates or matches the context when it was encoded (Duchek, 1984; Fischer & Craik, 1977). Hence information that was encoded semantically will be most effectively retrieved by a semantic retrieval cue (i.e., a category of animal) and information encoded nonsemantically will be best retrieved by a nonsemantic cue, (i.e., rhymes with "log").

A related phenomenon known as *state-dependent learning* further illustrates the importance of the encoding-retrieval interaction. State-dependent learning occurs when an individual is better able to recall the information because the physical or emotional state is the same as when the information was learned. In other words, one's physical or emotional state may also be part of the contextual information that is encoded along with the event. Research indicates that people will remember information better if they are in the same emotional state at both encoding and retrieval (Bower, Monteiro, & Gilligan, 1978) or the same physical setting (Smith, Glenberg, & Bjork, 1978). Thus, it is a good idea to schedule final exams in the same classroom where the class was held during the semester.

Retrieval. While encoding involves strategies used to organize and install information into memory, retrieval involves strategies used to reconstruct and pull the information out of memory. Any retrieval situation involves either a recall or recognition process. In a *recall situation*, information can be retrieved without the use of any cues. In a *recognition situation*, one must distinguish relevant information from other alternatives. Thus, an essay exam involves recall, whereas a multiple choice exam involves recognition.

The type of processing one uses in recall and recognition is somewhat different and has been referred as the *generate-edit theory of recall and recognition* (Anderson & Bower, 1973; Balota & Neely, 1980; Neely & Balota, 1981; Kintsch, 1970). Recall involves two steps, first generating the information and then editing the information to decide if it is correct. Recognition only involves editing information, since the information has already been generated. Some believe that recall is a more difficult retrieval task since it involves two stages, but it has been found that under certain conditions, recall can be better than recognition (Tulving & Thomson, 1973).

Recognition may also involve two stages. It often seems that we make our recognition judgements based upon familiarity (Atkinson & Juola, 1973; Balota & Chumbley, 1984). For example, when one takes a multiple choice exam, one is more likely to make a quick "yes" decision when the item is highly familiar and a quick "no" decision if the item is very unfamiliar. Yet if the item seems *somewhat familiar*, one must engage in a more careful search of memory. Thus, recognition may first involve a familiarity check, and if a decision cannot be made at this stage, then a slower search is initiated.

In our initial discussion of the structure of long-term memory, we proposed that these memories are permanently stored and our inability to remember something represents an accessibility or retrieval problem. I am sure you have experienced trying to remember something you are unable to even though you are sure you know it. For example, in trying to remember the title of a specific movie, you might remember the actors who played in the movie, when it was made, the story line, etc. Yet still you cannot remember the movie title itself. Then perhaps you think of another title that is the wrong one. Even though you know this is not the correct response, sometimes the incorrect response blocks the retrieval of the correct information and the more you think, the more this incorrect response leaps to mind. Finally, you stop trying to think about this movie and later you suddenly remember the correct title. This is known as the *tip-of-the-tongue phenomenon* (TOT) and represents an everyday example of retrieval blockage. This demonstrates how our memories are sometimes stored as packages of information. For example, the movie title was stored along with other contextual information, such as the actors and when the movie was first seen. The incorrect title actually served as a retrieval block or inhibitor, and the more one endeavors to think of the title, the stronger the block becomes. Abandoning the desperate attempts to remember the answer helps the block or inhibition to disappear and the correct answer surfaces seemingly without effort.

Automatic and Effortful Processing. Thus far we have discussed the memory processes of encoding and retrieval and their interaction. Hasher and Zachs (1979) presented another framework for memory processes: *automatic versus effortful.* **Automatic processes** are those processes that occur without much attentional effort while **effortful processes** require much attentional capacity. When we discussed attention, we saw how the once effortful process of reading

becomes automatic through extensive practice. Hasher and Zachs suggest that some types of information such as frequency, spatial and temporal information are coded automatically in the memory system. Automatic processes *are not* affected by the following: (1) learning instructions (intentional vs. incidental), (2) practice, (3) emotional states such as depression or anxiety, or (4) age. However, effortful processes are affected by all of the above. Any cognitive task can be viewed along this automatic-effortful continuum. Although, there has been some debate whether certain information can be encoded automatically (Kausler, Lichty, & Hakami, 1984; Naveh-Benjamin & Jonides, 1986; Williams & Durso, 1986), the automatic-effortful dimension has provided researchers with a framework for understanding memory processes.

Memory Deficits

Memory deficits can arise from several disorders such as head injury, chronic alcohol abuse, tumors, temporal lobe surgery, and Alzheimer's disease. Memory impairment is also seen in normal aging. Although the deficits associated with normal aging do not significantly interfere with daily functioning, it is still a frequent complaint of older adults.

There appears to be little or no age-related deficit in sensory or short-term memory (Craik, 1977) but there are deficits in some aspects of long-term memory functioning. Older adults often exhibit poor memory performance on episodic memory tasks (Balota & Duchek, 1989; Craik, 1977), whereas characteristics of semantic memory processing seem to be unaffected by age (Balota & Duchek, 1988; Burke, White & Diaz, 1987; Howard, McAndrews, & Lasaga, 1981). There is a larger age-related deficit in recall than recognition (Craik, 1977), and older adults exhibit more of a deficit on semantic processing tasks (Craik & Simon, 1980; Eysenck, 1974). It has also been shown that older adults show less of an encoding specificity effect than younger adults (Duchek, 1984; Rabinowitz, Craik, & Ackerman, 1982). It appears that age-related deficits are more related to cognitive tasks that involve effortful processing rather than automatic processing (Craik, Byrd, & Swanson, 1987), when the tasks require more cognitive resources or strategies.

Alzheimer's disease is a degenerative disorder which affects five to ten percent of the population over age 65 (Joynt & Shoulson, 1979). It is the most common form of dementia, and memory impairment is the hallmark clinical symptom of the disease. There appear to be deficits in both short-term and long-term memory. For example, digit span is greatly reduced in the later stages of Alzheimer's disease compared to normal aging (Botwinick, Storandt, & Berg, 1986; Storandt, Botwinick, Danziger, Berg, & Hughes, 1984). Large deficits are seen in episodic tasks where new information must be retained (Botwinick, Storandt, & Berg, 1986). Alzheimer's patients also show impaired performance on semantic memory tasks which involve effortful processing. For example, they exhibit poor performance on the Boston naming test (Knesevich, LaBarge, & Edwards, 1986) and word fluency tasks (Botwinick, Strorandt, & Berg, 1986; Storandt, Botwinick, Danziger, Berg, & Hughes, 1984).

Semantic memory performance involving automatic processing seems to be unaffected in Alzheimer's disease (Nebes, Boller, & Holland, 1986; Nebes, Martin, & Horn, 1984). There is evidence that procedural knowledge can be retained in some tasks (Dick, Kean, & Sands, 1988; Eslinger & Damasio, 1986; Knopman & Nissen, 1987).

The distinction between declarative and procedural knowledge has also been used in studying the memory deficits associated with certain forms of amnesia such as Korsakoff's syndrome. Korsakoff's syndrome results from chronic alcohol abuse and a subsequent severe thiamine deficiency. Although other aspects of intellectual functioning may remain intact (Talland, 1965), different components of memory functioning are impaired. STM deficits have been noted in Korsakoff patients (Butters, 1979; Kinsbourne & Wood, 1975). Butters and Cermak (1975) argue that Korsakoff patients have a semantic processing deficit and primarily engage in shallow processing at encoding. There is evidence that patients with amnesia can exhibit procedural learning such as mirror-drawing or pursuit motor tasks, yet show no episodic memory for learning the skill (Brooks & Baddeley, 1976; Cohen & Squire, 1980; Graf & Schacter, 1985; Squire, 1986; Starr & Phillips, 1970). It has also been suggested that amnesics show deficient automatic processing (Huppert & Piercy, 1978) and utilization of context at retrieval (Winocur & Kinsbourne, 1978), yet show normal semantic memory functioning (Baddeley & Warrington, 1970).

Milner (1959) reported the now famous case study of an amnesic who underwent bilateral medial temporal lobe resection to control seizures. After the surgery, this patient was virtually unable to learn any new information although his recall of events prior to the surgery was unimpaired. He was unable to transfer any new information from STM to LTM. However, he could acquire some new motor skills, yet showed no memory for learning these skills (Milner, Corkin, & Teuber, 1968). This case is often cited as strong evidence for the distinction between STM and LTM and declarative and procedural memory.

We can see from this discussion that theoretical frameworks of memory structures and processes have greatly advanced our understanding of memory deficits associated with different disorders. It is certain that a clearer understanding of the specific cognitive mechanisms involved in different memory disorders will lead to more fruitful remediation and therapy.

LANGUAGE

One of the most remarkable feats of humans is the ability to use language. It is this ability which allows us to precisely communicate our thoughts and sets us apart from other animals. There have been numerous attempts to teach some form of language to apes (Gardner & Gardner, 1969; Premack, 1971, 1976), however it has been argued that apes cannot learn or use language with the same complexity as that of humans (Terrace, Petitto, Sanders, & Bever, 1979).

There has been much debate in the literature on how language is acquired. According to Skinner's learning theory, language is acquired in the same way that any other behavior is acquired (Skinner, 1957). The apparent rules of grammar are simply learned through reinforcement and imitation. They can be shaped and conditioned just like any other behavior. A learning theory approach to language acquisition has been criticized for the following reasons: (1) A learning theory cannot explain the rapidity and ease with which children acquire language. (2) Children do not always imitate adult speech. For example, all children use over-generalizations of rules when first learning to speak that they clearly do not acquire from listening to adults, such as in the phrase, "I *goed* to grandma's." (3) If children acquired language through reinforcement, we would expect children to learn language in different ways given the differences in reinforcement contingencies across families. However, we find that there is considerable consistency in the sequence with which children acquire language.

A more cognitive approach to language acquisition has been proposed by Chomsky (1965). According to Chomsky, humans possess an innate predisposition for language. That is, the child already is equipped with an innate knowledge about the way language works. This innate knowledge is referred to as *linguistic universals*. For example, the child has some innate knowledge about the rules of syntax and thus can master proper syntax in a very short period of time. Through exposure to language and experience with language, this innate knowledge is verified and the child acquires a specific language.

Stages of Language Acquisition

Children acquire language in the same developmental sequence at approximately the same age. Although the exact age for a particular stage may vary across children, the ordering of the stages does not vary.

Crying and cooing represent the first stage of language

acquisition. During the first month of life the infant's cry is largely undifferentiated, and it is difficult to distinguish from the cry whether the baby is hungry, tired, or has a wet diaper. By the second month, the cry becomes differentiated and the mother and father can usually pinpoint the cause of distress by the sound of the cry. It is typically at this point that the baby starts to coo — much to the delight of the parents. Cooing sounds are vowel-like sounds, and it appears the infant is beginning to practice using his articulatory apparatus. Parents often make sounds in response to the infant's cooing and start setting the stage for the reciprocity of language.

By six months the infant starts babbling. Babbling occurs when a consonant sound is added to the vocalization (e.g, "da-da-da-da"). Mother might be disturbed that the first word sound her baby makes resembles the sound of "dad", however, it does not appear that babies attach any meaning to their babbling at this stage (Best, 1989). There is even evidence that congenitally deaf children babble, but language skills fall behind that of hearing children because they cannot benefit from the auditory feedback of their articulatory system (Lenneberg, 1967).

At about nine months of age, the babbling starts to take on the sounds of the infant's native tongue. This is referred to as *babbling drift*. The infant also starts to imitate adult speech sounds, which is referred to as *echolalia*.

At about one year of age, single word phrases are used to convey entire sentences and are referred to as *holophrastic phrases*. A single word is used to convey many different meanings dependent on the context. For example, the child uses the word "milk" to mean, "I want some milk," "I see the milk," or "I spilled the milk." These single words are typically nouns, adjectives or self-invented words that the parent can decipher due to their continued use in a particular context, such as "baba" for bottle (McNeill, 1970). Language comprehension exceeds language production at this stage. Vocabulary size increases dramatically from one to two years of age. At age two, the child may have a vocabulary of 300 words.

From 18 to 20 months of age, the child begins to use two-word phrases. Speech is referred to as *telegraphic speech* at this stage because the utterances are short yet convey meaning. Any nonessential words are not included such as articles and prepositions. Brown (1970) found that these two-word phrases typically have a certain structure in relation to meaning, such as phrases like "daddy shoe" for possession, "doll chair" for location, or "all gone" for agent-action.

Soon the child starts to extend these two-word phrases into three and four words. For example, "mommy read" becomes "mommy read book." Inflections in speech patterns and word order are used at this time to further

convey meaning. Over-generalizations of grammatical rules are also seen at this time, especially with irregular verb tenses and noun plurals. Sentences such as "He *runned* away" and "My *footses* hurt" are commonly heard at this stage and disappear when the child learns the exceptions to the rules (Berko, 1958).

The fundamentals of language are developed in an impressive four to five years. Later, language development includes an extension of vocabulary and more phonological and syntactic refinement.

Speech Comprehension

Speech perception involves those processes necessary to encode the acoustic signal. These processes transform the sound into the word.

When you listen to the news on the radio at home, you can easily perceive each word as completely distinct from the other words and have no difficulty understanding what the speaker is saying. But listening to the news in a foreign language sounds continuous, seemingly without boundaries between words. We are able to effortlessly understand our own language because we are able to segment the sounds into words. The problem we encounter in listening to a foreign language is that we do not know how to segment the sounds into words. Speech really does occur in a continuous stream, but we are able to distinguish breaks within words as between words. Somehow we are able to recognize patterns in this stream and extract meaning from them, and we are able to distinguish language across a variety of speakers and situations whether it is the speech of a four-year-old child or that of a college professor.

Knowledge of our language allows us to segment words according to phonemes. *Phonemes* are the most basic units of sound. Words are built from a number of phonemes. For example, the word "cat" is made up of three phonemes: [c], [a], and [t]. The word "light" also contains three phonemes: [l], [i], and [t]. There is not a direct correspondence between letters and phonemes. This makes learning to spell a difficult task for a child. In order to comprehend the spoken word, one must be able to identify and segment these phonemes. It is not entirely clear how this phoneme segmentation occurs, but it appears that speech perception is accomplished by a type of *feature analysis*.

Phonemes can be broken down into phonetic features. These features include the *consonantal feature, voicing,* and *place of articulation* (Chomsky & Halle, 1968). The *consonantal feature* is a consonant sound versus a vowel sound. *Voicing* is the vibration of the vocal cords when producing a phoneme. Some phonemes are voiced and some are unvoiced, for example, the phoneme [z] is voiced and the phoneme [s] is unvoiced. The distinction between voiced and unvoiced sounds can be easily demonstrated by placing one's hand on the vocal cords during pronunciation. *Place of articulation* is the location in the mouth that is constricted or closed in order to produce the phoneme. The place of articulation varies. For example, the place of articulation for [p] is at the lips and at the teeth for [t]. Once a phoneme is recognized, knowledge of phonological rules helps to segment the sounds into words, and then meaning is assigned to the words from stored information.

The exact manner in which speech is interpreted and meaning is extracted is obviously complex and remains largely unknown. It is evident that speech perception involves the interplay between bottom-up and top-down processing. **Bottom-up processing** occurs when the system encodes the physical signal and proceeds to identify the signal through a series of stages. Processing starts with the acoustic or visual signal and works up from the bottom. Bottom-up processing is also sometimes referred to as ''data driven.'' Phoneme identification and segmentation represent bottom-up processing.

Top-down processing occurs when the system generates expectations or inferences about the signal. Top-down processing is based upon a higher cognitive order of stored knowledge and is largely dependent upon contextual information. It is sometimes referred to as ''conceptually driven.''

Many times the acoustic signal in speech is distorted. Someone may slur their words at the end of a sentence or the speech signal may be embedded in a background of other noises. We use top-down processing to help interpret such speech. This is clearly demonstrated in what is known as the *phonemic restoration effect* (Warren, 1970). Warren and Warren (1970) demonstrated this effect by presenting the following series of sentences with a missing phoneme to subjects and substituting a non-speech sound for each missing phoneme (where the * appears):

> It was found that the *eel was on the axle.
> It was found that the *eel was on the shoe.
> It was found that the *eel was on the orange.
> It was found that the *eel was on the table.

Subjects reported hearing the words ''wheel'', ''heel'', ''peel'', or ''meal'' respectively in each sentence. Hence, they were using top-down processing to identify the missing word by making a contextual association with the last word in each sentence.

Speech perception involves an important interplay between bottom-up and top-down processing. Both types of processing most likely play a role in speech comprehension. The perception of speech would be quite slow without using top-down processing to generate expected words based on the context in addition to bottom-up processing that uses direct analyses of the stimulus features.

Speech Production

Not only do we comprehend speech, but we also spend a great deal of time producing speech. Researchers have developed theories of speech production based upon an analysis of speech errors and hesitations in speech. Garret (1982) has proposed a model of speech production which suggests that the stages of speech production occur in almost the reverse order of speech perception.

The first stage of speech production is at the *message level*. Here the representation of the message is in a thought and a nonlinguistic code. This message or thought is then translated into a language-specific code in the *functional level*. At the functional stage, certain decisions are made concerning the meaning to be communicated. The representation serves as an outline for speech production, and syntax is formulated at this time. The next stage is the *positional level* in which phrases are ordered and word forms are selected. In the *phonological level*, the actual sounds and phonetics are worked out. Finally, this code is passed on to the *articulatory level* in which the actual speech output occurs.

The production of speech involves some parallel processing in which a speaker is formulating and producing speech at the same time. In addition, a feedback mechanism operates as errors in speech are detected and revised. The speaker also makes adjustments in their productions depending upon the listener's needs (Balota, Boland, & Shields, 1989; Clark & Clark, 1977).

In summary, the use of language involves the interaction among different cognitive processes. Attention and perception are involved in many aspects of bottom-up processing, while the utilization of stored knowledge in memory is involved in top-down processing. Our ability to use language represents a higher-order cognitive skill which is mediated by the more basic components of cognition.

Language Deficits

Aphasia refers to a language disorder and can take many different forms. In 1860, Broca discovered that damage to a certain area in the frontal lobe of the brain resulted in a language deficit, now called Broca's aphasia. Patients with *Broca's aphasia* have difficulty in the production of speech, although comprehension seems intact. Speech is slow and telegraphic.

Damage to an area of the temporal lobe which lies posterior to Broca's area results in another type of aphasia known as Wernicke's aphasia. Patients with *Wernicke's aphasia* have no difficulty producing speech. Speech is fluent and syntactically correct but does not have any meaningful content. The two areas involved in Broca's and Wernicke's aphasia are connected by a band of tissue called the arcuate fasciculus. It has been suggested that the semantics or meaning of an utterance is first produced in

Wernicke's area and then passed along the arcuate fasciculus to Broca's area where the production of the utterance is formed (Geschwind, 1970). This theory of speech production has been virtually unchallenged until recently. There is now evidence from a series of positron emission tomography studies that Broca's area may be related to general motor programming rather than the specific programming of language output (Petersen, Fox, Posner et al., 1988). Furthermore, Wernicke's area has not been activated in these studies by a language task which requires semantic or comprehension processing.

Aphasia tends to be a general term used for many types of language deficits. A global aphasia may be reflected in a deficit in word retrieval and general language comprehension (Goodglass, 1987). Other forms of aphasia are more specific and thus may be more readily treated. *Anomia* is an inability to retrieve words from semantic memory during speech. It has been suggested that not only does the anomic patient have difficulty retrieving words from memory, but the conceptual representation of the word is also impaired (Whitehouse, Caramazza, & Zurif, 1978). *Agrammatism* represents the inability to use words in correct syntactic or grammatical form. Patients with transcortical motor aphasia have difficulty initiating an utterance although they can repeat phrases. A clear understanding of normal language processes and a particular patient's deficit and abilities are invaluable to the therapist's attempt to remediate function.

PROBLEM-SOLVING

Problem-solving is another higher order cognitive skill necessary for daily functioning. Problem-solving occurs when we engage in behavior in order to achieve a specific goal. When a goal is not readily obtainable, a problem exists. We encounter problems and engage in problem-solving on a daily basis, for example solving the problem of getting your child to clean her room or figuring out how to write a paper by tomorrow's class.

It seems logical that problem-solving occurs in a series of stages. Wallas (1927) identified four basic stages involved in problem-solving:

1. the *preparation stage*, in which one makes an initial attempt to understand the problem and starts to solve the problem.
2. the *incubation stage*, in which the person stops consciously thinking about the problem and moves on to other cognitive activities after the initial attempts to solve the problem have failed. However, the person is still unconsciously working on the problem.

3. the *illumination stage*, in which a solution suddenly comes to consciousness after the unconscious work is done (often described as the ''light-bulb'' phenomenon).
4. the *verification stage*, in which the solution is tested and verified.

Although we have all experienced some flashes of insight suddenly occurring, we clearly do not solve all problems in this manner. Polya (1957, 1968) has proposed a more general schema for problem-solving which incorporates some of the same stages of (1) understanding the problem, (2) devising a plan (3) carrying out the plan, and (4) checking the results.

Problem-solving does not necessarily occur in such a prescribed serial order where one stage is completed before another stage begins. Some activities are carried out in parallel.

Problem-solving generally involves some initial understanding of the problem. In order to come up with a solution, we must first have some mental representation for the problem. The adequacy of this representation will determine how much time it takes to find a solution as well as the correctness of the solution. Consider the following example (adapted from Maier & Burke, 1967):

You buy a horse for $60 and sell it for $70. Then you buy it back again for $80 and sell it for $90. How much money did you make in the horse business?

Now consider the same problem with a few changes in wording:

You buy a white horse for $60 and sell it for $70. Then you buy a black horse for $80 and sell it for $90. How much money did you make in the horse business?

The problem becomes much clearer in the second representation. By considering two horses, it is easier to see the problem in terms of two separate business deals. When subjects were given the first representation of the problem, only 40% reported the correct answer ($20), whereas 100% reported the correct answer with the second representation (Maier & Burke, 1967). This demonstrates that if a problem is incorrectly represented at the initial stage, then we are often led down an incorrect solution path.

Problem-solving not only involves the ability to adequately represent a problem but also the ability to reformulate the initial representation when a solution is not found or is incorrect. This requires some flexibility in thinking. Inflexibility in thinking is referred to as *functional fixedness*. Functional fixedness occurs when one is only able to visualize an object in one functional role. The following problem requires flexibility in thinking to solve the problem (Maier, 1931):

Problem: There are two strings hanging from the ceiling. Your task is to tie the two strings together. However, the two strings are so far apart that you cannot hold one and walk to the other to reach it. The following items are in the room: a chair, pliers, matches, and a piece of paper. Can you tie the two strings together with the help of those items?

Solution: Tie the pliers around the end of one string and set that string in motion like a pendulum. Take hold of the other string and take it to the center of the room. Wait for the pendulum to swing towards the center of the room and then tie the two strings together.

This problem is often difficult to solve because most people view the pliers only as a tool for twisting or loosening, not for any other functional use such as is needed in the above problem. In solving problems on a daily basis, it is often necessary to break out of these mental sets and see things in a different light. Otherwise, we find ourselves perseverating on the same incorrect solution paths.

There are many types of strategies to use for solving problems such as *algorithms* or *heuristics*. An *algorithm* is a procedure which follows a set of specific rules and will always lead to a solution. In contrast, an *heuristic* is more a general rule of thumb and will not always lead to a solution. Although algorithms always lead to a solution, they may be very time consuming to use. For example, in trying to solve the following anagram of ''HRYETAP'', you are not likely to use an algorithm which would require trying all permutations of letter ordering in order to solve the problem. It would be easier to use heuristics and the knowledge of letter combinations in order to solve the anagram. Knowing that the letters ''y'' and ''h'' are not likely to occur together but ''th'' and ''ph'' are common letter combinations will help one combine the correct letters to form the word ''therapy.''

More specific problem-solving strategies include subgoal analysis, working backward, and analogy. *Subgoal analysis* involves breaking down the final goal into various subgoals that will lead up to the final goal. The use of a subgoal analysis requires an understanding of the steps involved to achieve the final goal. A subgoal approach is often recommended in dealing with demented patients (Mace & Rabins, 1981). *Working backward* is a technique of moving from the goal backward through initial states to produce a solution. For example, if you have misplaced your keys, you may think about the last time you had them and retrace your steps from that point. *Analogy* is a technique of using the solution to another similar problem to solve the present problem.

It is evident that problem-solving is a complex cognitive skill which requires the interaction among many basic skills. We must be able to selectively attend to the relevant information to adequately represent the problem and produce a solution. We must be able to hold information about the problem in short-term memory and utilize stored knowledge from long-term memory to produce a solution. Problem-solving also requires an ability to formulate and initiate a plan of action and a feedback system which provides information about the correctness of the solution and the need for revision.

Problem-Solving Deficits

Problem-solving deficits are often associated with frontal lobe damage (Jouandet & Gazzaniga, 1979). Frontal lobe syndrome results in many types of cognitive-related deficits including deficits in sensory, attention, memory, motivation, and emotion (Goldstein & Levin, 1987). Any of these disturbances could have an impact on problem-solving ability, and any aspect of problem-solving could be impaired. The ability to understand the problem and formulate the goal may be impaired and/or the ability to initiate the plan and revise it during the process. Impulsivity and perseveration in responding are common behaviors in brain-injured patients and reflect an inability to think flexibly and to self-correct. The remediation program at New York University's Institute of Rehabilitative Medicine includes training programs in higher order skills such as reasoning and flexibility of thought (Ben-Yishay & Diller, 1983)

Impairment in goal formation and initiation often may not be apparent from more structured neuropsychological assessments (Goldstein & Levin, 1987). More unstructured tasks may be necessary to detect a disturbance (Lezak, 1983). Furthermore, a detailed analysis of a patient's basic cognitive skills as well as problem-solving deficits is necessary for implementing an appropriate and effective therapy.

NEURAL SUBSTRATES OF COGNITION

This chapter has presented several components of cognition in order to understand the basic cognitive mechanisms underlying performance. An ultimate goal would be to link these cognitive components to their corresponding neural substrates. Such an undertaking involves a great deal of interdisciplinary work and more knowledge of the relationship between cognition and the brain.

The work of Posner and his colleagues (Posner, Cohen, & Rafal, 1982; Posner, Walker, Freidrich, & Rafal, 1984; Posner, 1986; Posner & Rafal, 1987) reflects the importance of this approach. These researchers have proposed a neural model of spatial attention based on research with different patient populations and monkeys.

They argue that the control of spatial attention involves three cognitive components (engage, move, and disengage) which reflect different cortical substrates. The *engage operation* involves the pulvinar, the *move operation* involves the colliculus and surrounding midbrain areas, and the *disengage operation* involves the parietal lobe.

Theories of cognition and associated brain structures are often based on studies of different patient populations. By looking at the cognitive deficits produced by a lesion in a particular brain area, we assume that the missing cognitive ability is related to that damaged area of the brain. For example, damage to the hippocampus and temporal lobes often results in a memory impairment, hence we assume that these structures must somehow be involved in memory functioning. In addition, much of what we know about hemispheric specialization comes from studies of patients who have had the corpus callosum severed in order to prevent seizures (Gazzaniga & Sperry, 1967). A great deal has been learned about the relationship between cognitive components and neural substrates from lesion studies. However, these studies mostly involve a *post hoc* analysis in which the patient's premorbid abilities are often unknown and the extent of damage to interconnected brain fibers and the recovery of function by other areas are typically unknown.

Recent advances in *positron emission tomography* (PET) allow the study of on-line processing in the brain. It is possible to view which areas of the brain are activated when a specific cognitive activity is being performed, such as in the work of Petersen et al. (1988) who designated the brain areas involved in the processing of language. Such studies promise to greatly enhance our knowledge of both cognition and brain function.

SUMMARY

How can the study of cognition be incorporated into the practice of occupational therapy? In some ways, it is already incorporated. Views of development are largely influenced by Piaget's theory which is considered to be a theory of cognitive development. According to Piaget, children pass through a series of cognitive stages wherein they develop a mental representation of the world and appropriate ways of dealing with it. Recent evidence indicates that cognitive development is dependent on increased knowledge and development in memory and knowledge representation rather than increased cognitive abilities (Anderson, 1985).

Allen's (1985) theory of cognitive disability incorporates some of the basic cognitive components underlying performance. According to Allen, cognitive disability can be viewed as a hierarchy of functioning. The six levels of function represent differences in cognitive abilities, such as attention and problem-solving. Although there have not been many attempts to predict performance on different cognitive tasks based on Allen's levels of disability, Mayer (1988) did find significant correlations between Allen Cognitive Levels (ACL) test scores and various subtests of the WAIS-R. Clearly, further analysis and refinement of Allen's theory could be carried out with a better understanding of basic cognitive processes.

The goal of this chapter was to briefly examine some basic cognitive components underlying performance. In fact, certain topics in this enormous area of cognitive research, such as pattern recognition, decision-making, and artificial intelligence were not covered. Nearly all aspects of performance involve some form of cognitive processing, and most activities involve a complex interaction among these components. A clear understanding of basic cognitive skills can provide more detailed analyses of performance.

Consider again the patient who is experiencing difficulty in dressing. A detailed analysis of the potential cognitive mechanisms underlying performance will help guide therapy. For example, if the patient is having difficulty retaining the command in STM, then providing an external cue such as a written request in large bold letters will enhance function. If the patient is having difficulty in formulating and initiating a plan of action, then setting up subgoals for the desired behavior may enhance function. Unless the therapist understands the cognitive processes underlying a particular behavior, she/he will not truly understand the cognitive impairment and thus therapy may be misguided. Even though two patients may be performing at the same level, the underlying problem may not be the same. Thus, what is effective therapy for one patient may not prove effective for another.

In order to assess and remediate activities of daily living, it is necessary to understand the cognitive processes as well as the motor processes involved. The understanding of cognition should not be seen as a knowledge base outside the realm of occupational therapy, but should be seen as an additional knowledge tool the therapist uses to guide service and enhance patient functioning.

Study Questions

1. What are the basic assumptions underlying the information processing approach?

2. Describe the three components of attention.

3. Describe the interaction among the three memory stores and the function of each store.

4. How have the theoretical frameworks of memory structure and processes advanced our understanding of memory deficits?

5. What is the difference between bottom-up and top-down processing in speech perception?

6. How can the study of cognition be incorporated into the practice of occupational therapy?

Acknowledgment

The author acknowledges preliminary work performed by Donald A. Davidson and M. Laurita Fike in the preparation of this chapter.

References

Allen, C.K. (1985). *Occupational therapy for psychiatric diseases: Measurement and management of cognitive disabilities.* Boston: Little, Brown and Company.

Anderson, J.R. (1983). *The architecture of cognition.* Cambridge, MA: Harvard University Press.

Anderson, J.R. (1985). *Cognitive psychology and its implications.* New York: W.H. Freeman and Company.

Anderson, J.R., & Bower, G.H. (1973). *Human associative memory.* Washington, DC: Winston.

Anderson, J.R., & Ross, B.H. (1980). Evidence against a semantic-episodic distinction. *Journal of Experimental Psychology: Human Learning and Memory, 6,* 441-466.

Atkinson, R.C., & Juola, J.F. (1973). Factors influencing speed and accuracy of word recognition. In S. Kornblum (Ed.), *Attention and performance IV.* New York: Academic Press.

Atkinson, R.C., & Raugh, M.R. (1975). An application of the mnemonic keyword method to the acquisition of Russian vocabulary. *Journal of Experimental Psychology: Human Learning and Memory, 104,* 126-133.

Atkinson, R.C., & Shiffrin, R.M. (1968). Human memory: A proposed system and its control processes. In K. Spence & J. Spence (Eds.), *The psychology of learning and motivation,* Vol. 2, New York: Academic Press.

Baddeley, A.D., & Hitch, G.J. (1974). Working memory. In G.H. Bower (Ed.), *The psychology of learning and motivation,* Vol. 8, New York: Academic Press.

Baddeley, A.D., & Warrington, E.K. (1970). Amnesia and the distinction between long and short term memory. *Journal of Verbal Learning and Verbal Behavior, 9,* 176-189.

Balota, D.A., Boland, J.E., & Shields, L.W. (1989). Priming in pronunciation: Beyond pattern recognition and onset latency. *Journal of Memory and Language, 28,* 14-36.

Balota, D.A., & Chumbley, J.I. (1984). Are lexical decisions a good measure of lexical access? The role of word frequency in the neglected decision stage. *Journal of Experimental Psychology: Human Perception Performance, 10,* 340-357.

Balota, D.A., & Duchek, J.M. (1986). The influence of voice similarity on the 20 second delayed suffix effect. *Journal of Experimental Psychology: Learning, Memory, and Cognition, 12,* 336-345.

Balota, D.A., & Duchek, J.M. (1988). Age related differences in lexical access, automatic spreading activation, and simple pronunciation. *Psychology and Aging, 3,* 84-93.

Balota, D.A., & Duchek, J.M. (1989). Spreading activation in episodic memory: Further evidence for age independence. *Quarterly Journal of Experimental Psychology, 41*(4), 849-876.

Balota, D.A., & Neely, J.H. (1980). Test-expectancy and word-frequency effects in recall and recognition. *Journal of Experimental Psychology: Human Learning and Memory, 6,* 576-587.

Ben-Yishay, Y., & Diller, L. (1983). Cognitive rehabilitation. In M. Rosenthal, E.R. Griffith, M.R. Bond, J.D. Miller (Eds.), *Rehabilitation of the head-injured adult.* Philadelphia: F.A. Davis.

Ben-Yishay, Y., Piasetsky, E.B., & Rattok, J. (1987). A systematic method for ameliorating disorders in basic attention. In M.J. Meier, A.L. Benton, L. Diller (Eds.), *Neuropsychological rehabilitation,* New York: Guilford Press.

Ben-Yishay, Y., Rattok, J., & Diller, L. (1979). A clinical strategy for the systematic amelioration of attentional disturbances in severe head trauma patients. In Y. Ben-Yishay (Ed.), *Working approaches to remediation of cognitive deficits in brain damaged persons.* NYU Medical Center, Rehabilitation Monograph No. 60, pp. 1-27.

Berko, J. (1958). The child's learning of English morphology. *Word, 14,* 150-177.

Best, J.B. (1989). *Cognitive psychology,* St. Paul: West Publishing Company.

Botwinick, J., Storandt, M., & Berg, L. (1986). A longitudinal, behavioral study of senile dementia of the Alzheimer's type. *Archives of Neurology, 43,* 1124-1127.

Bower, G.H., Monteiro, K.P., & Gilligan, S.G. (1978). Emotional mood as a context for learning and recall. *Journal of Verbal Learning and Verbal Behavior, 17,* 573-587.

Brooks, D.N., & Baddeley, A.D. (1976). What can amnesic patients learn? *Neuropsychologia, 14,* 111-122.

Brown, R. (1970). *Psycholinguistics.* New York: Free Press.

Burke, D.M., White, H., & Diaz, D.L. (1987). Semantic priming in young and older adults: Evidence for age constancy in automatic and attentional processes. *Journal of Experimental Psychology: Human Perception and Performance, 13,* 79-88.

Butters, N. (1979). Amnesic disorders. In K.M. Heilman & E. Valenstein (Eds.), *Clinical Neuropsychology.* New York: Oxford University Press.

Butters, N., & Cermak, L. (1975). Some analyses of amnesic syndromes in brain damaged patients. In R.L. Isaacson & K.H. Pribram (Eds.), *The Hippocampus, Vol. 2,* New York: Plenum Press.

Cherry, R.S., & Kruger, B. (1983). Selective auditory attention abilities of learning disabled and normal achieving children. *Journal of Learning Disabilities, 16,* 202-205.

Chomsky, N. (1965). *Aspects of the theory of syntax.* Cambridge, MA: MIT Press.

Chomsky, N., & Halle, M. (1968). *The sound pattern of English.* New York: Harper & Row.

Clark, H.H., Clark, E.E. (1977). *Psychology and Language.* New York: Harcourt Brace Jovanovich.

Cohen, N.J., & Squire, L.R. (1980). Preserved learning and retention of pattern-analyzing skill in amnesia: Dissociation of knowing how and knowing that. *Science, 210,* 207-210.

Conrad, R. (1964). Acoustic confusions in immediate memory. *British Journal of Psychology, 55,* 75-84.

Cowan, N. (1984). On short and long auditory traces. *Psychological Bulletin, 96,* 351-370.

Craik, F.I.M. (1977). Age differences in human memory. In J.E. Birren & K.W. Schaie, (Eds.), *Handbook of the Psychology of Aging.* New York: Van Nostrand Reinhold.

Craik, F.I.M., Byrd, M., & Swanson, J.L. (1987). Patterns of memory loss in three elderly samples. *Psychology and Aging, 2,* 79-86.

Craik, F.I.M., & Lockhart, R.S. (1972). Levels of processing: A framework for memory research. *Journal of Verbal Learning and Verbal Behavior, 11,* 671-684.

Craik, F.I.M., & Simon, E. (1980). Age differences in memory: The roles of attention and depth of processing. In L.W. Poon, J.L. Fozard, L.S. Cermak, D. Arenberg, & L.W. Thompson (Eds.), *New directions in memory and aging: Proceedings of the George Talland memorial conference.* Hillsdale, NJ: Erlbaum.

Craik, F.I.M., & Tulving, E. (1975). Depth of processing and the retention of words in episodic memory. *Journal of Experimental Psychology: General, 104,* 268-294.

Crowder, R.G., & Morton, J. (1969). Precategorical acoustic storage (PAS). *Perception and Psychophysics, 5,* 365-373.

Darwin, C.J., Turvey, M.T., & Crowder, R.G., (1972). The auditory analogue of the Sperling partical report procedure: Evidence for brief auditory storage. *Cognitive Psychology, 3,* 255-267.

de Groot, A.D. (1966). Perception and memory versus thought. In B. Kleinmuntz (Ed.), *Problem-Solving.* New York: Wiley.

Dick, M.B., Kean, M.L., & Sands, D. (1988). The pre-selection effect on the recall facilitation of motor movements in Alzheimer-type dementia. *Journal of Gerontology, 23,* 127-135.

Duchek, J.M. (1984). Encoding and retrieval differences between young and old: The impact of attentional capacity usage. *Developmental Psychology, 20,* 1173-1180.

Duchek, J.M., & Neely, J.H. (1989). A dissociative word-frequency x levels of processing interaction in episodic recognition and lexical decision tasks. *Memory & Cognition, 17,* 148-162.

Eslinger, P.J., & Damasio, A.R. (1986). Preserved motor learning in Alzheimer's Disease: Implications for anatomy and behavior. *The Journal of Neuroscience, 6,* 3006-3009.

Eysenck, M.W. (1974). Age differences in incidental learning. *Developmental Psychology, 10,* 936-941.

Fisher, R.P., & Craik, F.I.M. (1977). The interaction between encoding and retrieval operations in cued recall. *Journal of Experimental Psychology: Human Learning and Memory, 3,* 701-711.

Fitts, P.M., & Posner, M.I. (1967). *Human performance.* Belmont, CA: Brooks Cole.

Gardner, R.A., & Gardner, B.T. (1969). Teaching sign language to a chimpanzee. *Science, 165,* 664-672.

Garrett, M.F. (1982). Production of speech: observations from normal and pathological language use. In A. W. Ellis (Ed.), *Normality and pathology in cognitive functions* (pp. 19-76). New York: Academic Press.

Gazzaniga, M.S., & Sperry, R.W. (1967). Language after section of the cerebral commissures. *Brain, 90,* 131-148.

Geschwind, N. (1970). The organization of language and the brain. *Science, 170,* 940-944..

Goldstein, F.C., & Levin, H.S. (1987). Disorders of reasoning and problem-solving ability. In M.J. Meier, A.L. Benton, & L. Diller (Eds.), *Neuropsychological Rehabilitation.* New York: Guilford Press.

Goodglass, H. (1987). Neurolinguistic principles and aphasia therapy. In M.J. Meier, A.L. Benton, & L. Diller (Eds.), *Neuropsychological Rehabilitation.* New York: Guilford Press.

Gopher, D., & Kahneman, D. (1971). Individual differences in attention and the prediction flight criteria. *Perceptual and Motor Skills, 33,* 1335-1342.

Graf, P., & Schacter, D.L. (1985). Implicit and explicit memory for new associations in normal and amnesic subjects. *Journal of Experimental Psychology: Learning, Memory, and Cognition, 11*, 501-518.

Hasher, L., & Zachs, R.T. (1979). Automatic and effortful processes in memory. *Journal of Experimental Psychology: General, 108*, 356-388.

Herrmann, D.J., & Harwood, J.R. (1980). More evidence for the existence of separate semantic and episodic stores in long-term memory. *Journal of Experimental Psychology: Human Learning and Memory, 6*, 467-478.

Hintzman, D.L. (1967). Articulatory coding in short-term memory. *Journal of Verbal Learning and Verbal Behavior, 6*, 312-316.

Howard, D.L., McAndrews, M.P., & Lasaga, M.L. (1981). Semantic priming of lexical decisions in young and old adults. *Journal of Gerontology, 36*, 707-714.

Huppert, F.A., & Piercy, M. (1978). The role of trace strength in recency and frequency judgements by amnesic and control subjects. *Quarterly Journal of Experimental Psychology, 30*, 346-354.

Jouandet, M., & Gazzaniga, M.S. (1979). The frontal lobes. In M.S. Gazzaniga (Ed.), *Handbook of Behavioral Neurobiology, Vol. 2.* New York: Plenum Press.

Joynt, R.J., & Shoulson, I. (1979). Dementia. In K.M. Keilman & E. Valenstein (Eds.), *Clinical Neuropsychology.* New York: Oxford University Press.

Kahneman, D. (1973). *Attention and effort.* Englewood Cliffs, NJ: Prentice-Hall.

Kahneman, D., Ben-Ishai, R., & Lotan, M. (1973). Relation of a test of attention to road accidents. *Journal of Applied Psychology, 58*, 113-115.

Kausler, D.H., Lichty, W., & Hakami, M.K. (1984). Frequency judgements for distractor items in a short-term memory task: Instructional variation and adult age differences. *Journal of Verbal Learning and Verbal Behavior, 23*, 660-668.

Kinsbourne M., & Wood, F. (1975). Short-term memory processes in the amnesic syndrome. In D. Deutsch & J.A. Deutsch (Eds.), *Short-term memory.* New York: Academic Press.

Kintsch, W. (1970). *Learning memory and conceptual processes.* New York: Wiley.

Knesevich, J.W., LaBarge, E., & Edwards, D. (1986). Predictive value of the Boston Naming Test in mild senile dementia of the Alzheimer type. *Psychiatry Research, 19*, 155-161.

Knopman, D.S., & Nissen, M.J. (1987). Implicit learning in patients with probable Alzheimer's disease. *Neurology, 37*, 784-788.

Kuehne, C., Kehle, T.J., & McMahon, W. (1987). Differences between children with attentional deficit disorder, children with specific learning disabilities and normal children. *Journal of School Psychology, 25*, 161-166.

LaBerge, D., & Samuels, S.J. (1974). Toward a theory of automatic information processing in reading. *Cognitive Psychology, 6*, 293-323.

Lenneberg, E.H. (1967). *Biological foundations of language.* New York: Wiley.

Lezak, M.D. (1983). *Neuropsychological assessment.* New York: Oxford University Press.

Mace, N. & Rabins, P. (1981). *The 36 hour day.* Baltimore: Johns Hopkins University Press.

Maier, N.R.F. (1931). Reasoning in humans: II. The solution of a problem and its appearance in consciousness. *Journal of Comparative Psychology, 12*, 181-194.

Maier, N.R.F., & Burke, R.J. (1967). Response availability as a factor in the problem-solving performance of males and females. *Journal of Personality and Social Psychology, 5*, 304-310.

Mayer, M.A. (1988). Analysis of information processing and cognitive disability theory. *American Journal of Occupational Therapy, 42*, 176-183.

Miller, G.A. (1956). The magical number seven, plus or minus two: Some limits on our capacity for processing information. *Psychological Review, 63*, 81-97.

Milner, B. (1959). The memory defect in bilateral hippocampal lesions. *Psychiatric Research Reports, 11*, 43-52.

Milner, B., Corkin, S., & Teuber, J.L. (1968). Further analysis of the hippocampal amnesic syndrome: A 14 year follow-up study of H.M. *Neuropsychologia, 6*, 215-234.

Morris, P.E., Jones, S., & Hampson, P. (1978). An imagery mnemonic for the learning of people's names. *British Journal of Psychology, 69*, 335-336.

Naveh-Benjamin, M., & Jonides, J. (1986). On the automaticity of frequency coding: Effects of competing task load, encoding strategy, and intention. *Journal of Experimental Psychology: Learning, Memory, and Cognition, 12*, 378-386.

Nebes, R.D., Boller, F., & Holland, A. (1986). Use of semantic context by patients with Alzheimer's disease. *Psychology and Aging, 1*, 261-269.

Nebes, R.D., Martin, D.C., & Horn, L.C. (1984). Sparing of semantic memory in Alzheimer's disease. *Journal of Abnormal Psychology, 93*, 321-330.

Neely, J.H., & Balota, D.A. (1981). Test expectancy and semantic organization effects in recall and recognition. *Memory and Cognition, 9*, 283-300.

Neely, J.H., & Durgunoglu, A.Y. (1985). Dissociative episodic and semantic priming effects in episodic recognition and lexical decision tasks. *Journal of Memory and Language, 24*, 466-489.

Neisser, U. (1967). *Cognitive psychology*. New York: Appleton-Century-Crofts.

Petersen, S.E., Fox, P.T., Posner, M.I., Mintun, M., & Raichle, M.E. (1988). Positron emission tomographic studies of the cortical anatomy of single-word processing. *Nature, 331*, 585-589.

Polya, G. (1957). *How to solve it*. New York: Doubleday Anchor.

Polya, G. (1968). *On understanding, learning, and teaching problem-solving*. New York: Wiley.

Posner, M.I. (1986). Probing the mechanisms of selective attention. Paper presented at the meeting of the Midwestern Psychological Association, Chicago, IL.

Posner, M.I., & Boies, S.W. (1971). Components of attention. *Psychological Review, 78*, 391-408.

Posner, M.I., Cohen, Y., Rafal, R.D. (1982). Neural systems control of spatial orienting. *Philosophical transactions of the Royal Society of London B298*, 187-198.

Posner, M.I., & Rafal, R.D. (1987). Cognitive theories of attention and the rehabilitation of attentional deficits. In M.J. Meier, A.L. Benton, L. Diller, (Eds). *Neuropsychological rehabilitation*. New York: Guilford Press.

Posner, M.I., Walker, J., Freidrich, F.J., & Rafal, (1984). Effects of parietal injury on covert orienting of visual attention. *Journal of Neuroscience, 4*, 1863-1874.

Premack, D. (1971). Language in chimpanzee? *Science, 172*, 808-822.

Premack, D. (1976). Language and intelligence in ape and man. *American Scientist, 64*, 674-683.

Rabinowitz, J.C., Craik, F.I.M., & Ackerman, B.P. (1982). A processing resource account of age differences in recall. *Canadian Journal of Psychology, 36*, 325-344.

Shoben, E.J., Wescourt, K.T., & Smith, E.E. (1978). Sentence verification, sentence recognition, and the semantic-episodic distinction. *Journal of Experimental Psychology: Human Learning and Memory, 4*, 304-317.

Skinner, B.F. (1957). Verbal behavior. New York: Appleton-Century-Crofts.

Smith, S.M., Glenberg, A., & Bjork, R.A. (1978). Environmental context and human memory. *Memory and Cognition, 6*, 342-353.

Sperling, G. (1960). The information available in brief visual presentations. *Psychological Monographs, 74*, (Whole No. 498).

Squire, L.R. (1986). Mechanisms of memory. *Science, 232*, 1612-1619.

Starr, A., & Phillips, L. (1970). Verbal and motor memory in the amnesic syndrome. *Neuropsychologia, 8*, 75-82.

Storandt, M., Botwinick, J., Danziger, W.L., Berg, L., & Hughes, C.P. (1984). Psychometric differentiation of mild senile dementia of the Alzheimer type. *Archives of Neurology, 41*, 497-499.

Talland, G.A. (1965). *Degraded memory*. New York: Academic Press.

Terrace, H.S., Pettito, L.A., Sanders, R.J., & Bever, T.G. (1979). Can an ape create a sentence? *Science, 206*, 891-902.

Tulving, E. (1972). Episodic and semantic memory. In E. Tulving & W. Donaldson (Eds.), *Organization of memory*. New York: Academic Press.

Tulving, E. (1983). *Elements of episodic memory*. Oxford: Clarendon Press/Oxford University Press.

Tulving, E. & Thompson, D.M. (1973). Encoding specificity and retrieval processes in episodic memory. *Psychological Review, 80*, 352-373.

Wallas, G. (1926). *The art of thought*. New York: Harcourt, Brace.

Warren, R.M. (1970). Perceptual restoration of missing speech sounds. *Science, 167*, 392-393.

Warren, R.M., & Warren, R.P. (1970). Auditory illusions and confusions. *Scientific American, 223*, 30-36.

Whitehouse, P.J., Caramazza, A., & Zurif, E.B. (1978). Naming in aphasia: Interactive effects of form and function. *Brain and Language, 6*, 63-74.

Williams, K.W., & Durso, F.T. (1986). Judging category frequency: Automaticity or availability? *Journal of Experimental Psychology: Learning, Memory, and Cognition. 12*, 387-396.

Winocur, G., & Kinsbourne, M. (1978). Contextual cueing as an aid to Korsakoff amnesia. *Neuropsychologia, 16*, 671-682.

CHAPTER CONTENT OUTLINE

Introduction

Overview of Major Psychosocial
Theorists

Factors Affecting Occupational
Performance

Psychological Factors and Healthy
Occupational Performance

Common Psychosocial Disorders

Summary

KEY TERMS

Ego

Epigenesis

Habituation subsystem

Id

Performance subsystem

Phylogenic

Schemas

Self-actualization

Superego

Symbols

ABSTRACT

This chapter explores the ways in which occupational performance is influenced
by psychosocial factors in the basic areas of self-identity, self-protection, and
motivation. These three basic areas are discussed from the perspective of the six
major theoretical views of human psychosocial function: psychoanalytic,
neo-Freudian, cognitive-behavioral, behavioral, meaning-in-experience, and
occupational performance. The chapter concludes with an examination of the
effects of specific psychosocial disorders on human performance.

Psychological Performance Factors

Elizabeth Depoy
Ellen L. Kolodner

"We cannot do justice to the characteristics of the mind by linear outlines like those in a drawing or in a primitive painting, but rather by areas of color melting into one another as they are presented by modern artists. After making the separation we must allow what we have separated to merge together once more."

—Sigmund Freud

OBJECTIVES

The information in this chapter is intended to help the reader—

1. organize basic concepts of psychosocial function through logical questions about individual behavior.

2. compare six major psychosocial theories in terms of common psychosocial factors.

3. understand key concepts and structures related to an individual's perception of self.

4. identify internal and external factors which explain motivation to act.

5. relate psychosocial disorders delineated in DSM III-R to occupational dysfunction.

6. understand basic psychosocial concepts related to self-maintenance and protection.

7. compare psychosocial theorists in terms of their emphasis on person or environment in explaining behavioral differences.

8. appreciate the relationship between psychosocial theories and the selection of intervention strategies for occupational therapy.

INTRODUCTION

Psychosocial aspects of human experience are essential determinants of competent occupational performance. These aspects of human function determine the nature of occupational behavior and the manner in which one perceives his/her functional abilities. Psychosocial factors include two major areas of focus regarding human existence: (1) what, how, and why an individual feels and thinks; and (2) how feelings and thought content are played out in behavior and relationships. This chapter will explore the ways in which occupational performance is influenced by psychosocial factors and examine the nature of psychosocial occupational dysfunction.

In this chapter, we first explore six major theoretical views of human psychosocial function: psychoanalytic, neo-Freudian, cognitive behaviorist, behaviorist, meaning-in-experience, and occupational performance. Each discussion of the six theories includes the basic tenets and the factors that influence occupational performance. It is important for occupational therapy clinicians to understand these views for a number of reasons: (1) occupational therapy intervention strategies are noted in these theoretical perspectives; (2) concepts of occupational performance emerge from a synthesis of information presented by these theorists; and (3) occupational therapists must be able to use an occupational performance perspective that espouses these theoretical approaches in their practice.

In the next section, the individual factors that effect occupational performance are discussed from the perspectives of these psychosocial theories and are organized around the three basic questions that are crucial to an understanding of all human behavior: Who am I and how do I know who I am? How do I maintain myself? and When and why do I act? Finally, the chapter presents the effects of psychosocial disorders on human performance including the occupational dysfunction exhibited in each major psychosocial disorder category of the *Diagnostic and Statistical Manual* (DSM III-R).

OVERVIEW OF MAJOR PSYCHOSOCIAL THEORISTS

Freud and the Psychoanalytic Theories

Freud may be classified as a predeterministic developmental theorist. He posited that one's life course is determined before birth and unfolds as one passes through stages of the life span. According to Freud, all human activity is directed at satisfying biological drives through the employment of a fixed reservoir of psychic energy. The biological urges can be separated into two instinctual categories: *Eros*, the life force, and *Thanatos*, the death force. Eros promotes survival, while Thanatos elicits destruction.

As a child grows, the finite amount of psychic energy is divided among the three personality structures: **id, ego,** and **superego.** At birth, an infant's id is the only existing element of the personality and is governed by the desire for pleasure (pleasure principle). As the child matures, the ego emerges in order to channel the child's instincts and desires that cannot be met by the id. The ego is focused on the *reality principle* and channels psychic energy into a means through which satisfaction can be achieved, such as delayed gratification, using *symbolism*, and creating mechanisms that will ultimately serve the id's pleasure principle. The *superego* is the last personality structure to develop. It functions as the moral arbiter of personality and operates to attain perfection. This structure is the internalization of parent discipline, which eventually serves as the individual's moral code. Essentially, the superego guards against and controls the undesirable sexual and aggressive instincts of the id by using such mechanisms as *guilt* and *shame* (Shaffer, 1985).

The interaction of the three personality structures forms the basis for personality dynamics. As the three main personality structures interact, material from each is relegated to one of the layers of consciousness depending on its acceptability. *Object cathexis* is the investment of psychic energy in objects external to the individual. Object cathexis serves to secure age-appropriate targets for investment of psychic energy. As the child grows, the focus of sexual fulfillment shifts from one erogenous zone to another, and these foci are played out through the different objects of cathexis at each stage.

To organize the development of human behavior and function, Freud theorized five psychosexual stages through which an individual passes during maturation. These developmental stages are classified as the oral, anal, phallic, latent, and genital stages. In each of these stages, the locus of sexual gratification shifts away from self and finally matures into sexual relations with others. Thus, in adulthood, the individual reaches the pinnacle of development engaging in love and work as primary tasks.

In summary, Freud emphasized that the early stages of development are the building blocks for the two major tasks of adulthood: love and work (Smelser & Erikson, 1980). In Freudian theory, order is seen as intrinsic homeostasis, and early childhood development is the foundation of that order. Disorder is conceptualized as a function of disruption in the early childhood stages of sexual maturation. This view of order suggests that if an individual reaches adulthood without significant childhood disorder then he/she remains stable throughout the rest of the life span. From the Freudian view of humans, the following factors emerge as influences on occupational performance:

1. nature of early experience
2. development of personality structures—id, ego, superego
3. dominance of Eros or Thanatos
4. defense mechanisms
5. management of anxiety and tension
6. reality testing
7. degree of real or symbolic sexual gratification
8. successful resolution of each developmental stage

Because order and disorder are viewed as intrinsic mechanisms, the focus for intervention is the individual. A shift from disorder to order can only be accomplished by the development of internal changes, promoted by a symbolic reexperience of early childhood stages (Woolman, 1982).

Carl Jung

Jung is classified as a psychoanalytic theorist because of the similarity of many of his constructs with Freudian theory. Jung views human behavior as motivated by the interaction of complex personality structures that represent not only the individual but all of biological history. Although the individual personality structures of Jung's conceptual framework are consistent with those outlined by Freud, a major point of departure from Freudian theory is the belief that humans are influenced by both the past and the future. Behavior is seen as purposeful, and the goal of unity of the personality is always an underlying motivation of behavior (Jung, 1964).

According to Jung, a number of interactive structures comprise the personality. These structures are categorized as either individual or collective. The individual structures are the *ego, personal unconscious,* and the *persona.* These personality components act in a similar fashion to the structures described in Freudian theory. *The ego* represents the conscious mind, *the personal unconscious* is where repressed material is stored, and the *persona* is essentially the social part of human personality that is known by others.

The collective structures are the *collective unconscious, shadow, anima,* and *animus* and are passed down from human **phylogenic** history, thus underscoring the importance of race and background in Jung's conception of humans. The inherited experience of the past is aggregated into universals or *archetypes* that exist in the collective unconscious and influence behavior.

In Jung's theory, the major life goal is the development of the self. The self is seen as a midpoint between the collective structures and the individual structures, and this life goal can rarely be fully achieved.

Within Jung's framework there are four major personality functions: thinking, intuiting, feeling, and sensing. Thinking and feeling are considered to be the rational functions in that they explore the environment through the intellect (thinking) and the value system (feeling). Sensing and intuiting are the irrational functions because they are seated in the perception of external events.

Like Freud, Jung postulates that conflict among personality structures gives rise to energy through the creation of tension. This energy does receive input from the environment, although this external input is limited. This view created the notion of the personality as a partially closed system. After life functions are conducted, whatever energy remains is channeled towards cultural and spiritual endeavors.

Although Jung does not identify discrete stages of development, he does suggest that humans develop according to age norms. Humans strive for **self-actualization** in order to achieve the ultimate balance between the collective and the individual world. Order is seen as a step in the process of development to achieve this balance. This balance cannot be addressed unless each of the personality structures is fully developed. Thus, Jung views disorder as immature development of individual and collective personality structures, and the inability to achieve balance. Similar to Freudian theory, the locus of intervention to promote order is intrinsic, because the individual is viewed as a partially closed system (Smelser & Erickson, 1980).

The Jungian conceptual framework suggests the following factors as major influences on occupational performance:

1. completeness and differentiation of each personality structure
2. movement towards or away from self-actualization
3. genetic background and past experience (collective unconscious)
4. degree to which energy is efficiently used
5. four basic personality functions: thinking, sensing, feeling, and intuiting

Neo-Freudians: Erik Erikson

Neo-Freudians can be characterized by their efforts to move Freudian constructs into the social, cultural, and interpersonal realm. Among the most famous are Erik Erikson, Alfred Adler, Karen Horney, and Harry Stack Sullivan. Although there are differences among the theories of these Neo-Freudians, certain common concepts place them in this category: (1) humans are viewed as social beings who are more strongly influenced by their relationships and environment than by their sexual drives, (2) there is a purposeful existence for humans, and (3) human behavior is viewed within a larger context.

Erikson is perhaps the most popular neo-Freudian theorist, thus we will use his theory as an example of neo-Freudian thought. Erikson supports the sequential development of humans and therefore is also frequently categorized as a developmentalist.

Erikson's theory of human development was based on many of Freud's constructs. He also believed that humans are motivated by biological needs; that the personality is made up of the id, the ego and the superego; that humans develop in a series of unfolding stages; and humans need to resolve particular issues at each developmental stage. However, in contrast to Freud, Erikson saw humans as more active in their own development and did not view one's emergence from each stage as invariant or unchangeable but responsive to modification at later stages in life. He also believed humans are influenced primarily by their social environment rather than by their sexuality.

Perhaps most valuable was Erikson's notion of the continuation of development in the aging process. A key concept is that of **epigenesis,** which is the observation that elements of each developmental stage are present in all other stages even when they are not the dominant focus. Therefore, unlike Freud who believed that personality was essentially set within the early developmental stages of life, Erikson believed that people could continue to influence their development by addressing issues at later stages. Erikson also believed that precursors to conflicts could also be seen in earlier stages.

Erikson proposed a developmental sequence of eight stages occurring throughout the entire lifespan. These stages are trust versus mistrust, autonomy versus shame and doubt, initiative versus guilt, industry versus inferiority, identity versus role confusion, intimacy versus isolation, generativity versus stagnation, and integrity versus despair. Within each stage, there is a crisis around which the majority of an individual's activity is centered. These stages are closely tied to Freud's first six stages of development. However, Erikson continues the developmental process into adulthood and old age by adding three stages of adult development. In these last three stages of the life-span,

individuals struggle to resolve crises that emerge from life events such as having children, contributing to society, and facing death.

Erikson's view of humans is one that acknowledges the interaction of the individual and his/her social milieu. Consequently, order is not only an intrinsic function, but is also in part dependent on the degree to which the individual personality adapts to the external environment. The results of these life stage conflicts can be an incomplete resolution, the dominance of the negative variable of the crisis dichotomy, or a balanced resolution. Order is seen as a balanced resolution. However, Erikson suggests that disorder experienced as a result of early childhood conflict may be reversed in adulthood through epigenesis and a renegotiation or reexperience of a crisis resolution.

Erikson does not directly address intervention, but his conceptual framework does suggest that the locus for intervention remains with the individual. The focus of order shifts away from intrapsychic mechanisms to the individual's ability to adapt to the social environment.

Erikson's perspective contributes these factors that affect occupational performance:
1. developmental sequence of eight life stages
2. balanced resolution of each life stage crisis
3. early childhood experience
4. renegotiation of negative crisis resolution
5. degree of independence reached at each stage
6. epigenesis

Here-and-Now Approaches

The here-and-now approaches view the primary determinant of psychosocial order in human psychosocial function as the present (here-and-now) rather than early childhood experience. Included in this category of theorists are the cognitive behaviorists, the ''meaning-in-experience'' theorists, and the behaviorally-oriented theorists.

Cognitive Behavioral Approach. Although there are many theorists associated with this approach, this chapter will focus on only two major theorists as examples: Albert Ellis and Aaron Beck. Although there are some differences between the two, both Beck and Ellis focus on the same basic constructs. They view behavior as a function of external input mediated by cognition. In other words, humans have control over their behavior if they approach the environment in a logical and rational manner. Disorder is therefore caused by faulty thought processes that may be conceptualized as irrational or disorganized thinking. Unlike the developmentalists, the cognitive behaviorists place their emphasis on therapeutic intervention such as the rational emotive therapy of Ellis and the cognitive therapy of Beck (Ellis, 1973; Beck, 1976).

Ellis, writing before Beck, listed a number of identifiable thought patterns that were common to neurotic patients. These patterns resulted in non-acceptance of the self. Therefore, therapeutic intervention was focused on challenging and replacing one's faulty beliefs with unconditional acceptance of the self.

Beck focused his therapeutic intervention on improving the patient's awareness of his/her own faulty thought patterns so that they could be recognized and changed even after therapy was terminated. This mode of therapy involved the identification of *misinterpretations of reality* and the *substitution of alternatives* that rendered the patient more able to achieve his/her own goals.

From the two cognitive behavioral perspectives these factors are suggested as major influences on occupational performance:

1. development of thought patterns
2. cognitive style
3. rationality of beliefs
4. rational control of emotions
5. logical goal-setting
6. perception or reality

Behaviorists. The behaviorists developed their theories based on the application of scientific method to the study of human behavior. These theorists' views expose a continuum of beliefs about the degree to which humans actively influence their behavior. Theorists such as Skinner and Watson saw humans as vessels that were totally molded by the environment. Others, like Bandura, suggested that although the environment was a major determinant of behavior, the individual still had intrinsic elements that mediated environmental input. The theories of Skinner and Bandura will be used as examples of the behavioral approach.

Unlike other theories, behavior is not viewed as a series of developmental states that can be differentiated from one another. According to B.F. Skinner, human behavior develops as a result of the degree to which it is reinforced. Reinforcement may be positive or negative, either strengthening a behavior or extinguishing it. Learning is totally controlled by the environment, and all human activity is therefore externally elicited. Skinner departed from some beliefs of the behaviorists before him. Skinner saw the human as fully molded by external occurrences. In this radical behavioristic approach, human behavior can be conceptualized as a series of observable and quantifiable cause-and-effect relationships between input and immediate output. This theory does not recognize any internal mediating factors influencing behavior (Skinner, 1971).

Bandura was not as extreme as Skinner and viewed learning as a process of interaction between intrinsic factors and environmental events. While he strongly espoused the notion of reinforcement and social learning, he also proposed that cognition was essential to the learning process. Perhaps the most valuable concepts in Bandura's work are the concepts of *modeling* and *novel learning*. According to Bandura, a behavior does not have to be present in order for learning to occur. An individual can learn new behaviors through a vicarious learning experience called novel learning that suggests that individuals can observe reinforced behaviors or modified behaviors and "model" their own behaviors after those observed. Reinforcement of observed behaviors and modification of observed behaviors may result in a vicarious learning experience called novel learning. These concepts support the notion of intrinsic mediation of external influence (Bandura, 1971).

Within the behavioral framework, it is clear that order and occupational performance are primarily determined by one's environment. The factors from this theory that affect occupational function are:

1. the external environment
2. the learning process

Meaning-in-Experience Theorists. The meaning-in-experience theorists depart from the constructs of both the developmental and behavioral approaches. Humanists, existentialist, and phenomenologists are included in this category. Among those who are well known are Carl Rogers, Abraham Maslow, Victor Frankl, and Stanley Hall (Evans, 1975; Frankl, 1975). Although each one has a different approach, there are some common characteristics that place each in the category. These theories maintain that each individual experiences the world differently, and develops a unique perception of his/her experience. Such perceptions are the major determinants of behavior. According to the meaning-in-experience theorists, humans are innately motivated to grow and to seek meaning for their own lives. Because each individual is considered free to choose his/her own destiny, it goes without saying that individuals are in effect alone and responsible for themselves. A further common element among meaning-in-experience theorists is a holistic emphasis in which humans are viewed not as discrete parts, but as a united whole.

Although each theory will not be addressed separately, the reader should be aware that there are major differences among therapists of this category. The theorists in this category differ from each other in the way that they interpret aloneness, existence, the nature of choice, and the development of an individual's subjective experience of the world. For example, Roger's humanistic theory suggests that parental acceptance of children is essential to the development of an individual's own positive self-regard, whereas Maslow takes a more socioeconomic view of what makes man satisfied with his existence (Evans, 1975).

Table 12-1
Major Psychosocial Theories View the Three Basic Questions

	IDENTITY Who am I? How Do I Know Who I Am?	SELF-PROTECTION How Do I Maintain Myself?	MOTIVATION When and Why Do I Act?
Psychoanalysts	Freud—Identity: Id, ego, superego Jung—Individual and collective identity	Freud—Defense mechanisms	Psychic energy demands from drives Energy and collective elements of personality
Neo-Freudians	Identity and social self	Through satisfying relationships Through a positive balanced crisis resolution	Intrapsychic mechanisms and energy mediated by socialization
Meaning-in-Experience	My experiences Who I make myself	I maintain a positive self concept I find meaning in life I experience I form positive relationships	Meaning—Search for relationships
Cognitive-Behavioral	Who I think I am	Rational thought and reason	My beliefs
Behavior	I am the environment	I respond to positive reinforcement	Environmental input
Occupational Performance	I am what I perform	I organize my skills into functional habits and routines I believe in myself I adapt to environmental demands	I am intrinsically motivated to act, explore, and master

According to most meaning-in-experience theorists, anxiety is experienced by all individuals when they become aware of their aloneness and their mortality. Finding meaning and self-acceptance in one's life may counteract this existential anxiety or poor self-concept.

The meaning-in-experience theorists view order as the ability to find meaning in life, to accept the nature of one's aloneness and ultimate death, and to find acceptance of the self. The focus of intervention is therefore on acknowledging the value of each individual's experience and on encouraging the individual to accept the self. Within this conceptual framework the following factors influence occupational performance:

1. quality of one's self-concept
2. degree to which one finds meaning in life
3. balance between healthy anxiety and dread
4. individual's ability to recognize subjective reality
5. measurement of self in light of others' perceptions

FACTORS AFFECTING OCCUPATIONAL PERFORMANCE

We will attempt to understand the concepts of each theory by organizing the information into three major areas

that affect occupational performance: self-definition or identity, self-protection, and motivation for action. These major areas are explained in each theory by how they answer the following questions: Who am I? (identity); How do I maintain myself? (self-protection); and When and why do I act? (motivation for action). These three questions are basic to the understanding of human behavior. Table 12-1 summarizes how each theory would answer the three questions.

An understanding of the effect of psychosocial factors on occupational performance is crucial to the determination of an occupational therapy intervention strategy. If one views the locus of psychosocial function as internal, strategies for promotion of competence in occupational performance would be directed at the individual. Conversely, if one views the locus of psychosocial competence as external, the focus of therapy becomes the environment in which the individual acts. Figure 12-1 demonstrates how each theory views the locus of control of individuals along an internal-external continuum.

Identity or "Who Am I?"

The question "Who am I?" addresses the basic structures of the self. In answering this question, the key concepts that must be understood are: psychological structures, self-concept, locus of control, well-being, emotion, environment, and performance (Figure 12-2). We can visualize the way these theories regard definition of self by placing them along an internal-external continuum. On this continuum, those at the internal extreme view the individual as defining himself/herself, and those at the external extreme, view the individual as defined by the environment in which he/she exists. Those theorists along the middle of the continuum view the self as an interplay of intrinsic and external variables (Figure 12-1). Furthermore, we can think of the way in which an individual comes to know the self in terms of the same continuum. Those who place themselves on the internal side of the continuum suggest that knowing the self is the responsibility of each individual, while those on the opposite end maintain that an individual comes to know the self through response to external feedback.

All psychological theorists concern themselves with the question of ''Who am I?'' in an effort to determine similarities and differences among personalities. In addition to identifying these similarities and differences, many of the theorists pose the related question ''How do I know who I am?'' The answers to both of these questions are determined by examining the theoretical concepts of psychological structures, self-concept, locus of control, well-being, and emotion.

Psychological Structures. Psychological structures are the anatomical elements or building blocks of human psychological function. The construct of personality structures first appeared in psychoanalytic theories. Freud and Jung each identified three elements of an individual's personality. Freud labeled the three basic elements as id, ego, and super-ego. Jung labeled these elements as ego, persona, and collective unconscious.

The neo-Freudians such as Erikson, Fromm, and Adler would answer the question, ''Who am I?'' differently from Freud. They would say one defines who one is by their interactions with humans and the non-human environment.

Thus they add the environment and interpersonal relationships as structural elements of the self, and they propose that basic personality structures are dynamic and capable of change throughout the life span.

When answering the question of ''Who am I?'', the here-and-now theorists move away from the internal personality structures of Freud. The cognitive approach sees **schemas** and cognitive structures as the mediating factors of human behavior. The behaviorists and learning theorists (in varying degrees) suggest that the external environment is responsible for the answer. For example, one defines oneself by identifying how biological needs could be met by the environment and by behaviors that are externally reinforced. The answer to ''How do I know who I am?'' would then be answered by acting and finding the reasons for actions in the environmental cues.

Meaning-in-experience theorists who see each individual as unique, might answer the question of ''Who am I?'' by suggesting, ''You are who you make yourself to be and who you believe yourself to be.'' In other words, our individual experiences and how we interpret them ultimately defines who we are.

Self-Concept. Self-concept may be defined as one's perception of oneself. Each category of major theorists views self-concept from a unique viewpoint.

The intrapsychic theorists define self-concept as one's identity, which unfolds throughout the life span, while the Freudian perspective holds that one's self-concept is fully formed and fixed by the time one reaches adulthood. Jung departs from Freud as he sees self-actualization and acquisition of self-knowledge as a vital, ongoing process throughout the life span. Additionally, Jung indicates that few people ever achieve self-knowledge, but those who do, achieve it through spiritual experience.

From the cognitive perspective, self-concept is divided into two elements: one's perception of the self, and the

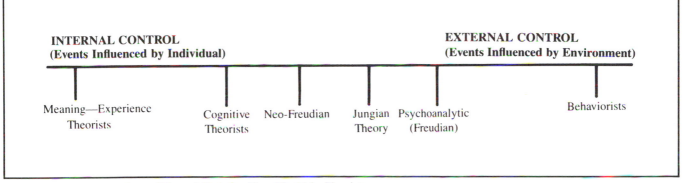

Figure 12-1. Continuum of Internal/External Control as Viewed by Major Theorists.

actual self. One can only know the self through subjective perceptions that may or may not be based on logical, rational thought patterns. Essentially, what one thinks, defines who one is.

The behaviorists do not conceptualize an internal representation of the self. The self is viewed as a product of the environment and is only manifested as a set of observable behaviors.

The meaning-in-experience theorists view the self as a unique perception of the self that is based on life's experiences. One comes to know the self through engaging in accepting relationships and meaningful, goal-oriented experiences.

Locus of Control.   Locus of control is defined as the perception of the degree of control one has in choosing the direction of his/her own life. Various theorists view this locus of control along the internal-external continuum. The more one sees life choices being governed by the external world, the closer the theory is located toward the externally-controlled end of the continuum (Figure 12-1).

Psychoanalytic theorists conceptualize locus of control as internal, although not necessarily conscious. Actions are prompted by the inherent drive of the organism to return to a state of equilibrium by reducing tension and satisfying biological needs. Since Freud believed the majority of one's life is determined before birth and the remainder of development parallels the experiences of early childhood, then he views the locus of control as more external than internal. Hence, one has little conscious control in selecting a life direction. Jung's psychoanalytic theory, although based on many of Freud's constructs, does allow a greater potential for internal control in the form of the individual's striving for self-actualization.

The theorists who suggest the greatest amount of external control are the behaviorists since they view the environment, not the individual, as responsible for behavior. Despite some differences in opinion about how the individual mediates external input, all behavioral theorists agree that control over acquired and repeated behaviors depends on how the environment reinforces those behaviors. This complete reliance on external influences places behaviorists at the external extreme of the continuum (Figure 12-1).

The meaning-in-experience theorists view the individual as being internally controlled, as they suggest that individuals choose behavior and select experiences which will define the meaning of their lives. The phrase, "You are responsible for your own happiness," characterizes the meaning-in-theory viewpoint of locus of control.

The Neo-Freudians view the individual as a product of the interaction between intrinsic factors, culture, and interpersonal relationships. As such, individuals are considered

to be more self-determining than the Freudians suggest. The degree to which an individual perceives that he/she may choose an environment and significant others, may determine the perceived locus of control.

The cognitive theorists move further to the side of internal locus of control. Although they acknowledge the influence of the environment on choice, they maintain that an individual's cognitive process is the major element in the selection of life goals and behavioral alternatives to meet those goals. Thus, the locus of control is internal because an individual can improve rational thinking and reasoning. As thought patterns become more appropriate, the behavior becomes more competent.

Well-being.   Well-being is defined as one's sense of contentment and order. Another term that is used to describe this concept when discussing occupational function is "order" (Kielhofner, Watts, & Barris, 1985). A sense of order or well-being occurs when one perceives a balance and sense of comfort in one's daily existence. Although health and stability are not essential characteristics of well-being, they are frequently present in those who perceive themselves as content.

Psychoanalytic theory proposes that well-being is achieved when the individual is in a state of homeostasis or balance in which tension is reduced and biological drives are satisfied. This view of well-being implies a circular and repetitive cycle that may be characterized in the following manner: increase in tension, resulting in a discharge of energy, resulting in a return to equilibrium. Freud addresses well-being as a state that results only from tension reduction in response to biological needs. Jung expands upon the Freudian concept by including the urge to achieve self-actualization in this cycle of homeostasis. Thus for Jung, a sense of well-being is gained as the individual becomes more self-actualized.

The neo-Freudians see well-being in close relation to human relationships and culture. These theorists view humans as essentially social beings, and therefore suggest that well-being is dependent on one's social function within a cultural context. Some suggest that well-being is achieved through a congruence between the real and ideal self; others maintain that well-being is determined by either the quality of an individual's interpersonal relationships or acceptance of the self. For example, according to Erikson, well-being is achieved through successful resolution of crisis at each of the eight stages of the life span. However, unsuccessful resolution of a crisis does not doom an individual to malcontent. Rather through epigenesis, an individual may restore well-being at any life stage by resolving a crisis with the added ingredients of maturity and experience.

The cognitive-behaviorists equate well-being with having

control over one's life through use of logical and rational thought. This concept promotes individual control over emotions, choice of relationships, and activities. One's sense of well-being is thus achieved through the development of an accurate set of beliefs about one's competence and self-worth.

The meaning-in-experience theorists conceptualize well-being subjectively and with great diversity. Some emphasize the role of interpersonal relationships on well-being. Others place the emphasis on acceptance of the self and acknowledgement and acceptance of death. However, over-all these theorists seem to agree that the ability to find meaning in one's life and to achieve a sense of belonging and acceptance are essential to achieving a sense of well-being.

Emotion.   Emotion is the affective component of psychological function. The concept of feelings is frequently used to explain emotion, implying that the individual physically perceives the presence of an emotion. Psychoanalytic theorists are not unified in their discussions of the concept of emotion. According to Freud, emotions are the investment of psychic energy in an external object (object cathexis). Individuals are viewed as being capable of investing energy in non-human as well as human objects, and as one passes through life, emotional investment is displaced from the self to expanding milieus. The ultimate investment of psychic energy is demonstrated in the form of adult sexual love. Jung discusses emotions as the subjective element of the four personality functions of thinking, intuiting, feeling and sensing. Feeling is an individual's method of subjectively experiencing the world as individuals evaluate their experiences through feelings such as love, hate, joy, sorrow, etc.

Consistent with their other theoretical constructs, the neo-Freudians view emotion as a function of human interaction within the sociocultural context. Erikson, for example, suggests that the mastery of each stage of development promotes a maturing of feelings and an investment of emotion in satisfying endeavors. Each of Erikson's eight crises is depicted as a conflict between two opposing feelings. In the ideal state, crisis resolution occurs through social interaction, leaving the individual with a dominant positive feeling.

The cognitive theorists acknowledge emotions, but value the domination of rationality over irrational beliefs. Thus, cognition is seen as the mediator of emotions.

Behaviorists do not directly address emotion because it is an intrinsic state. One can only demonstrate constructs such as happiness, sadness, and joy through observable behavior, thus these constructs are defined operationally rather than conceptually.

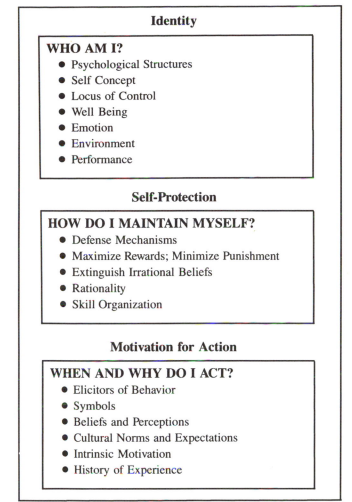

Figure 12-2. Major Factors Determining Identity, Self-Protection, and Motivation for Action.

According to the meaning-in-experience theorists, emotions are individual and subjective and must be accepted by both the one demonstrating the emotions and significant others in the individual's environment. Within this frame of reference, there are a variety of ways in which emotions might be interpreted. For example, some of the theorists such as Frankl (1975) describe the concept of existential anxiety. This is a feeling experienced when the meaning of life is unclear. The degree to which one allows this anxiety to dominate one's goal or purpose determines the quality of one's life. Other meaning-in-experience theorists, such as Maslow, maintain that emotions are consistent with how well one's needs have been fulfilled. However, in general, the meaning-in-experience theorists agree that subjective experience of emotions is based on an individual's unique accumulation of experience across the life span.

Self-Protection or "How Do I Maintain Myself?"

The question, "How do I maintain myself?" pertains to the psychosocial mechanisms by which one is able to achieve stability. A number of theorists have suggested that humans engage in practices to protect themselves from internal and external psychological harm. These devices can be thoughts, behaviors, and psychological functions that preserve one's image of self. Some of these mechanisms are productive, although a number of theorists suggest that an overabundance of protective devices place an individual into the realm of disorder.

Key concepts addressed by theorists when answering this question are: defense mechanisms, reward and punishment, irrational beliefs, rationality, and skill organization (Figure 12-2). This question is also answered from a wide variety of perspectives on the internal-external continuum. Those theorists whose perspectives lie toward the external side believe that an individual can maintain stability through appropriate response to environmental input, whereas those on the internal end view the individual as responsible for the degree of order in his/her own life.

Protective devices are a major influence on occupational performance. They mediate actions in order to facilitate the individual's need to view the self positively and/or the need to believe that others perceive him/her as engaging in socially acceptable behavior.

Freud viewed *defense mechanisms* as the protective maneuvers of the personality employed by the ego to relieve tension. These defense mechanisms are repression, projection, reaction formation, fixation, and regression (Hall & Lindzey, p.51). Although each performs a unique function, all have two common characteristics: they distort or change reality, and they are unconscious.

The Neo-Freudians have divergent views on protective mechanisms depending on how closely aligned they are with Freudian theory. However, as with the other psychological issues, the neo-Freudian protective mechanisms are expanded into the social and cultural environment. For example, according to Erikson, humans retain a healthy element of the less desirable conflict trait in order to protect themselves within the sociocultural context. Thus, a child who successfully resolves the trust vs. mistrust conflict still maintains a healthy proportion of mistrust as a protective mechanism.

The cognitive theorists, such as Beck and Ellis, hold still another perspective on the protective elements of human function. While they see the development of faulty beliefs as an immature reaction to negative social, environmental, and genetic influences, they do not view these reactions as self-destructive. The extinction of irrational beliefs and subsequent replacement with rationality is the only way a person is protected against self-doubt and non-fulfillment (Beck, 1976; Ellis, 1973).

According to the meaning-in-experience theorists, protection of the self is attained by one's ability to find meaning, to be accepted by significant others, and to accept the self. No one method of protection is common among individuals. Ultimately, one maintains an intact self-image in two ways: by accepting death and by identifying the meaning of one's life.

Within the behavioral frame of reference, there is no explicit discussion of protective mechanisms, as they are considered internal mechanisms. However, the behaviorist sees individuals as maintaining themselves through observing responses to environmental stimuli. They protect themselves by behaving in a manner that either maximizes reward or minimizes punishment. Without this implicit protective behavioral process, an organism would not be likely to learn.

Thus, the answer to "How do I maintain myself?" is obtained by examining aspects of both internal psychological function and the environment in which an individual exists. The degree to which emphasis is placed on either end of the internal-external continuum depends on the theoretical frame of reference (Table 12-1 and Figure 12-1).

Motivation for Action or "When and Why do I Act?"

For the practice of occupational therapy, perhaps the most critical and complicated psychosocial question is the one that explains why action takes place: "When and why do I act?" Actions are the link between the internal and external worlds of an individual. They are elicited from both internal and external sources and provide feedback to both others and the self. The factors that seem to motivate action include elicitors of behavior, symbols, beliefs and perceptions, cultural norms and expectations, intrinsic motivation, and history of experience (Figure 12-2). Once again, we see the answers to this question broadly distributed along the internal-external continuum. From the internal perspective, all humans are intrinsically motivated to act and possess the choice to initiate action at will; from the external perspective, action is initiated in response to environmental cues.

Elicitors of Behavior. Elicitors of behavior are those internal and external forces that prompt or initiate behavior. Freud believed that internal drives motivate action. Unsatisfied drives result in an increase in tension, and increased tension produces energy. The individual or organism constantly seeks homeostasis and attempts to return to a state of equilibrium through discharging this energy. Action results and the individual achieves equilibrium. The nature of the action is mediated by one's stage of life, the content of the unconscious material that surrounds drive satisfaction, and the dynamic interplay of personality structures.

Although Jung is considered to be a psychoanalytic theorist, he departs from Freud in answering this question. Jung views action as having an ultimate purpose or goal (teleological). That ultimate, long-term purpose in life is self-actualization, and therefore one acts to achieve this goal. Thus, Jung sees behavior as having a future-oriented goal, rather than the more immediate goals of Freud's physiological drive toward homeostasis. Furthermore, Jung sees action as influenced by the past experiences of individuals and the collective experiences of biological life forms.

On the other end of the spectrum, the behaviorists believe action is elicited by environmental stimuli. The initial motivation to act may be to fulfill biological needs, but as the organism grows and matures, it initiates action in response to external cues. An individual behaves for two reasons: to obtain reward or to avoid punishment. Therefore for behaviorists, human action is primarily reactive and no internal factors are identified as prompting action.

Cognitive theorists see the elicitors of behavior as internal. They propose that all behavior, even when a response to external cues, is preceded by thought and mediated by the nature of the cognitive content.

The neo-Freudians identify the social arena as prompting behavior. There are those who view human action as an attempt to define the self in relation to the perceptions held by others (Horney, 1967; Adler, 1972), on the other hand, sees human action as goal-oriented and related to realistic achievement in the larger cultural context. Overall, the neo-Freudians believe that action emerges from social and interpersonal relationships and is maintained by the continuation, growth, and meaning of these relationships. They suggest that responsibility for one's actions lies in the self.

The meaning-in-experience theorists also see action as intrinsically motivated and controlled. Although there are some differences among these theorists, most would agree that action is elicited by the search for meaning in one's life. Furthermore, actions are mediated by past experiences and one's subjective, unique perception of reality.

Symbols.   Abstract representations of reality are symbols. Many actions are symbolic and are performed to demonstrate personal perspectives or to conform to environmental expectations. The degree to which one shares the meaning of symbols with others will influence the type of action one performs. Also, the degree to which behavior is symbolic

may have an impact on how others understand and respond to one's actions.

Symbolic action is one of the cornerstones of Freudian theory. All of an individual's actions are viewed as being directly or symbolically aimed at sexual gratification. As an individual matures, his/her sexual fulfillment becomes increasingly symbolic through the cathexis of different and more socially acceptable love objects.

Within Jung's conceptual framework, an individual's life is viewed as symbolic from an historical as well as individual perspective. Jung's notions of collective unconscious and self-actualization represent a balance of the history of evolution and the future of mankind.

The meaning-in-experience perspective views symbols as specific to the individual, yet the degree to which these symbols are shared with others may enhance the meaning of one's life (Kielhofner, Barris, & Watts, 1985).

Neo-Freudians also look at symbolism from a social perspective, but they retain the construct of the unconscious and view action symbolically as tension reduction. Depending on the theorist, this action may take the form of seeking love (Fromm) or defining one's self-concept through engaging in interpersonal relationships.

In cognitive theory, actions symbolize the patterns of thought that an individual holds. The degree to which actions are effective in one's environment is dependent on the rationality of this underlying cognition.

Strict behaviorists do not acknowledge symbolism because it is not observable. However, there are those, such as Bandura, who do recognize the symbolic nature of behavior. According to Bandura, not only can behaviors be symbolically reinforced, but an individual may also learn and glean meaning from symbols represented in the environment.

Beliefs.   Beliefs are values and morals held by an individual. With the exception of the behaviorists, all psychological theorists view one's beliefs as playing a basic role in behavior, both by prompting action and resulting from actions.

According to Freud, values and morals are housed in the superego. The infant who has not yet developed a superego does not have a set of beliefs. However, as the infant is exposed to socialization from caretakers, the infant will develop beliefs that are consistent with those held by the parents. Further maturation allows differentiation of beliefs from those of the parents, as the superego broadens to internalize values and morals from the larger social arena.

Jung once again departs from Freud in his view of human action, and proposes that action emanates from beliefs stemming from both past collective experiences and the teleological or future-oriented nature of actions. Additionally, the extent to which an individual's values and morals are sociocentric is in part dependent on the amount of energy that remains after survival issues are addressed.

Neo-Freudians demonstrate a spectrum of thought about beliefs, ranging from those of Freudian theory to those which view beliefs as a product of one's sociocultural environment. For example, Erikson maintains that values and beliefs are functions of an individual's interaction with his/her milieu and culture. He also holds that development of beliefs unfolds throughout the life span and is dependent on the quality of crises resolution.

The cognitive theorists consider beliefs to be the anchor of all behavior. As previously stated, the degree to which beliefs are rational and logical will determine the nature and effectiveness of one's actions.

Behaviorists such as Skinner disregard the concept of beliefs because they are not observable and measurable. Bandura, however, places emphasis on internal beliefs as mediators for environmental input. He suggests that the unique mix of environmental cues and accumulated life experience contributes to an individual's ability to filter stimuli and respond in a unique manner.

In the meaning-in-experience tradition, values and morals are specific to the individual and are based on each person's unique experience. Those valued most highly are a sense of justice, meaning, and acceptance of the uniqueness of others. An individual with values and morals congruent with those of the social group will most likely find a more orderly existence than one who selects beliefs that are divergent from the majority. Nevertheless, each individual is perceived as equally worthy.

Perceptions of Experience. Perceptions of experience are subjective analyses that give one an understanding of life events and attach meaning to those events. They not only originate from action, but are arranged into patterns that mediate when and how when one acts.

According to Freud, the most critical experiences are those that occur in early childhood. The nature of these experiences and their subsequent storage in layers of consciousness determine the potential for one's actions to satisfy the individual.

Jung expands on Freud's concept of early experiences by incorporating a phylogenic approach, wherein an individual possesses not only his/her own perceptions of experience that mediate action, but also perceptions of earlier species. Additionally, heredity plays a critical role in the perceptions of experience and in the resultant actions.

The neo-Freudians view experience within the social arena in which events and perceptions arise from engaging in relationships. These perceptions are the essential building blocks for meaning in one's life. The extent to which

one's perceptions are congruent with those of the environment will influence the quality of one's actions and perceptions of self-worth.

The cognitive theorists are perhaps the group who most heavily focus on experience and perception. Experiences in early childhood may determine the extent to which rational and logical thought patterns develop. Rational perceptions of the self and the environment are essential for efficacious action; faulty perceptions decrease effective action. However, proper guidance can modify faulty perceptions into rational patterns at any life stage.

Although behaviorists do not directly address perception, experience is an important part of their conceptual framework. Behaviorists see experience as input from the environment. As one acts, one receives feedback from the environment that reinforces or decreases the likelihood of repeating that action. Thus, experience of environmental cues is both a precursor and a result of all actions performed by the individual.

Cultural Norms and Expectations. As revealed in Chapter 4, cultural norms and expectations are shared, common environmental elements that underpin behavior. These elements may be explicit, but are usually tacit. Culture can influence action in identifiable ways and in unrecognizable ways, unless systematically explored. An individual becomes a part of a culture as he/she matures through the process of *socialization*. Cultural norms and expectations dictate the boundaries of acceptable action, influence values and morals, define roles, and influence action in all spheres of life. All theorists address culture in some manner. Some believe that culture imposes little influence on behavior while others believe culture to be a dominant influence.

According to Freud, culture prompts action by influencing the way in which early childhood is experienced. Freud places little emphasis on culture in his writings, perhaps because he does not extensively address adulthood. Yet the notion of superego may be interpreted as Freud's notion of culture such that socializing influences beyond the parent are internalized as an individual matures. This personality structure can only be a product of one's general culture because it reflects the morals and values of one's social milieu.

Jung enlarges the role of culture in life by recognizing the individual's consciousness as a product of heritages and immediate surroundings. Furthermore, Jung suggests that an individual will invest energy in the larger cultural arena after survival needs are met. This indicates that the individual will shift focus beyond the self when energy permits.

The neo-Freudians are the group of theorists who shift the focus of psychology from intrinsic factors to the context in which people live. This context or milieu can include the social interactions as the dominant influence on action or may even include the whole, larger cultural arena as the essential impetus for action. Erikson seems to embody the total spectrum with his developmental view of humans. He suggests that as the individual grows, the milieu expands from limited social relationships with parents to interaction with the larger cultural context. The degree to which an individual is able to navigate these different levels of culture will influence the efficacy of action.

Cultural norms and expectations are relevant to the meaning-in-experience theorists who view people as defining themselves by measuring against these norms. However, unlike the behaviorists, they do not view conformity to these norms as essential to achieving order because there is an equal emphasis on the meaning of the experience.

The behaviorists do not recognize culture as an implied influence on behavior, however, they systematically explore the factors in the environment that precede and reinforce an individual's action. In essence, they suggest that culturization is the influence on action.

Although the cognitive behaviorists do not directly address cultural norms and expectations, the nature of rationality is defined by the culture in which the individual is living.

Thus, it can be seen that the question "When and why do I act?" is answered with much diversity. The internal and external forces that promote action are conceptualized by each theorist in his/her own unique manner (Figure 12-2).

PSYCHOLOGICAL FACTORS AND HEALTHY OCCUPATIONAL PERFORMANCE

Equipped with an overview of those psychological factors which affect performance, we now turn to a view of the individual which relates specifically to occupational therapy practice. It is convenient to use aspects of a model of human occupation advanced by Kielhofner, Burke and others (Kielhofner, 1982) as a perspective for considering the three identified questions (psychological areas) which influence occupational performance.

In that framework, three subsystems of occupational performance are identified. These are referred to as the volitional, habituation and performance subsystems. The **volitional subsystem** is embodied by the concepts of locus of control, well-being, and self-concept. The **performance subsystem** consists of the individual's abilities and skills which are reflected in observable behavior. The **habituation subsystem** embraces the manner in which an individual structures time and organizes activities into tasks and roles as well as habits and routines.

Identity: The "Who Am I?" Question

The answer to "Who am I?" seems to be a balance between internal and external self-definition. Most occupational performance is action motivated toward answering this question. Conversely, it appears that individuals are primarily defined by their occupational performance. Thus, the answer to this question is obtained by the dynamic interaction of an individual with the environment.

Central to occupational theory is the concept of humans as self-determining and intrinsically motivated towards action. External factors are seen as essential to occupational performance, and as inextricably intertwined with self-directed change. Thus, the answer to "Who am I?" may be viewed as a changing process, as individuals develop, experience the environment, and redefine themselves in relation to their function within their cultures.

Self-protection: The "How Do I Maintain Myself?" Question

The question rephrased in terms of the Kielhofner Burke framework would be: "How may I maintain the integrity of my performance subsystem and promote new skill acquisition to meet environmental demands?" Maintenance of performance takes three forms: (1) organization of abilities and skills into useful habits and roles, (2) belief in one's ability to control one's behavior and belief in the worth of one's activity, and (3) the potential of the human to adapt to environmental demands.

The development of organization may be seen once again as a dynamic interaction between the individual and the environment. Models and encouragement from one's sociocultural surroundings aide the individual in organizing performance elements into useful and effective occupational habits and routines (*habituation*). The degree to which habits and routines are consistent with environmental expectations determines the roles an individual fills. The organization of coping skills into orderly routines and habits provides additional protection of one's present and future performance skills.

From an occupational standpoint, humans are able to maintain themselves by controlling their habits, selecting their roles, and developing a sense of strengths and limitations (Miller, 1988). One's sense of control and self-worth (*volition*) governs the emergence of protective habits and routines and facilitates the individual's choice to adapt to environmental demands. Adaptation is the way in which humans ultimately protect themselves. Governed by volition, the healthy individual may choose to adapt to the environment through a number of strategies. He or she may use existing capacities but develop new routines, or may need to learn new skills to add to existing or new habits.

Table 12-2
Kielhofner & Burke's Subsystems of Occupational Performance and the Major Questions

	VOLITION (sense of self-worth and control)	HABITUATION (organization of activity through habits and roles)	PERFORMANCE (abilities and skills)
Who am I?	I am what I value I am what I control I am who I believe I am	I am my roles	I need process skill to think about who I am I am what I do I am what I communicate and what I hear about myself
How do I maintain myself?	I maintain control I believe in myself and my standards	I believe in a manner consistent with my accepted roles My habits organize my behavior into teleological action	I maintain my skills I develop new skills
When and why do I act?	I act when I believe I must I am my roles I act to maintain my standards I am intrinsically motivated to act	I act when I perform in my roles I organize my actions by my habits and routines	I possess the skills to initiate action process I possess the skills to perform musculoskeletal and communication/interaction I possess the skills to receive feedback from my actions

Adapted from Kielhofner G. (Ed.) (1982). Health through occupation. Philadelphia, PA: F.A. Davis.

Thus in occupational terms, the answer to the question "How do I protect myself?" may be found in the individuals' skill acquisition and organization and in their ability to adapt. This process of self-protection is a complex one that involves a mix of self-determination, environmental input, and action. Table 12-2 demonstrates how volition, habituation, and performance effect occupational performance in relation to the three basic questions.

Motivation for Action: The "When and Why do I Act?" Question

The answer to this question is central to understanding occupational performance. Equipped with the knowledge of identity and self-protection, answered by the first two questions, occupational therapists focus intervention around this last question.

Humans are viewed as intrinsically motivated to engage in activity. Human action is an essential element of the nature of humans of all ages. This internal force may be modified by external press, but it is a cornerstone of humanity. The nature of one's actions and their effectiveness in the environment are determined by the interaction of performance, habituation, volition, and the sociocultural milieu in which an individual functions.

The relationship of symbols to human performance is extremely important and involves three concepts: (1) that symbols are unique to the individual, (2) how the meaning of these symbols is shared within a culture, and (3) the degree to which the individual perceives the influence of symbols on his/her occupational performance. Action may be a response to an external or internal symbol. Because each individual is unique and places unique meanings on experience and objects, symbols can be idiosyncratic. However, they are shared within a culture and must also be evaluated from the sociocultural perspective. Individual and shared symbols may be extremely complex and tacit, therefore therapists should hold them unaccountable for action until they are analyzed and explicitly addressed in intervention.

The essential elements of action are the values that elicit it, the values that action holds for each individual, and the manner in which others interpret action through their own beliefs. Beliefs, morals, and values mediate action and create its meaning. Humans hold both individual and common beliefs, and occupational performance must be considered within the context of each. Although culture strongly influences an individual's beliefs, that individual still has the choice to examine and redefine morals and values. So we see that beliefs are dynamic and can be changed throughout life. These changing beliefs can provide new impetus for meaning in occupational performance.

As one engages in occupational performance, one builds a history of experiences. Within the framework of occupation, these experiences occur as a result of intrinsically-motivated engagement with one's environment. In turn, the repertoire of past experiences shapes the nature of new occupational performance as it organizes habits and provides the foundation for interpretation of the meaning of individual activity.

Culture dictates which skills are likely to be developed and provides the structure of norms. The organization of occupational performance is both implicitly and explicitly influenced by culture on the roles played. Individuals engage in a set of occupational behaviors that are characteristic of a recognized role, such as worker, family member, and player. Culture provides both the guidance for and acceptance of suitable role behaviors. In addition, individuals may develop expectations of their occupational performance skills based on the norms for a particular culture. For example, although an individual may possess a particular skill, the degree to which it is valued by the culture may influence the amount of effort the individual expends on enhancing and using that skill. Culture is a crucial determinant of the values that mediate occupational

performance by contributing to the shared meanings of occupational performance and ascribing a level of worthiness or value to one's actions.

COMMON PSYCHOSOCIAL DISORDERS

The following eight major diagnostic categories of psychological dysfunction taken from the *Diagnostic and Statistical Manual* (DSM III-R) have been selected as the focus for this section: organic mental disorders, schizophrenic disorders, affective disorders, substance abuse, personality disorders, anxiety disorders, adjustment disorders, and disorders usually first evident in childhood. These categories have been chosen because they are the disorders that are most commonly seen in occupational therapy practice. We will examine how each of these disorders/dysfunctions affects the psychological factors and impacts on occupational performance. Table 12-3 summarizes each psychosocial disorder in terms of the three major questions of identity, self-protection, and motivation. The definitions and explanations of disorders in this chapter

Table 12-3
Psychosocial Disorders and the Major Questions

	IDENTITY Who am I?	SELF-PROTECTION How Do I Maintain Myself?	MOTIVATION When and Why Do I Act?
Organic Mental Disorders	External locus of control	Deterioration of protective mechanisms	Unpredictable responses to internal and external stimuli
Schizophrenic Disorders	Idiosyncratic and changeable identity	Poor or absent protective mechanisms Ineffective adaptive strategies	Idiosyncratic beliefs and symbols
Affective Disorders	I am who I do not value I am what I feel	Poor or absent protective devices Adaptation mediated by mood	Action mediated by mood
Substance Abuse and Dependence	Influenced by degree of intoxication	Protective devices are influenced by intoxicant Intoxicant may be the protective device	The intoxicant
Personality Disorders	Immature development of self Distorted answer	Weak protective devices Immature adaptation	Response to external or environmental stimuli
Anxiety Disorders	Mediated by fear	Overactive protective mechanisms	Source of anxiety Avoidance of producer of anxiety
Adjustment Disorders	Confused identity	Impaired adaptive skill	Response to perceived imposed stimuli
Childhood Disorders	Immature personality structure Possible deterioration of personality structure	Immature protective and adaptive devices	Immature mechanisms

are by no means comprehensive. For complete and detailed descriptions of pathology and symptoms of specific disorders, the reader is urged to refer to the DSM III-R.

Organic Mental Disorders

Organic mental disorders are those caused by a chemical, structural, or electrical alteration of brain tissue. Examples include Alzheimer's disease, dementia, and intoxication. Organic mental disorders may be chronic, as in Alzheimer's disease, or they may only be temporary such as with drug intoxication. Regardless of the cause or time involvement, all organic mental disorders cause both behavioral and mental change. Motor dysfunction is not uncommon in these disorders because of central nervous system involvement. Because the organic mental disorders are too numerous to explore in this chapter, the focus will be on Alzheimer's disease for the purpose of analysis and discussion of occupational performance.

Alzheimer's disease is characterized by progressive deterioration of cognitive, motor, and ultimately, survival functions. It usually begins in the cognitive arena with complaints such as memory loss and the inability to learn new information and skills. As Alzheimer's progresses, the affected individual becomes increasingly disabled in all areas of occupational function. Alzheimer's disease is a disorder of the elderly, although symptoms may occur as early as midlife. Thus, the dysfunction caused by Alzheimer's may be complicated by other deleterious effects of aging.

Effects on Identity and Self-Protection. As an individual struggles with the progressive effects of Alzheimer's disease, his/her identity (the "Who am I?" question) becomes unclear. Personality structures become less recognizable by the victim, as well as by others around him/her. With one's identity changing and without the capacity to think clearly regarding it, self-concept is frequently affected early in the process. In other words, an individual becomes unsure of his/her identity and does not have the capacity to respond cognitively to internal changes taking place (Table 12-3).

When the individual loses skill, the locus of control moves outward. It is not surprising that people with Alzheimer's disease do not maintain a sense of well-being, particularly when they are aware of what is occurring. Whether due to organic or psychological causes, emotional liability is a common symptom of Alzheimer's. The answer to the question of, "Who am I?" loses an element of internal control. The individual responds less competently to both internal pathology and the external environment. Thus, the protective mechanisms of adaptation and routine are disrupted (Table 12-3). In the early stages of Alzheimer's, denial may be used as a protective mechanism by

the individual and by significant others. However, if needed structure is refused, denial of the disorder usually leads to less effective occupational performance.

Effects on Motivation. Answering the question, "When and why do I act?" is difficult for the individual with Alzheimer's disease because there seems to be no organization of behavior. The elicitors of behavior may be intrinsic or extrinsic, as the individual responds to stimuli in an unpredictable and seemingly random fashion. Furthermore, the decrease in the efficacy of skill does not permit one to act capably.

Although symbols may exist, the change in their meaning may be beyond the understanding of the individual or those around him/her. Because of cognitive deficits, the system of beliefs is no longer stable, nor can experience be organized into useful perceptions. As an individual deteriorates, he/she becomes less concerned with cultural norms and therefore becomes isolated from social surroundings. In short, as the disease progresses, the purposefulness of action decreases to a point where an individual may not be able to engage in even the simplest self-care activities.

Occupational performance in the patient with Alzheimer's becomes increasingly disorderly as the disease progresses. The primary locus of dysfunction in Alzheimer's, as in all organic mental disorders, is seated in the performance subsystem. Table 12-4 demonstrates the primary locus of dysfunction in each of the psychosocial disorders. Process skills demonstrate the most significant impairment early in the disease. Functions such as memory, new learning, and problem-solving become ineffectual without extensive external structure. As the disorder becomes more severe, these skills are lost even in the presence of environmental structure. Additionally, the individual's mobility is limited as motor deficits frequently accompany the process skill deficits.

With such significant loss in performance, habituation and volition follow as dysfunctional systems (Table 12-4). Within habituation it appears as if the organizers, such as habits and routines, are lost. This loss is based both on the poverty of capacities and on the individual's inability to organize existing skills into useful routines. Rapid loss of roles occurs as an individual is no longer able to regulate occupational performance. The individual is forced without choice to take on a dependent "sick role" (dysfunction in volition). Internal locus of control is forfeited because of the loss of skills, routines, roles, and habits. Thus, the Alzheimer's patient is in a position to respond only to external demands and to respond without adaptive capacities and purposeful occupational behavior.

Frequently depression accompanies the onset of Alzheimer's. One's sense of being able to control one's life and make contributions are negatively influenced by the inability to initiate competent occupational behavior. Values and interests that previously guided behavior and provided answers are no longer intact.

Schizophrenic Disorders

Schizophrenic disorders are usually pervasive and chronic, affecting all areas of function. However, with proper supervision and medication individuals with schizophrenia can often exhibit productive occupational performance. Nevertheless, schizophrenia is usually a chronic disability which includes recurrence of acute episodes. The majority of schizophrenic individuals must remain on psychotropic medications throughout their lifetimes. The DSM III-R categorizes and describes many types of schizophrenia. Although each type presents a different constellation of symptoms, there are common characteristics.

A diagnosis of schizophrenia must be based not only on presenting symptoms but also on careful history-taking, because acute episodes of schizophrenia are preceded by a *prodromal phase* in which deterioration of occupational performance can be seen. Thus schizophrenia is a disorder that is characterized by a history of long-term dysfunction that may exacerbate into acute episodes of psychosis. The onset of schizophrenia usually occurs in young adulthood, although "oddities" in childhood behavior of schizophrenics have been frequently noted (Kaplan & Sadock, 1988).

Schizophrenia is a psychotic disorder in which clarity of thought and goal-directed reasoning is interrupted. Furthermore, the ability to communicate and become involved in social relationships becomes impaired because of their idiosyncratic use of symbols and the unconnected and tangential speech patterns. Delusions and hallucinations are frequently associated with schizophrenia in its acute stage.

In addition to thought disorder and social dysfunction, inappropriate affect may also be exhibited in the form of *blunting of affect* (showing no emotion) or incongruity or inappropriate behavior within the present social situation. In recent literature, schizophrenic symptoms have been separated into two categories, negative and positive (Andreasen, 1985). Positive symptoms are those that can be described by their addition to one's functional repertoire, such as delusions and hallucinations. Negative symptoms are those that have been eliminated from function, such as lack of thought or roles. Recent literature (Kaplan & Sadock, 1988) has also suggested both biological and environmental causative factors, indicating that schizophrenia is a complex disorder that must be viewed from multiple perspectives.

Effects on Identity and Self-Protection. In schizophrenia, the answer to "Who am I?" is complicated and may change as the individual moves from one phase of the disorder to the next. In an acute episode, identity can only be determined by the individual and may be fraught with poor *reality testing,* idiosyncratic symbols, and delusions. Personality structures, such as cognitive schemes and ordered past experiences, are unstable. The self-concept is unrealistic because the individual is not able to reason effectively about his/her identity and perception of that identity.

Locus of control becomes a complicated issue. Although it may appear that a schizophrenic patient has an internal locus of control, this is not the case. Choice is dominated by the disorder, rather than by competent decision-making. The sense of well-being is also difficult to judge; it may be intact but based on disordered reasoning. Depending on the nature of how an individual is affected, emotions may be classified as positive or negative symptoms. Blunting of affect is a negative emotional symptom, whereas agitation or inappropriate affect indicates positive emotional disorder. Identity or stable characteristics of the individual are not observable. The answer to "Who am I?" changes with the severity and phase of the disorder.

Protective devices may be present or absent in schizophrenia. The psychoanalytic perspective suggests that an acute schizophrenic episode may be a protective device that is out of control (Kernberg, 1970). However, from the human occupation frame of reference, schizophrenia may be perceived as prompting poor or absent protective devices. Habits which organized skills are no longer present or adequate to promote adaptive functioning. Therefore, an individual is not capable of protecting the remaining skills by responding effectively to environmental demands.

Effects on Motivation. The answer to "When and why do I act?" is also complicated in schizophrenia. When considering activity, some generalizations can be found about the disorder itself, although each individual is unique. For instance, productive, goal-oriented activity is decreased or absent in an acute schizophrenic episode. Elicitors of behavior are mostly intrinsic, because the schizophrenic individual does not respond to the environment in a realistic manner. He/she may be responding to disordered thoughts that take the form of delusions and hallucinations. Idiosyncratic symbols may also be responsible for prompting action. Although beliefs may be systematic, as in delusions, they are not based in reality or coherently tied to each other. It is difficult to identify values or morals of an individual during an acute schizophrenic episode since they may not be articulated or acted on. Frequently, a schizophrenic individual will not act at all unless encouraged by external stimuli.

Table 12-4
Primary Locus of Dysfunction in Psychiatric Conditions
(Using Kielhofner & Burke's Model of Human Occupation)

	VOLITION SUBSYSTEM	HABITUATION SUBSYSTEM	PERFORMANCE SUBSYSTEM
Alzheimer's	External locus of control	Predominance of role deterioration	Process skill initially* All elements of performance ultimately impaired
Schizophrenic Disorders	External locus of control	Social role dysfunction Worker role dysfunction Patient role	Process skill*
Affective Disorders	External locus of control* Impaired sense of personal causation	Non-psychotic: none Psychotic: impaired role function	Non-psychotic: none Psychotic: process skill interaction/communication
Substance Abuse and Dependence	External locus of control	Substance becomes habit* Routines organized to obtain and take substance	All skill influenced by substance
Personality Disorder	External locus of control	Mediated by personality traits	Maladaptive development of process and communication interaction skill*
Anxiety Disorder	External locus of control* Impaired sense of personal causation	Potential role dysfunction	
Adjustment Disorder	External locus of control* Adjustment in personal causation	Shift in roles*	
Childhood Disorders Volition			Developmental distortion or delay in skills*

*Primary locus of dysfunction

This type of negative symptoms may be present because of poverty of thought or because of one's inability to initiate activity. The experiences and perceptions of a schizophrenic individual may be unorganized, confusing, and attached to bizarre meanings as a result of the disordered activity, nonproductive behavior, and unrealistic interpretation of action.

With disordered roles, it is not surprising to find the schizophrenic individual on the fringe of his/her culture. However, as noted by many professionals who work with schizophrenics, a culture of norms is visible within this disability group. Specific behaviors and values that may be attributed to frequent institutionalization, as well as to the disorder, may characterize the culture of the schizophrenic population. Cultural norms may include behaviors such as dependence, value of television time and cigarettes, and acceptable "patient" social behaviors tacitly communicated in institutions. It is clear that the schizophrenic individual's interaction with his/her culture is qualitatively different than the interaction of an individual with ordered occupational performance by way of two primary differences: (1) their elements of evaluation of norms and their choice to conform are dysfunctional and frequently not based on reality, and (2) the roles that characterize the institutional culture are dependent, nonproductive, and not serviceable in the larger culture.

Disruption in the Human Subsystems. Although schizophrenia significantly affects each human subsystem, the primary locus of the disorder lies in the performance subsystem (Table 12-4). By definition, schizophrenia is essentially a process-skill disorder in which reasoning is disrupted. Communication/interaction skills are also affected. Some theorists suggest that dysfunction of speech is caused by the underlying thought disorder (Haydon, 1980). Contemporary researchers are exploring the perspective that schizophrenia may be a communication disorder, shifting the primary locus of the dysfunction to the realm of communication/interaction. Motor deficiencies, such as impaired posture and psychomotor retardation or agitation, often accompany deficits in process and communication/interaction performance (Manschreck, Maher, Rucklos, et al., 1981).

With skills and abilities disrupted the foundation for organized behavior is unstable. The individual with schizophrenia often demonstrates poverty of roles, nonproductive habits, and inefficient routines. In addition, time usage is frequently poorly organized. The primary role for the schizophrenic individual is that of a dependent, chronic patient/client. Normal adult family roles and work roles are uncommon among the schizophrenic population.

Major volitional disorders exist within the schizophrenic adult. Within the acute phase of the disorder, locus of control is external, even if an individual is responding to internal stimuli, because the individual is not choosing action from among a set of realistically defined options. The chronic nature of the disorder places locus of control in the external realm throughout life. Although the schizophrenic may perceive a sense of personal causation, this perception is also unrealistic because the behavior is nonproductive and nonefficacious in the real world. For the most part, individuals with schizophrenia function poorly in unstructured settings. For the schizophrenic in remission, introducing structure to their environment may have positive effects on volition; values and morals are dictated from the external world but still provide some guidelines for occupational performance. Additionally, the impairment of performance may negatively influence interests and the potency of interests. It is not uncommon to find a lack of interests in people with schizophrenia. If an individual does state interests, he/she often cannot act on them because of the organizational and skill deficits.

In summary, schizophrenia is a pervasive and chronic disorder. Schizophrenics often exhibit an inability to formulate an identity that is functional in the adult world and may be incapable of independently initiating purposeful and goal-directed occupational performance. Although there have been cases of schizophrenia that have resolved, the majority of individuals with schizophrenia are considered to be chronically disordered and marginally functional throughout their life (Kaplan & Sadock, 1988). It affects all aspects of occupational performance throughout the affected individual's life.

Affective Disorders

Affective disorders are those that influence an individual's mood or feelings and include a spectrum of severity, from feelings of sadness to extreme depression. At some point in the life span, everyone experiences a mild form of affective disorder, sometimes commonly known as "the blues," in which symptoms include crying, lack of appetite, and decrease in activity or interests. However, such normal mood swings frequently triggered by an external event are not considered to be clinical disorders that require treatment. The distinction between a clinical and nonclinical affective disorder is whether it is severe enough to impair one's function in daily living tasks.

Individuals who receive treatment for affective disorders usually fall into two diagnostic categories: psychotic and nonpsychotic.

Nonpsychotic Affective Disorders. Nonpsychotic affective disorders usually include diagnoses such as depression and hypomania. Nonpsychotic depression is characterized by feelings of sadness and worthlessness. Some theorists and clinicians consider nonpsychotic depression to be exogenous or caused by a reaction to external stressors and events. For example, individuals seeking outpatient or inpatient treatment for physical illness frequently exhibit symptoms of situational depression (Davis & Moss, 1983). Theorists have suggested that the physical illness may act either as a mechanism that triggers depression in individuals with an underlying propensity toward affective disorder, or illness may promote the development of a depressive episode even in the absence of a history of depression. The individual's perception of the severity of the illness seems to be the key factor in triggering the development of depressive symptoms.

Hypomania is an elevated mood state that is present in the absence of causative external events. Pressured speech, high activity level, distractibility, and nonpurposeful behavior are commonly exhibited. Depression and hypomania are forms of mood exaggerations in which the person does not lose reality-testing. But although these individuals do not loose touch with reality, they do frequently experience an interruption in some areas of occupational performance. Individuals falling into these categories may receive treatment as outpatients or may experience a resolution to their disorder without intervention.

On the more extreme end of the spectrum are the major affective disorders. Major affective disorders are characterized by extreme mood swings during which an individual may loose touch with reality. There are a number of variations of major affective disorders including *bipolar disorder, major depressive disorder,* and *mania.*

Major depressive disorder is characterized by a loss of touch with reality. The individual sees no future for himself or herself. A pervasive, overwhelming feeling of despondency is accompanied by a thought disorder in which all experience is viewed through despair. It is not uncommon to see the presence of delusions and hallucinations, usually of the persecutory or self-degrading type. Major depressive disorder interrupts all areas of occupational performance to the extent that an individual is not able to fulfill role responsibilities. Major depressive disorder may be unipolar in nature, thereby not being followed by mania.

Mania is symptomatically opposite to depression. Mania rarely appears by itself but seems to occur in bipolar disorder where depression and mania appear in cycles. An individual with mania may exhibit extreme mood elevation, loss of touch with reality (frequently in the form of delusions of grandeur), pressured speech, inattention and distractibility, and high energy level. Mania may be described as being ''too happy'' in the absence of external events that would trigger such elation.

Not all affective disorders are considered to be chronic. People may often experience one or two episodes of depression during the course of their life. However, mania seems to recur in cycles and implies the need for ongoing supervision. During remission individuals with bipolar disorder may function normatively and may experience intact occupational performance as long as they remain on medication.

Disruption in the Human Subsystems. In depression or hypomania, the answer to ''Who am I?'' may still be intact, but unclear. Personality foundations are essentially intact, although the perception of those structures may be mediated by mood elevation or depression. The factors most affected by these mood disorders in formulating identity are locus of control, sense of well-being, and emotion.

In depression, one's sense of well-being is lost. The predominant emotions are sadness and despair. The depressed individual may feel that he/she has temporarily lost control over his/her life. There may be external events such as loss or failure that have contributed to the depression. As these events move further away in time, the depression may lift, leaving the individual with more of an internal locus of control. If the depression is endogenous, the likelihood of regaining an internal locus of control is not as great, because the mood cannot be attributed to an outside event.

In hypomania, feelings are of happiness. The individual may feel an internal locus of control, however, upon more thorough examination, it becomes evident that the locus of control is perceived improperly. The elevation in mood is

not controllable, nor is behavior that responds to that exaggerated mood elevation. Hypomanic individuals commonly report an unusual sense of well-being, which connotes excitement over contentment.

In both depression and hypomania, protective devices (from the occupational behavior perspective) are impaired. Because of the presence of a pervasive mood, an individual is not able to harness purposeful habits into useful and adaptive responses to environmental demands beyond routine daily activities and tasks (Table 12-3).

Depressed people frequently demonstrate a reduction in action, while hypomanic people exhibit hyperactivity, even if the hyperactivity is undirected and nonpurposeful. Nevertheless, both disorders decrease the efficacy of one's actions. In both disorders, the emotional tone dominates the elicitors of action (Table 12-3). In depression, one's negative beliefs about the self dampen action. In hypomania, excitement seems to add a frenzied mood to action.

Although symbols remain intact as elicitors of action, they are also influenced by the dominant emotion. Perhaps the factor most influenced by mood disorder is one's beliefs. In both the hypomanic and depressed individual, beliefs are distorted by the dominant mood. Although the individual maintains contact with reality, the distortion does influence the way in which an individual acts.

Regarding experiences, an individual who is able to maintain contact with reality may continue to be able to organize experience into meaningful patterns and use previous patterns to engage in occupational performance. However, the perceptions of experiences are significantly affected by mood. In depression, experience is evaluated from a negative perspective and is thus assigned a negative meaning. In hypomania, the opposite occurs. Experiences may be organized, but the meaning given to them may be inaccurate. In nonpsychotic mood disorders, individuals are capable of behaving in a compatible manner with cultural norms and expectations.

Locus of dysfunction in nonpsychotic mood disorders lies primarily in self-concept and control (Table 12-4). Personal causation and locus of control are most affected in depression because one loses belief in the self and the ability to modify one's direction in life. Interests may lose potency but values seem to remain intact. In hypomania, personal causation remains intact, perhaps inaccurately. Dysfunction can be seen in locus of control and in interest potency. Although stated interest may be increased, the extent to which one acts upon these interests in a purposeful way is impaired. Individuals with hypomania cannot control their activity level, thus experiencing an external locus of control.

Habituation is significantly affected in both disorders. Sleep is a common diagnostic criteria for both disorders, and it is common to hear reports of sleep disorders in both depressed and hypomanic patients. Although basic self-care routines are intact, other roles and routines are often interrupted, for example, roles of player or caregiver. Role function is impaired in both, but depressed individuals tend to withdraw from nonessential roles, while hypomanic individuals tend to take on too many roles, rendering their role behavior ineffective and fragmented. Abilities and skills in both disorders usually remain intact even though the disorder in other subsystems may temporarily decrease skill use.

Major Affective Disorders (Psychotic Disorders). The presence of a major affective disorder or psychosis greatly changes the factors that are involved and the picture of occupational performance. For an individual with major depressive disorder, answering the question, ''Who am I?'' takes on the complexity of poor reality-testing. Because thought structures are no longer intact, the answer to this question may be idiosyncratic and mediated by the dominant mood. Self-concept may, in turn, be based on impaired perception and reasoning. Psychosis intensifies the effects of dysfunctional subsystems. In a depressed psychotic individual, self-concept takes on the quality of despair, possibly exaggerated by loss of touch with reality, and the manic may exhibit extreme grandiose self-concepts. As in other psychological disorders, locus of control is external in that the disease process is responsible for choices. Well-being and emotion are affected by major affective disorders in a manner similar to nonpsychotic affective disorders, but again in intensified levels.

Protective devices in major affective disorders are less intact than in nonpsychotic disorders and render an individual that much more incapable of ordering occupational function in a adaptive manner (Table 12-3). Individuals with major affective disorders frequently must be institutionalized to be protected from environmental demands.

The actions of individuals with major affective disorders are difficult to understand. Elicitors of behavior are influenced by the mix of exaggerated emotion and mood-dominated cognition and are difficult to identify. The manic individual seems to act in a frenzied and agitated fashion, and the depressed patient frequently finds himself/herself immobilized.

The symbols that prompt behavior are often idiosyncratic because individuals with major affective disorder do not reason competently. Furthermore, the pervasive mood also distorts symbols and subsequent action. In examining beliefs, the dominant emotion that changes the beliefs of the depressed or manic individual is magnified by the severity of the disorder. Beliefs that are either self-deprecating or grandiose may find little basis in reality. Beliefs may be

organized into a set of delusions that elicit maladaptive behavior.

In the individual with a major affective disorder, experiences are shaped by unrealistic perceptions and extreme emotion. For example, the depressed patient may interpret a routine social encounter as disdain or deserved punishment from others. Experiences and the meanings attached to them are disordered and may be organized into a dysfunctional pattern that supports the cognitive and emotive tone being experienced by the individual.

As expected, individuals with major affective disorder cannot function in the larger culture when in an acute phase of the disease. They are unable to affect normal role behavior or meet cultural expectations and commonly must be under institutional care until medication and therapeutic intervention ameliorate the dysfunction.

Unlike nonpsychotic disorders, major affective disorders seem to affect function of the volition and performance subsystems (Table 12-4). In addition to the volitional issues discussed above, psychosis effects process skill and interaction/communication. These major affective disorders are often accompanied by motor symptoms such as psychomotor retardation or agitation. Organized behavior is also impaired to such a degree that an affected individual is unable to function in society in his/her normative roles.

Substance Abuse and Dependence

Substance abuse and dependence are two diagnostic categories that frequently accompany other psychiatric problems. Although for our purposes here we have chosen to discuss substance abuse and dependence independent of underlying psychopathology, please remember they often emerge in the presence of other disorders, and in many cases, may be symptomatic of those disorders.

A fundamental consideration in any discussion of substance abuse is the context in which the abuse occurs. For example, substance abuse can be a situational response to physical illness and may be seen in various health care settings and/or in an individual's home. Substances may include illicit drugs, alcohol, or even prescription drugs that were initially legitimately prescribed by the physician.

Substance abuse and dependence are terms that are relative and therefore difficult to clearly define. Diagnosis is in large part dependent on cultural norms and there is often a fine line between abuse and dependence. The DSM III-R has attempted to distinguish between abuse and dependence by their functional outcomes and by what occurs when the substance is not available. Hence, *abuse* involves the regular intake of a substance that may or may not be intoxicating but must in some way interfere with aspects of function. *Dependence* is more severe and interferes with most aspects of function, increases tolerance of the substance over time, and elicits withdrawal symptoms in the absence of the substance.

Substances that are typically abused include intoxicating drugs such as marijuana, cocaine, and alcohol, or nonintoxicating substances such as caffeine and tobacco. Although many of these substances are physically addictive, not all have been proven to promote physical dependence. However, psychological dependence might exist and should be considered when assessing those who abuse or are dependent.

Effects on Identity.   The ability for the substance-dependent or substance-abuser to answer the question "Who am I?" is greatly affected by the severity of the abuse or dependence. The recreational substance abuser may have intact personality structures and be fully capable of fulfilling adult roles. This person would most likely not be seen in treatment for substance abuse, nor would caffeine and tobacco abusers with no other psychiatric symptoms. At the other end of the continuum is the person who is fully dependent on alcohol or drug substances and whose entire personality is dominated by the substance; this person's identity becomes that of an addict or alcoholic.

Self-concept is another factor that may or may not be involved with substance abuse. It seems plausible that individuals may select certain substances such as alcohol to compensate for poor self-esteem. However, it is dangerous to make this generalization about all people who abuse substances without a full assessment of function. It is more logical to assume that individuals demonstrating severe dependence on intoxicating substances might have a poor self-concept for two reasons: (1) the intoxicant impairs judgement and cognition of the individual such that self-concept cannot be thought of in a competent manner, and (2) occupational performance is most certainly negatively affected in an individual who is fully substance-dependent and such a person cannot function in a capacity that will build self-esteem.

Locus of control is also affected, becoming more external as the individual becomes more dependent on a substance (Table 12-3). By definition, dependence is not voluntary. It would also seem that there is a relationship between well-being and substance use; however, the relationship probably complex. The intensity of substance use may be a barometer of well-being, but many variables must be considered when addressing sense of well-being as it relates to substance abuse. Once again a full assessment of function needs to be accomplished before drawing conclusions.

Effects on Self-protection.   The question of "How do I protect myself?" is also difficult to assess in substance abusers. Some individuals ingest substances with the intent

of protection. For example, the shy individual may take a drink of alcohol, believing the disinhibiting effects of the substance will promote confidence. Ultimately, clinical abuse and dependence are mechanisms that preclude self-protection in that individuals do not maintain control over their thoughts and actions when they are intoxicated (Table 12-3).

Effects of Motivation.   Regarding motivation for actions, one must continue to consider the severity and reasons for abuse and dependence. In extreme cases, the substance is primarily responsible for actions. The majority of the addict's life is spent not only in experiencing intoxication, but also in insuring access to the substance in order to avoid the effects of withdrawal (Table 12-3). With less severe abuse cases, the substance may only prompt action when under the direct influence of the substance.

Substances are closely tied to symbols that influence action. For example, teenagers may drink beer to show their friends that they are "cool." Furthermore, the beliefs about substances are instrumental in the meanings they hold and in their strength in influencing occupational behavior.

Intoxicating substances alter perception and thus give different meaning to the experiences one has while intoxicated. In many cases as the effects of the substance subside, reality-based perceptions are restored and become acceptable. However, individuals who find that experiences and perceptions are improved by a substance are more likely to continue to abuse a substance and may be at risk for dependence.

Perhaps of most concern is the cultural influence on substance abuse and dependence. In a culture where substances are accepted, individuals may feel pressured to conform to the norms of abuse. However, in a culture where substances are unacceptable, the abuser is perceived as deviant. Thus, the degree to which the abuser or dependent person is considered to be dysfunctional is relative to his/her surroundings.

Disruption of Subsystems.   In order to examine the effects of substance abuse on occupational performance, we consider the example of a cocaine abuser. Because of the habitual nature of substance abuse, the primary locus of the disorder seems to be seated in the habituation subsystem (Table 12-4). However, this may change depending on the severity of the abuse and the potential to develop additional psychological disorders. Cocaine abuse ritualistic, in that there is a set of "drug paraphernalia" needed to use the drug and a set of behaviors in which one engages in order to take the drug. The ritual becomes habitual as the abuser continues to use the drug over time. In the case of a severe abuser, the primary role may become that of a drug seeker and taker, to the exclusion of other productive and satisfying roles.

Abilities and skills are affected by cocaine abuse in a number of ways. First, intoxication alters process skills, communication/interaction, and possibly motor skills. If the abuse continues for prolonged period of time, more permanent physiological damage may occur, thereby weakening one's foundation of skill. Second, as the role of drug-taker increases and skills diminish, the individual may become unable to perform valued roles and manage time.

Substance abuse significantly influences volition as well. As the abuse becomes more severe, values are replaced by the importance of gaining access to the drug. It is quite common to see significant personal relationships dissolve as they become less valued by the drug abuser. Most significant in volition is the loss of internal locus of control (Table 12-4). The drug abuser gives up control to the substance that he/she seeks. It is difficult to comment on personal causation because as mentioned before, the individual may engage in abuse to improve a sense of personal causation regardless of the accuracy of the belief in self.

In summary, substance abuse and dependence are two diagnoses that are not clearly delineated. Exploration of these diagnoses reveals that there is a continuum of severity of substance use from recreational use to total dependence. Furthermore, the complexity of culture factors and additional psychological dysfunction that frequently accompany substance abuse renders these diagnoses difficult to analyze. Nevertheless, in clinical cases, occupational performance is affected by the continuous use of a substance and is a major concern in contemporary society.

Personality Disorder

Individuals with personality disorders "exhibit characteristic patterns of maladjustment in their social, interpersonal, and sexual relationships....A diagnosis of personality disorder is based upon recognition of typical behavioral patterns and the patient's inability to learn from experience" (Merck, 1980, pp. 1501, 1502). In other words, there is a clear pattern of disordered action that pervades an affected person's occupational performance and does not remit as he/she moves through life. Individuals with personality disorders usually have a history of odd behavior that goes undiagnosed until the personality decompensates in the face of a crisis. Without stress in the environment these individuals may function well, and for that reason, they usually seek help for some disorder other than the personality disorder.

The majority of personality disorders appear as exaggerations of human traits. For example, in paranoid personality disorder, mistrust becomes unwarranted suspicion, even in the absence of justifiable external cues.

Obsessive-compulsive personality disorder is characterized by rigidity and perfectionism and ultimately immobilizes the individual who is unable to act on obsessive thoughts. The antisocial personality is one in which an individual tends to live outside the norms and laws of society without regret. Thus, personality disorder is an underlying disorganization of the self in which individuals tend to respond poorly to stressful situations.

Most individuals with personality disorder are seen clinically for a diagnosis which is superimposed on the underlying personality deficit. Thus, it is difficult to treat personality disorder. The majority of treatment addresses acute concerns such as eliminating environmental stress as a preventative measure for further decompensation.

Effects on Identity. The answer to, "Who am I?" depends on the type of personality disorder. However, generally speaking, personality disorder is considered to be an immature or maladaptive development of personality structure. Thus an attempt to describe the cognitive and ego structures of an individual with personality disorder may be difficult because of the unstable nature of the ego. Because of lack of insight, the individual with a personality disorder may have a distorted self-concept (Table 12-3). For example, the individual who exhibits a narcissistic personality disorder may view the self as perfect and may not consider feedback from others in his/her self-assessment.

Although many personality disorders demonstrate an external locus of control, some types include more internal control than others (Table 12-4). Those with borderline personality disorder have a clear external locus of control because they impulsively respond to the environment and tend to change to suit a particular situation. Those with antisocial personalities are more complicated because they fight external control. The urge to indulge the self, regardless of how others are affected, seems to be a function of the disorder rather than a function of deliberate choice, and locus of control shifts as the environment presents demands. This shift seems to be characteristic of other types of personality disorders as well. For example, the individual with a paranoid personality disorder characteristically avoids intimacy. The choice to avoid closeness is deliberate, yet it is based on disordered reasoning that is not internally controlled.

Well-being and emotions are two other factors that seem to fluctuate in individuals with personality disorders. This is not surprising in light of the individual's vulnerability to stress, poor insight, and maladaptive social relationships.

Effects on Self-Protection. Individuals with personality disorders seem to be at the mercy of the environment without any personal protective devices. Because of the immature or incomplete development of personality structures, the foundations for adaptive occupational performance are weak and unstable (Table 12-3). The most effective protection for these individuals seems to be elimination of difficult environmental demands. This elimination can only occur with imposed external structure.

Just as the locus of control tends to be external in individuals with personality disorder, the elicitors of behavior seem to be seated in the environment. The likelihood of competent occupational performance increases in the presence of a sound and stable environmental structure. Conversely, in the absence of structure, ineffective occupational performance may result.

Because personality disorder does not involve thought disorder, symbols seem to remain intact. Symbols as elicitors of behavior, however, may have idiosyncratic meaning when interpreted through the exaggerated or poorly-developed cognitive schemes of personality disorder.

It is difficult to generalize about the influence of personality disorder on beliefs, but we do know that they are mediated through poorly-developed cognitive schemes. In some cases, such as in borderline personality, beliefs fluctuate with the environmental cues and norms. However, in other types of personality disorders, such as paranoid personality and obsessive-compulsive disorder, beliefs are rigid. The antisocial personality is frequently characterized as amoral. Thus beliefs, which form the structural foundation for normative occupational performance, are significantly affected by personality disorder.

Effects on Motivation. In examining how an individual with personality disorder functions within a culture, there are two interesting generalizations. First, personality disorders tend to shift with cultural change. Second, many individuals with personality disorders respond well to cultural norms that provide structure. For example, the individual with obsessive-compulsive personality disorder tends to be a high achiever as long as the environment does not demand flexibility.

Disruption of Subsystems. The locus of dysfunction in personality disorder appears to be in the performance subsystem. Essentially, personality disorder is viewed as the maladaptive development of skills such as process skills or communication/interaction skill (Table 12-4). The foundations for a mature personality have never formed, and the individual with a personality disorder is left with structural deficits which do not allow the individual to build sound habits and routines. In the presence of structure or comfort from the environment, an individual with a personality disorder may be capable of fulfilling productive and satisfying roles. However, these roles are inconsistent as they lack

internal stability. Volitional elements are equally changeable and vulnerable to external influence.

Anxiety Disorders

Disorders in this diagnostic category include phobias, panic disorder, post-traumatic stress disorder, and generalized anxiety disorder. They all have one common characteristic, the presence of anxiety. Although anxiety may accompany other diagnostic categories, in this category, anxiety is caused through fear or an attempt to avoid situations. The degree to which anxiety is experienced may be conceptualized as a continuum from mild discomfort to immobilizing fear.

The symptoms that are characteristic of anxiety disorders may be commonly observed in patients who are being treated for physical illness. The stressors of illness, treatment, and uncertainty may evoke feelings of uneasiness, uncertainty about one's future, and fear about mortality.

Effects on Identity. The individual with anxiety disorder may have intact personality structures unless the disorder is accompanied by another diagnosis. Self-concept may be impaired because of the struggle to maintain control over the environment and the self. The major difficulty in answering the ''Who am I?'' question seems to be in locus of control, which is external. Individuals with anxiety disorder have little voluntary control over the fears or physiological symptoms that elicit anxiety or little control over their anxiety responses (Table 12-3). It follows that the sense of well-being is impaired unless the anxiety can be prevented by avoiding the elicitor. Individuals with anxiety disorder seem to respond to negative situations with emotion rather than with rationality. Thus the anxious person is highly vulnerable to shifts in emotional tone based on the presence of the anxiety stimulus.

Effects on Self-protection. Protective devices are significantly affected in anxiety disorder. The locus of control is external, and individuals with anxiety disorder have impaired ability to moderate behavior to meet environmental demands. Because of the irrational fears and anxiety, the individual forms overactive protective devices such as *avoidance* and *withdrawal* (Table 12-3). For example, the two mechanisms of withdrawal and avoidance may be mistaken for lack of motivation in the patient who has experienced cerebrovascular accident and who is anxious about his/her recovery. The initiation of these devices also causes further impairment in occupational and role function as the need to avoid a stimulus becomes stronger.

Effects on Motivation. The answer to ''When and why do I act?'' is reasonably clear in this disorder. The elicitor of behavior is the stimulus that causes the anxiety and can range from mild to severe. The stimulus may prompt behavior either directly or indirectly. In the case in which exposure cannot be avoided, anxiety is likely to result. However, if indirectly stimulated, an individual may go to great ends to avoid a feared stimulus. An example is the condition of *agoraphobia* in which an individual may refuse to go out of the home in order to avoid the fear of open spaces.

Typical daily activity may symbolize discomfort to the individual with anxiety disorder. Although beliefs may not be impaired, perceptions and experiences are influenced by fear and avoidance.

The role of culture in anxiety disorders is twofold. The changing culture may alter the stimuli that elicit anxiety or induce discomfort with the unfamiliar. Also, as the severity of the disorder increases, an individual may not be capable of fulfilling normative cultural roles.

Disruption of Subsystems. In anxiety disorders, the primary problem appears to center around the individuals' sense of control or personal causation. Anxiety disorder seems to occur from a perception that one is externally controlled and that one cannot master the anxiety stimulus in a competent manner. As the severity increases, anxiety disorders may have an impact on roles, skills, and abilities.

Individuals will often develop rituals and inflexible behavioral patterns in order to avoid the noxious stimulus. Thus, the dysfunctional routines take the place of competent function in productive and satisfying roles. Performance seems to be most affected in process skill. Anxiety disorder seems to be seated in faulty perceptions and reasoning about feared situations and the solutions to addressing those fears.

In summary, anxiety disorders appear to be founded in an external locus of control and compounded by lack of belief in one's competence. Although most people have experienced anxiety to some degree, those who demonstrate anxiety disorder modify habits and roles to compensate for and avoid discomfort. Thus, although identity may be intact, the effect on well-being and occupational function is negative.

Adjustment Disorders

Adjustment disorders are a maladaptive response to an "identifiable psychosocial stressor" (DSM III-R, p. 299). When the stressor is no longer present, the disorder dissipates. The assessment of a maladaptive response is in large part dependent on norms. An individual may exhibit any number of symptoms in response to the stimulus that provokes the maladjustment. For example, a patient hospitalized for a physical disorder may react with agitation, fear, and inappropriate behavior in occupational therapy. However, when the patient returns home, he/she

may welcome the services of the same occupational therapist. In a case such as this, the hospitalization may be the situational condition to which the individual reacts in a disorderly manner.

Effects on Identity. Although a generalization regarding how the person with adjustment reaction defines himself/herself cannot be made, it may be surmised that adjustment reaction may be a response to a challenged identity. For example, the hospitalized patient may be uncomfortable assuming the dependent sick role that is a condition of institutionalization.

In adjustment reaction, the locus of control rests in the external realm in that the disorder is an incompetent response to an external stressor. Furthermore, the stimulus negatively influences well-being and seems to result in an emotional rather than reasoned response to stress. Perhaps the major area of dysfunction rests in the individual's inability to mobilize abilities into a competent strategy of response.

In adjustment reaction, the elicitor of behavior is the external stressor. The stressor may be one that is symbolic to an individual. The degree to which an individual responds to stress incompetently is strongly influenced by the perception or belief system that he/she employs to make sense of the stressful event or symbol.

Culture plays an essential part in a diagnosis of adjustment disorder. This disorder is essentially defined as a reaction in excess of the norm of responses. The degree of deviance of one's actions rather than the actions themselves is considered as the diagnostic criterion.

Adjustment reaction is short-lived and therefore seems not to affect performance. The primary locus of the disorder appears to be seated in habituation. The individual tends to respond to an external locus of control with a maladaptive organization of skill and behavior. Occupational performance is poorly organized and competent habits and roles are not employed to adapt to a stressor.

Disorders Evident in Infancy, Childhood, or Adolescence

Although children may be diagnosed with conditions that affect adults, the disorders that belong to this category are those that must emerge before adulthood. Because of the complex nature of development, disorders that occur before adulthood are diverse. The DSM-III-R has suggested five subcategories of pre-adulthood diagnoses: intellectual, behavioral, emotional, physical, and developmental.

Mental retardation is defined by subaverage intellect, impairment in function, and onset before 18 years of age. Development is delayed or prematurely halted but not distorted. Because of its similarity to dementia, the reader is referred to the section on organic mental syndrome for examination and analysis of the relationship among psychological factors and occupational performance.

Behavioral disorders are those that can be discerned by observing a child's activity including subcategories of attention deficit disorder and conduct disorder (DSM-III-R). Anxiety disorders in childhood are included under emotional disorders. Eating disorders and movement disorders are considered as physical disorders in that they are prompted by psychological disorder, but have negative physical outcomes as well. Developmental disorders are those in which there are distortions of the developmental sequence in areas of psychosocial function.

Because in childhood disorders development into adulthood is incomplete, we can also assume that the foundations for occupational performance are incomplete. Although the immediate effect may be on present function, the long-reaching consequences of childhood disorders may be severe. Because of the broad and diverse nature of childhood disorders, it would be impossible to address each separately here. Rather, this discussion will include an overview of general psychological factors and the effects on occupational function of these pre-adulthood disorders.

Effects on Identity. The age of onset and the severity of the disorder will determine the extent to which the "Who am I?" question can be answered. The answer to this question is always changing in childhood and adolescence, much more so than in adulthood. However, one of the fundamental traits of orderly adulthood is self-knowledge, which allows one to identify basic and well-established elements of one's personality. In childhood, the nature of one's identity changes significantly with the development of new skills and habits to organize those skills. If personality structures do not follow orderly development, an individual never experiences a solid foundation on which to know, feel, or anchor sound occupational performance. Thus self-concept, well-being, and satisfying emotions may be disorderly as well.

Effects on Self-protection. A child or adolescent may attempt to protect the self in many ways. From the occupational performance perspective, psychological disorder is accompanied by the inability to competently develop organization of skills or adapt to the environment. Thus, the individual lacks the skill and organization to protect himself/herself from psychological harm.

Effects on Motivation. Actions are equally as puzzling. Elicitors of behavior may be diverse, and the action that results from any source may not be based on an intact psychological structure. Thus, the meaning attributed to and emerging from action in the form of symbols, beliefs, or perceptions may be distorted or unserviceable to future growth and development. One very critical factor is that the child or adolescent becomes labeled as deviant when compared to cultural norms.

Disruption of Subsystems. Although disorders of childhood and adolescence affect all subsystems, the primary locus of the disorder is in abilities and skills. Due to the absence, delay, or distortion of skills, behavior is less organized and feelings of control and competence are diminished.

In summary, pre-adulthood disorders, although extremely diverse in nature, have one major characteristic in common: the lack of development of normative psychological structures and skills. Thus, the experience of competence in occupational performance is not likely to develop.

SUMMARY

The psychosocial dimensions of individuals have an inportant influence on their performance of everyday tasks and roles. A knowledge of psychological factors is therefore critical to understanding how thoughts and feelings shape behavior. In this chapter, six perspectives of psychological function have been considered in terms of their basic tenets, including the psychoanalytic, neo-Freudian, cognitive behaviorist, behaviorist, meaning-in-experience, and occupational performance perspectives. As a means of differentiating between these perspectives, explanations regarding three instrumental areas, including the *structures of self or identity* (including self concept, locus of control and sense of well-being), *protective-maintaining devices* (such as beliefs, defense mechanisms and rationality) and *motives for action* (such as symbols, perceptions, history, and intrinsic motivation) have been used as points of comparison. Additionally, common psychosocial disorders identified in eight diagnostic categories from the *Diagnostic and Statistical Manual* have been reviewed in terms of how these dysfunctions alter a persons sense of identity, feelings of stability and motivation to act.

Study Questions

1. What are the six major theories of psychosocial function? Who are the major theorists in each category?

2. What are the three major questions which all theorists address when discussing psychosocial factors? Define the key concepts used in answering each question.

3. Compare and contrast the cognitive-behaviorists' per-

spective with that of the behaviorists. What are the similarities in their approaches? What are the implications of each approach in terms of occupational performance?

4. What are the major differences between the psychoanalytic perspectives and the meaning-in-experience perspectives? How would you focus your general psychosocial program goals if you were using a psychoanalytic approach? How would your general goals differ if you were using a meaning-in-experience perspective?

5. Each major theoretical perspective uses a unique framework for discussing patient problems. In addition, each perspective has its own language or jargon. As an occupational therapist, you need to be able to frame patient problems using terminology that is congruent with the primary perspective of your environment while still maintaining the integrity of your unique professional program. Given this mission, how would you address the following scenarios:

a. You are the occupational therapist in a private psychiatric hospital. The psychiatrist and psychologist on your treatment team consider themselves to be behaviorists. The social worker describes himself as a Rogerian and the movement therapist is a Jungian. You want to design a program for young chronic schizophrenic patients. How would you describe the program so that all of the team members could understand what you are trying to accomplish? Consider the primary locus of the disorder as well as the theoretical perspectives and jargon of each team member.

b. You still work with the same team mentioned in scenario A, but there has recently been an influx of substance abuse patients to the unit. The team members do not understand why you can't just put them in the rest of your groups. You want to design a special program for these patients. How will you describe the problem areas so that the other team members can understand your perspective? How will your intervention focus differ from the one you used with the schizophrenics? What "buzz words" will you use in describing your new program so that the other team members will see your program as being congruent and complementary to theirs?

Recommended Readings

American Psychiatric Association (1987). *Diagnostic and statistical manual of mental disorders,* (3rd edition, revised.) Washington, DC: American Psychiatric Association.

Bandura, A. (1971). *A social learning theory.* New York: General Learning Press.

Bruce, M. & Borg, B. (1987). *Frames of reference in psychosocial occupational therapy.* Thorofare, NJ: Slack.

Erikson, E. (1950). *Childhood and society.* New York: W.W. Norton and Co.

Freud, S. (1961). The ego and the id. In *The complete psychological works of Sigmund Freud* (Vol. 9). London: Hogarth Press.

Jung, C. (1964). *Man and his symbols.* New York: Doubleday.

Smelser, N. & Erikson, E. (1980). *Work and love in adulthood.* Cambridge, MA: Harvard University Press.

References

Adler A. (1972). *Understanding human nature.* New York: Greenberg.

American Psychiatric Association (1987). *Diagnostic and statistical manual of mental disorders* (3rd edition, revised). Washington D.C.: American Psychiatric Association.

Andreasen, N. (1985). Positive and negative schizophrenia: A critical evaluation. *Schizophrenia Bulletin, 11*(3): 380-389.

Bandura, A. (1971). *A social learning theory.* New York: General Learning Press.

Barris, R., Kielhofner, G., & Watts, J. (1983). *Psychosocial occupational therapy: Practice in a pluralistic arena.* Laurel, MD: RAMSCO Pub Co.

Beck, A. (1976). *Cognitive therapy and emotional disorders.* New York: International Universities Press.

Bruce, M. & Borg, B. (1987). *Frames of reference in psychosocial occupational therapy.* Thorofare, NJ: Slack.

Davis, J.M. & Moss, J.W. (1983). *The affective disorders.* Washington, D.C: American Psychiatric Press, Inc.

Ellis, A. (1973). *Humanistic psychology: A rational emotive approach.* New York: McGraw Hill.

Erikson, E. (1950). *Childhood and society.* New York: W.W. Norton and Co.

Evans, R. (1975). *Carl Rogers: The man and his ideas.* New York: E.P. Dutton and Co.

Frankl, V. (1975). *The unconscious God.* New York: Simon and Schuster.

Freud, S. (1961). The ego and the id. In *The complete psychological works of Sigmund Freud* (Vol. 9). London: Hogarth Press.

Hall, C.S. & Lindzey, G. (1978). *Theories of personality.* (3rd ed.), New York: John Wiley and Sons.

Haydon, M.H. (1980). Schizophrenic dysfunction in verbal processing. *Dissertation Abstracts*, 40 (11) 5438-B.

Horney, K. (1945). *Our inner conflicts.* New York: Norton.

Jung, C. (1964). *Man and his symbols.* New York: Doubleday.

Kaplan, H.I. & Sadock, B.J. (1988). *Synopsis of psychiatry,* (5th ed.) Baltimore, MD: Williams and Wilkins.

Kernberg, O. (1976). *Object relations theory and clinical psychoanalysis.* New York: Jason Aronson, Inc.

Kielhofner, G. (ed.) (1982). *Health through occupation.* Philadelphia: F.A. Davis.

Manschreck, T.C., Maher B.A., Rucklos, M.E. Vereen, D.R., & Ader, D.N. (1981). Deficient motor synchrony in schizophrenia. *Journal of Abnormal Psychology,* 90(4): 321-328.

Merck & Co (Author) *Merck Manual of Diagnosis and Therapy*, (13th Ed.) Rahway NJ: Merck, Sharp & Dohm Research Labs, Rahway, NJ, 1977.

Miller, T.W. (1988). Advances in understanding the impact of stressful events on health. *Hospital and Community Psychiatry, 39*(6): 615-622.

Shaffer, D. (1985). *Developmental psychology.* California: Cole/Brooks.

Skinner, B.F. (1971). *Beyond freedom and dignity.* Toronto: Bantam.

Smelser, N. & Erikson, E. (1980). *Work and love in adulthood.* Cambridge, MA: Harvard University Press.

Wolman, B. (1982). *Handbook of developmental psychology.* Englewood Cliffs, NJ: Prentice Hall.

CHAPTER CONTENT OUTLINE

Introduction

Principles of Pharmacologic Management

Drugs and the Interaction of Systems

Drugs that Act on the Central Nervous System

Drugs that Act Outside the Central Nervous System

Sources of Drug Information

The Therapist's Role in Monitoring Drug Effects

Medication Case Studies

Summary

KEY TERMS

Adverse reactions

Analgesic

Antimicrobial

Antineoplastic agents

Anxiolytic

Enteral

Half-life

Metabolism

Neuroleptic

Opioid

Pharmacokinetics

Prophylactic

Receptor

Side effects

Target site

Tolerance

ABSTRACT

The use of pharmacological agents or drugs can affect performance both by intended, beneficial use and through side effects and adverse reactions that can interfere with or hinder performance. This chapter helps therapists understand the basic mechanisms of drug action, the major categories of chemical agents and their therapeutic purposes (both those that affect the central nervous system and those that affect other body systems), and identifies the known side effects and adverse reactions of various drugs. The therapist's role in monitoring drug effects is discussed along with the social and psychological factors that are associated with the use of medications.

Pharmacological Agents and Their Effect on Performance

Elizabeth Devereaux
James E. Berger
Charles Christiansen

"Human performance involves many functions, and drugs may selectively affect some of these even when others are unchanged."

—Broadbent, 1984

OBJECTIVES

The information in this chapter is intended to help the reader—

1. understand the basic mechanisms of drug action.

2. become familiar with major categories of chemical agents and their therapeutic purposes.

3. identify the known side effects and adverse reactions associated with various drugs.

4. appreciate social and psychological factors associated with the use of medications.

5. identify documented performance effects associated with the use of various agents in normal subjects.

6. appreciate the importance of careful monitoring and observation in identifying potential performance effects associated with various chemical agents.

7. identify sources of additional information about pharmacological agents.

INTRODUCTION

Pharmacological agents, or drugs, are chemicals used in the treatment of disease or prevention of illness. These chemical agents may be taken into the body through the gastrointestinal system by oral, rectal or nasogastric routes (**enteral**), parenterally as through injection or intravenous methods, and through percutaneous routes, which include inhalation, topical or sublingual routes of administration.

Drugs can affect performance through their intended actions as well as through **side effects** and **adverse reactions**. While intended effects may result in beneficial outcomes such as alleviating pain or reducing inflammation, the associated side effects may interfere with optimal function in other systems, thus affecting task performance. Side effects may range from nausea and headache to incoordination and vertigo. Moreover, the act of taking medication has psychological effects which may influence behavior totally independent of the chemical and physiological actions of the drug administered.

For these reasons, the effects of chemical agents on the performance of life tasks must be considered in terms of: (1) physiological changes affecting body systems, (2) changes in the mental or psychological state of an individual, and (3) the specific life tasks and responsibilities of the individual which must be performed. Since chemical agents are available for self-medication, contained in foods and beverages, and so widely prescribed in medical care, a basic knowledge of their intended and unintended effects on performance is essential for the practicing occupational therapist.

Pharmacokinetics is best described as the absorption, distribution, metabolism, and excretion of a specific chemical agent introduced to the body. Figure 13-1 illustrates several major points regarding the ability of a drug to reach its **receptors** or intended site of action. Drugs vary according to their routes of administration, rates of absorption, and their distribution through the circulatory system. Absorption refers to the process of getting the drug from the site of administration through the capillaries into the blood stream, where it can be distributed to the tissues. Once absorbed, the distribution of a drug, or how easily it diffuses through various body tissues, depends upon several factors, including its solubility. There are a number of factors that can affect the level of drug available and the amount of drug necessary to reach appropriate levels,

including the impairment of drug absorption, impairment of distribution (circulatory disorders), abnormal excretion (renal impairment), inappropriate **metabolism** (liver dysfunction) or the alteration of the receptor or **target site**.

PRINCIPLES OF PHARMACOLOGIC MANAGEMENT

Drugs affect tissues either in a specific fashion (specific receptors) or non-specifically (through membrane potential alteration). A selective drug activates a specific receptor and thus produces a cellular response; while a non-specific drug may depress membrane function and thus inhibit physiological function, such as through decreased respiration or heart rate. In order to understand pharmacologic management, three basic principles of pharmacokinetics must be considered:

Principle 1: Most drugs will affect both mental and motor functions to some degree if administered in levels sufficient to allow absorption and distribution.

Principle 2: A drug can only affect an existing physiologic system. The action of a drug attempts to return a system to normal (when diseased) and to affect the non-diseased system to produce desired results. It is not uncommon for the effect of a drug to be reflected in a change in the motivation or ability of a patient to perform specific activities. These changes may affect mood, memory, cognition, arousal, perception, or specific movements involving skeletal muscle. It is also possible for the smooth muscles of the body to be impeded, resulting in decreased sexual ability, diminished ability of the body to control blood pressure, constipation, or urinary difficulties.

Principle 3: The responses of individuals to a drug may vary greatly. The effectiveness of a specific dose of a drug will depend on the age, health status, size and sex of the person treated. The physical and psychological state of the individuals will also affect their response to a specific drug. Thus the effect of a specific drug is a complex phenomenon which requires careful monitoring and interpretation.

There are so many variables and subfunctions within each activity performed by an individual that few generalizations can be made regarding the effects of specific dose levels of particular drugs. Within the specialty known as behavioral pharmacology, research has employed many different techniques to assess the psychomotor skills and functions of individuals and their responses to various agents. However, the many variables which influence human performance have made controlled experimentation difficult, so that much of what we know about the effects of pharmacological agents is based upon relationships observed under non-experimental conditions (McKim, 1984). Therefore, causal relationships between various drugs and their observed effects have not been established conclusively and must be viewed as conjectural.

The inconclusive nature of most research involving the behavioral effects of chemical agents makes it important for health practitioners to be alert to performance changes in their patients who begin taking a medication for the first time. Because of their concern with the skills required for daily living, occupational therapists can play a vital role in providing feedback to physicians and other professionals interested in a patient's response to a particular pharmacologic agent.

Figure 13-2 illustrates the interactions that take place between the intrinsic and extrinsic components which contribute to performance when a specific pharmacologic agent is introduced. The introduction of such an agent involves a process of starting, slowing, or speeding up the movement of fluid through the many gateways in the human

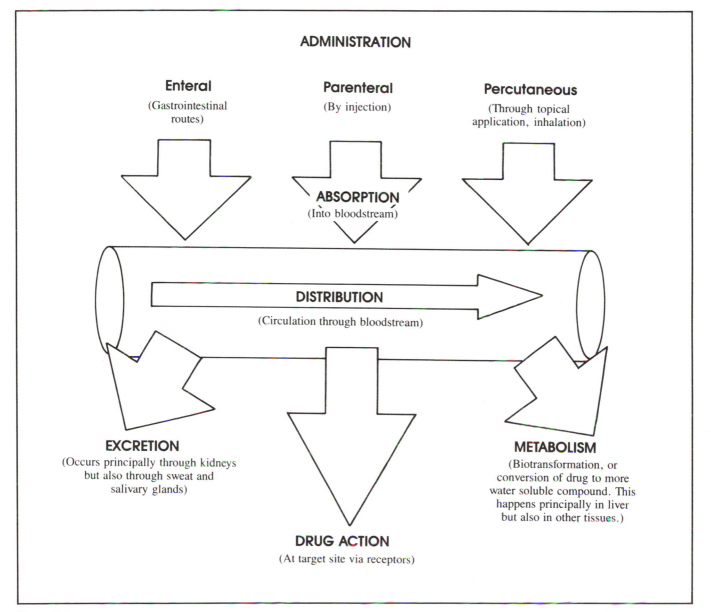

Figure 13-1. Process of Pharmacokinetics.

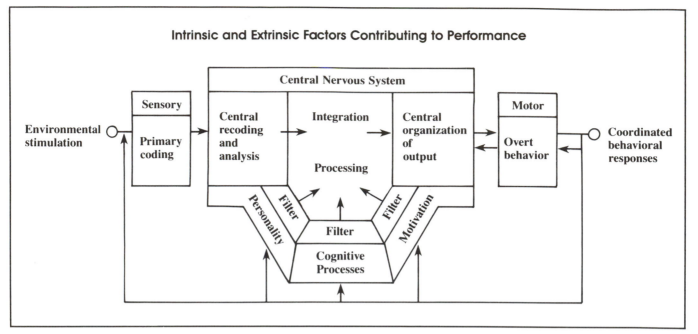

Figure 13-2. Performance occurs through the interaction of the individual's intrinsic components, including motor, sensory, cognitive, psychological, social/interpersonal and physiological characteristics; and extrinsic factors, including social, physical and cultural dimensions. *Adapted from Hindmarch, I. British Journal of Clinical Pharmacology, 10:189-209, 1980.*

body. Frequently, neither the site(s) of action nor the mechanism(s) of action are known for a specific agent.

Research on Pharmacologic Agents and Human Performance

For many years, scientists in the disciplines of psychology, psychopharmacology, and human factors engineering have had an interest in determining the effects of chemical agents on the performance of human tasks. These studies, which can be grouped under the heading of behavioral pharmacology, have become progressively more sophisticated in design and methodology.

An example of early work in this area is provided by Elkin, Fleishman, Van Cott et al. (1965). These scientists studied the effects of different drugs on various categories of human performance. Using standardized tasks that measured cognitive, perceptual, and motor areas, they found variable effects depending on the task performed. That is, some abilities in each area were more affected than others by the same dosage of the drug. The extent to which performance was affected as well as the number of trials necessary to attain maximum performance depended on the ability being measured. Additionally, the duration of the drug's effect also varied across abilities.

For example, in the area of motor performance, the drug scopolamine, which acts as a central nervous system depressant, had only slight negative effect on abilities

defined as dynamic flexibility and explosive strength in normal subjects. However, finger dexterity and multi-limb coordination as demonstrated on a two hand coordination task, were diminished markedly. Varying effects were also found with methylphenidate hydrochloride (Ritalin), which can be therapeutically prescribed to stimulate (in narcolepsy) or reduce (in attention deficit disorders) motor activity depending on the condition (Baker, Geist & Fleishman, 1967).

More recent studies have examined the effect of various drugs on psychomotor tasks under controlled conditions using comparison groups receiving placebos (Hindmarch, 1980; Johnson & Chernik, 1982). A review of 69 such studies, involving 18 tasks and 57 different drugs, has been provided by Wittenborn (1987). These studies used simple or repetitive laboratory tasks involving visual tracking, reaction time, nystagmus, attention, postural stability, digit copying and hand steadiness, among others, to determine the psychomotor effects of the drugs tested. Nineteen drugs were investigated by two or more of the studies, providing some implications based on similarity of findings. Interestingly, similar psychomotor effects were found for several drugs despite differences in their therapeutic use. For example, various drugs classified as hypnotic sedatives, antidepressants, or anxiolytics all resulted in impaired visual tracking, postural sway, and impaired reaction time. In constrast, tests of amphetamines actually yielded enhanced performance on four of the tasks in one study.

Because of the selectivity with which drugs appear to affect human function, it cannot be assumed that an agent which appears to diminish performance on simple tasks will also impair function during more complex activities. Thus, while the studies of psychomotor performance reviewed by Wittenborn provide information based on relatively simple or repetitive tasks in laboratory settings, other studies have attempted to use more complex tasks which simulate the task demands of everyday living.

Parrott (1987) has provided a useful review of many of these studies that have attempted to determine the impact of various drugs on driving, aircraft and space flight, various military tasks, and industrial and classroom situations. With the exception of automobile driving, most applied situations have not been studied in sufficient detail to permit conclusions or generalizations. Impaired driving, however, has been consistently demonstrated following administration or ingestion of alcohol, cannibis, diazepam, lorazepam, and many neuroleptics, barbiturates, antidepressants and sedative hypnotics (Betts, Clayton & McKay, 1972).

The studies described in the preceding paragraphs represent attempts by scientists to determine human performance effects of chemical agents under various laboratory and situational conditions. In contrast, studies by drug manufacturers during product development rely on laboratory animals, healthy volunteers and patients in controlled drug trials. The primary concern in these studies is to determine an agent's therapeutic effects and adverse reactions. Safety and efficacy, rather than affects on task performance, are of principal concern.

The ideal progression of research on the effects of pharmacologic agents in human performance would be to obtain information about a single drug studied under controlled conditions with laboratory animals, in clinical trials, in human studies with laboratory tasks, and in real life situations. Unfortunately, this rarely occurs, so conclusions and generalizations about the effects of specific drugs on performance must be viewed cautiously.

Research findings have permitted us to make some general observations about drugs and human performance, as follows:

1. Performance represents the complex interaction and integration of numerous components. Hence, performance assessment requires the evaluation of multiple subfunctions (Hindmarch & Stonier, 1987).
2. It is not appropriate nor possible to determine the total effect of a single pharmacologic agent through the evaluation of a single test of functional ability (Broadbent, 1984).
3. When developing a profile of effects, it is best to evaluate pharmacological effects by conducting a simulation or a battery of analytical tests (Broadbent, 1984).
4. The individual's motivation to perform a particular task can have a major impact on outcome and can affect the drug action (Hindmarch, 1980).
5. Over time, individuals will develop tolerance to drug effects, and psychological and biochemical changes which are likely to occur will alter the effect of a drug as it is used (Thompson & Trimble, 1982).

Current research is focused on developing refined methods for studying performance-related drug effects using microcomputer technology and exploring the effects of drugs on information processing. Cull and Trimble (1987) have described many of the advantages of using computers in this research, including the ability to present stimuli in a standardized, accurate and error-free manner that assures the accurate recording of behavioral responses. Wesnes, Simpson and Christmas (1987) emphasize the value of examining the effects of drugs on attention, cognition, and memory. This has important implications for research on age-related conditions and the treatment of cognitive dementia in elderly persons. However, older persons present unique challenges in such studies because of changes in their physiological systems, their prevalent need to take multiple medications, and their variability in psychological adjustment to the aging process (Moyes & Moyes, 1987). Fortunately, as the proportion of elderly persons in society increases, interest in the performance-related effects of pharmacological agents is likely to grow. Such increased public attention can only have a beneficial effect on the future development of research in behavioral pharmacology.

DRUGS AND THE INTERACTION OF SYSTEMS

Because of the complex nature of the human organism, we do not have the ability to introduce pharmacological agents which only impact and affect a single or isolated system within the body. As described in Chapter 1, the human is an "open system" in which a change affecting one system resonates to other systems. This dyamic complexity does not permit the identification of specific cause and effect relationships between drugs and specific behavioral changes. Such an "open system" viewpoint helps avoid the pitfall of viewing reactions to drugs in isolation and thus rendering a distorted picture of pharmacologic impact on an individual.

Somewhat paradoxically, despite the complexities of systems and the difficulty associated with determining whether behavioral changes are the result of a specific chemical agent, the action of a drug typically reflects functional specificity. That is, one skill or function may be diminished while others show no apparent impact. In this regard, Broadbent (1984, p. 5) has written that "more generally we have to regard human performance as made up of a number of separate functions. Conditions that cause a deterioration in one of these functions may leave others unaffected." From a practical standpoint, what matters is how a particular chemical agent influences the safe and satisfactory completion of the tasks a given individual must perform. Fortunately, many occupational therapists are in situations which permit them to provide the careful clinical observation necessary to discern both intended and unintended effects of chemical agents from this perspective.

In the sections to follow, specific pharmacologic agents will be reviewed, beginning with those acting on the central nervous system and followed by those acting outside the central nervous system. Within each category and subcategory, specific drugs, their therapeutic purposes, and their possible performance-related side effects and adverse reactions have been identified. Drugs are classified according to generic names and specific brand names (trademarks) used by manufacturers. In each section, the generic name is followed by the brand names, which appear in parentheses. (See Table 13-1) Where they differ, Canadian trade names of described therapeutic agents have been italicized.

DRUGS THAT ACT ON THE CENTRAL NERVOUS SYSTEM

Drugs that affect the central nervous system are more likely to interfere with the performance of the individual than are drugs that affect other organ systems. One group of drugs that depresses the cortical neurons has a hypnotic or sedative action, depending upon the dose taken by the patient. Another group of drugs, also acting to depress the sub-cortical neuron, has an antidepressant or an **anxiolytic** action, depending upon the chemical make-up of the drug. A third category of compounds has the ability to stimulate cortical as well as sub-cortical nuclei resulting in excitatory behavior (Katzung, 1987).

Hypnotic Agents

Drugs can produce cortical depression through nonspecific mechanisms involving slowing of membrane functions. As a result of this depression, the electrical activity of the brain's functioning cells decreases. If a low dose is given, the decrease is mild, resulting in a sedating or calming effect. An increased dose causes a more intense decrease in electrical activity, resulting in a hypnotic or sleep effect.

The barbiturates are classic examples of such drugs. These include secobarbital (Seconal, *Novosecobarb*), pentobarbital (Nembutal, *Novopentobarb, Pentogen*) and

	Table 13-1 Drug Names	
Classification	**Example**	**Explanation**
Chemical Name	4 dimethylamino-1,4, 4a,5,5a, 6,11, 12a ocathydro 3, 6,10, 12,12a-pentahydroxy -6- methyl-1, 11, dioxo-2-naphthcenecarboximide	Used by chemists to describe chemical composition.
Generic Name	tetracycline	The generic name may be used by all countries and by any manufacturer. It is not capitalized. In the United States generic names are provided by the U.S. adopted names council. (See note below)
Official Name	tetracycline, USP*	In the U.S., the official name is the name under which the drug is listed by the U.S. Food and Drug Administration. (See note below)
Brand Names	Achromycin Panmycin Tetracin	Manufacturers often register (trademark) official drugs and market them under trade or proprietary names. These names are capitalized.

*United States Pharmacopeia—a recognized standard for preparation and dispensation of drugs in the U.S. prepared by a national committee of scientific personnel in the U.S. and updated regularly since 1906.

Note: In Canada, an official drug is a drug for which a standard has been prescribed in the Food and Drug Regulations or one that has been listed in an official publication in the Food and Drugs Act. The proper name for a drug in Canada is the generic or non-proprietary name. In some cases, the brand or proprietary name of a drug in Canada differs from that used in the United States.

butabarbital (Butisol, *Day-Barb, Neo-Barb*). Other non-barbiturate hypnotic agents include chloral hydrate (Noctec, *Novochlorhydrate*), glutethimide (Doriden), and ethchlorvynol (Placidyl). These drugs are of some benefit in producing sleep in a person suffering from sleep disorders, but side effects include sluggish behavior the next day with headache and fatigue. These side effects are quite similar to the hangover seen with alcohol which produces its effects by similar activity in the brain tissues. Known performance-related effects include diminished visual acuity, impaired visual tracking, impaired postural stability, impaired reaction time, and decreased ability to perform tasks requiring divided attention. Such effects impose safety risks in the use of mechanical devices, impair driving ability, and may interfere with other aspects of daily functioning (McKim, 1984, p. 97). Several thousand persons die annually in the United States from barbiturate overdose.

Some drugs produce sleep by depression of sub-cortical nuclei via specific receptors. This result is a slowing of the activity within the reticular activating system (RAS). The RAS is thought to be responsible for sleep-wake patterns of daily living and functions to arouse the cortex. The receptor depressing action at the RAS may result in a number of different pharmacological effects, one of which is hypnosis. Drugs acting at this site, and thus reducing cortical arousal, include those of the benzodiazepine class of compounds, including flurazepam (Dalmane, *Apo-Flurazepam, Somnol*), triazolam (Halcion), and temazepam (Restoril)— all useful for treating insomnia. Studies have shown that flurazepam can impair function in complex tasks (such as driving) which require vigilance and the simultaneous performance of two or more subtasks (Moskowitz, 1984). Stone (1984) found significantly impaired performance on paper and pencil tasks requiring arithmetic letter cancellation and digit symbol substitution following adminstration of triazolam. These drugs may also cause hangover, but usually of a much less severe form than that seen with the barbiturates or ethanol. They also may result in confusion and disorientation in persons with head injury or in elderly persons. Fatigue is a common complaint with continued use of these agents (Hamor & Martin, 1983).

Benzodiazepines which are sometimes prescribed to treat seizures are chlorazepate (Tranxene) and clonazepam (Klonopin). Anticonvulsant drugs commonly used include phenobarbital, phenytoin (Dilantin, *Epanutin, Eptoin*), or carbamazepine (Tegretol, *Apo-Carbamazepine, Mazepine*). Patients taking these medications may experience selective depressive action in areas of the brain, which can result in drowsiness, dizziness, with occasional visual disturbances and depression (Eadie, 1984). Some evidence has been found that benzodiazepines can have anterograde amnesic effects, disrupting both short-term and long-term memory

function (Vogel, 1979). However, this side effect is thought to be due to the action of benzodiazapines in producing rapid sleep onset. Betts, Clayton & McKay, (1972), found significant driving impairment after administration of a 50 mg dose of chlordiazepoxide, and Linnoila & Hakkinen, (1974) found that a 10mg dose of diazepam could significantly impair performance on a simulated driving task. In the latter study, the impairments were increased in combination with alcohol.

Other drugs which can be purchased over-the-counter may result in depression of the central nervous system. Antihistamines are one category of these over-the-counter drugs, including two of the most common: chlorpheniramine and diphenhydramine. While antihistamines are used to combat the symptoms of hay fever, allergy, or the common cold, they also cause drowsiness, dullness, confusion and/or fatigue, especially in large doses or in elderly persons. Many of these over-the-counter antihistamines are in liquid form and contain up to 12% alcohol, which may contribute to the undesirable side effects.

Stimulants

Some drugs act as non-specific cortical stimulants to the CNS including the amphetamines, such as methylphenidate (Ritalin) and pemoline (Cylert), cocaine, and caffeine that is found in food, beverages and in many over-the-counter products. These stimulants have an immediate effect on improving the mood and decreasing fatigue. They may also result in symptoms of nervousness, insomnia, loss of appetite, emotional volatility, and irritability.

Ritalin and Cylert are used mainly in children to combat attention deficit disorder (with or without hyperactivity) or in adults as an appetite suppressant or to control symptoms of anxiety on a short-term basis. Caffeine has many CNS effects and affects voluntary skeletal musculature by increasing the force of contractions and decreasing fatigue (Kihlman, 1977). The amphetamines as well as cocaine can eliminate the effects of fatigue on most cognitive and perceptual tasks and on athletic activity (Smith & Beecher, 1959; Weiss, 1969). At high doses, they can also produce psychotic episodes, and result in sexual dysfunction (Siegel, 1982; Smith, Buxton & Dammann, 1979).

Drugs that Act on the Subcortical Level

Drugs that act at the sub-cortical level of the central nervous system include antiparkinson agents, anxiolytics, antidepressants, antimanics, antipsychotics, **analgesics**, and skeletal muscle relaxants. Their effects depend upon two major factors: the chemical nature of the drug and the site of action for the drug. Antiparkinson drugs act to overcome the imbalance of dopamine and aceytlcholine in neurotransmitters within the basal ganglia. This imbalance is thought to cause the tremors, shuffling walk, drooling and hesitant speech seen commonly in persons with Parkinson Disease. The side effects seen with these drugs include dry mouth, blurred vision and muscle weakness that is clinically observed as fatigue. Adverse reactions with these medications can include impaired concentration, depression and mood changes. Drugs in this category include levodopa (L-dopa, Dopar, Larodopa) levodopa-carbidopa (Sinemet), benztropine (Cogentin), and amantadine hydrochloride (Symmetrel) (USPC, 1988).

Anxiolytics

Anxiolytics are widely used agents for calming the anxious person, and may be prescribed as preoperative medication, for alcohol withdrawal, and for seizure disorders. They are also prescribed as an adjunct medication to reduce muscle spasms associated with neuromuscular conditions. Anxiolytics are classified as benzodiazepines and include the drugs diazepam (Valium, *Apo-diazepam*), clonazepam (Klonopin, *Rivotril*), chlordiazepoxide (Librium, *Apo-chlorax*), oxazepam (Serax, *Ox-Pam, Zapex*), alprazolam (Xanax), Lorazepam (Ativan, *Apo-lorazepam*), and clorazepate (Tranxene, *Novoclopate*). Although the exact mechanism of action is unknown, they appear to act on selected receptors of the sub-cortical nuclei of the limbic system and result in a decrease in neuroactivity which produces a calming effect. Frequent side effects include depression, fatigue, and confusion or disorientation. Studies have also shown increased postural sway following administration of diazepam (Swift, 1984), while diazepam and lorazepam have been associated with impaired performance in several psychomotor tasks, including simple reaction time, tracking, and saccadic eye movements (Vogel, 1979). The occupational therapist should be aware of the potential of patients who are taking benzodiazepines to be more vulnerable to accidents than those not taking these dugs. This potential increases with patients taking the longer acting tranquilizers (such as Valium, Dalmane and Librium), although those with a shorter **half-life** (Xanax, Atrian and Serax) still carry this risk. Very young and old persons are extremely sensitive to these drugs (USPC, 1988). Drugs in this class (benzodiazepines) are addictive.

Antidepressants

Antidepressants are drugs that alter amine neuro-transmitters and act to increase the activity of nuclei in select areas of the brain for improving mood, appetite, and alertness in depressed patients. Tricyclic or multicyclic antidepressants have become the most widely used medications of this therapeutic classification and include amitriptyline (Elavil, *Apo-amitriptyline, Levate*),

amoxapine (Ascendin), nortriptyline (Aventyl, Pamelor), imipramine (Tofranil, *Impril*), maprotiline (Ludiomil), and fluoxetine (Prozac). While these agents are useful in overcoming depression, side effects are produced, including dry mouth, blurred vision, constipation, and occasional apprehension. Mental confusion and hesitation may cause an uncooperative behavior in these patients (Thompson & Trimble, 1982). Older patients can have increased sensitivity to these drugs which produces exaggerated effects.

Linnoila, Johnson, & Dubyoski et al. (1984) studied amitriptyline and other antidepressants in healthy male volunteers. They found increased body sway, impaired tracking, and a diminished ability to process information. When combined with ethanol (alcohol), the impairments in performance were even more pronounced.

In cases where depression is resistant to the tricyclic and multicyclic drugs described above, Monoamine Oxidase Inhibitors (MAOIs) are frequently prescribed. MAOIs are capable of blocking or diminishing the activity of MAO, a metabolic regulator, thus resulting in increased amine levels in the brain. MAOIs also block amine uptake, which is thought to account for their clinical usefulness, in antidepressive, antineoplastic, antibiotic, and antihypertensive purposes. Examples of MAOI antidepressants include phenelzine sulfate (Nardil), isocarboxazid (Marplan) and tranylcypromine sulfate (Parnate). These drugs can result in dizziness when changing positions (orthostatic hypotension), tremors, blurred vision, and impaired sexual function. Drowsiness is a common side effect during initial stages of therapy with these drugs, so activities requiring coordination and alertness should be avoided during this period (McHenry & Salerno, 1989).

Antimanics

The affective disorder, mania, results in speech and motor hyperactivity, aggressiveness, poor judgment, elation, and grandiose thinking. This condition may be seen with recurring manic symptoms or in conjunction with depression, in the bipolar affective disorders which have both an acute manic phase and a hypomanic phase, or in alternating periods of mania and depression. In these cases, lithium is frequently prescribed. Lithium is theorized to work by accelerating presynaptic destruction of catecholamines, thus helping to correct the overactive catecholamine systems characteristic of these disorders. Lithium (Lithonate, Eskalith, *Carbolith, Lithizine*) can result in slight tremors of the hands, increased weakness, and respiratory difficulties on exertion.

Antipsychotic or Neuroleptic Agents

Over the past forty years, the evolution of drugs to

control symptoms associated with severe mental disturbance or psychosis has revolutionized psychiatric treatment. About two-thirds of all antipsychotic drugs are derived from phenothiazine (McHenry & Salerno, 1989, p. 311). These agents, thought to derive their effect through blockage of dopamine receptors in the subcortical and basal ganglia areas of the brain, are commonly divided into three chemical subgroups: the aliphathic, piperidine and piperazine compounds. Among the phenothiazines are chlorpromazine (Thorazine, *Chlorpropamide, Lagactil*), thioridazine (Mellaril, *Novoridazine, Apothioridazine*), mesoridazine (Serentil), trilfluoperazine (Stelazine, *Soloazine*), fluphenazine (Permatil, Prolixin, *Apo-Fluphenazine*) and prochlorperazine maleate (Compazine, *Stemetil*). Other frequently prescribed antipsychotic medications are structurally different than phenothiazines but yield similar effects, including haloperidol (Haldol, Apo-Halperidol, *Novoperidol*), thiothixene hydrochloride (Navane) molindone (Lidone, Moban) and loxapine succinate (Loxitane, Daxolin, *Loxapac*) .

Side effects of antipsychotic medications include sleepiness, dizziness, constipation and blurred vision (Kane, 1986). Adverse reactions can include Parkinson-like effects, including shuffling gait, imbalance, masklike facial expressions, tremors, and muscle spasms. Restlessness and insomnia have also been reported with several of the medications. One very serious reaction to these medications is tardive dyskinesia, a potentially irreversible neurologic disorder that results in unwanted facial grimacing, eyelid spasms, lateral jaw movements, and choreoathetoid movements of the extremities. Unfortunately, there is no known effective treatment for this disorder. Approximately 10 to 20% of patients are at risk for this adverse effect, with the risk increasing with total dosage and length of administration (Simpson, Pi & Sramek, 1986).

Analgesics

Analgesics are pain controlling medications that include the salicylates and the non-steroidal anti-inflammatory agents (NSAIAs) as well as the opiate-derived and synthetic opiate drugs. The salicylates, which include aspirin, are beneficial for minor aches and pains. Higher doses can result in salicylate intoxication, resulting in lethargy, dizziness and mental confusion. NSAIAs, which are classified as ''aspirin-like'' drugs, include Fenoprofen (Nalfon), Ibuprofen (Motrin, *Novoprofin*) and Piroxicam (Feldene). These are typically prescribed for mild to moderate pain, particularly with chronic conditions such as rheumatoid arthritis and osteoarthritis and can result in dizziness and lethargy in a small percentage of patients. Acetaminophen (Tylenol, Datril) and propoxyphene (Darvon) are other synthetic agents frequently prescribed

for mild pain which can be used as aspirin substitutes (USPC, 1988).

The analgesics which have the greatest effect on severe pain act centrally on the cortex and include morphine and the opiate synthetic drugs, referred to as **opioids**. Morphine (Roxanol, Morphine Sulfate), and Codeine (Codeine Sulfate, Paveral) are direct derivatives of opium used in clinical medicine today. Meperidine (Demerol, *Pethodine hydrochloride*), Hydromorphone (Dilaudid), and Oxycodone (Percodan, *Supeudol*) are synthetic analgesics frequently prescribed for severe pain. The side effects seen h these drugs include mental cloudiness, hangover, lethargy, and blurred vision. Some alteration of gait may be present with dizziness (Warfield, 1986).

Skeletal Muscle Relaxants

Skeletal muscle relaxants (SMR) have a tendency to depress cortical function by decreasing the activity of nerve transmission in the spinal cord. Skeletal muscle relaxants include baclofen (Lioresal), diazepam (Valium, *Apo-Diazepam, E-Pam*), carisoprodol (Rela, Soma), chlorzoxazone (Paraflex, Parafon), cyclobenzaprine (Flexeril) and metaxalone (Skelaxin). Side effects include feelings of drowsiness and fatigue and hangover after taking the medications for several days. Usually drug therapy for relaxing skeletal muscles has a duration of three weeks or less, thus limiting the degree of impaired performance likely to be observed by the occupational therapist as a result of these drugs (Esenbass, 1980).

DRUGS THAT ACT OUTSIDE THE CENTRAL NERVOUS SYSTEM

Drugs with target sites outside the central nervous system can also produce significant side effects that influence performance. These include the cardiovascular agents, including those that act directly to influence heart rate and rhythm and those designed to influence blood pressure through action on the vascular system.

Cardiovascular Agents

Many cardiovascular agents have the potential for affecting purposeful activity. Some of the most commonly used cardiovascular drugs include quinidine, digoxin, propranolol, atenolol, thiazides, enalapril, and clonidine. Quinidine (Quinidex, Quinaglute, *Apo-Quinidine*) is an antiarrhythmic agent that attempts to control the heart rate. In addition to slowing the activity of the heart, it will also slow skeletal muscle contraction and produce some CNS changes such as tinnitus, blurred vision, and dizziness.

There is also a tendency for these drugs to cause gastrointestinal upset resulting in diarrhea. Because of this, patients taking these drugs may sometimes appear disgruntled and somewhat uncooperative in the tasks assigned by the occupational therapist.

Digoxin (Lanoxin, Manoxin) is prescribed with a therapeutic aim to strengthen the heart beat in congestive heart failure. Due to its long half-life, the drug may accumulate in a patient until overt side effects occur, such as anorexia, nausea, vomiting, headache, dizziness, weakness, and even apathy.

Propranolol (Inderal, *Apo-Propanolol*) and atenolol (Tenormin) are agents used to treat myocardial infarctions as well as high blood pressure. They are known as beta-adrenergic blocking agents. These agents block a select area of the sympathetic nervous system that controls heart rate, thus slowing the heart rhythm. In addition, they act on the myocardial tissue to reduce the risk of a re-infarction. Hypertensive patients also respond to these drugs by a gradual lowering of blood pressure to normal limits. These drugs produce a few side effects. The most bothersome are those affecting the central nervous system, including light headedness, mental depression (with insomnia), lassitude, muscle weakness, fatigue and short-term memory loss. Complaints of decreased libido are fairly common with these drugs.

Thiazide diuretics are widely used to control blood pressure. While these drugs are too numerous to list, it will be useful to discuss a few of those which are most commonly prescribed. These include hydrochlorothiazide, abbreviated HCTZ (Hydrodiuril, *Diuchlor H*), furosemide (Lasix, *Furoside*), and a combination product with the trade name Dyazide. The most frequent complaint following use of these agents is that of muscle fatigue. This is caused by excessive loss of potassium from the body which accompanies the fluid loss which results from their diuretic action and a failure to replace the lost potassium through supplement, such as MicroK or Klotrix tablets. Anorexia, nausea, and vomiting, dizziness and paresthesias of fingers or hands have also been reported. Such side effects can significantly affect the patient's occupational performance.

Enalapril (Vasotec) is an *ACE Inhibitor* in medical jargon, which is a drug that reduces blood pressure by inhibiting select enzyme activity in the body that results in hypotension. Side effects include an altered sense of taste, nausea and vomiting. Clonidine (Catapres) is a drug that decreases activity of the sympathetic nervous system and helps reduce hypertension. Its pharmacological classification is that of an alpha-2 blocking drug, which results in a centrally-induced decrease in blood pressure. Dry mouth and sedation are frequent side effects. In addition, mental depression may be unmasked by this drug. Complaints of decreased libido have been associated with the use of clonidine (Katzung, 1987).

Antimicrobial Agents

These medications are designed to treat bacterial, fungal, and viral infections. The majority of the antimicrobial drugs are relatively safe for the patient while quite toxic to the target organism. **Antimicrobial** drugs typically act through inhibiting the synthesis of the cell wall, protein, or essential metabolites, or through disruption of membrane permeability. It is important to note that antimicrobial drugs do not kill all organisms but rather work against a specific group or particular spectrum of organisms. Some antibiotics do not destroy existing organisms (bactericidal), but rather prevent the development of additional bacterial organisms within a colony (bacteriostatic).

Adverse reactions to antimicrobial agents may include superinfections as well as allergies and hypersensitivity. Superinfections are clinical infections which result from the proliferation of resistant strains of bacteria during antimicrobial therapy for therapeutic or prophylactic reasons. Such infections, which occur in approximately 2% of persons treated with antibiotics, are identified and treated through discontinuation of the initial drug and administration of other appropriate antimicrobial agents.

Reactions due to hypersensitivity are more common and include nausea, vomiting, diarrhea, and skin rashes of a non-allergic nature. The allergic reactions to the penicillins are well noted and range from uticaria (hives) to anaphylactic shock. Anaphylaxis is the most serious type of antimicrobial allergic reaction and can occur anywhere from a few seconds to 30 minutes following an injection. The syndrome begins with diffuse flushing, itching and warmth, followed by generalized body edema. As the reaction progresses, upper airway edema can occur causing possible obstruction and respiratory difficulty from pulmonary involvement. Antihistamine treatment is administered to reverse the vascular effects of anaphylaxis.

The cephalosporins, in particular, Mefoxin, have been known to produce a disulfiram-like (Antabuse) reaction resulting in a sensitivity to alcohol causing nausea and vomiting. Tetracycline antibiotics, such as demeclocycline (Declomycin), can cause photosensitivity, thus making it advisable for patients undergoing chemotherapy with such agents to avoid prolonged exposure to the sun. Reactions to photosensitivity may cause some degree of itching and mental distraction in some patients. Dizziness and vertigo have occurred with minocycline (Minocin), especially at high doses.

Antifungal drugs include flucytosine (Ancobon, *Ancotil*),

and ketoconazole (Nizoral). Side effects for these drugs include headaches, nausea, and dizziness. Use of the antiviral agents acyclovir (Zovirax) and amantadine hydrochloride (Symadine, Symmetrel) can be accompanied by loss of appetite, dizziness, and insomnia (McHenry & Salerno, 1989).

Antineoplastic Agents

The rate of reported instances of cancer has increased 74% since 1971, with a 40% increase in mortality from these diseases (American Cancer Society, 1986). The fact that mortality has not climbed proportionately to incidence reflects the progress that has been made in treating cancer. Some of this progress is related to advancements in chemotherapy, particularly the development of antineoplastic drugs which act to destroy cancerous cells or inhibit their proliferation. One significant advancement has been the use of combinations of agents that can act collectively against specific cancers at different sites of action without increasing the adverse effects of toxicity.

Side effects of most **antineoplastic agents** include alopecia (hair loss), nausea, loss of appetite, and stomatitis. Adverse effects include bone marrow suppression and the destruction of blood cells which can have life threatening consequences. Liver, kidney, and cardiac function can be impaired at toxic doses of some drugs, as well as various neurological reactions, such as tingling of the distal extremities, ataxia, confusion and personality changes.

Psychological problems, aside from those that derive from the threat of serious illness, may accompany bodily changes resulting from chemotherapy. Alopecia can have a dramatic effect on body image, despite the availability of cosmetic aids or the realization that the condition is temporary. Hormonal changes may occur which affect the sex related characteristics of both men and women.

Of considerable importance are the hematologic changes that can place the individual at serious risk should infection or tissue damage occur, since infection-fighting or clotting mechanisms may be impaired. For this reason, care must be taken to ensure safe environments for patients in these risk categories (Ristuccia, 1985).

Sociopsychological Considerations in Drug Use

As reflected in Chapter 4, the cultural belief systems of individuals have a profound effect on their roles and behaviors, including their health-related practices. These influences are also reflected in an individual's responses to drugs, since their symbolic meaning can have a psychological effect that works in conjunction with the psychodynamic action of a particular agent. Studies have shown that attitudes toward medications may influence their effectiveness.

The impact of beliefs on the action of drugs is dramatically illustrated in placebo studies. Placebos include any therapeutic procedure that elicits a response because of its perceived intent rather than its known properties or ingredients. The medical literature contains abundant documentation of positive physiological changes with placebo therapy, including the relief of post surgical pain. Moreover, subjects who report placebo effects have included well-educated persons whose personality characteristics do not suggest increased gullibility or neuroticism.

Medications may be viewed as symbols of help or danger to the individual using them, depending upon their previous experience, current situation, and mental state. Drugs may symbolize the dependent state of someone under care, thus challenging their feelings of control and independence. If there are secondary gains associated with an illness, the patient may feel some ambivalence at the prospect of improvement and may exaggerate side effects in order to avoid taking the medication or in order to gain the additional attention or freedom from responsibility accorded to those in the *sick role*.

Attitudes about the effectiveness of a particular drug may also influence compliance behaviors. Patients who have experienced adverse side effects may act to reduce the amount and frequency of a recommended dosage, thus diminishing its effectiveness. Conversely, in the belief that a prescribed dosage is too weak, some patients may increase their intake of a particular medication or continue taking it beyond the prescribed period. These behaviors can lead to habitual usage or adverse reactions due to toxic overdoses in some drugs (Brown, Wright & Christensen, 1987).

In concluding this section, mention should be made of over-the-counter drugs (OTCs) and the potential danger of self-medication practices. Various age-related and socio-cultural factors can foster misuse of these medications. The inability or unwillingness to read and understand packaged product information due to visual or cognitive impairment, language barriers, or casual attitudes toward medication, can individually or collectively lead to dangerous practices. These can include overdose, lack of awareness concerning potential drug interactions, and the masking of symptoms indicating serious conditions (Wilkinson, Darby & Mant, 1987).

SOURCES OF DRUG INFORMATION

Drug effects can include those which have a beneficial effect as well as alteration of human function. It is impossible for health professionals to know all of the different reactions that may occur due to the various pharmacologic therapies. Sources of information which can be used by the practicing professional are described in the following paragraphs.

Sources of Information about Drugs in the United States

American Hospital Formulary Service is published annually by the American Society of Hospital Pharmacists in Bethesda, Maryland. This reference has been adopted by the U.S. Public Health Service and the Veteran's Administration as an official reference and approved by several professional societies, including the American Hospital Association and the American Pharmaceutical Association. Updated quarterly, the volume contains monographs on every drug available in the United States. Each monograph has sections on chemistry, administration, dosages, drug interactions and toxicity.

The Physician's Desk Reference (PDR) is a widely used source for drug information, providing product information supplied by the manufacturer including that contained in the product circular. Color coded sections provide indexes and information on manufacturers, product names, product classifications, generic and chemical names, product identification, product information, and diagnostic product information. This information includes the drug's pharmacology, indications for use, contraindications, warnings and precautions concerning adverse reactions as well as the appropriate dose to be used to provide therapeutic effects. The section on adverse reactions typically includes those that are most commonly reported as well as those that are reported as being seen infrequently. Through use of the PDR, occupational therapists can become quickly informed about possible adverse effects of the specific medications prescribed for their patients.

Facts and Comparisons is a drug compendium that is much more exhaustive than the PDR. Whereas the *Physician's Desk Reference* is somewhat selective and does not include many older and generic drugs, *Facts and Comparisons* is updated monthly and provides a comparison of many drugs based on data from Food and Drug Administration (FDA) approved package inserts. The format for *Facts and Comparisons* is a loose leaf compendium with twelve chapters, each containing a detailed table of contents. Updated supplements for the entire book are provided on a monthly basis.

Package Inserts are a comprehensive but concise description of drugs which are developed by manufacturers and approved by the FDA as a requirement of federal law. These printed descriptions include indications and precautions for clinical use, contraindications, recommendations for dosage, and known adverse reactions,

and must be included with each package of the product distributed by the manufacturer.

The *Handbook of Non-Prescription Drugs* is published by the American Pharmaceutical Association and is a comprehensive guide to over-the-counter medications. Information is organized by individual chapters on product categories, including antacids, cold and allergy products, vitamins and minerals, nutritional supplements, and feminine hygiene products. Each chapter contains information useful for the evaluation of symptoms, suggested treatments with recommended dosages, and a list of medications with their ingredients.

Sources of Information About Drugs in Canada

The *Compendium of Pharmaceuticals and Specialties (CPS)* is an annual publication of the Canadian Pharmaceutical Association. Its six color coded sections provide information on specific brands, manufacturers and distributors of pharmaceutical products in Canada, and useful tables and guidelines for conversions. Also included are sections which contain standards, reporting procedures, product recognition information, and medical abbreviations.

Canadian Self Medication (CSM) is also published by the Canadian Pharmaceutical Association. As its title suggests, it provides comprehensive information on nonprescription drug products available in Canada. Chapters are organized by therapeutic category, including sunscreens, eye care, laxatives, common cold, and allergies. Each chapter reviews the conditions suitable for self-medication, presents alternatives, and suggestions for general as well as pharmacologic management. An interesting feature is the product ingredient index, which identifies the brands containing a specific substance.

Other Information Resources

Basic pharmacology texts can be used to supplement the specific information provided in references listed above. Pharmacology texts are designed to provide general and specific information concerning classes and particular types of agents.

The practicing clinician may have a tendency to become overwhelmed with the number of adverse side effects listed in the various publications. It is wise for the clinician to be cautious when interpreting patient behaviors which could indicate drug effects, such as confusion or lack of cooperation (Physician's Desk Reference, 1989). A pharmacist can be a valuable resource to the occupational therapist in gaining understanding about individual patients and specific drugs.

THE THERAPIST'S ROLE IN MONITORING DRUG EFFECTS

Occupational therapists are in an excellent position to observe and assess drug-related performance deficits, whether they are readily apparent or reflected in the more subtle qualitative dimensions of task performance. While many medications produce side effects, it is difficult to establish with certainty that a single chemical agent is responsible for observed symptoms or behaviors. For this reason, therapists should consider the following information prior to concluding that a given behavior is the result of a chemical agent:

1. A wide range of chemical agents, ranging from those included in foods and beverages to over-the-counter and prescribed medications, can have some effect on performance.
2. The specific effect of any agent on performance cannot currently be determined because of the complexity of factors influencing performance.
3. The effect of chemical agents on performance cannot be generalized across tasks. Tasks requiring certain skills may be affected, while those requiring other skills are not.
4. Changes in a patient's performance thought to be the result of chemical agents should be reported to the attending physician, as appropriate.
5. Since knowledge about drugs and their effects and interactions is constantly changing, it is important to consult reliable sources of information. Resources can include pharmacists and other health professionals as well as drug-related references and current textbooks on pharmacology.

Clinical Implications of Drug Effects

Table 13-2 provides a summary of the major categories of drugs reviewed in this chapter and their effect on various areas of performance. The actual effects an individual may experience depend, of course, on many variables such as age, dosage level, possible interactions with other chemical agents being taken concomitantly, and possible interactions with disease processes other than that for which the medication is primarily prescribed. For example, if a patient diagnosed as having mild to moderate hypertension, becomes clinically depressed and begins taking a tricyclic antidepressant (such as amitriptyline (i.e., Elavil, Apo-Amitriptyline), it is possible that the patient's blood pressure will be lowered. Often, it may be sufficiently decreased for the patient to stop taking any anti-hypertension medication as long as he/she is receiving the anti-depressant.

Occupational therapists treat patients with both acute and chronic illnesses, so that short-term as well as long-term medication effects will be observed. These may alter patients' performance in many areas, including psychomotor functioning, perceptions, speech, coordination, level of arousal, attention span, memory and behavior. The occupational therapist typically has a broader scope of interaction with a patient, and thus a greater opportunity than other health care providers to recognize alterations in performance that may be due to medications. Accurate descriptions of these effects are valuable to physicians. Observations must be clearly described and communicated in order to aid the physician in making adjustments in medication or therapy to improve the overall quality of care for the patient (Lerfald, 1988).

MEDICATION CASE STUDIES

The following case examples describe patients who are receiving psychotropic medications. They illustrate the types of behavioral and performance effects to which the occupational therapist should be alert.

Case Study 13-1

Mrs. Gray is a 35-year-old mother of three children. She is very devoted to maintaining predictable family rituals. Her children, ages 6, 8, and 11, know that on Saturday night they eat dinner at a pizza place and then go home to watch VCR movies. Even though other evenings are fragmented with meetings, lessons and practices, Saturday evening is a whole-family event.

Mrs. Gray became depressed about a month after school started and was tearful. Her appetite and energy diminished, and eventually she began experiencing panic attacks. She was evaluated at a local Mood Disorders Clinic and was diagnosed as having major depressive disorder with associated panic attacks. The MAO inhibitor, Nardil, was prescribed. She was given extensive education about the drug and was particularly alerted to its potential interaction with substances in food that could produce a serious, even life-threatening hypertensive crisis. Mrs. Gray, a conscientious woman, carefully avoided foods that might be dangerous to her. She decided to give up the Saturday night pizza dinner because of the abundance of cheese and the other foods that were on the list of dietary restrictions for persons taking Nardil.

When Mrs. Gray first became depressed, the children had been alarmed at the changes in their mother, but as her mood normalized and she became more energetic and more like the mom they knew, they were reassured that she was once again okay. However, as time went on, the youngest child

Table 13-2
Effects of Selected Chemical Agents

Category	Antidepressants	Stimulants	Benzodiazeprines	Barbiturates	Methylxanthines	Opioids
Types	MAO inhibitors Tricyclic antidepressants Second generation antidepressants	d-amphetamine l-amphetamine Cocaine	Drugs in this category evolved from the development of chlordiazepoxide, marketed in 1958 as Librium.	Drugs in this category evolved from barbituric acid. They differ in their speed of action and duration, ranging from 5 minutes to 12 hours.	Drugs in this category are also known as xanthine stimulants and are derived from plants. These chemical agents are found in coffee, tea, & chocolate.	Drugs in this category include natural opiates, synthetic opiates, and opiate antagonists, which block the effects of the opioids
Generic Examples	tranylcyropromine imipramine amitryptyline magnesium pemoline	methylphenidate piprodol methamphetamine ephidrene	diazepam flurazepam oxazepam chlorazepate	phenobarbitol pentobarbital secobarbitol thiopental hexobarbitol	caffeine theobromine theophylline	heroin meperidine methadone morphine naxolone
Therapeutic Purposes	Prescribed for the treatment of depression.	Prescribed for weight reduction, narcolepsy, asthma. OTC as stimulant.	Prescribed for anxiety, muscle relaxation, insomnia and for controlling seizures.	Prescribed for anxiety, insomnia and for controlling seizures, as in epilepsy.	Prescribed for asthma, neonatal respiratory difficulties, and used in OTC cold and headache remedies.	Prescribed as analgesics for the relief of severe pain.
Physiologic Effects	Can cause dry mouth, constipation, dizziness, drowsiness, muscle twitches, tremors, blurred vision, arrythmia.	Can cause dry mouth, headache, anorexia, insomnia, gastrointestinal disturbances, dizziness, palpitations.	Reduce muscle tone, increases appetite, and reduce the time required to fall asleep. Can result in hangover effect on days following administration of single doses.	Reduce respiratory rate and blood pressure. Decrease the amount of time required to fall asleep. Effects are similar to those of alcohol.	These agents relax smooth muscles, strengthen striated muscles, constrict blood vessels in the brain, increase spinal reflexes, increase respiratory rate and can produce insomnia.	Usually result in nausea and vomiting on initial administration. They can result in increased sweating, constricted pupils, constipation, decreased libido and decreased fertility.
Effects on Behavior and Performance	These drugs improve the mood. They can result in apprehension and occasionally result in uncooperative behavior. Impaired visual tracking, postural instability, and information processing have been reported.	These drugs can improve the state of alertness and elevate the mood. Temporal awareness is diminished, endurance is increased, and reaction time is improved. Continued use can lead to stereotyped behavior or aggression.	Can decrease visual acuity, impair reaction time, and diminish performance on tasks involving calculation, and figure tracing. They can also cause feelings of fatigue and confusion as well as increased aggressive behavior.	These drugs distort the perception of time, decrease visual acuity and increase postural sway. They have also been shown to impair athletic performance and driving ability. With extended use, short term memory is impaired.	These drugs can increase the perception of alertness and enhance performance on perceptual tasks and physical activities reduced by fatigue. Some studies have shown subjective improvements in mood and attitude.	May produce feelings of euphoria. In higher doses can produce lethargy. Among elderly persons, they can produce confusion and other CNS effects.
Special Notes	Exaggerated effects are found when these drugs interact with alcohol. Mood effects are long lasting.	Ritalin, a methylphenidate, has a paradoxical effect in children with attention deficit disorder.	Some studies have shown that these drugs impair driving ability.	With continuous use at high doses, these drugs can cause neglect of self care and intellectual impairment.	High levels of caffeine can result in "caffeinism," increasing anxiety. Caffeine can also interfere with the effects of psychotropic drugs.	One of the unique features of opioid drugs is the rapid and extensive development of tolerance to them.

became withdrawn and clinging. While comforting the child, Mrs. Gray discovered that the child's fears of changes and her mother's illness were compounded when they eliminated the Saturday night pizza ritual.

This case demonstrates that prescribed drugs (and their potential interactions) while pertaining to individual patients, also affect families. It serves as a vivid illustration of both the socio-psychological dimensions of pharmacology, as well as the nature of systems theory. Recall that changes in one component of a system (in this case an individual family member) have an influence on other components (in this case, other members of the family).

Case Study 13-2

Mr. Carl was seen at a mood disorder clinic after months of decreasing function that involved dysphoria, sleep disturbance, loss of appetite, loss of energy, decreased interest in sex, and contemplation of suicide. Following the initial assessment, his symptoms were diagnosed as a single episode of major depression. He was placed on Pamelor (nortriptyline), an antidepressant medication with fewer side effects than Elavil.

Although Mr. Carl noticed a slightly dry mouth and very mild daytime sedation as side effects of his medication, within two weeks he reported improvement in all symptoms. Mr. Carl was a successful businessman, and about three weeks after treatment began his employees noticed he was becoming much more energetic. Each day he planned changes in the organization of the business and soon announced that henceforth he would share all profits with the employees. He purchased an expensive new car and began to be seen daily in the company of several young women. His family, friends, and co-workers were pleased that he no longer appeared depressed, but were alarmed as his actions became more grandiose.

It was discovered that Mr. Carl was experiencing a phenomenon known as "switching". The antidepressant drug therapy had revealed a patient with bipolar (manic-depressive) illness, and Mr. Carl was switching from the depressive phase into the manic phase of his disorder. Once his condition was accurately diagnosed, the tricyclic antidepressant he had been receiving was discontinued, and lithium, an antipsychotic drug often used for bipolar affective disorders, was prescribed.

SUMMARY

This chapter has provided an overview of the basic mechanisms of pharmacokinetics. Major categories of chemical agents that are used for therapeutic purposes have been reviewed, with particular consideration given to the effects of these substances on the performance of tasks required for everyday living. In many cases, it has been emphasized that the methods through which various chemical agents accomplish their therapeutic purposes is unkown. This is due both to the complexity of the human organism as well as our incomplete knowledge regarding the chemistry of physiological processes, particularly in the central nervous system. The principles of systems theory are useful for providing a conceptual framework in which these complexities can be viewed. However, much research is needed to expand and refine our knowledge of these mechanisms. The increasing sophistication provided by the technical advances in brain imagery will lead to a greater appreciation of the mechanisms of action by chemical agents and will ultimately allow us to predict, with some reliability, their effects on performance.

Occupational therapists can make an important and special contribution to pharmacological research and patient care by monitoring behavioral performance changes which occur with various drug regimens. In addition, through their knowledge of the psychosocial factors, side effects, adverse reactions and precautions associated with prescribed and over-the-counter medications, therapists can contribute to improved compliance and an awareness of the safety factors associated with pharmacological treatment.

Study Questions

1. Identify five variables that influence the action of a specific chemical agent.

2. Describe major elements in the process of pharmacokinetics.

3. Differentiate between the generic and proprietary names of drugs.

4. Distinguish between side effects and adverse reactions.

5. List common sources of drug information.

6. Describe social and cultural factors which influence medication use and compliance.

7. Identify and describe side effects you have experienced.

Acknowledgment

Grateful acknowledgment is made to Carolyn Baum and Terry Malone, who made extensive contributions to the development of this chapter.

Note to the Reader

The authors, editors and publisher have made a conscientious effort to ensure that the information about drugs cited in this chapter is accurate at the time of publication. However, advances in pharmacology occur rapidly, so readers should consult literature provided by manufacturers for the most current information on a given drug. Because this chapter is presented as an overview of selected pharmacologic information viewed as relevant to occupational therapists, only selected examples of drugs, their intended therapeutic effects, known side effects, and adverse reactions have been provided. Accordingly, readers are advised that the inclusion of a listed drug or brand name should not be construed as an endorsement of that drug or a particular product or brand. Similarly, the omission of a particular drug does not indicate that the product has been judged to be unacceptable.

Recommended Readings

American Pharmaceutical Association. (1982). *Handbook of Nonprescription Drugs,* (7th ed) Washington, D.C.: Author

American Society of Hospital Pharmacists (1987). *Drug Information.* Bethesda, MD: Author.

Asperheim, M. K. (1987). *Pharmacology, an introductory text.* (6th ed). Philadelphia: Saunders.

Gilman, Alfred & Goodman, Louis S.(Eds) (1985). *The Pharmacological Basis of Therapeutics* (7th Ed). New York: MacMillan Company.

Hansten, P.D., & Horn, J.R. (1989). *Drug Interactions: clinical significance of drug-drug interactions.* (6th ed) Philadelphia: Lea & Febiger.

Iversen, S.D. (1981). *Behavioral pharmacology.* (2 Ed). New York: Oxford University Press.

Katcher B.S., Young L.Y., & Koda-Kimble M.A. (1983). *Applied Therapeutics: The Clinical Uuse of Drugs.* (3rd ed) San Francisco: Applied Therapeutics

Katcher, B.S. (1988). *Prescription Drugs: An Indispensible Guide for Persons Over Fifty.* New York: Atheneum

Katzung, B.G. (1988). *Clinical Pharmacology.* Norwalk, CT: Appleton and Lange

Levine, R.R. (1983) *Pharmacology: Drug Actions and Reactions* (3rd Ed), Boston: Little, Brown and Company.

Malone, T.R. (ed.). (1989). *Physical and Occupational Therapy: Drug implications for practice.* Philadelphia: J.B. Lippincott

McKim, W.A. (1986). *Drugs and Behavior. An Introduction to Behavioral Pharmacology.* Englewood Cliffs, NJ: Prentice Hall.

Rakel, R.E. (1987) *Conn's Current Therapy.* Philadelphia, W.B. Saunders.

References

American Cancer Society. (1986). *Cancer facts and figures.* New York: The Society.

Baker, W.J., Geist, A.M., & Fleishman, E.A. (1967). *Effects of cylert (magnesium-permoline) on physiological, physical proficiency and psychomotor performance measures.* Washington, D.C.: American Institutes for Research.

Betts, T.A., Clayton, A.B., & McKay, G.M. (1972). Effects of four commonly used tranquilizers on low-speed driving performance tests. *British Medical Journal, 4,* 580-584.

Broadbent, D.E. (1984). Performance and its measurement. *British Journal of Pharmacy, 18*: 5-9 (supplement).

Brown, C.S., Wright, R.G., & Christensen, D.B. (1987). Association between type of medication instruction and patients' knowledge, side effects, and compliance. *Hospital and Community Psychiatry, 38*(1), 55-60.

Cull, C., & Trimble, M.R., (1987). Automated testing and psychopharmacology. In I. Hindmarch & P.D. Stonier (Eds). *Human psychopharmacology. Measures and methods.* (Volume 1). (pp. 113-154) Chichester, England: John Wiley & Sons.

Eadie, M.J. Anticonvulsant drugs: An update. *Drugs. 27*(4) 328-363.

Elkin, E.H., Fleishman, E.A., Van Cott, H.P., Horowitz, H., & Freedle, R.O. (1965). *Effects of drugs on human performance: Research concepts, test development, and preliminary studies.* Washington, D.C.: American Institutes for Research.

Elenbaas, J.K. (1980). Centrally acting oral skeletal muscle relaxants. *American Journal of Hospital Pharmacy, 30*(10), 1313-1323.

Hamor, T.A., & Martin, I.L. (1983). The benzodiazeprines. *Progress in Medicinal Chemistry, 20,* 157-223.

Henderson, G., & Primeaux, M. (1981). *Transcultural health care.* Menlo Park, CA: Addison-Wesley.

Hindmarch, I. (1980). Psychomotor function and psychoactive drugs. *British Journal of Clinical Pharmacology, 10,* 189-209.

Hindmarch, I., & Stonier, P.D. (1987). *Human psychopharmacology. Measures and methods.* Chichister, England: John Wiley & Sons.

Johnson, L.C., & Chernik, D.A. (1982). Sedative hypnotics and human performance. *Psychopharmacology, 76,* 101-113.

Kane, J.M. (1986). Neuroleptics in the treatment of schizophrenia. *Hospital Therapy, 11*(9) 111-117.

Katzung, B. (1987). *Basic and clinical pharmacology,* (3rd Edition) Los Altos, California: Appleton and Lange.

Kihlman, B.A. (1977). *Caffeine and chromosomes.* Amsterdam: Elsevier.

Linnoila, M., & Hakkinen, T. (1974). Effects of diazepam and codeine alone and in combination with alcohol, on simulated driving. *Clinical Pharmacology and Therapeutics, 15,* 368-373.

Linnoila, M., Johnson, J. Dubyoski, K., Buchsbaum, M., Schneinin, M., & Kilts, C. (1984). Effects of antidepressants on skilled performance. *British Journal of Clinical Phamacology, 18,* 109-120 (Supplement).

Lerfald, S. (1988). Personal communication.

McHenry, L.M., & Salerno, E. (1989). *Pharmacology in nursing.* St. Louis: C. V. Mosby.

McKim, W.A. (1986). *Drugs and behavior. An introduction to behavioral pharmacology.* Englewood Cliffs, NJ: Prentice Hall.

Medical Economics Company. (1988). *Physicians desk reference,* (43rd Edition). Oradell, NJ: Charles Baker.

Moskowitz, H. Attention tasks as skills performance measures of drug effects. *British Journal of Clinical Pharmacology, 18,* 51-61 (Supplement).

Moyes, I.C.A., & Moyes, R.B. (1987). Problems of assessment of function in the elderly. In I. Hindmarch & P. D. Stonier (Eds). *Human psychopharmacology. Measures and methods.* (Volume 1). (pp. 213-230) Chichester, England: John Wiley & Sons.

Parrott, A.C. (1987). Assessment of psychological performance in applied situations. In I. Hindmarch & P.D. Stonier (Eds). *Human psychopharmacology. Measures and methods.* (Volume 1). (pp. 213-230) Chichester, England: John Wiley & Sons.

Ristuccia, A.M. (1985). Hematologic effects of cancer chemotherapy. *Nursing Clinics of North America, 20*(1), 235-239.

Siegel, R. K. (1982). Cocaine and sexual dysfunction: the curse of mama coca. *Journal of Psychoactive Drugs, 14,* 71-74.

Simpson, G.M., Pi, E.H., & Sramek, J.J. (1986). An update on tardive dyskinesia. *Journal of Hospital and Community Psychiatry, 37*(4) 362-369.

Smith, G.M., & Beecher, H.K. (1959). Amphetamine sulfate and athletic performance. *Journal of the American Medical Association,* 542-549.

Smith, D.E., Buxton, M.E., & Dammann, G. (1979). Amphetamine abuse and sexual dysfunction: Clinical and research considerations. In D.R. Smith (Ed). *Amphetamine use, misuse, and abuse* (pp. 228-248). Boca Raton, FL: CRC Press.

Stone, B.M. (1984). Paper and pencil tests-sensitivity to psychotropic drugs. *British Journal of Clinical Phamacology, 18,* 15-20 (Supplement).

Swift, C.G. (1984). Postural instability as a measure of sedative drug response. *British Journal of Clinical Pharmacology, 18,* 87-90 (Supplement).

Thompson P.J., & Trimble M.R. (1982). Non MAOI antidepressant drugs and cognitive functions: a review. *Psychological Medicine, 12,* 539-548.

United States Pharmacopeia Convention (1988). *Drug information for the health care provider* (8th Ed), Rockville, Maryland: United States Pharmacopeia Convention, Inc.

Vogel, J. R. (1979). Objective measurement of human performance changes produced by anti-anxiety drugs. In J. Fielding & S. Lal (Eds) *Anxiolytics.* (pp. 343-374) New York: Futura.

Warfield, C.A. (1986). Psychotropic agents for pain control: Clinical guidelines. *Hospital Practice, 20*(5), 141-143.

Weiss, B. (1969). Enhancement of performance by amphetamine like drugs. In F. Sjoquist & M. Tottie, (Eds). *Abuse of central stimulants.* (pp. 31-60). Stockholm: Almqvist & Wiksell.

Wesnes, K., Simpson, P., & Christmas, L. (1987). Problems of assessment of function in the elderly. In I. Hindmarch & P.D. Stonier (Eds). *Human psychopharmacology. Measures and methods.* (Volume 1). (pp. 79-92). Chichester, England: John Wiley & Sons.

Wilkinson, I.F., Darby, D.N., & Mant, A. (1987). Self-care and self-medication: An evaluation of individuals' Health care decisions, *Medical Care, 25*(10), 965-978.

Wittenborn, J. R. (1987). Psychomotor tests in Psychopharmacology. In I. Hindmarch & P.D. Stonier (Eds). *Human psychopharmacology. Measures and methods.* (Volume 1). (pp. 69-78). Chichester, England: John Wiley & Sons.

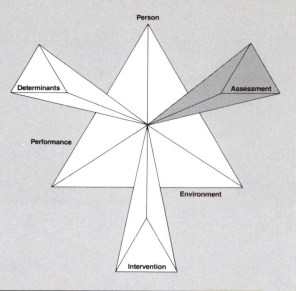

Section Three

Assessment
of Performance

CHAPTER CONTENT OUTLINE

KEY TERMS

Assessment

Construct

Criterion-referenced test

Efficacy

Mean score

Median score

Mode

Norm-referenced test

Raw score

Reliability

Test sensitivity

Specificity

Standardized test

Standard deviation

Standard scores

Validity

ABSTRACT

This chapter identifies the principles of informed decision-making, ethical and philosophical considerations in selecting appropriate assessment instruments, and the categories of assessments and assessment strategies. The chapter also provides a critical analysis of assessment tools and defines terminology associated with tests and measurements. The therapist's role in assessment and clinical decision-making is discussed, particularly the importance of assessment in communicating and resolving performance problems, careful consideration of ethical concerns, and the therapist's responsibility to continually question the nature of performance problems while providing occupational therapy.

Assessment and Informed Decision-Making

Karin Joann Opacich

"In the terrain of professional practice, applied science and research-based technique occupy a critically important though limited territory, bounded on several sides by artistry. These are an art of problem framing, an art of implementation, and an art of improvisation—all necessary to mediate the use in practice of applied science and technique."

—Schön, 1987

OBJECTIVES

The information in this chapter is intended to help the reader—

1. recognize the importance of assessment in communicating and resolving performance problems.

2. become aware of the important elements involved in the process of informed decision-making.

3. understand the meaning and importance of reliability and validity in assessment.

4. understand the terminology associated with tests and measurements.

5. gain the knowledge to critically analyze assessment strategies and tools.

6. comprehend the impact of assessment in shaping occupational therapy intervention.

7. realize the responsibility to question the nature of performance problems in order to provide effective occupational therapy.

INTRODUCTION

Assessment is a process by which data are gathered, hypotheses formulated, and decisions made for further action. In occupational therapy, assessment of performance assets and deficits guides the establishment of treatment goals and interventions. The effectiveness of the selected interventions is determined by subsequent assessment. When incorporated as an integral part of the process, assessment influences clinical reasoning and action. Additionally, assessment may be necessary to substantiate insurance claims, facilitate school placement, determine independent living status, support litigation, document need for a specific program, or establish competence on the job.

Without assessment, goal-directed therapy becomes impossible. Assessment provides the vantage point for constructing a rational approach to problem resolution. Carefully selected assessment strategies and instruments enhance the quality of clinical decisions. The American Occupational Therapy Association and the American Occupational Therapy Foundation Committee on Standardized Assessments/Evaluations developed a hierarchy of competencies related to the use of instruments and evaluation techniques to guide the preparation of occupational therapy practitioners (Maurer, Barris, Bonder & Gillette, 1984). These guidelines underscore the importance of the assessment process on clinical decision-making. According to Ottenbacher (1987), a respected occupational therapy researcher:

> A large part of our task as an emerging profession is to establish the importance of planned scientific inquiry to the practice of occupational therapy . . . .We educate ourselves and our colleagues by generating, refining, and testing new ideas and treatments, that is, by expanding our existing knowledge base. To expand our knowledge base, we must be actively involved in scientific inquiry relevant to occupational therapy. To avoid the apathy generated by scientific dependency, we must all be involved, at some level, in the systematic questioning and refining of existing intervention methods designed to advance the science of occupational therapy (pp. 214, 215).

Assessment provides the scientific foundation for decisions which in turn allow practitioners to demonstrate artistry in the therapeutic process.

PRINCIPLES OF INFORMED DECISION-MAKING

Terminology

An *assessment strategy* is a process which yields information about the nature of an identified problem. The term, *evaluation,* is often used interchangeably but implicitly adds the element of judgment regarding the problem or condition. In most cases, occupational therapists employ more than one assessment strategy to profile a problem. Assessment strategies are assessment techniques, instruments, or tests designed to gather data which enable the practitioner to formulate a comprehensive understanding of the problem. They are intended to provide discrete evidence of the existence of the problem under scrutiny and may address the questions: how much? how often? under what circumstances? and in what proportion to other phenomena? Because the data rendered may refer to quantity, assessment strategies are sometimes called *measurements*. For instance, a measurement of 35 pounds of grip allows the occupational therapist to make some decisions about strength and hand function. A subsequent measure of 50 pounds indicates progress in terms of increasing grip strength.

The *test procedure* refers to the protocol which is established for administering an instrument or strategy. Consistent procedures facilitate communication as well as interpretation of data. Assessments variously yield scores, measurements, and descriptive observations. Once the results have been compiled, it is necessary to consider the data within the context of a conceptual framework to render an interpretation. This interpretation leads to an hypothesis addressing the cause and nature of the target problem. If the hypothesis is based upon ''intuition'' rather than actual assessment, it is likely founded upon clinical lore rather than objective inquiry. While clinical lore may provide potentially verifiable concepts, it does not suffice as a basis for clinical decision-making.

Clinical decision-making entails systematic conceptualization and examination. According to social scientist, Donald A. Schön (1983):

> In real-world practice, problems do not present themselves to the practitioner as givens. They must be constructed from the materials of problematic situations which are puzzling, troubling, and uncertain. In order to convert a problematic situation to a problem, a practitioner must do a certain kind

of work. He [or she] must make sense of an uncertain situation that initially makes no sense. It is the sort of situation that professionals are coming increasingly to see as central to their practice. They are coming to recognize that although problem-setting is as necessary a condition as technical problem-solving, it is not itself a technical problem. When we set the problem, we select what we will trust as the "things" of the situation, we set the boundaries of our attention to it, and we impose upon it a coherence which allows us to say what is wrong and in what directions the situation needs to be changed. Problem-setting is a process in which, interactively, we name the things to which we will attend and frame the context in which we will attend to them (p. 40).

The assessment process addresses the "naming and framing" to which Schön refers. Assessment not only focuses on a particular problem or problems, but it also facilitates the selection of strategies and instruments to "frame" the problem, thereby determining the realm of potential clinical decisions. Without critical attention to the assessment process, the relevance of ensuing action may be questioned.

Assessment, after all, is a communication mechanism. Conscientious assessment should lend clarity to thought, enabling therapists to share ideas with peers and to convey their reasoning to patients/clients. Rigorous conceptualization should foster therapists' confidence in their decisions and should improve their ability to account for clinical decisions. Such scientific inquiry is necessary to amass professional credibility and to demonstrate the **efficacy** of specific therapeutic interventions. Measurable improvement in human performance will generally serve to increase consumer satisfaction and to underscore the value of occupational therapy.

Problem Setting

Before proceeding, it is necessary to understand the preliminary phase of assessment or "problem-setting", as Schön termed it. Logically, the practitioner begins by gathering information about events or conditions which marked the onset of dysfunction. The course and nature of dysfunctional performance provide the examiner with additional clues. Adding information about the patient/client's current status, the practitioner should begin to set assessment priorities and settle on the focal problems, which are those problems that have been deemed to be the highest priorities for remediation and which are within the domain of concern of occupational therapy. Identifying such problems necessarily entails collaborating with the client.

Although the parameters of assessment might seem obvious, the practitioner should pay conscious attention to such factors. For instance, who is qualified to assess the

identified problem? What exactly will be evaluated and how will the data be used? When, where, and under what conditions will the assessment take place? How much information will be necessary to enable clinical decisions? Why is it important to delineate the problem? Answering such questions will guide the practitioner in selecting instruments and strategies appropriate to the situation.

Essentially the practitioner makes a commitment at some point during the problem-setting phase which leads to the "name it" phase. "*Naming*" is actually identifying the constructs which become the target of assessment. A **construct** is an abstract quality or phenomenon which accounts for behavior. For example, when a person considered to be healthy begins to pant, feel fatigued, and sweat after twenty minutes of aerobic exercise, it appears that a lack of endurance accounts for these behaviors. In this case, the panting, fatigue, and sweating are observable manifestations of a construct: endurance. If a person with normal sensation and perception is asked to pick up ten pennies from a table, a different construct is the focus of performance, the construct of dexterity.

Constructs of concern to occupational therapists are often complicated. It may be difficult to discern whether a performance deficit can be attributed to one construct or a number of constructs. The more discrete the instruments and strategies used in the assessment, the better able therapists are to make clinical decisions likely to improve performance. For example, if a single measure simultaneously indicates strength, dexterity, and peripheral sensation, it may be difficult to determine which construct is responsible for poor hand function.

Another dilemma which occupational therapists face is assessing ability or potential in addition to current behavior. Assessing human performance deficits entails judgement or projection of a person's capability after intervention. For example, the current behavior of a recent stroke patient reveals that the patient is unable to move from bed to chair, from toilet to standing, or from chair to bathtub without physical assistance. At present these behaviors would preclude the patient from living independently. However, the therapist must also assess the patient's ultimate capacity or ability to overcome these performance deficits. The therapist must exercise clinical judgement based upon the assessment in order to facilitate attainable performance goals.

In reality, assessment and resultant clinical decisions occur throughout treatment. Critical examination, hypothesis formulation and modification, and goal setting occur dynamically. This flow of data allows the therapist to check his/her theoretical understanding of the problem and the selected course of treatment. Figure 14-1 is a schematic diagram of the clinical reasoning process. Schön (1983) refers to such introspection as "*reflection in action*."

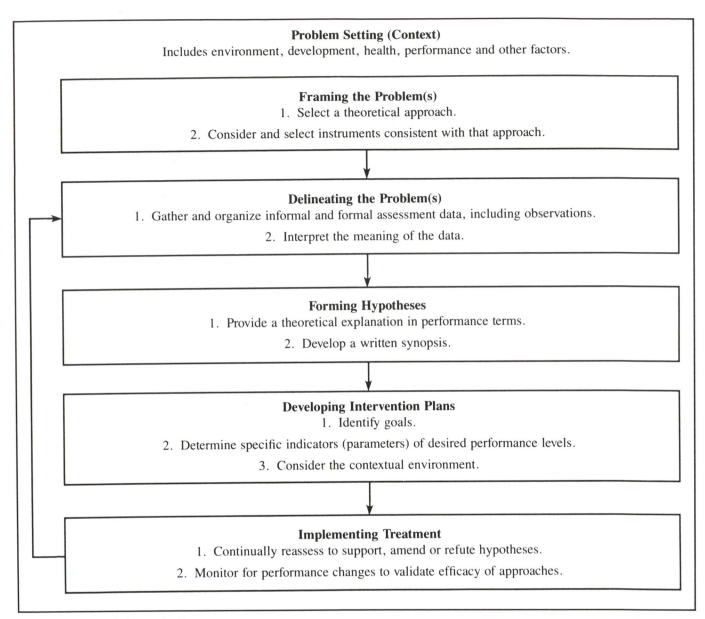

Figure 14-1. The Clinical Reasoning Process

In assessment, a practitioner simultaneously collects information and makes decisions. Learning to reflect on observed phenomena, to relate those observations to conceptual frameworks, and to generate new questions leads to heightened awareness and potential effectiveness. The occupational therapy assessment marks the beginning of reflective action which culminates in the resolution of human performance deficits. (See Figure 14-1.)

The Process of Informed Decision-Making

Once the problem has been named, the therapist engages in clarifying or characterizing it. Not only must one attend to the specific dysfunction, but one must also consider the problem in context. In what environment is the client expected to perform? How does the dysfunction reflect the developmental work of the client? How does the client's state of health contribute to the identified problem? These questions are likely to necessitate further investigation.

Framing is the process of illuminating the problem(s) in context. Framing the problem requires the practitioner to seek instruments or strategies which render information relating to the identified problem. According to Schön (1983, p. 269), "... inquiry, however it may initially have been conceived, turns into a frame experiment. What

Table 14-1
Standards Pertaining to Testing People With Handicapping Conditions

14.1   People who modify tests for handicapped people should have psychometric expertise available to them. In addition, they should have available to them knowledge of the effects of various handicapping conditions on test performance, acquired either from their own training or experience or from close consultation with handicapped individuals or acquired from those thoroughly familiar with such individuals.

14.2   Until tests have been validated for people who have specific handicapping conditions, test publishers should issue cautionary statements in manuals and elsewhere regarding interpretations based on such test scores.

14.3   Forms of tests that are modified for people who have various handicapping conditions should generally be pilot tested on people who are similarly handicapped to check the appropriateness and feasibility of the modifications.

14.4   Interpretive information that accompanies modified tests should include a careful statement of the steps taken to modify tests in order to alert users to changes that are likely to alter the validity of the measure.

14.5   Empirical procedures should be used whenever possible to establish time limits for modified forms of timed tests rather than simply allowing handicapped test takers a multiple of the standard time. Fatigue should be investigated as a potentially important factor when time limits are extended.

14.6   When feasible the validity and reliability of tests administered to people with various handicapping conditions should be investigated and reported by the agency or publisher that makes the modification. Such investigations should examine the effects of modifications made for people with various handicapping conditions on resulting scores, as well as the effects of administering standard unmodified tests to them.

14.7   Those who use tests and those who interact professionally with potential test-takers with handicapping conditions (e.g. high school guidance counselors) should: (a) possess the information necessary to make an appropriate selection of alternate measures, (b) have current information regarding the availability of modified forms of the test in question, (c) inform individuals with handicapping conditions, when appropriate, about the existence of modified forms, and (d) make these forms available to test-takers when appropriate and feasible.

14.8   In assessing characteristics of individuals with handicapping conditions, the test-user should use either regular or special norms for calculating derived scores, depending on the purpose of the testing. Regular norms for the characteristic in question are appropriate when the purpose involves the test-taker's functioning relative to the general population. If available however, special norms should be selected when the test-taker's functioning is being considered relative to their handicapped peers.

From Standards for Educational and Psychological Testing. Copyright © 1985 by the American Psychological Association. Reprinted with permission. Further reproduction without the express written permission of the APA is prohibited.

allows this to happen is that the inquirer is willing to step into the problematic situation, to impose a frame on it, to follow the implications of the discipline thus established, and yet to remain open to the situation's back-talk. Reflecting on the surprising consequences of his [or her] efforts to shape the situation in conformity with his initially chosen frame, the inquirer frames new questions and new ends in view.'' Careful selection of instruments, then, increases the likelihood of useful, accurate, clarification of the identified performance problems.

Each instrument has its unique characteristics, strengths, and weaknesses which must be carefully weighed. In weighing instruments, the therapist needs to acknowledge a conceptual approach or frame of reference compatible with his/her beliefs about the identified problem to facilitate the aforementioned reflective action. When instruments and strategies under consideration are reviewed, the therapist should be able to determine the philosophy and rationale around which each was constructed. Theoretical bias is inherent in all instruments, and the practitioner should choose the test or

strategy most congruent with the desired frame of reference and most relevant to the clinical problem.

Decisions about assessment tools require analysis of many aspects of the instruments. (These aspects will be explained in a later section.) Practitioners must recognize that they are consumers of tests and measurement instruments and are accountable for their choices. The *Standards for Educational and Psychological Testing* (American Educational Research Association, American Psychological Association, National Council on Measurement in Education, 1985) have been established by three cooperating organizations to help guide therapists in their choice of tests and measurements. Of particular interest to the occupational therapist are the standards pertaining to testing those with handicapping (disabling) conditions, which include standards for the publishers of the tests and measurements, the examiners, and the tests. These standards are listed in Table 14-1.

Delineating the Problem
After the practitioner has decided upon a strategy or

instrument(s), he/she then proceeds to implement them. It should be noted that frequently a single test or strategy will not address the entire scope of an identified problem. Using multiple measures of performance is common in clinical practice.

Adherence to prescribed or standardized procedures influences the credibility of the data in an assessment and this will be discussed later in the chapter. Implementation of tests and other measures yields valuable information. To enhance the picture rendered by the data, practitioners should take care to organize and categorize results before interpreting them. These data along with clinical observations, which are more subjective in nature, provide the basis for significant clinical decisions. Clinical observations are important in qualifying and substantiating numerical data. Interpretation entails a good deal of reflection. The practitioner should compare and contrast findings with theory and precedents to make a sound clinical judgment. Once the therapist arrives at conclusions about the targeted problem, he/she can formulate an hypothesis which will serve as the vantage point for subsequent clinical decisions.

Formulating an Hypothesis for Treatment

For a reflective practitioner, the work of formulating an hypothesis is a creative and intellectual challenge. It becomes a description of the therapist's beliefs regarding the nature and effect of the target problem(s), and allows the therapist to articulate and apply his/her theoretical understanding of the problem. It allows the therapist to think both expansively and specifically to develop a new synthesis of information and insight. In order to test this hypothesis, the therapist must return to initial phases of assessment and validate his/her hypothesis with observable manifestations of the human performance deficit(s).

The hypothesis serves as the cornerstone of therapy, but is subject to change and alteration during the course of treatment. The assessment process continues during treatment and may reveal new information which necessitates modification of the initial hypothesis. Therefore, it is imperative that the therapist write down the initial hypothesis. Concrete evidence of the initial decision-making process will facilitate the reflection that follows.

Case Study 14-1

Forming an Hypothesis for Treatment: Mr. Smith is a 75-year-old man who suffered a right hemisphere cerebrovascular accident (CVA). He was assessed by the occupational therapy department upon admission to a rehabilitation unit two weeks after his CVA. Although he was alert and articulate, he was disorganized in his approach to all tasks including dressing and hygiene. He conveyed little emotion when discussing his CVA and subsequent difficulties. Physical function was within normal limits, but Mr. Smith required considerable assistance for activities of daily life, and his safety awareness was poor. He expressed a desire to return to his home to live independently.

After synthesizing these data, Mr. Smith's occupational therapist hypothesized that right hemisphere structures had been damaged resulting in inaccurate spatial perception and adaptation, flattened affect, and impaired praxis. The hypothesis logically led to the following initial treatment goals:

1. Use environmental cues for spatial orientation.

2. Express feelings verbally while engaged in activity.

3. Efficiently sequence simple ADL tasks (i.e., putting on a shirt, making a pot of coffee).

4. Institute safety procedures (i.e., calling ambulance, correctly taking prescribed medicines) with necessary adaptations.

The findings from a CT scan provided addidtional insight and during the course of treatment, it was discovered that reminiscence triggered a greater range of affective responses in Mr. Smith. The therapist then amended the hypothesis to include this new information and stated: Right parietal lobe infarct has resulted in impaired spatial and organizational performance. General affect is dull but can be altered by capitalizing on long-term memory and association. Praxis is improved if sufficient spatial cues are provided, and if the treatment activity holds some historical appeal.

Reflecting back to the general goals, such new discoveries about the nature of the problem can be incorporated in selecting and implementing activities.

Developing an Intervention Plan

Assessment results and interpretations are certainly key to developing intervention plans, but there are other factors that influence treatment outcomes that must be considered. Of particular importance to the identification of meaningful activity is clarification of the client's values. Even a superb intervention plan based upon thorough initial assessment will not effect change if it cannot be valued by the patient. Thus, once again, it is necessary for the therapist to gather information.

Therapists must also consider the potential effect of the client's environment on the expected outcome of intervention. For example, a client who gets around in a wheelchair may be independent in toileting and bathing in a clinical facility. If the wheelchair does not fit through the bathroom door of his home, such expectations are meaningless. Support systems within the environment merit attention as well. If a client lives with family members, will they follow through with therapeutic recommendations? In a work environment, is an employer willing to allow the client the recommended worksite modification? Other significant factors or circumstances must be assessed in the course of treatment planning such as the client's motivation, medical prognosis, emotional status, and financial status.

The therapist must consider a wide range of enabling factors when making decisions about the goals and parameters of therapy. This attitude is summed up by Gillette and Mattingly (1987):

> The occupational therapist, however, is committed philosophically to viewing the patient as a whole person —not as someone with an injured part—and as one whose life should be considered in the context of a satisfying living environment. Such a phenomenological view necessarily requires an understanding of motivation, behavior, life-styles, values, and roles that extends far beyond the constraints of medical diagnosis (p. 400).

The practitioner at this point must decide upon the goals of treatment. Attending to all the information at hand, he/she must ensure that the established goals are congruent with the frame of reference selected earlier in the process. If the therapist wishes to modify the hypothesis and/or change the conceptual approach during the course of treatment, he/she will have a firmer basis for doing so.

Another step in the planning process which is frequently overlooked is identifying indicators of successful intervention. This is an information-gathering strategy which should aide the practitioner in making subsequent decisions about the treatment hypothesis and implementation. Ultimately, the indicators will help the therapist to make decisions about the termination of therapy.

Consideration of enabling factors and establishment of treatment goals leads to yet another set of clinical decisions—the practical parameters of treatment. The practitioner must establish the frequency of therapy and the scheduling and duration of each session. He/she must also delineate any specific conditions for treatment such as the client's attendance, punctuality, and financial reimbursement. For example, if the therapist has established family education as a goal, a condition of treatment may be that at least one family member be consistently present. It is also at this time that the therapist should establish a set interval for formal reassessment of the original dysfunction and should project the expected duration of treatment. Setting these practical parameters of treatment provides the practitioner and the client with a clear sense of direction.

Specific occupational therapy interventions will be addressed in subsequent chapters. But as we have seen, information-gathering and decision-making do not stop

with the initial assessment and establishment of treatment goals. As described in Chapter 1 data and clinical observations regarding changes in human performance are continually collected in the course of therapy. The information serves to support, refute, or amend the treatment hypothesis and allows the clinician to make informed decisions. Furthermore such evidence, systematically collected, can help determine the efficacy of treatment. If the therapy is not beneficial, the practitioner can decide to alter or terminate therapy.

SELECTION OF ASSESSMENT INSTRUMENTS

Before examining the myriad of choices of assessment tools and strategies, it is necessary to identify various features which characterize them. If the therapist understands the concepts behind the assessment tools it becomes easier to analyze the instruments to determine their value and utility in a given situation. The following section is by no means an exhaustive account of test characteristics, but it should impress upon the reader the forethought necessary to both design and to choose an appropriate assessment strategy.

We have already introduced the term, **construct.** Gronlund (1977), an acknowledged education and test construction expert, defines construct as a hypothetical quality which is assumed to account for behavior in many different specified situations. When surveying available assessment tools, the practitioner must first ask whether the tool addresses the constructs which are under scrutiny in the clinical problem. Some constructs are relatively simple to examine and others extremely complicated. Intelligence is an example of a multifaceted, complex construct made up of many contributing factors such as factual knowledge, judgement, and intuition. Estimates of intelligence must be based on indirect evidence, collected from observations of behaviors hypothesized as reflecting that attribute. This might include a score from an intelligence test, an assessment of problem-solving, or indications of academic achievement.

In contrast, the comparatively simple construct of strength can be directly observed and measured through mechanical means that measure torque or work. When analyzing instruments and strategies, the practitioner should note whether the evidence of the target construct is direct or indirect, since this will effect how construct validity is established (see construct validity later in this section).

Philosophical Base

All tests and measures reflect a philosophical bias, and

practitioners must be able to ascertain the philosophical perspective of the author of the test when choosing a test or measurement. Such insight allows the practitioner to decide whether the instrument will yield the kind of information that would facilitate treatment planning and intervention. Philosophical congruence in information gathering and clinical decision-making facilitates sound treatment planning and implementation.

Pelland (1987) states that all treatment planning begins with the selection of organizational structures to guide the collection of data. Clinicians often rely on forms used in a clinic or treatment setting for collecting the data needed for treatment planning. Students and new therapists should remember to consider the frame of reference or model of practice used in developing forms they are using, since they are based upon the designer's conscious or unconscious selection of specific models of practice. A therapist's philosophy of the purpose and focus of occupational therapy is the basis for the selection of models used in clinical problem-solving (Pelland, 1987).

Ideally, the practitioner should be able to access pertinent background materials of tests and measurements. Sometimes philosophical issues are addressed or at least referenced in manuals that accompany the instrument. If not, it may be necessary to write manufacturers, publishers, or test authors to obtain such information. The availability of background materials may influence the decision of whether or not to use the instrument.

Characteristics of Instruments: Validity and Reliability

The **validity** of an instrument is of utmost concern to practitioners, researchers, and test authors. *Validity* is the statistical descriptor that indicates whether or not the instrument or strategy truly measures what it claims to measure. The several types of validity are explained in the following:

Logical validity may be established when the practitioner directly observes the behavior under scrutiny. As in an earlier example, strength is a construct which may be directly observed. When an occupational therapist uses a dynamometer to measure grip strength, this assessment strategy may be said to be logically valid. When constructs become more complex, reflect ability, or require indirect observation, then validity must be established differently.

Content validity indicates how well the items included on the test represent the universe of possible responses. This is a matter of judgment. Both professional literature and experts are generally called upon to establish content validity. For instance, if a particular instrument uses block configurations to determine a client's ability to perceive and organize objects in space, one should question whether block configurations actually represent the ''universe'' of spatial awareness. If both the literature and the experts agree that they do represent one's abilities of spatial awareness, then it is likely that the content of the assessment strategy is valid. Numerical evidence of consensus might be collected and reported as an index of content validity.

Construct validity is critical to clinical decision-making and is also related to the issue of predictive validity. In order to establish construct validity, it must be demonstrated that performance is attributable to the identified constructs. Thus, all factors which may influence the target performance must be carefully examined to determine the possible contribution of each to differences in performance. Construct validity is established by gathering empirical evidence based upon testable hypotheses about the given constructs. Such studies contribute to the theoretical understanding of the behavior(s) in question and guide interpretation of data (Nunnally, 1978).

It may be important for a practitioner to make decisions based upon his/her projections of a client's future performance. If that is necessary, then the assessment strategy selected should have *predictive validity*. Predictive validity is established by empirical evidence that demonstrates the instrument is related to a specific criterion about which the practitioner is concerned. Predictive validity may also be associated with concurrent validity. *Concurrent validity* compares the relationship of the scores obtained on the focal instrument to those of another criterion or measure obtained at the same time. For example, assume that a practitioner finds that the scores on a test of motor development are below the norm for a four year old child. Additionally, in the clinic, the child is unable to competently perform coordination and dexterity tasks consistent with developmental milestones for that age. This clinical observation provides evidence of concurrent validity for the test of motor development, in that the data provided by two sources of assessment information are consistent.

The **reliability** of a test is important because it tells the practitioner how accurately the scores of data obtained from any assessment strategy reflect the true performance of the client. Just as there were many facets of validity, there are several aspects of test reliability (Kerlinger, 1973). Table 14-2 demonstrates the types of reliability and acceptable levels of reliability coefficients.

Test-retest reliability refers to the stability of the instrument. It is an indication of how consistent results are from one administrtaion of the test to another. Some variance in scores is likely, but ideally these should be minimized to enhance decisions related to the data. The longer the interval between measurements, the more score variance is likely to occur. This is especially true when a practitioner is examining a behavior which is affected by development or learning. If behaviors targeted by a particular assessment strategy are unstable, it is likely that a shorter interval between administrations will be recommended. Some tests and measures are not designed to be compared between long time intervals.

Another measure of reliability is *internal consistency*. This can be a statistic that describes the success of the instrument in terms of how consistently each item tests the construct. This can be done by arbitrarily dividing the test items into halves and comparing the results of each half. If the test results of the two halves are similar, there is a high measure of internal consistency which lets the practitioner know that he/she can rely on the entire instrument to measure the constructs in basically the same way.

The issue of *inter-rater reliability* is extremely important to occupational therapists and indicates how likely it is that test scores will be the same regardless of who the examiner is. Strict adherence to established protocol for a given assessment strategy increases the likelihood that test behaviors will be related to the target constructs and that the same results could be obtained by another examiner. When practitioners arbitrarily deviate from an established protocol, they introduce factors that are not accounted for in interpreting results and that may influence observed performance. These unpredicted factors are sometimes referred to as ''contaminants'', and they may well affect the validity of the assessment.

The concepts of validity and reliability should become clearer in subsequent chapters as the reader applies the principles to specific clinical situations. It is possible for an assessment strategy to be reliable, but not valid. If an instrument or method is not valid, reliability is of no consequence because the information is virtually useless. Reliability is a necessary but not sufficient attribute of an assessment instrument, and an unreliable instrument cannot be valid. Reliability and validity considered together indicate the degree of confidence a practitioner can have in making clinical decisions based upon the information collected in the assessment.

Two other concepts deserve attention when considering test results: sensitivity and specificity. **Test sensitivity** implies that the instrument will identify all of those who possess the behavior or characteristic in question. If a test or strategy is sensitive it will minimize false negatives and is able to identify what it is designed to detect in subjects. **Specificity** implies that only those manifesting the target behavior or characteristic will be identified. A specific instrument will minimize the number of false positives rendered by a test and will not identify subjects who clearly do not demonstrate the behavior or characteristic being

---

Table 14-2
Reliability Types and Desirable Reliability Coefficients for Decision-Making*

Type	Procedure	Coefficient
Stability (Test-retest)	Correlation between two administrations of test after defined interval	.70 or above
Inter-rater	Extent of agreement between different raters or evaluators	.90 or above
Equivalent forms	Correlation between two forms of same test	.80 or above
Internal consistency	Correlation among items, includes split-half, KR-20, coefficient alpha	.80 or above

* There is disagreement about the minimum level of accuracy that is permissible under given circumstances. For research purposes, standards slightly lower than these might be acceptable. Ultimately, the test user must decide how much measurement error can be tolerated in a given decision-making situation.

---

scrutinized. These terms relating to precision will become more meaningful as they are used later to describe certain kinds of assessment strategies (Mausner & Kramer, 1985).

Several terms are used in conjunction with reporting assessment results or scores. The **mean score** is the arithmetic average of all of the subjects' scores. The **median score** refers to the actual score value at which 50% of the observed scores were higher and 50% were lower. When considering all the subjects' scores, the **mode** is the score which occurred most frequently.

The **raw score** is the score from a test before it is mathematically manipulated for comparative purposes. Because a score on one test or subtest cannot be equated to the score on another and are not easily compared, raw scores are subjected to mathematical processes which allow them to be compared to other tests by way of standard scores. **Standard scores** are expressed in terms of standard deviation units. **Standard deviation** relates the performance of the subject to the mean. The standard deviation is determined by calculating the square root of the variance of all subjects' scores. Each standard deviation represents a fixed number of raw score units.

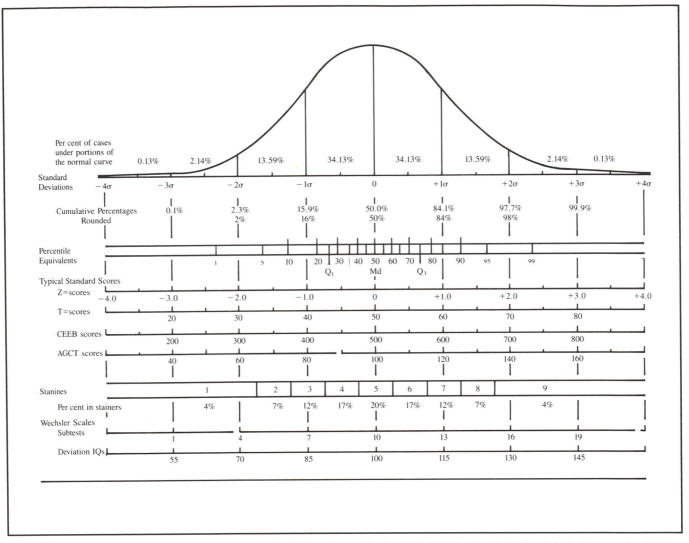

Figure 14-2. Various Test Scores and Their Correspondence to Each Other. *Source: Test Service Bulletin Number 48, The Psychological Corporation, 304 East 45th Street, New York, NY 10017. Reprinted with permission from the Psychological Corporation.*

For example, a standard deviation may equal fifteen raw score units. If the mean score is 100, then a score of 85 would be reported as: minus 1.0 standard deviation below the mean.

In general, a score within a range of plus or minus one standard deviation in relation to the mean represents performance that is within normal limits. Scores can be reported in terms of standard deviations or standard scores such as z-scores or stanines. See Figure 14-2 for a comparison of these scores.

Statistical processes and formulae are mathematical functions which must be understood to correctly interpret the meaning of scores derived from measurement instruments. Like any other technology, statistics and statistical operations expand with new theory and understanding. Appropriate application of statistics lend credibility to assessment results and clinical decisions.

Attending to Format

An important practical aspect of assessment design is the format. Webster's dictionary defines format as "the shape, size and arrangement of a book or the arrangement or plan of a presentation" (Webster's II, 1984). When referring to assessment strategies, format includes the test manuals, the testing protocol, the equipment, and the test environment.

When selecting a test instrument or strategy, the therapist

considers the clarity, completeness, and organization of the manual. The complexity and ease of understanding of administration procedures is also important. Equipment should be evaluated in terms of safety, utility, and durability. An important question to consider is whether the equipment can be repaired or replaced if broken or lost? Finally, the therapist must consider the recommendations set forth for the test environment. Certain instruments or strategies require an environment that may not be available to the practitioner, so such approaches are ruled out.

If a test specifies the need for particular training, certification, or credentialing, the practitioner should adhere to those specifications. Such recommendations are established to foster inter-rater reliability and to encourage theoretical understanding and accurate interpretation of performance. While some assessment strategies are self-explanatory and require little practice to administer or interpret them, others require extensive training, supervision, and practice.

Because many of the strategies employed in occupational therapy assessment include psychomotor skills, therapists often learn from each other. Strict attention to prescribed protocol is necessary to achieve and maintain inter-rater reliability. Today, many test authors produce training videotapes to provide a visual standard for test administration.

The Test Construction Process

When evaluating potential assessment strategies, the practitioner should be aware of the process which the completed test represents. If that process has been thorough, it is more likely that the end product reflects good quality. If the process has been haphazard, the instrument might reveal serious deficiencies.

Test development should begin with an hypothesis and examination of the state-of-the-art through the existing literature. When establishing the need for a new instrument, a test author identifies the void and states his/her own philosophy and rationale. Philosophical and theoretical inclinations become apparent at this point.

Once the target constructs are defined, the author begins to select items or devise methods which yield clear evidence of those constructs. There are many more items generated than those that appear in the final instrument. These items comprise the *item pool*. Pilot studies are conducted to refine items and procedures. The items selected for the final instrument are selected by a process known as *item analysis* and are those which statistically demonstrate that they are the strongest indicators of the target constructs. Such items are called *good discriminators*.

If an instrument is to be a **standardized test**, a detailed statistical design is generated for collecting data. This includes planning the *stratification sample* which is a numerically limited sample that is representative of the target population of the test and the most recent census data. Normative data collection entails the training of testers to obtain test data from a representative population. Validity and reliability studies may be conducted concurrently with the standardization effort to support the instrument and enable interpretation.

Additionally test development efforts frequently require expert consultation for highly specialized functions outside the scope of the test author. Considerable attention must be paid to both funding and marketing. Even a simple instrument undergoing standardization could be costly in terms of personnel, time, and data analysis. It is not unusual for test development efforts to take several years. The impact of this process and related skills upon occupational therapy will be discussed at the end of the chapter.

CATEGORIZING ASSESSMENTS AND ASSESSMENT STRATEGIES

When choosing any assessment instrument or strategy, a practitioner should be well informed and discriminative. There are many types available, and therapists need to be able to distinguish and choose well-designed, credible tests in order to sufficiently guide clinical decisions. If the instrument or strategy is poor, then clinical decisions based upon the data yielded by the test will be no better. It is the responsibility of every practitioner to analyze potential instruments and strategies for their suitability to a particular clinical problem.

Informal, Formal, and Standardized Instruments and Strategies

Occupational therapists have long been familiar with informal assessment mechanisms. These are usually intuitive methods or simple approaches one devises to delineate problems, a sort of "home grown" method. Although these methods may be inherently valuable, they cannot be generalized. Interpretation of data yielded by these methods stands to be idiosyncratic or highly contingent upon the theoretical understanding and clinical experience of the practitioner using such methods.

A formal assessment strategy or instrument specifically outlines what is to be examined, how it will be examined, the manner in which the data will be communicated, and how the information will be applied in clinical problem-solving. Formal tests lend themselves to critical analysis and duplication. However, formal tests may or may not be reliable or valid, and literature or research may not be

Table 14-3
Comparison of Norm-Referenced and Criterion-Referenced Assessment

Norm-Referenced	Criterion-Referenced
Scores are interpreted in terms of a specified normative group through percentile ranks, grade equivalents, etc.	Scores are interpreted through comparison to a specified criterion or standard of mastery.
Content domain tends to be broad in scope. Emphasis is on content validity and item discrimination.	Content domain tends to be narrow and specific. Emphasis is on content validity.
Usually standardized with high reliability.	May be standardized. Reliability may be difficult to establish.
Less sensitive to the effects of instruction or intervention.	More sensitive to the effects of instruction or intervention.

available to support interpretation or necessary clinical decisions.

Standardized assessments represent even more sophistication on the continuum of clinical reasoning. Although standardized assessments do not insure the high quality of an instrument, they reflect the process of scientific inquiry and describe performance in quantifiable terms and additionally provide normative (or criterion-referenced) data as a standard of comparison. Statistical representations of both validity and reliability of an instrument can help guide the practitioner in clinical decisions. If the standardized instrument is determined to be of high quality, it can be safely assumed that the targeted performance is a valid representation of the underlying constructs, that the tests results are sufficiently reliable, and that the normative standards may be generalized to interpret the observed performance. Two standardized instruments authored by occupational therapists are the *Miller Assessment for Preschoolers* (MAP) (Miller, 1982) and the *Sensory Integration and Praxis Tests* (SIPT) (Ayres, 1988).

Norm-Referenced versus Criterion-Referenced Strategies

Norm-referenced tests are those in which an individual's performance is compared and/or ranked relative to a broad typical sample (the normative sample) to which the test has previously been administered. If subsequent studies expand on the meaning of the scores by applying them to special populations, the information may facilitate the practitioner's understanding of the performance deficit and foster a resolution. Normative data are expressed numerically, so the interpretation of norm-referenced tests requires quantitative analysis.

Criterion-referenced tests employ descriptive standards by which to measure performance. Rather than comparing individual performance to a sample group, performance is judged in terms of a desired outcome. Since few norm-referenced tests address the unique behaviors and characteristics of concern to occupational therapists, criterion-referenced tests are more useful in clinical practice. Criterion-referencing is particularly useful when the practitioner is trying to determine performance competency or mastery. An example of a performance criterion would be: "functional dishwashing" as defined as immaculately cleaning and drying five plates, ten glasses, twenty pieces of silverware, and two bowls in fifteen minutes with no breakage. In criterion-referencing, the client's performance would then be measured against this criterion. Table 14-3 compares norm-referenced and criterion-referenced assessment.

Primary, Secondary, and Tertiary Assessment Strategies

Paralleling the classifications of levels of health care is yet another way to analyze assessment strategies. *Primary strategies* are screening devices that are relatively simple and cost effective enough to be implemented with large numbers of subjects. Screening involves less time and less examiner training than secondary or tertiary strategies. Screening tools should be sensitive and identify all subjects with the disorder or condition of concern. The conclusions generally associated with primary level assessments are classified as normal, abnormal, or questionable. It follows that clinical decisions based upon abnormal or questionable findings generally warrant further assessment. Some examples of primary tools used by occupational therapists are: the *Denver Developmental Screening Test*, group manual muscle testing, and the *Mini Mental Status Test*.

Secondary assessment strategies yield more information about the nature of a performance deficit. Once the existence of a problem is identified, the secondary strategy serves to diagnose or describe the problem. Such description leads to additional options in clinical decision-making by affording more numerous or expansive clinical hypotheses. Diagnostic tests usually require more time and training on the part of the practitioner. Interpretation entails comparable theoretical understanding and clinical judgement. Secondary assessment strategies include the *Jebson-Taylor Hand Function Test*, the *Allen Cognitive Test*, the *Bay Area Functional Performance Evaluation*, the *Purdue Pegboard*, and the *Bruininks-Oseretsky Test of*

Motor Performance.

Tertiary assessment strategies are highly specialized, very specific tests or measurements. Such instruments have a narrow, in-depth focus and yield detailed information about particular kinds of performance dysfunction. Such strategies require clinical expertise. To administer a tertiary test, advanced training or perhaps even special certification or licensing may be required. Interpretation of these instruments is likely to be complicated and to call for sophisticated theoretical understanding. Complex clinical decisions are inherent in tertiary level assessments. An example of such an instrument used by occupational therapists is the *Sensory Integration and Praxis Tests* (SIPT) battery.

Formative and Summative Assessment Strategies

When used in reference to assessment, the terms formative and summative refer to the nature of the

---

Comparative Chart Method for Analysis of Assessments

Features	Strengths	Weaknesses
Philosophy & Rationale		
Design		
Format		
Validity Issues		
Reliability Issues		
Other Statistical Features		
Practicality or Applicability		

Figure 14-4. Comparative Chart Method for Analysis of Assessments. *Developed by K.J. Opacich, Department of Occupational Therapy, Rush University.*

New Test Entry

Miller Assessment for Preschoolers. Ages 2-9 to 5-8; 1982; MAP; screening tool to identify children who exhibit moderate developmental problems; 6 scores: foundations, coordination, verbal, non-verbal, complex tasks, total; individual; 1 form; 6 developmental levels (ages 2-9 to 3-2, 3-3 to 3-8, 3-9 to 4-2, 4-3 to 4-8, 4-9 to 5-2, 5-3 to 5-8); record booklet (4 pages); drawing booklet (4 pages); item score sheet (2 pages) for each developmental level; examiners manual (220 pages); 1983 price data: $225 per complete kit in carrying case; $6.25 per 25 item score sheets; $6.25 per 25 record booklets; $6.25 per 25 drawing booklets; $2.50 per labels for kit box; $22.50 per examiner's manual; (20-30) minutes; Lucy Jane Miller; The Foundation for Knowledge in Development.

Key to information in MMY listings: Title; Descriptions of the groups for which the test is intended; Date of publication; Acronym; Special comments; Part scores; Whether individual or group test; Forms, parts and levels; Number of printed pages in test booklets and manuals; Availability of machine scoreable answer sheets; Costs of test packages or individual elements; Approximate length of time required to administer the test; Author of the test; Publisher of the Test.

Note: Tests which have been previously listed in a Buros Institute Publication have a final paragraph with cross references for reviews excerpts, and references for the test in that volume. The addresses of test publishers are listed in a section entitled "Publisher's Directory and Index."

Figure 14-3. New Test Entry. *Source: Mental Measurements Yearbook, 1985. Courtesy of Gryphon Press.*

---

associated clinical decisions. *Formative assessment strategies* are ongoing and shape the course of further gathering of information and intermediate decisions. Occupational therapists engage in formative assessment in all client encounters. Formative assessment allows the practitioner to alter the hypothesis guiding treatment, upgrade treatment activity, modify the activity, or to respond to changes in performance(Anderson, Ball & Murphy et al, 1975).

In contrast, *summative assessment strategies* occur at pre-determined intervals and focus on outcomes and final decisions. One of the first summative decisions facing the practitioner stems from the initial assessment when the practitioner must decide whether or not the performance problem warrants intervention. Other summative decisions within the course of treatment might be to continue the intervention, to escalate treatment, to reduce treatment, or to discontinue intervention. Unless the practitioner has contemplated treatment outcome and established discharge criteria, the decision regarding termination of intervention can provoke much anxiety. Therapists establish the treatment outcome and discharge criteria early in the

Table 14-4
Standards Pertaining to Clinical Testing

7.1 Clinicians should not imply that interpretations of test data are based on empirical evidence of validity unless such evidence exists for the interpretations given.

7.2 When validity is appraised by comparing the level of agreement between test results and clinical diagnoses, the diagnostic terms or categories employed should be carefully defined or identified, and the method by which a diagnosis was made should be specified. If diagnosis was made based on judgments, information on the training, experience, and professional status of the judges and on the nature and extent of the judges' contacts with the test takers should be included.

7.3 When differential diagnosis is needed, the user should choose, if possible, a test for which there is evidence of the test's ability to distinguish between the two or more diagnostic groups of concern rather than merely to distinguish abnormal cases from the general population.

7.4 Test users should determine from the manual or other reported evidence whether the construct being measured corresponds to the nature of the assessment that is intended.

7.5 Clinicians should share with their clients test results and interpretations, as well as information about the range of error for such interpretations when such information will be beneficial to the client. Such information should be expressed in language that the client (or client's legal representative) can understand.

7.6 Criterion-related evidence of validity for populations similar to that for which the test will be used should be available when recommendations or decisions are presented as having an actuarial, as well as a clinical, basis.

From Standards for Educational and Psychological Testing. Copyright © 1985 by the American Psychological Association. Reprinted with permission. Further reproduction without the express written permission of the APA is prohibited.

therapeutic process, so that the decision of when to terminate intervention is not dictated by external factors such as the exhaustion of funds, injury litigation, or family disinterest.

Interpretation of Assessment Data

Interpretation of data is the culmination phase of assessment. The practitioner must translate scores and observations into a meaningful explanation of performance assets and deficits. If results are to be compared to normative data, the practitioner relates the examinee's performance to that of the sample subjects. For criterion-referenced strategies, results are compared against the established standard and described in relation to that standard. In any situation, the formal data are then weighed

in light of the clinical observations. In most cases, scores reflect the end products or outcomes of test tasks while clinical observations elucidate the manner or process in which the task was accomplished.

Many assessments include data from more than one instrument in addition to clinical observations and historical or interview information. Interpreting the data obliges the practitioner to evaluate and weigh the various data and information in order to render a profile of the client's performance which will lead to the formulation of a viable treatment hypothesis. Interpretation is, in large part, superimposing the delineated problem onto a conceptual framework. The practitioner can distinguish behavior that is typical of or different from those phenomena explained by theory and supported by research. Interpretation calls upon the practitioner's ability to synthesize knowledge and experience and to decide upon a therapeutic course of action.

The confidence placed in any clinical decision is directly proportional to the quality of the assessment strategy used to obtain the data. A well-designed tool subjected to rigorous field testing should afford a solid opportunity to plan efficacious treatment, whereas tools that are not accurate and effective in gathering information, leave the practitioner vulnerable in making clinical decisions.

CRITICAL ANALYSIS OF ASSESSMENT TOOLS

The discussion of systematic analysis of assessment tools will help to illustrate the principles presented in this chapter. Although there is no one best method of accomplishing this analysis, each practitioner will probably have a preference. The crucial issue is that the decision to use any instrument or strategy should be conscious and well-informed. A good way to begin researching an instrument is to check the *Mental Measurements Yearbook* which gives a description of the instrument, the purpose for which the test was designed, the materials included with the test, and cost of materials. Figure 14-3 gives an example of a new test entry in the *Mental Measurements Yearbook* and the key to information included in this reference.

One way of analyzing a potential assessment is to list the strengths and weaknesses on a chart like the one in Figure 14-4. Consistently examining instruments along the same parameters will help the practitioner to build a repertoire of assessment options. Utilizing this method requires a reasonable understanding of test characteristics and the test construction process.

A new practitioner might feel more comfortable with a detailed checklist of test features so that the features are already listed. In the *Standards for Educational and Psychological Testing* (AERA, AMA, NCME, 1985), test features are presented as primary, secondary, or conditional. A checklist pertinent to an assessment tool could easily be compiled from these standards. The publication provides detailed explanations and serves as an excellent resource for both novice and experienced practitioners. (See Table 14-4).

A third approach to test analysis is the critique method which includes writing a narrative of both positive and negative features of an instrument. This summary of test instruments can help the practitioner when faced with an assessment decision. It might be helpful to the practitioner to develop his/her own set of questions for critically analyzing assessment strategies. Both composing and answering the questions help the practitioner to discover the salient features of a given assessment instrument. Table 14-5 is a list of sample questions for critical analysis.

Still another way to systematically review assessment strategies is to compile an annotated bibliography of the various tools as they are encountered. This method provides a helpful filing system to easily access materials. Figure 14-5 presents an example of an information sheet to be filled out for each assessment tool.

OCCUPATIONAL THERAPY CONCERNS IN ASSESSMENT AND CLINICAL DECISION-MAKING

The assessment process, assessment tools and strategies, assessment data, and clinical decisions are inextricably linked. Professional credibility depends on the ability of occupational therapists to make sound decisions supported by empirical evidence.

Examination of current assessment options demonstrates the paucity of standardized instruments that have been developed by occupational therapists. Assessment is fundamental to clinical problem-solving, and occupational therapists certainly have a vested interest in assessment of performance dysfunction. Unfortunately, developing such instruments requires not only tremendous effort and commitment on the part of the author, but also advanced levels of education and research skill. Hopefully, more occupational therapists will become involved in the development of sound assessment instruments that are sensitive to occupational performance constructs. These endeavors would certainly be a needed and worthy contribution to the profession.

Assessment strategies and tools are critical to the determination of efficacy of intervention. The profession has identified efficacy research as a leading priority. Without

---

Table 14-5
Sample Questions for Critical Analysis of Assessment Instruments or Strategies

1. Are the philosophy, rationale, and frame of reference used in constructing the instrument evident and accessible?

2. Are guidelines set forth for potential examiners in terms of training, credentials, or theoretical background?

3. Is adequate information available regarding the method of standardization (or formalization), the standardization sample, or field testing?

4. Are the statistics and statistical methods appropriate and understandable?

5. What evidence exists for the instrument's validity?

6. Are reliability values acceptable?

7. Is the training process explicitly presented or offered to insure inter-rater reliability?

8. Do test scores reasonably lend themselves to interpretation?

9. Is the instrument under consideration designed and/or standardized for the population on which you wish to use it?

10. Is the manual complete, well organized, and easy to use?

11. Is the complexity of administration congruent with the levels of required training and potential clinical decisions?

12. Are administration procedures clear and precise?

13. Does the assessment take a reasonable amount of time to conduct?

14. Is the test format organized, logical, and appealing?

15. Is all the necessary equipment included? Is it safe, durable, manageable, and replaceable?

16. Would you consider this a cost effective assessment strategy?

17. Is this test or strategy of a quality that would be respected by other health professionals?

18. Were references and corollary studies cited or conducted?

19. Does the assessment represent the highest state of the art in its target area?

Developed by K.J. Opacich, Department of Occupational Therapy, Rush University.

Synopsis of Test or Measurement Used in Occupational Therapy

Assessment Tool: _____   Presented by: _____

Vendor: _____

        Address: _____

                _____

        Phone: _____

Cost of Assessment Tool: _____

Test Materials & Characteristics:

Required Test Environment:

Standardization Sample, Statistics, & Issues:

Format/Procedures:

Scoring/Interpretation:

Strengths:

Weaknesses:

References:

Figure 14-5. Synopsis of Test or Measurement Used in Occupational Therapy. *Developed by K.J. Opacich, Department of Occupational Therapy, Rush University.*

the necessary instrumentation, practitioners are frustrated in their attempts to illustrate the effect of occupational therapy on restoring or improving human performance.

In this age of economic accountability, occupational therapists must be able to link performance with fiscal benefit. Proper instrumentation is needed to conduct cost-benefit analyses of treatment. We need to be able to demonstrate the cost-effectiveness of treatment in relation to the benefits of enhancing clients' ability to live independently at home and in work, play, and leisure (Baum, 1987; Christiansen, 1983).

Ethical Considerations in Assessment

One of the foremost ethical concerns pertaining to assessment concerns credentialing. In many instances, test authors provide potential users with guidelines regarding theoretical background, testing skill, and interpretation requirements. Some instruments require special training, reliability checks, and even certification of competence. If

such recommendations are made, it serves the interest of both the practitioner and the consumer to adhere to the recommendations. Where such guidelines are not provided or are deemed unnecessary, the practitioner must assume the responsibility for determining his/her own competence to implement and interpret the assessment.

Another concern is that tests and measures be applied to populations for whom they were designed. If a test is standardized for a particular population and used on another, the resulting data may not be valid for that unintended subgroup. If a practitioner feels that a test is appropriate for a particular population although the test was not designed for that population, he/she should try to scientifically establish the validity of such an hypothesis. Using a test on an unintended population becomes subjective rather than objective analysis and hence scores should not be reported.

When assessment strategies or tools have been formalized or standardized, the practitioner should strictly adhere to the procedures and testing protocol. Deviation from the protocol affects reliability and possibly validity of the test. If it is absolutely necessary to alter the protocol, the practitioner must develop a written rationale for doing so. This decision may preclude the reporting of scores.

Caution should be exercised when interpreting and applying data. The practitioner should avoid conclusions which exceed the data. Any decisions based upon the data should be congruent with the constructs to which the instrument is addressed. Whenever possible, clinical decisions should be supported by the professional literature.

Practitioners should make every effort to observe copyright laws in using test instruments. In many cases, duplication of test equipment, manuals, or protocols is forbidden. Such practices could affect reliability and validity of assessment findings and certainly invite legal action.

Writing reports raises both ethical and professional issues. Practitioners should take special care that reports are accurate, succinct, and professionally presented. Reports are tangible evidence of clinical reasoning. Therapists should always keep in mind the target audience when writing reports. Unnecessary jargon and superfluous information should be avoided in consideration that reports function as documents of communication and public relations.

All client information should be handled with discrimination. Occupational therapists are expected to respect confidentiality. Written permission should be obtained to share confidential information, including test results. It is also important for practitioners to take special caution to avoid using labels or terminology which might be easily misconstrued or damaging to the client.

SUMMARY

Assessment is a complex dynamic process requiring the practitioner to gather information and to make clinical decisions. Exercising sound clinical judgement entails critical analysis. The goal of the occupational therapist in assessment is to identify and resolve human performance deficits. This reflective action requires a theoretical perspective, empirical testing, and clinical skill. In this context, assessment becomes an integral and critical component of occupational therapy.

Study Questions

1. Why is assessment critical to clinical decision-making?

2. If you were aware that you were treating a client whose case was under litigation, what test characteristics would you analyze when selecting assessments?

3. What are the differences between norm-referenced and criterion referenced tests? How do these differences affect occupational therapists?

4. If you are an occupational therapist developing a clinical assessment strategy, how might you envision establishing reliability? validity?

5. What are the differences and limitations associated with screening instruments versus diagnostic instruments? How do they influence clinical decisions?

6. Describe the process of standardization. Why are standardized instruments desirable?

7. What are some of the ethical issues associated with assessment and clinical decision-making?

8. Define a construct. Why are constructs of sometimes difficult to test or measure for occupational therapists?

9. How are the data obtained from clinical assessments applied to the following: patient treatment? determination of clinical efficacy? research? documentation?

10. Describe the cyclical process of clinical decision-making. What is meant by "reflection in action"?

Recommended Readings

Benson, J., & Clark, F. (1982). A guide for instrument development and validitation. *American Journal of Occupational Therapy, 36*, 789-800.

Eden, G. (1986). *The skilled helper: A systematic approach to effective helping.* Belmont, CA: Brooks/Cole, Inc.

Gilette, N. & Mattingly, C. (1987). Clinical reasoning in occupational therapy. *American Journal of Occupational Therapy, 41*(6), 399-400.

Hasselkus, B. and Safrit, M. (1976). Measurement in occupational therapy. *American Journal of Occupational Therapy, 30*(7) pp. 429-436.

Mauer, P., Barris, R., Bonder, B., & Gilette, N. (1984). Hierarchy of competencies relating to the use of standardized instruments and evaluation techniques by occupational therapists. *American Journal of Occupational Therapy, 38*(12), 803-804.

Rogers, J.C. (1983). Clinical reasoning: The ethics, science and art. *American Journal of Occupational Therapy, 37*(9), 601-616.

Rogers, J.C., & Masagatani, G. (1982). Clinical reasoning of occupational therapists during the initial assessment of physically disabled patients. *Occupational Therapy Journal of Research, 2*, 195-212.

Schön, D.A. (1983). The reflective practitioner: How professionals think in action (pp. 40, 49-69). New York: Basic Books

References

American Educational Research Association, American Psychological Association, National Council on Measurement in Education (1985) *Standards for educational and psychological testing*, Washington, D.C.: American Psychological Assocation.

Anderson, S.B., Ball, S., Murphy, R.T. et.al. (1975) *Encyclopedia of Educational Evaluation.* San Francisco: Jossey-Bass

Ayres, A.J., (1988) *Sensory integration and Praxis Tests.* Santa Monica, CA: Western Psychological Association.

Baum, C. (1987). Research: Its relationship to public policy. *American Journal of Occupational Therapy, 41*(3), 143-145.

Christiansen, C.H. (1983). Research an economic imperative. *Occupational Therapy Journal of Research, 3*(4), 195-198.

Gillette, N. & Mattingly, C. (1987). Clinical reasoning in occupational therapy. *American Journal of Occupational Therapy, 41*(6), 399-400.

Gronlund, N. (1977, 1968). *Constructing achievement tests,* 2nd edition. Englewood Cliffs, NJ: Prentice Hall, Inc.

Kerlinger, F.N. (1973). *Foundations of behavioral research* (2nd Ed.) New York: Holt Rinehart and Winston.

Mauer, P., Barris R., Bonder, B. & Gilette, N. (1984). Hierarchy of competencies relating to the use of standardized instruments and evaluation techniques by occupational therapists. *American Journal of Occupational Therapy, 38*(12), 803-804.

Mausner, J.S. & Kramer, S. (1985). *Epidemeology: An Introductory Text.* Philadelphia, PA: W B Saunders.

Miller, L.J., (1982). *The Miller Assessment for Pre-Schoolers.* Littleton, CO: Foundation for Knowledge in Development.

Nunnally, J.C. (1978). *Psychometric theory.* (2nd Ed.) New York: McGraw-Hill.

Ottenbacher, K.J. (1987). Research: its importance to clinical practice in occupational therapy. *American Journal of Occupational Therapy, 41*(4), 213-215.

Pelland, M.J. (1987). A conceptual model for the instruction and supervision of treatment planning. *American Journal of Occupational Therapy, 41*(6), 351-359.

Schön, D.A. (1983). *The reflective practitioner: How professionals think in action* (pp. 40, 49-69). New York: Basic Books.

Schön, D.A. (1987). *Educating the reflective practitioner* (p. 13). San Francisco: Jossey-Bass.

CHAPTER CONTENT OUTLINE

KEY TERMS

ADL

Battery

Characteristic behavior

Checklist

Domain

Domain specificity

Dysfunctional hierarchy

History

Reactivity

ABSTRACT

This chapter reviews assessment strategies that provide information on an
individual's ability to perform role-related tasks. General issues relevant to
assessing occupational performance are identified, including capability versus
characteristic performance, reactivity bias, and problems related to numerical
scoring. Assessment tools are categorized according to the three major
occupational performance areas of self-maintenance, play/leisure, and work,
with an additional category for those instruments which are multi-dimensional in
nature. Descriptions and reliability and validity data are presented for each
instrument reviewed.

Occupational Performance Assessment

Charles Christiansen

"The inherent complexity of rehabilitation is itself mirrored in the complexity of assessment issues. As our early concepts of rehabilitation were concerned with a narrow pathology-oriented view of the individual, so too were our concepts of assessment. However, our current views of rehabilitation have changed, and they now focus attention more clearly on problems associated with environmental functioning and adaptation."

— William D. Frey, 1984

OBJECTIVES

The information in this chapter is intended to help the reader—

1. appreciate the dysfunctional hierarchy as a means of classifying assessment approaches.

2. distinguish between capability and characteristic behavior.

3. explain "reactivity" as an assessment issue.

4. identify appropriate instruments for assessing self-care, work, and play/leisure.

5. appreciate the measurement of satisfaction as a means of deriving information relevant to performance.

6. identify appropriate global or multi-domain assessment approaches.

7. appreciate the complexity of performance assessment.

OVERVIEW

Assessment is the process of gathering sufficient information about individuals and their environments so as to be able to make informed decisions regarding intervention. Such information may be gathered using both formal and informal screening and evaluation strategies that include chart reviews, direct observation of behavior, interviews, standardized tests, and various clinical assessment procedures.

Because occupational therapy is concerned with functional performance, it is appropriate that many of the assessment strategies relevant to the field involve the performance of tasks. Task-oriented approaches can provide valuable information about an individual's level of function in the various domains of occupational performance. Reference to performance domains reflects a concern for both the breadth and the purpose of functional abilities. In contrast, attention to the level of assessment provides a means for ordering information about function as it relates to role performance. Thus, assessment strategies can be classified on the basis of their domain of concern as well as the level at which they provide performance-oriented information.

Dysfunctional Hierarchy

To speak of levels of information in human performance assessment is to suggest the existence of a hierarchy of dysfunction. The concept of a **dysfunctional hierarchy** in rehabilitation was introduced in chapter one, and will be summarized briefly here. Dysfunctional hierarchy refers to the distinction among the terms impairment, disability, and handicap as originally developed by Nagi (1976) and Wood (1980). At the lowest level of this framework, the function of organs can be evaluated. Here, a deficit is referred to as an *impairment*, which may or may not affect a person's ability to accomplish tasks. This is important to recognize, since some early approaches to functional assessment were based on the assumption that impairment was equated with disability.

The next level of dysfunction is termed a *disability,* in which task accomplishment is affected. If weakness or paralysis in a forearm and hand renders a person unable to turn a key and open a locked door, disability is present for that task. The use of an adaptive device to help one to unlock the door would negate the presence of disability, despite the presence of impairment. If performance of that task (turning keys to open a lock) was instrumental to one's role as a worker (e.g., night watchman), then a *handicap* would be demonstrated. At this highest level of dysfunction or handicap, an inability to satisfactorily perform tasks often hinders successful role performance and results in social disadvantage.

Independent task performance is not by itself a condition of role competence, although some cultural biases do exist in favor of autonomy and self-sufficiency. Halpern and Fuhrer (1984) were among the first to use the dysfunctional hierarchy as a means of classifying assessment instruments in rehabilitation. While it has been argued that the ultimate purpose of rehabilitation is the elimination of handicap, the focus of many assessment strategies in occupational therapy practice has tended to occur at the levels of impairment and disability.

Many of the assessment strategies addressed in the following chapters provide information about deficits related to specific performance factors, such as sensory, neuromotor, social, cognitive, psychological, and social areas of functioning. Impairment within a specific factor may have a marked impact on an individual's occupational performance or ability to satisfactorily perform important life tasks in the domains of self-care/maintenance, play/leisure or work/education.

Domain Specificity

Role performance takes place within or across the occupational performance **domains** of self-maintenance, play/leisure, and work. For example, to perform competently in the worker role, one must not only be able to perform tasks required for a particular job, but must be able to perform tasks of self-maintenance as well. The role of head of household might require competence in all three domains, including competence and independence in self-maintenance, the ability to provide for economic needs (which suggests competence in the world of work), and the ability to engage in the recreational or leisure activities of a family unit.

Some assessment approaches in occupational therapy are domain-specific, in that they seek information on task performance in a defined area of occupational performance. For example, traditional **activities of daily living (ADL)** scales provide information specifically on self-care while other assessments provide information on vocational or work-oriented skills. Some assessment strategies are more global in nature and provide useful information on a person's performance in two or more areas of human occupation.

In this chapter, attention will be paid to assessment strategies which provide information on an individual's ability to perform role-related tasks. Some instruments used in occupational therapy yield information at more than one level of the dysfunctional hierarchy. However, the focus here will be on assessments that yield information at the level of disability or handicap. With these assessment strategies, information is most often provided through task performance as observed by the rehabilitation professional or reported by the patient or others.

Occupational performance assessments can be organized according to (1) the occupational domain to which they are directed, (2) the level of focus in the dysfunctional hierarchy, and (3) whether they are norm-referenced or criterion-referenced (See Figure 15-1). Within these general categories, there are instruments designed for populations with special characteristics, such as children, older persons, those in long-term care facilities, or individuals with mental retardation. Strategies developed for persons with severe hearing and/or visual impairment are not included because they are used less frequently within the profession of occupational therapy. In addition, this is not an all-inclusive coverage of assessment approaches, but rather a selective discussion of those instruments which are readily available and for which evidence of acceptable reliability and validity has been established or is being actively pursued.

Approaches to Obtaining Information about Occupational Performance

For the instruments described in this chapter, there are several approaches used to derive information about functional performance: (1) by direct observations of specific (or *criterion*) behaviors by the client in structured or unstructured situations, (2) by self-administered questionnaires, (3) by structured interviews, or (4) by clinical judgment. Each of these approaches has its advantages and disadvantages.

Instruments which are designed for direct observation of a client's performance under standardized conditions can be highly reliable and valid, but such approaches are also costly since they require the time and judgment of skilled personnel. These requirements limit the utility of the direct observation approach for assessing performance in natural environments. Less direct approaches to performance assessment, such as client self-report, questionnaires, and structured interviews, involve more subjectivity and hence result in diminished reliability. However, they are less costly and thus more practical for the assessment of performance in complex situations. Moreover, they have

been shown to have sufficient validity to justify their use in clinical situations (Brown, et al., 1982; Garrard & Bennet, 1971; Kivela, 1984).

One type of self-report strategy, the *measurement of satisfaction*, deserves special mention here. Although not behavioral in focus, this type of strategy is useful in assessing function because it reflects the patient/client's perception of functional inadequacy. Kielhofner (1985, p. 65) has identified dissatisfaction as a component of inefficacy, one of three identified levels of maladaptation or dysfunction in occupation. (See Chapter 1)

It has been argued that all approaches to performance assessment must be administered under standardized conditions in order to ensure maximum reliability and validity. To obtain standardized conditions, one must specify the conditions under which performance will be observed. However, this creates formidable difficulties if one is concerned with getting an accurate picture of the characteristic level of functional performance under everyday living circumstances, which will vary from one person to the next.

Assessing Capability versus Characteristic Behavior

The process of assessment should be viewed as a means of gathering information to provide the best possible picture of an individual's level of functional performance. For this reason, it is important that function not be viewed in isolation from its environmental context. As Alexander and Fuhrer (1984) have noted, a distinction should be made between a

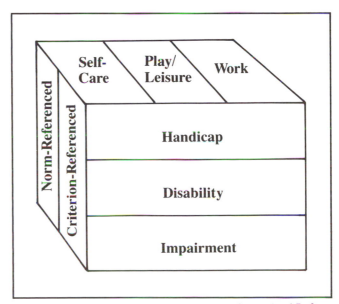

Figure 15-1. Classifying Instruments for Assessing Occupational Performance.

person's capability as demonstrated during the assessment process and the **characteristic behavior** or performance demonstrated by the person in a natural context.

For example, an individual might be able to perform a self-care task within a rehabilitation environment but unable to perform the task to satisfaction at home. Some studies have shown an apparent decline in the functional abilities of patients following discharge from the treatment setting. This may be due to the differences between the two settings. Hence, the physical and social environment in which assessment takes place must be carefully considered so that conclusions about functional ability accurately reflect characteristic performance.

Unfortunately, very few instruments have been designed to assess individuals within their natural environments. Because such assessments must be designed to permit maximum flexibility in the choice of items and the conditions under which items are presented, these approaches are very difficult to standardize. As a consequence, efforts to establish their reliability and validity are also hindered. Nevertheless, it can be argued that valid assessment of role performance is difficult to achieve outside the daily living context of an individual, and efforts to focus on role performance must rely more on client self-report or interviews with observers in the environment rather than on direct observation of standardized tasks.

Reactivity Bias

Specialists in behavioral measurement have long been concerned with the issue of reactivity. **Reactivity** refers to the process whereby the very act of observing or evaluating an individual introduces an environmental condition which itself influences or changes performance. For example, when children at play are assessed using direct observation, there is danger that the addition of a camera or observer might create sufficient distraction so as to change the very nature of the activities being observed. During assessment of work or self-care performance, reactivity might be a factor because of provoked anxiety that could influence a person's failure to attain criterion levels. As the assessment becomes more obtrusive and the patient becomes more aware of being observed or evaluated, the situation becomes less typical, and generalizations about the patient's performance within a natural context are more difficult to justify.

Numerical Scoring and Weighting of Assessments

Many of the functional status instruments to be reviewed in this chapter yield numerical scores. Such scores easily convey a summary of detailed information, and thus permit easy comparison of a patient's performance over time. Numerical scores also facilitate the comparison of

performance between diagnostic groups or intervention programs for research purposes. Functional assessment scores are typically derived from the assignment of a single digit rating on an ordinal or ranked scale (often 1 through 5) for each item. Total performance scores for the assessment are then based upon the cumulative total of item scores. A higher total score usually reflects greater functional performance and independence.

Scoring systems for functional assessment instruments are generally based upon implicit assumptions about the value of a particular performance item or category. In most instruments, items are weighted equally so as to avoid the difficulties associated with assigning values to various functional categories. However, in some instruments, items reflect different weighting based upon the developers' judgment that one activity is more important than another. For example, an item related to mobility might earn a higher value than an item pertaining to grooming.

Jette (1985) asserts that explicit weighting schemes should be developed for all functional assessments so as to permit more precise and valid discrimination of functional performance levels. This can be accomplished through the use of experts and various weighting methods. Explicit weighting schemes have been developed for some global health status instruments (addressed later in this chapter).

Noting that the regular use of rating scales tends to give them credibility, Merbitz, Morris, and Grip (1989) have pointed out that many scales used to assess performance in rehabilitation employ ordinal (ranking) scales and treat the resulting scores as though they had the properties of more precise levels of scaling (i.e., as though they were interval or ratio level scales). Such treatment, they argue, leads to invalid inferences and could result in flawed decisions regarding resource allocation in rehabilitation.

Readers are encouraged to refer to a discussion of this issue by Wright and Linacre (1989), who have observed that the Rasch measurement model permits the design of instruments which translate observations into linear and ratio measures. This method accounts for the variability that occurs across situations when persons with varying circumstances are subjected to a given measuring instrument (Rasch, 1980).

ASSESSMENT OF SELF-CARE/MAINTENANCE

One of the more traditional areas in which role performance has been assessed is in the area of self-maintenance, which includes self-care. Historically, assessment of self-care has meant establishing the degree to which an individual was independent in those tasks related to toileting, bathing and grooming, eating, dressing, transferring, and mobility. However, a review by Kellman and Willner in 1962 found that scales tended to vary considerably in the degree to which they yielded consistent or valid scores largely because of the lack of specific performance criteria in scoring, lack of standardization, and failure to consider the influence of the setting on performance. There were also problems in comparing the approaches because scales varied in the tasks covered, and scores seldom could be translated easily into a clear picture of a patient's level of independence.

Kaufert (1983) has identified the following factors which make it difficult to validate measures of independence in self-care: (1) the level of assistance needed, (2) the use of adaptive aids and devices, or even the use of helpers, (3) the professional orientation of evaluators, and (4) the motivation and role expectations of the patient. All of these factors can substantially influence performance and should be considered in the assessment of functional independence.

In reviewing the characteristics of an ideal self-care scale, Christiansen, Schwartz, and Barnes (1988) suggested that in addition to reliability, validity, standardization, and scalability, an instrument should be comprehensive, performance-based, and practical. Few basic ADL scales developed over the years have been able to approach these rigorous standards.

History of Self-Care Instruments

Despite their shortcomings, the rehabilitation literature has reflected general acceptance of several self-care scales over the years. These include the *PULSES* profile, the *Katz Index of ADL*, the *Barthel Index*, and the *Kenny Index of ADL*. Each of these scales is characterized by an interpretable score and at least minimal evidence of reliability and validity. Thus, they can be considered among the better basic ADL scales that have become widely used during the past 40 years.

The PULSES Profile. This profile, published by Moskowitz and McCann in 1957, actually began as a means of classifying military personnel in the 1940's and was designed to measure physical condition, performance using the upper extremities, mobility as permitted by lower extremity function, communication and sensory performance, bowel and bladder or excretory performance, and psychosocial status. The acronym PULSES is formed from letters from these areas of assessment: **P**hysical condition, **U**pper extremities, **L**ower extremities, **S**ensory, **E**xcretory, psychosocial **S**tatus.

The original PULSES lacked carefully defined criteria and was based on the assumption that impairment equated

with disability. However, it subsequently was revised and improved by Granger and associates in 1975 and has shown evidence of reliability and validity in several published studies since that time. It appears to be most useful in detecting change prior to discharge and lacks sensitivity, so that only substantial changes in function, such as those occurring in patients with cerebrovascular accident or spinal cord injury, tend to be reflected through its scoring system.

The Index of Independence in Activities of Daily Living. This index was developed by Katz, Ford, & Moskowitz, (1963) to study the results of treatment and prognosis in elderly and chronically ill persons. The Katz Index of ADL, as it is commonly known, is unique in that it yields an alphabetical rating from "A" through "G" that reflects a progressive loss of independence, with "A" being independent and "G" being dependent. The individual is scored in the following six subscales: bathing, dressing, toileting, transferring, continence, and feeding. The overall grade of independence is determined from the scores of the six subscales. Therefore, a person who is *independent* in all the subscale areas would receive an overall rating of "A," whereas an overall rating of "G" would indicate *dependency* in all six of these categories.

Studies have shown the scale to be consistent between raters and valid as a tool to accumulate information about recovery following stroke (Gibson, 1974), as well as to indicate care needs in other disorders (Brorsson & Asberg, 1984; Katz, Downs, Cash, et al., 1970). As a true Guttman scale, the Katz index of ADL has been found to correctly classify the functional abilities of patients 86% of the time.

The Barthel Index. This index has been perhaps the most studied of basic ADL scales and shows sensitivity to change over time and the ability to predict rehabilitation outcome. It includes ten items: feeding, transfers, personal grooming and hygiene, bathing, toileting, walking, negotiating stairs, and controlling bowel and bladder (Mahoney & Barthel, 1965). Scoring of items is based on a weighted system that considers assisted performance. An individual with a maximum score of 100 on the scale is defined as continent, able to feed and dress independently, walk at least a block, and climb and descend stairs. The developers of this index cautioned that independent performance of these tasks would not equate with the ability to live alone in the community, since important instrumental skills related to self-maintenance are not assessed. (See Table 15-1)

The Barthel Index has been studied widely and has demonstrated good reliability as well as predictive and concurrent validity. Test-retest reliability coefficients were estimated at .89 in one study (Granger, Dewis & Peter, 1979), and interrater reliability coefficients were above .95.

Table 15-1
Barthel Index

	With Help	Independent
1. Feeding (If food needs to be cut up = help)	5	10
2. Moving from wheelchair to bed and return (includes sitting up in bed)	5-10	15
3. Personal toilet (wash face, comb hair, shave, clean teeth)	0	5
4. Getting on and off toilet (handling clothes, wipe, flush)	5	10
5. Bathing self	0	5
6. Walking on level surface (or, if unable to walk, propel wheelchair) (*score only if unable to walk)	0*	5*
7. Ascend and descend stairs	5	10
8. Dressing (includes tying shoes, fastening fasteners)	5	10
9. Controlling bowels	5	10
10. Controlling bladder	5	10

A patient scoring 100 BI is continent, feeds himself, dresses himself, gets up out of bed and chairs, bathes himself, walks at least a block, and can ascend and descend stairs. This does not mean that he is able to live alone: he may not be able to cook, keep house, and meet the public, but he is able to get along without attendant care.

Reprinted with permission: Mahoney, F.I., Barthel, D.W. (1965). Functional evaluation: The Barthel index. Maryland State Medical Journal 14(2), 61-65.

The Barthel Index has consistently shown positive correlations with other scales of ADL (concurrent validity), while also demonstrating significant relationships with various rehabilitation outcome measures (Hertanu, Demopoulous, Yang, et al., 1984; and Wade, Skilbeck, & Hewer, 1983).

The Kenny Index of ADL. This index developed by Schoening, Anderegg, Bergstrom, and colleagues in 1965 has not been studied as widely as previous scales mentioned here, but has shown impressive sensitivity to change. It measures six categories of self-care: bed movement, transfers, locomotion, dressing, personal hygiene, and feeding. The 17 items of the Kenny Index of ADL are rated on a five-point scale, and the averages for each of the six categories are summed.

Researchers have found significant correlations between total independence scores and the amount of time required for transfers performed on a rehabilitation unit (Schoening, & Iverson, 1968). One study found the Kenny Index of ADL to be more sensitive to change than either the Barthel Index or the Katz Index of ADL (Donaldson, Wagner, & Gresham, 1973). Table 15-2 gives a summary comparison of the characteristics of the PULSES, Katz, Barthel and Kenny scales.

No historical account of developments in ADL measurement would be complete without mentioning the efforts of M. Powell Lawton at the Philadelphia Geriatric Center. Lawton recognized that activities of daily living consisted of more than self-care tasks such as feeding, grooming, bathing, dressing, and mobility. He conceptualized that other tasks, such as telephone use, housekeeping, laundry, transportation, food preparation, medication management, and the handling of finances were necessary to function independently, particularly if a person is to remain within a typical home or community. These instrumental activities of daily living require higher neuropsychological organization, and therefore represent a higher level of independent functioning.

With this in mind, Lawton and his colleagues (Lawton & Brody, 1969) developed two scales designed to assess the self-care performance of older persons. These scales were the *Physical Self Maintenance Scale* (PSMS) and the *Instrumental Activities of Daily Living Scale* (IADL). The notions behind these scales were incorporated into a broader assessment of the overall well-being of elderly persons known as the *Multilevel Assessment Instrument* (Lawton, Moss, Fulcomer, et al., 1982), which is discussed in the section on comprehensive assessment approaches.

Contemporary Developments in Assessing Self-Care Performance

Since the mid-1970's, there has been a great deal of additional effort in the development of tools to assess independence in ADL or self-care. As a result, several promising instruments have emerged, most notably the *Klein-Bell ADL Scale*, the *Kohlman Evaluation of Living Skills* (KELS), the *Milwaukee Evaluation of Daily Living Skills* (MEDLS), the *Functional Status Index*, and the *Functional Independence Measure* (FIM) along with its counterpart for children, the *Wee FIM*. In the following sections, each of these instruments will be examined with respect to their development, design, reliability, validity and practicality.

Klein-Bell ADL Scale. This scale was developed with the objective of overcoming various shortcomings of the traditional and widely used ADL scales, including inconsistency in assigning point values, a lack of differentiation between the levels of assistance needed to perform tasks, and the lack of applicability of some scales' items to all patients. In selecting items for the scale, the developers analyzed basic categories of self-care tasks in order to identify critical and easily observable components of these behaviors which would be necessary for independent functioning.

The resulting scale included 170 items which relate to dressing, mobility, elimination, bathing/hygiene, eating, and emergency communication. Each item on the scale is scored as either "achieved" or "failed," depending upon whether the person needs either physical or verbal assistance in order to perform the task. The performance of an item with the use of adaptive equipment is scored as "achieved" because the purpose of such equipment is to increase independent functioning.

Scoring for items on the Klein-Bell ADL Scale was derived empirically using a panel of rehabilitation professionals who were asked to rate potential items along four dimensions for subsequent weighting: (1) importance of the activity to health of the individual, (2) difficulty of an item for an able-bodied person to perform, (3) the time required to perform the item, and (4) difficulty of an item if performed by an able-bodied person for someone else (assistance). Successful performance or achievement of an item yields the total number of points possible for that item, and unsuccessful performance results in a score of zero. The total points achieved within each ADL area are totaled and combined to yield an overall ADL independence score. Score totals are designed to be used to measure change in an individual's performance.

Total raw scores on the Klein-Bell ADL scale can range from zero to 313, but are expressed as percentages of the total points possible. An advantage of the scale is the ease

---

Table 15-2
Summary of Widely Used ADL Scales

	PULSES Moskowitz & McCann 1957	**Index of ADL** Katz et al., 1963	**Barthel Index** Mahoney & Barthel, 1965	**Kenny** Schoening et al., 1965
Domain/ Tasks Assessed	• Physical Condition • Upper extremity • Lower extremity • Sensory components • Excretory (bowel and bladder) • Status of patient (mental and physical)	• Bathing • Dressing • Going to toilet • Transfer • Continence • Feeding	• Feeding • W/C Transfer • Grooming • Toilet transfer • Bathing • Level walking • Stairs • Dressing • Bowel control • Bladder control	• Bed • Transfers • Locomotion (walking, stairs, W/C) • Dressing (UE, LE, Feet) • Personal Hygiene (incl. bowel/bladder) • Feeding
Scoring	Numerical 4 point scale. Range 0-24. Adapted version relates upper and lower extremity function to ADL tasks and mobility.	Ordinal ranking A-G based on descending levels of independence.	Adapted version is based on weighted numerical scale yielding mobility and self care score. Range 0-100.	Overall score derived from rating (0-4) among all items within each category. Range 0-24.
Reliability/ Validity	Reported Coefficients: Test/retest = .87 Interrater = >.95 Evidence of predictive and concurrent validity.	Coefficient of scalability = .89. Some evidence of predictive and concurrent validity.	Reported test-retest reliability .89, interrater reliability >.95. Evidence of predictive and concurrent validity.	Formal reliability coefficients have not been reported. Some evidence of predictive and concurrent validity.
Strengths/ Limitations	Widely used among varying patient populations. Lacks subscore detail in discrete ADL variables.	Derived score yields specific information about patient's functional independence.	Comprehensive and widely used in U.S. Adapted versions permit distinction between levels of independence.	Sensitive to patient change in overall function. Has not been extensively validated.

Adapted with permission from: Christiansen, C.H., Schwartz, R.K. & Barnes, K.A. (1988). Self care: Evaluation and Management. In Delisa, J., et al. (Eds.). Rehabilitation Medicine: Principles and Practice. Philadelphia: J.B. Lippincott (p. 104).

Items from the Klein-Bell ADL Scale					

A. Bed Mobility

(Date of assessment placed above appropriate column.)

89. Turn from supine to one side for 30 seconds	(3)					
90. Turn from side to prone	(3)					
91. Turn from prone to side	(3)					
92. Go from supine to at least 70 degrees sitting for one minute	(3)					

Figure 15-2. Example of Mobility Items from the Klein-Bell ADL Scale. (Item value is in parentheses.) *Reprinted with permission: Klein, R.J. and Bell, B.J. (1979).*

with which it can be used to instruct family members about a patient's need for assistance on specific activities. The small, observable behaviors comprising each area of self-care can be used to readily document or communicate the specific needs or level of performance of each person who is evaluated. Analysis of failed items can also give important data about deficits in performance subsystems, and thus can also serve as a convenient basis for determining treatment plans.

Interrater reliability was estimated during development of the scale using six pairs of raters. Across all items on 20 patients, a 92% agreement was achieved. Evidence of predictive validity also exists. A high degree of correlation was found between scores on the scale and the number of hours per week a person required assistance during a five- to ten-month period after discharge (Klein & Bell, 1982). A study by Smith, Morrow & Heitman, et al. (1986) found that use of the Klein Bell Scale within a clinical setting improved documentation and communication of the self-care needs of patients, and thereby enhanced the effectiveness of the rehabilitation team (see Figure 15-2).

Kohlman Evaluation of Living Skills. The Kohlman Evaluation of Living Skills is an evaluation of basic living skills which combines interview and task performance techniques. Suitable for a variety of settings and populations, the KELS originally was developed for use with psychiatric patients at Harborview Medical Center in Seattle, Washington (McGourty, 1988). It is intended to be administered easily and scored within 30 to 45 minutes.

The KELS assesses 18 living skills grouped within five major categories of self-care, safety and health, money management, transportation and telephone, and work and leisure. Some items require use of props, such as a bar of soap, a bill, local phone number cards, a local phone book, and a telephone. Other items including some in the Safety

and Health section, use pictures which are included in the administration and scoring manual (see Figure 15-3).

Instructions to be given by the examiner and the method of presenting the necessary equipment items have been standardized. No performance feedback is given to the patient during administration. Scoring criteria have been formulated to indicate the minimum standards required for living independently within the community. Independence is viewed by the author (McGourty, 1979) as the ability to perform basic living skills in a healthful and safe manner without the assistance of others.

Items scored as "needs assistance" are given a score of one point except those in the work/leisure category which are assessed one-half point. Special provisions are made for those items in which the assignment of points is not appropriate. They are designated as "not applicable" or "see note," and assigned a score of zero. A score of zero is also assigned to all items labeled "independent." A total score of five and one-half or less indicates the patient is capable of living independently. A score of six or more indicates the person being evaluated would need assistance in order to live in the community.

The examiner is encouraged to gather additional information about the individual's skills and abilities during the administration process. For example, pictures regarding safety and health have been designed to evaluate the presence of figure-ground skill, which is a factor related to environmental safety. Other opportunities exist during administration for determining cognitive abilities, such as memory, attention span, and comprehension. Information about the patient's use of time is observed during administration of the work and leisure section. A summary note of findings related to these areas is placed at the bottom of the KELS score sheet.

Several studies have been completed which address the reliability and validity of the KELS. A study of interrater reliability involving psychiatric patients was conducted by Ilika and Hoffman in 1981 with significant correlations reported. Percentage of rater agreement ranged from 74% to 94%. Evidence of the scale's validity is also available, including reported correlations of .78 to .89 (p<.001) with scores on the *Global Assessment Scale* (Ilika & Hoffman, 1981), and a correlation of .84 with the *Bay Area Functional Performance Evaluation* (BaFPE) (Kaufman, 1982).

In a study of the scale's discriminate validity, Tateichi (1984) found that the scale was able to correctly differentiate persons living in a sheltered setting versus those living independently with an accuracy rate of 90%. The same study demonstrated interrater reliability of 84% to 94%. A later study by Morrow (1985) demonstrated that the scale

predicted the discharge situations of 20 inpatients on a geriatric unit with 72% accuracy.

In summary, the KELS appears to be a reliable and easily administered scale for determining the capacity of patients to live independently. While more research is needed to establish its validity, early studies have been encouraging. The scale is suitable for use by various types of patients in different settings.

Milwaukee Evaluation of Daily Living Skills. The Milwaukee Evaluation of Daily Living Skills (MEDLS) was developed for long-term psychiatric patients with the purpose of assessing behavioral performance in the skill areas of basic communication, medication management, personal

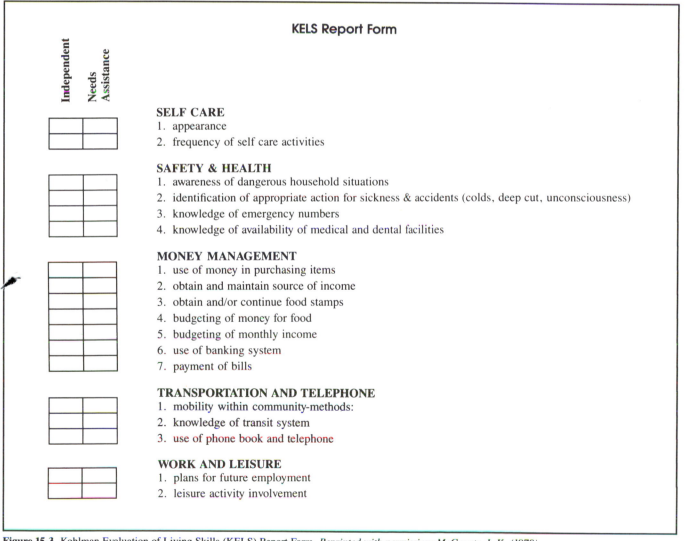

Figure 15-3. Kohlman Evaluation of Living Skills (KELS) Report Form. *Reprinted with permission: McGourty, L.K. (1979).*

care and hygiene, time awareness, dressing, eating, personal health care, safety in the home, use of telephone, and transportation. The present version is considered a research version since validation has not been completed (Leonardelli, 1987). The scale is designed for individual evaluation. Group administration is not recommended.

The focus of MEDLS is assessment of the skills needed for adequate functioning in the client's anticipated living situation. Evaluation is conducted through 21 subtests which can be administered individually or in any combination (see Figure 15-4). There are four major components to the scale: a screening form, equipment list, subtests with administration procedures, and a reporting form.

The MEDLS screening form is used to determine skill areas appropriate for evaluation. Subtests are selected based on the evaluator's review of information from the medical record, input from family and other health care workers, client observations and interview, and professional judgment.

The 21 subtests of the MEDLS, which may be used individually or in any combination, are scored separately according to the number of subskills needed to demonstrate competence in the respective skill area. Performance on a subtest is measured in comparison to the overall possible

---

Subtests of the Milwaukee Evaluation of Daily Living Skills (MEDLS)

- Basic communication skills
- Eating
- Maintenance of clothing
- Medication management
- Toileting
- Brushing teeth
- Denture care
- Bathing
- Use of make-up
- Shaving
- Nail care
- Hair care
- Eyeglass care
- Personal health care
- Safety in community
- Safety in home
- Time awareness
- Use of money
- Use of telephone
- Use of transportation

Figure 15-4. Subtests of the Milwaukee Evaluation of Daily Living Skills (MEDLS).

---

score for that subtest. Score values are assigned to reflect the proportion of observed skill deficits for each subtest. There is no cumulative or total score for this instrument.

The MEDLS offers a flexible, performance-based approach to gathering assessment information about important life skills related to independent functioning. Self-report is kept to a minimum and appropriate discretion is left to the professional caregiver to select relevant subtests for administration. At the present time, no reliability or validity studies have been completed for the MEDLS. However, the instrument shows promise in being able to provide baseline data for establishing treatment objectives and providing a quantifiable measure of change.

Functional Independence Measure. The Functional Independence Measure (Hamilton, Granger, Sherwin, et al., 1987) evolved from a task force of the American Congress of Rehabilitation Medicine and the American Academy of Physical Medicine and Rehabilitation. This task force was charged to develop a uniform data system for describing and communicating about disability. Its efforts led to grant support from the National Institute of Disability and Rehabilitation Research of the United States Department of Education. The funded project sought to develop a measure which would provide information that was reliable and valid, discipline-free, and both practical and acceptable to practitioners.

Following a review of 36 functional assessment instruments, the task force selected the most common and useful functional assessment items and developed a rating scale that would permit the assessment of severity of disability in a consistent manner. It was determined that the FIM would assess the areas of self-care, sphincter management, mobility, locomotion, communication, and social cognition. Provision was also made for the documentation of demographic information, diagnoses, impairment groups, length of hospital stay, and hospital charges.

The FIM is intended to serve as a basic indicator of the severity of disability and thus measures disability rather than impairment. It is designed to measure what the patient actually does, rather than what he or she is capable of doing. The underlying rationale for rating items on the scale relates to the amount of assistance needed by the patient to complete the activities being measured. This permits the FIM to provide data that reflect both the social as well as economic costs of disability, as was the intended purpose.

No inference is made by the developers of the scale that the FIM is a comprehensive clinical assessment instrument. Practitioners are encouraged to include additional items viewed as relevant to the patient during the assessment process. Consequently, the FIM should be viewed as an infrastructure which provides sufficient information to result in valid conclusions about severity of disability or level of independence. It also provides uniform terminology and procedures which permit the collection and analysis of data for nationwide samples of patients in rehabilitation.

The FIM consists of 18 items, each of which has scoring levels ranging from one to seven (see Table 15-3). Thus, a patient who could not be tested or who needed total assistance would score a one on every item, yielding a minimum score of 18. Similarly, the highest possible total score for an individual who demonstrated complete independence on all 18 items of the FIM would be 126. Levels for each item on the FIM have carefully constructed behavioral criteria to assist in scoring.

Since 1984, data have been gathered at several sites using the FIM for the purpose of refining the instrument and establishing its reliability and validity. Interrater reliability, assessed during the pilot phase over a version of the measure that had only four levels of precision, yielded an average intra-class correlation (Kappa) of .54. Further refinements in the instrument are expected to result in improved interrater reliability (Hamilton, Granger, Sherwin, et al., 1987).

Face validity for the FIM was assessed by asking experienced clinicians who administered the scale to identify items that were ''difficult to understand,'' ''unnecessary,'' or ''additional items,'' and to rate the FIM as a measure of the severity of disability on a five-point scale representing poor to excellent. Data from 114 clinicians at 11 separate rehabilitation facilities were collected. Results indicated that the FIM was perceived as an acceptable measure with relevant items of reasonable difficulty (Granger, Hamilton, Keith, et al., 1986).

Self-Care Instruments for Special Populations

Several measures of ADL have been developed for specialized populations, including children, persons with chronic disease such as rheumatoid arthritis, and elderly persons. A few of these instruments are summarized in the following sections.

Functional Independence Measure for Children (WeeFIM). A version of the Functional Independence Measure, known as the ''WeeFIM,'' has been developed for children from the ages of 6 months to 6 years of age (Granger, 1989). The developers are attempting to standardize the instrument for specific age groups, so that the measure of disability yielded by the WeeFIM will be age-appropriate. The research version of the WeeFIM duplicates the FIM in terms of content except that the social cognition items have been omitted. Later versions of the instrument are expected to

---

Table 15-3
Abilities Assessed on the Functional Independence Measure (FIM)

Self Care
Feeding
Grooming
Bathing
Dressing—upper body
Dressing—lower body
Toileting

Sphincter Control
Bladder management
Bowel management

Mobility
Transfers: Bed, chair, wheelchair
Transfers: Toilet
Transfers: Tub or shower

Locomotion
Walking or using wheelchair
Stairs

Communication
Comprehension
Expression

Social Cognition
Social interaction
Problem solving
Memory

---

include this category when suitable definitions relevant to children of the appropriate age group have been developed. Once field testing has been completed, the authors hope to be able to provide reliability and validity data on this children's version of the FIM.

The developers of the WeeFIM have carefully described the relationship between developmental assessment and functional assessment as overlapping and complimentary to each other. The authors state that developmental assessment analyzes patterns of limitations in a child's functioning within specified categories (gross motor, fine motor, personal-social, language, and adaptive or problem-solving behavior), whereas functional assessment measures the burden of care imposed by disability and aids an efficient allocation of rehabilitation resources to achieve functional competence.

Functional Status Index

Activity	Assistance (1 → 5)	Pain (0 → 7)	Difficulty (0 → 7)	Comment
Mobility				
Walking inside	———	———	———	
Climbing up stairs	———	———	———	
Transferring to and from toilet	———	———	———	
Getting in and out of bed	———	———	———	
Driving a car	———	———	———	
Personal care				
Combing hair	———	———	———	
Putting on pants	———	———	———	
Buttoning clothes	———	———	———	
Washing all parts of the body	———	———	———	
Putting on shoes/slippers	———	———	———	
Home chores				
Vacuuming a rug	———	———	———	
Reaching into high cupboards	———	———	———	
Doing laundry	———	———	———	
Washing windows	———	———	———	
Doing yardwork	———	———	———	
Hand activities				
Writing	———	———	———	
Opening containers	———	———	———	
Turning faucets	———	———	———	
Cutting food	———	———	———	
Vocational				
Performing all job responsibilities	———	———	———	
Avocational				
Performing hobbies requiring hand work	———	———	———	
Attending church	———	———	———	
Socializing with friends and relatives	———	———	———	

Key: Assistance: 1 → 5; **1** = independent; **2** = uses devices; **3** = uses human assistance; **4** = uses devices and human assistance; **5** = unable to do. Pain: 0 → 7; **0** = no pain and **7** = extremely severe pain. Difficulty: 0 → 7; **0** = not difficult and **7** = extremely difficult. Time frame, on the average, during the past seven days.

Figure 15-5. Functional Status Index. *Reprinted with permission: Jette A: The Functional Status Index: reliability of a chronic disease evaluation instrument. Arch Phys Med Rehab 61:395, 1980.*

Functional Status Index. The Functional Status Index (FSI) is a self-report measure of basic and instrumental activities of daily living. It is designed to evaluate functional outcomes among chronically disabled populations living in non-institutional environments (Jette, 1980a, 1980b). It was derived from the original Katz Index of ADL for use in a pilot program for older persons with rheumatoid arthritis. The most recent version of the scale includes 17 representative activities, selected from an earlier pool of 44 (see Figure 15-5). These items are grouped into subscales of basic ADL, instrumental ADL, social/role function, and emotional function.

Early versions of the scale assessed three dimensions of function in the performance of selected daily activities: dependence, pain, and perceived difficulty. However, subsequent revisions have omitted use of the pain dimension. Functional dependence is assessed using a five-point scale ranging from independence to dependence (0 = completely dependent, and 4 = complete independence). Level of difficulty is measured on a separate four-point ordinal scale ranging from "no ·difficulty" to "severe difficulty" in performing daily activities.

The FSI has demonstrated inter-observer reliability in the range of .61 to .78 (Jette & Deniston, 1978) with slightly higher values reported in a study of adults with rheumatoid arthritis (Jette, 1980b). Deniston and Jette (1980) found that scores in the FSI dimensions of pain, difficulty, and independence were correlated positively with client reports of joint condition, their ability to deal with arthritis, and their number of "good days." The same study failed to show relationships between scale scores and professional assessments of joint condition or the client's ability to deal with the attendant problems of arthritis.

More recently, the FSI was used in a study of patients recovering from hip fracture (Harris, et al., 1986; Jette, et al., 1986). Criterion validity for the scale items was established by comparing patient responses to direct observation of the criterion performance for nine physical activities. Levels of agreement using the five-point scale ranged from .71 to .95 for the nine items.

The FSI is a unique clinical tool that measures both perceived difficulty with activity and independent function through self-report. Although originally designed for use with patients having rheumatoid arthritis, the scale seems clinically useful for all patient populations with chronic disease. The scale has demonstrated acceptable reliability and has shown evidence of validity in several studies.

Performance Test of ADL. The Performance Test of ADL (PADL) was developed by Kuriansky and Gurland (1976) as part of a study involving geriatric patients with organic mental problems in the United States and Great Britain. The PADL consists of 16 basic self-care tasks, ranging from drinking from a cup to removing a jacket. For each task, the patient is asked to demonstrate performance under standardized conditions. The use of props permits control of these performance variables for the test (see Table 15-4).

Scoring for the PADL is based upon observed performance on each of the items or for each component of more complex items. A zero is assigned for reasonable completion (with or without assistance) and a rating of one is given for unsatisfactory performance. Items are rated as "9" if they cannot be scored or are not applicable. An overall score is based on the proportion of tested functions completed satisfactorily, with 100% indicating independence, 75% to 99% indicating moderate dependence, and scores below 75% indicating dependence.

The PADL has demonstrated interrater reliability levels of greater than .90 when an interviewer and independent observer were used to collect data for geriatric psychiatric patients. Kuriansky and associates (1976) have demonstrated the ability of the PADL to correlate positively with physical health status, mental status and survival or discharge from the hospital.

The scale appears to be useful as a measure of basic ADL, especially with patients who may have cognitive impairments. Its main weakness seems to be a dependence on rater judgment in determining whether or not an activity is completed at a satisfactory level due to the fact that behavioral rating criteria are not well defined.

Satisfaction with Performance Scaled Questionnaire. The Revised Satisfaction with Performance Scaled Questionnaire (SPSQ) is designed to measure individuals' levels of satisfaction with their performances of independent

---

Table 15-4
Performance ADL Test: Items
(and Required Props)

1. Drink from a cup. (Cup)
2. Use a tissue to wipe nose. (Tissue box)
3. Comb hair. (Comb)
4. File nails. (Nail file)
5. Shave. (Shaver)
6. Lift food onto spoon to mouth. (Spoon with candy on it)
7. Turn faucet on and off. (Faucet)
8. Turn light switch on and off. (Light switch)
9. Put on and remove a jacket with buttons. (Jacket)
10. Put on and remove a slipper. (Slipper)
11. Brush teeth, including removing false ones. (Toothbrush)
12. Make a phone call. (Telephone)
13. Sign name. (Paper and pen)
14. Turn key in lock. (Keyhole and key)
15. Tell time. (Clock)
16. Stand up and walk a few steps and sit back down.

Reprinted with permission. Kuriansky, J., Gurland, B. (1976). The Performance Test of Activities of Daily Living. International Journal of Aging and Human Development, 7, 343-352.

Satisfaction with Performance Scaled Questionnaire

Name _____ During the last six months have you performed the following activity in such a way that you have felt happy, pleased, or contented with what you have done? In other words, how much of the time have you felt satisfied with the way you

Date: _____ have done these activities?

I. Home Management This item does not apply to me (check)	All (100%) of the time	Most (75%) of the time	Some (50%) of the time	Almost none (25%) of the time	None (0%) of the time
1. Scrape/stack dishes					
2. Wash pots and pans					
3. Remove/put away utensils/dishes in cupboards over sink/counters					
4. Set/clear table					
5. Load/unload washing machine					
6. Dust high surfaces					
7. Remove/put away utensils/dishes in cupboards under sink/counters					
8. Use a floor mop					
9. Make a bed					
10. Use stove top elements					
11. Put clothes on hangers					
12. Clean a bathtub/shower					
13. Reach high cupboards					
14. Dispose of garbage					
15. Sort clothes for washing					
16. Open screw-top lids					
17. Put clothes away in drawers/closet rod					
18. Handle a milk carton					
19. Use a vacuum cleaner					
20. Clean up counter/cooking surfaces					
21. Get objects off top store shelves					
22. Clean vegetables					
23. Carry hot foods to table					
24. Stir against resistance in a bowl					

Figure 15-6. Satisfaction with Performance Scaled Questionnaire. *Reprinted with permission. Yerxa, E.J., Burnett-Beaulieu, S., Stocking, S., & Azen, S.P. (1988). Development of the Satisfaction with Scaled Performance Questionnaire (SPSQ). American Journal of Occupational Therapy, 42(4), 215-221.*

living skills (Yerxa, Burnett-Beaulieu, Stocking, & Azen, 1988). In this scale, satisfaction is defined as the subjective opinion of the one being evaluated in regard to being pleased or contented with their level of performance on selected daily living activities.

The SPSQ includes two subscales, containing a total of 46 items. The subscales include home management (24 items) and social/community problem-solving (22 items). (See Figure 15-6). Each item is scored on a five-point scale based on the percentage of time during the previous six months the subject has felt satisfied with his/her perform-

ance of an identified activity. As a clinical tool, the SPSQ is felt to be useful as a means of identifying treatment goals related to independent living.

ASSESSMENT OF PLAY AND LEISURE

The assessment of play and leisure (the adult form of play) has received much less attention in the scientific literature than have assessments within the other occupational domains

Satisfaction with Performance Scaled Questionnaire (continued)

II. Social/Community Problem Solving This item does not apply to me (check)	All (100%) of the time	Most (75%) of the time	Some (50%) of the time	Almost none (25%) of the time	None (0%) of the time
1. Socialize with other persons					
2. Have friends					
3. Explore training requirements					
4. Assert your thoughts and feelings with others					
5. Go on an interview					
6. Find and use social activities					
7. Find and use financial assistance programs					
8. Meet new people					
9. Find and use educational programs					
10. Talk with partner about sex and problems					
11. Get the most for your money					
12. Find a job					
13. Understand class material					
14. Make decisions					
15. Talk with teacher about class problems					
16. Pay bills and balance account					
17. Plan for future savings/expenses					
18. Budget your income					
19. Take a trip/sightsee					
20. Talk and participate in class					
21. Plan recreational activities					
22. Find resources/help					

Note. Scoring: Each item is scored 1 to 5 points: None (0%) = 1, and All (100%) = 5. Factor I has 120 possible points; Factor II has 110 possible points.

Figure 15-6. Continued.

of work or self-maintenance. As Kielhofner and Barris (1984) point out, this may reflect a cultural bias that productive occupations of self-maintenance or work represent a more valuable use of time than activity described as play or leisure. It may also reflect the inherent difficulties associated with the assessment of activities which are largely subjective in nature, often spontaneous, and greatly influenced by their environment. While the subjective characteristics of play and leisure complicate efforts to assess them, several instruments can provide valuable information about maturation, development, and competent role performance. We begin this section with a review of several approaches to the assessment of play.

Approaches to Assessing Play

The field of occupational therapy has viewed the domain of play as an important source of experience that facilitates and enriches childhood development. Play serves as a medium for learning the skills and roles necessary for competence in adolescence and adulthood. Thus, the assessment of play can serve as an index of developmental progress. Additionally, because play is viewed as an integral part of a child's daily life, play assessment can provide information on the current nature and quality of living circumstances.

Because play is perhaps more greatly influenced by environmental factors than either work or self-care, it is more subject to the problems of reactivity during assessment. However, this dynamic interplay between the player and the environment also creates difficulties with the interpretation of observations. It is difficult to be certain whether the behavior being observed is a product of the player's intrinsic characteristics or instead is due to the characteristics of the environment in which the play occurs. Furthermore, the spontaneous and personal nature of play makes it difficult to determine when or if an adequate sampling of the behavior has taken place.

Despite these difficulties, several approaches have been developed to assess play from various dimensions. Some are observational in nature (e.g., the Preschool Play Scale), while others depend upon parental reports (e.g., the Play History). Descriptions and reviews of some of these instruments are provided below.

Preschool Play Scale—Revised. The Preschool Play Scale is an observational tool designed to provide a description of play behavior for children from birth to six years of age (Knox, 1974). The scale is based on the supposition that the manner in which children play provides important information about their development, learning, and ability to cope with the world around them.

Sixteen categories of play behavior are identified within four general play dimensions: space management, material management, imitation, and participation. Space management concerns the manner in which a child learns to manage the body and the surrounding space through exploring and manipulating the environment. Material management reflects the manner in which a child explores objects through manipulation and the use of oral and tactile senses. Imitation reflects the child's understanding of the social world through mimicking the actions of others and learning to express and control feelings. Participation is defined by the nature of the child's interaction with other persons in the environment and the amount of independence and cooperation demonstrated in play interactions.

In using the scale, free play is observed for 15 to 30 minute periods, and the observed behaviors are compared with expected behaviors for specified age groups, which were formulated based on developmental principles of play. This results in a calculated ''play age'' score. It is recommended that persons using the scale have some experience in observing children at play and a reasonable familiarity with the literature on childhood play.

The reliability of the Preschool Play Scale was examined in a study of 90 children by Bledsoe and Shephard (1982). Interrater reliability was estimated at .99 for the overall play age score and was above .98 for each of the four dimension scores. Test-retest stability following a one-week interval ranged from .86 to .97 for the dimensions and total play age.

The study also provided some evidence for the scale's validity. Correlations of .62 to .85 were obtained between the 16 categories of the scale and chronological age. Relationships between the child's age and the scores for the four dimensions and total play age were higher, ranging from .85 to .96. The Preschool Play Scale also correlated positively with two other scales of play behavior, thus yielding evidence of concurrent validity.

Play History. The Play History (Takata, 1969, 1974) is designed to determine the developmental level and adequacy of play environments and experiences for children or adolescents. As originally developed, the instrument consisted of a semi-structured interview to be conducted with the parents or caretakers of individuals being assessed. A revision completed in 1981 by Rogers and Takata added additional structure with the purpose of assuring that the elements of materials, actions, people, and environmental characteristics were considered for each of five epochs of play. According to the theory underlying this assessment, a *play epoch* is a developmental period during which one of five types of play occurs, beginning with the sensorimotor play of infancy and extending through the stage of recreation attained during adolescence and continued through adulthood. Underlying the interview is the assumption that knowledge of a child's play history will increase understanding of current play.

In 1984, Behnke and Menarchek-Fetkovich further revised the Play History and developed a manual for standardized administration and a scoring system for assigning values to historical data based on developmental levels experienced by the child and the adequacy of play experiences within each level. Using this scoring system, estimates of the reliability of the scale could be derived.

An interrater reliability of .91 was found for adequacy of play in a study of 30 children which included both disabled and able-bodied individuals from one to seven and one-half years of age. Coefficients for individual dimensions of play ranged from .58 to .84 for the total sample. Test-retest reliabilities were slightly lower for the play elements and .77 for the overall play score.

Concurrent validity for the Play History was examined through comparing obtained scores on the sample with scores on the Minnesota Child Development Inventory, which assesses language, self-help, comprehension, and motor skills. Correlations between the two instruments were .97 for able-bodied and .70 for disabled subjects. Correlations between the children's chronological ages and the developmental score on the Play History were .94 for the able-bodied children and .79 for disabled subjects. The scale also showed a sensitivity to differences between the two groups on their developmental level of play.

Other Instruments for Assessing Play Behaviors. Examples of other scales which have been developed to provide information about the play behaviors of children include the *Organization of Play Behavior Scale* (Holme & Lunzer, 1966), the *Social Play Scale* (Parten, 1933), and the *Standardized Clinical Play Observation* (Kalverboer, 1977). Because of their limited evidence of validity and/or clinical value to occupational therapists, complete reviews have not been provided here.

Leisure Assessment

Leisure activity in adulthood is viewed as an important means of facilitating social transition during the maturational process. As one ages, leisure activities may be instrumental in providing continuity with the past and giving one a satisfying use of discretionary time during retirement. Leisure engagement during adulthood is also viewed as a means of balancing one's lifestyle so as to promote health and life satisfaction through the physical, psychosocial, and emotional benefits.

Within occupational therapy, approaches to the assessment of leisure have included the occasional use of interviews to determine one's history of leisure participation (Potts, 1969) or the determination of leisure interests (Matsusuyu, 1967; Rogers, et al., 1978). Several activity indexes have been developed and used as interviews or questionnaires for deriving information on levels of participation in leisure and the associated meaning and/or satisfaction of such participation.

Activity Index (Revised) and Meaningfulness of Activity Scale.

The Activity Index (Revised) was developed to determine the extent of participation in leisure activities. It consists of a scoreable self-report questionnaire with 23 leisure activities. Space is provided for respondents to list up to three additional leisure pursuits on the index. Gregory (1983) adapted this instrument from an earlier version by Nystrom (1974) for a study of leisure participation and satisfaction during retirement. His revision changed the format to that of a self-report questionnaire, which yields a score range of 0 to 52 (see Figure 15-7).

Test-retest reliability for the revised Activity Index was reported as .70 (Gregory, 1983, p. 550). While this index has reasonable face validity, no specific validity studies have been reported. Scores on the Activity Index correlated significantly (r = .43) with life satisfaction scores in the life satisfaction study.

The Meaningfulness of Activity Scale (Gregory, 1983) is used in conjunction with the Activities Index and is designed to gather information on the enjoyability, autonomy, and competency of leisure activities. Adapted from a scale developed by Whiting (1975), the instrument consists of three subscales yielding a potential score range of 78 to 234. This scale asks respondents to rate their degree of enjoyment, autonomy (why they do it) and competency (how well they do it) for each leisure activity in which they participate on a consistent basis (more than once a week). Likert-type scales are provided for responses to each of the three dimensions (see Figure 15-7). An overall meaningfulness of activity score is derived from summing the subscale scores.

Test-retest reliability for the Meaningfulness of Activity Scale was reported (Gregory, 1983, p. 550) as .87. No validity data were reported. However, significant correlations were reported between each of the subscales and the overall meaningfulness of activity score and life satisfaction; the autonomy subscale score achieved the highest correlation value.

When used together, the Activity Index and the Meaningfulness of Activity Scale can provide a convenient means of gathering useful information on leisure activities and the meaning of these activities. Although they were designed for use by retired persons, the instruments could be used by other adult populations capable of responding to the questionnaire items. The short, scoreable nature of the combined instruments increases their utility as research tools.

Leisure Diagnostic Battery.

The Leisure Diagnostic Battery (LDB) (Witt, Compton, Ellis, Howard, et al., 1982) was developed to measure leisure function and provide a basis for determining remediation programming. The **battery**, comprised of eight subscales, is based on the belief that freedom is the essential element in leisure and that leisure is a state of mind. As a consequence, the battery yields information on the outcomes of leisure experiences as well as the motivational and situational demands which lead to these outcomes rather than emphasizing the structure or performance demands of activities.

The Leisure Diagnostic Battery measures the current level of leisure functioning and gathers information to direct remediation efforts. Section I of the scale is directed toward leisure functioning and consists of five scales, each based on a theoretical structure presumed to be related to perceived freedom in leisure functioning. Section II provides information related to perceived barriers, individual leisure preferences, and knowledge of leisure opportunities. Versions of the scale have been developed for children and youth ages 9 to 14 with normal cognitive functioning (Version A) and those of the same age groups who are categorized as educably mentally retarded (Version B).

Reliability and validity data for the LDB has accrued from several studies (Witt, Ellis, Aquilar, et al., 1982). In initial studies by the developers involving four separate samples, both stability and internal consistency data were analyzed. Retest coefficients for the diagnostic scales ranged from .77 to .89. Coefficients for the remediation scales ranged from .38 to .82. Internal consistency (Cronbach's Alpha) ranged from .88 to .96 for the diagnostic scales and from .61 to .91 for the remediation scales.

To determine if evidence of validity could be found for the battery, two samples were administered—the Piers-Harris Self-Concept Scale and the Crandall Social Desirability Scale—along with the LDB. It was found that neither self-concept nor social desirability accounted for a significant portion of the variance in the LDB scores. At

Modified Activities Index

For each activity on this page, place a check (✔) in one of the four columns that best describes the activity.

Be sure that, for every activity, there is a check in one of the four columns.

ACTIVITY	Don't Do/ Not Interested	Don't Do/ Would Like To	Do at Least Once a Week	Do at Least Three Times a Week
Takes Rides				
Cards/Bingo				
Movies				
Group Singing				
Visit/Entertain Relatives				
Write Letters				
Theater/Lecture/ Concerts				
Phone Friends/ Relatives				
Work (for pay)				
Work (volunteer)				
Read				
Needle Arts/Small Handcrafts				
Watch Television				
Radio/Listen to Music				
Hobby				
Take Care of Plants				
Repair Things in Apartment/Home				
Social Clubs				
Clubs for Older People				
Church Groups				
Women/Men Clubs				
Lodge				
Other (specify):				

Column annotations: each check valued 0 (Don't Do/Not Interested), each check valued 0 (Don't Do/Would Like To), each check valued 1 (Do at Least Once a Week), each check valued 2 (Do at Least Three Times a Week).

Figure 15-7a. Modified Activities Index. *Reprinted with permission. Gregory, M.D. (1983). Occupational behavior and life satisfaction among retirees. American Journal of Occupational Therapy, 35(8), 548-553.*

the same time, the diagnostic scales were found to be highly correlated, and observed relationships were generally viewed as supportive of the theoretical structure underlying the diagnostic scales. Data were less supportive of the remediation scales, and the authors advised caution when planning intervention programs based on data from those scales.

Dunn (1987) sought to generalize the LDB to young adults. Both reliability and validity data were examined using a sample of 513 university students. While reliability coefficients were generally similar to those obtained in earlier studies by the developers, Dunn found that with the adult sample used, the playfulness subscale had higher stability and the depth of involvement in leisure experi-

Meaningfulness of Activity Scale

ACTIVITY	How Much You Enjoy It (check 1 of the 4 boxes)				Why You Do It (check 1 of 2 boxes)		How Well You Do It (check 1 of 3 boxes)		
	Enjoy Doing It Very Much	Enjoy Doing It Somewhat	Enjoy Doing It Very Little	Do Not Enjoy It at All	Want to Do It	Have To Do It	Do It Very Well	Do It Well Enough	Do Not Do It Well
Takes Rides									
Cards/Bingo									
Movies									
Group Singing									
Visit/Entertain Relatives									
Write Letters									
Theater/Lecture/ Concerts									
Phone Friends/ Relatives									
Work (for pay)									
Work (volunteer)									
Read									
Needle Arts/Small Handcrafts									
Watch Television									
Radio/Listen to Music									
Hobby									
Take Care of Plants									
Repair Things in Apartment/Home									
Social Clubs									
Study Group									
Clubs for Older People									
Church Groups									
Women/Men Clubs									
Lodge									
Other (specify):									

Scoring annotations (diagonal labels across columns):
- Enjoy Doing It Very Much: each check valued 4
- Enjoy Doing It Somewhat: each check valued 3
- Enjoy Doing It Very Little: each check valued 2
- Do Not Enjoy It at All: each check valued 1
- Want to Do It: each check valued 2
- Have To Do It: each check valued 1
- Do It Very Well: each check valued 3
- Do It Well Enough: each check valued 2
- Do Not Do It Well: each check valued 1

Figure 15-7b. Meaningfulness of Activity Scale. *Reprinted with permission. Gregory, M.D. (1983). Occupational behavior and life satisfaction among retirees. American Journal of Occupational Therapy, 35(8), 548-553.*

Leisure Diagnostic Battery (LDB)

Instructions: For each statement below, fill in the circle over the number on the enclosed response sheet to indicate how much you think that statement sounds like you.

1=Sounds like me
2=Sounds a little like me
3=Doesn't sound like me

1. I'm good at almost all recreation activities I do.
    1 2 3

15. I'm able to play outdoor sports as well as I want to.
    1 2 3

28. I usually decide who I can do recreation activities with.
    1 2 3

44. I like to do recreation activities which involve surprises.
    1 2 3

49. When I'm tired, doing recreation activities helps me to relax.
    1 2 3

71. I usually have fun when I'm involved in recreation activities.
    1 2 3

109. It's easy for me to start a new activity.
    1 2 3

Figure 15-8. Sample items from the leisure diagnostic battery. *Reprinted with permission: Witt, P.A., Compton, D.M., Ellis, G., Howard, G., Aguilar, T., Forsyth, P., Niles, S., & Costilow, A. (1982). The leisure diagnostic battery: Background, conceptualization and structure. Denton, Texas: North Texas State University, 1982, North Texas State University.*

ences scale had lower stability than found with earlier samples.

Factor analysis of the data by Dunn (1987) validated the presence of a perceived freedom factor for the diagnostic scales and confirmed the factor structure obtained in earlier studies by the developers. However, Dunn recommended that additional revision of the scale be accomplished and that the perceived freedom score be used as an overall score of leisure functioning in making therapeutic programming decisions. (Figure 15-8)

Leisure Satisfaction Questionnaire. The Leisure Satisfaction Questionnaire (Beard & Ragheb, 1980) was designed to provide a measure of the extent to which individuals perceive that their personal needs are met through participation in leisure. Items in the scale are clustered according to one of six need categories: psycho-

logical, educational, social, relaxation, physiological, and aesthetic. These categories are based on factor analysis of item responses by subjects who participated in field tests of the instrument and are consistent with areas of satisfaction provided by leisure activities previously reported in the play/leisure literature.

Subjects are asked to respond to 51 statements using a five-point Likert-type degree of agreement scale. Scoring is done by adding the values assigned to each statement in a given need category. Table 15-5 provides sample items for each of the six subscales.

Reliability of the Leisure Satisfaction Scale (LSS) was estimated using a measure of internal consistency, coefficient alpha. Coefficients were .96 for the total scale and ranged from .85 to .92 for the six components. To obtain evidence of its validity, the authors distributed a form of the scale to 160 professionals in the area of leisure/recreation and reported general satisfaction. On this basis, they claimed evidence of face validity. Factor analyses have supported the independence of the six scale components, and intercorrelations of the component scores ranged from .38 to .66.

The authors of the LSS suggest that the scale is suitable for use in counseling situations as a means of examining the use of an individual's free time or discussing ways in which leisure activities could be altered to better serve their needs. The scale may also serve as a useful tool for exploring the validity of theories of leisure participation.

Minnesota Leisure Time Physical Activity Questionnaire. There is a tendency to view and thus assess leisure in terms of its use as a vehicle for contributing to life satisfaction through social/psychological contributions. However, as the relationship between lifestyle and health has generated increased attention, researchers have begun looking at the physical benefits of leisure involvement in a systematic way. One of the tools developed for this purpose is the Minnesota Leisure Time Physical Activity Questionnaire or Minnesota LTPA. It is included here because it holds promise of potential benefit for research or clinical use for therapists involved in stress reduction, health promotion, or cardiac care situations.

The Minnesota LTPA was developed to determine the energy expenditure of individuals during leisure time activities (Taylor, Jacobs, Schucker, et al., 1978). The questionnaire is designed to be used as a structured interview rather than self-report tool. The purpose is to gather physical activity information which would be of value in determining pre-morbid levels of exertion and in studying the relationship between levels of physical activity and weight control, cardiovascular fitness, disease, and general health.

A standard interview and a list of 63 physical activities is used to determine the activities that have been performed by

---

Table 15-5
Subscales from the Leisure Satisfaction Scale and Sample Items

Subscale and Meaning	Sample Item
Psychological—A sense of freedom, enjoyment, involvement, and intellectual challenge.	(2) My leisure activities are very interesting to me.
Educational—Intellectual stimulation, self-learning and awareness of surroundings.	(18) My leisure activities increase my knowledge about things around me.
Social—Rewarding relationships with other people.	(27) I have social interaction with others through leisure activities.
Relaxation—Relief from the stress and strain of life.	(38) My leisure activities help to relieve stress.
Physiological—A means to develop physical fitness, stay healthy, control weight, and otherwise promote well-being.	(44) My leisure activities help me to stay healthy.
Aesthetic—Leisure activities are viewed as being pleasing, interesting, beautiful, and generally well-designed.	(49) The areas or places where I engage in my leisure activities are beautiful.

Note: Responses to each item are on a 5 point graphic response scale where 1 = Almost never true, 2 = Seldom true, 3 = Sometimes true, 4 = Often true, and 5 = Almost always true. *Reprinted with the permission: Beard, J.G., & Ragheb, M.G. (1980). Measuring leisure satisfaction. Journal of Leisure Research, 12, 20-33.*

---

the respondent within the previous 12 months. Subjects report the number of months of involvement in each leisure activity selected and the average number of occasions and duration per occasion per month. Work activity is excluded. An activity metabolic index is derived for total leisure activity plus categories of light activity, medium activity, and heavy activity. This is done by multiplying the intensity code times the number of months, number of occasions, and duration for each activity. This score provides an estimate of the average caloric expenditure per day for the previous year (see Table 15-6).

Values from the Minnesota LTPA Questionnaire for 175 men were correlated with performance at various levels of exertion on a treadmill test. Clear and statistically significant relationships were found between an exercise endpoint and energy expenditures during leisure time physical activity indicated by the questionnaire data.

ASSESSMENT OF PERFORMANCE IN THE DOMAIN OF WORK

The third major domain for assessment of occupational performance is work. Because work refers to one's participation in socially purposeful and productive activities, it rightfully can include such endeavors as education and volunteer work. The majority of assessment instruments available to occupational therapists are vocational in nature, and many focus on performance components, such as cognitive ability or motor strength and dexterity. Others focus on motivational components such as aptitudes, interests, or personality factors.

In this section, those instruments or batteries that focus on the ability of a patient or client to accomplish work-related tasks in a situational or role-oriented context will be reviewed. These include approaches that derive information from an

---

Table 15-6
Selected Activities and Intensity Codes from the
Minnesota Leisure Time Physical Activities Questionnaire

Code	Activity	Intensity	Code	Activity	Intensity
010	Walking for pleasure	3.5	510	Touch football	8.0
040	Cross country hiking	6.0	600	Raking lawn	4.0
200	Running	8.0	540	Carpentry outside	3.0
310	Scuba diving	3.0	660	Fishing from river bank	3.5
400	Volleyball	4.0	710	Hunting large game	6.0

Adapted from the Minnesota Leisure Time Physical Activities Questionnaire.

individual's self-report or through observation by a rater or evaluator, either through role-playing or simulated conditions or in the context of actual or on-the-job performance. A short section on commercial systems is also included.

For purposes of organization, instruments in this domain have been grouped into the categories of self-report inventories and questionnaires, situational approaches, direct observation, and commercial evaluation systems.

Self-Report Inventories and Questionnaires

Loma Linda University Medical Center (LLUMC) Activity Sort. The Activity Sort is a self-report assessment procedure designed to ascertain the degree to which an individual feels capable of participating in any of a number of household tasks using common domestic tools and

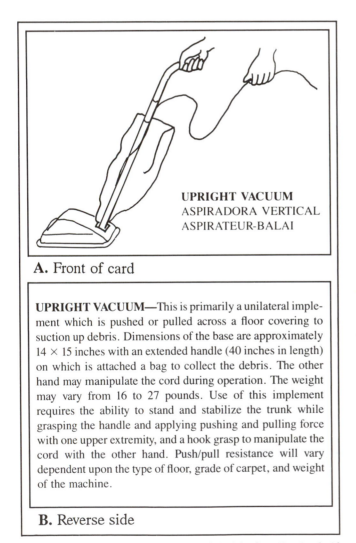

UPRIGHT VACUUM
ASPIRADORA VERTICAL
ASPIRATEUR-BALAI

A. Front of card

UPRIGHT VACUUM—This is primarily a unilateral implement which is pushed or pulled across a floor covering to suction up debris. Dimensions of the base are approximately 14 × 15 inches with an extended handle (40 inches in length) on which is attached a bag to collect the debris. The other hand may manipulate the cord during operation. The weight may vary from 16 to 27 pounds. Use of this implement requires the ability to stand and stabilize the trunk while grasping the handle and applying pushing and pulling force with one upper extremity, and a hook grasp to manipulate the cord with the other hand. Push/pull resistance will vary dependent upon the type of floor, grade of carpet, and weight of the machine.

B. Reverse side

Figure 15-9. Example of card from LLUMC Activity Sort. *Reprinted with permission: West Evaluation Systems Technology.*

implements. The assessment is administered through a standard card sorting technique, whereby each activity or implement included in the assessment is graphically depicted on one side of a 5 x 8 inch card. The entire stack of cards comprising the instrument is given to subjects to be evaluated with instructions to sort through them and select those tools which they are able to use at the time of evaluation. Subjects then place the cards into one of five categories or beneath title cards placed on the table in front of them according to how they perceive their ability to use the tool. The categories range from A through D, with A being "no decrease in ability to work" to D which is "unable to use." A fifth category (don't know) is provided for when subjects do not know whether they are able to use the tool/implement either because of unfamiliarity with the tool or its usage or their inability to predict symptom responses from usage of the tool.

Once the cards have been sorted, the evaluator records the responses on an evaluation record. This provides documentation of the responses and serves as a basis for an interview session in which the evaluator seeks clarification of the reasons for placement of various cards. During this debriefing stage of the assessment process, the evaluator identifies various work function themes and asks the subject to list and describe tools pertinent to his or her work which have not been included in the sort. A task matrix, furnished with the card sort kit, provides easy identification of factors associated with the 65 stimulus cards.

Cards can also be sorted on the basis of 28 functional characteristics or requirements of the tool. The cards in the activity sort are punched in a manner that permits use of a keyhole-sort procedure. Thus, cards related to specific factors (such as bilateral control, elbow flexion/extension, or light physical demand characteristics) can be identified quickly. This permits an analysis of the sorted cards for particular functional themes.

The activity sort contains three pairs of validity cards which permit a determination of the consistency of the subject's responses. Once the sort has been completed, discrepancies in the placement of these cards provide a basis for eliciting clarifying information from the subject. Additionally, the assessment procedure can include verification of tool use during the debriefing, at which time the subject is observed using a specific tool.

Although no reliability or validity studies have been published, the content of the LLUMC Activities Sort has been based on careful analysis of tool use and performance criteria. Since the card-sort technique is essentially a means of gathering interview information in a structured format, and the tools depicted are used commonly in vocations requiring light physical activity, the procedure must be viewed as having satisfactory face validity.

WEST Tool Sort	
1. PICK, Mattock	34. BRUSH, Paint
2. PICK, Clay	35. BROOM, Household
3. SHOVEL, Flathead	36. SAW, Portable-Reciprocating
4. POST HOLE DIGGER	37. SAW, Portable/Circular
5. HOE, Garden	38. TWEEZERS
6. RAKE	39. SCREWDRIVER, Slotted (Small)
7. BROOM, Street/Pushbroom	40. WHEELBARROW
8. SHOVEL, Round	41. SCRIBER
9. DRILL, Hand	42. MICROMETER
10. CHISEL, Wood	43. SCREWDRIVER, Optician's
11. CHISEL, Cold	44. NIPPERS
12. SCRAPER	45. SHEARS, Pruning
13. BOLT CUTTER	46. SHEARS, Hedge Trimming
14. SAW, Hand	47. DRILL, Bit Brace
15. HACKSAW	48. PLIERS, Diagonal Cutting
16. HAMMER, Sledge	49. PLIERS, Locking/Channel Lock
17. WRENCH, Pipe	50. SCREWDRIVER, Ratchet
18. FILE, Round	51. BRUSH, Scrubbing/Scouring
19. PLIERS, Long Nose	52. WRENCH, Box (Straight & Offset)
20. PLIERS, Lineman's	53. WRENCH, Open-End (Straight & Offset)
21. PLIERS, Crimping	54. WRENCH, Crescent/Adjustable
22. SCREWDRIVER, Slotted	55. SOLDERING IRON
23. PLIERS, Locking/Visegrip	56. SHEARS, Scissors
24. HAMMER, Claw	57. CLAMP, "C"
25. WRENCH, Torque	58. PLIERS, Brake
26. PRY BAR	59. PLIERS, Electronic
27. FILE, Flat	60. DRILL, Electric
28. NUTDRIVER	61. SANDER, Vibrating
29. CALIPERS	62. HAMMER, Hand Drilling
30. PLIERS, Hog Ring	63. HOE, Garden
31. PLIERS, Wire Stripping	64. HACKSAW
32. STAPLE GUN	65. PLIERS, Wire Stripping
33. PLIERS, All Purpose	

Figure 15-10a. Tool List for WEST Tool Sort. *Reprinted with permission: WEST Evaluation Systems Technology.*

WEST Tool Sort. The WEST Tool Sort is a clinical procedure designed to provide information about the ability to perform work tasks (West Evaluation Systems Technology, 1986). This procedure includes 65 cards depicting tools used primarily in industrial, construction, and commercial areas. Each card is titled in English, Spanish, French, German, Japanese and Vietnamese and also includes information on minimum grip strength and the size and weight of the tool. There are six validity check cards used as part of the assessment procedure.

The WEST Tool Sort is administered in exactly the same manner as the LLUMC Activity Sort (described earlier) and has several different applications: (1) evaluation of treatment effect, (2) easy determination of the vocational consequences of functional limitation, (3) identification of individuals who suffer from symptom magnification syndrome, (4) identification of critical work demands to suggest necessary tool modifications, and (5) identification of appropriate vocational alternatives.

One useful feature of the WEST Tool Sort is identification of the factors related to the ability to use each tool. Twenty-eight such factors have been selected from a larger pool of over 100 such factors. These sort factors pertain to the controlling hand for tools that are unilateral and to both hands for bilateral tools. Figure 15-10a lists the tools included in the WEST Tool Sort.

Situational Approaches

Situational approaches include those assessment instruments which rely upon direct observation of work-related behaviors in controlled environments such as in role-playing or within sheltered workshop settings.

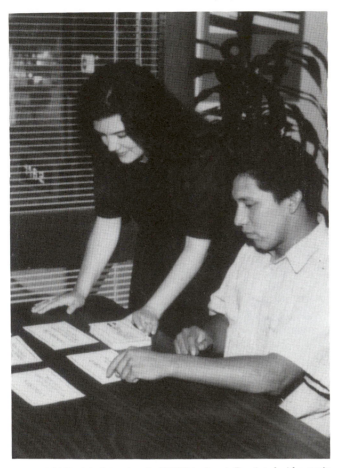

Figure 15-10b. Administering the WEST tool sort. *Reprinted with permission: Ogden-Niemeyer, L. and Jacobs, K., Word Hardening, . SLACK Inc., 1989.*

Social and Prevocational Information Battery—Revised (SPIB-R). This battery represents the outcome of additional development of the original Social and Prevocational Information Battery (SPIB) developed at the University of Oregon Research and Training Center in the 1970's (Halpern, Raffeld, Irvin, & Link, 1975). The battery consists of nine true-false tests to be administered orally during three 90-minute testing sessions to students at the junior high or high school level who can be classified as mildly retarded. Items are designed to measure knowledge of skills and competencies regarded as important for successful community adjustment (Halpern, Irvin, & Munkies, 1986).

The nine tests of the SPIB-R are job-search skills, job-related behavior, banking, budgeting, purchasing habits, home management, physical health care, hygiene and grooming, and functional signs. These tests relate to five long-range goals of employability, economic self-sufficiency, family living, personal habits, and communication.

The entire battery consists of 277 items (see Figure 15-11). Separate scores are obtained for each test, and a

total battery score is derived from the aggregated subtest scores. A standardization sample used for the original SPIB forms the basis for percentile ranking norms constructed for the SPIB-R. Absolute performance of subjects can be determined through tables which reflect the percentage of items correct on each subtest. A student profile sheet has been developed which facilitates the interpretation and use of information derived from the battery.

The SPIB-R has been carefully designed to serve as a basis for planning instructional programs through the development of instructional and enabling objectives. The authors of the battery point out that the SPIB-R results can be used to identify high priority/low performance areas. Attention has been devoted in the instructional manual to using the SPIB-R results to facilitate Individual Educational Plan (IEP) documentation for programming which falls under the aegis of Public Law #94-142 and subsequent legislation in the United States.

The original standardization sample consisted of 906 students from approximately 30% of all junior high (grades 7 to 9) and from senior high schools (grades 10 to 12) in the state of Oregon. Students were educable mentally retarded adolescents ranging in age from 14 to 20 years (average IQ of 68, standard deviation of 8).

Reliability for the SPIB-R was estimated using an internal consistency formula and gathering test-retest data. A median reliability coefficient of .75 was found for internal consistency of the nine subtests with the overall battery yielding coefficients of .94 for the junior high students and .93 for the senior high sample. Stability (test-retest) coefficients were .94 for the junior high and .91 for the senior high sample with a testing interval of two weeks.

The SPIB-R examiner's manual describes various studies conducted by the developers in an attempt to determine the battery's validity. The original research during development of the SPIB showed relationships between scores on that instrument and community adaptation following completion of schooling. Concurrent validity of the original SPIB was demonstrated using a five-scale counselor rating instrument and correlating these ratings with student performance on the SPIB. Modest intercorrelations were found.

Subsequent studies have provided additional data on the reliability and validity of the SPIB and SPIB-R (Halpern, Irvin, & Landman, 1979; Irvin & Halpern, 1977; Irvin, Halpern, & Landman, 1980). These data have suggested that while the SPIB may be useful for assessing personal-social adjustment in training programs, it has not been successful in predicting later employment status. Additional study with the SPIB-R is needed to provide further information about its predictive validity.

Occupational Skills Assessment Instrument. This instrument is designed to determine a client's actual level of skills in a variety of job-related situations (Mathews, Whang, & Fawcett, 1980). The instrument includes both role-playing and a written criterion test situation. Skills assessed through role-playing pertain principally to job related social interaction skills, such as telephoning a potential employer, participating in an interview, and accepting suggestions or criticism from a supervisor. Criterion test situations include writing letters in response to specific situations and completing a federal income tax return.

This instrument is organized in a checklist format and is scored according to the proportion of task elements performed correctly. The instrument was designed to be used in vocational training situations for adolescents with learning disabilities. Evidence of satisfactory reliability and preliminary validity data were reported in a study by Mathews, Whang, & Fawcett (1982).

Direct Observation of Work Behaviors

Another approach to gathering work-related performance information involves direct observation of a person's performance while on the job. Emphasis is typically placed on specific behaviors, known as work behaviors, that enable a person to meet the demands of a job in accordance with employment standards such as attendance, punctuality, cooperation, and teamwork. When this approach is used in controlled settings such as sheltered workshops, it is commonly called situational assessment.

Vocational Adaptation Rating Scales. This scale tests six general domains in a vocational context: verbal manners, communication skills, attendance and punctuality, interpersonal behavior, respect for property, rules and regulations, and grooming and personal hygiene. Administration can be accomplished by any competent professional who has observed the subject during a specified observation period (usually 30 days) and who has had a minimum of 70 hours of face-to-face contact with the worker.

Using a self-scoring rating booklet, items which represent maladaptive behaviors are reviewed and rated according to their frequency of occurrence or severity. A four-point scale is used to indicate frequency, while severity scores for each item have been predetermined based on the likelihood that the maladaptive behavior would result in termination of a worker's employment. These scores were derived from 31 employment supervisors' ratings of each frequency category for each item on a nine-point scale.

Items for the Vocational Adaptive Rating Scales (VARS) were developed from an initial list of over 220 maladaptive behaviors reported by workshop supervisors and teachers. (Table 15-7) Factor analysis of individual items remaining after determining the item/total score correlations yielded

the six scales. Scale scores tend to be only moderately intercorrelated, indicating factorial independence.

The VARS exhibit satisfactory interrater reliability and internal consistency estimates, with coefficients generally in the .50 to .70 range for interrater reliability and .80 to .90 for internal consistency. Scores show only negligible correlations with sex, IQ, and age, with the highest coefficient of correlation being .44 (p<.01) between the Communication Scale score and IQ.

The concurrent and predictive validity of the VARS were studied through administration of the instrument to 125 retarded adolescents and adults (Malgady, Barcher, Towner, & Davis, 1980). These individuals had been screened and placed into sheltered workshop programs based upon a seven-level classification system. Scores for the total scale and four of the six subscales predicted concurrent workshop placement significantly. However, the scales for "verbal manners" and "respect for property, rules, and regulations" were uncorrelated with concurrent placement. Multiple correlation analyses of data from the same study demonstrated that the six scales collectively were able to predict concurrent and follow-up placement of workers with a high level of validity. These data permitted the development of tables for seven placement levels based on frequency and severity scores for each scale.

A study by Malgady, Barcher, Towner, and Davis (1979)

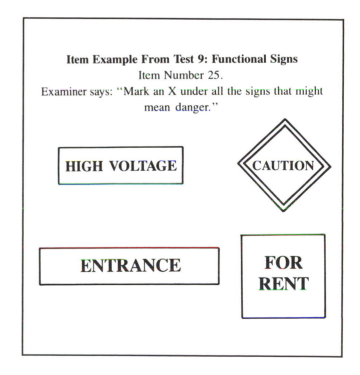

Figure 15-11. Social and Prevocational Information. *Examiner's Manual. Social and Prevocational Information Battery-Revised, 1986, by Andrew S. Halpern, Larry K. Irvin and Arden W. Munkres. Distributed by CTB/ McGraw-Hill, Monterey, CA. Reprinted with permission.*

also demonstrated concurrent validity of the VARS. Individual scale scores and total scale scores showed significant correlations with the *AAMD Adaptive Behavior Scales* (reviewed later) and the *San Francisco Vocational Competency Scale*.

Vocational Behavior Checklist. The Vocational Behavior Checklist (VBC) is a comprehensive list of 344 employment-related skills which have been carefully assembled to serve as a guide to assessment and training in programs for special populations (Walls, Zane, & Werner, 1978). Over 200 checklists from facilities of varying types across the nation were reviewed to produce the VBC. The **checklist** is specifically designed for professionals in work adjustment, prevocational and vocational training, vocational evaluation, and Individualized Education or Written Rehabilitation Programs. The VBC is organized into seven categories. Table 15-8 lists these categories along with their corresponding number of identified skills.

Behavioral definitions or skill objectives have been written for each skill. Each skill objective includes specifications for the behaviors desired to demonstrate the skill, the conditions under which the behavior is to occur, the instructions to be given to the client to elicit the desired behavior, and the standard of performance necessary to achieve the objective (see Table 15-9).

Summary charts provided in the VBC manual list the skills in each area and provide a means of recording the client's performance and training progress. Also provided

Table 15-8
Vocational Behavior Checklist Item Categories

Category	Number of Items
Prevocational	194
Job Seeking	20
Interview	21
Job Related	21
Work Performance	47
On-the-Job/Social	19
Union-Financial Security	22

are optional data sheets or forms upon which daily training data can be recorded for each skill objective. The skill objectives profile allows for a quick survey of a client's progress in all seven skill categories. This profile allows for an indication of the percentage of skill objectives which have been mastered in each category.

The developers of the VBC emphasize that the items with each categorical checklist can be used as formulated or selected specifically to meet the needs of individual clients or programs. Tablets containing both itemized and blank forms accompany the VBC package.

To determine the reliability and validity of the VBC, the developers conducted several studies. To estimate the stability and inter-observer reliability of the items, vocational trainees were videotaped in work (training) and testing situations. Five skill objectives were randomly selected from each category and used to assess five individual clients. Two weeks later, the same skill objectives were again assessed from the same videotapes by the same observers. Stability across all seven categories ranged from 92% to 100% using two observers. The mean stability of the VBC was .97.

Inter-observer reliability was computed by comparing the scores across observers for the first observation period. Reliability ranged from .92 to 1.0 across the seven scales. The overall inter-observer reliability of the VBC was 95%.

Because items on the VBC were selected from a comprehensive array of related checklists at facilities across the country, the authors assert that content validity for the VBC must be considered high. To estimate the criterion or predictive validity of the VBC, the authors reviewed studies of skills identified by employers to determine their correspondence with skills included on the VBC. Based on the data presented in four studies, they estimated the criterion-related validity of the items on the VBC. Across the four studies, the VBC items and skills identified as ''essential,'' ''vital,'' ''important,'' or ''related to success'' corre-

Table 15-7
Sample Scale Items from the Vocational Adaptation Rating Scales

Item #	Description	Scale
5	Heckles other workers	Verbal Manners (VM)
15	Speech is echolalic.	Communication Skills (CS)
43	Is absent from job.	Attendance and Punctuality (AP)
53	Laughs Inappropriately.	Interpersonal Behavior (IB)
95	Writes on walls.	Respect for Property, Rules, and Regulations (RP)
121	Is unshaven.	Grooming and Personal Hygiene (GP)

Reprinted with permission: Western Psychological Services.

sponded to retention in competitive employment on an average of .97. On this basis, the developers assert that the VBC includes the most relevant and important skills necessary for vocational success.

Commercial Vocational Evaluation Systems

Although there are many systems available commercially which purport to provide work-related assessment information, their utility, validity, and quality vary greatly. These systems can be grouped into several categories based upon their format, administration, conceptual basis, or target population. For example, many are designed to provide vocational exploration through determination of skills, interests, and/or aptitudes and are targeted toward persons with special needs or mental retardation. The APTICOM, CES, KEVAS and McCarron Dial Systems are examples of this type of system. (See Figure 15-12).

Another approach involves the use of work samples which include the tasks, materials, and tools required in a specific job or cluster of jobs. Data from these systems frequently correspond directly to job requirements identified in the Dictionary of Occupational Titles. The TOWER, VALPAR, VES (Singer) and VIEWS systems are examples of this type of approach.

Unfortunately, despite their wide use and relatively high cost, very few of these commercial systems have objective data on reliability and validity. Figure 15-13a provides summary information on the systems cited. The reader is referred to an excellent and comprehensive review of commercial work assessment and evaluation systems authored by Botterbusch (1987).

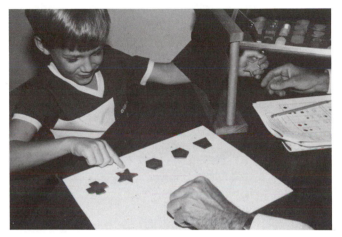

Figure 15-12. Administration of the Haptic Visual Discrimination Test Shape Subtest of the McCarron Dial Work Evaluation System. *Photo courtesy of McCarron-Dial Systems, Dallas, Texas.*

GLOBAL PERFORMANCE ASSESSMENT

Global assessment approaches are those which provide for assessment in several domains of occupational performance and/or at several levels of the functional hierarchy. The evolution of more comprehensive assessment approaches reflects a growing concern with quality of life issues in rehabilitation, including the need to address the multiple role requirements of everyday living. Assessment approaches are also reflecting increased awareness of the importance of gathering information based upon characteristic performance patterns in natural settings or, at least, they are reflecting a sensitivity to the importance of environmental factors in performance.

In the following sections, global instruments and approaches are grouped into two major categories: (1) interviews and self-reports and (2) strategies involving direct observation or longitudinal activity time samples. In some cases, assessment systems may involve both observation and self-report strategies or may present an option for use of either strategy.

Interviews and Self-Report Approaches

AAMD Adaptive Behavior Scale. The American Association on Mental Deficiency (AAMD) Adaptive Behavior Scale was originally developed in 1969 and revised in 1975 as a means for describing how individuals maintain their personal independence in daily living and how they meet the social expectations of their environments (Nihira, Foster, Shellhaas, & Leland, 1975). It is designed for use with mentally retarded, emotionally maladjusted, and developmentally disabled individuals. However, the administration manual points out that the

---

Table 15-9
An Example of a Skill Objective from the Pre-Vocational Skills Index of the Vocational Behavior Checklist

SHIRT HANGERS (153)

Condition	Given five shirts and five wire hangers.
Instruction	"Hang the shirts."
Behavior	Client will put one shirt on each hanger and button the top button.
Standard	Behavior, within five minutes on three of four occasions. Each hanger must be inside the shirt sleeves and the top button buttoned.

Reprinted with permission: Walls, R.T., Zane, T., and Werner, T.J., 1978, The Vocational Behavior Checklist, West Virginia Research and Training Center, Dunbar, WV.

Comparison of Selected Commercial Vocational Assessment Systems

	APTICOM	Career Evaluation System (CES)	Key Educational Vocational Assessment System (KEVAS)	McCarron-Dial Work Evaluation System
Sponsor	Vocational Research Institute Philadelphia Jewish Employment and Vocational Services (JEVS)	Career Evaluation Systems, Inc.	Key Education, Inc.	McCarron-Dial Systems, Inc.
Target Group	English or Spanish Speaking Disadvantaged Job Applicants	Each division intended for a different population, including able bodied, disabled, and persons with mental retardation.	Designed for disabled and able-bodied populations with a wide range of abilities.	Designed for special education and rehabilitation populations at any level of intellectual functioning.
Descriptive Summary	Assessment unit consists of a dedicated computer and other testing devices. Aptitudes, Interests and Skills are assessed. Aptitude portion consists of 11 tests. Occupational Interest Inventory is based on USES Measure. Language and Math Skills are evaluated.	Consists of a battery of psychological tests and ratings designed to relate aptitudes to Data-People-Things Hierarchy of the Dictionary of Occupational Titles. Each of three "series" of the system uses a different combination of written and apparatus tests and ratings.	System consists of a combination of apparatus, achievement, interest, and personality tests designed to test underlying perceptual skills which are fundamental for learning. There are 20 work samples.	Based on a neuropsychological framework. Consists of six tests which provide information on 5 factors: Verbal-Spatial-Cognitive, Sensory, Motor, Emotional, and Integrative-Coping. Data from other tests can be factored into analytical model.
Norms	Selected samples.	Under development.	Three nationwide norm studies have been conducted.	Excellent norms.
Reliability/ Validity	Aptitude and interest components have acceptable reliability. Correlates with U.S. Dept. of Labor Tests.	Test-retest for individual tests ranged from .72-.95. Little validity data.	Reliability coefficients in .80's Some validity data.	Reliability estimates in .80's and .90's. Several validity studies have shown utility as diagnostic instrument.
Address	Vocational Research Institute 1528 Walnut Street, Suite 1502 Philadelphia, PA 19102	Career Evaluation Systems 7788 Milwaukee Avenue Niles, IL 60648	Key Education Inc. 673 Broad Street Shrewsbury, NJ 07701	McCarron-Dial Systems P.O. Box 45628 Dallas, TX 75245

Figure 15-13a. Comparison of Selected Commercial Vocational Assessment Systems. *Adapted with permission from: Botterbusch, K.F. (1987) Vocational assessment and evaluation systems. Menomonie, WI: Materials Development Center, University of Wisconsin-Stout.*

scale can be used with other disabled and handicapped persons.

The AAMD Adaptive Behavior Scale consists of two parts. The first part is organized developmentally and is designed to assess skills and habits in ten behavioral domains regarded as important in the development of personal independence in daily living. These include independent functioning, physical development, economic activity, language development, numbers and time, domestic activity, vocational activity, self-direction, responsibility, and socialization.

Part two of the scale measures maladaptive behavior related to personality and behavior disorders in 14 domains. The fourteenth domain provides information on the client's use of medications, and is therefore not a means for classifying maladaptive behavior as are the other domains. The developers of the scale describe the following purposes: (1) to facilitate placement in training programs, (2) to determine necessary changes in a curriculum or training program based upon documented changes over time, (3) to determine how environmental factors influence an individual's performance. (4) to understand the relationship be-

	The TOWER System	Valpar Component Work Sample Series	Vocational Evaluation System (VES)	Vocational Information and Evaluation Work Samples
Sponsor	International Center for the Disabled	Valpar International	New Concepts Corp. (Originally developed by Singer Educational Division)	Vocational Research Institute Philadelphia Jewish Employment and Vocational Service
Target Group	Persons with all types of disabilities.	Suitable for general population but has been used extensively with industrially injured persons. Adaptations for visual and hearing impairments are available.	Intended for socially and educationally disadvantaged populations. Can also be used with able-bodied persons.	Designed especially for moderately and severely mentally retarded adults.
Descriptive Summary	Originally developed by the U.S. Vocational Rehabilitation Administration, TOWER is the oldest complete work evaluation system. The system contains 93 work samples arranged in 14 job training areas ranging from clerical and drafting to welding and workshop assembly. Used for vocational exploration and for recommendation in areas tested.	System consists of 19 work samples designed to be used as individual components, including use of small tools, numerical sorting, size discrimination, clerical comprehension, drafting, money handling, dynamic physical capacities, and others. Performance is related to worker trait groups as well as to specific occupations.	System consists of 28 work samples designed to be used independently. These include cosmetology, welding, machine trades, cook and baker, auto body repair, plumbing, information processing, bench assembly and others. Can be used for vocational exploration as well as recommendations.	Consists of 16 work samples organized according to worker skill groups, or groups of activities requiring similar task demands. Skill groups include materials sorting, machine feeding, routine tending, and fabricating. Samples yield data on 10 well defined work performance factors and several work behaviors.
Norms	Normed on clients at the International Center for the Disabled. Size and characteristics of sample are unknown.	Data have been collected on a large number of norm groups with various characteristics.	Norm groups are varied and adequate.	Normed on 452 mentally retarded persons.
Reliability/ Validity	No data are available on reliability. Validity research has been inconclusive.	Reliability has been estimated for each work sample. Coefficients are generally high. No validity data are available.	Test-retest reliabilities of .61 and .71 have been reported for an EMR sample.	No reliability or validity data are available.
Address	International Center for the Disabled 320 East 24th Street New York, New York 10010	Valpar International Corp. P.O. Box 5767 Tucson, Arizona 85703-5767	New Concepts Corporation 2341 Friebus Avenue Suite 14 Tucson, Arizona 85713	Vocational Research Institute 1528 Walnut Street, Suite 1502 Philadelphia, PA 19102

Figure 15-13a. Continued.

tween a client and various raters, (5) to provide a standardized reporting system to facilitate information exchange, (6) to stimulate research and the development of new training programs, and (7) to promote realistic administrative decision-making with respect to staffing and programming needs.

The scale has been designed to be administered by either professional or non-professional staff, including parents. Administration can be performed by first person, third party, or interview methods. The portions of the scale which are not relevant to a particular client or situation can be ignored, but norms cannot be used when these omissions

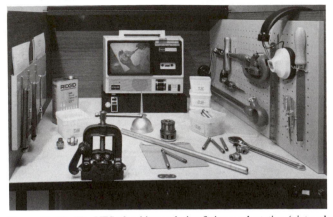

Figure 15-13b. The VES plumbing and pipe fitting work station (pictured above), explores and assesses interest and ability for performing plumbing tasks. *Photo courtesy New Concepts Corporation, Tucson, Arizona.*

have been made because normative data were developed on administration of the entire scale. Table 15-10 illustrates sample items from Part One of the AAMD Adaptive Behavior Scale.

Scoring of the AAMD Adaptive Behavior Scale includes the assignment of values to items based on either criterion definitions, cumulative responses, or frequency of occurrence. Item scores are then totalled to yield domain scores, which can be compared to tabled percentile norms and recorded using a Profile Summary Sheet.

The reliability of the revised version of the AAMD Adaptive Behavior Scale was obtained by administering the test to a total of 133 residents, ages 4 to 69, at three state training schools for mentally retarded persons. Reliability estimates for Part I domain scores were derived from pairs of independent ratings from ward personnel on different shifts. The mean reliabilities for these administrations ranged from .93 for physical development to .71 for self-direction. Average reliability across all domains was .86. For Part II, domain reliabilities ranged from .84 to .40 with a mean reliability of .67.

Factor analysis of domain scores yielded three major dimensions of personal independence, social maladaptation and personal maladaptation. The factor of personal independence is defined by the individual's skills and abilities that are required to maintain his/her personal independence and by the presence of autonomy or motivation to manage his/her personal affairs (Nihira, 1969a, 1969b).

A limited number of studies have been conducted which support the validity of the AAMD Adaptive Behavior Scale. In one study, domain scores on Part I were correlated with previous ratings of adaptive behavior based on clinical judgment (Leland, Shellhaas, Nihira, & Foster, 1967). A study by Greenwood and Perry (1968)

showed that the Part I domain scores and several of the domain scores in Part II significantly discriminated among clients who had been placed into homogeneous administrative units. A third study, involving 260 retarded clients with psychiatric disorders, showed that six of the domain scores in Part II of the scale significantly discriminated between impairment groups (Foster & Nihira, 1969). Finally, a study by Foster and Foster (1967) showed that several domain scores from both Part I and Part II showed significant improvement for an experimental group receiving operant training, while no changes in score were observed for a control group.

Assessment of Occupational Functioning. The Assessment of Occupational Functioning (AOF) is a screening tool specifically developed for use with residents of long-term treatment settings who have physical and or psychiatric problems. The purpose of the tool is to provide a brief overview of the overall functioning of the patient or resident and to identify areas for further assessment and intervention. Based on the human occupation model developed by Kielhofner and colleagues, the AOF assesses six variables related to functional capacity: values, personal causation, interests, roles, habits, and skills. (See Table 15-11)

The AOF is administered as a self-report instrument which consists of a series of questions asked of the client

---

Table 15-10
Sample Item from Part One, Independent Functioning, Section VI of the AAMD Adaptive Behavior Scale

VI. DOMESTIC ACTIVITY
A. Cleaning

[44] Room Cleaning (Circle only ONE)

Cleans room well, e.g., sweeping, dusting and tidying	2
Cleans room but not thoroughly	1
Does not clean room at all	0

[45] Laundry (Check, <u>ALL</u> Statements which apply)

Washes clothing	___
Dries clothing	___
Folds clothing	___
Irons clothing when appropriate	___
None of the above	___

Reprinted with permission from the AAMD Adaptive Behavior Scale for Children and Adults, (1974 Revision). Copyright 1969, 1974, 1975. American Association for Mental Deficiency, p. 8.

Table 15-11
Questions on the Assessment of Occupational Functioning (AOF) Screening Instrument

Instructions: Please interview the resident following this format. You may use a few follow-up questions or rewordings to elicit further information. Note responses on this form. Responses from this interview will provide input for you to make ratings on the assessment form. For use in research, investigators are to rely only on information collected from these interview questions to determine ratings.

VOLITION SUBSYSTEM

Values

What activities are important to you? Name at least five.

Do you have certain ideas about how you should carry out your daily activities? Do you think about what others expect of you?

What were you doing last year at this time? Do you have plans for one year from now? For five years? What are they?

Do you think about the future? Do you have goals for the future? What are your goals?

Personal Causation

Do you feel in control of your life? For example, do you make your own decisions? Do other things or people (for example, family, health, age, institutional rules, etc.) interfere with your life? Was it your decision to come to this program (facility)?

Are you able to do the different things you want to do (go different places, meet different people, try different activities)? List these things.

Can you do the things that you need to do each day? Can you do them well?

Do you believe you will be able to do the things you need and/or want to do in the future?

Interests

Name the things you like to do. Which of these do you like best? How often do you do each of these things?

Are there things that you would like to do that you are not doing now? List them.

HABITUATION SUBSYSTEM

Roles

How do you spend most of your time? What do you do? With whom? How often?

What are your major roles in life? What does that mean you have to do?

How would you describe your involvement here in this program (facility) as a hobbyist, volunteer, active participant, patient, participant in social activities, friend, client, student, worker, or in another role?

Habits

What is a typical weekday like for you? Weekend day? Do you have enough time to do the things you need to do? Do you have too much time?

Do you feel you are flexible when the situation requires a change in your routine? How do you act when things change?

Do you depend on encouragement or reminders from others to accomplish routine daily tasks?

PERFORMANCE SUBSYSTEM

Skills

Do you have trouble moving or getting around? Does it interfere with the things you need and/or want to do?

If you run into problems, can you usually figure them out for yourself? Do you ask others for help to figure out a problem?

Do you feel you get along well with others? Do you ever have trouble understanding what others want you to do? Do you ever have trouble making others understand you?

---

through a semi-structured interview. Following this interview, the therapist completes a rating form by using a five-point scale ranging from ''absent'' to ''fully adaptive'' to describe the client's function. A total score between 6 and 30 is possible. The developers describe the interview as providing useful qualitative data on the person, while the ratings are designed to summarize and quantify the therapist's judgment about the patient's level of functioning (Watts, Kielhofner, Bauer, et al., 1986).

In a published study of its reliability and validity, the

Table 15-12
Factors and Items on the Functional Assessment Inventory

Factor Name	Item Descriptor
Adaptive Behavior	Congruence of behavior with rehabilitation goals
	Judgment
	Persistence
	Accurate perception of capabilities and limitations
	Effective interaction with people
	Work Habits
	Social Support System
Motor Functioning	Hand Function
	Coordination
	Upper Extremity Function
	Motor speed
Cognition	Learning ability
	Ability to read and write
	Memory
	Perceptual organization
Physical Condition	Endurance
	Loss of time from work
	Capacity for exertion
	Stability of condition
	Mobility
Communication	Speech
	Hearing
	Language
Vocational Qualifications	Acceptability to employers
	Access to job opportunities
	Work history
	Economic disincentives
	Personal attractiveness
	Skills
Vision	Vision

developers reported satisfactory test-retest reliability (r = .70 to .90) and interrater consistency of .78. The validity of the AOF was estimated by determining whether scores on the instrument would discriminate between health community subjects and subjects in institutional settings. Out of a total of 249 classifications made through use of the instrument using three raters' scores, there were 14 errors. However, the raters were aware of the actual situations of the clients and could have been been influenced by this knowledge. The findings did show that the scores derived from the AOF were correlated significantly with both the *Life Satisfaction Index-Z*, a self-report measure of life satisfaction, and the *Geriatric Rating Scale*, a measure of functional performance.

Functional Assessment Inventory and Life Functioning Index. The Functional Assessment Inventory (FAI) (Crewe & Athelstan, 1979, 1984) is a brief, yet comprehensive scale of functional limitation and a checklist of ten special strength areas. Developed at the University of Minnesota, the FAI is designed specifically to help those involved in vocational rehabilitation to effectively organize and use information about the problems of severely disabled clients. In addition to physical functioning, other variables that affect employability are included. The inventory consists of 30 behavioral scales of functional limitation, each rated on a four-point scale ranging from "no significant impairment" to "severe degree of limitation." Each rating alternative has an accompanying behavioral referent which was selected specifically for its vocational relevance.

The FAI also includes a checklist of special strengths and provisions for identifying areas of expected change. The scales are intended to apply to all disability groups and are completed by the evaluator based upon interview data, medical charts, and diagnostic evaluations without requiring the client to be present.

Reliability estimates for the FAI, derived from two separate studies (Crewe & Athelstan, 1981; Crewe, Athelstan & Meadows, 1975), estimated interrater reliability to be satisfactory. One study yielded 97% agreement (within one point of the total number of items between pairs of raters), while the other study yielded average item reliability coefficients of .79 and .80 for counselor ratings of videotaped interviews with accompanying background material. The reliability of the LFI was also estimated in the second study, yielding average coefficients of .74 and .79 respectively for the two videotaped sessions.

Factor analysis of the FAI, performed on data from three field tests, yielded a consistent underlying structure of seven factors (Crewe & Turner, 1984). Table 15-12 demonstrates these seven factors and the item descriptors which principally define them.

The Life Functioning Index (LFI) (Crewe & Turner, 1984) was developed to assess significant change in the life status of clients as part of a project in 1980 to develop a state/federal management information system for vocational rehabilitation programs. This instrument measures change in vocational areas and relevant areas of adjustment related to vocational success. The LFI is designed to complement the FAI.

Six categories of life function were selected for the LFI: vocation, education, self-care, residence, mobility, and communication. Each category consists of a series of descriptions that represent different status levels. The status levels, in turn, are arranged ordinally so that client progress or deterioration of function can be interpreted.

Concurrent validity of the FAI was demonstrated through data reflecting significant correlations between the FAI and vocational counselors' ratings of the severity of disability and likelihood of employability. Similar results were obtained for the LFI.

The FAI was also able to discriminate between disability groups on the basis of score differences for the instrument's seven factors. For example, individuals with mental retardation had scores indicating the most impairment in the cognitive category, while persons with orthopedic problems or amputations yielded higher impairment scores on the motor functioning factor than did individuals from other groups.

Finally, the ability of the FAI to predict client outcomes such as successful service closure, earnings at closure, work status and service costs was tested. Both total FAI scores as well as specific items were correlated with these dependent variables. The results were mixed with the total FAI score and 17 of the items failing to show significant relationships with service outcome. On other variables, such as work status and cost of rehabilitation services, larger numbers of FAI scales showed significant relationships.

In summary, it appears that the FAI is a reliable, valid, and useful assessment tool for identifying the nature of an individual's functional limitations. Its companion instrument, the LFI, is useful for describing the consequences of those limitations as manifested in important areas of living. Using both the FAI and LFI together can provide a promising combination of functional scores which can describe an individual's capabilities and relate them to important areas of life function.

Functional Status Questionnaire. The Functional Status Questionnaire (FSQ) is a brief, self-report scale which can be administered in a clinic or home situation. The FSQ is designed for use by ambulatory, mentally competent patients as a tool to screen for functional disability and to monitor change in function. The questionnaire consists of 34 items grouped into six subscales of basic activities of daily living, instrumental activities of daily living, a mental health subscale, work performance, social activity, and quality of interaction subscale. These six subscales test the physical function dimension, the psychological function dimension, and the social-role function dimension.

A unique aspect of the FSQ is its computer scored algorithm, which produces six summary scale scores and six single item scores. Transformed scale scores range from 0 to 100, with a score of 100 indicating the absence of any functional disability. Computerized patient reports provide summary data through visual analog scales and highlight "warning zones" or scores which indicate important functional disabilities.

In a study of its reliability, the FSQ demonstrated internal consistency coefficients of .64 to .82, with the two ADL scales and the mental health subscale achieving the highest reliabilities. Intercorrelations among subscale scores for several hundred ambulatory patients in the Boston area were computed to provide evidence of convergent validity. Observed relationships were consistent with predictions. Evidence of construct validity was obtained through determination of relationships between FSQ scale scores and independent health related variables (Jette, Davis, & Cleary, et al., 1986).

Although early evidence suggests that the FSQ has satisfactory reliability for its use as a research tool to provide group comparisons, higher coefficients would be desirable for its use in individual comparisons. However, as a clinical tool for screening and monitoring, its self-administered format and computerized scoring and reporting are useful.

Multilevel Assessment Instrument. The Multilevel Assessment Instrument (MAI) was developed at the Philadelphia Geriatric Center to measure the well-being of elderly persons through analysis of four major sectors, including behavioral competence, psychological well-being, perceived quality of life, and objective environment (Lawton, Moss, Fulcomer, & Kleban, 1982). Underlying the scale is a conceptual model developed by Lawton (1971) which suggests that behavioral competence involves a hierarchy of complexity of several domains, each of which must be assessed appropriately using adequate psychometric standards. These domains include physical health, cognition, activities of daily living, time use, and social interaction. In keeping with this broad view of behavioral competence, the MAI also provides information on an individual's psychological well-being and perceived environmental quality.

The format of the MAI consists of a series of behavioral checklists that are completed by an interviewer. With the exception of time use, which is intended to assess a person's noninstrumental uses of time, each of the behavioral domains of the MAI consists of two or more subscales or indices. The entire instrument consists of 135 items.

To determine the reliability and validity of the Multilevel Assessment Instrument, a total of 590 individuals were interviewed. These included older persons living independently, those who were recipients of high intensity in-home services, and 65 persons who were on a waiting list for admission to a public nursing home. Intra-class correlations ranged from .58 to .88 across the seven domains for two raters. Internal consistency coefficients were reported as satisfactory across all scales except those attenuated by too few items. Stability coefficients ranged from .73 to .95 across domains.

Evidence of both predictive as well as concurrent validity for the MAI have been provided. In one study, MAI scale scores correlated with independent ratings on subjects done by a clinical psychologist and a housing administrator. Coefficients ranged from a low of .23 for cognition to .69 for personal adjustment. Using a dummy variable approach, an attempt was made to compare subjects whose living situations could be described as independent versus those whose situations were more dependent. Resulting categorization was correlated with MAI scale scores and yielded coefficients ranging from .04 to .56.

Occupational Performance History Interview. The Occupational Performance History Interview was developed to gather useful information on an individual's work, play, and self-care performance (Kielhofner & Henry, 1988). The semi-structured interview consists of 39 questions about the client's past and present behavior with respect to the five content areas of daily living routines, life roles, interests values and goals, perceived ability and responsibility, and environmental influences.

Interviewers using the scale are encouraged to modify, delete or adapt questions as clinically appropriate during the course of the interview. Reported function for items individually referenced is quantified using a five-point rating scale ranging from ''totally adaptive'' to ''totally maladaptive.'' Responses regarding environmental influences are also rated with a five-point scale ranging from ''conditions which maximize function'' to ''conditions which pose significant obstacles to function.'' Since each item is rated in terms of both past and present behaviors, the interviewer must establish a convenient point of historical demarcation which can be a change of roles, living circumstances, or a significant change in health status.

A narrative form is used to report qualitative information, and a five-item nominal scale is used to describe the overall pattern of behavior suggested by the responses and scoring of items. Five categories of life **history** patterns are identified: (1) chronic maladaptation, (2) adaptation recently interrupted by acute onset of maladaptation, (3) variable periods of both adaptation and maladaptation, (4) adaptation followed by gradual progressive maladaptation, and (5) other. The interview process, including rating and narrative report, requires approximately 90 minutes.

The Occupational Performance History Interview was developed with the purpose of building upon previous interview instruments while maintaining compatibility with a wide range of frames of reference for practice. Items were selected and reviewed by a panel of experts for flexibility,

relevance to different age and disability groups, and ease of use.

Studies of the instrument's stability were conducted using 153 subjects, of which 129 provided data for interrater reliability estimates. For two administrations of the test to the total group, correlations ranged from .55 to .68 for past ratings and .31 to .49 for present ratings. Stability coefficients for total scale scores for the entire subject group were reported to be .73 for past and .53 for present. Interrater reliability estimates based on the total score were .60 for the individual total and .63 for the scale total.

Since these data are based on an early version of the scale, it is likely that future revisions will result in improvemented reliability coefficients. Additional data are anticipated with respect to evidence of the scale's validity. Even in the absence of validity data, the focus and design of the instrument should be useful to therapists who routinely gather historical information on performance variables through clinical interview procedures.

Role Activity Performance Scale. The Role Activity Performance Scale (RAPS) was developed to measure role-functioning for diagnostic purposes, treatment planning and outcome research (Good-Ellis, Fine, Spencer, & DiVittis, 1987). The format of the instrument is a semi-structured interview and rating scale designed to gather information concerning an individual's role performance history over a period of up to 18 months. Areas of functional skill assessed include: work or work equivalent, education, home management, family of origin and extended family relationships, mate relationship, parenting, social relationships, leisure activities, self-management, health care, hygiene and appearance, and rehabilitation treatment settings.

The RAPS has been designed so that evaluators can select those role areas that are relevant to the patient undergoing assessment. Interview questions elicit background information about the perceived importance and long-term performance history of a specific role. Additional information is sought regarding role environment, responsibilities, and difficulties and changes in functioning within the role. Data are also sought regarding the individual's methods of coping and adapting to these difficulties and the perceptions of the individual and others regarding how he/she performed in the role. Thus, the RAPS is designed to collect data not only from the individual being evaluated, but also from significant others, other members of the treatment team, and the individual's medical record.

Approximately 90 minutes are required for completion of the scale, including interview activities, data collection, and scoring. A rating scale for each area permits assignment of score values ranging from one to six based upon operational definitions for each point on the scale. Provisions are made for assigning scores between identified criteria for a given score value.

The rating system is designed so that changes in the individual's functional level are identified through comparison of time-segment ratings. An overall performance rating is also derived for each role during the entire period for which data were collected. This permits both an overall score and a summary of the individual's best and worst functioning and frequency of change.

Reliability of the RAPS was estimated using two pairs of raters who evaluated 30 patients. The resulting coefficients, derived from the intra-class correlation coefficient, were greater than .82 for all subscales and .98 for both unweighted and weighted total scores. These estimates may be high because of rater interaction following evaluation of some subjects.

Validation data were collected through a review of items by experts in occupational therapy, through correlation with related scales, and through examination of the scale's ability to discriminate successfully between different patterns of role functioning in two diagnostic groups. Several subscales of the RAPS were found to correlate significantly with related role areas on the Social Adjustment Scale-II (Weissman, Sholomskas, & John, 1981). On 35 subscale pairings between the two scales, 17 showed significant correlation coefficients, ranging from .50 to .82. Additional significant relationships have been reported between various subscales of the RAPS and DSM III, Axis V, the Levels of Functioning Scale, the Katz Adjustment Scale, and the Global Assessment Scale.

In summary, the Role Assessment Performance Scale provides a structured method for gathering information on role functioning in a broad spectrum of roles. It covers a longer time period than most scales and has the advantage of offering a flexible system for defining the segments of time for which behavior is rated. This permits the identification of change in patient behaviors, so that periods of lower and higher levels of functioning can be described and quantified. The scale has shown evidence of adequate reliability, and preliminary validation efforts are encouraging. The primary disadvantages appear to be the amount of time required for gathering information and the complex scoring system.

Role Checklist. One of the first role-oriented instruments developed for clinical use by occupational therapists was the Role Checklist (Barris, Oakley, & Kielhofner, 1987). This self-report instrument is designed specifically to assess the patient's involvement in various roles, the perceived importance of each role, and whether the patient's current role involvement is balanced. The instrument also provides information about the expectations of individuals regarding future role involvement.

The Role Checklist consists of two parts. Part I assesses major roles, which can serve as an organizing influence on a person's life. Ten roles are listed: student, worker, volunteer, caregiver, home-maintainer, friend, family member, religious participant, hobbyist/amateur, and organizational participant. There is also a space for the subject to insert a relevant unlisted role. Roles in this section were chosen specifically because of their implication for productive use of time. Other roles such as cousin or uncle were purposely omitted. For each role listed in Part I, patients are asked to indicate their previous, current or expected performance of a given role by checking columns labeled "past," "present," or "future."

Test-retest reliability was estimated in a study of 124 adults without dysfunction who were living in the community. Kappa and percent agreement were used to estimate consistency between two administrations of the instrument. Estimates of weighted kappa for each role across temporal categories were moderate for past and future and substantial for the present. Percent agreement for each role averaged 87%, with a range of 77% to 93%. Analysis of data showed that stability was higher for older subjects, perhaps reflecting role uncertainty regarding the future for those in the 18 to 30 age group. For the value component (Part II), the weighted estimate of kappa for all roles indicated moderate concordance, with the composite estimate of percent agreement at 79%. These data suggest acceptable stability for the instrument, although reliability data have not been published on use of the scale with dysfunctional clients.

Sickness Impact Profile. The Sickness Impact Profile (SIP) was developed over several years at the University of Washington to provide a measure of perceived health status that is sensitive enough to detect changes occurring over time (Bergner, Bobbitt, Pollard, Martin, & Gilson, 1976). The final form of the SIP contains 136 statements regarding health-related dysfunction in twelve areas of activity across three dimensions (Bergner, Bobbitt, Carter, & Gilson, 1981). Items consist of descriptive statements which may be completed by self-report or administered by an interviewer within 20 to 30 minutes (see Table 15-13).

Each category results in a percentile score based upon the number of items checked or endorsed by a respondent as applicable to their current situation. Additionally, there is an overall or global percentile score representing the dysfunctional effect of a given illness.

To determine the reliability and validity of the SIP, a large field trial was conducted on a random sample of patients seen in a group practice and smaller trials were conducted on samples of patients with hip replacement,

Table 15-13
Sickness Impact Profile Categories and Selected Items

Category	Items Describing Behaviors Involved in or Related to	Selected Items	Scale Values
A	Social interaction	I make many demands, for example, insist that people do things for me, tell them how to do things	7.7
		I am going out less to visit people	5.2
B	Ambulation or locomotion activity	I am walking shorter distances	3.3
		I do not walk at all	9.2
C	Sleep and rest activity	I lie down to rest more often during the day	4.6
		I sit around half-asleep	8.1
D	Taking nutrition	I am eating no food at all, nutrition is taken through tubes or intravenous fluids	12.3
		I am eating special or different food, for example, soft food, bland diet, low-salt, low-fat foods	5.6
E	Usual daily work	I often act irritable toward my work associates, for example, snap at them, give sharp answers, criticize easily	7.1
		I am not working at all	8.6
F	Household management	I have given up taking care of personal or household business affairs, for example, paying bills, banking, working on budget	6.9
		I am doing less of the regular daily work around the house that I usually do	3.9
G	Mobility and confinement	I stay within one room	9.9
		I stop often when traveling because of health problems	4.2
H	Movement of the body	I am in a restricted position all the time	13.6
		I sit down, lie down, or get up only with someone's help	10.4
I	Communication activity	I communicate only by gestures, for example, moving head, pointing, sign language	11.3
		I often lose control of my voice when I talk, for example, my voice gets louder, starts trembling, changes pitch	6.4
J	Leisure pastimes and recreation	I am doing more physically inactive pastimes instead of my other usual activities	3.9
		I am going out for entertainment less often	2.8
K	Intellectual functioning	I have difficulty reasoning and solving problems, for example, making plans, making decisions, learning new things	8.3
		I sometimes behave as if I were confused or disoriented in place or time, for example, where I am, who is around, directions, what day it is	11.2
L	Interaction with family members	I isolate myself as much as I can from the rest of the family	8.9
		I am not doing the things I usually do to take care of my children or family	6.8
M	Emotions, feelings, and sensations	I act irritable and impatient with myself, for example, talk badly about myself, swear at myself, blame myself for things that happen	5.4
		I laugh and cry suddenly for no reason	8.1
N	Personal hygiene	I dress myself, but do so very slowly	4.6
		I do not have control of my bowels	11.2

Reprinted with permission: Bergner, M., Bobbitt, R.A., Carter, W.B., & Gilson, B.S. (1981). The Sickness Impact Profile: Development and final revision of a health status measure. Medical Care, 19(8), 787-805.

rheumatoid arthritis, and hyperthyroidism. Test-retest reliability was estimated at .92, while the coefficient for internal consistency was .94.

Interviews yielded higher reliability than data collection through self-administration. Evidence of validity was based on relationships between SIP scores, self-assessments of dysfunction, and other measures of dysfunction. Correlations were moderate to high and established the ability of the scale to distinguish between patients of varying levels of dysfunction either due to illness type or severity. Other studies have demonstrated the ability of the SIP to distinguish between the functional status of patients with end-stage renal disease (Hart & Evans, 1987) and chronic low back pain (Follick, Smith, & Ahern, 1985). A shortened version of the SIP was found to work nearly as well as the full scale in estimating the functional status of patients with low back pain (Deyo, 1986).

Unfortunately, the SIP seems to function less effectively as a measure of change within patients (MacKenzie, Charlson, DiGioia, & Kelley, 1985). A study comparing SIP scores with patient self-ratings over time showed that the scale was unable to equally detect improvements and deteriorations in condition.

In summary, the SIP is a useful measure of general health status with satisfactory evidence of reliability and validity. It is one of very few such instruments appearing as outcome measures in clinical trials reported in the medical literature. However, the failure of the instrument to indicate change within the same patient may limit its use as a tool for clinical management.

Vineland Adaptive Behavior Scales. The Vineland Adaptive Behavior Scales (VABS) is described as a newly introduced version of the Vineland Social Maturity Scales and includes a survey or short form of 297 items and an extended form offering 572 items (Sparrow, Balla, & Cichetti, 1984). The following information pertains to the survey or short form.

Designed to be administered as a semi-structured interview, the scales are appropriate for age levels from birth to 18 years and low functioning adults. The VABS provide information on function in four domains, including communication, daily living skills, socialization, and motor skills. Thirteen scores are provided, as summarized in Figure 15-14. Items contributing to the adaptive behavior measures are arranged within domains with five possible scores for each (2, 1, 0, "no opportunity," or "don't know"). Another section of 36 items allows assessment of problem or maladaptive behaviors. With training, a professional interviewer can administer the VABS in less than one hour.

Standardization of the VABS involved a sample of 3,000 normal children and a supplemental sample of 2,202

retarded and disabled children and adults (including those with emotional disturbance, hearing, and visual impairments). Each of the subtests of the VABS and the composite score can be expressed in standard scores, percentile ranks, and age equivalents.

The median split-half and test-retest reliability coefficients for the domain and composite scores range from .83 for the motor skills domain to .94 for the composite. Interrater coefficients ranged from .62 to .78, with considerable variation within subdomains.

The administration manual reports some studies of construct validity. For example, some standardization subgroups were compared to the original *Vineland Social Maturity Scales*, the *Kaufman Assessment Battery for Children* and other scales. Low to moderate correlations were found. These findings were interpreted as generally supportive of the construct validity of the VABS.

Observation/Longitudinal Approaches

Bay Area Functional Performance Evaluation. The purpose of the revised Bay Area Functional Performance

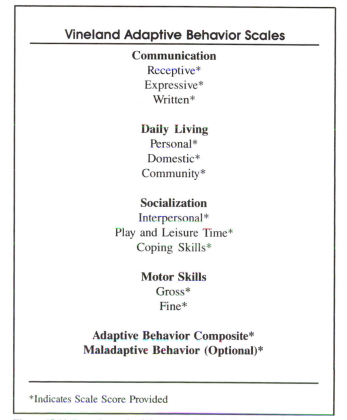

Vineland Adaptive Behavior Scales

Communication
Receptive*
Expressive*
Written*

Daily Living
Personal*
Domestic*
Community*

Socialization
Interpersonal*
Play and Leisure Time*
Coping Skills*

Motor Skills
Gross*
Fine*

Adaptive Behavior Composite*
Maladaptive Behavior (Optional)*

*Indicates Scale Score Provided

Figure 15-14. Domains and subdomains of the Vineland Adaptive Behavior Scales.

Evaluation (BaFPE) is "to assess general components of functioning that are needed to perform activities of daily living" (Williams & Bloomer, 1987, p. 1). The revised BaFPE has two parts, the Task-Oriented Assessment and the Social Interaction Scale.

The Task Oriented Assessment or TOA consists of the following five specific tasks which the developers claim provide information about twelve functional parameters: a task of sorting shells according to size, shape, and color, a money management task (labeled money/marketing) consisting of totalling the cost of several grocery items and writing a check; a task of drawing a floor plan for a home; a task of copying a design with blocks from memory with a visual cue; and a task of drawing a person engaged in some activity.

A client's performance on each task is rated according to cognitive, affective, and performance components. Within each component, specific characteristics (termed "symptoms" by the test developers) are rated on a four-point scale (see Table 15-14). Each of the five tasks also presents the evaluator with an opportunity to note observations of performance related to expressive language, comprehension, hemispatial neglect, memory, and abstract thinking, and to indicate the presence of itemized task-specific observations. These task-specific observations, under the heading of qualitative signs and referral indicators, are not scored. They serve as a means of gathering clinical information that may indicate the need for further testing.

Scores on the Task Oriented Assessment can be interpreted by examination of parameters or components across tasks, by examination of specific task scores, or through comparison with norms. A special scoring routine has been designed to draw the examiner's attention to the possibility of organic involvement and the need for further evaluation or consultation.

The second major component of the BaFPE is the Social Interaction Scale (SIS). In this scale, seven categories of verbal and non-verbal interaction which reflect normal interaction patterns are assessed across five situations in which there is opportunity to observe the client's social interaction. These situations include an interview with the evaluator at mealtime, in group unstructured activity, in structured group activity, and during structured verbal group settings. The seven categories assessed during these situations include verbal communication, psychomotor behavior, socially appropriate behavior, response to authority figures, independence/dependence, ability to work with others, and participation in group or program activities. Scores in each category are determined by ratings on a five-point scale and each point has specific behavioral definitions. An optional client self-report of social interaction can also be used to provide additional clinical information.

Reliability studies on the revised BaFPE have been conducted by the instrument developers and have included examinations of its interrater reliability and internal consistency (Bloomer & Williams, 1987). For the Task Oriented Assessment, the total score and cognitive component correlations exceeded .90 for three of four rating pairs, and correlations for the affective component ranged from .72 to .96. Correlations for specific tasks ranged from .75 to .97, with the sorting shells task demonstrating the most variability. Intercorrelations of functional parameters and component areas ranged from .29 to .84 with an average correlation of .60.

Reliability data for the revised Social Interaction Scale showed interrater correlations of .56 to .94 across the seven parameters for two of six groups. Correlations for the observation situations ranged from .74 to .94. Intercorrelations among SIS parameters ranged from .38 to .81.

In general, the reliability data for the revised BaFPE show improvements over the initial instrument, but there is some indication of a lack of consistency among some component items. Thus these limitations should be considered.

Evidence of the validity of the revised BaFPE is limited. However, a study by Thibeault and Blackmer (1987) found significant correlations between three subscales of the *Wechsler Adult Intelligence Scale* and the total score for the Task Oriented Assessment, thus providing evidence of the convergent validity of that subscale of the BaFPE. In the same study, the researchers also found strong correlations among the three component subscores of the BaFPE and sought to determine whether evidence of discriminate validity existed within their study sample of 60 patients. The TOA total score and three task scores were able to discriminate between patients who had and had not received electroconvulsive therapy within two years prior to the study. Total scores on the TOA did not differentiate between subjects who had received higher doses of neuroleptic medications, despite the hypothesis that these individuals should exhibit diminished functional performance. Other correlations supported the validity of the BaFPE, including no relationship between either gender or diagnostic classification (depression versus schizophrenia) and functional performance as reflected in the TOA. As expected, significant relationship between performance and age was found for these scores. In this study, no information was collected using the Social Interaction Scales.

In a study of the relationship between cognitive level and performance on the TOA, Newman (1987) found a significant correlation of .63 for 21 patients using the revised Allen Cognitive Level Test. In the same study, both measures were found to correlate significantly with the Global Assessment Scale.

In a comprehensive report of the development and standardization of the original and revised BaFPE (Houston, Williams, Bloomer, & Mann, 1987) the need for further validation studies was acknowledged. In the same report, the authors conceded the difficulties imposed by the absence of national normative data. Noting that therapists have reported reducing the length of the TOA for use in acute care settings, they emphasized that such *ad hoc* revisions are not comparable to the full scale version and thus cannot be compared with preliminary standardization results. Further validation efforts with the full scale version were encouraged.

Longitudinal Functional Assessment System. The Longitudinal Functional Assessment System (LFAS) represents a comprehensive approach to the measurement of functional performance and health status in rehabilitation (Norris-Baker, Stephens, Rintala, & Willems, 1981). One of its unique attributes is its ability to provide direct measurement of client performance across time and in different settings. The principal strength is that it permits assessment of the behaviors that are most relevant to the long-term adjustment of patients with severe disabilities.

The LFAS has three components: (1) the Self-Observation and Report Technique (SORT), (2) two instruments to measure activity level, including the Rest/Time Sit/Time Monitor (RTM/STM) and a wheelchair odometer, and (3) the Environmental Negotiability Survey (ENS). The SORT results in a quantitative record of an individual's activities and provides documentation of what they did, with whom, where, and how the activities were performed. The activity level measures are used to measure mobility and activity level, respectively. The Environmental Negotiability Survey provides an objective measure of the accessibility of environments used by persons with physical disabilities.

Although all three components of the LFAS together provide an integrated and comprehensive assessment of life functioning, the SORT is the most useful from the standpoint of providing a rich array of information on an individual's performance of daily activities. SORT information is gathered through an interview technique that seeks to quantify an individual's activity for a defined period of time, usually 24 hours. During the interview process, which usually lasts less than an hour, the client provides descriptions of all activities that occurred during the assessment period, including the duration and locations of the activities and the roles of those involved. During the process, the role of the interviewer is to record the sequence of activities and to facilitate recall. (See Figure 15-15) Activities are translated into behavioral units according to specified criteria based on discernibility, client involvement, duration, and observability. Behavioral units are then analyzed according to four basic measures of frequency, accumulated time, proportion of activities performed independently, and diversity. Activity diversity is based on the number of locations, types of activity, and companions involved.

In studies of the SORT, the reliability of client self-reports of activity was compared with independent, direct observations. For a 24-hour reporting period in which reported events were matched with observed events based on context rather than time of occurrence, the extent of agreement was 76% when clinical staff were used as interviewers (Uttermohlen, Alexander, and Willems, 1982). A study using family members of clients as informal observers found a level of 80% agreement for reported activities (Rintala, 1982). The same study showed that the mode of interview was independent of reliability, so that gathering data for the SORT is possible through telephone interviews. The developers recommend that a regular system of reliability checks be used to increase reporting accuracy when the SORT is used on a routine basis.

Using the variables of independence, behavioral diversity, number of active behaviors, and changes of location or mobility derived from SORT data, researchers have been able to predict the following functional behaviors at three months after discharge: community involvement, productivity as measured by vocational or educational activity, and social support as measured by the diversity of companions. These data were derived from patients with spinal cord

---

Table 15-14
Component Abilities Rated on Bay Area Functional Performance Evaluation Tasks

Cognitive Components	Affective Components	Performance Components
• Memory for Written/Verbal	• Motivation & Compliance	• Task Completion
• Organization of Time & Materials	• Frustration Tolerance	• Errors
• Attention Span	• Self-confidence	
• Evidence of Thought Disorder	• General Affective & Behavioral Impression	

				Assistance					
Patient Name: Robert Jones				Patient #: 46		Protocol #: 063		Date: 04/06/82 (DD/MM/YY)	
Interviewer Name: Carol Smith - 063				Week #: 9 (In-Hospital)		Month #: (Post-Hospital)		Time Period: 24 hrs.	

#	Begin Time	Activity Description	Code	Assistance — Any	Assistance — ½ or More	Companions	Locations	S
09	15 30	Sitting in lobby	1 4 1	∅ / 3 0	∅ / 3 0	friend / 5 1	lobby 0 2 0	1
10	16 20	Transporting to Room	0 5 1	friend / 5 1	∅ / 2 9	friend / 6 1	lobby 0 2 0 · ward 0 1 0	1
11	16 25	Reading magazine	0 7 0	∅ / 2 9	∅ / 2 9	∅ / 3 0	ward 0 1 0	1
12	17 00	Talking with Social Worker	1 3 2	∅ / 3 0	∅ / 3 0	sw / 1 4	" 0 1 0	1
13	17 25	Watching TV	1 4 2	∅ / 3 0	∅ / 3 0	∅ / 3 0	" 0 1 0	1
14	18 15	Eating Dinner	0 4 1	NA / 1 2	∅ / 2 9	NA / 1 2	" C 1 0	1
15	18 45	Talking on Phone	1 3 3	∅ / 2 9	∅ / 2 9	mother / 4 3	" 0 1 0	1
16	19 15	Playing Cards	2 2 2	∅ / 2 9	∅ / 2 9	other patient / 6 5	" 0 1 0	1

Figure 15-15. SORT Data Collection Form. *Reprinted with permission: Rintala, D.H., Uttermohlen, D.M. & Buck, E.R., et al. (1984). Self-observation and report technique (SORT). In A.S. Halpern & M.J. Fuhrer, (Eds). Functional Assessment in Rehabilitation. Baltimore: Paul H. Brookes (pp. 205-222).*

injury and indicate that the SORT could be useful for predicting poor adjustment after discharge.

The instrument can be used with other populations as well because variables of interest can be selected from daily activities according to their relevance to particular client types. For example, Buck (1983) studied cardiac patients using the SORT. In this study, behaviors of interest included exercise, smoking, and dietary habits. Adaptation of the SORT requires only that the questions used in the interview be modified to address the specific information sought.

Parachek Geriatric Rating Scale. The Parachek Geriatric Rating Scale evolved from a longer scale and is designed to serve as a quick screening instrument (Miller & Parachek, 1974; Plutchik, Conte & Lieberman, et al., 1970). It includes ten items directed toward physical condition, general self-care, and social behavior (see Figure 15-16). Each item is scored on a five-point scale and lower scores indicate greater difficulty. Items can be completed and charted on a graph within three to five minutes by any caregiver familiar with the patient's level of function.

Based on obtained scores from the Parachek Geriatric Rating Scale, patients are classified into one of three groups. Patients scoring 10 to 24 points (Group I) are considered sufficiently impaired so as to warrant substantial nursing care. An intervention program based on positioning, sensory stimulation and group work is recommended for this group. Individuals scoring from 25 to 39 points (Group II) are responsive, participative, and semi-independent in self-care activities. Recommended treatment for these patients includes extensive group-oriented social stimulation. Patients scoring 40 to 50 points (Group III) are generally independent in self-care and self-motivated. Accordingly, they are viewed as candidates for return to their family setting or foster placement.

A study of 150 patients hospitalized with deteriorative neurological disorders at a state facility provided the basis for some evidence of the scale's validity (Miller & Parachek, 1974). The Paracheck scale correlated .88 with a

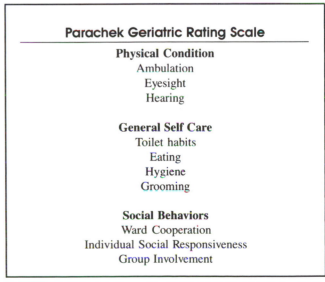

longer, previously validated scale used by the National Institute of Mental Health (the Plutchik Geriatric Rating Scale). Criterion-related validity was estimated at .77 for the scale's ability to correctly predict initial diagnostic classification, and a correlation of .73 was obtained for predicting final diagnostic classification.

Rehabilitation Indicators. Rehabilitation Indicators (RI's) is a term representing a cluster of functional assessment instruments which can be used individually or in combination. These instruments were developed over a period of time at New York University as part of a federally funded project (Diller, Fordyce, Jacobs, et al., 1983).

The Rehabilitation Indicators cluster of assessment approaches were based on an underlying philosophy that recognized the importance of considering ecological factors in providing valid documentation of what clients do in their actual environments, rather than describing behaviors which may be assessed in less representative settings, such as hospitals or rehabilitation centers. Underlying this view is a realization that competencies, *per se*, do not completely predict day-to-day functioning. For example, the ability to maneuver a wheelchair independently can be a useful skill, but it does not predict actual function in a setting where the physical dimensions of doorways impede its use or where family members insist on pushing the wheelchair.

The four component instruments of the RI battery have been designed to provide complementary information about a client's functioning. Three of these instruments have been completed, while a fourth remains under development. The instruments include skill indicators, status indicators, activity pattern indicators, and environmental indicators. Each of these components will be summarized below.

Skill Indicators (SKI's) are designed to document a client's areas of strength and weakness in various areas of functioning, such as self-care, mobility, social behavior, communication, vocational activity, and homemaking. Thus, they are most like traditional approaches to functional assessment. However, they differ in that specific skill indicators are listed in a taxonomy from which the evaluator selects relevant items. This permits the assembly of an assessment package that includes only those skills that are most relevant to a given intervention program or set of outcomes. This approach results in client profiles that include only that level of detail viewed as appropriate for the identified purposes of the assessment activity.

Status Indicators (SI's) represent one of two tools in the RI instrument cluster that describe what the person does. SI's describe a person's position in the sociocultural environment by summarizing the key resources available to them which could influence their overall level of life performance. SI's are facts that note characteristics which clearly impact the person's overall functional status in the sociocultural environment, such as employment status, income, or living arrangements. SI's are derived from interviews, written self-reports, or by reviewing an individual's records.

A third component, *Activity Pattern Indicators* (API's), also describes behavioral output by documenting an individual's typical patterns and temporal characteristics of activity engagement. API's are based on research that shows that such activity dimensions relate consistently with levels of impairment and disability.

API data may include such details as the amount of time spent in travel, the location of activity, percentage of time spent working or in school, community involvement, the diversity of activity, the proportion of time spent in social activities, and related characteristics. Data can be gathered by the individual's completion of an activity diary or by an interview, questionnaire, or observation.

The level of detail regarding activity participation may vary from simple frequency counts to information on an activity's duration, location, social content, and amount of assistance required for participation. While administration of the API's varies according to format and level of detail, the range is from 10 to 60 minutes.

Environmental Indicators is the final component of the RI's and is a set of tools designed to document extrinsic factors which influence optimal performance. This portion of the assessment strategy is viewed as an important part of shifting the focus of assessment from the client to one of perceiving the client within an environment that supports or inhibits performance. The organizing model for the Environmental Indicators includes settings such as community,

Parachek Geriatric Rating Scale

Physical Condition
Ambulation
Eyesight
Hearing

General Self Care
Toilet habits
Eating
Hygiene
Grooming

Social Behaviors
Ward Cooperation
Individual Social Responsiveness
Group Involvement

Figure 15-16. Behaviors assessed by the Parachek Geriatric Rating Scale.

work, and home, and each has physical, social, legal, and economic elements. Examples of relevant dimensions for these settings would be availability, accessibility, and negotiability.

Because of the design of the Rehabilitation Indicators approach, no single reliability or validity statement would be appropriate. However, while noting the various logistical difficulties associated with gathering reliability and validity data in community environments, Brown, Gordon, & Diller (1984) have reported on some attempts to determine these characteristics of the Rehabilitation Indicators Instruments.

One study conducted by O'Neill, Gordon, & Brown (1983) showed very high reliability coefficients for a single SKI measurement tool in a study of community-based patients. The SKI data have been used to successfully forecast performance differences among patients with different types of disability, thus demonstrating predictive validity.

The Status Indicators reflect high reliability as a result of attention to this during item development. Each item was designed to be clear with respect to content and context and to require little discretionary judgment. Items were revised until perfect test-retest and interrater relia-

---

Table 15-15
Abbreviated Outline of OT FACT Assessment Categories

I. Role Integration

II. Functional Activities of Performance
  A. PERSONAL CARE ACTIVITIES
    1. Cleanliness Hygiene and appearance
    2. Medical and Health Management Activities
    3. Nutrition Activities
    4. Mobility Activities
    5. Communication Activities
  B. OCCUPATIONAL ROLE RELATED ACTIVITIES
    1. Home Management Activities
    2. Consumer Activities
    3. Studentship Activities
    4. Employment and Volunteer Preparation Activities
    5. Caregiving Activities
    6. Employer Activities
    7. Community Activities
    8. Avocational Activities

III. Functional Integration Skills of Performance
  A. MOTOR INTEGRATION SKILLS
    1. Functional Motor Skills
    2. Postural Control
    3. Activity Tolerance
  B. SENSORY INTEGRATION SKILLS
    1. Perceptual
    2. Perceptual-Motor

  C. COGNITIVE INTEGRATION SKILLS
    1. Problem Solving
    2. Generalization of Learning
    3. Sequencing
    4. Concept Formation
    5. Categorization
    6. Intellectual Operations in Space
  D. SOCIAL INTEGRATION SKILLS
    1. Peer Interactions
    2. Authority/Subordinate Interactions
    3. Family Interactions
  E. PSYCHOLOGICAL INTEGRATION SKILLS
    1. Situational coping/Stress Management
    2. Time Use/Planning

IV. Components of Performance
  A. NEUROMUSCULAR COMPONENTS
    1. Muscle tone
    2. Reflexes
    3. Range of Motion
    4. Strength (pinch, hand, muscle)
    5. Endurance
    6. Soft Tissue integrity
    7. Skeletal integrity
  B. SENSORY AWARENESS COMPONENTS
    1. Tactile
    2. Proprioceptive
    3. Ocular control & vision
    4. Vestibular
    5. Auditory
    6. Olfactory
    7. Gustatory

  C. COGNITIVE COMPONENTS
    1. Level of arousal
    2. Memory
    3. Orientation
    4. Attention Span
    5. Recognition
    6. Thought processes (form and content)
  D. SOCIAL COMPONENTS
    1. Group Interaction
    2. Dyadic Interaction
  E. PSYCHOLOGICAL COMPONENTS
    1. Personal Responsibility Motivation
    2. Initiative
    3. Termination of action
    4. Body Image
    5. Value Identification
    6. Interest Identification
    7. Goal Setting

V. Environment
  A. SOCIAL CULTURAL ENVIRONMENT
    1. Social Support system
    2. Financial resources
    3. Medical resources
    4. Educational resources
  B. PHYSICAL ENVIRONMENT
    1. Transportation Accessibility
    2. Architectural Accessibility
    3. Special Equipment

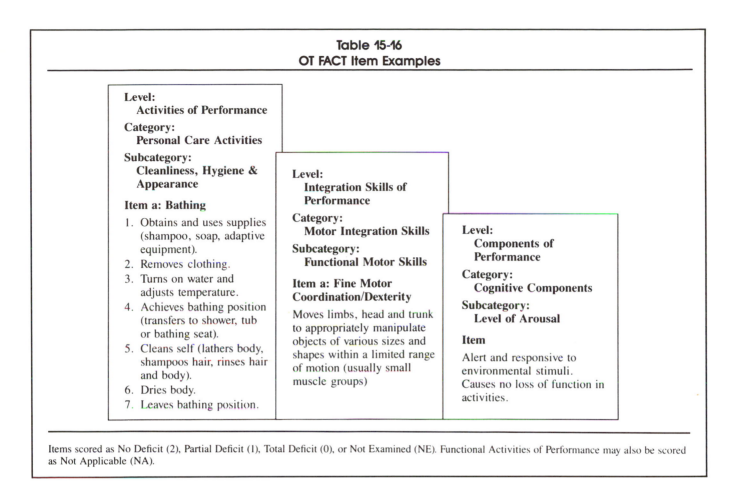

Table 15-16
OT FACT Item Examples

Level:
  Activities of Performance
Category:
  Personal Care Activities
Subcategory:
  Cleanliness, Hygiene & Appearance

Item a: Bathing

1. Obtains and uses supplies (shampoo, soap, adaptive equipment).
2. Removes clothing.
3. Turns on water and adjusts temperature.
4. Achieves bathing position (transfers to shower, tub or bathing seat).
5. Cleans self (lathers body, shampoos hair, rinses hair and body).
6. Dries body.
7. Leaves bathing position.

Level:
  Integration Skills of Performance
Category:
  Motor Integration Skills
Subcategory:
  Functional Motor Skills

Item a: Fine Motor Coordination/Dexterity

Moves limbs, head and trunk to appropriately manipulate objects of various sizes and shapes within a limited range of motion (usually small muscle groups)

Level:
  Components of Performance
Category:
  Cognitive Components
Subcategory:
  Level of Arousal

Item

Alert and responsive to environmental stimuli. Causes no loss of function in activities.

Items scored as No Deficit (2), Partial Deficit (1), Total Deficit (0), or Not Examined (NE). Functional Activities of Performance may also be scored as Not Applicable (NA).

bility was achieved with ten respondents. Validity of the SI's was obtained from an analysis of over 100 clients' self-reports that were compared with chart documentation indicating their actual ability. Over 95 percent of the cases showed agreement in this study.

The reliability of Activity Pattern Indicators was more difficult to establish because of the natural variability of activity patterns in daily life. However, the developers noted work done by others that showed that the reliability of activity data can be quite high for summary measures. Studies have also demonstrated the validity of such approaches, finding high correlations between data derived from self-reports and those derived from observation (Brown, 1982).

In the final report of the Rehabilitation Indicators Project, the authors noted that reliability and validity studies for the RI instruments are encouraging but not complete. Potential users may need to conduct studies in their own settings prior to use of the instruments for important decision-making regarding clients. However, since their development, many of the tools have been used for such purposes as program evaluation, case management, identifying and documenting unmet needs, and counseling. Although federal funding was terminated in 1982, further development of the Rehabilitation Indicators has continued.

MANAGING ASSESSMENT DATA

Because of the complexity of occupational performance assessment, it is not unusual for therapists in some settings to use several instruments during the course of intervention. In many cases, these assessments may be repeated, thus producing a large amount of assessment information which must be organized and analyzed for purposes of decision-making and documentation. The need for increased efficiency and the advent of affordable microcomputer technology has made it possible to design automated systems for integrating and reporting assessment information. While many facilities have developed 'in-house' software to serve their unique settings, commercial systems are also becoming available. One of these systems, OT FACT, is described in this section.

OT FACT

OT FACT, an acronym for Occupational Therapy Functional Assessment Compilation Tool (Smith, 1990), is designed to provide an efficient means for summarizing and documenting client performance. The system has been developed to facilitate the progression and recording of functional assessment data from general to specific.

Available in computer software and paper and pencil versions, OT FACT is based on a hierarchy of function, and yields information on levels of function that include role integration, functional activities of performance, functional integration skills of performance, and performance components and environment (See Table 15-15). Functional activities of performance include personal care activities and occupational role-related activities. The evaluation of functional integration skills of performance includes categories for motor, sensory, cognitive, social, and psychological integration skills. For example, fine motor coordination and dexterity are subskills under the general category of motor integration skills (See Table 15-16).

OT FACT consists of a scoring guide and scoresheet for manual use. Based on observed or tested performance in each of the categories, the evaluator assigns a rating (2 = no deficit, 1 = partial deficit, or 0 = total deficit) for each item. Scoring provisions have been made for items which are not applicable to a given individual.

Features of OT FACT include the comprehensive scope and the appreciation for the role of the environment in affecting functional performance. The instrument examines performance at the level of role-related activity, yet also simultaneously gives attention to deficits in underlying performance subsystems. Thus a clear distinction is made between impairment and disability with respect to functional performance. The individual who is able to perform a personal care activity such as grooming with an adapted device does not have a deficit. However, the inability to perform task components without the device might reflect deficits in neuromuscular components, such as range of motion. This approach permits ready identification of the relationship between deficits in performance subsystems and disability, thus facilitating treatment planning.

An unusual and desirable feature of OT FACT is the built-in decision tree. Because the system's 213 scoring categories do not pertain to all individuals, 42 hierarchical decision nodes have been incorporated to adjust the degree of functional performance detail needed if certain performance levels are met. Although a paper format is available,

the complexity of the system is best suited for use with electronic data processing equipment.

Since OT FACT is designed as a criterion-based instrument, scores are plotted as a percentage of needed performance. This permits the identification of both intervention needs and the documentation of improvement over time. The system focuses on documenting functional performance by providing guidelines for sequencing the evaluation process in an efficient, yet comprehensive format. It is not designed to replace the use of more focused assessment instruments in use within specialized areas of practice.

SUMMARY

As Frey has suggested in the introductory quotation for this chapter, assessment in rehabilitation has been profoundly influenced by the diagnostic, impairment-oriented view of medical practice. However, a growing appreciation for the importance of the assessment of function at the level of disability and role performance has led to the development of several useful instruments and approaches.

This chapter has presented approaches to assessing the client's ability to perform role-related tasks of living in the domains of self-care/maintenance, play/leisure, and work. Several more global instruments and approaches have been described which provide information across two or more functional domains. Evolving assessment approaches that provide for the consideration of environmental factors that influence performance have also been reviewed.

As further advances are made in the assessment of occupational performance, several issues will need to be addressed, including the practicality and cost, representative performance, relative task value, and generalization of instruments and approaches. Where appropriate, additional work must also be done to provide reliability and validity data on established instruments. It is clear that occupational therapists can benefit from their knowledge of functional assessment approaches being developed in occupational therapy as well as in other disciplines across the health, social, and behavioral sciences.

Study Questions

1. Construct a matrix of occupational domains and levels of dysfunction. Can you identify an assessment approach for each cell of the matrix?

2. List three major issues of concern to those developing assessment approaches in rehabilitation. How are these issues being confronted?

Identify environmental factors which might influence performance. Can you cite an example of an assessment where efforts were made to control (or hold constant) environmental factors?

4. Identify 5 self-care tasks commonly assessed by early basic ADL scales.

5. What is meant by Instrumental Activities of Daily Living?

6. Why is play behavior difficult to assess through direct observation approaches?

7. Cite examples of (1) a global screening tool developed for geriatric patients, (2) a global screening tool developed for mentally retarded persons, and (3) a global tool designed for severely disabled clients.

8. Discuss the advantages and disadvantages of direct observation versus self-report approaches in functional assessment.

Recommended Readings

Benson, J. & Clark, F. (1982). A guide for instrument development and validation. *American Journal of Occupational Therapy, 36*, 789-800.

Bolton, B. (1987). *Handbook of measurement and evaluation in rehabilitation*. Baltimore: Paul H. Brookes.

Botterbusch, K.F. (1987). *Vocational assessment and evaluation systems*. Menomonie, WI: Materials Development Center, Vocational Rehabilitation Institute, University of Wisconsin-Stout.

Christiansen, C.H., Schwartz, R.K., & Barnes, K.J. (1988). Self-care: Evaluation and management. In DeLisa, J., et al., (Eds.). *Principles of rehabilitation medicine*. (pp. 95-115). Philadelphia: J.B. Lippincott.

Halpern, A.S. & Fuhrer, M.J. (1984). *Functional assessment in rehabilitation*. Baltimore: Paul H. Brookes.

Hemphill, B.J. (Ed.). (1988). *Mental health assessment in occupational therapy*. Thorofare, NJ: Slack, 1987, 133-146.

Jette, A.M. (1985). State of the art in functional status assessment. In Rothstein, J. (Ed.). *Measurement in physical therapy*. (pp. 137-168). New York: Churchill-Livingstone.

Kaufert, J.M. (1983). Functional ability indices: Measurement problems in assessing their validity. *Archives of Physical Medicine & Rehabilitation, 64*, 260-267.

McDowell, I. & Newell, C. (1987). *Measuring health: A guide to rating scales and questionnaires*. New York: Oxford University Press.

References

Alexander, J.L., Fuhrer, M.J. (1984). Functional assessment of individuals with physical impairments. In Halpern, A.S., & Fuhrer, M.J.: *Functional assessment in rehabilitation*. Baltimore: Paul H. Brookes.

American Association for Mental Deficiency. *AAMD adaptive behavior scale for children and adults* (revised 1974).

Barris, R., Oakley, F., & Kielhofner, G. (1987). The role checklist. In Hemphill, B.J. (1987). *Mental health assessment in occupational therapy*. Thorofare, NJ: Slack.

Beard, J.G., & Ragheb, M.G. (1980). Measuring leisure satisfaction. *Journal of Leisure Research, 12*, 20-33.

Behnke, C.J. & Menarchek-Fetkovich, M. (1984). Examining the reliability and validity of the play history. *American Journal of Occupational Therapy, 38*(2), 94-100.

Bergner, M., Bobbitt, R.A., Carter, W.B., & Gilson, B.S. (1981). The Sickness Impact Profile: Development and final revision of a health status measure. *Medical Care, 19*(8) 787-805.

Bergner, M., Bobbitt, R.A., Pollard, W.E., Martin, D.P., & Gilson, B.S. (1976). The Sickness Impact Profile: validation of a health status measure. *Medical Care, 14*(1) 57-67.

Bledsoe, N. & Shephard, J. (1982). Reliability and validity of a preschool play scale. *American Journal of Occupational Therapy, 36*, 783-788.

Bloomer, J.S. & Williams, S.K. (1987). *The Bay Area Functional Performance Evaluation* (Research Ed.). Palo Alto, CA: Consulting Psychologists Press.

Botterbusch, K.F. (1987). *Vocational assessment and evaluation systems*. Menomonie, WI: Materials Development Center, Vocational Rehabilitation Institute, University of Wisconsin-Stout.

Brayman, S., Kirby, T., Misenheimer, A., & Short, M. (1976). Comprehensive occupational therapy scale. *American Journal of Occupational Therapy, 30*, 94-100.

Brockett, M.M. (1987). Cultural variations in Bay Area Functional Performance Evaluation Scores—Considerations for Occupational Therapy. *Canadian Journal of Occupational Therapy, 54*(4), 195-199.

Brorsson, B. & Asberg, K.H. (1984). Katz index of independence in ADL: reliability and validity in short term care. *Scandinavian Journal of Rehabilitation Medicine, 16*, 125-132.

Brown, M.M., (1982). Actual and perceived differences in activity patterns of able-bodied and disabled men. Unpublished doctoral dissertation. New York University.

Brown, M., Gordon, W.A., & Diller, L. (1982). Functional assessment and outcome measures: An integrative review. *Annual Review of Rehabilitation, 3,* 93-120.

Brown, M., Gordon, W.A., & Diller, L. (1984). Rehabilitation indicators. In Halpern, A.S. & Fuhrer, M.D. (Eds.) *Functional assessment in rehabilitation.* Baltimore: Paul H. Brookes. (pp. 187-203)

Bruett, T. & Overs, R. (1969). A critical review of 12 ADL scales. *Physical Therapy, 49,* 857-862.

Buck, E.L. (1983). The utilization of the self-observation and report technique in cardiac rehabilitation. Unpublished master's thesis. University of Houston.

Christiansen, C.H., Schwartz, R.K., & Barnes, K.J. (1988). Self-care: Evaluation and management. In DeLisa, J., et al., (Eds.). *Principles of Rehabilitation Medicine.* Philadelphia: J.B. Lippincott. (pp. 95-115).

Crandall, R. (1980). Motivations for leisure. *Journal of Leisure Research.*

Crewe, N.M. & Athelstan, G.T. (1979). Functional assessment in vocational rehabilitation. *International Journal of Rehabilitation Research, 2,* 535-536.

Crewe, N.M. & Athelstan, G.T. (1981). Functional assessment in vocational rehabilitation: A systematic approach to diagnosis and goal setting. *Archives of Physical Medicine and Rehabilitation, 62,* 299-305.

Crewe, N.M. & Athelstan, G.T. (1984). *Functional assessment inventory manual.* Menomonie, WI: Materials Development Center, University of Wisconsin-Stout.

Crewe, N.M., & Athelstan, G.T. & Meadows, G. (1975). Vocational diagnosis through assessment of functional limitations. *Archives of Physical Medicine and Rehabilitation, 56,* 513-516.

Crewe, N.M. & Turner, R.R. (1984). A functional assessment system for vocational rehabilitation. In Halpern, A.S. & Fuhrer, M.D. (Eds.). *Functional assessment in rehabilitation.* Baltimore: Paul H. Brookes. (pp. 223-238.)

De Grazia, S. (1962). *Of time, work, and leisure.* New York: Twentieth Century Fund.

Deniston, O.L. & Jette, A. (1980). Validity of a functional status assessment instrument. *Health Services Research, 15,* 21-34.

Deyo, R.A. (1986). Comparative validity of the sickness impact profile and shorter scales for functional assessment of low back pain. *Spine, 11,* 951-954.

Diller, L., Fordyce, W., Jacobs, D., Brown, M., Gordon, W., Simmens, S., Orazem, J. & Barrett, L. (1983). Final report, Rehabilitation Indicators Project. National Institute of Handicapped Research, U.S. Department of Education, Grant G008003039.

Donaldson, S.W., Wagner, C.C., & Gresham, G.E. (1973). A unified ADL form. *Archives of Physical Medicine and Rehabilitation, 54,* 175-180.

Driver, B. & Tocher, S. (1970). Toward a behavioral interpretation of recreational engagements, with implications for planning. In Driver, B. (Ed.). *Elements of outdoor recreational planning.* Ann Arbor: University of Michigan Press.

Dunn, J.K. (1987). Generalizablity of the leisure diagnostic battery. Unpublished doctoral dissertation. University of Illinois at Urbana-Champaign.

Follick, M.J., Smith, T.W., & Ahern, D.K. (1985). The sickness impact profile: a global measure of disability in chronic low back pain. *Pain, 21,* 67-76.

Folsom, A.R., Jacobs, D.R., Jr., Casperson, C.J., Gomez-Marin, O., & Knudsen, J. (1986). Test-retest reliability of the Minnesota Leisure Time Physical Activity Questionnaire. *Journal of Chronic Diseases, 39*(7), 505-511.

Foster R. & Foster, R. (1967). The measurement of change in adaptive behavior. A paper presented at the Region 5 meeting of the American Association of Mental Deficiency. Wichita, KS, October, 1967.

Foster, R. & Nihira, K. (1969). Adaptive behavior as a measure of psychiatric impairment. *American Journal of Mental Deficiency, 74*(3), 401-404.

Frey, W.D. (1984). Functional assessment in the 80's: A conceptual enigma, a technical challenge (pp. 11-93). In Halpern, A.S. & Fuhrer, M.D. (Eds.). *Functional assessment in rehabilitation.* Baltimore: Paul H. Brookes.

Garrard, J. & Bennet, A.E. (1971). A validated interview schedule for use in population surveys of chronic disease and disability. *British Journal of Preventive and Social Medicine, 25,* 97-104.

Gibson, C.J. (1974). Epidemiology and patterns of care of stroke patients. *Archives of Physical Medicine and Rehabilitation, 55,* 398-403.

Good-Ellis, M.A., Fine, S.B., Spencer, J.H., & DiVittis, A., (1987). Developing a role activity performance scale. *American Journal of Occupational Therapy, 41*(4), 232-241.

Gordon, C., Gaitz, C., & Scott, J. (1976). Leisure and lives: Personal expressivity across the lifespan. (pp. 310-341) In Binstock, R. & Shanas, E. (Eds.). *Handbook of aging and the social sciences.* New York: Van Nostrand Reinhold.

Granger, C. (1989). *Guide for the use of the functional independence measure for children.* Buffalo: State University of New York at Buffalo.

Granger, C.V., Hamilton, B.B., Keith, R.A., Zielezny, M., & Sherwin, F.S. (1986). Advances in functional assessment for medical rehabilitation. *Topics in Geriatric Rehabilitation, 1*(3), 59-74.

Granger, C.V., Dewis, L.S., Peters, N.C., (1986). Stroke Rehabilitation: Analysis of repeated Barthel Index measures. *Archives of Physical Medicine & Rehabilitation, 60,* 14-17.

Greenwood, D. & Perry R. (1968). Use of the adaptive behavior checklist as a means of determining unit placement in a facility for the retarded. Paper presented at the Rocky Mountain Psychological Association, Denver, Colorado, May, 1968.

Gregory, M.D. (1983). Occupational behavior and life satisfaction among retirees. *American Journal of Occupational Therapy, 8,* 548-553.

Halpern, A.S. & Fuhrer, M.D. (Eds.). (1984). *Functional assessment in rehabilitation.* Baltimore: Paul H. Brookes.

Halpern, A., Irvin, L., & Landman, J. (1979). Alternative approaches to measurement of adaptive behavior. *American Journal of Mental Deficiency, 84,* 304-318.

Halpern, A.S., Irvin, L.K., & Munkies, A.W. (1986). *Social and prevocational information battery—revised.* Monterey, CA: CTB/McGraw-Hill

Halpern, A., Raffeld, P., Irvin, L., & Link, R. (1975). Measuring social and prevocational awareness in mildly retarded adolescents. *American Journal of Mental Deficiency, 80,* 81-89.

Hamilton, B.B., Granger, C.V., Sherwin, F.S., Zielezny, M., & Tashman, J. S. (1987). A uniform national data system for medical rehabilitation. In Fuhrer, M.J. (Ed.). *Rehabilitation outcomes: Analysis and measurement.* Baltimore: Paul H. Brookes

Harris, B.A., Jette, A.M., Campion, E.W., & Cleary, P.D. (1986). Validity of self-report measures of functional disability. *Topics in Geriatric Rehabilitation, 1,* 31-41.

Hart, L.G. & Evans, R.W. (1987). The functional status of ESRD patients as measured by the sickness impact profile. *Journal of Chronic Diseases, 40,* Suppl. 1, 117S-130S.

Hertanu, J.S., Demopoulos, J.T., & Yang, W.C., et al. (1984). Stroke rehabilitation: Correlation and prognostic value of computerized tomography and sequential functional assessments. *Archives of Physical Medicine and Rehabilitation, 65,* 505-508.

Holme, I. & Lunzer, E.H. (1966). Play, language and reasoning in subnormal children. *Journal of Child Psychiatry, 7,* 107-123.

Houston, D., Williams, S.L., Bloomer, J., & Mann, W.C. (1989). The Bay Area functional performance evaluation: Development and standardization. *American Journal of Occupational Therapy, 43*(3), 170-183.

Ilika J. & Hoffman, N.G. (1981). Reliability study on the Kohlman Evaluation of Living Skills. Reported in McGourty, L.K. (1987). Kohlman Evaluation of Living Skills. (pp. 133-146) In Hemphill, B.J. (Ed.). (1987). *Mental health assessment in occupational therapy.* Thorofare, NJ: Slack.

Irvin, L. & Halpern, A. (1977). Reliability and validity of the social and prevocational information battery for mildly retarded individuals. *American Journal of Mental Deficiency, 81,* 603-605.

Irvin, L., Halpern, A., & Landman, J.T. (1980). Assessment of retarded student achievement. *Journal of Educational Measurement, 17,* 51-58.

Jette, A.M. (1980a). Functional capacity evaluation: An empirical approach. *Archives of Physical Medicine and Rehabilitation. 61,* 85-89.

Jette, A.M. (1980b). Functional status index: Reliability of a chronic disease evaluation instrument. *Archives of Physical Medicine and Rehabilitation, 61,* 395-401.

Jette, A.M. (1985). State of the art in functional status assessment. In Rothstein, J. (Ed.). *Measurement in physical therapy.* (pp. 137-168). New York: Churchill-Livingstone.

Jette, A.M., Davis, A.R., Cleary, P.D., et al. (1986). The functional status questionnaire: Reliability and validity when used in primary care. *Journal of General Internal Medicine, 1,* 143-149.

Jette, A.M. & Denniston, O.L. (1978). Inter-observer reliability of a functional status assessment instrument. *Journal of Chronic Diseases, 31,* 573-580.

Kalverboer, A.F. (1977). Measurement of play: Clinical applications. In Tizard, B. and Harvey, D. (Eds.). *Biology of play* (pp. 100-122). Philadelphia: J.B. Lippincott.

Katz, S., Ford, A.B., & Moskowitz, R.W. (1963). Studies of illness in the aged. The Index of ADL: a standardized measure of biological and psychosocial function. *Journal of the American Medical Association, 185,* 914-919.

Katz, S., Downs, T., Cash, H., & Grotz, R. (1970). Progress in development of the Index of ADL. *Gerontologist, 10,* 20-30.

Kaufert, J.M. (1983). Functional ability indices: Measurement problems in assessing their validity. *Archives of Physical Medicine & Rehabilitation, 64,* 260-267, 1983.

Kaufman, L. (1982). Concurrent validity study on the Kohlman Evaluation of Living skills and the global assessment scale. Unpublished master's thesis, University of Florida.

Kelman, H.R. & Willner, A. (1962). Problems in measurement and evaluation of rehabilitation. *Archives of Physical Medicine and Rehabilitation, 43,* 172-181.

Kielhofner, G. (1985). Occupational function and dysfunction. In Kielhofner, G. (Ed.). *A model of human occupation: Theory and application* (pp. 63-75). Baltimore: Williams and Wilkins.

Kielhofner, G. & Barris, R. (1984). Collecting data on play: A critique of available methods. *Occupational Therapy Journal of Research, 4*, 150-181.

Kielhofner, G. & Henry, A.D. (1988). Development and investigation of the occupational performance history interview. *American Journal of Occupational Therapy, 42*(8), 489-498.

Kivela, S.L. (1984). Measuring disability—do self-ratings and service provider ratings compare? *Journal of Chronic Diseases, 37*(2) 115-123.

Klein, R.M. & Bell, B. (1982). Self-care skills: behavioral measurement with Klein-Bell ADL scale. *Archives of Physical Medicine and Rehabilitation, 63*, 335-338.

Knox, S. (1974). A play scale. In Reilly, M. (Ed.). *Play as exploratory learning* (pp. 247-266). Beverly Hills, CA: Sage Publications.

Kuriansky, J. & Gurland, B. (1976). Performance test of activities of daily living. *International Journal of Aging and Human Development, 7*, 343-352.

Kuriansky, J., Gurland, B., Fleiss, J., & Cowan, D. (1976). The assessment of self-care capacity in geriatric psychiatric patients. *Journal of Clinical Psychology, 32*, 95-102.

Lawton, M.P. (1971).The functional assessment of elderly people. *Journal of the American Geriatric Society, 14*, 65-481.

Lawton, M.P. & Brody, E. (1969). Assessment of older people: Self-maintaining and instrumental activities of daily living. *Gerontologist, 9*, 179-186.

Lawton, M.P., Moss, M., Fulcomer, M., and Kleban (1982). A research and service oriented multilevel assessment instrument. *Journal of Gerontology, 37*, 91-99.

Leland, H., Shellhaas, M., Nihira, K., & Foster, R. (1967). Adaptive behavior: A new dimension in the classification of the mentally retarded. *Mental Retardation Abstracts, 4*(3), 359-387.

Leonardelli, C. (1987). The Milwaukee evaluation of daily living skills (MEDLS). In Hemphill, B.J. (Ed.). *Mental health assessment in occupational therapy* (pp. 151-162). Thorofare, NJ: Slack.

MacKenzie, C.R., Charlson, M.E., DiGioia, D., & Kelley, K. (1985). Can the sickness impact profile measure change? An example of scale assessment. *Journal of Chronic Diseases, 39*(6), 429-438.

Mahoney, F.L. & Barthel, D.W. (1965). Functional evaluation: The Barthel index. *Maryland State Medical Journal, 14*, 61-65.

Malgady, R.G., Barcher, P.R., Towner, G., & Davis, J. (1979). Language factors in vocational evaluation of mentally retarded workers. *American Journal of Mental Deficiency, 83*, 432-438.

Malgady, R.G., Barcher, P.R., Towner, G., & Davis, J. (1980). Validity of the Vocational Adaptation Rating Scale: Prediction of mentally retarded workers' placement in sheltered workshops. *American Journal of Mental Deficiency, 84*, 633-640.

Mathews, R.M., Whang, P.L., & Fawcett, S.B. (1980). Development and validation of an occupational skills assessment instrument. *Behavioral Assessment, 2*, 71-85.

Mathews, R.M., Whang, P.L., & Fawcett, S.B. (1982). Behavioral assessment of occupational skills in learning disabled adolescents. *Journal of Learning Disabilities, 15*, 38-41.

Matsutsuyu, J. (1967). The interest checklist. *American Journal of Occupational Therapy, 32*, 628-630.

McGourty, L.K. (1979). *Kohlman evaluation of living skills*. Seattle, WA: KELS Research.

McGourty, L.K. (1988). Kohlman evaluation of living skills. In B. Hemphill, (Ed.). *Mental health assessment in occupational therapy* (pp. 133-146). Thorofare, NJ: Slack.

Merbitz, C., Morris, J., & Grip, J.C. (1989). Ordinal scales and foundations of misinference. *Archives of Physical Medicine and Rehabilitation, 70*, 308-312.

Miller, E.R. & Parachek, J.F. (1974). Validation and standardization of a goal-oriented, quick screening geriatric scale. *Journal of the American Geriatrics Society, 22*(6), 1974.

Morrow, M. (1985). A predictive validity study of the Kohlman evaluation of living skills, Master's thesis, University of Washington.

Moskowitz, E. & McCann C.B. (1957). Classification of disability in the chronically ill and aging. *Journal of Chronic Diseases, 5*, 342-346.

Nagi, S.Z. (1976). An epidemiology of disability among adults in the United States. In Health and Society. *Milbank Memorial Fund Quarterly, 54*, 439-467.

Newman, M. (1987). Cognitive disability and functional performance in individuals with Chronic Schizophrenia. Unpublished masters thesis. University of Southern California.

Nihira, K. (1969a). Factorial dimensions of adaptive behavior in adult retardates. *American Journal of Mental Deficiency, 73*(6), 868-878.

Nihira, K. (1969b). Factorial dimensions of adaptive behavior in mentally retarded children and adolescents. *American Journal of Mental Deficiency, 74*(1), 130-141.

Nihira, K., Foster, R., Shellhaas, M., & Leland, H. (1975). *AAMD adaptive behavior scale-revised*. Los Angeles: Western Psychological Services.

Norris-Baker, C., Stephens, M.A.P., Rintala, D.H., & Willems, E.P. (1981). Patient behavior as a predictor of outcomes in spinal cord injury. *Archives of Physical Medicine and Rehabilitation, 62,* 602-608.

Nystrom, E.P. (1974). Activity patterns and leisure concepts among the elderly. *American Journal of Occupational Therapy, 28,* 337-345.

O'Neill, J., Gordon, W., & Brown, M. (1983). The impact of a community-based residence on skill levels and patterns of daily activity.

Parten, M. (1933). Social participation among pre-school children. *Journal of Abnormal and Social Psychology, 28,* 136-147.

Plutchik, R., Conte, H., Lieberman, M. et al. (1970). Reliability and validity of a scale for assessing the functioning of geriatric patients. *Journal of the American Geriatrics Society, 18,* 491-500.

Potts, L. (1969). Toward a developmental assessment of leisure patterns. Unpublished master's thesis. Department of Occupational Therapy, University of Southern California.

Rasch, G. (1980). *Probabilistic models for some intelligence and attainment tests.* Copenhagen: Danish Institute for Educational Research, 1960; and Chicago: University of Chicago Press, 1980.

Rintala, D.H. (1982). Forecasting behavioral outcomes: Posthospital adjustment of spinal cord injured persons. Unpublished doctoral dissertation, University of Houston.

Rintala, D.H., Utlermohlen, D.M., Buck, E.R., et al. (1984). Self-observation and report technique (SORT). In Halpern, A.S. & Fuhrer, M.J. (Eds.). *Functional assessment in rehabilitation.* (pp. 205-222). Baltimore: Paul H. Brookes.

Rogers, J.C., Weinstein, J.M., & Figone, J.J. (1978). The interest checklist: An empirical assessment. *American Journal of Occupational Therapy, 32,* 628-630.

Rogers, J.C. & Takata, N. (1981). The play history as an assessment tool. Unpublished paper. Chapel Hill: University of North Carolina.

Schoening, H.A., Anderegg, L., Bergstrom, D., et al. (1965). Numerical scoring of self-care status of patients. *Archives of Physical Medicine and Rehabilitation, 46,* 689-697.

Schoening, H.A. & Iversen, I.A. (1968). Numerical scoring of self-care status: a study of the Kenny self-care evaluation. *Archives of Physical Medicine & Rehabilitation, 49,* 221-229,

Smith, R.O. (1990). Administration and Scoring Manual. *OT FACT (Occupational Therapy Functional Assessment Compilation Tool.* Rockville, Maryland: The American Occupational Therapy Association, Inc.

Smith, R.O., Morrow, M.E., Heitman, J.K., Rardin, W.J. Powelson, J.L., & Von, T. (1986). The effects of introducing the Klein-Bell ADL scale in a rehabilitation service. *American Journal of Occupational Therapy, 40*(6), 420-424.

Sparrow, S.S., Balla, D.A., & Cichetti, D.V. (1984). Vineland adaptive behavior scales. Circle Pines, MN: American Guidance Services.

Takata, N. (1969). The Play History. *American Journal of Occupational Therapy, 23,* 314-318

Takata, N. (1974). Play as prescription. In Reilly, M., (Ed.). *Play as exploratory learning.* Beverly Hills: Sage Publications.

Tateichi, S. (1984). A concurrent validity study of the Kohlman evaluation of living skills. Master's thesis. University of Washington.

Taylor, H.L., Jacobs, D.R., Jr., Schucker, B., Knudsen, J., Leon, A.S., & Debacker, G. (1978). A questionnaire for the assessment of leisure time physical activities. *Journal of Chronic Diseases, 31,* 741-755.

Thibeault, R. & Blackmer, E. (1987). Validating a test of functional performance with psychiatric patients. *American Journal of Occupational Therapy, 41*(8), 515-521.

Uttermohlen, D.M., Alexander, J.L., & Willems, E.P. (1982). Functional independence: Measurement by the self-observation and report technique. *Archives of Physical Medicine and Rehabilitation, 63,* 513 (Abstract).

Wade, D.T., Skilbeck, C.E., Hewer, R.L. (1983). Predicting Barthel ADL score at six months after an acute stroke. *Archives of Physical Medicine and Rehabilitation, 64,* 24-48.

Walls, R.T., Zane, T., & Werner, T.J. (1978). *The vocational behavior checklist.* Dunbar, West Virginia Research and Training Center.

Watts, J.H., Kielhofner, G., Bauer, D.F., Gregory, M.D., & Valentine, D.B. (1986). The assessment of occupational functioning: A screening tool for use in long-term care. *American Journal of Occupational Therapy, 40*(4), 231-240.

Weissman, M., Sholomskas, D., & John, K. (1981). The assessment of social adjustment: an update. *Archives of General Psychiatry, 38,* 1250-1257.

West Evaluation Systems Technology. (1986a). *WEST tool sort.* Long Beach California: Publisher.

West Evaluation Systems Technology. (1986b). *LLUMC activity sort.* Long Beach California: Publisher.

Whiting, N. (1975). Meaningful activities in life satisfaction. Unpublished master's thesis, Virginia Commonwealth University.

Williams, S.L. & Bloomer, J. (1987). *Bay Area functional performance evaluation administration and scoring manual.* (2nd ed.). Palo Alto: Consulting Psychologists Press.

Witt, P.A., Compton, D.M., Ellis, G., Howard, G., Aguilar, T., Forsyth, P., Niles, S., & Costilow, A. (1982). *The leisure diagnostic battery: Background, conceptualization and structure*. Denton, Texas: North Texas State University.

Witt, P.A., Ellis, G., Aguilar, T., Niles, S., & Costilow, A. (1982). *User's manual for the leisure diagnostic battery: Version A*. Denton, Texas: North Texas State University

Wood, P.H.N. (1980). Appreciating the consequences of disease—The classification of impairments, disabilities and handicaps. *The WHO Chronicle, 34*, 376-380.

Wright, B. & Linacre, J.M. (1989). Observations are always ordinal; measurements, however, must be inter-val. *Archives of Physical Medicine and Rehabilitation, 70*, 857-860.

Yerxa, E.J. & Baum, S. (1986). Engagement in daily occupations and life satisfaction among people with spinal cord injuries. *Occupational Therapy Journal of Research, 6*, 271-283.

Yerxa, E.J., Burnett-Beaulieu, S., Stocking, J.S., & Azen, S.P. (1988). Development of the satisfaction with per-formance scaled questionnaire. *American Journal of Occupational Therapy, 42*(4), 215-221.

CHAPTER CONTENT OUTLINE

Decisions Regarding Assessment

The Total Environment

Social Groups, Systems, and Networks

Socially-Defined Activity Patterns, Beliefs, and Expectations

Physical Space and Objects

Summary

KEY TERMS

Activity pattern analysis

Environment

Environmental assessment

Ergonomics

Exchange relationship

Person-environment fit

Physical environment

Programming

Social environment

Social systems

Temporal environment

Work setting

ABSTRACT

In order to address the changing aspects of the social environment and help provide the optimum person-environment fit for clients and patients, occupational therapists must be familiar with the assessment tools that include elements of both the physical and social environment. This chapter reviews specific assessment tools that help evaluate the physical and social aspects of the environment. Some are comprehensive, but others are more specifically focused on (1) social groups, systems, and networks, (2) socially defined activity patterns, beliefs, and expectations, or (3) physical spaces and objects.

Assessing Environmental Factors

Harriett Davidson

"Systematic strategies for assessing environments provide important groundwork on which sound environmental interventions can be planned . . . A wise choice of methods to be used for environmental assessment depends heavily on careful clarification at the outset of the purposes for which the assessment is undertaken and clear specification of questions one is seeking to answer. For therapists, this often hinges on identifying features of an environment that are potentially alterable by therapeutic intervention in order to improve client functioning."

—Spencer, 1987

OBJECTIVES

The information in this chapter is intended to help the reader—

1. identify and discuss selected variables which might be important for an occupational therapist to examine in the client's environment.

2. describe assessments currently available which might measure the variables under consideration.

3. describe the data yielded by environmental assessments.

4. discuss limitations and strengths of environmental assessments.

5. indicate situatinos in which it would be valuable to use environmental assessments.

DECISIONS REGARDING ASSESSMENT

What to Assess: Determining Measurement Variables

A comprehensive **assessment** of the **environment** will include consideration of both physical and social aspects. Although in practice the therapist uses a holistic model which considers all factors related to environment and person, the therapist will often search for an assessment tool that will yield very specific information. Sometimes such assessment tools are very narrow in focus and sometimes they are very broad, depending upon the client and the setting.

After deciding to assess environments, the therapist must first ask the question: What do I want to assess? Each discipline has a slightly different way of framing the environmental system. The occupational therapist is biased toward looking for ways that the system can support performance of valued roles with their related occupations. This chapter is organized to examine **environments** from three perspectives: (1) as **social** groups, **systems** and networks, (2) as socially defined activity patterns, beliefs, and expectations, and (3) as **physical** spaces and objects, as suggested by Spencer (1987). As we will see, many assessments easily fit into more than one of these categories.

How to Assess: Development of Reliable and Valid Measurement Tools

The second question the therapist asks is: How should I assess? Examination of the assessments currently being used reveals some of the problems in developing a theoretically sound and useful tool. There are a number of methods for assessing environments. Spencer (1987) identifies five ways of **assessing environments**: measurement of physical properties, naturalistic observations, respondents' self-reports, users' perceptions, and interpretive analysis.

Each method used for securing data presents its own set of problems. The following are examples. Gathering data by objective means, such as counting people in the social network, or number of contacts, limits the richness of the data obtained, and ignores the meaning and symbolism that are central to understanding the environment. Assessments in naturalistic settings may not permit the control of extraneous variables; however, strategies for careful observation, coding and recording can enhance reliability.

Measurement in artificial settings (e.g., the laboratory or clinic) changes the nature of the environmental context so that individuals' responses may not be typical. However the ability to control variables in artificial settings makes this desirable for certain kinds of data-gathering. Observer bias can also cause faulty inferences, but careful training of observers can minimize bias. Self-report must assume that the memory of the informant is intact, that the informant has the necessary information, and that there is no reason for the informant to avoid truthful answers; a carefully designed questionnaire can help minimize the possibility of errors.

The development of assessments of environments is in its early stages. A major problem is definition of certain basic constructs. For example, there is no universally agreed-upon definition of social support upon which to base measurement. (It has been suggested that some purported measures of **social environment**, such as social support, are really measures of personality.) Once a definition is decided upon and an instrument designed, one must establish its validity, which requires long and painstaking work. High reliability (stability, internal consistency) is essential to the presumption of validity. As described in Chapter 14, other important factors are content validity, criterion-related validity, and construct validity. Sometimes there are no measures with which the variable under study can be correlated to determine criterion validity. Construct validity is the most critical concern in the development of an assessment--that is, how it fits into a theoretical system with other variables to form a coherent rationale for practice.

Where to Assess: The Context of Assessment

The third question the therapist might ask is: Where shall I assess? Although the clinician is accustomed to using the controlled clinical environment for assessment of the individual client's performance, there are obvious limits to the information to be gained in the constructed environment of the clinic. For example, a patient who may be able to simulate purchasing a bar of soap in the clinic may not be able to negotiate the same task in a large supermarket. An intermediate step might be to make a purchase in the small hospital store. Thus, the therapist can provide an assessment environment designed to elicit the best response from the patient. If the assessment environment is rich and naturalistic, it is more likely that the therapist has correctly approximated the client's real or expected environment, and thus more likely to provide a more accurate prediction about the client's ability to function in that environment.

THE TOTAL ENVIRONMENT

A comprehensive assessment of the total environment would attempt to measure the system (**person-environment**) across all situations and would provide some information about the **fit** between the person and the environment. Because most therapists are concerned with specific client populations in specific situations, they often prefer an assessment designed for a certain aspect of the environment or for a limited population, such as an assessment of the home environment of the developmentally delayed child rather than a general assessment of all possible environments. However, comprehensive assessments of the total environment have obvious value in a variety of situations and treatment programs. The following sections describe instructions which can be useful to occupational therapists.

Environmental Assessments

Arousal and Environmental Layers Assessment. Barris, Kielhofner, Levine, and Neville (1985) provided the framework for a person-environment assessment and presented an exercise for students and therapists that has potential as a tool for clients. Individuals are asked to visualize the environment as composed of concentric layers of objects, tasks, social groups and culture and to examine their own environment in terms of the properties of these layers. Arousal refers to feelings of excitement and stimulation generated by an interaction between a person's previous experiences and features of the environment. Conditions often contributing to increased levels of arousal are those that present novelty, complexity or unfamiliar situations. Figure 16-1 presents part of an exercise related to social groups which helps people explore the concept of arousal and how social groups (one part of the environment) can contribute to arousal. Examination of the environment by the client could improve understanding of the **person-environment** fit and lead to helpful modifications involving physical and social elements.

Relationship to Occupational Performance. The authors of the Arousal and Environmental Layers Assessment have established the theoretical relationships among the variables they examined. For example, if a social environment is undermanned with too few people in it, the individual is more likely to become involved in the group's tasks, even with less skill to offer. However, there are no data on normative responses or indications for intervention based upon specific findings.

Strengths and Limitations. Eight such exercises are included to create all the necessary information for an occupational performance assessment. Although these exercises generate assessment data, they are not classified as an assessment, but simply exercises. This has potential merit as a framework for an assessment, but has the following three disadvantages: (1) It is written at the level of a college student's reading comprehension and would need to be reworded for some clients, (2) To administer the exercises in their entirety would be time-consuming and therefore less practical, (3) It has not been tested in terms of its reliability, validity, or utility.

Example of Application to Occupational Therapy. The therapist is working with a group of juvenile offenders in a detention center and designs a group activity in which the individuals assess the environment of their own social group. They explore reasons for how these groups provide ''arousal,'' how the groups influence their behavior, and how that behavior is perceived by the community.

The therapist then develops a board game called ''Street Life'' in which the environmental factors are embedded into the game and influence the course of the game-player's route through the environment. Players throw dice and move their ''men'' down the ''street.'' If they land on certain ''blocks,'' they draw cards which can be used to prevent ''going to jail.'' The cards are labeled with social strategies such as ''talk to a friend.'' The clients enjoy the game, and it prompts them to discuss things they might do differently to avoid detention.

Implications for Treatment/Environmental Consultation. In the hands of a skilled clinician, this assessment would be a useful guide for interview and problem-solving with the client. It would provide an excellent basis for environmental consultation in terms of questions to ask, but gives no specific guidelines for interpretation of the data that it yields.

The Environmental Grid Description Assessment. Dunning (1972) designed a semi-structured interview in which questions are asked about space, people, and tasks. The questions regarding space are directed at the individual's perceptions of the physical properties of home, neighborhood, and larger community. The questions about people (or the **social environment**) relate to social role relationships of marriage, nuclear family, extended family, friends, peers and neighbors. Also questions are asked about patterns of nearness and distance between the individual and others, about the client's perception of the possibility for change in the social relationships of patterns of interaction, and about the client's preference for change in the current social environment. Task information includes the environment's task expectancies, sources of task stimulation, availability of objects,

---

Excerpt from Social and Environmental Layers

Compare two organizations or groups of which you are a member. Choose groups that differ in the degree of arousal they induce in you. To determine why one group is more arousing than the other, fill in the following chart.

Social Groups Table

Description	Arousing group	Unarousing group
How many people belong?		
What is its function?		
What do you do to become a member?		
Is this group highly vulnerable to things that happen outside it?		
What kinds of networks exist among members?		

Figure 16-1. In comparing the two groups, consider the following questions: Is the size of the group a source of arousal for you? Is the function? Was the group difficult to join, thereby making membership a source of arousal? Does this group expect members to be similar? If so, do your expectations of not being like other members lead to your arousal? Is the group vulnerable to outside forces, thus making its activities more consequential and arousing? Are the networks in the group complex, making it difficult to "learn the ropes"? *Reprinted with permission from: R. Barris (1985). Workbook: Applying model of human occupation. In G. Kielhofner (Ed.), Model of human occupation (p. 421). Baltimore, Williams & Wilkins.*

the spatial behavior related to task performance, and the satisfaction received from task accomplishment.

Relationship to Occupational Performance. Family and social roles are examined in this assessment, and those are related to task expectancies and availability of task stimulation as well as spatial variables. The theoretical relationships are established by the author.

Strengths and Limitations. This assessment is designed for a psychiatric population and has not been widely applied to other populations. Besides having the obvious shortcomings of a self-report instrument, it has not gone through a rigorous instrument development process. Dunning pretested her questionnaire with 10 psychiatric patients. From the trends she observed, she developed certain propositions which would need to be tested. Although other assessments have been based upon her work, her instrument has yet to be further developed and methodically tested.

Examples of Application to Occupational Therapy. A therapist working on discharge planning with a patient with a diagnosis of chronic schizophrenia is helping the patient identify preferences and possibilities for change in the home. The therapist wants to help the patient decrease dependency and to become more actively involved in decision-making when considering options. The therapist asks the patient about the home situation. The patient answers that he does not like the feelings of dependency, but he is not sure of his ability to cope with the responsibilities of living outside the home. The therapist asks him to consider whether it might be possible to change some arrangements in the home so he could feel more independent. She makes some very specific suggestions when she discovers that the client cannot envision possibilities of change. For example, the client agrees that he would prefer to take the bus, but his parents insist that he ride with them in the car. The client also says that he would prefer staying in the home and trying new arrangements rather than moving into a residential setting. The therapist agrees to support his efforts in talking about this with his parents.

Implications for Treatment/Environmental Consultation.   One of Dunning's propositions suggests that psychiatric outpatients who live in the community tend to be dependent and to see limited possibilities for change. Use of this instrument allows the therapist to assess the environment in terms of the patient's perception and also to assess his preference and expectancy for change. Choice and expectancies are two concepts that are particularly related to performance.

SOCIAL GROUPS, SYSTEMS, AND NETWORKS

Family and Home Environments

Assessment of Home Environments (Yarrow, Rubenstein & Pedersen, 1975).   Most developmentalists identify the mother as the significant environmental agent for the infant, although recently the importance of other people has been acknowledged. The home is still considered the most important socializing site, although many children spend a substantial amount of time away from home soon after birth.

In their study of home environments, the authors used an assessment intended to identify factors that contributed to early cognitive and motivational development. Subjects were five- to six-month-old infants. Their methods provide a model for assessing the home environment of infants. They used a time-sampling method with a 30-second observation and 60-second recording through 120 cycles on two separate days. Frequency counts and ratings were recorded on a data sheet. Measures were taken of the following: infant behavior, social stimulation, inanimate stimulation, context, and responses to problem-solving and novel situations. Variables assessed in the infants' social environment included kinds of attentiveness (hold, look, touch, vocalize, move), contingency measures (responses of the caregivers to the infants' positive vocalizations and to signs of distress), affect (expression of positive affect, smiling, and play), social mediation to stimuli (including minimal social reinforcement, and reinforcement with smiles and vocalizations), maternal mediation of inanimate objects (caregiver positioning of objects or showing the child their stimulus properties), and general characterization of the social environment (level and variety of play interaction between caregiver and infant). Inanimate environment was assessed on the infants' responsiveness to

objects (extent to which parts move, image is reflected, or changes in shape) and the complexity of their response.

Relationship to Occupational Performance.   The authors' basis for this study is that the groundwork of adult competency is established in infancy. The authors suggest implications for treatment by demonstrating statistical relationships between environmental variables and measures of infant functioning. Infant competency is measured in terms of ability to respond adaptively to a number of human and nonhuman environmental elements. The human caregiver is seen as the mediator between the infant and the physical environment. The measures of infant functioning addressed by this assessment are: general status, social responsiveness, language, motor development, cognitive-motivational goal directedness, object permanence, exploratory behavior, and preference for novel stimulus. (This research is discussed in further detail in Chapter 5, The Physical Environment and Performance.)

Strengths and Limitations.   This assessment was used in a limited study, therefore the only reliability scores available are an inter-rater range of .75 to .99. Further work needs to be done on a wider and more heterogeneous sample before its general utility is established. Because this assessment was designed as a research tool using observations in a naturalistic setting, evidence is lacking to support its wide-range applicability. It is time-consuming to administer and assumes that the assessor has a knowledge of human development. One advantage is that it forms the basis for a way to view the infant in a home environment that is structured and specific and which has potential for further development and testing. There is also a potential for expanding the use for infant day care environment or even to other adult populations, such as adults with physical or psychosocial disability.

Examples of Application to Occupational Therapy.   Therapists working with high risk neonates or infants with failure-to-thrive could use this assessment to help to prepare a checklist for mothers of such infants to guide them in providing an environment that stimulates growth for their child.

Implications for Treatment/Environmental Consultation.   Early identification of competencies and deficits is considered a keystone to intervention for optimal development. This finding of Yarrow and associates supports the notion that specific kinds of environments foster specific adaptive behaviors and suggests that the clinician can potentially specify particular kinds of treatment to foster specific kinds of growth.

The Home Observation for Measurement of the Environment (HOME).   This inventory (Bradley, & Caldwell, 1979; Elardo, Bradley, & Caldwell, 1975) was designed to assess the quality of the social, emotional and cognitive support available to the child in the home environment from birth to three years of age. Scoring is based on observation using a rating form that consists of 45 items regarding six aspects of the environment that are believed to support social, emotional, and cognitive development: emotional and verbal responsiveness of mothers, avoidance of restriction and punishment, organization of the physical and **temporal environment**, provision of appropriate play materials, maternal involvement with the child, and opportunities for variety in daily stimulation. The assessment yields a total score and six subscale scores. There is also a version for preschoolers 3 to 6 years of age and for children ages 6 to 19 (Bradley, Caldwell, Rock, Hamrick, et al., 1988; Elardo, Bradley, & Caldwell, 1977).

Relationship to Occupational Performance. The authors have done longitudinal studies to examine the relationship of scores on the HOME assessment to mental test performance as measured by the Stanford-Binet. They concluded that organization of the environment by the parent appears more important than age. Also the following correlations were found for subscale scores between certain age pairings: age six months and three years (.54), twelve months and three years (.59), and twenty-four months and three years (.72). They also longitudinally studied the relationship between HOME scores and language development. Examining 91 families, they found significant relationships between scores on the HOME and on the *Illinois Test of Psycholinguistic Ability*. There were some differences observed between these tests for males and females; for males, emotional and verbal responsiveness of mothers and provision of appropriate play materials were related to language development, whereas for females the areas were maternal involvement with the child, emotional and verbal responsiveness of mothers, and opportunities for variety in daily stimulation. Thus, early data indicate that this assessment might identify specific parental behaviors that could lead to improved cognitive and language performance.

Strengths and Limitations. The HOME appears to be a relatively popular assessment to use in research and such studies will continue to generate more data about its usefulness as a tool. Advantages include its ease of administration and its reliance upon observation in a naturalistic setting. The presence of the observer/assessor may influence the behavior of the parent(s) to some degree, but observational data may be compared with interview data to identify possible errors in perception. Content validity has been supported by a study of empirical data, developmental theory, and expert opinion. The instrument was standardized using 176 families in central Arkansas. The authors found inter-rater reliability of .90 and internal consistency coefficients ranging from .44 to .89 for the subscales and .89 for the total scale. Concurrent validity

was tested by studying relationships to language and mental development As detailed in the previous section, results were encouraging.

Example of Applications for Occupational Therapy. The following is an example in which the occupational therapist might find the HOME assessment useful. The occupational therapist practicing in home health is referred to a home in which a premature infant with pulmonary problems is being discharged following three weeks in neonatal intensive care. The infant's APGAR scores were low, and there is concern of possible developmental compromise. The mother is fearful of caring for the infant and is asking for assistance in parenting skill development. The HOME would be useful to help the therapist assess the home and help the mother identify ways in which she can design the environment to foster competence in the infant.

Implications for Treatment/Environmental Consultation. Recognizing its importance as the preferred site for intervention, occupational therapists have traditionally evaluated the home environment. The HOME provides a standardized method of assessing the home environment and yields information useful to occupational therapists as the basis for treatment planning and education of the parents and other health care workers.

Contexts for Play

Many of the play assessments focus on how the child acts upon the environment or the way in which he/she assimilates or accommodates to the play situation. The Play History described below is such an instrument. The playground assessment looks at the variables in the playground, including the children's play behavior which is a part of the social environment as well as a result of it. There are some analyses of play environments that provide the groundwork for a play assessment such as the *Play Agenda* (Michaelman, 1974) which is described in more detail in Chapter 6.

The Play History Assessment. The Play History is an interview with the mother or caretaker that was developed by Takata (1969) and revised by Behnke & Fetkovich (1984). It examines four elements of the play situation: materials, action, people, and settings. It also examines the play behavior in the context of four of the following five major epochs through which the child is assumed to move: sensorimotor (independent gross motor play), symbolic and simple constructive (social play with peers with symbolization becoming more apparent), dramatic and complex constructive, and the game epoch. The fifth epoch or the recreation epoch is the one in which team participation and organized sports occur and is not examined in the assessment. The Play History is a "semi-structured qualitative questionnaire aimed at identifying play experiences, inter-actions, environments, and opportunities'' (Behnke & Fetkovich, 1984, p. 94).

Relationship to Occupational Performance. The Play History assessment offers the opportunity to examine the child's play using an historical approach in the context of the development of performance components from one step to the next. It provides quantitative and qualitative data which help the therapist examine the play behaviors and the play environment. This provides the opportunity for the therapist to consider the ''goodness-of-fit'' between the child's performance and the qualities of environmental press and arousal.

Strengths and Limitations. Although limited, a study by Behnke and Fetkovich suggested both reliability and valid-ity for the instrument. They studied 30 children of ages one to seven and one-half, both handicapped and nonhandi-capped. They found inter-rater correlations from .58 to .76; however coefficients were lower for the handicapped chil-dren. Test-retest reliability was .77 for a subsample of ten children. Concurrent validity studies demonstrated the following correlations with the *Minnesota Child Develop-ment Inventory*: .97 for nonhandicapped children and .70 for handicapped children. They also give evidence that the assessment may discriminate between disabled and able-bodied children in developmental play level. Further re-search needs to be done to confirm these findings.

Strengths of the Play History include the fact that it engages the parent in examining the play behavior and environment of the child, thus increasing the parent's awareness and potential for being involved in the enhance-ment process, and that behavior is observed in a natural setting which increases the possibility of validity. One possible limitation of the Play History Assessment is that the ability to obtain, interpret and use the qualitative informa-tion therapeutically is dependent upon the therapist's level of skill in application of the theoretical base and understand-ing of child development. This assessment has the potential to be a valuable tool in occupational therapy, but continued research needs to be done involving larger and more diverse populations.

Example of Application to Occupational Therapy. The therapist is working with a young child with spina bifida whose mobility is limited to wheelchair ambulation. Lately the child has become a behavior problem. The therapist uses the Play History to assess play patterns and identifies a play environment with few other children and primarily adults for playmates. The therapist helps the mother explore ways to enrich the child's play environment and introduce other children into the environment as through behavior models.

Implications for Treatment/Environmental Consulta-tion. The disabled child has been identified as being at risk for play deficits which compound the risk of having limited adaptive capacity. In addition to its use as a clinical assessment tool, the Play History might be also useful in research to establish the effects of different play environ-ments on the disabled child's play behaviors. The particular value of this assessment is to provide information to aid the therapist in designing an individual assessment, but it can also provide useful information for the parent or caretaker when developing ways to enrich the play environment.

Neighborhood Community Network Assessments

Network analysis borrows from mathematical graph theory in which it is assumed that any individual can be represented as a dot, and any interaction or **exchange relationship** can be represented by a line that links the dots. Thus, by identifying people with whom the individual interacts, a picture of the personal network can be constructed. These analyses are used traditionally by sociologists and anthropologists.

The Personal Network Map Assessment. This process of describing networks, consists of identifying the individu-als in the network and how they are linked by drawing them on a chart (Attneave, 1981; Pilisuk and Parks, 1986, p. 121). Four lists of people are generated and placed on a circular chart with four zones: Zone I – members of the household, Zone II – people with whom the subject has significant ties, Zone III – people with whom the subject maintains casual relationships, and Zone IV – people with whom they have distant relationships or people whom they see only on special occasions. The circle is bisected with one hemisphere representing the family and the other hemisphere representing nonfamily. In addition, there is a separate space for those persons whom the individual dislikes or with whom he/she feels discomfort. The male figure is represented by a square and the female by a circle. Lines are drawn to link people who are connected to each other as well as to the subject. (See Figure 16-2.)

The information is gathered through interview and obser-vation. The patient or client is asked to draw the network if possible. This drawing can be a very personal experience and can help the person realize that there is some sort of support system available. Also requesting that the client explain the drawing to someone else can clarify the exact nature of relationships and potential support.

If the patient or client is unable to fill out the chart, the therapist can do so using data that have been collected. The therapist can then view the present relationships, and determine the nature of the relationships by further inter-view and observation. The relationships may be ones of supportive caring, of responsibility for the client, of reci-

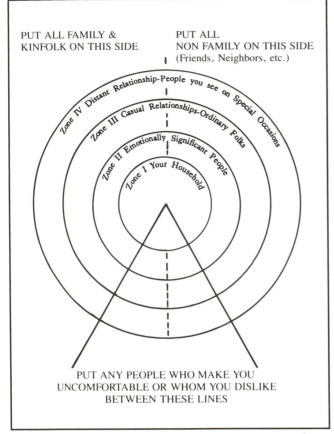

PUT ALL FAMILY &
KINFOLK ON THIS SIDE

PUT ALL
NON FAMILY ON THIS SIDE
(Friends, Neighbors, etc.)

Zone IV Distant Relationship–People you see on Special Occasions
Zone III Casual Relationships–Ordinary Folks
Zone II Emotionally Significant People
Zone I Your Household

PUT ANY PEOPLE WHO MAKE YOU
UNCOMFORTABLE OR WHOM YOU DISLIKE
BETWEEN THESE LINES

Figure 16-2. Personal Network Map. *Reprinted with permission from: Pilisuk, M. and Parks, S.H. (1986). The healing web (p. 121). Hanover, NH: University Press of New England and Carolyn Atteneave, Department of Psychology, University of Washington.*

procity with the client, or ones in which someone controls power (either positively or negatively) over the client's best interests.

Relationship to Occupational Performance. The expectations, values, support, and demands and challenges of the network operate in very complex ways to influence functional or dysfunctional behaviors. Assessment of the network allows the therapist to examine the negative relationships as well as the positive, and to look at reciprocity, power, and status in relation to the individual's behaviors.

Strengths and Limitations. The personal network map is designed as a semi-structured interview or pencil-and-paper exercise and is not intended to be developed further as a test. The strategy can provide a framework for an occupational therapist to develop a standardized assessment. The limitations might be that the method is time-consuming to administer and depends upon the respondents' accuracy and honesty. This method permits the therapist to explore the client's near and distant relation-

ships, positive and negative ones, and the nature of kinships and friendships.

Example of Applications for Occupational Therapy. The therapist is helping in a difficult decision about whether a male patient can maintain residency in the community after having a stroke with appreciable loss of endurance, some memory lapses, and a moderate aphasia. The therapist asks the patient to assess social resources for independent living in the community by using the personal network map. From this information, the therapist discovers that although no one else lives in the household, there are five people in Zone II who are resources, including a neighbor who checks every day to see that the patient has picked up his newspaper, a couple living two blocks away with whom he plays dominoes twice weekly, and a son and daughter-in-law who live five miles away, visit him every Sunday and buy his groceries and medications. The therapist recommends that with those support systems in place, the client can still live independently with some modifications in the home environment to accommodate for the low endurance and memory loss.

Implications for Treatment/Environmental Consultation. The therapist can use the data to identify needs or gaps in the patient's social resources that may need to be filled by formal services. The Map should be charted periodically since the measure represents a point in time which can be expected to change, particularly with significant life events such as moving, illness, births, deaths, marriage or divorce. One should also expect that the Map will change at different stages of the client's life. For example, very young children and very old individuals would be expected to have smaller networks.

The Kinship Network Analysis (Zisserman, 1981). The family tree model is used to identify members of the family who act in significant ways in relation to the network. Information is recorded in a genogram in which conventionally the male is on the left, female on the right, and children are arranged by age left to right. Figure 16-3 presents a sample of a summary of the medical kinship analysis form.

Types of information obtained from this kinship network that the therapist can use in therapy and discussions include:

1. first-order family roles of the patient, such as roles of mother, grandmother, or expected breadwinner (even though the dysfunction precludes the ability to act out the roles)
2. supportive family members
3. available alternatives for resources
4. those individuals who can receive and carry out therapeutic tasks or roles for the patient
5. those who are close enough to help out occasionally

6. family interactions that are likely to be strained by the illness or dysfunction.

Relationship to Occupational Performance. The focus during the interview is on roles and tasks and the responses are specific to the client's expected environment and the kinds of support needed. A network that is too dense may increase the demand for conformity to group members' standards for performance and may not give the person the freedom to change or try new behaviors. A network with gaps may not provide the support needed for optimal performance. The network may include various linkages which can also specifically influence performance. The size of the network will influence the ability of the individual to move flexibly and freely through time and space without having to take out time and energy to develop networks for each task.

Strengths and Limitations. A kinship analysis provides a macrocosmic perspective for the occupational therapist. It

fully acknowledges the importance of social environments and also the idiosyncratic nature of each individual's social environment.

Limitations include the fact that it is time-consuming for the therapist to develop an accurate network map if the patient cannot provide the data, and reliability and validity remain problematic. Another limitation of the Kinship Analysis is that it is limited to relatives of the patient and may omit important individuals who are not related. Also since reports are subjective, it may be difficult to obtain accurate information if the client has memory problems or if the client's perception of a relationship reflects that of the other person. The interpretation of the data is dependent upon the clinical skills of the occupational therapist.

Examples of Applications for Occupational Therapy. The therapist is hoping that the patient with spinal fractures related to osteoporosis will be able to return to her apartment where she has been living alone. Using the

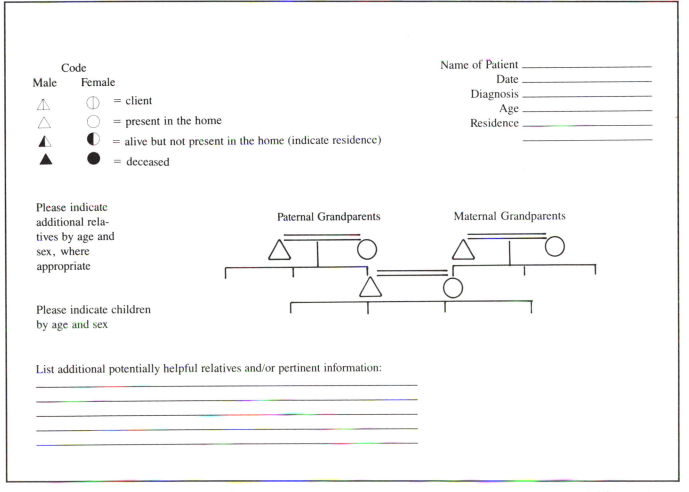

Figure 16-3. Summary of Medical Kinship Analysis Form. *Reprinted with permission from: L. Zisserman (1971). The modern family and rehabilitation of the handicapped: A macrosociological view. American Journal of Occupational Therapy, 35, 18.*

kinship network, the therapist is able to assess the potential for relatives helping her with heavy household tasks, shopping, etc. The kinship network reveals that her relatives have cut off relationships with her because of her excessive demands and her tendency to complain a great deal. The therapist refers the client to the social worker to identify formal services for helping her to live independently.

Implications for Treatment/Environmental Consultation. This analysis has broad applications for a variety of clinical settings and community settings, and could be useful as one of several assessments in discharge planning.

Social Support Systems

These are special cases of social networks. Some theorists have argued that the whole network must be assessed to understand all the dynamics and interrelations of the situation; others argue that the social support system is a more relevant unit for intervention (Pilisuk & Parks, 1986).

Occupational Role History (ORH) Assessment. Florey and Michelman (1982) have designed a psychiatric screening tool in the form of a semi-structured interview assessment consisting of 34 questions relating to occupational role performance. It includes questions about the significant influences of the social environment upon work and play activities. For example, one question is, "Did your parents have any influence on your choice of occupation?"

Relationship to Occupational Performance. The authors conclude that this interview provides information about the patient's adaptive function (social relations, occupational functioning, and the use of leisure time, as defined by tne DSM-III). They state that the instrument permits the information to be categorized according to two dimensions: role status (functional, temporarily impaired, and dysfunctional) and role balance.

Strengths and Weaknesses. Data on the reliability and validity of the instrument are not included, but the authors state that they are in the process of further development of the assessment. It is assumed that the therapist conducting this interview is trained and knowledgeable about the occupational behavior frame of reference.

Examples of Application to Occupational Therapy. This assessment might be used by a therapist who has a patient with a major depressive episode whose occupational skills seem superficially intact. The therapist may wonder whether this person has any performance deficits in roles in the expected environment or whether the symptoms of depression are the primary presenting problem. The ORH helps explain the context in which the performance takes place and gives the therapist a basis for initiating further assessments or therapy.

Implications for Treatment/Environmental Consultation. The authors suggest that this tool could be used as a screening tool by highly trained clinicians for making decisions about further assessment and treatment and give specific examples of how this might be done. Used for this purpose, it lacks evidence of reliability or validity in categorizing and in predicting outcomes and invites further research.

Arizona Social Support Interview Schedule (ASSIS) Inventory of Socially Supportive Behavior (ISSB). Two assessments developed by Barrera (1981) examine different aspects of social support. *The Arizona Social Support Interview Schedule* (ASSIS) documents the perceived need for certain kinds of support, the patient's current satisfaction with support that exists in six areas (private feelings, material aid, advice, positive feedback, physical assistance, and social participation), and characteristics of support-providers. The respondent is first asked to name and give information about people who performed certain functions of social support in the six areas. Then they are asked to respond on a three-point scale to the question of whether they wanted or needed more of each type of support. Finally, the respondent is asked to list people with whom they have had negative interactions (see Figure 16-4).

The *Inventory of Socially Supportive Behaviors* (ISSB) assesses the frequency of certain supportive behaviors within the past four-week period. The person is asked to respond to 40 items (regarding the areas of assisting others in mastering emotional distress, sharing tasks, giving advice, teaching skills, and providing material aid) using a five-point Likert-type scale that ranges from "not at all" to "about every day." Sample statements include the following: "Talked with you about some interests of yours," "Gave you over $25," and "Said things that made your situation clearer and easier to understand."

Relationship to Occupational Performance. When Barrera used both the ASSIS and the ISSB assessments with a population of pregnant adolescents, he found that satisfaction with the support was more important than the frequency or kind of support. Those with more stressful life events were receiving more social support, but this did not necessarily relate to better adjustment. Those individuals who have more severe stressors need more social support, but just the existence of more social support does not necessarily act directly to improve adaptation or performance. Barrera emphasizes the importance for therapists to understand this relationship and to assess both the negative and positive interactions in the social environment.

Barrera and associates developed these assessments with college age students and studied their use with pregnant

Arizona Social Support Interview Schedule (ASSIS).

In the next few minutes I would like to get an idea of the people who are important to you in a number of different ways. I will be reading descriptions of ways that people are often important to us. After I read each description I will be asking you to give me the first names, initials, or nicknames of the people who fit the description. These people might be friends, family members, teachers, ministers, doctors, or other people you might know.

I will only want you to give me the names of people you actually know and that you have actually talked to during the last month. It's possible, then, that you won't get a chance to name some important people if for one reason or another you haven't had any contact with them in the last month.

If you have any questions about the description after I read each one, please ask me to try and make it clearer.

A. PRIVATE FEELINGS

1. If you wanted to talk to someone about things that are very personal and private, who would you talk to? Give me the first names, initials, or nicknames of the people that you would talk to about things that are very personal and private.

PROBE: Is there anyone else that you can think of?

2. *During the last month,* which of these people did you actually talk to about things that were personal and private?

PROBE: Ask specifically about people who were listed in response to #1 but not listed in response to #2.

3. During the last month, would you have liked:
   1 = a lot more opportunities to talk to people about your personal and private feelings
   2 = a few more opportunities
   3 = or was this about right?

4. During the past month, how much do you think you needed people to talk to about things that were very personal and private?
   1 = not at all
   2 = a little bit
   3 = quite a bit

B. MATERIAL AID

1. Who are the people you know that would lend or give you $25 or more if you needed it, or would lend or give you something (a physical object) that was valuable? You can name some of the same people that you named before if they fit this description, too, or you can name some other people.

PROBE: Is there anyone else that you can think of?

2. *During the past month,* which of these people actually loaned or gave you some money over $25 or gave or loaned you some valuable object that you needed?

PROBE: Ask about people named in response to #1 that were not named in response to #2.

3. During the past month, would you have liked people to have loaned you or to have given you:
   1 = a lot more
   2 = a little more
   3 = or was it about right?

4. During the past month, how much do you think you needed people who could give or lend you things that you needed?
   1 = not at all
   2 = a little bit
   3 = quite a bit

C. ADVICE

1. Who would you go to if a situation came up when you needed some advice? Remember, you can name some of the same people that you mentioned before, or you can name some new people.

PROBE: Anyone else?

2. *During the past month,* which of these people actually gave you some important advice?

PROBE: Inquire about people who were listed for #1 but not for #2.

3. During the past month, would you have liked:
   1 = a lot more advice
   2 = a little more advice
   3 = or was it about right?

4. During the past month, how much do you think you needed to get advice?
   1 = not at all
   2 = a little bit
   3 = quite a bit

D. POSITIVE FEEDBACK

1. Who are the people that you could expect to let you know when they like your ideas or the things that you do? These might be people you mentioned before or new people.

PROBE: Anyone else?

2. *During the past month,* which of these people actually let you know that they liked your ideas or liked the things that you did?

PROBE: Ask about individuals who were listed for #1 but not for #2.

3. During the past month, would you have liked people to tell you that they liked your ideas or things that you did:
   1 = a lot more often
   2 = a little more
   3 = or was it about right?

4. During the past month, how much do you think you needed to have people let you know when they liked your ideas or things that you did?
   1 = not at all
   2 = a little bit
   3 = quite a bit

E. PHYSICAL ASSISTANCE

1. Who are the people that you could call on to give up some of their time and energy to help you take care of something that you needed to do—things like driving you someplace you needed to go, helping you do some work around the house, going to the store for you, and things like that? Remember, you might have listed these people before or they could be new names.

PROBE: Anyone else you can think of?

2. *During the past month,* which of these people actually pitched in to help you do things that you needed some help with?

PROBE: Ask about people who were named in response to #1 but who were not named in response to #2.

3. During the past month, would you have liked:
   1 = a lot more help with things that you needed to do
   2 = a little more help
   3 = or was this about right?

4. During the past month, how much do you feel you needed people who would pitch in to help you do things?
   1 = not at all
   2 = a little bit
   3 = quite a bit

Figure 16-4. Arizona Social Support Interview Schedule (ASSIS). *From M. Barrera (1981). Social support in the adjustment of pregnant adolescents: Assessment Issues. In B.H. Gottlieb (Ed.). Social networks and social support. Beverly Hills, CA: Sage Publications, 1981.*

adolescents. Other researchers have applied them to other populations.

Strengths and Limitations. Reliability of the ASSIS was tested using 45 university students. The test-retest correlation of the total network size was .99 and conflicted network size was .54. The support satisfaction measure had a test-retest correlation of .69, but a low internal consistency (coefficient alpha = .33). The support need showed .80 test-retest correlation and an internal consistency of .52.

The ISSB was tested with 71 university students and was found to have high internal consistency of .92 and .94 and a test-retest correlation coefficient of .88. The ISSB was found to correlate modestly with the total network size of the ASSIS.

One of the problems with assessing social support is the difficulty of factoring out the variable of personal or interpersonal competency. Also bias and error are built into such a questionnaire. Some questions may be unacceptable to individuals and so the answers may be guarded or inaccurate. The responses may also have cultural biases regarding social support, yet this is not well-explored. Much of the research done using this assessment has attempted to relate social support to general health indicators rather than performance. Further studies are needed to relate social support to performance.

Example of Applications for Occupational Therapy. The therapist has just received a referral for an oncology patient who will be going back home to live with her husband who has partially recovered from a cerebrovascular accident. Although limited home health services are available, the therapist is concerned about the needs for support for both the husband and his wife. The therapist administers the ASSIS and the ISSB to ascertain the resources available, the client's perceived adequacy of those resources, and to identify major negative relationships that might hinder the patient's recovery. The results of the assessments reveal that the wife has never felt that she could depend upon her husband for emotional support and has always relied upon her extended family, although the husband provides adequate financial support. The therapist concludes that with both the home health services and family support, both husband and wife will be able to continue performing their family roles.

Implications for Treatment/Environmental Consultation. Therapists involved in discharge planning are committed to aiding the patient in returning to and remaining in the community and in performing daily life roles. Sound instruments such as the ASSIS and the ISSB help to assess all aspects of the expected environment, which is essential in preparing the client for return to the community.

Cost of Care Index (CCI). This instrument was developed by Kosberg and Cairl (1986) as a case management tool to help health care professionals identify real or perceived problems experienced by families in caring for their elderly relatives. It consists of 20 items with four questions regarding each of the following five dimensions: (1) personal and social restrictions, (2) physical and emotional health, (3) value placed upon caregiving, (4) care recipient as "provocateur" or characteristics of the recipient of care that may provoke negative responses, and (5) economic costs of caregiving. Responses are given in Likert-type categories of "strongly agree" to "strongly disagree." The following are examples of items: "I feel that my elderly relative is (will be) an overly demanding person to care for" or "I feel that caring for my elderly relative is causing me (will cause me) to dip into savings meant for other things." Scores range from a low score (low cost) of 20 to a high score (high cost) of 100. Subscores are examined to determine specific problem areas currently being experienced or which are anticipated.

Relationship to Occupational Performance. Availability of a caretaker may make it possible for the client to perform roles in a home or community setting rather than in a more restricted environment and may help by freeing a family member to perform a greater variety of occupational roles. Many primary caretakers in the home are people who are still trying to remain in the workplace outside the home. If other caretakers are hired for periods of time, this can greatly aid those who wish to work outside the home while remaining a primary caretaker. In cases of severe disabilities, often the caretaker burden may be perceived as severe and unrelenting. Assessments such as the Cost of Care Index may help to identify levels of perceived burden so that intervention may permit deterioration of the role behaviors.

Strengths and Limitations. The five categories in this index were developed from a factor analytic study of a larger pool of items. The authors report high internal consistency (coefficient alpha of .91). Work is in process by the authors to determine predictive validity and the value of using the assessment repeatedly to evaluate the effectiveness of intervention by health care workers. The instrument has been developed and tested for caregivers of elderly persons and evidence is not available to demonstrate its generalization to other populations.

Example of Applications to Occupational Therapy. The occupational therapist has already used the Kinship Network Analysis to determine whether the client has possible care available on a part time basis from any family members. The therapist discovers only two possible persons, one of whom is a sister who is almost as frail as the client and the other is a niece who says she is willing to have the client move into her home and take on the primary responsibilities. Because of the paucity of support people for this client, the occupational therapist uses the Cost of

Care Index to measure the niece's perceptions of the true extent of the perceived burden and to gain an idea of what specific burdens this would create for the niece.

Implications for Treatment/Environmental Consultation. The CCI might be used as a tool for the occupational therapist in educating community members about policy decisions that provide community resources for elderly and disabled persons. The CCI would also be useful in teaching groups of caretakers preventive measures for avoiding burn-out. With careful selectivity, the CCI could be used to educate the disabled and elderly persons about ways to manage their human environments by reducing the kind of behaviors that increase the burdens of the caretaker.

Workplaces

Measure of Social Support in the Workplace (House and Kahn, 1985). This instrument provides guidelines and methodology for defining social support in the workplace; indicating supportive acts and the possible supporters on a grid. The supportive acts are placed on the vertical axis and include the following:

1. emotional concern (empathy, caring, and concern) which is considered the most important area,
2. instrumental aid (such as giving money or assistance),
3. information (advice, suggestions, directions), and
4. appraisal (feedback or social comparison relevant to a person's self-evaluation).

The horizontal axis lists the set of possible supporters including spouse or partner, other relations, friends, neighbors, work supervisor, co-workers, service or caregivers, self-help groups, and health/welfare professionals.

The cells created in this grid are then filled with information including both general and problem-focused and objective and subjective. For example, in the cell relating to emotional concern by friends, the general information might be that the friends provide day-to-day emotional support versus the specific support needed for stress on the job. Objective information might include evidence that the friend spends a certain amount of time listening to the person's complaints concerning the job versus the subjective feeling by the client that this friend is emotionally supportive.

Relationship to Occupational Performance. There is ample support in the literature for the relationship between social support and health (D'Auguelli, 1983; DiMatteo & Hays, 1981; Blythe, 1983; & Gottlieb, 1981). There is also evidence of a relationship between social support and performance, although this is a more complex relationship to demonstrate. House and Kahn (1985) studied the differential effects of givers of support upon the health of workers. They found that work-related sources of support were generally considered more important in the work setting, although spouses were also important. This study did not demonstrate a substantial effect for friends and relatives. The importance of different sources of support varied with work settings, such that it appeared that the supervisor is more important in settings in which the worker is relatively isolated, but co-worker support becomes more important to health and function in settings in which peers work together.

Strengths and Limitations. Social support is not a well-defined or clearly measurable variable, hence instruments used to measure it cannot be used as the sole indicator of support networks. It may be equally important to measure the negative support or other kinds of relationships. The work setting is very complex and this instrument assesses only a single set of variables, so there are questions regarding the validity of a social support measure. Other possible causal factors of positive findings could be job satisfaction, social status, or ego strength.

The primary value of this assessment is to provide a guide for the assessment of social support in the workplace. Used in combination with other sources of information, this assessment can be helpful in discriminating sources of barriers to performance in the workplace.

Example of Applications for Occupational Therapy. The client is a nurse working in a trauma center. She identifies her work as highly stressful and has problems of increased anxiety, sleeplessness, and overuse of various medications to help her function. The therapist, in helping the client to understand the nature of the stress, might use this assessment to determine to what extent the lack of a social network contributes to her level of perceived stress.

Implications for Treatment/Environmental Consultation. The occupational therapist working in business or industry might use this measure in combination with other assessments to develop a profile of the work setting. A therapist who has a client with any dysfunction who has work-stress related problems (physical or psychosocial), might use information from this assessment to specify the locus of stress or dissatisfaction.

SOCIALLY DEFINED ACTIVITY PATTERNS, BELIEFS, AND EXPECTATIONS

Assessing Attitudes Toward Disabled Persons

Collective attitudes toward individuals with differences or disabilities create a social environment that sets a level of expectation for what the individual can and will do. The measurement of such attitudes is complicated by the fact that the phenomenon in question is assumed to be multidimensional and a number of facets must be considered, and by the fact that attitudes can be measured only indirectly by overt behavior. Although a number of measures have been devised, most of them are situation-specific and validation studies are limited. There are notable exceptions in the work of Linkowski (1971), Siller (1969), Makas, et al. (1988), and Yuker, Block & Young, 1970). A review of the issues involved in assessing attitudes toward disabled persons is found in Antonak (1988).

The Attitude Toward Disabled Persons Scale (ATDP) (Yuker, Block & Campbell, 1960; Yuker, Block & Young, 1970).

The ATDP was designed to assess individuals' attitudes toward persons with disabilities. It consists of a pencil-and-paper questionnaire with 20 to 30 questions (depending upon the form that is used) to which the person responds on a Likert-type six-point scale from ''I agree very much'' to ''I disagree very much.'' A sample statement would be: ''Disabled persons are usually easier to get along with than other people.'' Higher scores tend to indicate that the person views disabled persons as being similar to himself/herself while low scores may reflect prejudice or suggest that the person views the disabled person as inferior.

Relationship to Occupational Performance. Social expectations, however subtle, influence the individual's and others' expectations of subsequent performance. Attitudes are assumed to correlate with expectations and, if these expectations are widespread, they may determine what roles and tasks are tolerated and valued. If expectations are ambiguous, individuals may have difficulty in developing a clear definition of social roles or, in contrast, they may have the latitude to develop a greater variety of social roles.

Strengths and Weaknesses. Yuker and associates (1970) report that the ATDP has a median stability coefficient of .73 and ranging of split-half reliability coefficients from .75 to .85. The authors and others have found inconclusive correlations between attitudes and demographic and experiential variables (Antonak, 1981a). A person's general attitude toward disabled persons may be different from those of a specific instance, such as one's own child; hence the multidimensional nature of attitudes toward disabled persons may not be addressed by this instrument.

Testing attitudes toward disability is difficult because disability is a broad term and means different things to different people. For example, functional deficits that are less obvious (or invisible) to observers may not be considered to be disabilities by some people, such as juvenile rheumatoid arthritis that is in remission. It is also difficult to determine whether peoples' responses on such a questionnaire is an accurate indication of how they would really act in relation to disabled persons.

The clinical utility of the ATDP has not been widely tested. It has been used in a number of studies to establish relationships between attitudes and behavior. Some studies seem to support the instrument's ability to reflect attitudinal changes, but others are less positive. The ATDP appears to address primarily physical disability. In addition, some critics have suggested that there is a difference between a general view of disability and the perception of a specific disabled individual's function or worth.

Examples of Applications for Occupational Therapy. A therapist is interested in designing an educational program to help parents of disabled children change their attitudes toward disability. In needing to establish a baseline of the parents' attitudes to identify educational needs, the therapist administers the ATDP. After the educational program is completed, the therapist notices positive changes in the performance level of these parents' children and thus concludes that her educational program has produced a desired effect.

Implications for Treatment/Environmental Consultation. The instrument could be useful to indicate attitudes of individuals and groups toward disabled persons. It is important to assess the attitudes of people who may interact with a client or patient because their expectations may influence performance. Such assessments can help identify and change expectations based upon the disability rather than the person.

Therapists are also interested in creating climates for establishing realistic expectancies for disabled children who have been ''mainstreamed'' back into the regular classroom. Thus therapists might want to use the ATDP to measure attitudes of both teachers and students to determine need for change.

The Scale of Attitudes Toward Disabled Persons (SADP) (Antonak (1981a; 1981b).

The SADP contains three subscales of optimism/human rights, behavioral misconceptions, and pessimism/hopelessness. The respondent answers questions on a Likert-type scale and scores range from 0 (negative) to 144 (favorable).

Strengths and Weaknesses. The author reports acceptable reliability and an alpha index of internal consistency of .88. More work needs to be done to validate the instrument, but it appears conceptually to tap some of the attitudes that concern occupational therapists in their education and advocacy for disabled and handicapped persons.

Application to Occupational Therapy. A program director for an occupational therapy school is having difficulty placing students with visible disabilities in internships, even when students give evidence that they can fulfill the work expectations. In order to make a decision about future admission of disabled students, the therapist uses the SADP to survey attitudes of occupational therapists, physicians, and patients. Subscale scores are examined to determine where these attitudinal problems occur. The feasibility of educational programs to effect attitude changes is studied.

Assessing Treatment Settings

Ward Atmosphere Scale (WAS). The Treatment Settings Ward Atmosphere Scale (WAS) is a well-researched set of assessments developed for a variety of institutional, treatment, and community settings by Rudolf Moos and his associates at the Social Ecology Lab in Palo Alto, California. Ward staff and patients are asked to respond to 100 true-false items (40 in the short form) in terms of the real ward, ideal ward, and expectation. Categories include: involvement, support, spontaneity, autonomy, anger and aggression, order and organization, program clarity, staff control personal problem orientation, and practical orientation. These categories cluster into three major dimensions of relationships, treatment program dimensions, and administrative or systems maintenance dimensions. Profiles can be constructed to indicate the relationship between patient and staff perceptions and differences and similarities among wards.

Relationship to Occupational Performance. Moos (1974) and others have demonstrated relationships between certain dimensions of ward environment and certain behaviors; for example, cohesion, resident influence, and physical comfort have been shown to lead to functional performance and social competence.

Strengths and Limitations. The assessments have been well researched by Moos and his colleagues. One of the potential difficulties with obtaining truthful information on this self-report instrument is the possible reluctance of the patient or client to be honest about his perceptions while still in the care of the staff upon whom he is dependent. The staff also may be reluctant to state their perceptions for fear of offending their supervisors. This assessment has been widely used for research, and acceptable reliability has been established. Some work has been done to establish construct validity.

Example of Application to Occupational Therapy. The occupational therapist is a part of a team in a psychiatric hospital which sees many patients with a diagnosis of borderline personality disorder. The staff has been uncomfortable with the way patients are responding to the environment of the treatment ward and acknowledge that the social climate of the ward may not be supportive of appropriate behavior of the patients. As a result of use of the WAS, staff and patients develop a picture of the elements of the ward atmosphere that they believe may be contributing to the problem. They institute changes in several dimen-

Environmental Assessment Scale	
Item #	**T-F Statement**
3.	Laughing and joking are often heard in occupational therapy.
7.	There is much excitement around here when a patient completes a project that is a work of art.
11.	In Occupational Therapy patients try to hide their anger even though they might feel better if they talked about it or expressed it through crafts.

Figure 16-5. Sample items from Kannegieter's Environmental Assessment Scale (EAS).

sions that are identified as less than ideal. Upon reevaluation of the program, they find a decrease in disruptive incidents and in staff frustration.

Implications for Treatment/Consultation in Occupational Therapy. The occupational therapist who consults with a hospital or other treatment setting may use this instrument to assess activity patterns and social and physical environments. The results would identify areas that need modification to create an environment that fosters recovery of health and function.

The Environmental Assessment Scale (EAS). Kannegieter (1987) developed the EAS based upon the work of Moos and associates. It is designed to provide a profile of the atmosphere of treatment clinic settings. Four scales are included that measure environmental interactions, personal interactions, involvement, and treatment approaches. The instrument consists of a self-report questionnaire of 80 true-false questions which measure the patient's perception of the psychiatric occupational therapy clinic (see Figure 16-5).

Relationship to Occupational Performance. The assumption is made that treatment can best be accomplished if the treatment environment can be tailored to the patient's personal characteristics and diagnosis. Such environmental variables as autonomy, spontaneity, and personal concern for patients are believed to enhance general treatment effectiveness in a psychiatric setting and to enhance performance.

Strengths and Limitations. The author of this scale has limited her work to psychiatric treatment settings, and applicability may not generalize. This assessment has been piloted in 12 treatment settings involving 242 patients. It was examined for internal consistency, retest reliability, reading level, and validity. Concurrent validity was examined by correlating scores with the *Ward Atmosphere Scale* and the *Minnesota Multiphasic Personality Inventory.* Correlation with the WAS was moderate and diagnosis was not related to EAS scores. More research is needed and the author recommends the assessment be limited to research usage.

Examples of Application to Occupational Therapy. Through a quality assurance process, the occupational therapist has identified rates of functional achievement for patients with a diagnosis of major depression that are slower than expected. The occupational therapist wishes to design an environment to foster active, assertive behavior. Using assumptions from Moos and Kannegeiter, the therapist assesses the clinic atmosphere and finds that opportunities for spontaneity, autonomy and personal interaction are deficient. She institutes an educational program to change certain staff behaviors and reassesses the clinic atmosphere to see whether these changes have been made. She then follows up with a review to see whether expected changes in activity and assertiveness occur in the patient groups.

Implications for Treatment/Environmental Consultation. If elements of the therapeutic clinic can be identified, then certain environmental elements can be introduced into the treatment setting. The EAS can be used to verify the presence of these elements. The therapist can then continue to refine the theory about environment and treatment through further research.

The occupational therapist can also investigate the applicability of this assessment to other treatment settings, including acute care, intensive care, and physical rehabilitation, and then offer advice on how to match treatment environments or living environments with patients' needs.

Social Interaction Scale of the Bay Area Functional Performance Evaluation (Williams & Bloomer, 1987). This scale was designed to assess functional skills in daily living of adult patients in a psychiatric treatment setting. It consists of a Task-Oriented Assessment (TOA) and a Social Interaction Scale (SIS). In the original version, the therapist could not score and use the two parts separately. This can be done in the revised version, although the therapist is cautioned that scores of both parts should be considered together in order to obtain an accurate measure of functional ability.

In the SIS, the patient is observed and rated in five kinds of settings: in a one-to-one situation (interview with staff), during mealtime, in an unstructured group setting, during a structured activity group, and during a structured verbal group. For each setting, each of seven parameters is rated on a scale of 1 to 5 ranging from "unable to assess" to "almost always functional or appropriate." The seven parameters include verbal communication, psychomotor behavior, socially appropriate behavior, response to authority figures, independence/dependence, ability to work with others, and participation in group or program activities. The assessment attempts to take into account the interaction between social behavior and the social environment. A score can be calculated for each situation and for the total assessment. Scores are compared to mean scores for patients in a similar setting.

Relationship to Occupational Performance. Social and psychomotor behavior is assessed within the context of the role of a psychiatric patient. The patient's ability to participate appropriately in the situation depends partly upon adaptive capacity and partly upon the social expectations. Although there are differences in expectations for performance in various treatment settings, the scores may confirm the patient's ability to read the social climate and respond accordingly.

Strengths and Limitations. Preliminary findings show that inter-rater correlations were modest for some parameters (participation in group activities, ability to work with others) to good in others (verbal communication, response to authority figures). Internal reliability among parameters and situations was low to moderate, thus they are considered to be different aspects of social interaction. A patient self-report form is included but correlations with therapists' ratings proved low and thus its use is recommended primarily as a measure of patient insight. There is no information available about the predictive validity of the instrument, but the individual's behavior should generalize to the extent that the treatment environment approximates the conditions of the patient's expected environment. A limitation of interpretation of the data is that test data are available from a limited number of patients in four different kinds of psychiatric settings, thus to interpret a patient's score, the therapist must select the setting most like his/her own and then compare the patient's score with the mean score of that group.

Example of Application to Occupational Therapy. The therapist is engaged in goal-setting with Sam, a young single male patient who has identified problems in getting along with people in the work setting and in socially meeting young women. Therapist and patient both individually fill out the SIS, and they compare and discuss their findings together. They agree that in the one-to-one setting with the therapist and in the structured activity setting, Sam functions comfortably and adequately, but during mealtime and in verbal group activities, he sets himself apart and shows a low level of energy and involvement, so that others tend to ignore him. The therapist and Sam plan some activities and interactions that he will initiate during the day in informal settings. These will then be discussed and evaluated in the verbal group sessions.

Implications for Treatment/Environmental Consultation. By using the SIS to help identify the type of situations in which a patient functions with relative strength it might become possible to recommend settings in which certain kinds of learning or therapeutic change could take place easily. The patient could be given adequate support or guidance for interacting in the more difficult settings. This could allow the therapist to use the existing structure of the treatment setting to optimize patient learning.

PHYSICAL SPACE AND OBJECTS

Assessing the Physical Environment in the Home

Descriptive Home Evaluation (The Rehabilitation Institute, Kansas City, MO). Occupational therapists have devised assessments to record information about the home environment for use in treatment and discharge planning. These assessments are completed by the therapist during a home visit. The instruments are descriptive, have face validity, and have not been subject to reliability testing. Figure 16-6 is an example of a home evaluation used at The Rehabilitation Institute, Kansas City, MO.

Relation to Occupational Performance. Maintaining an occupational role with a physical, psychosocial or cognitive deficit requires the support of a functional and safe environment. The occupational therapist functions as a consultant in recommending changes in the environment to support performance.

Strengths and Limitations. The observational descriptive approach is very individualized. The instrument would benefit from reliability studies.

Examples of Application to Occupational Therapy Consultation. The therapist usually performs these assessments for individual clients in preparation for discharge. The changing nature of our population with an increase in the relative numbers of disabled and elderly persons living in the community makes the occupational therapists role in assessing the physical environment more important to governmental officials and private investors. For this reason, it is envisioned that the occupational therapists' consultative role in assessing the physical environment will become more visible in the next decade.

Assessing Play Settings

Assessment of Playground Characteristics. The variables to be examined in an assessment of playgrounds are suggested in a study by Wolff (1979) in which he compared conventional playgrounds to that of ''adventure'' playgrounds by measuring the following variables: (1) number of facilities available, (2) type of facilities available, specifically the extent to which the children could effect change in the facilities, (3) administrative structure of the rules guiding play in this setting, and (4) the adult role in the

setting, whether supervisor, disciplinarian, or a supportive, friendly resource person. Wolff compared the play of able-bodied and disabled children and also examined the type of play in which these children engaged (described as solitary, parallel, positive or negative interaction with another child, or positive or negative interaction with an adult).

Relationship to Occupational Performance. There is evidence that disabled children have play deficits and that they engage in different kinds of play experiences and different relationships with the children and adults in their play settings (Behnke & Fecktovich, 1984; Gralewicz, 1973). To be able to offer an environment to foster play development as proposed by Michaelman (1974), occupational therapists should be able to assess playground environments in order to identify the level of desirable elements. Elements in the play setting that are considered precursors to successful role performance include the relative freedom to play, adults who model a spirit of playfulness as well as provide nonjudgmental support for successful play experiences, and peers who engage in a variety of relationships and who reflect group norms.

Strengths and Weaknesses. Wolff has not developed a standardized assessment, but has suggested a method of observation and analysis. Validity of the findings from the assessment of playground characteristics greatly depends upon the skill of the therapist.

Example of Application to Occupational Therapy. A therapist in a school for the blind is modifying the current playground area for the students. The therapist wants to determine which of the existing elements of the playground design and guidelines for use would be helpful to retain and which need changing. Wolff's assessment of playground elements could be used as a basis for analysis of the setting.

Implications for Treatment/Environmental Consultation. Occupational therapists may need to assess playground environments for their young clients in their neighborhood or in special settings. Occupational therapy consultants who treat young psychosocially or physically dysfunctional individuals in residential settings can also use these elements as guidelines for parents, teachers, and others who are involved with designing or altering children's play environments.

Assessing Institutions

Environmental Humanization Assessment (Bowker, 1982). In studying the concept of the total institution as described in Goffman's (1961) work, Bowker (1982) collected data using naturalistic observation and interview from four residential institutions for elderly persons (three

Home Evaluation

Patient:
Address:
Phone:

Please give information on items checked.

I. Physical Environment
  A. Location of Home
   1. Urban _____
   2. Suburban _____
   3. Rural _____

  B. Type Housing _____
   1. Apartment _____
   2. Private house _____
   3. Floor or floors occupied by patient (number) _____
   4. Type of heating _____
   5. Plumbing: Yes ___ No ___ Hot Water _____

  C. Entrance
   1. Steps
      a. Front   b. Back
         1) how many _____   1) how many _____
         2) with rails _____   2) with rails _____
         3) without rails _____   3) without rails _____

   2. Width of doors (inches)
      a. Front _____ b. Back _____

   3. Sill or step at door (if so, give height)
      a. Front _____ b. Back _____

   4. Distance from entrance to street or road _____

  D. Plan of House
   1. Number of rooms _____

   2. Location of patient's room in relationship to bathroom, kitchen or dining area, living room, etc. _____

   3. Bathroom: Yes ___ No ___
      a. Width of door (inches) _____
      b. Tub: Yes ___ No ___
         1) Shower over tub ___
         2) Stall shower ___
      c. Type of tub:
         1) Built in ___ Leg ___
         2) Height from rim to floor ___
         3) Height from inside bottom of tub to rim ___
         4) Which side is open _____

      d. Amount of space between all bathroom fixtures, and arrangement of these fixtures _____
         _____
         _____
         _____

         1) Will patient be able to manipulate wheelchair (26″ wide) between fixtures _____

Figure 16-6. Home Evaluation. *Used with permission from The Rehabilitation Institute, Kansas City, MO.*

Home Evaluation

e. Height of commode seat from floor _____

f. Does door have sill? If so, how high? _____

Bedroom: Private _____ Shared _____ If shared, with how many others? _____

a. Description of bed _____
_____

b. Type mattress _____ Thickness _____

c. Height of bed and mattress from floor _____

d. Does door have sill? If so, how high? _____

e. Size of bedroom _____

5. Dining area

   a. Height of table from floor to underneath surface _____

6. Kitchen

   a. Stove

      1) Type _____ If electric, height of stove and location of switches _____
_____

         a) Oven: Height of oven from floor _____

   b. Refrigerator: Yes ___ No _____

      1) Door open to right _____ left _____

   c. Sink

      1) Type: Cabinet _____ Open _____ None _____

      2) Height sink rim to floor (inches) _____

      3) Rim to inside bottom of sink _____

   d. Cabinets

      1) Height from floor to first shelf _____

      2) Height from floor to second shelf _____

      3) Other _____

      4) Height of work surface _____

   e. Size of kitchen _____

7. Miscellaneous information

   a. Telephone: Yes ___ No ___

      Location _____ Height _____

   b. Automobile: Yes ___ No ___ Model _____

   c. Electricity _____ If so, list and describe electrical appliances: _____
_____
_____
_____

   d. Kitchen stool _____ Type _____ Height _____

II. Social Environment

Preface: Please use the reverse side of the interagency referral form enclosed to include the following information:

A. Please list the members of the family living in this home, and include approximate ages, relationship, occupation, and scheduled hours away from home.

B. Are members of the family in good health? Please describe briefly the condition of those who are not.

Figure 16-6. Continued.

were nursing homes and one was a community-based residential home). From an analysis of extensive data, Bowker developed a typology of roles and recurrent themes from which he identified 33 variables representing humanistic principles that can be used as a framework for observation and analysis of an institution's environment. He categorized these variables as having four dimensions: (1) structural design, (2) general administrative policies, (3) programming, and (4) social relationships. The following are examples of variables in each category: A *structural design variable* includes use of color coding and use of living things to humanize physical structures. A *general administrative policy* is the presence of flexibility of scheduling to meet the human needs of the residents. **Programming** includes such factors as defining and developing rituals for holidays, birthdays, and other potentially humanizing events. *Social relationships* include permanent assignment of staff to specific areas and training staff in humanistic social relations such as the use of touch and aspects of terminal care.

Relationship to Occupational Performance. This model considers varying backgrounds and needs of both staff and residents. It operationalizes concepts which are known in theory to foster performance and self-efficacy in human groups. It addresses factors that enable institutions to support the role definition for a nursing home resident as someone who is active, involved, and valuable.

Strengths and Limitations. This set of variables has yet to be developed into a standardized assessment. An observer in an institutional setting would need to be well-trained and sensitive to environmental information and would need to spend considerable time interacting in order to make a valid assessment. This assessment certainly fosters the concept that a humanistic environment is not just one in which the individual is physically well-accommodated but one in which diverse human needs are addressed.

Example of Application to Occupational Therapy. An occupational therapist has been engaged as a consultant to a nursing home program. She interviews various staff members at various levels and residents using the items in Bowker's assessment as a framework. From the assessment, the therapist discovers that the nursing home is physically well-equipped, but there appears to be a deficiency regarding the following item: ''Special focus on humanizing activities in the early months of each resident's institutionalization.'' Knowing that the residents are at risk if they are not actively engaged in the relocation process, the therapist recommends setting up a program which will include not only the first months, but also planning with the family and resident before the relocation process. These recommendations are presented to the administration and

then the therapist proceeds to establish guidelines for the process.

Implications for Treatment/Environmental Consultation. This assessment might be extended to live-in group homes for children, adolescents, and mentally ill or mentally retarded persons. There is a clear need for research to validate the relationship between the presence of these variables and the client's performance.

Multiphasic Environmental Assessment Procedure (MEAP) (Moos & Lemki, 1984). This procedure assesses the physical and social environments of such sheltered care settings as nursing homes, residential care facilities and congregate apartments. This is a rather detailed and lengthy assessment consisting of five parts which can be used individually or as a whole:

1. The *Physical and Architectural Features* Checklist (PAF) has eight subscales focused on the following: community accessibility (e.g., convenience of grocery store, public transportation), physical amenities (attractiveness and comfort), social-recreational aids (e.g., furnished for resting or casual conversation), prosthetic aids (barrier-free), orientational aids (color-coded, etc.), safety features (e.g., call buttons in bathrooms), staff facilities (e.g., staff lounge), and space availability (e.g., space for special activities).

2. The *Policy and Program Information* (POLIF) includes questions about the types of rooms or apartments available, the way in which the residence is organized, and the services that are provided.

3. The *Resident and Staff Information Form* (RESIF) includes characteristics of residents such as social backgrounds, functional abilities and the way in which they use services or participate in activities and characteristics of staff and volunteers.

4. The *Sheltered Care Environment Scale* (SCES) assesses residents' and staff members' perceptions of seven characteristics of the social environment of the facility, including coercion, conflict, independence, self-exploration, organization, residents' influence, and physical comfort.

5. The *Rating Scale* (RS) taps independent observers' impressions of the physical environment and of resident and staff functioning.

Relationship to Occupational Performance. The work of Moos and associates (1983) has shown correlations between functional ability and social competence of residents in sheltered living settings and environmental variables such as cohesion, residents' influence, and physical comfort of residents. Furthermore, there are relationships which suggest that certain physical amenities, opportunities for social-recreational activities, and space can foster the emergence of these variables.

Strengths and Limitations. This instrument was developed from a conceptual framework and tested in 93 facilities in northern California, revised and then tested in 151 facilities in 20 states in a representative sampling. Psychometric analyses have been done to show moderate to high internal consistency of all of the parts of the assessment (.62 to .95) with the exception of the staff functioning dimension of the Rating Scale component which has since been revised. Test-retest reliability was moderate to high on all scales (.61 to .95). The data generated in these studies can be used to characterize findings from different kinds of settings (e.g., private vs. public setting or nursing home vs. community setting) in terms of means and standard deviations. A nice feature of the instrument is a handbook for users which includes detailed, clear guidelines for use of the instrument.

This instrument shares with other self-report assessments the problems of administering it to residents who lack the cognitive capacities to respond accurately or to those who may be reluctant to say anything negative about their caretakers. The entire assessment is long and time-consuming; however, individual parts can be quite useful to the occupational therapist. The PAF takes about two hours, and includes a thorough examination and measurement of the physical facilities. The SCES, which is a 63-item yes/no questionnaire, takes 15 to 20 minutes to complete and should be done in a group setting.

Example of Application to Occupational Therapy. The occupational therapist consulting with the nursing home identifies poor participation by residents in the activity available and a rather passive attitude among residents. Some of them had poor nutritional status. The therapist used the PAF and the SCES to determine the physical and social climate of the nursing home. The findings revealed that the activity areas were poorly arranged, preventing residents from being able to naturally cluster together to visit, and the dining room was unattractive with barriers to easy mobility. The therapist also noticed that residents did not often take charge of activities and were not often allowed to make choices such as selecting meal menus. The therapist made the following recommendations to the administration: (1) activity areas arranged to encourage visiting, (2) activities offered that residents could initiate, (3) the dining room made more attractive and accessible (4) residents to be more actively involved in choices of menus (including ethnic foods and personal preferences), and (5) that staff not feed residents who can feed themselves although it takes longer and is more "messy." The occupational therapist reassesses activity level and indicators of nutritional status six months later and finds them both improved.

Implications for Treatment/Environmental Consultation. Occupational therapists who are consultants to nursing homes or community residential agencies need a method to assess total systems, not just individuals. This assessment takes into account a variety of aspects of the environment. Moos suggests that the use of this assessment in a nursing home encourages staff and administration to consider a variety of ways in which change can occur, rather than the traditional focus of moving from "bad care" to "good care."

Information obtained from administration of the MEAP could also be useful to the therapist advising clients in suitable nursing home placement. The instrument developers invite the therapist to use it as a research tool and to test its usefulness in other settings.

Assessing Neighborhoods and Communities

Cantor's Neighborhood Assessment (Cantor, 1979). This neighborhood assessment contains four categories of information: extent of residents' life-space, perceptions of their neighborhoods and the availability of needed goods and services, the social support systems used by the residents, and their views of the advantages and disadvantages of city life. (More information on the total assessment can be found in Chapter 5.) It is mentioned here because the interview includes a set of questions about the social environment. Questions are asked about social support systems components including those of children, close friends, and neighbors. Residents are asked how frequently and where these individuals are contacted and to describe the types of services or assistance exchanged, such as crisis intervention, assistance in chores of daily living, giving advice, and gift giving.

Relationship to Occupational Performance. This assessment acknowledges that performance of certain life tasks and life roles may be hampered by the inavailability of certain human and nonhuman resources. It also acknowledges that the ability to exchange support functions fosters further motivation and continued ability to give and receive. The ability to exchange support services is related to continued active engagement in occupational roles.

Strengths and Limitations. The strengths of this assessment are several. First, it attempts to quantify the relationships between the individual and human resources. Second, it looks at the fit between individuals and the immediate daily environment in which they usually meet basic and independent daily living needs. Third, and very importantly, it measures the exchange between the individuals in the social network rather than just looking at support received.

The instrument has not been tested with different kinds of populations and in different parts of the country, and is not limited to just the social environment. Some validity data are available from Cantor's study, but these data apply to a certain area and a certain aging population in New York City. The data alone do not tell us whether function or dysfunction or deficit or adequacy exists in performance of daily activities; this is determined in the context of the neighborhood and the person's individual skills. The self-report is also subject to the biases of the individual reporting and to the effects of clients' depression, psychosis, or other distortions of reality.

Example of Applications for Occupational Therapy. A therapist is preparing an elderly patient recovering from cerebrovascular accident to return home. The patient is concerned about his mobility in relation to meeting his daily needs. The therapist assesses his endurance and finds that he can walk three blocks without undue fatigue. The therapist uses Cantor's assessment to specify his mobility sphere and discovers that there is a pharmacy and a small grocery store within three blocks. When he needs to leave the neighborhood, he usually rides with a neighbor or relative. He has a rich set of exchange relationships with individuals including sharing vegetables from his backyard garden with the neighborhood pharmacist, volunteering with a foster grandparents' program, and taking a young grandson fishing and teaching him woodworking skills in his small shop attached to the house. The therapist identifies these exchange relationships as strengths and recommends that he return to this supportive environment.

Implications for Treatment/Environmental Consultation. Cantor's neighborhood assessment can help the therapist in assessing and planning for social and physical resources in the community when returning patients to the community setting. It allows the therapist to consider the importance of the need for clients to find meaning in life by giving support as well as receiving it. The neighborhood assessment can be used as a tool for collecting information for advocacy of better allocation of community resources.

Community Assessment Wheel (Anderson and MacFarlane, 1988). The community health wheel is a circle equally divided into eight segments representing physical environment, education, safety and transportation, politics and government, health and social services, communication, economics and recreation. Data about each of the segments is gathered and analyzed to make a "diagnosis" of the community to form the basis for health program planning. This is a very thorough process which includes document review, personal contact, and a "windshield survey" in which one drives through a community and looks for information on 15 variables, such as open space, availability of "commons", and service centers. The one

making this community assessment is expected to be knowledgeable about community systems although the checklist provides the needed data.

Relationship to Occupational Performance. The client is identified as the community and the occupational therapist can view the community as a configuration of roles, tasks and activities, for which a measure of total performance can be developed. However, such an assessment can also be used to view an environment which can influence the performance of an individual client.

Strengths and Limitations. The authors have made no attempt to standardize this assessment; instead they have refined it through use by a number of graduate students in community nursing. The validity of the findings relies upon the skill of the investigator in becoming integrated into a community so that the necessary data become available. The boundaries of a community must be identified, and the one administering it must be willing to invest a substantial amount of time in the assessment process.

Example of Application to Occupational Therapy. The occupational therapist is working with a team of individuals who are planning to provide outpatient and community health services for high risk infants and their parents in a barrio of a large city. The team uses the Community Assessment Wheel to identify resources and deficits in the eight segments of the wheel. They identify a need for early prenatal identification of risk factors and for post-natal support and education. They identify a school, a YMCA, and several churches as resources. Using volunteers who act as translators, they develop classes in risk-monitoring and health practices for the pregnant women and new mothers.

Implications for Treatment/Environmental Consultation. As occupational therapists move out of the clinic and into the community, they need perspectives and tools to guide them in program planning and in involvement in influencing public policy. This community assessment wheel provides such a perspective.

Assessing Work Settings

Model Assessment Guide for Nursing in Industry (Anderson & McFarlane, 1988). This Assessment Guide identifies several components that might influence the health and performance of workers: the company, the plant, the working population, the industrial process, the health program, and stressors. The format is both observational and interview. The guide provides a detailed series of questions for data-gathering. An example of a question the evaluator asks to investigate the stressors is: "What stressors are identified by employees as pressures felt on the job?" The evaluator also gathers data about what problems the health providers perceive as stressors.

Relationship to Occupational Performance. Successful performance in the **work setting** is the most difficult to achieve for many populations involved with occupational therapists, and hence it is often not even attempted. But today the developing field of **ergonomics** has focused much attention upon the physical environment of the workplace. The occupational therapist is in a unique position to combine knowledge of physical manipulation of the environment with social manipulation to enhance the worker's ability to maintain the worker role. For some populations, such as mentally retarded persons, the social design of the workplace is as important as the physical one.

Strengths and Limitations. There is no evidence of attempts to standardize this instrument. The authors make the assumption that someone highly trained in community assessment and systems analysis will gather valuable data from this method. It is time-consuming and requires obtaining data from a number of sources and implies that those sources will be willing and able to give the needed data. The usefulness of the data gathered depends upon the clinical skill of the therapist.

These questions could form the framework for assessments in several work settings, such as a wellness program to assist management in understanding the role that social support can play in maximizing their workers' health and their level of performance on the job.

Example of Application to Occupational Therapy. The therapist is seeing a client who is planning to return to work after hospitalization for coronary thrombosis. The therapist is helping him develop a health profile. He has identified his work as generally "very stressful" but has been unable to pinpoint the source of the stress. The therapist has identified the physical aspects of his job, but would like to measure the level of social support which is believed to have beneficial effects upon his health. The therapist hypothesizes that much of the stress he feels at work is self-imposed rather than a response to external demands. This model assessment guide for nursing in industry could help determine the level of support at work which the client might use to more effectively counterbalance the perceived stresses.

Implications for Treatment/Environmental Consultation. There is a clear application to the expanded role of occupational therapy into the industrial work setting. The broad scope of the assessment data suggests the wide range of knowledge and skills required of an occupational therapist working in the community. The assessment can form the framework for an assessment strategy or a specific tool to help the therapist address all components of the industrial setting.

Analysis of Design Standards and Human Performance. Meister (1985) describes the following necessary elements as a knowledge base for designing physical work environments:

1. design standards for equipment and features which describe the relationship between a system characteristic (such as a control mechanism on a machine) and human performance. There should be information about what occurs when the design is not optimal and principles for incorporating such a characteristic into a design.

2. a human performance database that when given specific characteristics can predict what the range of human performance can be. Clearly, this complete body of knowledge does not exist, although human factors engineers and ergonomic experts have produced some useful information. A simple example will illustrate how such knowledge is accumulated.

In a certain workplace there was a high incidence of repetitive strain injuries believed to be induced by the use of one primary tool: a pair of conventional straight-handled, long-nosed pliers. These pliers forced the worker to markedly flex the wrist with each use. A redesign of the pliers resulting in a bending and lengthening of the handles, reduced the incidence of injuries markedly. These standards may be found in Pheasant (1987), American National Standards Institute (1980), Architectural and Transportation Barriers Compliance Board (1985), and other documents.

Relationship to Occupational Performance. The performance of a job requires a setting that is safe and that has certain environmental conditions that allow an individual to respond optimally such as proper illumination, temperature, noise control, workspace design and structure, and communication patterns. In order for an individual to achieve competence in the work setting, there must be a match of individual characteristics, task performance, and design of the work setting. The assessment should address the task performance and the work setting design so that the therapist can then find the best match for individuals' capacities.

Strengths and Limitations. This approach offers the careful research methods of measurement and control for individual mechanics of a distinct aspect of the work setting, such as the physical and cognitive aspects of computer usage. The weakness lies in the lack of a coherent system of organization for application of these principles.

Example of Application to Occupational Therapy. The therapist is assisting a child with cerebral palsy to use a rocker switch to operate a computer for classroom activities. Because excessive resistance increases associated movements, the therapist is looking for the optimal resistance of the rocker switch for control. The therapist designs an evaluation device which uses a force gauge to measure resistance of rocker switches and uses a counter activated by a movement detector attached distally to an arm or leg to measure associated movement. Then the therapist selects the rocker switch with the resistance level that elicits the least associated movement.

Implications for Treatment or Environmental Consultation. The occupational therapist helping the severely physically disabled person interface with the environment meshes data about the physical capacity of the client with data about the performance demands of the work or community setting of the client. Then the therapist recommends tool adaptation and positioning of client or equipment involved in the work. In addition, the therapist may also work with preventive programs in the workplace.

SUMMARY

Occupational therapists have typically addressed the physical and social environment in their assessments. However, it has been only recently that they have approached the task in a systematic and theoretical way. Recently they have begun the process of standardizing and validating such assessments and using those assessments developed by other practitioners in the field in an attempt to provide the optimum person-environment fit for their clients and patients.

The contexts studied include a combination of physical, social, cultural, and psychological phenomena. It is impossible to separate the physical from the social and cultural environments; however, there are sometimes benefits from conceptually separating them so that the phenomena can be examined in detail.

Study Questions

1. A number of current assessments focus on the measurement of social support. What are some of the problems that interfere with the reliability and the validity of data collected by these assessments?

2. Which of the following methods would you use to assess social support for your client: (a) measuring the objective environment (numbers of individuals available and support function that they perform) or (b) measuring the client's perception of the adequacy of the support? Why?

3. What are some ways that you can assess the environment of the infant or child in the home without interfering with the typical responses of the infant or the mediating functions of the mother?

4. The occupational therapy clinic is an important environment for therapists to assess, yet the only environmental assessment for an OT clinic presented in this chapter is

designed for a psychiatric clinic. How would you assess a clinic in a rehabilitation setting? Would the same assessment be applicable or would you need to modify this assessment or design a new assessment?

5. A social environment is dynamic and fast-changing, in contrast to a more predictable physical environment. Which of the assessments presented in this chapter address the changing (temporal) aspects of the social environment?

6. In your work with a community agency for elderly persons, you are asked to evaluate a day care setting for individuals with Alzheimer's and related diseases. Which assessment(s) would you select for this process? Why?

7. In planning for discharge of your patient who has suffered cerebrovascular accident, what would be the important environmental variables to assess? Which assessment presented in this chapter would you select?

References

American National Standard Institute. (1980). *Specifications for making buildings and facilities accessible to and usable by physically handicapped people.* New York: Author.

Anderson, E.T. & McFarlane, J.M. (1988). *Community as client.* Philadelphia: J. B. Lippincott.

Antonak, R.F. (1981a). Developmental and psychometric analysis of the Scale of Attitudes Toward Disabled Persons. Unpublished manuscript, University of New Hampshire, Durham.

Antonak, R.F. (1981b). Prediction of attitudes toward disabled persons: A multivariate analysis. *The Journal of General Psychology, 104*, 119-123.

Antonak, R.F. (1988). Methods to measure attitudes toward people who are disabled. In H.E. Yuker (Ed.). *Attitudes toward persons with disabilities* (pp. 109-126). New York: Springer Publishing Company.

Architecture and Transportation Barriers Compliance Board (1985). *Uniform federal accessibility standards.* Washington, D.C.

Attneave, C. (1981). Interdependence unbound by time and space. Commencement Address, May 9, Saint Vincent College, PA.

Barrera, M. (1981). Social support in the adjustment of pregnant adolescents: Assessment issues. In B.H. Gottlieb (Ed.), *Social networks and social support* (pp. 69-96). Beverly Hills: Sage Publications.

Barris, R., Kielhofner, G., Levine, R.E. & Neville, A.M. (1985). Occupation as interaction with the environment. In G. Kielhofner (Ed.), *A model of human occupation:*

Theory and application (pp. 42-62). Baltimore: Williams & Wilkins.

Behnke, C. & Menarcheck-Fetkovich, M. (1984). Examining reliability and validity of the play history. *American Journal of Occupational Therapy, 38,* 94-100.

Blythe, B.J. (1983). Social support networks in health care and health promotion. In J.K. Whittaker, J. Barbarino, et al. (Eds.) *Social support networks: Informal helping in the human services* (pp. 107-131). New York: Aldine Publishing Company.

Bowker, I.H. (1982) *Humanizing institutions for the aged.* Lexington, MA: D. C. Heath and Company.

Bradley, R.H., & Caldwell, B.M. (1979). Home observation for measurement of the environment: A revision of the preschool scale. *American Journal of Mental Deficiency, 84,* 235-244.

Bradley, R.H., Caldwell, B.M., Rock, S., Hamrick, H.M., et al. (1988). Home Observation for measurement of the environment: Development of a home inventory for use with families having children 6 to 10 years old. *Contemporary Educational Psychology, 13,* 58-71.

Cantor, J.H. (1979). Life space and social support. In Byerts, T.O., Howell, S.C. & Pastalan, L.A. (Eds.). *Environmental context of aging: Lifestyles, environmental quality, and living arrangements.* New York: Garland STPM Press.

D'Auguelli, A. (1983). Social support networks in mental health. In J.K. Whittaker, J. Barbarino, et al. (Eds.), *Social support networks: Informal helping in the human services* (pp. 71-106). New York: Aldine Publishing Company.

D'Matteo, M.R. & Hays, R. (1981). Social support and serious illness. In B.H. Gottlieb (Ed.). *Social networks and social support* (pp. 177-148). Beverly Hills, CA: Sage Publications.

Dunning, H. (1972). Environmental occupational therapy. *American Journal of Occupational Therapy, 26,* 292-298.

Elardo, R., Bradley, R., & Caldwell, B. (1975). The relation of infants' home environments to mental test performance from six to thirty-six months: a longitudinal analysis. *Child Development, 46,* 71-76.

Elardo, R., Bradley, R., & Caldwell, B. (1977). A longitudinal study of the relation of infants' home environments to language development at age three. *Child Development, 48,* 595-603.

Florey, L.L., & Michelman, S.M. (1982). Occupational role history: A screening tool for psychiatric occupational therapy. *The American Journal of Occupational Therapy, 36,* 301-308.

Goffman, E. (1961). *Asylums: Essays on the social situation of mental patients and other inmates.* New York: Doubleday.

Gottlieb, B.H. (1981). Social networks and social support in community mental health. In B.H. Gottlieb (Ed.). *Social networks and social support* (pp. 11-42). Beverly Hills, CA. Sage Publications.

Gralewicz, A. (1973). Play deprivation in multihandicapped children. *The American Journal of Occupational Therapy, 27,* 70-72.

House, J.S., & Kahn, R.L. (1985). Measures and concepts of social support. In S. Cohen & S.L. Syme (Eds.). *Social support and health* (pp. 83-108). Orlando: Academic Press, Inc.

Kannegieter, R.B. (1987). The development of the environmental assessment scale: Final report. Rockville, MD: The American Occupational Therapy Foundation.

Kosberg, J.I., & Cairl, R.E. (1986). The Cost of Care Index: A case management tool for screening informal care providers. *The Gerontological Society of America, 26,* 273-278.

Linkowski, D.C. (1971). A scale to measure acceptance of disability. *Rehabilitation Counseling Bulletin, 14,* 236-244.

Makas, E., Finnerty-Fried, P., Sigafoos, A., & Reiss, D. (1988). The Issues in Disability Scale: A new cognitive & affective measure of attitudes toward people with physical disabilities. *Journal of Applied Rehabilitation Counseling, 19,* 21-29.

Meister, D. (1985). The two worlds of human factors. In R.E. Eberts & C. G. Eberts (Eds.). *Trends in ergonomics/human factors II* (pp. 3-11). Amsterdam: North-Holland.

Michaelman, S.S. (1974). Play and the deficit child. In F. Reilly (Ed.), *Play as exploratory learning* (pp. 157-208). Beverly Hills, CA: Sage Publications.

Moos, R.H. (1974). *Evaluation of treatment environments: A sociological approach.* New York: John Wiley and Sons.

Moos, R.H. (1983). Supportive residential settings for older people. In I.A. Altman, J. Wohlwill & P. Lawton (Eds.), *Human behavior and the environment: The elderly and the physical environment.* New York: Plenum Press.

Moos, R.H., & Lemke, S. (1984). *Multiphasic environmental assessment procedure hand scoring booklet.* Palo Alto: Stanford University.

Pheasant, S.T. (1987). *Ergonomics—standards and guidelines for designers.* PP7310. Milton Keynes: British Standards Institution.

Pilisuk, M. & Parks, S.H. (1986). *The healing web: Social networks and human survival.* Hanover: University Press of New England.

Siller, J. (1969). The general form of the disability factor scales. Unpublished manuscript, New York University, New York.

Spencer, J.C. (1987). Environmental assessment strategies. *Topics in Geriatric Rehabilitation, 3*(1), 35-41.

Takata, N. (1969). The play history. *American Journal of Occupational Therapy, 23*, 314-318.

Tichauer, E.R. (1978). *The biomechanical basis of ergonomics*. New York: Wiley Interscience.

Williams, S.L., & Bloomer, J. (1987). *Bay Area Functional Performance Evaluation* (2nd edition) Palo Alto, CA: Consulting Psychologists Press.

Wolff, P. (1979). The adventure playground as a therapeutic environment. In D. Canter & S. Canter (Eds.), *Designing for therapeutic environments*. Chichester, Great Britain: John Wiley and Sons, Ltd.

Yarrow, L.J., Rubenstein, J.L., & Pederson, F.A. (1975). *Infant and environment: Early cognitive and motivational development*. New York: Wiley and Sons.

Yuker, H.E., Block, J.R., & Campbell, W.J. (1960). *A scale to measure attitudes toward disabled persons*. Albertson, NY: Human Resources Center.

Yuker, H.E., Block, J.R. & Young, J.H. (1970). *The measurement of attitudes towards disabled persons*. Albertson, NY: Human Resources Center.

Zisserman, L. (1981). The modern family and rehabilitation of the handicapped: A macrosociological view. *American Journal of Occupational Therapy, 35*, 13-20.

CHAPTER CONTENT OUTLINE

Introduction

Body Composition

Muscle Endurance

Muscle Strength

Flexibility

Cardiorespiratory Function

Summary

KEY TERMS

Arm Crank Ergometer

Bicycle Ergometer

Borg Scale of Rating of Received Exertion (RPE)

Graded Exercise Test

Isokinetic Strength Testing

Isometric Muscular Endurance

Isotonic Muscular Endurance

Maximal Oxygen Consumption

Maximum Voluntary Contraction (MVC)

Repetitive Maximum

Step Test

ABSTRACT

To understand the effect of activity on general health and the rehabilitation process, it is necessary to use meaningful methods of measuring and expressing the physiologic and performance changes associated with activity. This chapter discusses the various methods of assessment and the rationale for using them in the five fitness areas of cardiorespiratory function, muscle strength, muscle endurance, flexibility, and body composition. Information is provided on the procedures and equipment, the subject population, the validity and reliability statistics, and the strengths and limitations of each measure in order to better help therapists select appropriate assessment measures, administer the tests correctly, and appropriately interpret and apply the results.

Assessing the Physiological Enablers of Performance

Marian A. Minor

"Exercise testing is directed toward measurement of the individual components of the system; the symptoms experienced by a patient when he performs a certain activity depend on the way the whole person responds to the environment."

—Jones, 1988

OBJECTIVES

The information in this chapter is intended to help the reader—

1. discuss advantages and disadvantages of hydrostatic weighing and skin fold measurement for assessment of body composition.

2. understand the clinical implications of results from absolute and relative endurance tests.

3. describe major differences in isokinetic, isometric and isotonic muscle strength testing.

4. discuss the clinical usefulness of assessment of dynamic flexibility.

5. describe the clinical applicability of information gained from a graded exercise test.

6. briefly outline testing procedures for body composition, muscle strength, muscle endurance, flexibility and cardiorespiratory fitness that would be possible in a clinical setting.

INTRODUCTION

The study of the physiologic components of human performance traditionally has been the domain of exercise physiology, which began with interests rooted in athletic training. The science has expanded to include studies of physiologic response to activity and exercise in a variety of populations other than the young and athletic male. Therapists benefit from increased knowledge of the effect of exercise on many populations including well and elderly persons, cardiac patients, individuals using wheelchairs, people with diabetes or arthritis, obese people, and clinically depressed individuals.

To understand the effect of activity on general health and the rehabilitation process, it is necessary to have meaningful ways to measure and express physiologic and performance changes associated with activity. As in the chapter on Physiologic Dimensions of Performance, physical fitness will be used as the organizational concept for this discussion, looking at the five components of health-related physical fitness: *cardiorespiratory function, muscle strength, muscle endurance, flexibility* and *body composition.* Each component includes factors that can be objectively measured, and various tests and measurements have been devised to measure these factors. In some instances, norms have been established based on large population studies. As clinicians, our ability to assess the components of physical fitness is made difficult not by a scarcity of measurement tools, but by the choices and decisions we must make to insure that the tests used are appropriate, reliable and safe for the intended purpose. The aim of this chapter is to present various methods of assessment along with the rationale for using them in all five fitness areas. Additionally, it will provide information which will allow you to select measures appropriate to your needs, administer them correctly, and interpret and apply the results in a meaningful fashion. There is no one test that is always best in all situations. The goal is to be able to make good choices. Using even an informal checklist as shown in Table 17-1 will facilitate selection of the best measurement tools for each situation.

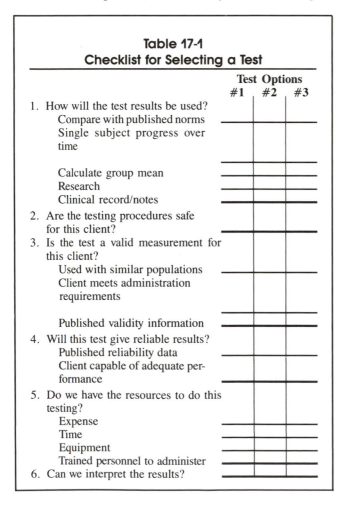

Table 17-1
Checklist for Selecting a Test

BODY COMPOSITION

The assessment of body composition is the estimation of the proportion of body fat to total body weight. This assessment can be used to determine percent body fat of an individual, current lean body weight, and to project an ideal body weight. Percent body fat of an individual can be compared to normative data to assess obesity. It can be used as a repeated measure to indicate the effectiveness of fat reduction interventions such as dietary restriction and/or exercise regimens.

The two most common ways of estimating body composition are *hydrostatic* (underwater) *weighing* and *skinfold measurement.* Hydrostatic weighing is the procedure of choice for research studies and is confined to laboratories equipped to perform this procedure and subjects who are motivated to endure it. Skinfold measurement is used clinically and in field test situations. This procedure requires only skinfold calipers and a trained administrator to estimate percent body fat. Less common methods include calculation of body fat from equations based on circumference measurements, arm roentgenogram for fat width measurements, computerized tomography (CT) assessment, ultrasound, and a variety of biochemical techniques.

Hydrostatic Weighing

Fat floats because it is less dense than water. Fat is also less dense than muscle, bone and other lean body tissues. The theoretical basis of hydrostatic weighing for calculating percent body fat rests on using Archimedes' principle to find the volume of a human body underwater. Knowing body volume allows calculation of body density. Once density is determined, formulae are available for converting body density to percent body fat. These formulae were developed from research done on cadavers to test for body density and chemically analyze fat content. An excellent description of theory and protocol of hydrostatic weighing can be found in McArdle, Katch & Katch (1986).

The subject is weighed in air (WA) and then residual lung volume (RLV) is determined. The subject is then submerged and weighed underwater (WW) while attempting to expel as much air as possible by forceful exhalation. The underwater weighing is repeated 8 to 12 times, and an average of the last few trials is used as the value for underwater weight. Underwater weighing requires a scale and chair assembly of known weight which is suspended in a pool or tank. It is also important to know the temperature of the water at the time of weighing to determine water density (DH_2O). Once the measurements have been taken, the equations shown in Table 17-2 are used.

Validity. Hydrostatic weighing is considered the most accurate means to assess body composition of living subjects. It serves as the "gold standard" for other techniques such as skinfold measurement. The equations used to calculate body fat from measured body density were developed through direct chemical analysis of cadavers and have been validated in subsequent laboratory tests of the density range of adipose and lean tissue (McArdle, Katch & Katch, 1986).

Reliability. Body volume scores derived from hydrostatic weighing show a high test-retest reliability ($r = .94$) (McArdle, Katch & Katch, 1986) for measurements taken several times on the same day or on consecutive days. Reliability is subject to accuracy of measurement of weight, residual lung volume and water temperature. A difference of

---

Table 17-2

Formulas for Determining Body Composition from Hydrostatic Weighing

1. **Body Density** =
$$\frac{WA \times DH_2O}{(WA - WW) - (RLV \times DH_2O)}$$

2. **Percent Body Fat**

   Siri equation:

   % Fat = (495/Body Density) − 450

   Brozek equation:

   % Fat = (457/Body density) − 414

   Having calculated percent body fat, it is now also possible to calculate total body fat weight, lean body weight, and ideal body weight as follows:

3. **Fat Weight** = WA × % Fat/100

4. **Lean Weight** = WA − Fat Weight

5. **Ideal Body Weight** = Lean Weight/1.00 − % fat desired

Note: WA = weight in air; WW = weight in water; RLV = residual lung volume; DH_2O = density of water (corrected for temperature)

---

100 ml in the residual volume value results in a 0.7% difference in the calculated percent body fat.

Subjects. Hydrostatic weighing is appropriate for subjects who are not afraid of water, capable of following directions and able to forcefully exhale and hold their breath underwater for 5 to 15 seconds. Individuals who are extremely obese may require a weight belt to stay adequately submerged.

Strengths and Limitations of the Method. The strength of this method is its high validity and reliability for accurately assessing body composition. The limitations lie in the cost and availability of equipment, procedural time per subject, and high level of cooperation needed on the part of the subject.

Skin Fold Measurement

The measurement of skin fold thickness to assess body composition is based on knowledge that approximately 50% of the store of human body fat is located just below the skin. Thus, people with more body fat have thicker skin folds. To go beyond this relative statement of fatness and use actual skin fold measurements to estimate per cent of body fat, researchers have used the technique of multiple regression to develop equations that use various combinations of skin fold measurements to predict results obtained from hydrostatic weighing. The aim has been to identify the

---

Table 17-3
Examples of Estimation of Percentage Body Fat by Skinfold Measurement

A = triceps skinfold measurement (mm)
B = subscapular skinfold measurement (mm)

Women, 17 to 26 years:
Per cent body fat $= .55(A) + .31(B) + 6.13$
Men, 17 to 26 years:
Per cent body fat $= .43(A) + .58(B) + 1.47$

From: Katch, F.I., and McArdle, W.D. (1973). Prediction of body density from sample anthropometric measurements in college-age men and women. Human Biology 45, 445.

---

number and location of skin fold measurements at body sites that most closely predict the results achieved by hydrostatic weighing.

There are now a number of equations and tables from which to choose. The regression equations that have been developed to predict body fat from skinfold thickness are specific to populations. This means that the person being assessed must be similar to the population of subjects that was used to derive the equations. If you measure skin folds on a 60-year-old woman and insert them into an equation developed from data on 20-year-old men, the results of your calculations of body composition will not be valid. Equations that are population specific and correction factors are available.

Procedures and Equipment. Special skinfold calipers are required. The procedure involves firmly grasping a fold of skin and subcutaneous fat between the thumb and forefinger and pulling it away from the underlying muscle layer. The calipers are applied to this fold and a reading of thickness is taken directly from the caliper dial. The ideal caliper will have parallel jaw surfaces and a constant spring tension. The calipers exert constant tension on this fold of skin and subcutaneous fat. The reading should be taken within two seconds of maximum caliper tension. Usually two or three measurements are taken for an average value at each site.

Measurements are performed on the right side of the body with the subject standing. The five most common sites of measurement are at the triceps, subscapular, anterior suprailiac, abdominal and anterior thigh. The choice of site and number of skin fold measurements is determined by the particular protocol or methodology being used to determine body fat from the skin fold measurements.

Age and sex specific equations, tabled data, and no-

mograms are available in the exercise physiology and physical fitness literature (deVries, 1980; Lamb 1984; Sharkey, 1984; and Winnick, 1985). Some equations directly calculate body fat from skin fold measurements; others are based on body density and further calculations are performed using the Siri or Brozek equations (see Table 17-2) to derive per cent body fat from body density. Examples of body composition equations using skinfold thickness to calculate percent body fat are given in Table 17-3.

Validity. The validity of skinfold measurement to assess body composition rests on the assumption that there is a predictable relationship between subcutaneous fat and internal fat and body density. This relationship has been tested using statistical techniques to derive regression equations using skinfold measurements to predict body density/ percentage body fat that was calculated from hydrostatic weighing. Predictive ability has been shown to be as high as $r = .95$ to $.82$ when the equations are applied to subjects who are similar in age, sex and fatness to the population of subjects from whom the original data was taken.

Reliability. In practice, the reliability of skinfold measurements for assessing body composition depends upon using calculations derived from appropriate population data and minimizing measurement error with accurate calipers and skilled measurement technique. Katch and Katch (1980) say that measurement error can produce body fat estimates that vary as much as 200% for the same person. Dehydration can decrease skinfold thickness by as much as 15%, which will result in a change in the percent body fat figure. Thus, time of day and preceding activity which affect hydration could impact on body fat assessment.

Subjects. Participation by the subject is minimal for this procedure, making it possible for most people. The use of this measurement is not limited to subjects because of their age, sex, and health status in the actual caliper application, but by the availability of appropriate equations to use for the body fat calculations.

Strengths and Limitations of the Method. The strengths of this method are that it requires very little equipment and many people can be measured in a short period of time. It is useful for screening procedures and field tests. If proper equations and protocols are chosen and measurements taken accurately, validity and reliability can be reasonably good with a minimal investment of resources.

Limitations of this method are the potential for large measurement errors arising from technicians who are inexperienced in the proper measurement technique, the relative insensitivity of the method to detecting changes in body composition following weight loss (Brooks 1984), and the constraints of equations that must be population specific for accurate results.

MUSCLE ENDURANCE

There are many ways to measure muscular endurance. The first decision is whether to measure endurance of an isometric or isotonic contraction. Most often the criterion for assessing isotonic endurance is the number of repetitions of the movement that can be performed in a fixed period of time. The greater the number of repetitions, the greater the endurance. Another criterion that can be used for assessing muscular endurance, both isometric and isotonic, is the length of time that a contraction or motion can be sustained at a given, constant workload. The longer the activity can be sustained without a decrement in performance, the greater the endurance.

The difficulty that arises in assessing muscular endurance in clinical settings is in controlling the confounding variables of muscular strength, cardiorespiratory function, and motivation of the subject. The most effective way to control these variables is to use testing procedures that can be individualized and/or graded to achieve a balance between the load placed on the muscle and the test time period. If the load is too heavy, test results will be more representative of strength than endurance. If the load is too light and/or the timed period is too long, test results may be affected by cardiorespiratory fitness or how motivated the subject is to continue for an extended period of time.

Isometric Endurance

Testing **isometric muscular endurance** is most effectively done by timing how long the individual can maintain the tension of a **maximum voluntary contraction (MVC)**. Strain gauges, dynamometers, and the some isokinetic equipment can be used to measure MVC and indicate onset of fatigue by reductions over time in force exerted. The longer the MVC can be maintained, the greater the muscular endurance for isometric contraction. Holding time (endurance) increases as percent of MVC decreases. When testing isometric endurance, tension should be greater than 60% MVC or there may be no appreciable fatigue produced (deVries, 1980).

Isotonic Endurance

Most timed tests of **isotonic muscular endurance** count repetitions for 0.5 to 1.0 minute to avoid the cardiorespiratory and motivation effects. If one chooses to set up muscle endurance protocols, this is a good time frame to use. The other concern is determining the muscle load that will achieve a balance between muscle strength testing and result in a meaningful range of intersubject scores in a 0.5 to 1.0 minute time period. Too great a load tests strength more than endurance. Too small a load will yield test scores so similar that they will be neither discriminating nor sensitive.

Testing muscular endurance for an isotonic contraction is most often done by counting the number of repetitions of the contraction/relaxation cycle that can be performed in 0.5 to 1.0 minute. Current thought suggests that this testing should be done with a load that is 70% of the subject's maximum strength for that movement, that is one **repetition maximum** (1 RM) (Pollock, Wilmore & Fox, 1984). For example, if 1 RM for knee extension is 35 pounds, one would use 24.5 pounds as the load on the quadriceps and count the number of knee extensions that could be completed in 30 seconds with this load. There are no norms yet established for this testing procedure; however, research to date suggests that the healthy, active adult should be able to perform 12 to 15 repetitions at 70% of maximum strength while competitive athletes are closer to 20 to 25 repetitions at 70% of maximum (Pollock, Wilmore & Fox, 1984). By testing each person at the same percentage of their own maximum strength, the strong influence of absolute strength on endurance is minimized.

Endurance Tests in a Fitness Battery

Physical fitness test batteries designed for the healthy population most commonly use timed tests of push-ups, pull-ups and sit-ups as assessments of muscular endurance. These tests have published norms by age and sex. Although the use of these tests is probably fairly limited in the rehabilitation setting, an explanation of procedure and use of normative values is available in Pollock, Wilmore and Fox (1984). Testing procedures and comparative data for disabled children are available in *Physical Fitness Testing of the Disabled* (1985) by Winnick and Short.

Measuring Clinical Endurance

The most pertinent clinical information regarding muscular endurance is generally not found in comparing client scores to populations norms, but in monitoring individual client progress through a treatment program. By applying the principles of the timed test of repetitions at a submaximal workload, one can evaluate and quantify endurance performance.

Another method that is clinically applicable to assessing changes in endurance and activity tolerance is to monitor the client's perception of how hard he/she is working or how

---

Table 17-4
Borg Scale of Perceived Exertion

0	Nothing at all
0.5	Very, very slight (just noticeable)
1	Very slight
2	Slight
3	Moderate
4	Somewhat heavy
5	Heavy
6	
7	Very heavy
8	
9	Very, very heavy (almost maximal)
10	Maximal

For exercise testing, the Borg Scale can be applied to common symptoms of muscle fatigue, general fatigue, difficulty breathing (dyspnea), and chest pain. *From Borg, GV (1982). Med Sci Sports Exercise, 14:377-387.*

---

tired he/she is after a given amount of time at a specified workload. As endurance improves, the client will perceive that he/she is not working as hard to complete the task or that the onset of fatigue is delayed. A simple, valid and reliable method for gathering this information is to systematically use the **Borg Scale of Rating of Perceived Exertion (RPE)** (Noble, Borg, Jacobs, et al., 1983).

Borg Scale of Rating of Perceived Exertion (RPE)

The original Borg scale was developed by Swedish exercise physiologist, Gunnar Borg, during the 1950's. His intent was to create a system which people could use to describe the intensity of the work that they perceived they were doing and that would correlate with the objective physiologic measures of exercise exertion. The original 15-point scale has since been modified into a 10-point category-ratio scale. The scale ranges from the category of "no work at all" (0 on the scale) to the category of "very, very heavy work" (10 on the scale). See Table 17-4.

Procedures and Equipment. It is useful to have a visual representation on display in the clinic so that clients may refer to the scale numbers and descriptors as often as they wish. Reference to the scale and recording of the response should be done consistently on a pre-determined schedule or following a specific task or activity. The client responds to the question, "On this scale of 0 to 10, how much work do you feel that you are doing?" Clients able to use the scale for self-monitoring of

fatigue and endurance should be encouraged to do so both in and out of clinic. The Borg scale is an easily understood concept and a meaningful measure of changes in endurance and activity tolerance for both documentation as well as client encouragement and motivation.

Validity. This perceptual rating scale is a valid psychophysical method of assessing exertion. Subject self-ranking correlates highly with well accepted objective measures of exercise intensity and exertion. Correlations ranging from .80 to .90 have been reported between RPE scores and exercise heart rate, oxygen consumption, and blood lactate levels (Carton and Rhodes, 1985).

Reliability. Test-retest reliability coefficients are reported most frequently above .90 (Carton and Rhodes, 1985).

Subjects. The RPE scale has been successfully used with a wide variety of age groups performing a variety of exercise activities. The scale is often used during exercise testing in cardiac rehabilitation programs to assess not only self-perceived exertion, but also dyspnea and anginal pain. The concept of rating on a 0 to 10 scale appears to be easy for most people to understand.

Strengths and Limitations of the Method. The strengths of using this method for monitoring changes in perception of exertion are that it requires no equipment and a bare minimum of staff training. It can be used successfully in self-care programs where level of exertion and/or onset of fatigue are important parameters.

The limitations of this method are that it has all the difficulties inherent in any self-reporting assessment technique. To be most effective as a measurement tool, it should be used in a consistent manner.

MUSCLE STRENGTH

Muscle strength is the maximum force that a muscle or muscle group can generate over a brief period of time. There are several methods of measuring this force. Although strength can be measured for all types of contractions, measurements are usually confined to the strength of isometric (static) contractions and concentric isotonic (shortening) contractions. Muscle strength tests can be categorized into three basic methods:

1. tests of a single maximum isometric contraction
2. tests of a single maximum dynamic weight lift, and
3. tests of force exerted through the entire range of motion.

Choice of measurement method depends on the type of contraction being tested and how the strength information will be used. There is no one method that is always the best. Each of these methods have been tested for reliability specific to that method of measurement; however, the general amount of individual variability in strength from day to day can be as high as 9% to 12% (deVries, 1980).

Single Maximum Isometric Contraction

Traditionally single maximum isometric contraction has been the most widely used method for testing muscle strength. Cable tensiometers, strain gauges and dynamometers are the instruments used to measure the force or tension generated in the isometric contraction. Batteries of tests measuring cable tension strength have been developed to measure the static force of muscles of the fingers, thumb, wrist, forearm, elbow, shoulder, trunk, neck, hip, knee, and ankle (McArdle, Katch & Katch, 1984). Dynamometry is typically used for hand-grip and back-lift strength measurements. The *manual muscle test*, widely used in the therapeutic setting, makes use of this method of assessing the strength of an isometric contraction at a specified point in the range of motion. The difference is in the objectivity of scoring test results. *Cable tensiometry* and *dynamometry* yield quantifiable scores. Manual muscle testing yields a subjective assessment and more qualitative information of muscle function (Daniels and Worthingham, 1986). Published norms are available for a wide variety of tensiometer and dynamometer tests (Baumgartner & Jackson, 1982; McArdle, Katch & Katch, 1984; Pollock, Wilmore & Fox 1984) and information regarding strength in relation to ideal body weight and muscle balance is available also.

Procedures and Equipment. The *cable tensiometer,* originally used to measure the tension on steel cables linking various parts of an airplane, is a lightweight, portable, durable and relatively inexpensive device. It measures muscular pulling force exerted on a cable during an isometric contraction. The subject is positioned for the desired movement, and the tensiometer is placed on the cable between the body part and cable anchor point. The force that the muscular contraction exerts on the cable is read from the tensiometer dial. *Dynamometers* are specifically designed to measure force of a particular muscle group. The *hand-grip dynamometer* is the most common example. The principle of dynamometry is that external force compresses a steel spring and moves a pointer. The amount of force needed to move the pointer a certain distance is the reading given on the dynamometer dial. Dynamometry equipment can be as simple and portable as the hand-grip model or can involve stationary equipment that is used for testing all major muscle groups including the trunk.

Validity. The validity of isometric strength testing is based on construct validity of muscle strength of the muscle group being tested. This procedure is not necessarily a valid test of isotonic strength of the same muscle group. Correlation with dynamic strength measurements have been shown to range from .90 (Baumgartner & Jackson, 1982) to .62 (deVries, 1980). Tests of the same muscle group at different joint angles will produce different scores.

Reliability. The objectivity coefficients of cable tensiometry can frequently be .90 and above when the testing procedures are done by trained personnel (deVries, 1980). Manual muscle testing is more subjective and affected by rater bias and technique.

Subjects. These measurement techniques are widely applicable and require that the test administrator be able to communicate the desired muscular action to the subject. The motivation of the subject to give a maximal effort is crucial for meaningful results.

Strength and Limitations of the Method. The strengths of the single maximal isometric contraction method are that the testing requires very little time, is not demanding of the subject, can be inexpensively performed, and renders highly objective results. Cable tensiometry allows great versatility in testing many muscle groups at almost any joint angle desired.

The two major limitations of this method are that results do not necessarily generalize to dynamic strength training and measurement, and that there may be limited correlation with functional ability.

Single Maximum Dynamic Weight Lift

Testing muscular strength with a single dynamic contraction is done with the one **repetition maximum** or 1 RM method. The maximum amount that the person can correctly move through the full range of motion one time, but no more than one time, is 1 RM. The weight (lb/kg) of this resistance is the test result.

Procedures and Equipment. The resistance can be applied with free-weights or floor exercise equipment. The procedure is trial and error. A weight that is judged to be close to 1 RM is attempted. Weight is either added or removed until the subject can perform one lift with that resistance, but can not perform a second lift.

Validity. This method has construct validity of muscle strength for the muscle group being tested; however, use of the results as a clearly objective finding should not be assumed. The method of arriving at 1 RM can be lengthy and factors such as fatigue and poor motivation can affect the results. This is particularly true if the subject and/or the test administrator are inexperienced and many lifts are required. Fitness test batteries use only one or two specific muscle groups to make an assessment of general body strength. In a test of college men, it was found that the 1 RM bench press (r = .84) was a good predictor of total dynamic strength when measured by seven separate tests (Pollock, Wilmore & Fox, 1986).

Reliability. Test-retest reliability is within the expected range of subject variability.

Subjects. The 1 RM method is widely applicable. The length of the trial and error process to arrive at 1 RM should be kept as short as possible. For subjects who are easily fatigued or if fatigue is undesirable, extreme care should be taken.

Strengths and Limitations of the Method. The strengths of this method are that it tests strength throughout the full range of motion, not just at one joint angle (as in isometric tests) and that it can be performed with a great variety of resistive equipment. Results are easy to understand and useful for client motivation and reinforcement.

The major limitation in this method is the variability in the number of lifts preceding determination of 1 RM, making fatigue an important yet inconsistent factor. It is not as objective as some other methods, although it is more objective than manual muscle testing.

Tests of Strength Throughout the Range of Motion

Isokinetic strength testing allows measurement of muscular force being exerted throughout the range of motion. Specialized electromechanical equipment, linked to computer systems, is capable of supplying precise counterforces to voluntary muscle contraction while regulating the voluntary contraction at a constant speed. Isokinetic equipment is used for both strength training and strength testing. NASA has pioneered in the use of isokinetic equipment to measure the effect of weightlessness and space flight on muscle strength (Baumgartner, 1982). The measure of muscle force being exerted throughout the full range of motion is recorded graphically as a force curve and yields information about muscle dynamics that is not available from the other testing methods. This methodology measures force output in three ways: (1) force output at any specified joint angle through the range, (2) peak force achieved in the contraction, and (3) total force applied (the measurement under the force curve).

Procedures and Equipment. The equipment needed for isokinetic testing is highly specialized and expensive. The apparatus is an *isokinetic dynamometer* interfaced with a computerized system for almost instantaneous readouts (McArdle, Katch & Katch, 1986). Three of the best known manufacturers of isokinetic equipment are Cybex, Hydra-Fitness and Nautilus. Thorough training is necessary prior to use of this equipment.

Validity and Reliability. Data relating to validity and reliability of isokinetic testing procedures are specific to the test and population of subjects.

Subjects. Equipment is applicable to most people. At this time, the primary constraints are availability of equipment and trained personnel for administration and interpretation of strength testing.

Strengths and Limitations of the Method. Strengths of this method are objectivity, detailed information of actual muscle dynamics, and versatility of testing formats. Isokinetic measurement is the method of choice for data collection for research purposes.

Limitations of this method include the expense of the equipment and the special training of personnel needed for proper maintenance and use of equipment and interpretation of results.

FLEXIBILITY

Flexibility is the extent of joint range of motion and the ease with which that motion is accomplished. The concept of flexibility contains both a static and a dynamic component. Dynamic flexibility can be thought of as the "looseness or stiffness" of a joint. With specific instrumentation this looseness/stiffness quality can be quantified as the amount of force (torque) needed to move a joint through a specified range (Byers, 1985; and deVries, 1980). Although dynamic flexibility is not normally assessed, technology is available to do so. Static flexibility is the range of movement in a joint or series of joints. It can be measured directly or indirectly.

Direct assessment of flexibility is done by actual measurement of the angle of the joint with instruments such as the *goniometer, Leighton flexometer* or *electrogoniometer* (elgon) or by filming sequential movement that allows joint angles to be measured and compared from pictures. Assessment of range of motion of the spine is most accurate when done by measuring angles from roentgenograms. Indirect assessment is done by measuring how closely two body segments can be brought together or how far a body part is from some external reference point.

Direct measurement of flexibility is performed for clinical and research purposes. *Indirect measurement* is the method most often used for screening and field testing. Since assessment of joint range of motion is an integral skill in the professional competencies of health professionals, and choice of methodology is determined by clinical need and experience, this chapter will not attempt to review range of motion assessment methodologies. Detailed descriptions of procedures and their reliability are available and should be carefully studied (e.g., see Trombly, 1989)

Flexibility is joint and activity specific. There is no single, valid test for general flexibility (Baumgartner, 1982). Physical fitness test batteries usually have only one flexibility measure. The inclusion of a particular measure should be performed based on a rationale for why flexibility of that particular body segment is important for the population for whom the test battery was developed. It is incorrect to assume that a single flexibility measure in a test battery is providing information about general flexibility. The only flexibility information it provides is about the specific body segment or joint tested.

Sit-and-Reach Test

The Sit-and-Reach test is a test for low back and posterior thigh flexibility. It is the test most often included in current physical fitness test batteries for both adults and children. The rationale for this measurement is based on research that poor flexibility in these areas contributes to low back pain and dysfunction. Since low back disorders are a major source of disability in this country, the choice of this particular flexibility measure seems most appropriate.

The description of the original procedure was described by Wells and Dillon in 1952 (Jette, 1978). Since that time the original procedure has been slightly modified and used extensively in fitness testing batteries throughout the United States and Canada. Normative data are published for this test; however, due to the modifications in equipment, it is imperative that you match equipment specifications with the normative data. Descriptions of method and resulting normative data can be found in widely used physical fitness test batteries (AAHPERD, 1980; Golding, Meyers, & Sinning, 1982). Only a general description of method and use follow here.

Procedures and Equipment. Equipment for the Sit-and-Reach test usually includes a wooden box with an attached measuring scale (usually a yard or meter stick) extending out from one edge. The subject to be tested removes shoes

and sits down on the floor or other firm surface in the straight leg sitting position with feet shoulder width apart and soles of the feet flat against the box. Knees must be fully extended. The measuring scale is directly in front of the subject. The test is performed by placing the hands together and extending the arms forward, flexing the hips and trunk, reaching as far forward on the measuring scale as possible without bouncing or flexing knees. The test score is the number on the measuring scale that the subject is able to touch and hold for at least one second.

Testing variations include the unit of measurement on the scale (inches or centimeters), the point on the scale where it is attached to the box (14″, 15″, 23 cms, etc.), the specification for how many trials are allowed, and the amount of warm-up that is allowed. It is easy to understand how these variations in method can produce different scores.

Validity. This test has been validated using other flexibility measures with resulting correlation coefficients ranging between .80 and .90 (Baumgartner, 1982). Validity can be improved by a consistent procedure for practice and warm-up prior to actual testing. The Sit and Reach test is considered a logically valid measure of low back, hip and posterior thigh flexibility, but results cannot be generalized beyond these body segments.

Reliability. Reliability coefficients for this test range above .70 (Baumgartner, 1982).

Subjects. This test has been used and normative data established for people from 5 to over 80 years of age. It should not be used by anyone for whom extreme hip or lumbar flexion is contraindicated. Knee flexion contracture will limit the usefulness of the test score for comparison with published norms; however, by recording the degrees of knee flexion, the procedure can still be useful for following progress of an individual over time.

Strengths and Limitations of the Method. The strengths of the Sit and Reach test are its wide use and the availability of age and sex-matched norms and percentile scores, the ease of administration in a wide variety of settings, and inexpensive equipment. The major limitation of this method is the fact that the single score does not indicate the locations and extent of ranges in the complex motion that is used to achieve the Sit-and-Reach score. Lack of adequate range in shoulders and elbows can lower the score. Even if the score achieved is in the acceptable range, it is possible that the motion was gained through mobility in the hip and posterior thigh despite relatively little lumbar flexion. Body build can also limit the measurement.

CARDIORESPIRATORY FUNCTION

Cardiorespiratory function is assessed by monitoring the responses of the cardiorespiratory system to exercise stress. This assessment is done by administering a *graded exercise tolerance test* (GXT). There are several reasons to test cardiorespiratory function with a GXT (ACSM, 1986):

1. To identify and diagnose coronary heart disease in asymptomatic or symptomatic individuals.
2. To assess safety for exercise prior to starting an exercise program.
3. To assess cardiorespiratory fitness of apparently healthy or diseased individuals.
4. To provide a basis for developing an exercise prescription for improving cardiorespiratory fitness.
5. To monitor the course of known coronary or pulmonary disease.
6. To assess the efficacy of treatment procedures and the rehabilitation program.

The great variety of GXT protocols available reflects the fact that this test is used in many different settings. The basic assumption underlying the use of exercise stress testing for assessment of cardiorespiratory function is that the capacity of the heart, lungs and circulation to deliver adequate oxygen to the working muscles is the principal limiting factor of *aerobic exercise* (exercise that requires sustained and rhythmical activity of the large muscle groups of the body). By applying graded stress to the cardiorespiratory mechanisms with exercise demands of known workloads, it is possible to monitor cardiorespiratory responses during exercise and determine the maximal functional capacity of the cardiorespiratory system.

Maximal functional capacity is stated in terms of **maximal oxygen consumption** (max VO_2). Max VO_2 is the greatest difference between the rate of oxygen inspired and oxygen expired. The difference between these two values is the amount of oxygen taken up and used by the active muscles to produce energy to sustain activity (Lamb, 1984). The greatest difference occurs when the individual is sustaining activity with a large proportion of body muscle mass at a maximal level of intensity. Max VO_2 is considered the gold standard for assessing cardiorespiratory fitness (or functional capacity), however, it is not necessary to directly measure oxygen consumption during maximal exercise to estimate the max VO_2 of a person. There are many GXT protocols for assessing cardiorespiratory fitness. A test can be either maximal or submaximal, and can either directly measure or estimate oxygen consumption.

The modality for providing graded exercise stress may be a motor driven treadmill, **bicycle ergometer, arm crank ergometer** or **step test.** Choice of measurement devices may yield minimal or exhaustive information of coronary re-

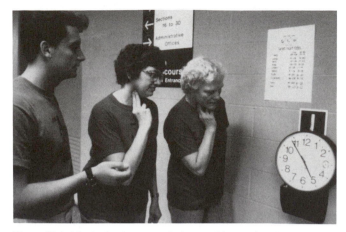

Figure 17-1. Monitoring heart rate during aerobic exercise class.

sponse. The choice of GXT protocol is based on age, health status and level of physical activity of the person to be tested and information required by the tester. The purpose of this section is not to present a detailed procedure for performing a particular GXT protocol, but to supply the basic principles and terminology of exercise testing and the information that can be obtained.

Maximal or Submaximal Testing

A true maximal oxygen consumption test requires an intensity of effort that is exhaustive. Attainment of maximal capacity can be objectively determined. Among the criteria for determining achievement of max VO_2 are plateaus in heart rate and oxygen consumption values in spite of increasing workloads, indication of reaching the ventilatory breaking point, respiratory quotient (RQ) above 1.05, and blood lactate levels of 8 mmol or above.

A *true maximal exercise test* occurs only with a highly motivated subject who is willing and able to exercise to exhaustion. It should only be attempted with carefully screened subjects and under close supervision by experienced exercise test personnel. It is important to recognize that a ''maximal effort'' by the subject does not ensure that true maximal oxygen uptake was achieved. For example, if a subject stops the test because of local muscle fatigue, it is a test of their maximal effort, but it is not a measure of max VO_2.

Outside the exercise physiology research lab, maximal GXT's are performed as subjective maximal tests or symptom-limited tests. This means that the test is terminated when the subject requests it, or the examiner stops the test due to abnormal responses of heart function or blood pressure. Subjective maximal or symptom-limited GXTs with continual electrocardiogram and blood pressure monitoring are considered diagnostic tests for coronary

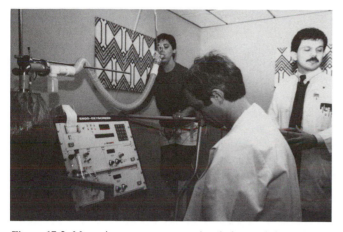

Figure 17-2. Measuring oxygen consumption during graded exercise test on treadmill.

health. The correct term for oxygen consumption data obtained from symptom-limited or subjective maximal exercise tests should be "peak oxygen consumption" to differentiate the results from a true max VO_2.

When evaluating cardiorespiratory fitness testing results presented as max VO_2, it is essential to know the criteria for GXT termination. Oxygen consumption can either be directly measured during an exercise test or it can be estimated from the exercise heart rate or distance/time performance on a standardized GXT protocol. Direct measurement of oxygen consumption is the most accurate method of assessing max VO_2. Estimating or predicting max VO_2 can result in errors of 5% to 10% with reliability coefficients of .70 to .90. (Pollock, Wilmore & Fox, 1984). Errors much larger than this can occur. It has been shown that overestimation of max VO_2 can be as much as 30% particularly in testing older women (Shephard, 1978).

New computerized, automated systems for collecting metabolic data during exercise testing are now available. This equipment and the technical expertise required for maintenance, operation and interpretation of results add to the financial and time cost of a GXT. By applying good standardization to testing procedures, errors have been shown to be consistent over time, and estimation of oxygen consumption without direct measurement can be a valid indicator of cardiorespiratory fitness.

A *submaximal exercise test* terminates when a predetermined end point is reached. This end point may occur when the subject attains a certain percentage of age-predicted maximal heart rate or when a particular exercise intensity is reached. Submaximal tests are used for fitness evaluation and are not considered as diagnostic tools for coronary health. Submaximal and maximal oxygen consumption can be estimated from submaximal exercise heart rate or distance/time of test performance on certain standardized test protocols.

There is increased error in estimating max VO_2 from submaximal heart rate or performance variables. However, submaximal testing with max VO_2 estimation is the most popular method of describing cardiorespiratory fitness. Changes over time in cardiorespiratory fitness of an individual can be assessed by comparing exercise heart rate at the same submaximal workload. As an individual becomes more fit, heart rate at a given workload will decrease as the exercise becomes less stressful. Therefore, lower submaximal heart rates over time indicate improved cardiorespiratory fitness.

Exercise Test Modality

The most common modalities used for exercise testing are the *motor driven treadmill* and the *bicycle ergometer*. Originally, exercise testing was done by having the subject step up and down from steps of varying heights. There are still step test protocols being used, especially adapted to field test environments. Arm crank ergometers are also used when lower extremity exercise is not possible. All of these modalities allow workloads to be measured and intensity of work to be gradually increased in stages. Specific protocols for each modality have been developed with accompanying data regarding populations tested and standardized data regarding oxygen consumption and fitness categories (Jones and Campbell, 1982; ACSM, 1986).

Choice of test modality is usually dictated by available equipment and personnel. The treadmill is the most popular modality, followed by the bicycle ergometer. The bicycle is increasing in popularity. It can be less expensive to purchase and maintain, requires less room for operation and makes electrocardiogram and blood pressure recording easier and more stable during exercise.

The major disadvantage to the bicycle as a test modality in the United States is that most adults are not accustomed to cycling and local fatigue of leg muscles may lead to test termination before cardiorespiratory limits are reached. This situation is particularly evident in testing older subjects (Shephard, 1978). Also, max VO_2 achieved on the bicycle tends to be slightly lower than that achieved on the treadmill due to the smaller active muscle mass involved in cycling.

The treadmill is the most widely applicable modality. Workload is determined by adjusting combinations of treadmill speed and slope. Speed can vary from slow walking (less than 2 mph) to running, and slope can vary from 0% to more than 20% grade. Oxygen consumption (ml/kg/min) requirements at various stages can be determined. The latitude for varying speed and intensity makes the treadmill a versatile modality for exercise testing subjects over a wide range of fitness and abilities. Since walking is a common activity, treadmill work does not require unique muscular efforts. The movement of the upper body that occurs with treadmill walking or running does make electrocardiogram and blood pressure recordings

---

Table 17-5
Contraindications and Indications for Stopping Exercise Testing

Exercise testing should NOT be performed when an individual has:

a. an illness with an acute fever
b. pulmonary edema
c. myocarditis or pericarditis
d. uncontrolled hypertension (above 250 systolic, 120 diastolic)
e. uncontrolled asthma
f. unstable angina
g. uncontrolled heart failure

Exercise testing should be performed WITH EXTREME CAUTION UNDER MEDICAL SUPERVISION ONLY when an individual has:

a. had a recent myocardial infarction (within four weeks)
b. aortic valve disease
c. a resting heart rate above 120 beats per minute
d. resting EKG abnormalities
e. epilepsy
f. cerebrovascular disease
g. respiratory failure
h. poorly controlled diabetes
i. electrolyte disturbances

Exercise Testing Should be STOPPED when an individual:

a. experiences severe chest pain
b. has extreme difficulty breathing
c. feels faint or dizzy
d. demonstrates confusion, apprehension, or incoordination
e. has sudden onset of pallor or sweating
f. becomes pale
g. shows abnormal EKG signs
h. has systolic blood pressure higher than 300 systolic or 140 diastolic
i. shows a drop of more than 20 mmHg in systolic pressure after a normal exercise rise
j. shows any decline in systolic pressure below the resting value

---

Adapted from Jones, N.L. and Campbell, E.J.M. (1988). Clinical Exercise Testing. Philadelphia: W.B. Saunders Company, pp. 90-91.

---

a bit more difficult to perform, but adequate results are obtainable.

There are also field tests of cardiorespiratory fitness. These tests are applicable only to apparently healthy individuals who are not at risk for heart disease. The usefulness of this mode of testing is that large numbers of people can be assessed at the same time, they are inexpensive to perform, have norms established, and may be used by individuals as self-assessments. These tests involve measuring distance travelled within a specified period of time or the time that is required to cover a specified distance. The results of the field test are used to estimate max VO_2 and/or cardiorespiratory fitness level from normative data. The validity of this method rests heavily on adherence to test protocol procedures and the similarity of the test subject to the population used for developing the norms.

General Principles of Exercise Testing

1. The test should begin at a level of intensity considerably below the anticipated maximal level.
2. Exercise intensity should be gradually increased in stages with observations made at each stage.
3. Contraindications for testing and indications for stopping should be closely observed (see Table 17-5).
4. If there is any doubt as to the benefit of testing or the safety of testing, the test should not be performed.
5. Heart rate, blood pressure, patient appearance, rating of perceived exertion (RPE), and symptoms (either observed or verbally reported) should be monitored regularly.
6. All observations should be continued for a 7- to 10-minute recovery period, unless abnormal responses occur which would require a longer post-test observation.
7. Exercise tolerance (oxygen consumption in ml/kg/min or METs) should be calculated from the test protocol used or measured directly if oxygen uptake is obtained.
8. Temperatures in testing area should be 22° Centigrade (72° F) or less and the humidity 60% or less if possible.

SUMMARY

Traditionally, only those occupational therapists involved with general fitness programs, cardiac rehabilitation, and work hardening have had involvement with assessing the majority of the physiological components of performance described in this chapter. However, it is clear that physiologic factors, including body composition, muscle strength and endurance, flexibility and cardiorespiratory function, represent an important dimension that should be understood by therapists, since general health and fitness are fundamental to all activity. Therapists with a basic knowledge of the various approaches to measuring physiologic factors will find themselves better prepared to communicate with professionals in exercise physiology and better able to determine the fitness levels of their patients. Moreover, they will have at their disposal an additional array of approaches for measuring performance related factors in research. This should lead to improved understanding of the relationship between various activities and tasks and the selected physiological enablers described in this chapter.

Study Questions

1. What are the differences between cardiorespiratory endurance and muscular endurance? Is it possible to increase muscular endurance without increasing cardiorespiratory endurance? Is it possible to increase muscle endurance without increasing cardiorespiratory endurance?

2. What factors would you consider in choosing a muscle strength test: isometric, isotonic or isokinetic?

3. What are the advantages and disadvantages of bicycle ergometry and the treadmill for cardiorespiratory testing?

4. What is the Perceived Exertion Scale? Discuss possible clinical uses.

5. What factors need to be considered before using skinfold measurements as a measure of percentage of body fat?

6. What are some methods for assessing dynamic (extent) flexibility? When would this assessment be important?

Recommended Readings

American College of Sports Medicine (1986). *Guidelines for exercise testing and prescription* (3rd ed). Philadelphia: Lea and Febiger.

Jones, N.L. & Campbell, E.J.M. (1982). *Clinical exercise testing* (2nd ed). Philadelphia, PA: W.B. Saunders Company.

Pollock, M.L., Wilmore, J.H. & Fox, S.M. (1984). *Exercise in health and disease*. Philadelphia: W.B. Saunders Company.

Sharkey, B.J. (1984). *Physiology of fitness* (2nd ed). Champaign, IL: Human Kinetics Publishers, Inc.

Winnick, J.P. & Short, F.X. (1985). *Physical fitness testing of the disabled*. Champaign, IL: Human Kinetics Publishers, Inc.

References

American Association of Health, Physical Eduction Recreation Department (AAHPERD) (1980). *Health related physical fitness manual*. Washington, D.C.: AAHPERD.

American College of Sports Medicine (1986). *Guidelines for exercise testing and prescription* (3rd ed). Philadelphia: Lea and Febiger.

Baumgartner, T.A. & Jackson, A.S. (1982). *Measurement for evaluation in physical education* (2nd ed). Dubuque, Iowa: Wm C. Brown Publishers.

Brooks, G.A. & Fahey, T.D. (1984). *Exercise physiology: Human bioenergetics and its applications*. New York: John Wiley and Sons.

Byers, P.H. (1985). Effect of exercise on morning stiffness and mobility in patients with rheumatoid arthritis. *Research in Nursing and Health, 8*, 275-281.

Canadian Association for Health Physical Education and Recreation (1977). *Canadian Home Fitness Test*. Ottawa, Author.

Carton, R.L. & Rhodes, E.C., (1985). A critical review of the literature on ratings scales for perceived exertion. *Sports Medicine, 2*, 198-222.

Daniels, L. & Worthingham, C. (1986). *Muscle testing, techniques of manual examination* (5th ed). Philadelphia: W.B. Saunders Company.

deVries, H.A. (1980). *Physiology of exercise for physical education and athletics* (3rd ed). Dubuque, Iowa: Wm C. Brown.

Golding, L.A., Meyers, C.R., & Sinning, W.E. (Eds) (1982). *The Y's way to physical fitness* (revised). Chicago: The YMCA of the USA.

Jette M. (1978). The standardized test of fitness in occupational health, a pilot project. *Canadian Journal of Public Health, 69*, 431-438.

Jones, N.L. & Campbell, E.J.M. (1982). *Clinical exercise testing* (2nd ed). Philadelphia, PA: W.B. Saunders Company.

Katch, F.I. & Katch, V.L. (1980). Measurement and prediction errors in body composition assessment and the search for the perfect prediction. *Research Quarterly for Exercise and Sport, 51*, 249.

Lamb, D.R. (1984). *Physiology of exercise, responses and adaptations*. New York: MacMillan Publishing Company.

McArdle, W.D., Katch, F.I., & Katch, V.L. (1986). *Exercise physiology, energy nutrition and human performance* (2nd ed). Philadelphia: Lea and Febiger.

Noble, B.J., Borg, G.A.V., Jacobs, I, et al. (1983). A category-ratio perceived exertion scale: relationship to blood and muscle lactates and heart rate. *Medical Science and Sports Exercise, 15,* 523-528.

Pollock, M.L., Wilmore, J.H. & Fox, S.M. (1984). *Exercise in health and disease.* Philadelphia: W.B. Saunders Company.

Sharkey, B.J. (1984). *Physiology of fitness* (2nd ed). Champaign, IL: Human Kinetics Publishers, Inc.

Shephard, R.J. (1978). *Physical activity and aging.* London: Crooms Helm Ltd.

Trombly, C. (1989). *Occupational therapy for physical dysfunction* (3rd Ed.). Baltimore: Williams & Wilkins.

Well, K.F. & Dillon, E.I. (1952). Sit-and-reach. A test for back and leg flexibility. *Research Quarterly of the American Association of Health and Physical Education, 23,* 115-118.

Winnick, J.P. & Short, F.X. (1985). *Physical fitness testing of the disabled.* Champaign, IL: Human Kinetics Publishers, Inc.

CHAPTER CONTENT OUTLINE

KEY TERMS

Acuity

Dermatome

Distractibility

Perception

Postrotary nystagmus

Praxis

Receptive field

Responsivity

Stereognosis

ABSTRACT

This chapter reviews the standardized assessments and clinical methods which can be used to assess the sensory components of an individual's performance. The chapter identifies sensory components of tasks required for self-maintenance, work, and leisure and gives recommendations on how to conduct a skilled observation of task performance. There is also a discussion of the sensory elements of assessment methods commonly used by other professionals, including intelligence tests, psychoeducational tests, and neuropsychological tests.

Assessing Sensory Performance Enablers

Winnie Dunn

"In dealing with sensory disturbance in man after injury to cutaneous nerves, the first thing to be considered is what kind of sensations belong to the normal skin and to the underlying tissues . . . It is, therefore, right to say that the localization of a given stimulus and the intensity with which it is felt depends not only on the physical properties of the stimulus and on the number and quality of the terminal organs engaged, but also on the conditions existing in the central nervous system . . . I am quite aware that the explanation that I propose . . . is more or less a hypothetical one. Still it has the advantage, as I believe, of being consistent with all the observations as yet known. Of course, every hypothesis is by itself transient and has to be changed as experience grows. That is the reason why I have wished to bring the matter before you, hoping that your experience will show me how far my conclusions are right and where I have missed the point. I am quite convinced that physiology alone, unaided by clinical observation, would be very slow in unraveling the mysterious functions of the nervous system."

—von Frey, 1906

OBJECTIVES

The information in this chapter is intended to help the reader—

1. create a plan for sensory assessment as part of a comprehensive assessment.

2. identify sensory components of underlying occupational performance in self-maintenance, work, and leisure.

3. appreciate the sensory information available within data gathered by others.

4. summarize major tests available which provide data on sensory performance in whole or in part.

5. evaluate the level of responsivity of each sensory system and its potential contribution to functional performance.

INTRODUCTION

As discussed in Chapter 9, Sensory Dimensions of Performance, sensation is an important correlate of human performance. Sensation supplies the system with information and in turn allows the organism to develop accurate and reliable maps of both self and environment. Therapists must not only understand the theoretical constructs underlying sensation but must also be equipped to assess performance in relation to sensory processes. The purpose of this chapter is to review standardized assessments and clinical methods which can be used to assess the sensory components of an individual's performance.

GENERAL PRINCIPLES OF SENSORY ASSESSMENT

The assessment of sensation requires both technical skill and artful observation. For all sensory systems, these skills and observations are based on several basic principles.

The first basic principle is that *therapists observe the individual's responses to stimuli*. Direct knowledge about the processing of sensation is only possible through various recording devices used in laboratory procedures. Since it is not feasible to conduct these procedures in the therapist's daily routine, therapists must develop skills to interpret observable responses in the context of possible sensory involvement. Human responses fall into three categories: *autonomic, motor*, and *affective*, with affective or emotional responses primarily observed as one of the first two types. So in order for therapists to observe effectively, they must have a clear knowledge about the output systems, the behaviors produced by them, how the nervous system produces them and which behaviors may be signals of poor sensory processing.

The second principle is that *responsible judgments about sensory processing are only made when multiple assessment procedures have been employed to make those decisions*. All decisions regarding sensory involvement are based on several opportunities to gather information including skillful review of the available data base, informal and formal evaluation procedures, well planned interviews, and careful observation of performance. It is the congruity or incongruity of these multiple pieces of information that

enables therapists to determine the integrity of the sensory system in question.

The third principle is that *knowledge regarding the integrity of sensory systems is only important in the context of task performance*. Investigation of sensory processing which merely serves the academic purpose of gathering and recording information is considered inadequate for contemporary occupational therapy practice. Potential relationships among sensory system actions, task performance, and role actualization must be clearly defined in order to justify the collection of sensory information. Since most behavior is driven by memories of sensory experiences, presently occurring stimuli, or sensation that is anticipated, the therapist can evaluate an individual's sensory systems in the context of task performance through careful planning.

A fourth principle is that *interdisciplinary team members can be a very important source of information regarding sensory processing*. Information gathered by other team members from their own philosophical perspectives can provide additional data which enables therapists to make accurate decisions about the integrity of an individual's sensory systems. When members of the team act collaboratively, the individual benefits from a more integrated program.

ASSESSMENT METHODS

Assessment takes many forms. For this review, assessments will be discussed within four categories for each sensory system: (1) collection of the initial data base, (2) formal assessment procedures, (3) clinical assessment procedures, and (4) interview procedures.

The initial data base can include the referral complaint, the description surrounding the referral complaint, medical records, and information regarding the exact location of lesions. This information is analyzed for its potential contribution to occupational therapy assessment.

Formal assessment procedures are available to occupational therapists to evaluate aspects of sensory processing. Since therapists observe external behavior, most of these tools assess more than sensory processing. Therefore, multiple observations will be required to isolate the functions of a sensory system. A number of formal assessments routinely used by occupational therapists contain sensory components even though they evaluate other components. Table 18-1 provides a brief overview of the sensory components of selected instruments. As can be seen in Table 18-1, there are only a few formal assessments designed and tested on adults. Thus, occupational therapists who work with adults must rely more heavily on other types of data collection.

In addition to formal assessment procedures, there are a number of *clinical assessment techniques* and skilled observations that can be used to identify the sensory components of performance. The therapist can determine the individual's ability to notice various sensations by only requiring simple responses to isolated input. In this chapter, these direct sensory evaluation procedures will be outlined for each system. But this in itself is not a sufficient level of data collection. Skilled observational techniques will also be presented as an effective method of obtaining sensory data. Participation in daily life tasks presents many opportunities for receiving and responding to sensation. Examples will be presented to elucidate the components of task performance which can indicate sensory involvement. Please refer to Table 18-2 for examples of the sensory components of daily life tasks.

Nelson (1984) describes the observational process:

> "Evaluation through activity analysis and activity synthesis demands strong observational skills. Observation is not just a passive process. It is a dynamic process involving an interplay between taking in information and questioning the meaning of what is taken in. The questioning part of the process helps shape subsequent observations, and the subsequent observations lead to new kinds of questions. The observer must strike a balance between an ability to look at the phenomena in a directed way and a willingness to take in new information or to be surprised by unanticipated data" (p. 117).

Nelson (1984) goes on to suggest that the therapist must consider the objective properties and the purpose of the task for normal individuals in order to interpret both the typical reactions of diagnostic groups and the responses of a specific individual.

A final method for obtaining sensory data is through the *interviewing process.* Although this is not a direct evaluation technique, the information provided from good interviews can be invaluable in planning an intervention program that will be effective for the individual and the family members. The information gathered from an interview enables the occupational therapist to determine not only the individual characteristics, but also the style and preferences of the family members and other professionals who may be dealing with this individual. Teachers, clients, family members, and other team members are all appropriate persons from whom to gather interview data.

Throughout this chapter, behaviors are described as indicators of the integrity of the sensory systems. The same behaviors can also be indicative of other problems, including motor dysfunction; poor motivation or attention; perceptual, cognitive or language problems; or even lack of experience. Therefore, it is imperative that hypotheses regarding any system be confirmed with multiple assessments and skilled observations. Corroboration of problems across settings and tasks strengthens the therapist's decisions for intervention planning.

ASSESSMENTS FOR SPECIFIC SENSORY SYSTEMS

The Olfactory and Gustatory Systems

The olfactory and gustatory systems are primitive sensory mechanisms which contribute to similar task performance areas, and therefore will be discussed together in a more generalized format. It will not be common for a referral complaint to focus specifically on the olfactory or gustatory systems. When trauma has occurred to these systems, other problems are frequently more prominent.

From a neurological standpoint, the olfactory system is at-risk for damage if the base of the frontal lobe has been injured or if the area around the eyes or nose has been traumatized. The olfactory system has connections with the hypothalamus and the arousal mechanisms of the limbic system. The gustatory system is at-risk for dysfunction if involvement includes brain stem lesions, as the cranial nerves that serve taste have their connections in the pons and medulla.

Olfactory assessment procedures are gross in nature and the therapist expects a generalized response. To detect general responsiveness to smell, therapists generally use small containers of very strong odors such as oil of peppermint, smelling salts, or vinegar. Even comatose patients can produce a reflexive postural shift in response to very strong odors. Stimuli such as these should be used with caution while carefully observing the individual's reactions. Ability to arouse to a strong olfactory stimulus indicates some, albeit a very low, level of **responsivity** in the central nervous system (CNS).

Researchers have long recognized the specific taste patterns for the tongue, with sweet, salty, sour, and bitter tastes most densely represented on specific portions of the tongue. Additionally, people lose many of the taste receptors (as many as 60%) in the senior years leading to reports of taste differences (Coren, Porac & Ward, 1984). However, testing for the presence of this pattern on the tongue is usually inappropriate, since it has no direct relationship to functional performance (Coren, Porac & Ward, 1984).

Table 18-1
Summary of Sensory Components of Tests Used by Occupational Therapists

Test Name	Sensory/Perceptual Subtest	Sensory Areas Addressed*							Age Group	Diagnosis	Validity	Reliability	Norms
		O	G	A	Vis	S	Ves	P					
Balcones Sensory Integration Screening	finger to nose standing balance visual motor forms arm postures stereognosis tactile graphics				X X X	 X X	X	X X X	primary grades	learning neuro- logical behavior			130 children 6-9 years
Beery Developmental Test of Visual Motor Integration					X				2-15 yrs	develop- mental neuro- logical LD	construct	interrater	1039 normal
DeGangi-Berk Test of Sensory Integration	postural control items						X	X	3-5 yrs	develop- mental delays	construct	test-retest	101 normal 38 delayed
Marianne Frostig Developmental Test of Visual Perception	all subtests				X				4-8 yrs	learning problems	predic- tive	test-retest	100 normal
Miller Assessment for Preschoolers	Foundations Index Coordination Index Complex Task Index Behaviors & Observations				X X	X X	 X	X X X X	2 yrs 9 mo-5 yrs	develop- mental at-risk	criterion- relation	test-retest	1200 normal
Motor free Visual Perception Test	all subtests				X				4-8 yrs	all types	construct	test-retest	881 normal 22 states
Sensory Integration and Praxis Tests	visual subtests somatosensory subtests				X	 X		 X	4-9 yrs	learning & behavior problems	construct criterion content	test-retest interrater	1997 children

Therapists usually identify problems with olfactory or gustatory centers through behavioral observations at meal time, including frequent complaints from the individual that the food is bland or observing the person over-seasoning food. Table 18-2 gives a list of observations that reflect both olfactory and gustatory components of daily life tasks.

Ayres & Tickle (1980) report on a study with autistic children in which they constructed a test for reactivity to sensory stimuli. One olfactory and one gustatory reaction were observed within the test of 14 items. Orange peel, vanilla bean, and vinegar were used to test olfaction. They observed the children to determine whether they: (a) did not notice the stimuli, (b) noticed it only some, or (c) displayed a negative reaction to any of the stimuli. To test gustatory response, the therapists interviewed parents to determine the children's response to the taste of specific foods. This represents a simple method designed by therapists to evaluate sensory responsiveness.

The Somatosensory System

Initial Data Base. Since the somatosensory system path- ways travel from all body surfaces into the spinal cord and up through the brain stem to the cortex, this system can be at-risk with peripheral or central nervous system dysfunc- tion at any level. The initial data base may describe behaviors which trigger the therapist's thinking toward a somatosensory-based problem. For example, hypersensitiv-

Table 18-1 (continued)
Summary of Sensory Components of Tests Used by Occupational Therapists

Test Name	Sensory/Perceptual Subtest	O	G	A	Vis	S	Ves	P	Age Group	Diagnosis	Validity	Reliability	Norms
Quick Neurological Screen Test	figure recognition and production palm form recognition sound patterns double simultaneous stimuli arm & leg extension stand on one leg behavior irregularities			X X	X X	X X X	X	X X	5 yrs+	neuro-logical	interrater	test-retest	1231 normal 1008 LD
Southern California Postrotary Nystagmus Test							X		5-9 yrs	learning problems		interrater	226 normal
Southern California Sensory Integration Tests	visual subtests somatosensory subtests				X	X		X	4-8 yrs 11 mo for sensory tests	learning problems		test-retest	somato 953 normal visual 240 normal
Test of Visual Motor Skills					X				4-12 yrs 11 mo	learning problems	content criterion	internal consis-tency	1000+ normal
Test of Visual Perceptual Skills (non-motor)	all subtests				X				4-12 yrs 11 mo	learning problems	content criterion	internal consis-tency	962 normal

* O=Olfactory G=Gustatory A=Auditory Vis=Visual S=Somatosensory Ves=Vestibular P=Proprioceptive
This information was compiled from the following sources: Keyser, D.J. & Sweetland, R.C. (Ed.) (1984) *Test critiques*. Test Corporation of America, Kansas City; Sweetland, R.C. & Keyser, D.J. (1986) *Tests*. Test Corporation of America, Kansas City; Mitchell, J.V. (Ed.) (1985). *The Ninth mental measurement yearbook*. The Buros Institute of Mental Measurements, Lincoln, NB; King-Thomas, L. & Hacker, B.J. (Eds.) (1987). *A therapist's guide to pediatric assessment*. Little, Brown & Co., Boston; Compton, C. (1984). *A guide to 75 tests for special education*. Fearon Education, Belmont, CA; Sattler, J.M. (1982). *Assessment of children's intelligence and special abilities* (2nd Ed.). Allyn and Bacon, Inc., Boston. Ayres, J. (1989). *Sensory integration and praxis tests manual*. Los Angeles: Western Psychological Services. Test manuals were used when they could be obtained.

ity to touch may be noted in the person's agitated, hyper-reactive or distractible behavior in situations. At the other extreme, the individual may be unresponsive to touch experiences; this may be reported as a lack of responsiveness to or awareness of environmental conditions such as closeness of others or clothing.

Formal Assessment. Five of the tests presented in Table 18-1 contain specific somatosensory subtests. The *Quick Neurological Screening Test* (QNST) contains three somatosensory items: palm-form recognition, double simultaneous stimuli, and behavioral irregularities. *Palm-form recognition* requires the individual to recognize numbers drawn on the hand. *Double simultaneous stimuli* asks the individ-

ual to recognize stimuli to the hand and face at the same time. *Behavioral irregularities* include perseveration, tactile defensiveness, fidgeting, and **distractibility.** Each of these is an adaptation of the classic sensory tasks used in clinical neurological assessment. The therapist obtains a gross measure of responsiveness to stimuli with these items.

The Southern California Sensory Integration Test Battery (SCSIT) contains the following five somatosensory subtests, which tap several types of touch stimuli. *Finger identification and localization of tactile stimuli* require the child to find the place being touched and are a more gross awareness of input through light-touch receptors. *Double tactile stimuli* (DTS) perception requires the child to simultaneously identify touches to hands and face (in all

Table 18-2
Summary of General Considerations When Observing Sensory Components of Daily Life Tasks

R = Response
T = Tolerance
W = Willingness

	General	Personal Hygiene	Dressing
Somatosensory	R to touch W to touch/be touched R to types of tactile experiences	R to water T of washcloth/towel R to hairwashing/hair drying R to toothbrush/paste W to wipe self after toileting	R to clothing items R to textures variety of clothing worn R to donning/removing clothing T for accessories (e.g., bracelets, scarves)
Proprioceptive	T for prolonged activity Presence of joint stability Use of external support Ability to accurately reach and grasp	T for standing at sink T for standing in shower Presence of propping	T for task completion Presence for anti-gravity movements T for manipulating heavy objects (e.g., boots)
Vestibular	R to movement W to choose movement R to types of movement Presence of postural stability T for variety of positions	W to bend over sink W to use lower drawers W to bend down to wash legs	W to bend down for socks W to use lower drawers Presence of variety of movement
Visual	R to light, colors R to busy visual environment T for high contrast or low contrast environment	Ability to locate items in drawer T for disarray on sink Ability to place toothpaste on brush	Ability to position clothing on body Ability to find buttons Ability to find clothing in closet Ability to find items in drawers T for disarray in drawers
Auditory	R to sounds T for background noise R to various voices Ability to carry on conversation while engaged in tasks	T for sound of hair dryer T for running water T for flushing	T for accessories which produce sound (e.g., bracelets, necklaces) T for squeaky shoes
Olfactory/Gustatory	R to tastes R to smells T of tastes/smells Attention to odors	R to toothpaste/mouthwash R to soap smell T for cologne Ability to notice body odors	Ability to notice dirty clothes (odors)

This table provides a general framework for skillfully observing the sensory components of daily life tasks. The items included represent examples of the behaviors that might be observed. Keep in mind the category within which the behavior is listed to determine why you are watching the performance. For example, "response to toothpaste" in the somatosensory category refers to the texture of the paste in the mouth, while in the olfactory/gustatory category it refers to the taste and smell of the paste. Abnormal behavior can occur at either extreme; an individual can over react to stimuli or seem unresponsive to stimuli. Record behaviors accordingly. Also remember that all behaviors can indicate a number of problem areas; multiple observations enable accurate conclusions.

Table 18-2 (continued)
Summary of General Considerations When Observing Sensory Components of Daily Life Tasks

R = Response
T = Tolerance
W = Willingness

Eating	Home Making	School Work/ Job Performance	Play/Leisure Activities
R to food textures/temperatures R to utensils in mouth W to eat fingerfood W to use utensils R to food on face	W to use hands to prepare food W to clean surfaces T of dirt/food on skin T of various household cleaners on skin	T for position of writing utensil T of glue, tape on skin T for sitting at desk R to closeness of others R to pats for reinforcement R to textures in environment Ability to type without watching hands	Pattern of task choices Presence of textures T for group activities Appropriate use of objects
Presence of leaning on table T for completion of meal Ability to cut meat T for lifting heavy objects	T for lifting heavy objects T for standing to work Presence of leaning/propping at work space Ability to pour T for task completion	Presence of leaning, propping T for task completion T for carrying books T for strength/endurance activities T for prolonged position	T for task completion Pattern of task choices T for running, jumping T for strength, endurance
W to bend head down to eat Ability to stay in chair	T for bending to dust/vacuum T for learning to empty dishwasher Ability to perform bilateral tasks	Presence of consistency in work Ability to negotiate body in space Ability to remain stable in chair W to engage in movement Presence of coordinated movement W to use stairs	Presence of organized movement Pattern of task choices Presence of postural control W to engage in movement W to jump off stable surface W to roughhouse W to climb
Ability to locate items on table T for same color foods and plate	Ability to find items in drawer Ability to notice dust/dirt T for disorder/disarray	T for clutter Ability to keep place on page Ability to remember what is seen Ability to follow map Ability to follow visual plan Ability to find way T for written work, directions	Pattern of task choice T for multiple images T for clutter
R to requests to pass foods Ability to track conversations T for extraneous sounds	T for sound of vacuum W to play radio or TV during tasks R level to others during tasks	T for background noise R to specific noises T for unexpected sounds Ability to accurately follow conversation Ability to follow oral directions T for quiet or mumbled talking	Pattern of task choice T for completing auditory environment
R to taste of food W to season food Ability to identify food being cooked	Ability to identify cooking food Ability to notice household odors Ability to properly season foods T for household cleaners	Ability to notice work/school odors R to *scratch-n-sniff* stickers Interest in smells/tastes of non-food objects T for strong odors R to glue on envelopes	Pattern of task choices Presence of odors/tastes Appropriate use of smell/taste to explore objects

possible combinations) and seems to tap another gross, protective function of the central nervous system. *Graphesthesia* (GRA) and *Manual Form Perception* (MFP) are more complex tasks, requiring an integration of somatosensory, visual, and motor skills. For GRA, the child retraces shapes drawn on the back of the hand without vision. Although the initial stimulus is somatosensory, the child must have some mechanism for capturing a mental image of the form and figuring out how to recreate it in motor movements. Failure on this subtest alone would be insufficient evidence to conclude the origin of the problem. MFP utilizes **stereognosis** in requiring that children manipulate geometric forms without seeing them and asking them to identify a matching visual image. The complexities of the requirements of GRA and MFP also make these subtests more applicable to learning tasks which require integration of input for a well-designed response.

Ayres (1986) reviewed the neuroscience literature on **praxis** and identified a number of approaches to assessing praxis. This and other material have been used to design a revision of the SCSIT, called the *Sensory Integration and Praxis Tests* (SIPT). Many of the sensory components from the original SCSIT have been retained, but several were improved to facilitate administration or broaden subtest focus. In relation to somatosensory subtests, DTS was eliminated because of the gross nature of its results and poor discriminatory ability with older children. MFP was expanded significantly to include a second section in which the child matches one tactile form with another by touch instead of vision. This expansion enables the therapist to compare visual and somatosensory searching. The combination of refined sensory subtests and expanded testing of several types of praxis on the SIPT will enable occupational therapists to investigate the relationship between sensory processing and task performance in a more systematic way.

The Miller Assessment for Preschoolers (MAP) contains two subtests and supplemental observations of somatosensory responsiveness. Stereognosis requires the child to identify objects placed in the hand without vision. Finger localization requires the child to identify the finger that has been touched. These two items contribute to the Foundations Index. Response to touch is a skilled supplemental observation.

The Balcones Sensory Integration Screening (Balcones) was designed to identify those children who might have sensory integration difficulties prior to a full diagnostic assessment. The somatosensory contributions to this screening test include tactile graphics, a subtest similar to graphesthesia on the SCSIT, SIPT, and stereognosis.

Clinical Assessment and Skilled Observations. There is some controversy regarding the appropriate use of clinical

assessment of the somatosensory system. Some authors have reported very detailed methods for assessing and recording somatosensory integrity, especially in relation to the hand (e.g., Callahan, 1984). However, Dellon (1981) states that somatosensory testing should be limited to those procedures that are related to function, a philosophy which is quite compatible with occupational therapy philosophy. It is useful to know the classic methods of somatosensory assessment so that one might apply this knowledge to functional assessment.

Assessment of Skin Integrity. Skilled observations of skin surface integrity can provide initial data regarding sensibility. Callahan (1984) reports on sympathetic nervous system reactions which affect skin integrity and correlate to sensory innervations. Skin temperature, color, and edema that differ from intact regions are warning signals; more obvious changes occur longer after the injury such as rosy-colored to mottled skin or warm to cool skin. Sweating may be diminished and the skin may feel less elastic, and have less texture. Hair may fall out or may change in relation to intact areas. Skin may be more susceptible to injuries.

Assessment of the somatosensory system using the **dermatome** map has been widely discussed in the literature (e.g., Heimer, 1983; Noback & Demerest, 1981; Chusid, 1985). In this procedure, the clinician applies a variety of stimuli to the surface regions of the skin to identify which regions are responsive to which stimuli. Originally professionals used dermatome testing as partial evidence for localization of a spinal cord injury since the dermatomes generally correspond to spinal nerve levels. All body surfaces respond to all types of sensation, so complete dermatome testing would include temperature, light touch, two-point discrimination, localization of touch, and sharp-dull perception. For example, if an individual demonstrates paralysis on a portion of the upper extremity, dermatome testing would be completed along the entire upper extremity to determine at what level each sensation can or cannot be processed. Bell (1984a) and Callahan (1984) provide an excellent introduction to sensibility testing of the hand, which contains more detail than is possible to include in this presentation.

For *temperature* testing, the therapist can use two test tubes, one containing hot water and the other containing cold water, alternating the use of each stimulus while asking the individual to report the hot or cold sensation. The therapist must be sure to keep the stimulus on the body surface long enough to allow a temperature change to occur on the skin; Callahan (1984) suggests a one-second time period.

The *Ninhydrin* test and the wrinkle test seem to correlate with pain and temperature findings, suggesting that all these functions are supported by the same neurological processes (Dellon, 1981). The Ninhydrin test requires the therapist to take an impression of a clean hand onto bond paper. The paper is then treated with chemicals to reveal presence of sweat on the impression (Callahan, 1984). In the wrinkle test, the hand is submerged in warm water to observe whether wrinkling will occur. Denervated regions are thought not to wrinkle or sweat, but there is conflicting evidence regarding this finding (Callahan, 1984). Suggested uses include testing of children and unreliable persons who may be poor reporters.

Sharp and dull sensations can be tested with an open safety pin, using the tip as the sharp stimulus and the head as the dull stimulus. Pain from a pinch may be an early sign of sensory recovery (Callahan, 1984). Callahan (1984) suggests that the sharp-dull dichotomy is a more accurate test than merely testing for pain. As with the temperature testing, the individual is given alternating stimuli and asked to identify which one is felt.

Light touch stimuli can be produced with soft bristles of a brush or with a cotton ball, eraser, or therapist's fingertip to the surface of the skin (Callahan, 1984). The individual reports when the sensation is felt. Bell (1984a) reports that hand function can still remain intact when light touch processing is diminished. More complex somatosensory processing skills can still be intact (e.g., graphesthesia and stereognosis). Deep pressure sensation falls along this continuum, being stimulated by more firm application of stimuli. These tests are imprecise because calibration has not been reliably identified across examiners (Callahan, 1984). The most objective currently available instrument for testing light touch and deep pressure is the *Semmes-Weinstein Pressure Aesthesiometer Testing Set* (Research Designs, Inc., 7320 Ashcroft, Suite 103, Houston, TX 77081) (Bell, 1984a; Callahan, 1984). The 20 filaments are varying sizes and are therefore variably resistant to pressure. The tester presses the tip of the filament directly into the skin surface until the filament bows, and responsivity to the stimulus is noted. Early correlations with functional outcomes are promising (Bell, 1984b).

Basic somatosensory reactivity of autistic children has been tested using four types of stimuli (Ayres & Tickle, 1980). Light touch was evaluated in two ways. First, researchers recorded whether these children reacted to the stimulus of an air puff to the back of the neck. Then they recorded the children's reaction to touch from persons or objects in the environment. Defensive reactions to these encounters was considered hyper-reactive. Touch-pressure was evaluated by placing a large bolster or mat over the children and pressing down firmly. Avoidance of this stimulation was considered hyper-reactivity and seeking out deeper pressure and more frequent experiences of this

nature was considered hypo-reactivity. Pain was evaluated through judgments regarding children's reactions to bumps and falls. These observations provide an example of a simple framework for assessing somatosensory responses in a population that does not respond well to structured formal assessment.

An object with blunt tip(s) such as the unfolded ends of a paper clip have been frequently used for both *localization* and *two-point discrimination*, but Callahan (1984, pp. 420-421) does not recommend this procedure, describing it as imprecise. She recommends the Boley gauge or the DeMayo 2-point discrimination device because they are calibrated for more accurate reporting. In localization testing, the individual must identify one location that has been touched. In two-point discrimination, the individual must distinguish between the presence of one or two stimuli. The therapist asks the individual to report whether one or two stimuli are present, while alternating the single stimulus and the double stimuli. Stimuli are provided with pressure light enough to produce initial skin blanching (Callahan, 1984).

In order to refine two-point discrimination data, the therapist adjusts the distance between the double stimuli during testing, to identify the amount of distance needed between the two stimuli before the individual perceives that two are present. Two-point discrimination addresses the sensitivity of overlapping **receptive fields** on the body surface. One expects a very small distance between the two points on the hand, fingertips, and face because of the great overlap of receptive fields, while one would expect a larger distance between the two points on the back where there is small overlap of receptive fields. (Refer to Chapter 9 for an explanation of the neurological constructs which underlie this testing method.) Chusid (1985, p. 475) reports that an individual normally can perceive a 0.3 to 0.6 centimeter distance on the finger tips, 1.5 to 2 centimeters on the palms of the hands and soles of the feet, and 3 to 4 centimeters on the dorsum of the hand and the shin area of the leg. Callahan (1984) describes another device, the *sensitometer*, which measures tactile responsivity by asking the individual to report when a ridge of increasing depth is felt on the skin surface. This test seems to correlate with the two-point discrimination (Callahan, 1984).

When examining the hand, Dellon (1981) suggests using a vibration test and a *moving two-point discrimination* test, stating that they are reliable measures related to recovery of functional hand skill. The vibration test requires that one tine of the vibrating tuning fork be placed on the tip of the finger to identify whether this vibratory sense is being received by the nerve cells. Please note that this procedure is somewhat different than vibratory testing over the body which recommends placing the base of the tuning fork on bony prominences (Chusid, 1985). There is greater vibration on the ends of the tuning fork, increasing the possibility of response through the fleshy tissue of the fingertips. By identifying where the vibration is felt and at what point it can be processed correctly, the clinician can identify how the neurons are recovering in that region. Vibration seems quite sensitive to any type of nerve trauma, and so can be an indicator of both initial loss and level of recovery.

The moving two-point discrimination test is similar to the classic two-point discrimination test except that the stimuli are simultaneously moved along the surface of the skin. Bell (1984a) reports that the moving two-point discrimination test suffers from the same uncontrollable variable as other surface tests: pressure control is difficult to maintain which makes interpretation more complicated. The therapist cannot be sure whether findings are related to two-point discrimination or pressure changes which occur as the therapist applies stimuli to the skin. The moving stimuli enable a variety of receptive fields to identify the sensation. When different nerves are stimulated at the same time, (across dermatomes) the brain intercepts the input as spatially oriented (e.g., where it is on the body surface). When successive receptive fields of the same nerve are stimulated, the brain interprets the input as temporally oriented. Dellon (1981) reports that in a normal hand one can discriminate the two moving stimuli when they are 2 millimeters apart.

Stereognosis is another form of sensory testing. In this test, a common object is placed in the individual's hand and the individual is asked to explore the object without vision and then identify the object. This skill requires not only somatosensory processing, but also perceptual organization and language. If an individual has difficulty with stereognosis, all the variables which comprise this complex task must be further analyzed. In this case, the individual may have a language problem which prohibits the production of the correct word to name the object, or there may be perceptual disorganization which precludes correct identification of the object. Alternative methods of testing can be used to narrow these possibilities. Photographs of the items can be provided so the individual can point to the correct item instead of naming it; several objects can be placed within reach so the individual can find the one that matches the item being tested. Documentation of procedural changes helps to isolate the exact nature of the problem. Dellon (1981) adapted Moberg's picking-up test by requiring motor skill to manipulate the small common objects and language skills to identify them. This is another version of a stereognosis measure that utilizes manipulation skills and language.

Bell (1984a) describes the functional implications of sensory integrity of the hand. She outlines five levels of sensory integrity: normal touch, diminished light touch, diminished protective sensation, loss of protective sensation, and untestable. Individuals whose performance would fall into the first two categories (normal touch and diminished light touch) have good hand function because more complex sensory abilities such as stereognosis and graphesthesia are intact. Hand use will be difficult for those in the third category (diminished protective sensation); the person will drop objects, complain of weakness, and need sensory re-education. Persons in the fourth and fifth categories (loss of protective sensation and untestable) will have extreme difficulty using the hands. Vision will be required for object use; extra safety procedures are necessary due to loss of temperature sensation.

Functional Application of Assessment Principles. Although *dermatome testing* certainly outlines the capability of processing somatosensory information, some experts question the need for this level of detail in testing for most rehabilitation circumstances. Dellon (1981), who discusses the recovery of function in the hand, suggests that sensory evaluation only be done in relation to the individual's ability to use that body part for functional activity. This author further comments that it is a poor use of an individual's time and financial resources to complete a somatosensory evaluation, if that information will have no impact on knowledge of functional ability as an outcome.

For example, one might question the utility of an assessment which merely identifies sensory change without relating it to task performance. Occupational therapists strive to improve task performance for functional life activities, and so must also consider appropriate assessment situations which link the integrity of sensation with task performance (Callahan, 1984). There may be situations in which classic dermatome testing is appropriate, such as just after an injury for the purpose of determining sensory loss, prognosis, and course of recovery. Later in the recovery process dermatome testing may aid in determination of disability compensation (Callahan, 1984).

Many times it is necessary to compare the integrity of the sensory and motor systems to determine the appropriate therapeutic intervention. If motor systems are functioning poorly while sensation remains intact, intervention is directed at such factors as coordination, control, and endurance. But if sensation appears to be the source of performance problems, adaptations in environmental conditions or activities to facilitate sensory processing would be more important. Moberg (1966) describes the clinical criteria for hand function in relation to *precision sensory grip* and *gross sensory grip* both of which require constant contact of hand surfaces with objects in the environment and a motor action. Precision sensory grip would include movements such as screwing on a bolt, sewing with a needle, or buttoning.

Gross sensory grip would include holding a handle of a cart, turning a doorknob, carrying a bucket or basket, or holding onto a bottle or can. Moberg (1966) found that two-point discrimination was closely aligned with these grip skills.

The *face and oral motor structures* also depict an interdependent sensorimotor system. The fifth cranial nerve (trigeminal) serves sensation for the face and has the same components as the sensory nerves that serve the body, for example. When an individual has difficulties with language, questions arise about the type of problem that exists. The problem can involve internal central nervous system structures which are unable to process language effectively, the motor systems which produce the sounds, or the sensory systems which provide input and feedback from the oral motor structures.

When the sensory areas of the oral motor structures are involved, the motor systems are technically intact, but functionally the individual has difficulty forming speech sounds. When the dentist administers anesthesia the sensory neurons of the face and jaw are paralyzed. The actions of the motor system are significantly altered during this time; movements of the mouth become labored and deliberate, and speech becomes more difficult to understand. The sensory mechanisms within the oral structures greatly influence the ability to produce correct speech and language.

Direct sensory evaluation of the outside of the mouth can include dermatome testing because the mouth is extremely well innervated and therefore very sensitive to various types of stimuli. Evaluation of the mouth internally includes identifying the individual's capacity for receiving objects into the mouth, including straws, spoons, and food. One can also observe during eating to determine whether certain textures or temperatures are aversive, whether the food is moved around in the mouth effectively, and whether proper closure of the mouth is achieved for these tasks. Poor mouth closure can be related to poor sensory integrity of the lips and tongue which in turn can affect muscle tone and motor control (sensorimotor system, see Chapter 9). If one does not move food around in the mouth or avoids textures, the individual may be avoiding these touch experiences. Additional information about the sensory mechanisms of the mouth can be obtained through good interviewing techniques which will be discussed in the next section.

The earliest movements of infants are in response to touch. Primitive reflexes enable the infant to have beginning interactions with the environment. Touching the face elicits the *rooting reflex*, which is the reflex of the infant searching for the nipple to suck. Touch to the palm and plantar surfaces of the hands and feet elicits a grasping response. As the infant grows older, these patterns of movement become integrated into goal-directed behavior.

Assessment of reflex responses in comparison to chronological and developmental ages contributes to the sensory picture, especially in infants and young children.

Many self-care and personal hygiene activities provide an opportunity to observe responses to tactile input (Ayres, 1980; Royeen, 1986). The individual may avoid or display discomfort with water splashing on the body, especially the face. The textures of the soap, washcloth, or towel might elicit a negative reaction. Both hair washing and hair brushing can be especially upsetting due to both the intensity and variety of stimuli provided during this activity and the high ratio of innervation to the head area. The individual may also react negatively to ear cleaning.

During dressing, the texture and fit of clothing are often important. Pulling socks on may be uncomfortable and texture may be a significant variable, with fuzzier socks being less desirable. The individual may insist upon wearing the same clothing over and over again, even when they don't fit well. Frequently, individuals with poor ability to process tactile input tend to wear clothing which decreases opportunities for random, unpredictable sensation such as long-sleeved shirts, extra jackets (even when hot) and long pants, all of which decrease the amount of accessible skin surfaces. Kitchen activities also provide opportunities to observe somatosensory responsiveness. Responses to hand-washing and to various textures of foods and utensils allow the therapist to observe defensive reactions. It is frequently difficult for the individual to complete food preparation without many interruptions as defensive reactions continuously interfere with ongoing task performance. For example, if the individual is preparing cookies, the activity may be stopped each time dough gets on the individual's hands, so that the dough can be wiped off. This would significantly increase the time taken to finish making the cookies and might even lead to a very agitated, hyperactive state. Other life tasks specific to the individual might also be observed.

Many leisure activities involve somatosensory processing, such as gardening and sewing. The therapist can observe during these tasks as well to detect any negative reactions to tactile input. These observations are most significant when they clearly interfere with task performance. Table 18-2 lists examples of somatosensory components of daily life tasks.

Interviewing. A number of interviewing strategies have been designed which provide helpful information regarding somatosensory processing. Callahan (1984) cautions that questions should be phrased in such a way as to avoid leading the individual to the desired answer.

Ayres (1980) constructed a checklist of behaviors which indicate tactile defensiveness. Royeen (1986) refined this information and designed a self-reporting touch scale for

---

Table 18-3
Touch Scale for Tactile Defensiveness

Responses: no, a little, a lot.

1. Does it bother you to go barefooted?
2. Do fuzzy shirts bother you?
3. Do fuzzy socks bother you?
4. Do turtleneck shirts bother you?
5. Does it bother you to have your face washed?
6. Does it bother you to have your nails cut?
7. Does it bother you to have your hair combed by someone else?
8. Does it bother you to play on a carpet?
9. After someone touches you, do you feel like scratching that spot?
10. After someone touches you, do you feel like rubbing that spot?
11. Does it bother you to walk barefooted in the grass and sand?
12. Does getting dirty bother you?
13. Do you find it hard to pay attention?
14. Does it bother you if you cannot see who is touching you?
15. Does fingerpainting bother you?
16. Do rough bedsheets bother you?
17. Do you like to touch people but it bothers you if they touch you back?
18. Does it bother you when people come from behind?
19. Does it bother you to be kissed by someone other than your parents?
20. Does it bother you to be hugged or held?
21. Does it bother you to play games with your feet?
22. Does it bother you to have your face touched?
23. Does it bother you to be touched if you don't expect it?
24. Do you have difficulty making friends?
25. Does it bother you to stand in line?
26. Does it bother you when someone is close by?

From Royeen, C.B. (1986). The development of a touch scale for measuring tactile defensiveness in children. American Journal of Occupational Therapy, June, 40(6), p. 417.

---

tactile defensiveness. Table 18-3 lists the 26 items on this scale. She originally designed a 49-item scale and administered it to 80 normal and 22 tactually-defensive children. Twenty-six items remained after item analysis, and this scale classified the children correctly 85% of the time. As can be seen in Table 18-3, a large variety of tasks were included in the scale. More recently, Royeen (1987) reported good test-retest reliability with a pilot sample of children.

Melendez (1978) designed both a child and an adult neuropsychological questionnaire which includes a number of items that tap sensory processing. He suggests that information be gathered regarding the onset, progression, and frequency of pain; the presence of numbness; and uncontrollable excitability. This information would be used as baseline data to determine what further assessment might be necessary. Questions such as these are directed more towards diagnosis of central nervous system problems than towards determination of functional ability.

Additional behaviors might be reported by caregivers or other professionals. *Avoidance* behaviors might be elicited by messy material such as sand in a sandbox, food on dirty dishes in the sink, or lotion for skin. There may be reports from others' observations of aggression without apparent cause, thus suggesting that fight or flight responses are occurring more frequently than one would expect. There may be reports of an inordinate number of bumps and bruises, or the individual may seem overly concerned about very small or "invisible injuries." Oral-motor region sensitivity may be reflected in reports of eating problems, especially in regard to textures and temperatures, or in complaints regarding oral hygiene or dental work.

Individuals who are hyposensitive to touch will fail to notice or seek tactile input. Family members, caregivers and teachers may notice behaviors that indicate a craving for input. They may report that many objects go into the mouth, or that the individual touches or rubs on certain surfaces. Hands may be very active in exploration of objects in the immediate environment. The individual may become bothersome to others by getting too close to people or by remaining in physical contact too long. At extreme levels, high thresholds for touch may be manifested in more aggressive actions such as head banging or self-biting.

All of the behaviors reported by caregivers and professionals as described above are important because they interfere with ongoing goal-directed activity. When an individual seeks or avoids touch (a constant source of stimulation in our environment), interruptions in task performance are inevitable. The occupational therapist organizes both direct intervention and suggestions to others to minimize the effects of somatosensory interference and improve the individual's ability to respond appropriately to touch experiences during functional activities.

The Proprioceptive System

Initial Data Base. When the initial data base includes comments about poor tolerance for activity, the proprioceptors may be dysfunctional. It may be reported that the individual tires easily or has a difficult time maintaining a singular posture for a period of time. This can include simple postures such as sitting at a desk or propping on forearms. These types of observations suggest that muscle tone cannot support normal activity, which can be due to poor proprioceptive feedback from the joints and muscles. If work samples are provided as part of the referral complaint, the occupational therapist can analyze this material for its sensory components. For example, written work may reveal very light or extreme pressure on the paper as indicated by the texture of the line. There may be a change in the quality of the writing from the beginning to the end which might indicate rapid fatigue for the task.

Formal Assessment.   The formal assessments which contain proprioceptive components include both position in space and postural control items. Motor performance is a significant parameter for observation of proprioceptive integrity because the sensory receptors are responsive to changes in muscle, tendon, and joint activity. The *De-Gangi-Berk Test of Sensory Integration* (Berk & DeGangi; 1983a, 1983b) contains postural control items which can indicate both proprioceptive and postural integrity. As discussed above, hypermobility at the joints or inability to maintain postures can indicate poor proprioceptive feedback, but these observations must also be consistent with referral complaints and other skilled observations to lead to that conclusion.

The *Quick Neurological Screening Test* contains two items from which proprioceptive information can be gleaned. Arm and leg extension requires ongoing tension in the muscles which is supported by proprioceptive feedback. Standing on one leg is a balance test which also requires efficient proprioceptor action to maintain the position.

The SCSIT has a number of motor subtests which might be related to proprioceptive function, but this battery also contains a subtest called *kinesthesia* (KIN) which was designed specifically to assess proprioception. In this subtest, the examiner moves the child's pointed finger through the air from one location to another with vision occluded. The child must then return to the first location without assistance. This task requires memory of the arm and hand positions that represented the original location. Accuracy of location is recorded for scoring. The SIPT also uses the KIN subtest to evaluate proprioception. The *Miller Assessment for Preschoolers* contains four items in the Foundations Index and supplemental observations which evaluate proprioceptive feedback: (1) the child is asked to move finger to nose, (2) to stand still with feet together, (3) to maintain the supine flexion position, and (4) to maintain the kneel-stand position. Supplemental observations include reporting of quality of movement patterns. Each of these items requires ongoing feedback from the muscles,

joints, and tendons. Poor ability to position the body correctly is thought to be related to poor proprioceptive feedback. The Balcones contains similar items described on other tests (arm postures and standing balance).

Clinical Assessment and Skilled Observations.   Body position testing assesses the individual's ability to identify limb position in space without vision. The individual is either blindfolded or asked to keep the eyes closed while the limbs are placed in various positions in space; the individual is then asked to identify the limb position. Fingers and toes can also be positioned by holding the sides between joints and moving the finger or toe up and down. The therapist can suggest target words such as "up," "down," "in front of," "over," and "behind." These cueing words are helpful to clarify the request while minimizing the effects of language on the task. When one positions a limb in space, the receptors within the joints, tendons, ends of muscles and skin surfaces fire to allow recognition of the limb in space. Dellon (1981) suggests that the cutaneous receptors that respond to skin stretching and repositioning also play a critical role in body position **perception.** Knowledge of body position has also been shown to correlate with two-point discrimination.

A number of clinical tests reported in the literature for equilibrium and cerebellar function provide another means for observation of both proprioceptive and vestibular processing. DeQuiros and Schrager (1978) report on the tests of Romberg and Mann as methods for identifying separation of two body sides. In *Romberg's test*, the individual is asked to stand with arms crossed, feet together and eyes closed. In *Mann's test*, which is sometimes called "sharpened" Romberg, the individual is asked to stand with one foot in front of the other and arms crossed on the chest (Montgomery, 1985a). These two tasks demand continuous feedback from the proprioceptors on both sides of the body and from the vestibular organs.

The *finger-to-nose test* requires the individual to hold the arms out to the side and bring the fingertips in to touch the nose without vision. Smooth performance of this movement is traditionally associated with adequate function of the cerebellum, whereas shaky, choppy, or inaccurate movements are associated with cerebellar dysfunction (Chusid, 1985). As a proprioceptive indicator, the individual may demonstrate quick fatigue or inability to hold the arms out to the sides.

Schilder's arm extension test requires that the individual hold the arms out in front with eyes closed. This position is to be maintained even when the head is rotated side to side, demonstrating integration of postural reflexes associated with the head and neck (Ayres, 1973). Dunn (1981) showed that normal kindergartners are not yet able to completely separate head and body movements on this test. This clinical observation also requires integrity within the proprioceptive system to maintain the required positions. Other clinical observations of neuromuscular development also contain underlying proprioceptive features, such as the ability to assume positions of prone extension and supine flexion, but seem to be more strongly associated with other aspects of central nervous system processing (Ayres, 1973; Harris, 1981). The constellation of results from skilled observations will assist the therapist to determine the reason for the problems and to direct the course of intervention.

Proprioception tasks and *vibration* (a sensation which travels in the same pathways) tasks were used to assess autistic children (Ayres & Tickle, 1980). Traction was provided to limb joints, and those who sought more of this stimulation were considered hypo-reactive. Response to vibration was evaluated by observing the children's acceptance of a vibrator applied to body surfaces. Prolonged interest was considered hypo-reactivity, and avoidance was considered hyper-reactivity.

Playing wheelbarrow can elucidate the integrity of proprioceptive feedback. The individual assumes the prone position on the floor, and the therapist takes hold of the lower body and asks the individual to walk on hands across the room. The therapist holds onto the trunk, pelvis, thighs, shins, or ankles, providing necessary support for the task. More distal holding positions place greater postural control demands on the individual. School-aged children should be able developmentally to play wheelbarrow with support provided at the shins or ankles. A great deal of co-contraction is necessary to play wheelbarrow (Dunn, 1986). The therapist observes the individual's ability to assume the initial position supporting the upper trunk on the hands and the patterns of stability and mobility as the individual "steps" with the arms. The therapist also notes the functional components of the task, such as whether the individual uses proximal or distal stability. When an individual demonstrates distal stability, the hands become "planted," and movement can be observed in the trunk region which mitigates against hand movements. As with other skilled observations, proprioceptive support underlies functional ability on this task.

The therapist also can observe the individual during other movement and holding patterns to determine the effect of muscle tone and joint stability on task performance. The proprioceptors constantly monitor actions around the joints to keep the brain apprised of the exact body position in space and time. This, in turn, allows the planning of subsequent movements to match environmental demands. Ayres (1980, p. 98) uses the example of drinking a hot cup of coffee while blindfolded, in which proprioceptive feedback enables the individual to lift the cup with the correct amount of force. If the proprioceptors improperly reported that the cup was filled with something heavier, such as lead, then the force generated would cause the individual to fling the cup across the room. This individual may have difficulty with tasks that require co-contraction such as lifting pots and pans or carrying books.

The therapist might also observe the person having difficulty anticipating movements, such as reaching for a glass or door knob. The individual may be observed locking joints for stabilizing rather than exercising control over the neuromusculoskeletal system. Poor proprioceptive feedback may interfere with the postural background patterns required for these simple movements.

Frequently individuals with poor vestibular and proprioceptive processing rely on visual input to orient them in the environment, and removal of vision or lack of access to visual orientation (as in a crowded place) leads to poor postural control and stability. It is important for therapists to examine the individual's dependence on visual guidance during movements within the environment. The therapist observes movements with and without visual guidance as a method of determining the integrity of the proprioceptive system and how much the person is able to rely on proprioception as background support for task performance. Table 18-2 lists examples of the proprioceptive components of daily life tasks.

Interviewing. Caregivers may report that the individual demonstrates poor activity tolerance, rapid fatigue, or lethargic behavior. In an effort to provide stability, the individual may lock the joints in extreme ranges which causes the family or other professionals to report unusual posturing. Walking patterns may be affected and will be noticeable to others; for example, the individual may lock hip or knee joints for stability. Usually persons can describe the movements if the therapist asks questions which categorize the joint and limb positions.

There may be reports of frequent accidents during activities requiring heavy work, such as carrying groceries or lifting a casserole dish. This is because poor proprioceptive feedback may prohibit the individual from stabilizing across the joints. Alteration of the environment to decrease heavy work components is likely to improve safety. For example, the family can use plastic dishes instead of the heavier stoneware or can bake in individual dishes instead of one large dish. Family members intuitively may make alterations such as these and careful questioning by the therapist can reveal them.

Children sometimes have developmental histories which suggest proprioceptive involvement. The child may avoid crawling or only crawl for short distances in comparison to other children. The child may "tummy-crawl" rather than using strong proprioceptive stabilization to remain on hands and knees during crawling. Some children walk on their toes, a posture which places the joints and muscles in extreme positions for stabilization, and perhaps to increase proprioceptive feedback (Montgomery, 1985b). Parents and teachers will frequently report that the child is destructive with toys (Ayres, 1986). Poor modulation of stability and mobility is likely to contribute to this outcome.

Falling, bruising and other accidents also are reported commonly. Teachers complain that these children cannot sit up in their desks, are constantly leaning on walls and cabinets, and cannot hold their books up during reading sessions. Since proprioceptive feedback provides a background for task performance, it is important for therapists to ask questions regarding all the areas suggested above. Although caregivers may be aware of these behaviors, they may not recognize their importance for therapeutic assessment and treatment planning.

The Vestibular System

Initial Data Base. The *vestibular organ* is located in the inner ear; the neurons travel into the brain stem to synapse at the pontomedullary junction and the cerebellum. Thus, the vestibular system is at-risk if the lower brain stem has been damaged or if certain regions of the cerebellum have been affected. The initial data base may report behaviors such as frequent falls, or an extreme amount of mobility in the trunk. These behaviors can be observed because the descending vestibulospinal pathways control trunk and neck posture. There may also be comments regarding rigidity in posture with an unwillingness to move about. These behaviors indicate an avoidance of vestibular input, perhaps because the individual is unable to process the input effectively.

Formal Assessment. The assessment of the vestibular system is complex because it is difficult to isolate the functions of vestibular organ and nuclei. The brain stem connections are multisensory and divergent, so that loss of specific vestibular input leads to compensation by other systems.

One test available to occupational therapists which directly assesses vestibular responsiveness is the *Southern California Postrotary Nystagmus Test* (SCPNT). In this test, the examiner places the child in a standardized body and head position and spins the child on a rotating platform ten times in 20 seconds. Left and right trials are performed to yield a total score. The score is based on the number of seconds that nystagmus is observed after abruptly stopping the child facing a blank wall. The blank wall precludes focus on a specific object which inhibits nystagmus. Nystagmus is related to vestibular function because the vestibular nuclei have direct connections with the cranial

nerves which serve the extraocular muscles (cranial nerves III, IV, and VI). Individuals can have an underreaction, a normal reaction, or an overreaction to the spinning. Results from this test frequently corroborate other skilled observations and comments in the referral complaint. Although Ayres (1975) provides normative data on the SCPNT, other authors have also reported additional normative data (Crowe et al., 1984; Dunn, 1981; Kimbal, 1981; Morrison & Sublett, 1983; Potter & Silverman, 1984). Ayres (1975) hypothesizes that hypo-responsive nystagmus indicates overinhibition of the vestibular nuclei or inadequate excitation reaching the vestibular nuclei. Overreactivity may indicate insufficient inhibition from higher centers to the vestibular nuclei. Ayres (1978) found that learning disabled children with hypo-reactive and hyper-reactive postrotary nystagmus responded differently to sensory integration treatment.

Montgomery (1985a) suggests that reliance on SCPNT as the overall indicator of vestibular function is short-sighted. She proposes that multiple observations, including assessment of the postural control system, are necessary to obtain a complete picture. Dutton (1985) reviewed the literature on the SCPNT and identified a number of important variables. He found that normal subjects demonstrated reliability across time and there was more variability present in dysfunctioning populations. This is consistent with expectations, since Ayres has hypothesized that some children's problems are based on sensory processing deficits.

Arousal state may also play an important role in SCPNT outcome, and some studies reported adequate relationships between SCPNT and *electro-nystagmography* (ENG) which is another test that elucidates vestibular function. The ENG records activity at the eyeball during stimulation. Speed of slow and fast components of nystagmus are recorded and are considered sensitive measures of vestibular activities (Montgomery, 1985a). Montgomery and Capps (1980) found that ENG responses differed significantly in normal children in a relaxed state versus those in an aroused state. *Brainstem-evoked potentials* also render information about vestibular function. The evoked potential is a test to determine whether normal patterns of brain stem response occur during stimulation through surface electrodes. A formal test available through specialized laboratory procedures is the *caloric test*. In this measure, water or air is forced into the ear canal, which triggers the vestibulo-ocular response of nystagmus (Montgomery, 1985a). This test is more accurate than the SCPNT (Montgomery, 1985a) but also is not available routinely to occupational therapists. However, when they are available, these tests can be used to corroborate test and observational findings.

Many of the balance and posture items with proprioceptive components also contain vestibular components. Standing on one foot not only requires proprioceptive feedback from the muscles and joints of the body, but also requires monitoring by the vestibular mechanism to maintain head and neck position against gravity. When vision is occluded, as in the Standing Balance-Closed subtest on the SCSIT and the Standing and Walking Balance items on the SIPT, vestibular and proprioceptive mechanisms are more challenged. Postural control is clearly linked to the vestibular system via the descending vestibulospinal pathways to the muscles.

Clinical Assessment and Skilled Observation. Clinical methods for assessing the integrity of the vestibular system frequently include motor observations because of the close neurological connection between the vestibular and postural systems. The *prone-extension position* is the postural item most commonly associated with vestibular functioning (Ayres, 1980). The individual is asked to lift head, arms, chest, and legs off the floor from the prone position and hold it for 20-30 seconds. Harris (1981) found that by six years of age, children can hold this position for 30 seconds. The strong influence of the vestibular centers on this extended position is via the descending vestibulospinal pathways. Bundy and Fisher (1981) demonstrated that performance on equilibrium sitting and kneeling, eye-midline crossing, and teacher reports of academic performance could be used to predict prone extension performance.

Romberg's test (see description in the proprioceptive section) relies heavily on vestibular feedback as well. Persons with vestibular deficit cannot hold this position, whereas normal persons can stand for at least 30 seconds (Montgomery, 1985a). Schilder's test (described earlier) also elicits vestibular processing when the head is moved side to side. All movements of postural control, especially those which include head movement, have underlying vestibular support for the muscle tone required for the action. For example, Montgomery and Gauger (1978) investigated a relationship between toe-walking and sensory processing deficits. They hypothesized from their findings that vestibular processing may be an underlying factor in toe-walking.

Dynamic relationships with gravity may be more appropriate assessments for vestibular processing. A number of researchers have designed dynamic measures, some quite simple and others very complex (Montgomery, 1985a). DeQuiros and Schrager (1978) designed a board that appears to be solid but has soft and hard parts on the surface. Therapists use equilibrium boards and moveable equipment. Black, Wall and Nashner (1983) designed a testing unit to alter and control somatosensory, visual, proprioceptive, and vestibular input. By careful manipulation, these researchers provided congruent or conflicting messages among the systems. While normal people seem to resolve conflicts by attending to vestibular input, immature children and adults with vestibular deficits do not appear to be able to handle the sensory conflict, and fall (Black, Wall, and Nashner, 1983).

Montgomery (1985a) suggests that the vestibular system may resolve conflict among sensory systems. Although professionals separate vestibular, proprioceptive and somatosensory systems for discussion, these systems naturally function in unison to allow normal interaction to occur. Hence, separating these systems when observing behavior is artificial. Montgomery (1985a) states that vestibular input in isolation is insufficient to maintain posture and found that the combination of visual, somatosensory and vestibular input led to improved performance on an orientation task (Montgomery, 1985b). In this study, adults were better able to perform without vision than kindergartners or fourth graders, but fourth graders and adults performed equally well when all sensory input was available.

Two classic tests designed by Fukada are used to assess vestibular-postural control (Montgomery, 1985a). The *stepping test* records deviations from the center of a circle when the individual marches with eyes closed and arms raised overhead. It has been hypothesized that deviations occur toward the person's dysfunctional side. The *writing test* requires the individual to write capital letters on a vertical surface with the preferred hand with eyes both open and closed. The arm is extended forward so that no support on the body or table is possible. It is hypothesized that with vestibular dysfunction, there will be greater than 10° deviation with eyes closed. Preliminary relationships have been identified between these tests and more precise tests (e.g., ENG), but researchers continue to suggest that these clinical observations only be used in concert with other measures (Montgomery, 1985a).

Bundy et al. (1987) investigated the concurrent validity of various equilibrium tests including the tilt board and reaching, standing, and walking balance items. They confirmed the initial findings of earlier research (Fisher & Bundy, 1982) that multiple tests are necessary to access all aspects of equilibrium. They made five recommendations to therapists who clinically are assessing equilibrium:

1. include vision and vision-occluded items,
2. consider placement or movement of non-weight bearing extremities in maintaining equilibrium,
3. consider whether the individual is able to use visual fixation as a benefit to equilibrium performance,
4. consider the position and amount of work required on the weight-bearing extremity,
5. consider whether displacement movements are controlled by the therapist or individual being assessed when completing the task.

Although these five variables were not consistently high or low across the learning disabled children tested, these seemed to be the variables that triggered variance in performance. Although Bundy et al. (1987) provide a helpful initial framework for designing clinical assessment procedures, further research is necessary to clarify the relationships among types of equilibrium problems and task performance.

More recently, Fisher, Wietlisbach and Wilbarger (1988) reported on three tests of equilibrium given to adults, the *tilt board tip* (TBT), *tilt board reach* (TBR), and the *flat board reach* (FBR). Their findings suggest that some tests of equilibrium differentiate between male and females as was found on earlier tests with children (TBT). They hypothesize that experiences may play a part in performance of equilibrium. The vestibular organ sends information directly to both the vestibular nuclei and the cerebellum. Therefore, many cerebellar signs also relate to vestibular system functions. When vision is occluded with both cerebellar and vestibular dysfunction, swaying and falling occur. There are also direct connections with the extraocular muscles, making the observation of smooth eye movements another feature of clinical observations. Concordance of head and eye movements allows the individual to remain oriented against gravity and in the spatial environment.

For young children, vestibular responsiveness can be assessed during handling. The therapist can note responsiveness of very young children when they are repositioned with displacement of the trunk and head. Children from toddler age upward can be normally expected to respond to displacement with protective extension or with righting responses of body and head. The righting responses allow the head to remain properly aligned with both the pull of gravity and the vertical orientation of the visual environment. Quick displacement or inversion are more likely to produce protective responses due to the speed of the stimulus.

In adults, other types of observations are made, since it is not as easy to manipulate an adult's body. For example, one can observe the adult's responsiveness to wheelchair movements when being transported. This can include fast direction changes, back tilting of the wheelchair to negotiate stairs, or patterns of starting, stopping or turning that occur during transport. Transfers from bed to chair, chair to toilet or tub, and chair to mat also provide appropriate opportunities to observe responses to vestibular input. The individual will normally use righting and protective responses during these activities. When an individual demonstrates intolerance for activity at the very beginning of a treatment session, the therapist might question whether too much vestibular input was provided in transit making the system already overloaded with input. Since any movement

of the head is an adequate trigger for the vestibular organ, any functional activity which moves the head is an appropriate activity during which to observe vestibular responsiveness (Dunn, 1988). All of these activities produce a large amount of vestibular input and so can be used easily in the assessment process. Table 18-2 lists examples of the vestibular components of daily life tasks.

When vestibular input is not processed correctly, a number of behaviors can be observed. When displaced, the individual may not react at all to the stimulus and thus fall, using no protective responses. When behavioral response is not observed, the therapist must then question whether the vestibular input is being recognized within the central nervous system. If the response is visible but delayed, this might infer slow or inefficient processing of sensory input in producing a motor response. One should remember that if there is obvious central nervous system damage of the motor systems (e.g., cerebral palsy or stroke), slow responsiveness may also be related to poor motor output.

Sometimes the person with *vestibular dysfunction* may act to avoid movement, since movement is the stimulus which triggers the vestibular organ. This person appears rigid and stiff especially in the trunk and neck regions. The individual may also display fear regarding movement. It is hypothesized that this is due to poor ability to process the vestibular input produced when the head is displaced in relation to gravity, hence it has been termed *gravitational insecurity* (Ayres, 1980). Both children and adults may display gravitational insecurity; it may be associated with a variety of central nervous system and developmental dysfunctions. This avoidance of movement can have a serious effect upon task performance because all purposeful activity requires delicate balance of stability and mobility of the head, trunk and limbs.

Some authors hypothesize that self-stimulating behaviors such as rocking or head-shaking are an attempt to provide vestibular input (Freeman, Frankel & Ritro, 1976; Ornitz, 1978). The threshold for registering input may be very high, making the increased stimulus intensity necessary to reach thresholds (Damasio & Maurer, 1978; Gold & Gold, 1975). Further clinical research involving the effects of providing high intensity sensory input imbedded into purposeful activity will clarify this relationship.

Ayres & Tickle (1980) provide a simple model of clinical assessment of vestibular processing by combining skilled observations and test scores to assess children with autism. They observed: (1) response to movement on therapeutic equipment (2) general responses to movement, (3) anxiety reactions to sudden, unpredictable movement, and (4) ability to engage in a visual-vestibular task. They also recorded reactions to movement; avoiding movement was considered overreactive and seeking movement with great intensity was considered underreactive. The SCPNT was administered to obtain a postrotary nystagmus score. Optokinetic nystagmus was evaluated by spinning a striped disk in front of the children and measuring the length of visual regard. Brief regard (approximately 3 seconds) was considered normal.

Interviewing. Teachers, family members and other professionals frequently observe behaviors that are helpful in determining the integrity of the vestibular system. One can inquire about the types of activities that increase energy level or calm the individual. Teachers will report poor performance in school, which is commonly the reason the child becomes involved with occupational therapy. Problems with reading in some learning disabled children are thought to be related to poor vestibular processing (Ayres, 1980). Further questioning can often reveal other important information. The teacher may report clumsiness in the classroom both in negotiating space between furniture and in handling materials for seat-work. Inquiry about the child's ability to stay in the desk might produce comments such as ''he just falls out of his desk suddenly'' or ''none of the seats seem to fit him; he leans, rocks and squirms a lot.'' The child may display unusual behavior in transition periods, such as returning to classroom tasks after recess or gym class. The teacher may comment that the child has a hard time refocusing on the new task. Children who are intolerant of movement appear stiff and rigid. Teachers may report that it's hard to engage the child in activities at recess, or that free play choices are always sedate, controlled activities, such as playing with blocks.

Family members are very aware of the unusual behaviors exhibited, and frequently associate them with social-emotional problems. They may report that the individual becomes nervous or afraid at the suggestion of certain routine activities such as riding in the car, walking on uneven surfaces, stepping off curbs, or climbing stairs. Parents describe their disappointment that their child hates the neighborhood playground and has a very hard time learning to ride a bike. If the therapist inquires about home tasks, the family may report either that the individual is reluctant or that it takes an inordinate amount of time to carry out tasks requiring stooping or bending (e.g., emptying the dishwasher or reaching under the bed). This reluctance or difficulty may stem from poor ability to process the vestibular input produced during these tasks. Family members will often describe the fear or discomfort the individual demonstrates during family outing activities such as jumping into a swimming pool or riding a merry-go-round at an amusement park. All of these comments can indicate other problems as well, re-emphasizing the need to have multiple sources of data before creating a hypothesis.

Occasionally, family members will report autonomic reactions such as nausea, sweating, or dilated eyes in response to movement. At the other end of the continuum, comments may suggest that the individual craves movement such as rocking or swaying in the seat, or in extreme cases, self-stimulating behaviors may be reported. Since many of the behaviors indicative of poor vestibular processing are interpreted (incorrectly) as emotional problems, it is important to explain the possible reasons for the behaviors as the interviews take place. This helps the family and others to cope with their situation and plan appropriate environmental adaptations.

The Visual System

Initial Data Base. The visual system is unique because its pathways travel from front to back in the cortex. The visual system is at risk if initial assessment information reports involvement of any portion of the optic nerve, chiasm or tract, midbrain region, optic radiations, or occipital lobe. Behaviors which might be reported in the file would include tiring very quickly when reading or looking at things, ignoring significant parts of self or environment, or being easily distracted by visual stimuli.

Formal Assessment. Occupational therapists frequently assess components of visual processing. Table 18-1 includes ten tests which contain visual components with five of them only evaluating visual processing. Additional assessment procedures that are considered to be more cognitively-oriented are not included in this discussion.

The Beery Developmental Test of Visual Motor Integration (VMI) is a form-copying instrument. The person is expected to copy increasingly complex forms, and performance is evaluated on specific parameters addressing the quality of the form. Examiners obtain a visual motor age equivalent score. A more recent type of visual-motor test is the *Test of Visual-Motor Skills* (TVMS) which also requires form-copying. The scoring criteria are more clearly defined on this test.

The *Marianne Frostig Developmental Test of Visual Perception* was designed to evaluate children's perceptual skills. Interpretation of visual-perceptual performance can be complicated because this is a paper and pencil test which requires motor skills to indicate responses. More recent tests have been designed to assess visual perception more thoroughly and omit motor skill from the test. The *Motor-Free Visual Perception Test* (MVPT) is an example of such a test. Individuals point to their item choice from a selection of four answers for the 36 items. The examiner computes a perceptual quotient to compare an individual's score to the normative group. An even more recent test, the *Test of*

Visual Perception Skills (TVPS) not only omits motor skill from testing, but also divides visual perception into seven subgroups. The examiner obtains a score for each subtest and for the composite test. This breakdown of scores is very useful for program planning. Since it is a newer test, further validation will be necessary to clarify relationships. Menken, Cermak and Fisher (1987) found significantly different outcomes on the TVPS when comparing normal children and children with cerebral palsy.

The *Quick Neurological Screening Test* (QNST) contains two items that include visual components: figure recognition and production, and behavioral irregularities. In the first, the individual is asked to name and copy several geometric forms; this item contains both motor and language components. Distractibility and perseveration are relevant observations that could be made. As with all items on the QNST, a gross measure of responsivity is obtained.

The SCSIT and the SIPT both contain visual perception subtests. As the updated test battery, the SIPT contains relevant changes. *Space visualization* requires the child to mentally rotate blocks to determine which will fit into a form board. The *Position-in-Space* test also requires form rotation in pictures; this subtest is on the SCSIT but was not included in the SIPT. *Figure-ground perception* requires the child to identify pictures which are imbedded within a visual image. *Design-copying* contains line drawings which the child must reproduce. The SIPT has expanded design copying to include not only a score of the finished product, but also qualitative measures of the way the drawing is made.

The *Miller Assessment for Preschoolers* contains two items which address basic visual responsiveness, although many of the cognitive tasks incorporate visual processing. The figure-ground subtest is part of the non-verbal index, and requires the child to find hidden pictures. Observations are also made of the child's response to visual stimuli in the environment as a gross estimate of attention and distractibility. The *Balcones* contains one item which assesses visual motor skills by a copying task, and another item, tactile graphics, which relies on visualization skill. Other factors also strongly influence these items.

Clinical Assessment and Skilled Observation. Although actual visual **acuity** (the ability of the sensory organ to receive the information correctly) is tested by other professionals, there are several areas therapists can assess to identify the integrity of components of the visual system. A primary area of assessment is the identification of visual field integrity.

Visual field deficits are a major source of difficulty for functional outcomes and are therefore very important for the occupational therapist. The visual fields are divided into quadrants for each eye. There are two upper and two lower quadrants and two left and two right quadrants for each eye. The left and right quadrants are frequently called temporal and nasal quadrants, depending on their positioning in relation to the temple or the nose. Each quadrant of the visual field is served by a certain area of the retina and corresponding neurons in the optic nerve, chiasm, tract, and higher centers of the brain including the occipital lobe (topographic organization). When specific parts of those nerve fibers are damaged, specific visual fields are lost (see discussion in Chapter 9).

A clinical method for assessing the visual field is to move a stimulus from outside of the visual field into the visual field and ask individuals to identify when they can see the object. For example, when testing the left visual fields of the left eye (both upper and lower left quadrants), one would place the object 12 to 18 inches laterally from the left ear. While the individual maintains a forward gaze, the therapist moves the stimulus forward and requests a response when the individual sees the object. If the peripheral fields are intact, the individual should comment that they see the stimulus when the object is parallel to the left cheek. Persons with a left *homonomous hemianopia* (loss of one side of the visual field; in this case, due to right occipital tract damage) will not identify the stimulus until it is approaching the center of the face as the therapist curves the stimulus around the face. The side ipsilateral to the injury (the right visual field and left occipital tract in this example) will have an intact visual field. The therapist must also assess the visual fields from top to bottom. A similar procedure can be used to identify if the entire top to bottom visual field is intact for both eyes, but in this case the stimulus is moved from above the head to the chest region.

The functional significance of visual field defects lies in the individual's ability to maintain contact with the external environment in an appropriate way. When a portion of the visual field is lost, the individual's task performance diminishes. For example, loss of a lower quadrant may affect mobility because the individual would not see objects on the floor; whereas loss of peripheral quadrants (*tunnel vision*) may lead to difficulty with daily living activities such as cooking or cleaning because the person might not see objects out of central vision.

The oculomotor system controls eye movements with the extraocular muscles, which are served by three cranial nerves (III oculomotor, IV trochlear and VI abducens). With brain stem trauma, these nerves can be affected. Dysfunction can also occur with vestibular deficits because of the direct connections between the vestibular nuclei and these cranial nerves. The therapist observes the subject's use of visual regard to complete tasks and the position of eyeballs both during tasks and at rest.

With oculomotor nerve involvement, the ipsilateral eye is pulled downward and outward, making binocular central vision difficult. Also, the eye is dilated and the eyelid droops (*ptosis*). The individual may tire easily with tasks requiring visual regard because only one eye will work when tasks are in the central field. With trochlear nerve involvement, the individual is unable to look downward with the contralateral eye. Eyes are normally aligned when looking forward or to the sides. This individual is likely to bump into or stumble over objects on the floor or may not notice furniture when passing through a room. Sometimes the individual adapts by holding the head down while walking, thus masking the eye movement difficulty. In this case, persons might misinterpret behavior as shyness or lack of social skill.

With abducens nerve involvement, the ipsilateral eyeball is pulled inward, producing double vision (*diplopia*) when looking forward. This situation can also lead to rapid fatigue or complaints of headaches. These individuals frequently adapt by either looking to the opposite side or turning the head toward the involved side. Both of these postural adaptations align the eyeballs and minimize the effects of the problem. Other persons might wrongly interpret these adaptations as being suspicious or strange, since the individual does not face forward.

The occupational therapist also identifies the individual's responsivity to visual stimuli. The therapist will want to determine answers to the following questions:

1. Does the individual notice or respond appropriately to visual stimuli?
2. Is the individual distracted by all or certain types of visual stimuli?
3. Are there types of visual stimuli that produce different responses in this person?

In addition to skilled observations made by the therapist, these questions can be answered through reports of direct care staff and family.

Initial observations might be made as the individual enters the environment; the therapist observes whether the individual is disoriented and notices what strategies the person uses to figure out this new place. Individuals with visual processing problems may either use looking behaviors (without seeming to profit from them) or may stand in one place making no attempt to orient visually, even if it happens to be in the doorway, blocking others. During physical therapy gait training, the individual may repeatedly make the wrong turns, even though the same pattern is used every day. The individual may become disoriented by slight changes in the path such as curbs or steps.

For tabletop tasks, the individual may display a whole range of behaviors indicative of various types of visual processing problems. Children will have difficulty with activities normally given to them for play or leisure such as block building, puzzles, and peg designs. Both children and adults will have characteristic problems with writing, drawing, and cutting. For example, tracing may be difficult, letters and numbers may be poorly formed and randomly placed on the page or reversed, and forms in pictures may be the wrong proportional size or may be unrecognizable. The individual may repeatedly lose materials on the work surface, especially when the items are similar in color to the work surface. If this problem is observed, intervention can include choosing work surface materials that produce a high color contrast, thus making objects easier to find. This can also be a problem when the individual tries to find objects on the shelves in cabinets in which depth, the presence of competing stimuli, and darkness add to the difficulty of the task. This person might be observed just standing in front of the cabinet, as if the object will present itself.

When a homonomous hemianopia is present, the individual may ignore or miss objects on that side. In this case, the therapist can either cue the individual to turn his head so that the lost visual field is over the person's shoulder or can place all items in the intact visual field. These problems can often manifest themselves during mealtime. Foods that match the table may be difficult to locate or the person might complain of not getting dessert on a meal tray, when a piece of pie is on the side of the tray corresponding to the lost visual field.

Sometimes it is appropriate to create special visual conditions to observe responsivity. For example, the therapist might clutter the kitchen or open cabinet doors to observe response to a distracting environment. It is especially important to assess these sensory components of daily life tasks (Table 18-2) if the individual will soon be placed in a mainstream and community environment or will be going home. Observations always occur within the individual's natural life environments.

Interviewing. Many activities of learning, work, home, and leisure are structured to take advantage of the functions of the visual system. Therefore, when difficulties arise in processing visual stimuli, the effect on task performance can be significant. As with other senses, difficulties can arise both in over- and under-responsiveness to environmental conditions. Families may report that the individual stares into space, avoids eye contact, or has more problems with behavior in busier environments. Attempts to retrieve items from cabinets, drawers, or closets are fruitless. The therapist should inquire about the person's orientation in space and whether the individual gets lost in familiar or unfamiliar surroundings. Other pertinent questions include: Do belongings get lost frequently? Are there patterns to these orientation problems?

If the individual is distracted by the visual environment, the family may report the person's frustration with getting ready in the morning, meal preparation, or house-cleaning because these activities place the individual in contact with very busy visual surroundings. When the individual is distracted by other stimuli, ongoing activity ceases.

Conversely, the person may become intensely interested in a very small part of the visual environment, examining it closely and for a period of time, or may observe his/her own hand as it flicks in front of lights or moves in a repetitive manner. These behaviors not only direct attention toward a non-goal directed stimulus, they also systematically shut out the rest of the environment. Such behaviors can be quite distressing to family members.

Other professionals and family members are likely to recognize the effect that poor visual guidance has on performance outcomes. The therapist can help direct their thinking by asking questions which clarify the observed behaviors. For example, the therapist can ask if the individual keeps working when not using vision to guide task performance. Persons might also report that the individual is distracted by visual stimuli in the environment (e.g., someone walking into the room, multiple items on a workspace). Other observations that are important to note include: losing one's place on a page; a poor ability to complete work in the order presented (e.g., rows of math problems, computer printouts); inability to find one's place in work that has been interrupted; reversals in writing; poor organization of parts (spatial relationships) in writing, drawing or construction tasks; and poor ability to copy from a model or the chalkboard. There may also be reports that the person gains very little information from pictures, charts or diagrams.

The Auditory System

Initial Data Base.   The auditory system functions to orient individuals with sound. The auditory system is at-risk when initial records have evidence of ear, brain stem, or temporal lobe damage. It is important to remember that when hearing is lost on one side of the auditory system, the major functional outcome is an inability to localize sound (see Chapter 9). The auditory system contains bilateral, central connections so both hemispheres will still receive input if the peripheral sense organ or the auditory nerve is only damaged on one side.

Behavioral comments that might trigger a hypothesis about poor auditory functioning would include comments about disorientation to sound, poor responsiveness to auditory stimuli, or an increased sensitivity to auditory stimuli in the environment.

Formal Assessment.   Therapists do not have primary responsibility for formal assessment of the auditory system, thus most of the tests listed in Table 18-1 do not contain auditory subtests. The *Quick Neurological Screening Test* contains a sound patterns subtest. The individual reproduces simple patterns demonstrated by the examiner. The *Miller Assessment for Preschoolers* contains items on the Communications index and Supplemental Skilled Observations of understanding sounds that require auditory processing especially for communication. These items contribute to a cursory view of the individual's overall performance and could not lead to conclusions without many other skilled observations.

Clinical Assessment and Skilled Observation.   The occupational therapist's responsibility is to identify the auditory system's contribution to functional performance. At a very basic level, the therapist can provide an obviously strong auditory stimulus and observe whether the individual responds, and if so, the therapist describes the characteristics of those responses. A startle reaction alone is a primitive arousal response. A startle reaction followed by a verbal utterance or a motor gesture to either remove the stimulus or oneself demonstrates rudimentary goal-directed behavior. A very simple adaptive response to auditory stimuli is looking up when one's name is called. More complicated responses are involved when the individual is asked to follow one simple or a series of oral directions. Such simple tasks can be incorporated into the initial few minutes of a visit with a client to identify whether the auditory system is going to interfere with performance (Table 18-2). As with the visual system, the therapist will also want to ask several questions including:

- *Is the individual responsive to auditory stimuli in the environment?*
- *Is the individual distracted by all or selected auditory stimuli?*
- *Does the individual recognize specific auditory stimuli?*
- *Can the person respond appropriately to auditory stimuli?*

Most of the answers to these questions are obtained during skilled observation of the individual's performance in functional tasks and from interviewing caregivers.

Distractibility to auditory stimuli is observed when the individual is in therapeutic, classroom, work, or community environments. These environments routinely contain many types of auditory stimuli including voices, physical, and mechanical sounds. By placing the individual proximally to or distally from these different stimuli, the therapist can

Table 18-4
Summary of Sensory Components of Tests Used by Team Members

Test Name	Sensory/Perceptual Subtest	O	G	A	Vis	S	Ves	P	Age Group	Diagnosis	Validity	Reliability	Norms
Bender Visual Motor Gestalt Test					X				3 yrs+	neurological behavior learning problems	interrater	test-retest	1,100 students
Benton Revised Visual Retention Test					X				8 yrs-adult		criterion discrim.	interrater alternate form split half	
Boston Diagnostic Aphasia Examination	word comprehension word picture meaning			X X	X				adult	neurological	construct	internal consistency	242 aphasic males
Carrow Auditory Visual Abilities	visual abilities battery auditory abilities battery			X	X				4-10 yrs	lang. problems learning prob.	content construct	split half	1032 children national dist.
Detroit Test of Learning Aptitude-2	oral directions word sequences design reproduction objective sequences			X X	 X X				6-18 yrs	learning neurological	construct	test-retest	150 at each age level
Flowers Auditory Test of Selective Attention				X					6-12 yrs	any		internal consist.	231 normal 231 EMR 218 mildly retarded 120 LD 3 states
Goldman Fristoe Woodcock Auditory Skills Test Battery	aural-oral visual-oral aural-written visual-written			X X	 X X				5.5 yrs-12 yrs	all	discrim.	test-retest	810 normal stratified sample
Halstead-Reitan Neuropsychological Test Battery	tactual performance test speech sounds perc. test rhythm test trail making test sensory perceptual tactile form recognition tactile finger recognition fingertip number writing matching figures test target test		 X X X		 X X X X X	X X X X			adult children 5-14 yrs (adapted subtests)	neurological	concurrent		
Hooper Visual Organization Test					X					neurological	concurrent	split half	
Illinois Test of Psycholinguistic Abilities-Revised	aud. perception subtests vis. perception subtests			X	 X				4-8 yrs	learning speech/language	concurrent	internal consistency	962 normal
Kaufman Assessment Battery for Children (KABC)	sequential proc. scale simultaneous proc. scale achievement scale			X X X	X X X				2.5 yr-12.5 yr	learning disabled minorities	construct content concurrent	split-half test-retest	2000 children 34 sites 24 states stratified
Learning Staircase	auditory-memory auditory perception spatial relationships visual memory			X X	 X X				1-7 yrs	any			criterion-referenced

Table 18-4 (continued)

Test Name	Sensory/Perceptual Subtest	O	G	A	Vis	S	Ves	P	Age Group	Diagnosis	Validity	Reliability	Norms
Leiter International Performance Scale and Leiter Adult Intelligence Scale	perceptual spatial imagery				X	X			2+ yrs adult	learning language CP MR cultural disadvantage	concurrent	split-half	80 children 256 men
Luria-Nebraska Neuropsychological Battery	rhythm tactile functions visual functions			X	X	X			15 yrs	neurological	discrim. construct		50 normal 30 neuro
Memory for Designs Battery					X				8.5 yrs-60 yrs	neurological		interrater	535 control 243 brain-disoriented
Minnesota Percepto-Diagnostic Test					X				5 yrs-adult	neurological learning behavior	discrim.	split half test-retest alternate form	4000 children 657 adults
Minnesota Spatial Relations Test-Revised					X				16 yrs+	any including normal	construct content	interrater consist. test-retest	various studies 46 normal
Perceptual Maze Test					X				adult	neurological	concurrent	test-retest alternate form	540 adults
Revised Minnesota Paper Forms Test					X				high school/adult	any	content	test-retest	
Stanford Binet Intelligence Test				X	X				2 yr-adult	all	edition	not reported in 1972 edition	2100 urban & rural students various locations
Test of Listening Accuracy in Children				X					K-6th grade	any	not reported in 1972	internal consist.	
The Single and Double Simultaneous Stimulus Test						X			18-75 yrs	neurological	discrim.		431 caucasians normal
Wechsler Scales: Wechsler Intelligence Scale for Children-Revised (WISC-R) Wechsler Preschool Primary Scale of I Intelligence (WPPSI) Wechsler Adult Intelligence Scale-Revised (WAIS-R)	performance subtests verbal subtests			X	X				4—adult	All	criterion concurrent predictive	test-retest odd-even split-half test-retest	2,200 children 1,200 children 115 centers 39 states
Woodcock-Johnson Psycho-Educational Battery	spatial relations visual and learning visual-matching			X	X X X				preschool-adult	all	content construct concurrent predictive	split half test-retest	Part I-III 4732 subj. from nat'l sample Part IV 1700 subj.

* O=Olfactory G=Gustatory A—Auditory Vis—Visual S=Somatosensory Ves=Vestibular P=Proprioceptive
This information was compiled from the following sources: Keyser, D.J. & Sweetland, R.C. (Ed.) (1984) Test critiques. Test Corporation of America, Kansas City; Sweetland, R.C. & Keyser, D.J. (1986) Tests. Test Corporation of America, Kansas City; Mitchell, J.V. (Ed.) (1985). The Ninth mental measurement yearbook. The Buros Institute of Mental Measurements, Lincoln, NB; King-Thomas, L. & Hacker, B.J. (Eds.) (1987). A therapist's guide to pediatric assessment. Little, Brown & Co., Boston; Compton, C. (1984). A guide to 75 tests for special education. Fearon Education, Belmont, CA; Sattler, J.M. (1982). Assessment of children's intelligence and special abilities (2nd Ed.). Allyn and Bacon, Inc., Boston, Ayres, J. (1989). Sensory integration and praxis tests manual. Los Angeles: Western Psychological Services. Test manuals were used when they could be obtained.

observe whether the individual is distracted by those stimuli and if so, what types of stimuli seem to be the most distracting. For example, the therapist might observe whether the individual is distracted by another therapist's directions in an adjoining treatment area.

Ayres and Tickle (1980) used two auditory stimuli to assess reactivity in autistic children. The first was two trials of ringing a bell out of view to determine whether the child could orient to the sound. The second stimulus was *white noise* (continuous, repetitive sound) provided for one minute. They recorded whether the children oriented quickly, after a short delay, or not at all. A variety of responses were obtained, suggesting that children with more sensitivity to sensory stimuli were also more responsive to their sensory integrative interventions.

Environmental sounds can interrupt task performance in individuals with auditory processing problems. The individual may complain of the loud noise of the dishwasher; announcements over intercom or public address systems may disrupt performance. The therapist may find that during meal preparation, instructions must be repeated if they are given when pots are banging or water is running. Inability to cope with competing auditory stimuli can severely impair an individual's ability to function in natural environments. During initial intervention one wants to avoid the distracting auditory (and visual) stimuli; as one moves into the later phases of intervention, controlled introduction to distracting stimuli becomes important in helping the individual to adjust to natural life environments.

Persons with auditory impairments may misinterpret what is said which leads to confusion. If the therapist is not aware that the client misunderstood a word or phrase, the therapist may make incorrect conclusions. For example, if the therapist says "We're going to work in the kitchen, let's go back there," the client may have perceived the phrase "Let's go pack there," responding with, "Where are we moving the stuff to?" Without consideration of the client's auditory processing problem, this response appears strange and inappropriate and could lead to the incorrect conclusion that the individual is confused and disoriented.

Interviewing. The observations that caregivers might make in association with the auditory system are subtle and often are regarded as poor attention or lack of interest. This misperception can lead to poor handling and improper structuring of the surroundings to support or protect the individual. When family members report feelings of frustration, the therapist inquires about the reasons for their frustrations. Reports may indicate that the person does not respond to his/her name when called, ignores requests, or constantly asks for things to be repeated. The individual

may mumble while others are talking or frequently may complain that others mumble. Teachers or other professionals commonly notice hypersensitivity to sounds because the associated behaviors are disruptive. Behaviors can include holding hands over ears, changing work space to move away from noise, frowning, or turning in the seat toward the person talking. Comments such as the following are commonly reported: "He tells me about sounds I'm not even aware of, like the toilet flushing down the hall," or "She continuously makes comments about other activities while we're trying to work, such as about who is outside in the hall or that the heat just turned on." These behaviors disrupt ongoing task performance, which prevents the individual from benefitting from therapeutic intervention.

Another observation that may be reported is that the individual produces a series of sounds over and over again, either with the mouth or with objects. Nelson (1984) describes many of these behaviors in persons with autism. This is not only bothersome to other persons, it allows the individual to block out the surrounding environment. Auditory stimuli are transient and temporally related, thus after the stimulus has occurred it is no longer available to the individual as with visual stimuli.

Collaboration with speech-language pathologists and audiologists regarding an individual's auditory processing problems is critical to the success of intervention strategies. Accurate information enables the therapist to organize a therapeutic environment which supports the evolution of adaptive behaviors.

ASSESSMENT METHODS OF OTHER PROFESSIONALS

When occupational therapists assess an individual, there are frequently other professionals involved in the overall assessment. In some environments such as the public schools, occupational therapy receives referrals through other professionals in order for the individual to be eligible for services. These other professionals produce diagnostic information from the philosophical viewpoint of their specific professions. This allows the team to have a complete picture of the individual when all the data are combined. By having a basic knowledge of the type of data collected by others and its relationship to occupational therapy data, therapists can create more cohesive intervention strategies. Table 18-4 summarizes the sensory components of tests frequently used by other professionals. It is advisable for therapists to obtain further information on those tests that are frequently used in their own settings.

Intelligence Tests

The most frequently used formal tests are the intelligence tests. Sattler (1982, 1988) provides an excellent review of intelligence testing, including information regarding interpretation of test data that is useful not only for psychologists but also for other team members. Dunn (1990) discusses the use of child assessment data in the occupational therapy program planning process.

Intelligence testing has changed a great deal through the years. In the early part of this century, heavy emphasis was placed on auditory-language skills. The *Stanford Binet Intelligence Test* was originally designed during this period. Unlike tests designed later, the Stanford Binet yields a mental age and an IQ score for the total performance, without subscale scores. The researchers that contributed knowledge to the formation of the Stanford Binet revolutionized the manner by which professionals would look at performance (Sattler, 1982).

The Wechsler Scales were designed after the Stanford Binet, and continue to be the most widely used intelligence tests for children and adults. The major change in content was to address perceptual skills as a separate and important problem-solving component of intelligence. All the Wechsler Scales contain a verbal scale (following the earlier traditions), a performance scale which tests perceptual organization, and a full scale score containing all subtest scores.

The *Wechsler Adult Intelligence Scale* (WAIS) was developed first and the *Wechsler Intelligence Scale for Children* (WISC) was designed in 1949 and was revised as the WISC-R in 1974. The *Wechsler Preschool and Primary Scale of Intelligence* (WPPSI) was developed in 1967 to evaluate children from 4 to 6 1/2 years old (Sattler 1982). Most subtests on the three scales are the same and the WPPSI has three of eleven subtests that are unique to younger ages. For our purposes here, these three scales will be discussed as one. Therapists are urged to investigate the individual properties of a specific Wechsler Scale instrument when used.

Table 18-5 contains a summary of the WISC-R subtests. Factor analytic studies revealed three primary factors in this scale. The most prominent are the verbal and the performace factors, which have been organized into scales. The *verbal scales* are comprised of six subtests (one is

---

Table 18-5
Individual Subtests for the Wechsler Intelligence Scale for Children-Revised (WISC-R)

Verbal Scale

1. **Information.** 30 questions requiring general knowledge and simple statements of fact (example: Where is Brazil?).
2. **Similarities.** 17 pairs of words that require the child to explain how the 2 items are similar (example: How are a mirror and a window alike?).
3. **Arithmetic.** 18 orally presented (timed) problems to which children must respond verbally without the aid of pencil and paper (example: If apples are priced at 2 for 25 cents, then how many can you buy for $1.00?).
4. **Vocabulary.** 32 words presented orally and requiring practical problem-solving ability (example: What is a garage?).
5. **Comprehension.** 17 problem situations requiring practical problem-solving ability (example: What should you do if someone steals your bicycle?).
6. **Digit Span.** Orally presented sequences of numbers requiring oral repetition (example: Please listen carefully and then say the following numbers: 5-1-6-9.).

Performance Scale

1. **Picture Completion.** 26 drawings of common objects in which children are requested to find an important part that is missing.
2. **Picture Arrangement.** 12 picture series similar to cut-up comic strips that the child is requested to place in correct order so that they make a sensible story.
3. **Block Design.** Picture of an abstract geometric design that the child is asked to replicate by using red and white blocks.
4. **Object Assembly.** Similar to a jigsaw puzzle in that the child is asked to assemble a number of puzzle pieces to make a common object, person, or animal.
5. **Coding.** Requires the child to copy symbols (e.g., vertical lines, circles) that are matched to numbers.
6. **Mazes.** 8 mazes requiring the child to find the most direct route out.

From Woodrich, D.L., & Joy, J.E. (1986). Multidisciplinary assessment of children with learning disabilities and mental retardation. Baltimore: Paul H. Brookes Publishing Co., p. 45.

Table 18-6
Some Hypotheses Regarding Verbal-Performance Discrepancies on the Wechsler Scales

VS>PS (Verbal scale score higher)

* language better than perceptual organization
* visual motor skills may be deficient
* visual perceptual skills may be deficient
* auditory processing may be better than visual processing
* manipulation tasks may be more difficult
* may "talk" way out of perceptual tasks

PS>VS (Performance scale score higher)

* perceptual organization better than language
* reading problems
* can't follow oral directions
* visual processing may be better than auditory processing
* talking, conversation may be more difficult
* may prefer drawing, constructing

From Dunn, W. (1991). Tests used by other professionals. In W. Dunn (Ed.), Pediatric occupational therapy: Facilitating effective service provision. Thorofare, NJ: SLACK Inc.

---

supplementary) which require the individual to respond verbally to questions. The questions differ in their degree of complexity and in the type of response required. Individuals with poor auditory processing, poor language skills, or lack of life experience are likely to have more difficulty with these items. The *performance scales* are comprised of six subtests (one supplementary) which require the individual to construct designs and patterns, sequence pictures and codes, and interpret visual images. Language is not required in giving directions or producing responses. Perceptual organization is assessed, allowing a non-language based view of the individual's ability to solve problems. Persons with poor visual processing skills will have difficulty with these subtests. Visual-motor ability can affect copying (coding) and construction tasks (object assembly). Much research has been done on the relationships between verbal scale and performance scale IQ scores. The research that suggests that differences greater than 15 points between the two scales (more than one standard deviation apart) is diagnostically meaningful requires further analyses (Sattler, 1982). Table 18-6 lists some of the hypotheses regarding the verbal scale and performance scale discrepancies.

Factor analytic studies also revealed a third factor, which was named Freedom from Distractibility. The subtests (arithmetic, digit span, and coding) require sustained attention, concentration, short-term memory, and the

ability to screen out extraneous influences for successful performance (Sattler, 1982). When all three of these subtest scores are low, one can hypothesize that the person will be distractible. Kaufman suggests that the mean of these subtests must be three or more scaled scores below the mean of both the performance scale and the verbal scale subtests to indicate a significantly different performance (Sattler, 1982). This comparison can add useful information to the diagnostic process.

Sattler (1982) provides an excellent discussion comparing each subtest to all the others on the Wechsler Scales, so that any pattern of individual subtest highs and lows may also be analyzed. Since intelligence tests are frequently available prior to occupational therapy assessment, these comparisons can help clarify the referral complaint and guide the course of assessment. For example, a high score on the block design and a low score on coding may indicate that visual organization skills are better than visual-motor skills (Sattler, 1982). In such a case, assessment directed at visual-motor performance may be indicated.

The *Kaufman Assessment Battery for Children* (KABC) is the most recently designed test of intelligence, coming into the marketplace in 1983. The authors are very experienced in test construction, and have designed a theoretically-based test for children ages 2 years, 6 months to 12 years, 6 months (King-Thomas and Hacker, 1987; Wodrich and Joy, 1986). The theoretical basis for this test arises from the work of Luria (neurology) and Das (cognitive psychology) (Wodrich and Joy, 1986; Kaufman and Kaufman, 1983). The test contains a sequential processing scale that requires a serial order use of stimuli, and a simultaneous processing scale that requires a Gestalt use of stimuli. The KABC also contains an achievement scale that measures school achievement. Table 18-7 contains a description of each subtest. Additionally, a non-verbal intelligence score can also be computed. Initial research demonstrates that this test discriminates between normal and disabled populations, especially those with learning problems (Wodrich and Joy, 1986). The dichotomy on this test reflects differences in problem-solving approaches and may have implications for teaching and intervention strategies (Kaufman and Kaufman, 1983). Table 18-8 provides examples of skills and problems that may be present with sequential and simultaneous processing discrepancies. Since this test focuses on the learning activities, occupational therapy must examine the component skills necessary for task performance to hypothesize relationships between process and product. The KABC Interpretive Manual (1983) provides in-depth presentations which analyze task performance and provide a framework for remedial planning. Case examples are presented and results of intervention studies are discussed. It is an excellent resource for all team members as planning proceeds.

The *Leiter Scales* provide an alternative to the language-based intelligence assessments. The individual places tiles in a tray to correspond with a model. In this test, perceptual skills are being tapped to measure problem-solving ability while minimizing the effects of language or culture. The test is not useful for those with severe physical limitations (King-Thomas and Hacker, 1987), but does minimize the cultural bias of language.

Psychoeducational Tests

The *Woodcock-Johnson Psychoeducational Battery* (WJPEB) is a comprehensive test battery that assesses cognitive ability, achievement, and interest in people ages three through adult. Table 18-9 provides a short description of the cognitive subtests and a list of the achievement and interest subtests. This test battery was designed to tap a full range of cognitive abilities to develop an accurate picture of the individual's problem-solving strategies and how they are

being used for achievement. The authors propose *cluster scores* (groups of subtest scores requiring similar strategies) as a method for examining strengths and deficits (Woodcock and Johnson, 1977). An example of a cluster score is the ''memory cluster'' which is comprised of ''memory for sentences'' and ''numbers reversed.'' These cluster scores have not been documented through factor analysis, but rather were designed by observing the inherent characteristics of each subtest performance (Sattler, 1982). The cognitive abilities subtests require adequate sensory processing in various forms, especially visual and auditory processing. As with other intelligence tests, analysis of the similarities in the individual's low or high scores can be helpful in further diagnostic work by narrowing the field of focus.

Recently a Part IV of the WJPEB has been published called the *Scales of Independent Behavior* which is a comprehensive measure of adaptive behavior and functional independence obtained by gathering information through structured

---

Table 18-7
Description of Individual Subtests of the Kaufman Assessment Battery for Children (KABC)
(Not all subtests are given to all age groups)

Sequential Processing Scale

1. **Hand Movements.** Performing a series of hand movements in the same sequence as the examiner performed them.
2. **Number Recall.** Repeating a series of digits in the same sequence as the examiner said them.
3. **Word Order.** Touching a series of silhouettes of common objects in the same sequence as the examiner said the names of the objects. More difficult items include an interference task between the stimulus and response.

Simultaneous Processing Scale

1. **Magic Window.** Identifying a picture that the examiner exposed by slowly moving it behind a narrow window, making the picture only partially visible at any one time.
2. **Face Recognition.** Selecting from a group photograph the one or two faces that were exposed briefly on the preceding page.
3. **Gestalt Closure.** Naming an object or scene pictured in a partially completed ''inkblot'' drawing.
4. **Triangles.** Assembling several identical triangles into an abstract pattern to match a model.
5. **Matrix Analogies.** Selecting the meaningful picture or abstract design that best completes a visual analogy.
6. **Spatial Memory.** Recalling the placement of pictures on a page that was exposed briefly.
7. **Photo Series.** Placing photographs of an event in chronological order.

Achievement Scale

1. **Expressive Vocabulary.** Naming an object pictured in a photograph.
2. **Faces and Places.** Naming the well-known person, fictional character, or place pictured in a photograph or drawing.
3. **Arithmetic.** Demonstrating knowledge of numbers and mathematical concepts, counting and computational skills, and other school-related arithmetic abilities.
4. **Riddles.** Inferring the name of a concrete or abstract concept when given a list of its characteristics.
5. **Reading/Decoding.** Identifying letters and reading words.
6. **Reading/Understanding.** Demonstrating reading comprehension by following commands that are given in sentences.

From Kaufman Assessment Battery for Children Interpretive Manual. A.S. Kaufman and N.L. Kaufman. American Guidance Service, Circle Pines, Minnesota, 1983. p. 3-5.

Table 18-8

Examples of Skills and Difficulties Which May Be Present When a Discrepancy Exists Between the Sequential and Simultaneous Processing Scales of the KABC

Sequence > Simultaneous Processing	Simultaneous Processing > Sequence
• ability to use stepwise math procedures (e.g., borrowing)	• good math concepts
• utilizes scientific method	• good overall comprehension
• understands chronology of events	• good use of picture cues
• good knowledge of grammar rules	• uses diagrams, flow charts
• rote knowledge of math facts	• uses shapes of letters/words to recognize
• poor space/time relations	• poor decoding skills/phonics
• poor sight vocabulary	• doesn't remember details of story
• phonetic speller	• can't recall order of story
• difficulty using context	• failure to understand rules
	• poor retention of math facts
	• poor use of steps to solve math problems
	• poor ability to follow oral directions

From Dunn, W. (1991). Tests used by other professionals. In W. Dunn (Ed.), Pediatric occupational therapy: Facilitating effective service provision. Thorofare, NJ: SLACK Inc.

---

interview (Bruininks et al., 1984). Table 18-10 summarizes the subscales of this scale. Such adaptive behavior scales are useful for teams because they provide a structured mechanism for examining the individual's ability to interact successfully with objects and persons in the environment. They can assist with placement decisions and can be helpful in determining when targeted functional outcomes have been achieved. *The Scales of Independent Behavior* was designed to correlate with findings on the Woodcock-Johnson Psychoeducational Battery to give a complete picture of an individual's function in all life tasks. There are other adaptive behavior scales which also comprehensively view functional performance (Sparrow et al., 1984; Nihira et al., 1975). Increased use of measures such as these is likely to facilitate team collaboration. + p. 500 →

Neuropsychological Assessments

Neuropsychological assessments were originally designed to assist in the diagnosis of brain injury through a battery of tests of sensory, motor, language, cognitive, and mental functions. Rather than providing a precise location of brain damage, neuropsychological assessments elucidate brain-behavior relationships.

The two most prominent figures in neuropsychological assessment are R. Reitan and A.R. Luria. Reitan contributed to the development of both the *Halstead-Reitan Neuropsychological Test Battery* and the *Reitan-Indiana Neuropsychological Test Battery* (Sattler, 1982). Luria's theoretical work led to the *Luria-Nebraska Neuropsychological Battery* (Wodrich and Joy, 1986). The components of these

batteries are summarized in Tables 18-11 and 18-12. The pattern of sensory components addressed on these tests most closely compares to the occupational therapy assessments summarized in Table 18-1 (pp. 474-475). These neuropsychological assessments and tests used by occupational therapists are based on similar literature and therefore are comparable in many areas. Neuropsychologists share concerns of occupational therapists regarding the process an individual uses to solve problems (See Chapter 11, Cognitive Dimensions of Performance). Collaboration between neuropsychology data collection and occupational therapy program planning and intervention can be fruitful.

SUMMARY

Sensory components of performance are often elusive because therapists must rely on outward behaviors to determine actions of an inward system. In this chapter, we have reviewed the assessment of the sensory components of performance from a variety of perspectives and given recommendations about how to conduct skilled observation of task performance. It is only through multiple findings that hypotheses regarding sensory components can be confirmed and used in intervention planning. Information provided through test data and observations of other professionals help to give a complete and accurate picture of the status of all performance areas, further enabling intervention to maximize independence for the individual.

Table 18-9
Woodcock Johnson Psychoeducational Battery—Subtests

Part One: Tests of cognitive ability

Subtest 1: **Picture Vocabulary** tests the subject's ability to identify pictured objects.

Subtest 2: **Spatial Relations** tests the subject's ability to compare shapes visually. The subject's task is to select from a series of component shapes those necessary to make a given whole shape. The shapes become progressively more abstract and complex. The test has a three-minute time limit.

Subtest 3: **Memory for Sentences** tests the subject's ability to remember material presented auditorily. In a task such as this, subjects make use of sentence meaning to aid recall.

Subtest 4: **Visual-Auditory Learning** tests the subject's ability to associate new visual symbols (rebuses) with familiar words in oral language and to translate series of symbols into verbal sentences. The subtest involves a controlled learning situation, presenting the subject with a miniature learning-to-read task.

Subtest 5: **Blending** tests the subject's ability to integrate and then verbalize whole words after hearing components (syllables and/or phonemes) of the words presented sequentially.

Subtest 6: **Quantitative Concepts** tests the subject's knowledge of quantitative concepts and vocabulary. No actual calculations or application decisions are involved.

Subtest 7: **Visual Matching** tests the subject's ability to identify two numbers that are the same in a row of six numbers. The task proceeds in difficulty from single-digit numbers to five-digit numbers. The test has a two-minute time limit.

Subtest 8: **Antonyms-Synonyms** tests the subject's knowledge of word meanings. Part A (Antonyms) requires the subject to state a word whose meaning is the opposite of the presented test word. Part B (Synonyms) requires the subject to state a word whose meaning is the same as the presented word.

Subtest 9: **Analysis-Synthesis** tests the subject's ability to analyze the components of an equivalency statement and reintegrate them to determine the components of a novel equivalency statement. Although this is not pointed out to the subject, the task is one of learning a miniature system of mathematics. The subject must be able to identify the colors yellow, black, blue, and red to take the subtest.

Subtest 10: **Numbers Reversed** tests the subject's ability to repeat a series of numbers in an order opposite to that in which they are presented. The subtest assesses the subject's ability to hold a sequence of numbers in memory while reorganizing that sequence. Numbers Reversed is more of a perceptual reorganization task than a memory task (in contrast to a numbers forward task).

Subtest 11: **Concept Formation** tests the subject's ability to identify rules for concepts when given both instances of the concept and non-instances of the concept. It can be considered a categorical reasoning task.

Subtest 12: **Analogies** tests the subject's verbal ability by requiring the subject to complete phrases with words that indicate appropriate analogies. It is largely a relational reasoning task.

Part Two—Tests of Achievement

Subtest 13: **Letter-Word Identification**
Subtest 14: **Word Attack**
Subtest 15: **Passage Comprehension**
Subtest 16: **Calculation**
Subtest 17: **Applied Problems**
Subtest 18: **Dictation**
Subtest 19: **Proofing**
Subtest 20: **Science**
Subtest 21: **Social Studies**
Subtest 22: **Humanities**

Part Three—Tests of Interest

Subtest 23: **Reading Interest**
Subtest 24: **Mathematics Interest**
Subtest 25: **Written Language Interest**
Subtest 26: **Physical Interest**
Subtest 27: **Social Interest**

From Woodcock, R.W., & Johnson, M.B. (1977). Woodcock Johnson Psycho-Educational Battery. Hingham, MS: Teaching Resources, p. 312-317.

Table 18-10
Subscales of the Scales of Independent Behavior

Subscale A: *Gross-Motor Skills.* The 17 tasks in this subscale sample skills from below one year, such as sitting without support, to mature adult fitness, such as using large muscles of the arms, legs, or the entire body in tasks involving balance, coordination, strength, and endurance.

Subscale B: *Fine-Motor Skills.* This subscale evaluates performance on 17 tasks that require eye-hand coordination using small muscles of the fingers, hands, and arms. The skills sampled range from those typically developed in infancy, such as picking up small objects, to those acquired after age 12, such as assembling objects with small parts.

Subscale C: *Social Interaction.* This subscale evaluates performance on 16 tasks that require social interaction with other people. Tasks range in difficulty from socialization appropriate in infancy, such as handing toys to another person, to more complex interactions involving entertaining and making plans to attend social activities outside the home.

Subscale D: *Language Comprehension.* This subscale evaluates performance on 16 tasks involving understanding of signals, signs, or speech and in deriving information from spoken and written language. The tasks included in this subscale range in difficulty from basic skills observed in infants, such as recognizing one's name, to more complex levels that include searching for and securing information through reading or listening.

Subscale E: *Language Expression.* This subscale evaluates performance on 17 tasks that involve talking and other forms of expression. Provision is made for assessing the skills of subjects who use non-oral methods of communication (sign language or language boards). The tasks range in difficulty from those typically mastered in infancy or early childhood, such as indicating "yes" or "no" and repeating common words, to the more complex skills involved in preparing and delivering formal reports to other people.

Subscale F: *Eating and Meal Preparation.* This subscale includes 16 tasks that evaluate performance in eating and preparation of meals. Initial tasks are appropriate for infants and assess simple eating and drinking skills; more advanced items test mastery of tasks involved in meal preparation.

Subscale G: *Toileting.* This subscale includes 14 tasks that evaluate performance in using the toilet and bathroom. The range of skills in this subscale is relatively more restricted than other subscales. The tasks range in difficulty from infancy and early childhood, such as staying dry or using the toilet regularly without accidents, to later childhood activities such as selecting and using appropriate bathroom facilities outside the home.

Subscale H: *Dressing.* This subscale includes 18 tasks that evaluate performance in dressing. These tasks range from simple levels for very young children, such as removing clothing, to complex skills requiring appropriate selection and maintenance of clothes.

Subscale I: *Personal Self-Care.* The 15 tasks in this subscale evaluate performance in basic grooming and health maintenance skills. The tasks range in difficulty from skills normally mastered by young children, such as using a toothbrush or wiping one's face with a washcloth, to adult skills of seeking professional assistance to treat illness or maintain health.

Subscale J: *Domestic Skills.* This subscale evaluates performance on 16 tasks needed in maintaining a home environment. The tasks range in difficulty from the early childhood level, such as putting a dish in or near the sink, to complex maintenance tasks, such as routine painting or repairs.

Subscale K: *Time and Punctuality.* This subscale includes 15 tasks that evaluate time concepts and use of time. The tasks range in difficulty from assessing the concept of time of day to keeping appointments.

Subscale L: *Money and Value.* This subscale evaluates skills on 17 tasks related to determining the value of items and using money. The tasks range in difficulty from skills generally mastered in early childhood, such as saving small amounts of money or selecting particular coins, to complex consumer decisions involving investments and use of credit.

Subscale M: *Work Skills.* The 16 tasks in this subscale evaluate work habits and selected prevocational skills. These skills are generally more developmentally advanced than most of the other subscales. They range from simple work tasks, such as indicating when a chore is finished, to prevocational skills, such as completing employment applications and job resumes.

Subscale N: *Home/Community Orientation.* This subscale evaluates performance on 16 tasks involving getting around the home and neighborhood and traveling in the community. Starting with very simple tasks that assess the subject's concept and use of space within the home environment, the subscale progresses to advanced tasks that assess more complex travel skills involving the location of important sites within the subject's home community.

Scale PB: *Problem Behaviors.* In addition to evaluating functional independence and adaptive behaviors, the SIB includes a scale for identifying problem behaviors that often limit personal adaptation and community adjustment.

From Bruininks, R.H., Woodcock, R.W., Weatherman, R.F., & Hill, B.K. (1984). Interviewer's Manual, Scales of independent behavior. Allen, TX: DLM Teaching Resources, p. 5 & 6.

Table 18-11
Description of the Halstead Neuropsychological Test Battery for Children
and the Reitan-Indiana Neuropsychological Test Battery

TEST	DESCRIPTION
Category Test[a]	Measures concept formation and requires child to find a reason (or rule) for comparing or sorting objects.
Tactual Performance Test[a]	Measures somatosensory and sensorimotor ability; requires child to place blocks with dominant hand alone, nondominant hand alone, and with both hands in appropriate recess while blindfolded.
Finger Tapping Test[b]	Measures fine motor speed and requires child to press and release a lever like a telegraph key as fast as possible.
Matching Pictures Test[b]	Measures perceptual recognition and requires child to match figures at the top of a page with figures at the bottom of the page.
Individual Performance Test[b]	
Matching Figures	Measures perception and requires child to match different complex figures.
Star	Measures visual-motor ability and requires child to copy a star.
Matching Vs	Measures perception and requires child to match "Vs."
Concentric Squares	Measures visual-motor ability and requires child (a) to connect a series of concentric squares.
Marching test[b]	Measures gross motor control and requires child (a) to connect a series of circles with a crayon in a given order with right hand alone and with left hand alone and (b) to reproduce examiner's finger and arm movements.
Progressive Figures Test[b]	Measures flexibility and abstraction and requires child to connect several figures, each consisting of a small shape contained within a large shape.
Color Form Test[b]	Measures flexibility and abstraction and requires child to connect color shapes, first by color and then by shape.
Target Test[b]	Measures memory for figures and requires child to reproduce a visually presented pattern after a three-second delay.
Rhythm Test[c]	Measures alertness, sustained attention, and auditory perception and requires child to indicate whether two rhythms are the same or different.
Speech Sounds Perception Test[c]	Measures auditory perception and auditory-visual integration and requires child to indicate, after listening to a word on tape, which of four alternative spellings represents the word.
Aphasia Screening Test[a]	Measures expressive and receptive language functions and laterality and requires child to name common objects, spell, identify numbers and letters, read, write, calculate, understand spoken language, identify body parts, and differentiate between right and left.
Trail Making Test (Parts A and B)[c]	Measures appreciation of symbolic significance of numbers and letters, scanning ability, flexibility, and speed and requires child to connect circles that are numbered.
Sensory Imperception[c]	Measures sensory-perceptual ability and requires child to perceive bilateral simultaneous sensory stimulation for tactile, auditory, and visual modalities in separate tests.
Tactile Finger Recognition[c]	Measures sensory-perceptual ability and requires child, while blindfolded, to recognize which finger is touched.
Fingertip Number Writing[c]	Measures sensory-perceptual ability and requires child, while blindfolded, to recognize numbers written on fingertips.
Tactile Form Recognition[c]	Measures sensory-perceptual ability and requires child to identify through touch alone various coins in each hand separately.
Strength of Grip[c]	Measures motor strength of upper extremities and requires child to use Smedley Hand Dynamometer with preferred hand and nonpreferred hand.

[a]This test appears both on the Halstead Neuropsychological Test Battery for Children and on the Reitan-Indiana Neuropsychological Test Battery.
[b]This test appears only on the Reitan-Indiana Neuropsychological Test Battery.
[c]This test appears only on the Halstead Neuropsychological Test Battery for Children.
From Sattler, J.M. (1982). Assessment of Children's Intelligence and Special Abilities (2nd Ed). Boston: Allyn and Bacon, Inc.

Table 18-12
Summary of Individual Scales of the Luria-Nebraska Neuropsychological Battery

INDIVIDUAL SCALE	DESCRIPTION	ITEMS	TECHNICAL REFERENCE
Motor Functions	Assesses a number of motor skills for left and right sides of body. Unilateral and simultaneous simple and complex motor movement.	51	Golden et al. (1978)
Acoustico-Motor (Rhythm Scale)	Evaluates similarity of tones, reproduces tones orally and motorically. Rhythmic patterns generated from verbal description.	12	McKay & Golden (1979)
Higher Cutaneous and Kinesthetic (Tactile Scale)	Without aid of vision requires identification of where touched, head and point of pin, direction of movement, geometric and alpha-numeric symbols traced on wrist, matching movements, and item identification.	22	Golden et al. (1982)
Spatial (Visual Functions)	Requires visual recognition of common objects, pictures with obscurity and disorganization. Matrices tasks and complex block count.	14	Golden (1981)
Receptive Speech Scale	Requires oral, written, and motoric response to spoken speech.	33	Golden (1981)
Expressive Speech Scale	Items involve orally repeated words, increasingly complex sentences; name, count, recite; offer missing words; and organize mixed-up sentence.	42	Golden (1981)
Writing Scale	Involves basic writing skills—spelling, copying words and letters from cards and memory. Writing words and letters from dictation and spontaneously.	13	Golden et al. (1978)
Reading Scale	Range includes reading letter sounds, syllables, words, sentences, and a short story.	13	Golden et al. (1978)
Arithmetic Scale	Involves simple number identification, writing and reading series of numbers; simple skills to more complex skills.	22	Golden et al. (1981)
Memory Scale	Requires learning word list, picture memory, rhythmic pattern, hand positions, sentences, story, and paired association task.	13	Golden et al. (1982)
Intellectual Scale	Involves sequencing pictures, identifying abstract theme of pictures, identifying picture absurdities, proverbs, definitions, opposites, analogies, and word problems.	34	Golden & Berg (1983)

From Dean, R.S. (in press). Perspectives on the future of neuropsychological assessment. In B.S. Plake and J.C. Witt (Eds.), The future of neuropsychological assessment. Hillsdale, NJ: Lawrence Erlbaum Associates.

Study Questions

1. Explain the four basic principles upon which sensory observations are made.

2. Name four categories of sensory assessment.

3. Summarize current thinking in regard to the use of dermatome testing.

4. Formulate a list of personal hygiene observations that would make you suspect poor processing of sensory input.

5. Describe a clinical observation that could be made to identify hypersensitivity and hyposensitivity to movement.

6. Although other team members formally assess auditory functions, describe two pieces of information that he occupational therapist contributes to this data base.

Recommended Readings

Ayres, A. J. (1980). *Sensory integration & the child*. Los Angeles: Western Psychological Services.

Bach-y-Rita, P. (Ed.). (1980). *Recovery of function: Theoretical considerations for brain injury rehabilitation*. Baltimore: University Park Press.

deQuiros, J.B., & Schrager, D.L. (1978). *Neuropsychological fundamentals in learning disabilities*. San Rafael, CA: Academic Therapy Publications.

King-Thomas, L. & Hacker, B.J. (1987). *A therapist's guide to pediatric assessment*. Boston: Little, Brown and Company.

MacWhinney, K., Cermak, S.A., & Fisher, A. (1987). Body part identification in 1- to 4-year-old children. *The American Journal of Occupational Therapy, 41*(7), 454-459.

Mitchell, J.V. (Ed.). (1985). *The Ninth Mental Measurements Yearbook*. Lincoln, NB: The Buros Institute of Mental Measurement.

Moberg, E. (1962). Criticism and study of methods for examining sensibility of the hand. *Neurology, 12*, 8-19.

Montgomery, P.C. (1981). Assessment and treatment of the child with mental retardation. *Physical Therapy, 61*(9), 1265-1272.

Montgomery, P.C. (1982). Effect of state on nystagmus duration on the Southern California Postrotary Nystagmus Test. *The American Journal of Occupational Therapy, 36*(3), 177-182.

Nelson, D.L. (1984). *Children with autism and other pervasive disorders of development and behavior: Therapy through activities*. Thorofare, NJ: Slack Inc.

Royeen, C.B., & Kannegieter, R.B. (1984). Factors affecting textural discrimination in normal children. *The Occupational Therapy Journal of Research, 4*(4), 261-270.

Royeen, C.B. (1986). The development of a touch scale for measuring tactile defensiveness in children. *The American Journal of Occupational Therapy, 40*(6), 414-419.

References

Ayres, A.J. (1973). *Sensory integration and learning disorders*. Los Angeles: Western Psychological Services.

Ayres, A.J. (1975). *Southern California postrotary nystagmus test manual*. Los Angeles: Western Psychological Services.

Ayres, A.J. (1978). Learning disabilities and the vestibular system. *Journal of Learning Disabilities, 11*, 18-29.

Ayres, A.J. (1980). *Sensory integration and the child*. Los Angeles: Western Psychological Services.

Ayres, A.J. (1986). *Developmental dyspraxia and adult onset apraxia*. Torrance, CA: Sensory Integration International.

Ayres, A.J., & Tickle, L.S. (1980). Hyper-responsivity to touch and vestibular stimuli as a predictor of positive response to sensory integration procedures by autistic children. *The American Journal of Occupational Therapy, 34*(6), 375-381.

Bell, J.A. (1984a). Sensibility testing: state of the art. In J.M. Hunter, L.H. Schneider, E.J. Mackin, & A.D. Callahan (Eds.), *Rehabilitation of the hand* (2nd Ed.). (pp. 390-398). St. Louis: C.V. Mosby Company.

Bell, J.A. (1984b). Light touch-deep pressure testing using Semmes-Weinstein monofilaments. In J.M. Hunter, L.H. Schneider, E.J. Mackin, and A.D. Callahan (Eds.). *Rehabilitation of the hand* (2nd Ed.). (pp. 399-406). St. Louis: C.V. Mosby Company.

Berk, R.A. & DeGangi, G.A. (1983a). *DeGangi-Berk Test of Sensory Integration*—Administration Manual. Los Angeles, CA. Western Psychological Services.

Berk, R.A. & DeGangi, G.A. (1983b). Psychometric Analysis of the Test of Sensory Integration. *Physical and Occupational Therapy in Pediatrics, 3*(2), 43-60.

Black, F.O., Wall, C., & Nashner, L.M. (1983). Effects of visual and support surface orientation references upon postural control in vestibular deficient subjects. *Acta Otolaryngologia, 95*, 199-210.

Bruininks, R.H., Woodcock, R.W., Weatherman, R.F., & Hill, B.K. (1984). *Interviewer's manual, scales of independent behavior*. Allen, TX: DLM Teaching Resources.

Bundy, A.C., & Fisher, A.G. (1981). The relationship of prone extension to other vestibular functions. *The American Journal of Occupational Therapy, 35*(12), 782-787.

Bundy, A.C., Fisher, A.G., Freeman, M., Lieberg, G.K., & Izraelevitz, T.E. (1987). Concurrent validity of equilibrium tests in boys with learning disabilities with and without vestibular dysfunction. *The American Journal of Occupational Therapy, 41*(1), 28-34.

Callahan, A.D. (1984). Sensibility testing: clinical methods. In J.M. Hunter, L.H. Schneider, E.J. Mackin & A.D. Callahan (Eds.). *Rehabilitation of the hand*: (2nd Ed.) (pp. 407-431). St. Louis: The C.V. Mosby Company.

Chusid, J.G. (1985). *Correlative neuroanatomy and functional neurology:* (19th Ed.). Los Altos, CA: Lange Medical Publications.

Compton, C. (1984). *A guide to 75 tests for special education*. Belmont, CA: Fearon Education.

Coren, S., Porac, C., & Ward, L.M. (1984). *Sensation and perception* (2nd (Ed.). Orlando: Academic Press, Inc.

Crowe, T.K., Dietz, J.C., & Siegner, C.B. (1984). Postrotary nystagmus response of normal four-year-old children. *Physical and Occupational Therapy in Pediatrics, 4*, 19-28.

Damasio, A.R., & Maurer, R.G. (1978). A neurological model for childhood autism. *Archives of Neurology, 35*, 777-786.

Dean, R.S. (In press). Perspectives on the future of neuropsychological assessment. In B.S. Plake and J.C. Witt (Eds.). *The future of neuropsychological assessment*. Hillsdale, NJ: Lawrence Earlbaum Associates.

Dellon, A.L. (1981). *Evaluation of sensibility and re-education of sensation in the hand*. Baltimore: Williams & Wilkins.

de Quiros, J.B., & Schrager, O.L. (1978). *Neuropsychological fundamentals in learning disabilities*. San Rafael, CA: Academic Therapy Publications.

Dunn, W. (1980). Evaluation of pre-schoolers. *Sensory Integration, Special Interest Section Newsletter, 3*(3).

Dunn, W. (1981). *A guide to testing clinical observations in kindergartners*. Rockville, MD: The American Occupational Therapy Association.

Dunn, W. (1986). Developmental and environmental contexts for interpreting clinical observations. *Sensory Integration, 9*(2), 4-7.

Dunn, W. (1988). Models of occupational therapy service delivery in public schools. *The American Journal of Occupational Therapy*.

Dunn, W. (Ed.) (1991). *Pediatric occupational therapy: Facilitating effective service provision*. Thorofare, NJ: Slack Inc.

Dutton, R.E. (1985). Reliability and clinical significance of the southern California postrotary nystagmus test. *Physical & Occupational Therapy in Pediatrics, 5*(2/3), 57-68.

Fisher, A.G., & Bundy, A.C. (1982). Equilibrium reactions in normal children and boys with sensory integrative dysfunction. *Occupational Therapy Journal of Research, 2*, 171-182.

Fisher, A.G., Nixon, J., & Herman, R. (1986). The validity of the clinical diagnosis of vestibular dysfunction. *The Occupational Therapy Journal of Research, 6*(1), 3-20.

Fisher, A.G., Wietlisbach, S.E., & Wilbarger, J.L. (1988). Adult performance on three tests of equilibrium. *The American Journal of Occupational Therapy, 42*(1), 30-35.

Freeman, B.J., Frankel, F., & Ritro, E.R. (1976). The effects of response contingent vestibular stimulation on the behavior of autistic and retarded children. *Journal of Autism and Childhood Schizophrenia, 6*, 353-358.

Gold, M.S., & Gold, J.R. (1975). Autism and attention: theoretical considerations and a pilot study using set reaction time. *Child Psychiatry and Human Development, 6*(2), 68-80.

Harris, N.P. (1981). Duration and quality of the prone extension position in four-, six-, and eight-year-old normal children. *The American Journal of Occupational Therapy, 35*(2), 26-30.

Heimer, L. (1983). *The human brain and spinal cord*. New York: Springer-Verlag.

Kaufman, A.S., & Kaufman, N.C. (1983). *Kaufman assessment battery for children interpretive manual*. Circle Pines, MN: American Guidance Service.

Keyser, D.J., & Sweetland, R.C. (Eds.). (1984) *Test critiques*. Kansas City: Test Corporation of America.

Kimball, J. (1981). Normative comparison of the Southern California Postrotary Nystagmus Test: Los Angeles vs Syracuse data. *The American Journal of Occupational Therapy, 35*, 21-25.

King-Thomas, L. & Hacker, B.J. (1987). *A therapist's guide to pediatric assessment*. Boston: Little, Brown and Company.

Melendez, F. (1978). *Revised manual for the adult neuropsychological questionnaire*. Psychological Assessment Resources, Inc.

Menken, C., Cermak, S.A., & Fisher, A. (1987). Evaluating the visual-perceptual skills of children with cerebral palsy. *The American Journal of Occupational Therapy, 41*(10), 646-651.

Moberg, E. (1966). *Methods for examining sensibility in the hand*. In J.E. Flynn (Ed.). *Hand Surgery*. Baltimore: Williams & Wilkins.

Montgomery, P. (1985a). Assessment of vestibular function in children. *Physical & Occupational Therapy in Pediatrics, 5*(2/3), 33-56.

Montgomery, P.C. (1985b). Sensory information and geographical orientation in healthy subjects. *Physical Therapy, 65*(10), 1471-1477.

Montgomery, P.C., & Capps, M.J. (1980). Effect of arousal on the nystagmus response of normal children. *Physical and Occupational Therapy in Pediatrics, 1*(2), 17-29.

Montgomery, P., & Gauger, J. (1978). Sensory dysfunction in children who toe walk. *Physical Therapy, 58*(10), 1195-1204.

Morrison, D., & Sublett, J. (1983). Reliability of the Southern California Postrotary Nystagmus Test with learning disabled children. *The American Journal of Occupational Therapy, 37*, 694-698.

Nelson, D.L. (1984). *Children with autism and other pervasive disorders of development and behavior: Therapy through activities*. Thorofare, NJ: Slack Inc.

Nihira, K., Foster, R., Shellhaas, M., & Leland, H. (1974). *AAMD adaptive behavior scale-For Children and Adults*. Washington, D.C.: American Association on Mental Deficiency.

Nihira, K., Foster, R., Shellhaas, M., & Leland, H. (1975). *AAMD adaptive behavior scale-Public School Version*. Washington, D.C.: American Association on Mental Deficiency.

Noback, C.R. & Demarest, R.J. (1981). *The human nervous system: Basic principles of neurobiology*: (3rd Ed.). New York: McGraw-Hill Book Company.

Ornitz, E.M. (1978). Neurophysiologic studies. In M. Rutter & E. Rutter (Eds.). *Autism: A reappraisal of concepts and treatment*. New York: Plenum Press.

Potter, C.N., & Silverman, L.N. (1984). Characteristics of vestibular function and static balance skills in deaf children. *Physical Therapy, 64*, 1071-1075.

Reitan, R., & Davison, L. (Eds.). (1974). *Clinical Neuropsychology: current status and applications*. New York: John Wiley & Sons.

Royeen, C.B. (1986). The development of a touch scale for measuring tactile defensiveness in children. *The American Journal of Occupational Therapy, 40*(6), 414-419.

Royeen, C.B. (1987). Test-retest reliability of a touch scale for tactile defensiveness. *Physical & Occupational Therapy in Pediatrics, 7*(3), 45-52.

Sattler, J.M. (1982). *Assessment of children's intelligence and special abilities*: (2nd Ed.). Boston: Allyn and Bacon, Inc.

Sattler, J.M. (1988). *Assessment of children* (3rd Ed.). San Diego, CA: Jerome M. Sattler.

Sparrow, S.S., Balla, D.A., & Cicchetti, D.V. (1984). *Vineland adaptive behavior scales*. Circle Pines, MN: American Guidance Service, Inc.

Sweetland, R.C., & Keyser, D.J. (1986). *Tests*. Kansas City: Test Corporation of America.

von Frey, M. (1906). The Distribution of Afferent Nerves in the Skin. *The Journal of the American Medical Association, 57*(9), 445-448.

Weschler, D. (1974). *Weschler Intelligence Scale for Children Revised*. New York: Psychological Corp.

Wodrich, D.L. & Joy, J.E. (1986). *Multi-disciplinary assessment of children with learning disabilities and mental retardation*. Baltimore: Paul H. Brookes Publishing Co.

Woodcock, R.W., & Johnson, M.B. (1977). *Woodcock Johnson Psycho-Educational Battery*. Hingham, MS: Teaching Resources.

CHAPTER CONTENT OUTLINE

KEY TERMS

Affective state

Apraxia

Balance

Coordination

Cortically programmed movements

Dexterity

Disinhibition

Epicritic senses

Muscle tone

Obligatory reflexive response

Protective extension response

Protopathic sensation

Sensory integration

ABSTRACT

This chapter identifies the various areas of neuromotor performance that should be evaluated and the general principles that should govern all neuromotor assessment. Various helpful references for locating a representative sample of neuromotor related tests are presented and pertinent evaluation tools are described.

Assessing Neuromotor Performance Enablers

19

Shereen D. Farber

"Man fathoms the nature of things by tracking their motion."

—Selim, 1982

OBJECTIVES

The information in this chapter is intended to help the reader—

1. appreciate the importance of continuous assessment when one is treating neuromotor pathology.

2. identify sources for locating appropriate neuromotor assessments.

3. identify those elements affecting neuromotor performance which typically need assessment.

4. become familiar with instruments appropriate for assessing the following areas of neuromotor performance: function, dexterity, the autonomic nervous system, reflexes, perceptual motor or sensory integrative ability, and motor development.

INTRODUCTION

This chapter will identify and describe the various areas of neuromotor performance that should be evaluated and describe general principles and evaluation concepts relative to these areas. Useful references for locating a representative sample of neuromotor-related tests will be described. Both qualitative and quantitative assessments provide valuable information regarding an individual's ability to perform fundamental movement patterns. Therefore, qualitative approaches for assessing neuromotor performance will be integrated into the chapter content.

GENERAL PRINCIPLES

Several general principles regarding assessment are pertinent to the determination of neuromotor function, as follows:

1. *Before incontestable evaluations can be done on patients, we must formulate operational definitions of important words and concepts to ensure consensus among therapists* (Rothstein, 1985). It seems obvious that preceding behavioral evaluations, therapists should agree on definitions for target behaviors and reach consensus regarding methods to be used to measure those behaviors, however, we have not yet reached consensus in definitions nor methods of evaluation. Efforts are being made to achieve uniform terminology, but there is still much nomenclature with variant definitions.

2. *Therapists must carefully select evaluations that most accurately assess the area of interest.* Standardized evaluations may be more appropriate for some situations, such as controlled research studies, but the therapist should avoid the misconception that all standardized evaluations are better than non-standardized ones. If a given test is outdated or if the equipment used for the protocol has been modified since the standardization process, the validity may be compromised; that is, the test may not assess what it is designed to do. Another problem with standardized tests is that the population may change over time and the norms may not reflect the current population. The decision to select a standardized or non-standardized evaluation should depend on a thorough review of the patient's needs, the therapist's goals, and the characteristics of the test. With operational definitions, the measurement process is clarified.

3. *Therapists must be knowledgeable in the interacting domains of neuromotor performance in order to achieve accurate neuromotor evaluation.* Chapter 10 contains a conceptual framework for understanding neuromotor performance. Proficiency in identification of neuromotor components assists the therapist in selecting the most appropriate evaluation tools for a particular patient, population, or age group. Once an assessment is selected, a therapist must scrutinize the tool in order to learn about its organization, objectives, purposes, testing protocol, scoring procedures, and interpretation of results. Several standardized evaluation tools can be ordered and used only by individuals who have taken a certification course sponsored by the test construction company. This practice attempts to ensure that the tester is qualified to administer and interpret the assessment according to the standardized procedures, thus increasing the reliability. Reliability is established when testing outcomes are consistent, when separate individuals use the same test, or one tester repeats use of a given test. Therapists modifying a standardized evaluation must analyze their findings with great care. Objectivity and well developed observational skills are also essential.

4. *An ongoing or continuous evaluation of a patient's progress is particularly crucial when one is treating individuals with neuromotor pathology.* If a patient demonstrates an adaptive behavioral response to therapeutic intervention, it is essential that the therapist immediately reinforce the response, allow the patient to consolidate the skill, and then adjust the intervention to provide gradual challenges to the patient. The therapist should perpetually evaluate all aspects of a patient's performance. Visually scanning a patient's whole body while that patient attempts a functional activity gives the therapist an increased awareness of the influence of that activity on the patient's performance. This practice allows the therapist to make rapid adjustments in the intervention to promote the best possible motor execution should the activity be inappropriate for the patient.

NEUROMOTOR ASSESSMENT RESOURCES

There are many books, usually located in the reference section of a medical library, that contain norms or lists of tests related to human behavior. Included below are several references that contain pertinent assessments.

- Roche, A.F. & Malina, R.M. (Eds.) (1983). *Manual of Physical Status and Performance in Childhood,* Vols. 1A, 1B and 2, New York, London: Plenum Press.

These volumes contain physical status and performance norms for children through adolescents for many types of behavior. An annotative bibliography catalogs specific studies and tests used to obtain the status and performance norms.

- Sweetland, R.C. & Keyser, D.J. (1983). *Tests: A Comprehensive Reference for Assessments in Psychology, Education and Business.* Kansas City, MO: Test Corporaton of America.

This text includes many assessments of development, motor skills, sensorimotor skills, and manual dexterity. For each test, the following information is provided: age range, purposes, description, scoring procedures, cost, and publisher.

- Keyser, D.J. & Sweetland, R.C. (1984). *Test Critiques,* Vol.1., Kansas City, MO: Test Corporation of America.

Each chapter of this book contains a detailed description of a given test including an introduction, overview, history of test development, practical applications, technical aspects, and a summary critique.

- Mitchell, J.V., Jr. (1985). *The Ninth Mental Measurements Yearbook,* Vols. I and II, Lincoln, Nebraska: The Buros Institute of Mental Measurements, The University of Nebraska.

This is one of the most comprehensive listings of tests, many of which relate to neuromotor performance. Detailed critiques are provided for each test.

EVALUATION AREAS: GENERAL CONCEPTS

The comprehensive assessment of neuromotor performance involves appraisal of many individual areas including: **affective state**, autonomic nervous system status, **balance**, body image, cognition, **coordination**, components of movement, developmental performance, **dexterity**, endurance, flexibility and range of motion, health status, motivation, motor planning, **muscle tone**, postural reflexes, rate and rhythm of movement, response to stress or motor challenge, sensory function, **sensory integration**, strength, and stereotypical behavior (perseveration). Each of these areas will be discussed

followed by a list of evaluation tools that relate to neuromotor performance.

Affective State

Detailed information regarding assessment of affective state is located in the chapter on Psychological Assessment, but one must consider how the affective state relates to neuromotor performance. For example, the depressed individual is not likely to walk with animation but the person suffering from a manic episode of manic depression may move very rapidly. Consider your own movement patterns when everything seems to be going wrong versus how you move when you are especially happy.

Autonomic Nervous System Status (ANS)

When an individual is dominated by the sympathetic division of the ANS, one consequence is an increase in muscle tone (Farber, 1982). This factor alone can change the quality of movement. Likewise, those who are parasympathetically dominated may show a reduced alertness with decreased muscle tone (Farber, 1982). It is important to establish a daily ANS baseline for each patient and continuously monitor the behavior throughout the treatment session (see Table 19-1). During the course of a treatment session, if a therapist inadvertently causes a patient to experience pain, the patient might then demonstrate sympathetic division ANS behavior. Pain is one of the most powerful stimulators of the sympathetic division of the ANS. A patient experiencing pain may demonstrate dilated pupils, increased muscle tone, nausea, diaphoresis, cool skin, erect hair, and other manifestations of the sympathetic division of the ANS. All these responses can block normal movement patterns. The procedure for ANS assessment will be discussed later in the chapter.

Balance

Neuromotor performance is governed by many inputs and components. Balance is similarly influenced by a variety of components (see Chapter 10). Balance reactions should be tested in all developmental postures, both qualitatively and quantitatively. Qualitative assessment require observation of the patient moving through alternate postures in which the center of gravity is statically and dynamically disturbed. The patient must be able to restore the center of gravity to the appropriate location within or near the body so that the posture can be maintained. Balance can be quantitatively measured by noting the amount of perturbation from the midline and the stimulus-response time. Videotaping is often helpful in quantitative assessment.

Carr and Shepherd (1980) emphasize that lateral weight shift and lateral flexion of the trunk and **protective extension responses** in the limbs are important to the regulation of

Table 19-1
Autonomic Nervous System Inventory

Organ	Sympathetic Response	Parasympathetic Response	Method of Measurement
Eye	Pupil dilated	Pupil contracted	Direct observation.
Nose	Vasoconstriction of nasal glands	Thin, copious secretion from nasal glands	Direct observation.
Mouth (Salivary Glands)	Dry mouth and thick saliva	Increased parotid gland stimulation, thin watery saliva	Examine oral cavity. Have patient spit into a cup. Examine saliva.
Sweat glands	Copious sweating	No response	Can be measured by galvanic skin resistance test. With increase in skin moisture, a decrease in resistance occurs. One can palpate the patient's skin for wetness, although this is less precise.
Apocrine glands	Thick odoriferous secretion	None	Body odor change can be detected.
Gut	Decreased peristalsis and tone with increased sphincter tone (constipation)	Increased peristalsis and tone with decreased sphincter tone (defecation reflex).	Palpate abdomen, question patient regarding bowel habits.
Skin temperature and color	Less than 31-33°C when room is 26-27°C. Skin color pale. Blood vessels constricted.	More than 31-33°C when room is 26-27°C. Skin color pink. Blood vessels dilated.	Skin temperature can be measured by temperature tapes or by biofeedback units.
Piloerector muscles	Hair standing on end. Goose pimples.	None	Direct observation.
Muscle tone	Increased tone and strength	Decreased tone and strength	Palpation of musculature; biofeedback (EMG) to measure tone and dynamometer to measure grip strength.
Mental activity	Increased activity, asynchronous cortical potentials, emotional excitement.	Decreased activity, synchronous cortical potentials. Relaxation.	Talk with patient. Ask questions. EEG can be used by qualified personnel.

balance. Cash (1977) recommends testing balance by placing a patient in a posture, asking him to hold that posture with and without vision. Tilt boards, balance beams, and one-foot standing tests are also used to assess balance. Specific tests for balance are listed in the next section of this chapter.

Body Image

Assessment of body image can give a therapist valuable clues as to a patient's functional movement patterns. Patients who have a sensory deficit may ignore part of their body (*body side disregard*). Patients with this problem often walk into walls or drive wheelchairs into walls and corners on the affected side of their body. For further discussion of this phenomenon, see Chapter 18, Assessing Sensory Performance Enablers.

Cognition

This vital area of cognition also impacts upon movement. It is easy to realize that an individual must be aware of the environment in order to be motivated to systematically

explore it, as demonstrated when we observe a profoundly retarded child who is unaware of the environment. Without cognition, movement may be random, stereotypic, or reflexive. For further discussion, see Assessing Cognition, Chapter 20.

Coordination

Although there are many standardized assessments to evaluate coordination, it is important to remember that qualitative observation can yield important findings as well. Anyone can observe a ponderous, bumbling individual who trips while walking upstairs or someone who hits himself in the head with a tennis racket while trying to serve and deduce that such people lack coordination. But it takes a professionally trained observer to look for specific findings and determine which aspects of neuromotor performance are deficient to produce such awkwardness in coordination.

Individual movement patterns should be observed to determine the degree of effort expended and the smoothness achieved. The highly skilled individual makes few extraneous

Table 19-1 (continued)
Autonomic Nervous System Inventory

Organ	Sympathetic Response	Parasympathetic Response	Method of Measurement
Blood pressure	Most experts agree that blood pressure greater than 140/90 is hypertension at any age and bears watching.	Lower blood pressure than normal.	Measured by sphygmomanometer with arm held at the level of the aorta. Blood pressure values vary for age and sex, getting progressively higher with age. 118/73 is normal for a teenage male. 125/78 is mean value for a 25-year-old male and 142/85 is mean value for a 60 to 65-year-old male.
Organ pulse	Sympathetic response is higher than normal	Parasympathetic response is lower than normal	Method of measurement is to palpate pulse at the wrist. Normal values vary with age (pulse rate/minute): Birth 122 2-5 114 range 5-9 103 range 9-12 89 range Adult 75 range
Respiration	Faster than normal; shallow pattern	Slower than normal	Count respiration cycles per minute. Normal values vary for each age: Birth 30 range 2-5 26 range 5-9 25 range 9-12 24 range Adult 17 range

The data in this table have been compiled from: Guyton, 1977; Peele, 1977; Adams and Victor, 1977; Altman and Dittmer, 1971; Sunderman and Boerner, 1949; Hurst, 1978.

movements, reducing energy expenditure as skill and coordination increase. Conversely, the clumsy individual uses nonessential movements that do not contribute to the overall movement pattern goal. Individuals who have poor coordination frequently cannot change the rate or rhythm of their movement, thus making transitions from stationary postures to movement sequences much more difficult.

Muscle tone should be assessed as part of a qualitative evaluation of coordination. Those who have the most precise and coordinated movements often demonstrate excellent proximal muscle tone throughout the trunk and proximal joints. This balanced tone allows them to operate from a stable base. In contrast, the poorly coordinated individual may have increased mobility where he/she should have stability. Proximal joints may be hypermobile and trunk tone may be decreased. Without a stable base, it is often impossible to make smooth, precise movements or to reproduce a given motor pattern reliably. This concept can be tested by asking an individual to do an activity that requires distal coordination and observing the response. Following this, the therapist

should assist the patient in maintaining a stable trunk and proximal joints and repeat the activity to judge whether improved distal coordination evolves. The patient may have good distal coordination without balanced proximal tone, but if he/she cannot place the extremity in the desired location, the skill may not be used.

Therapists should be aware that there are those who demonstrate poor coordination only when being examined. These individuals demonstrate poor coordination when stressed, challenged or when **cortically programming movement**; at other times they may not appear as uncoordinated. Emotions can significantly alter the degree of precision. See Chapter 10 for additional factors that may impair coordination.

Components of Movement

Every movement pattern consists of multiple components. Some of the simple constituents are flexion, lateral flexion, extension, lateral extension (or elongation), abduction, adduction, pronation, and supination. Other components combine several simple movements including rotation of limb, trunk, or neck. Other movement components are *weight shifts*, (loading and unloading of a limb, also called support and non-support postures), and reciprocal and diagonal movements that cross the body's midline. Movement components are generally assessed in developmental postures. For example, if an eight-month-old child cannot separate his upper trunk from his lower trunk (*decreased trunk segmentation*), he or she will have difficulty rotating his trunk over his hips while moving from sitting to prone.

Neurodevelopmental Therapy (NDT) specifically addresses assessment of movement components for the patient who has neurological involvement (Bobath, 1971; Bobath, 1974). Consideration of components of movement is valuable for individuals of all ages and diagnoses with movement pathology. When performance is compromised, the therapist should identify the missing movement components and plan therapy to incorporate those components.

Developmental Level

Most developmental testing profiles have motor performance sections. Developmental milestones must be considered as more than a serial set of behaviors. Motor developmental posture results from a highly complex integration of postural reflexes, motivation, cognition, autonomic nervous system status, integrity and maturation of the central nervous system, and response to sensation, all of which are expressed by the motor end organs.

Most developmental assessments are designed for children, therefore application to the adult population will require modification. For example, the therapist must assess common postures used by adults and determine the quality of movement components in each posture as well as the patient's ability to assume, maintain, move within and move out of a posture. It is also important to challenge the patient while in a given posture to see if the patient can function with the same quality of neuromotor performance while being stressed.

Dexterity

Dexterity is a type of fine coordination which is usually demonstrated in the upper extremity. Many standardized tests assess manual dexterity or fine motor coordination. Some of these tests are administered by personnel departments to determine if a candidate for a given position has the necessary manual skills. Erhardt (1982) reviews the development of hand function throughout the developmental continuum. She has created an assessment of developmental hand dysfunction (listed in the next section) based on these findings. The types of behavior generally tested in this area include: prehension patterns, grasp and release ability, hand posture and tone, speed of object manipulation, accuracy of movement during a small muscle task, tremor, writing, and pre-writing skills. Many of these tests are administered to the individual sitting with arm supported. It is also important to test these skills in a variety of postures and with the arm in both supported and unsupported positions.

Endurance

Endurance is a measure of stamina and fitness and should be assessed initially, before beginning treatment since it may determine the patient's tolerance for activity. Endurance may be compromised by the energy wasted during superfluous movements, poor motor planning skills, inappropriate muscle tone, and many other factors. In some cases, patients must build endurance to facilitate changes in position. Any patient who has been recumbent for long periods of time will experience weakness when moving from lower level postures to sitting and vertical postures. One of the most important reasons to monitor a patient's endurance is to protect that individual from injury. Many accidents occur when a person is fatigued and incapable of maintaining good joint alignment.

Flexibility and Range of Motion

Flexibility should be evaluated during active and passive movement and during movement patterns. Joint mobilization courses teach detailed assessment procedures for passive range. Cyriax and Cyriax (1983) recommend that passive range be tested with the body part totally relaxed. Passive range assesses joint capsules, ligaments, bursae, fascia and other inert structures. Detailed methods and norms for measurement of range of motion are described by Sullivan and Poole (1981) and Smith (1978). Goniometers are commonly used to measure the achieved range. Newer methods may employ videotaped performance with computerized assessment.

When measuring either passive or active range in a patient who has neurological damage, care must be taken not to stimulate primitive postural reflexes or hypertonicity, both of which may limit range. Too much flexibility or range can cause as many problems as reduced flexibility. Miller (1985) reviewed alternate range of motion evaluations and reported that there are variables in the methods of measurements that can affect the results, such as age, sex, and activity profiles of the subjects. Some joints are easier to measure than others and therefore have better reliability indices when compared to others.

Health Status

An individual's state of health can influence neuromotor performance. Patients often forget to mention some symptom or illness to their physicians when the medical history and physical examination is performed. After reviewing the history and physical performed by the physician, the therapist should ask the patient additional questions regarding his/her health status if indicated. Good communication among physician, patient, family, and therapy staff is essential. Therapists should also obtain a record of the patient's medications and consult with the physician and/or the *Physician's Desk Reference* to ascertain if the pharmacological regimen might modify the patient's neuromotor performance.

Motivation

There are few, if any, components of human performance that are not directly influenced by a person's level of motivation; thus it is important to determine whether the individual is motivated to improve neuromotor performance. Without motivation, patient cooperation and active participation is decreased. The methods for assessment of motivation are discussed in Chapter 21, Assessing Pyschological Performance Factors.

Motor Planning

Many individuals can execute specific components of movement but are completely unable to produce previously learned motor sequences or patterns after a traumatic injury or neurological impairment. It seems that when these people cortically direct their own movement, performance quality decreases. This behavior is typical in patients with the diagnosis of **apraxia**. It is vital that the patient be asked to perform motor acts that require planning in order to assess the extent of apraxia. If possible, it is helpful to determine if the patient can achieve success in the same activity when the therapist provides subcortical guidance and handling rather than structuring the activity so that cortical planning is required on the part of the patient. Once performance improves with subcortical guidance and practice, the therapist may again attempt cortical commands.

Muscle Tone

Assessment of muscle tone is difficult to accomplish with reliability and validity. Every method of tonal assessment has limitations. Physicians often use the stretch reflex and grade responses from zero to four. Low scores are used for no response to passive stretch (hypotonus) while high scores represent hypertonus. Barrows (1980) defined tone as resistance offered by a muscle to a stretch when a joint is passively moved. He recommended that tone be assessed in the limbs, trunk, and neck and that distal segments of limbs should be tested before proximal ones.

Physicians also use needle electrode electromyographs to assess muscle tone. Surface electrode electromyographs can be used to assess tone as well as for biofeedback and muscle re-education. Electrical interference can reduce the reliability of the data with this latter method. A subjective assessment is obtained by handling a limb or moving the trunk through its range. Some therapists assign grades from one to four based on the degree of tonus. This method may demonstrate reduced intertester reliability unless therapists are trained to assess tone using the same frame of reference. In addition, therapists must take great care when moving a patient's body part in order to avoid influencing the tone due to handling methods used. The extremity should be supported by its bony prominences, thus avoiding inserting pressure into either muscle or tendons that can modify tone. As one manipulates a patient's limb, both slow and fast stretch may be employed depending on the desired result, since hypertonic muscles are often velocity sensitive and will increase tone with fast movement.

An additional method of tonal assessment aspect involves determining if the tonus is appropriate for the activity in progress. If the patient generates too much tone, overflow or unwanted movement may appear. Overflow occurs in normal individuals when they are executing a new motor act or one that requires more skill than they possess. If a normal person is asked to cortically suppress overflow, supression is usually possible.

Postural Reflexes

Postural reflexes are commonly evaluated by therapists and provide insight regarding a patient's ability to move voluntarily. These reflexes are said to occur according to a developmental hierarchy, and many of them are subsequently integrated by higher motor centers in the nervous system. Postural reflexes serve as a foundation for tone and movement. They can re-emerge after being integrated if a motor challenge is too great for the individual or if brain damage yields **disinhibition** of higher integrating centers. Even when it is normal for a child to demonstrate a postural reflex, he or she is never dominated by it. Domination, also known as an **obligatory reflexive response**, indicates pathology. When patients are obligated to respond with a primitive postural response, movement is lock-stepped and non-flexible. Therapists must employ several principles in testing primitive reflexes: (1) *Reflexes and responses should be tested in all developmental postures.* A given reflex might not be present in prone and supine positions, but when the patient is placed in a more demanding posture like standing, positive responses may be elicited. (2) *Any stress can disinhibit (release) elements of the primitive postural reflexes.* These reflexes are often seen in the normal population. (3) *It is rare that a patient with chronic neuromotor pathology will demonstrate a given primitive postural reflex in its pure form.* More often, reflexes are combined so that patients demonstrate elements of several reflexes in one behavioral response.

Rate and Rhythm of Movement

Every person utilizes their own natural rate and rhythm of movement. When any illness disrupts a patient's functional movement patterns, the therapist must attempt to determine the most effective rate and rhythm to use in therapy for adaptive response production. A history from family members may help the therapist to learn about the patient's rate and rhythm prior to the illness or injury. For example, some families have videotapes or movies showing the patient ambulating before the illness. Once the condition prevents the patient from moving normally or independently, the therapist cannot expect to return immediately to the original rate and rhythm; however, progress toward that goal is helpful in triggering motor memories.

Response to Stress and Motor Challenge

Motor challenges and application of subtle stresses are constructive evaluation techniques to display what might happen to a patient's motor responses in the real world. Therapeutic settings are often sensory controlled, and a patient may move using a reasonable quality of movement when in those settings. It is vital to help prepare the patient to move in his/her typical environments with acccceptable movement quality. Therapists may be able to increase a patient's ability to handle stress with resultant improvement of neuromotor performance.

Sensory Function

One of the most important factors that influences motor function is a patient's level of sensory awareness. There are many sensory testing batteries available in neurology texts, occupational therapy references, and related literature. Areas that should be assessed include: (1) response to _protopathic sensations_ or protective sensations, also known as exteroceptive sensations because the receptors are primarily located in the skin; (2) **epicritic senses** or discriminative touch, also known as _proprioceptive senses_ because of contribution from stimuli from joints, tendons, deep skin receptors, muscles and deeper structures; (3) olfactory responses; (4) vestibular integrity; (5) gustatory senses; and (6) visual and auditory systems.

Care must be exercised to avoid sensory bombardment in susceptible patients during the evaluation of sensation. If bombardment is a possibility, the therapist should test only a few types of sensation per evaluation session.

Sensory Integration

Sensory integration is the ability of the brain to receive inputs from various sensory sources and to mix and prioritize those inputs in order to accelerate development of highly flexible, survival-oriented behavior (_adaptive behavior_). It is important for the therapist to determine if neuromotor performance is interrupted due to the brain's ability to integrate inputs from multiple systems. Several test batteries that are specifically designed to evaluate sensory integration are listed in the section below. This subject is also covered extensively in the chapter on sensory function.

Strength

Dynamic and static strength are assessed in various ways including use of _manual muscle testing_ (MMT), a Cybex machine (_isokinetic capacity_), or functional strength patterns. Lamb (1985) presents a complete discussion of various aspects of MMT including the variables of testing procedures, reliability and validity issues, and appropriate population. While various operational definitions exist for strength, it has yet to be determined whether all of the various measures of strength address the same features. There are also differences in methodology during MMT, such as application of force, stabilization, and positioning, and it has not been firmly established whether these variations make functional differences in strength determinations during controlled studies (Smidt and Roger, 1982).

Other factors that must be considered when doing MMT are the type of contraction characteristic of each tested muscle and the rate of tension generated during testing. Lamb (1985) believes that there is a degree of reliability in MMT when performed on the appropriate population by therapists who are knowledgeable in anatomy and kinesiology. In addition, MMT does have _face validity_, (measures what it purports to measure) and _content validity_, (reflects physiological and anatomical principles). Whether MMT has other types of validity is yet to be determined (Lamb, 1985). Manual muscle testing is rarely used for patients suffering from central nervous system pathology since application of resistance against hypertonic muscles does not yield a true picture of the baseline strength. Resistance may exacerbate abnormal tone. Technological advancements have provided therapists with new, expensive equipment that manufacturers claim quantitate measurements to a high degree. Rothstein and associates (1985) describe some pieces of equipment and completed studies that test the reliability and validity of measures gathered with them. Many types do not demonstrate _intra-equipment reliability_ (rendering the same values when tested at different times) nor _inter-equipment reliability_ (rendering the same values when two different pieces of the same type of equipment are used). Much research is needed to ensure that such methods and equipment do measure what we expect them to measure, rather than just generating meaningless data.

Stereotypic Behavior

Many brain-injured or mentally retarded individuals

motor behavior that grossly interferes with the quality and quantity of neuromotor performance. Perseveration is a type of stereotypical behavior that inhibits an individual's functional exploration capabilities within a given environmental setting. Stereotypical behavior is also seen at certain time periods in the normal development of children. See Chapter 10, Neuromotor Dimensions of Performance, for more information on this subject. When evaluating a patient who demonstrates stereotypical behavior, the critical factor is to determine whether such behavior is adaptive or maladaptive.

EVALUATIONS RELATED TO NEUROMOTOR PERFORMANCE

Autonomic Nervous System Inventory

Source: Farber, S.D. (1982). Neurorehabilitation evaluation concepts. In Farber, S.D. (ed.): *Neurorehabilitation: A Multisensory Approach.* Philadelphia, W.B. Saunders Company.

Comments: This is a non-standardized assessment compiled from numerous neurobiology texts. It contains methods of measurement of ANS behavior and norms for all age groups.

Developmental Assessments

Bayley Scales of Infant Development.
Source: The Psychological Corp., A subsidiary of Harcourt Brace Jovanovich, Inc., 7500 Old Oak Blvd., Cleveland, Ohio 44130

Comments: This well-known test screens all aspects of development in babies from 2 to 30 months of age. The motor scale contains tests of general body control, and coordination. It is scored by the examiner.

Comprehensive Developmental Scale.
Source: El Paso Rehabilitation Center, 2630 Richmond, El Paso, Texas 79930.

Comments: This assessment battery was developed by a multi-disciplinary team and measures a wide range of behaviors including gross motor and fine motor coordination, muscle tone, reflexes, and other related behaviors.

The Gesell Developmental Tests.
Source: Programs for Education, Box 85, Lumberville, Pennsylvania 18933.

Comments: This comprehensive developmental scale was standardized for children ages 5 to 10. A motor behavioral scale is included in the battery.

Reynell-Zink Developmental Scales for Young Visually Handicapped Children.
Source: NFER-Nelson Publishing Co., 1120 Birchmount Road, Scarborough, Ontario, Canada M1K 5G4

Comments: This is an unusual test for a special population, the visually impaired. It looks at sensorimotor behavior, environmental exploration and other related behaviors and provides comparisons between the visually impaired and age-matched controls.

Dexterity Assessments

Crawford Small Parts Dexterity Test.
Source: The Psychological Corporation, A Subsidiary of Harcourt Brace Jovanovich, Inc., 7500 Old Oak Blvd., Cleveland, Ohio 44130.

Comments: The purpose of this assessment tool is to determine if an individual possesses the manual dexterity necessary for certain professions such as dentistry, jewelry construction, etc. It was designed for teenagers and adults.

The Erhardt Developmental Prehension Assessment.
Source: RAMSCO Publishing Co., A subsidiary of RAM Associated, Ltd., P.O. Box N, Laurel, Maryland 20707

Comments: This prehension test is part of a text entitled, *Developmental Hand Dysfunction Theory Assessment Treatment* by Rhoda P. Erhardt, OTR. The text provides a conceptual frame for understanding the development of prehension, information regarding the development of the assessment tool, and treatment information.

Fine Dexterity Test.
Source: Educational and Industrial Test Services Ltd., 83 High St., Hemel Hempstead, Herts. HP1 3AH, England.

Comments: This test was specifically designed to assess the fine finger movements of the adult population.

The Grooved Pegboard Test.
Source: Lafayette Instrument Co., P.O. Box 5729, Lafayette, IN 47903

Table 19-2
Sensory System Inventory

Sensory System	Stimulus	Response	Possible Significance or Implications
Spinothalamic-spinoreticular system	*Maintained pressure: A. To perioral region	Head hyperextending away from stimulus	Aversive response. Use maintained pressure on abdomen, palms or soles of feet first. Retest.
	B. To other body surface areas, including abdomen, palms, soles of feet, or skin over specific muscles.	Generalized calming	Proceed with appropriate other sensory testing such as light moving touch.
		Specific calming of underlying muscle	Proceed to functional test of specific muscle function. (An example is to apply maintained pressure to the masseters, resulting in a relaxation of spasticity. Chewing function or jaw jerk should then be tested.)
		Clawing of toes or reflexive grasp response	Hypersensitive skin in the palmar or plantar surface needing normalization.
	Light moving touch: A. To perioral midline	Total flexor pattern with the palmar surface out	More primitive response. Repeat light moving touch stimulus with rolling to assist pattern.
		Total flexor pattern with palms to face	More adaptive response. Proceed to activities using hand-mouth pattern.
	B. To T10 dermatome (adult)	Flexion of homolateral side leg	Proceed to activities using dorsiflexion and flexion of the leg (rolling, creeping, walking).
Vestibular system	Inversion	Reduction of hypertonicity, facilitation of midline trunk extensors, soleus, extensor carpi ulnaris and radialis, gastrocnemius, biceps femoris (long head), vasti, rectus femoris, triceps, gluteus maximus, deltoid. Good co-contraction pattern at the neck	Desired responses. Proceed to appropriate developmental pattern. Reinforce components of pattern with proprioceptive stimulation.
		Aversive response: flushed face, excessive sweating, other sympathetic responses	Carotid sinus may not be properly functioning. Discontinue inversion.
		Hyperextension of the neck	Reflexive neck extension pattern instead of desired co-contraction pattern. Place visual stimulus on the floor to direct patient's visual responses.
	Anteroposterior motion in each developmental pattern Slow, even movement→	Generalized relaxation→	Desired response, proceed to appropriate developmental or facilitation pattern.
	Fast, irregular motion→	Generalized increase in tone→	Desired response for patients with systemic hypotonia. Add proprioceptive stimuli to pattern when appropriate.
	Side-to-side movement in a slow even pattern	Weight shifting	Desired response. Add resistance to pattern if appropriate, then proceed to diagonal pattern.

Table 19-2
Sensory System Inventory (continued)

Sensory System	Stimulus	Response	Possible Significance or Implications
Vestibular system (cont.)	Diagonal rocking	Weight shifting	Desired response. Proceed to appropriate developmental pattern to reinforce movement (crawling, creeping, walking).
	Rotating: A. Rolling	Log-rolling response	Primitive reflex level. Need to do slow rolling pattern or other inhibitory handling to assist in integration of the primitive response. Follow with facilitation of segmental rolling.
		Segmental rolling response	Adaptive response. Proceed to next appropriate developmental pattern.
	B. Facilitory rotation in any developmental pattern	No change in muscle tone, no post-rotatory nystagmus	Patient may have sensory integrative dysfunction. Do comprehensive testing and carefully monitor vestibular input.
		Post-rotatory nystagmus and appropriate change in muscle tone	Adaptive response.
Olfactory	Banana/vanilla	Reflex sucking	As an initial response, this would be considered an adaptive response. If the patient does not progress, the continued reflex sucking is no longer considered adaptive. More advanced behavior includes changes in facial expression, muscle tone, movement patterns, verbalization following stimulation.
	A variety of common odors	Patient is able to identify the odor	Advanced, adaptive response.
Gustatory	Sweet, sour, bitter, salt stimuli to appropriate tongue areas	Change in facial expression; changes in muscle tone; reflex sucking; increased salivation; movement of tongue and lips; swallowing	Progressive adaptive responses.
Epicritic function	Quick stretch to a given muscle	Normal contraction of that muscle	Monosynaptic reflex (muscle stretch reflex) working properly.
		Hypertonicity of muscle stretched	Disinhibition of higher centers secondary to an upper motor neuron lesion.
	Vibrating tuning fork applied to bony prominences	Perception of vibration	Adaptive response; dorsal columns/medial lemniscus system intact.
	Vibration of a specific muscle with an electric vibrator	Appropriate contraction of muscle and relaxation of antagonist	Tonic vibratory response intact
	Placement of an object in hand for tactile discrimination without visual clues	Stereognosis	Adaptive response of epicritic system and development of association areas of brain.
		Astereognosis	Lesion in dorsal columns, medial lemniscus, or higher centers associated with stereognosis

Table 19-2
Sensory System Inventory (continued)

Sensory System	Stimulus	Response	Possible Significance or Implications
Epicritic function (cont.)	Move patient's body part while asking him to identify direction of movement	Correct identification of movement direction	Adaptive response (kinesthetic sense)
	Move body part to a specific position then ask patient to identify position	Correct identification	Adaptive response (position sense)
Temperature	Cold or warm water in tubes applied to various skin surfaces	Lack of identification	Deficit in protopathic sensation. Instruct patient in compensation techniques until protopathic sense improves.
Auditory	Ring a bell 12 inches from patient's ear	Patient turns head to the sound or can identify stimulus	Adaptive response.
	Present a sequence of numbers	Patient cannot repeat sequence	Possible receptive problem or memory deficit. Assess further.
	Alternately stimulate each ear with tones of different pitches and volumes	Patient cannot hear many of the tones	Refer the patient to an audiologist for further evaluation.
Vision	In a dark room, press on patient's eyeballs (see Chap. 3); coma sequence	Patient changes facial expression, vocalizes, opens eyes, moves a body part	Adaptive response.
	In a dark room, move flashlight across visual fields	Patient does not track stimulus	Possible vestibular problem or cranial nerve lesion.
		Patient tracks stimulus in all directions, demonstrating conjugate eye movement	Adaptive response.

* It is recognized that maintained pressure is an epicritic stimulus. In this case, it is used to determine whether the patient is demonstrating tactile defensiveness.

Comments: This standardized test is designed to measure finger dexterity and eye-hand coordination. It only takes approximately five minutes to administer.

Moore Eye-Hand Coordination and Color Matching Test.
Source: Joseph E. Moore and Associates, Perry Drive, RFD 12, Box 309, Gainesville, Georgia 30501.
Comments: This test was developed to measure speed of eye-hand coordination and color matching for all age groups.

Purdue Pegboard Test.
Source: Science Research Association, 155 North Wacker Drive, Chicago, Illinois 60606.
Comments: This test of dexterity provides norms for adults and children, 5 years to 15 years, ll months.

General Motor Function Assessment Batteries

Bruininks-Oseretsky Test of Motor Proficiency.
Source: American Guidance Services, Publishers Blvd., Circle Pines, Minnesota 55014.
Comments: This comprehensive test battery is standardized to test individuals from the ages of 4 years, 6 months to 14 years, 6 months. The primary purpose is to assess various motor functional components in order to make the correct educational placement. The areas tested include: gross and fine coordination, dexterity, upper limb speed, visual motor control, strength, running speed and ability, balance, and coordination.

Devereux Test of Extremity Coordination.
Source: The Devereux Foundation, 19 S. Waterloo Road, Devon, Pennsylvania 64112.
Comments: This standardized test was developed for children from the ages of 4 to 10. The test assesses static balance, motor attention span, body image, fine motor activity, and sequential motor activity.

Gardner Steadiness Test.
Source: Lafayette Instrument Co., P.O. Box 5729, Lafayette, IN 47903.
Comments: This test measures various types of behavior including hyperactivity, tremors, choreiform movement patterns, and motor impersistence. This test is standardized for children from the ages of 5 years to 14 years, 11 months.

Lincoln-Oseretsky Motor Development Scale.
Source: Stoelting Company, 1350 S. Kostner Ave., Chicago, Illinois 60623.
Comments: This test was designed to assess 36 motor tasks in children ages 6 to 14. Some of the activities tested include: one foot standing, deep knee bend while on tiptoes, tapping rhythms, walking backwards, static and dynamic coordination, speed of movement, eye-hand coordination, gross hand activities, and finger dexterity.

Miller Assessment for Preschoolers.
Source: Kid Foundation, 8101 Prentice Ave., Suite 518, Englewood , CO, 80111
Comments: This screening test for the preschool-aged population was developed by Lucy Jane Miller, MS, OTR. It contains 27 core items in the sensory and motor areas and is standardized. Some of the activities tested include walking a line, hand-to-nose test, stepping, vertical writing test, touch sense, components of normal movements, gross motor assessment, and the Romberg test.

The Quick Neurological Screening Test.
Source: Academic Therapy Publications, 20 Commercial Blvd., Novato, California 94947.
Comments: This comprehensive test screens neurological integration in subjects 5 years of age through the adult age. Areas that are tested include: attention, cerebellar-vestibular function, balance, spatial organization, rate and rhythm of movement, motor planning, coordination, and level of maturity of the nervous system.

The Rail-Walking Test.
Source: S. Roy Heath, Ph.D., 1193 S. East Street, Amherst, Massachusetts 01002.
Comments: The primary function of this test is to assess locomotor coordination and balance of individuals ages six through adult. The test kit contains detailed instructions and norms.

The Riley Motor Problem Inventory.
Source: Western Psychological Services, 12031 Wilshire Blvd., Los Angeles, California 90025.
Comments: This test battery screens gross and fine motor behavior and takes approximately 5 to 10 minutes to administer. It has been standardized for children ages 4 through 9.

Sequin-Goddard Formboards.
Source: Stoelting Co., 1350 S. Kostner Ave., Chicago, Illinois, 60623.
Comments: The major purpose of this test is to measure tactual performance, including the areas of spatial perception, recognition of forms, manual construction, and motor coordination. This test has been standardized for individuals ages 5 through 14.

The Test of Motor Impairment (Henderson Revision).
Source: Brook Educational Publications Ltd., Box 1171, Guelph, Ontario, Canada, N1H 6N3.
Comments: The purpose of this test is to assist in diagnosis of motor deficits. The areas tested include static and dynamic balance, manual dexterity, eye-hand coordination, speed of movement, and manner of coping or problem-solving. The test is designed for children ages 5 to 14 years.

Perceptual Motor or Sensory Integration Tests

Bender Visual Motor Gestalt Test.
Source: American Orthopsychiatric Association, 1775 Broadway, New York, New York 10019.
Comments: This comprehensive assessment analyzes several visual motor activities. It was designed for a wide range of ages from children of age three years through adults.

Purdue Perceptual Motor Survey (PPMS).
Source: Charles E. Merrill Pub. Co., 1300 Alum Creek Drive, Box 508, Columbus, Ohio 43216.
Comments: The PPMS is a comprehensive motor assessment battery designed for children from preschool through 8th grade. The following behaviors are tested: walking board performance, balance and posture, jumping, body image, imitation of movements, obstacle course, Krauss Weber Test, angels in the snow, and rhythmic writing.

Southern California Sensory Integration Tests.
Source: Western Psychological Services, 12031 Wilshire Blvd., Los Angeles, California 90025.
Comments: This test is widely used by occupational and physical therapists and was developed by A. Jean Ayres, Ph.D., OTR. There are many sub-tests in the battery which was standardized for children from the ages of 4 to 10 years. Certification in testing and interpretation is required to administer this test.

Sensory Integration and Praxis Tests.
Source: Western Psychological Services, 12031 Wilshire Blvd., Los Angeles, California 90025.
Comments: This carefully standardized test battery is based on earlier work of the late A. Jean Ayres, Ph.D. There are 17 subtests which are used to generate a computerized score profile. Formal training is highly recommended for administration and interpretation.

Reflex Assessments

Bender Purdue Reflex and Training Manual.
Source: Academic Therapy Publications, 20 Commercial Blvd., Novato, California 94947.
Comments: This publication contains a testing protocol for some of the primitive postural reflexes and treatment suggestions to reduce the effect of these reflexes on neuromotor performance. It was designed for children between the ages of 6 and 12.

Neurophysiological Basis of Patient Treatment. Vol. 2: Reflex Testing.
Source: Crutchfield, M.R., Barnes, C.A. and Heriza, C.B., Stokesville Publishing Company, Morgantown, West Virginia. 1978.
Comments: This manual provides background information on the development of individual reflexes and includes testing instructions and charts. The authors demonstrate the testing of given reflexes in a variety of developmental postures.

Reflex Testing Methods for Evaluating CNS Development.
Source: Fiorentino, M.R., C.C. Thomas Publishing Company. Springfield, Illinois, 1973.
Comments: This standard text contains methods to test primitive postural reflexes and higher level postural reflexes.

Sensory Assessments and Resources

Barrow's Guide to Neurological Assessment.
Source: Barrows, H.S., M.D., J.B. Lippincott Company, East Washington Square Philadelphia, Pa, 19105.
Comments: This is an excellent, concise text originally developed for medical students and house staff in neurology. Many of the sensory tests provided in this neurological examination are appropriate for use by occupational therapist.

Sensory System Inventory.
Source: Farber, S.D. (1982). Neurorehabilitation: A Multisensory Approach. Published by W.B. Saunders Company, Philadelphia, pages 111-113.
Comments: This sensory inventory was designed to use with patients having neurological impairments. The inventory addresses each sensory system, suggests appropriate stimuli, identifies the desired responses, and includes the possible significance or implication for therapy.

SUMMARY

Consistent with the perspective taken in this text, assessment neuromotor performance enablers should be considered as part of a comprehensive assessment approach which considers both intrinsic as well as environmental factors. Competent movement is a complex phenomenon which results from the contributions of many areas, which include the person's affective state, autonomic nervous system status, balance, cognition, coordination, dexterity, endurance, and other factors.

In this chapter, approaches to assessing the various neuromotor factors have been summarized. Rather than providing in-depth information on the available approaches for each factor, the reader has been referred to a list of resources about specific tests, batteries, and clinical methods which are viewed as helpful to assessing fundamental movement patterns. While much emphasis has been placed on standardized tests in the past, the importance of qualitative information should not be overlooked; particularly that which can be derived from careful observation of the patient in activities which place varying postural and movement demands. To derive the most complete picture of the patient's level of function and permit appropriate adjustments in intervention, assessment should be viewed as an ongoing process which provides continuous information to the therapist over time.

Study Questions

1. Why should endurance testing be conducted early in the assessment process?

2. What factors might influence one's gross coordination?

3. Why is continuous patient assessment vital to effective intervention with an individual having neuromotor problems?

4. Why is manual muscle testing seldom used in patients having hypertonicity?

5. Why might dexterity be decreased in an individual with decreased proximal stability?

References

Barrows, H.S. (1980). *Guide to neurological assessment.* Philadelphia: J.B. Lippincott Co.

Bobath, B. (1971). Motor development, its effect on general development, and application to the treatment of cerebral palsy. *Physiotherapy, 57,* 526-532.

Bobath, K. (1974). *The motor deficit in patients with cerebral palsy.* Suffolk: Lavenham Press.

Boyle, A.M. & Santelli, J.C. (1986). Assessing psychomotor skills: the role of the Crawford Small Parts Dexterity Test as a screening instrument. *Journal of Dental Education, 50,*176-179.

Campbell, S.K. (1985). Assessment of the child with CNS dysfunction. (pp 207-228) In Rothsetin J. M. (Ed): Measurement in physical therapy. New York: Churchill Livingstone.

Carr, J.H. & Shepherd, R.B. (1980). *Physiotherapy in disorders of the brain.* London: Wm. Heinemann Medical Books Ltd.

Cash, J. (1977). *Neurology for physiotherapists.* 2nd ed. Philadelphia: J.B. Lippincott Co.

Cyriax, J. & Cyriax, P. (1983).*Illustrated manual of orthopaedic medicine.* London: Butterworths.

Daniels, L. & Worthingham, C. (1980).*Muscle testing: Technique of manual examination* (4th ed). Philadelphia: W.B. Saunders.

Erhardt, R.P. (1982). *Developmental hand dysfunction: Theory, assessment, treatment.* Laurel, MD: RAMSCO Publishing Company.

Farber, S.D. (1982). *Neurorehabilitation: A multisensory approach.* Philadelphia: W.B. Saunders Co.

Haines, C.R., Brown, J.B., Granthan, E.B., Rajagopalan, V.S., & Sutcliffe, P.V. (1985). Neurodevelopmental screen in the school entrant medical examination as a predictor of coordination and communication difficulties. *Archives of Diseases of Children, 60,* 1122-1127.

Haley, S.M. (1986). Postural reactions in infants with Down syndrome. Relationship to motor milestone development and age. *Physical Therapy, 66,* 17-22.

Kendall, H., Kendall, F., & Wadsworth, G. (1971). *Muscle testing and function* (2nd ed). Baltimore: Williams and Wilkins.

Lamb, R.L. (1985). Manual muscle testing. (pp. 47-102) In Rothstein, J.M. (Ed.): *Measurement in physical therapy.* New York: Churchill Livingstone.

Mann, A.H. (1985). The clinical relevance of psychometric testing. *European Journal of Clinical Pharmacology, 28* (Suppl): 31-34.

Mayhew, T.P., Rothstein, J.M. (1985). Measurement of muscle performance with instruments. (pp. 57-102). In Rothstein, J.M. (Ed.) *Measurement in physical therapy.* New York: Churchill Livingstone.

Miller, P.J. (1985). Assessment of joint motion. (pp 103-136). In Rothstein, J.M. (Ed.): *Measurement in physical therapy.* New York: Churchill Livingstone.

Rothstein, J.M. (Ed.) (1985). *Measurement in physical therapy.* New York: Churchill Livingstone.

Selim, R.D. (Ed.). (1982). *The human body: Muscles: The magic of motion.* New York: Torstar Books. (p. 1).

Smidt, G. & Roger, M. (1982). Factors contributing to the regulation and clinical assessment of muscle strength. *Phys Ther 62,* 1283.

Smith, H.D. (1988). Specific evaluation procedures. (pp. 217-245) In Hopkins. H.L., Smith, H.D.: *Willard and Spackman's occupational therapy.* (7th ed) Philadelphia: J.B. Lippincott.

Sullivan, J. & Poole, S. (1981). Range of motion. (pp. 9-21) In Abreu, B.C. (Ed): *Physical disabilities manual.* New York: Raven Press.

CHAPTER CONTENT OUTLINE

Introduction

Standardized Batteries

Comprehensive Neuropsychological
Batteries

Specialized Batteries to Access
Cognitive Deficits

Computerized Assessment

Behavioral Assessment

The Role of the Occupational
Therapist in Cognitive Assessment

Summary

KEY TERMS

Standardized battery

Comprehensive battery

Specialized battery

Computerized assessment

Behavioral assessment

ABSTRACT

A clear understanding of the nature of a cognitive deficit will help the occupational therapist interpret the impact of the deficit on daily living skills. This chapter describes some of the basic neuropsychological assessments for cognitive functioning, including some general standardized batteries for brain dysfunction, specialized tests for specific cognitive deficits, computerized assessment, the use of behavioral assessment, and the role of the therapist in cognitive assessment.

Assessing Cognition

Janet Duchek

"Psychological tests are simply a means of enhancing (refining, standardizing) our observations. They can be thought of as extensions of our organs of perception—the seven-league boots of clinical behavioral observation. If we use them properly, as extensions of our observational end-organs, like seven-league boots they enable us to accomplish much more with greater speed. When tests are misused as substitutes for rather than extensions of clinical observation, they can obscure our view of the patient much as seven-league boots would get in the way if worn over the head."

—Muriel Lezak, 1987

OBJECTIVES

The information in this chapter is intended to help the reader—

1. develop an understanding of the criteria for a standardized test.

2. become familiar with some of the comprehensive batteries to assess cognition.

3. become familiar with some of the specialized tests for different components of cognition.

4. become familiar with computerized and behavioral assessment techniques.

5. develop an understanding of the role of the occupational therapist in the assessment of cognition.

INTRODUCTION

The assessment of cognitive function is often associated with the field of neuropsychology and the use of standardized tests. Neuropsychology is a discipline dealing with "the behavioral expression of brain dysfunction" (Lezak, 1983). The term itself is relatively new and represents the interaction between psychology and neurology. Neuropsychological assessment combines the neurologist's knowledge of brain-behavior relationships and the psychologist's knowledge of behavior and the psychometric properties of standardized instruments.

According to Lezak (1983), neuropsychological assessment serves three major purposes: diagnosis, treatment, and research. Neuropsychological assessment is most often used for diagnostic purposes. Assessment tools provide behavioral data which are used in diagnosing the presence of brain damage as well as discriminating among different neurologic or psychiatric disorders. In addition to providing a diagnosis, neuropsychological assessment can be invaluable in planning patient treatment. A clear understanding of the patient's disability will guide and facilitate careful rehabilitative programs. Finally, the use of standardized assessments fosters the understanding of different neurologic conditions and their corresponding impact on behavior. For example, the natural course of a specific disease can be followed with the longitudinal use of various neuropsychological tests (Berg, Storandt, Miller, Duchek, Morris, Rubin, Burke, and Coben, 1988).

Why should the occupational therapist be concerned with standardized cognitive assessment? Occupational therapists are confronted daily with the issue of the cognitive status of the patient. They are involved in assessing the integrity of cognitive function and ways of helping the patient and family adjust to the level of cognitive function/dysfunction. The occupational therapist often works closely with the neurologist in both the assessment and treatment of cognitive dysfunction. In Chapter 11, the importance of understanding the basic cognitive components underlying performance was emphasized. It was determined that effective intervention requires a clear comprehension of the nature of cognitive deficits and their basic elements. Because neuropsychological assessments are often used in the diagnosis of cognitive dysfunction, it is also vital that the therapist has a good working knowledge of the commonly used assessments designed to measure cognitive deficits. If the therapist has both knowledge of the basic components of cognition and the common standardized assessments of cognitive dysfunction, he/she can readily interact with the other members of the treatment team in developing the most effective treatment plan for the specific patient.

STANDARDIZED BATTERIES

Many **standardized batteries** for the assessment of cognitive dysfunction are now available. A standardized battery consists of a number of tests which assess performance in various functional areas. Tests of cognitive dysfunction often provide measurements of attention, memory, language, and problem-solving. The battery is standardized in the sense that the testing procedure is fixed. That is, the content or test items always remain the same for a given battery, and all tests in the battery should be administered. The instructions for administration should remain the same across all people and situations. The scoring of the test is well-defined and fixed, and the interpretation of the test involves the comparison of an individual's score with standardized norms. These norms serve as a frame of reference for determining the extent and nature of dysfunction.

Although standardized tests are often criticized as being too rigid and lengthy, they do serve three important functions in relation to patient treatment. (1) They provide an evaluation reference for comparing how impaired the patient is in relation to the normal population (normative data). This is crucial information for the therapist in determining educational and employment opportunities for the brain-damaged patient (Goldstein, 1987). (2) Standardized tests require that the tester make every effort to administer all the tests included in the battery which provides valuable information regarding not only deficits but also assets in performance. For example, even if a patient is not exhibiting attentional problems, tests of attention are still given as part of the entire test battery. Clearly, both the patient's assets and deficits should be used in planning and implementing treatment. (3) The quantitative nature of standardized tests allows precise examination of their psychometric properties. A test is useful only if it is both reliable and valid. Recent

---

Table 20-1
WAIS-R Subscales

WAIS-R Verbal Scale	WAIS-R Performance Scale
1. Information	1. Picture Completion
2. Vocabulary	2. Picture Arrangement
3. Comprehension	3. Digit Symbol
4. Similarities	4. Object Assembly
5. Arithmetic	5. Block Design
6. Digit Span	

technological advances in the neurosciences can provide strong criteria for the concurrent validity of standardized assessments. As described in Chapter 14, the predictive validity of a test can be determined by following the course of the illness over time, and the reliability of standardized batteries can be determined by examining test-retest scores. However, relatively little work has been done on the reliability of many neuropsychological tests (Goldstein, 1987).

COMPREHENSIVE NEUROPSYCHOLOGICAL BATTERIES

Neuropsychological tests can be described as comprehensive or specialized (Goldstein, 1987). A comprehensive assessment includes a battery of tests which measure different components of cognitive functioning and perceptual and motor functioning. A specialized assessment includes different tests which measure a more specific component of cognitive functioning, such as attention or language. The following are discussions of **comprehensive test batteries** that are highly standardized and commonly used in the assessment of brain damage.

Wechsler Adult Intelligence Scale

The *Wechsler Adult Intelligence Scale* (WAIS) was originally developed by Wechsler (1945) as a test of intelligence, which measured both the ability for abstract thought and the ability to respond to practical situations. The WAIS has been revised in recent years (Wechsler, 1981) and the WAIS-R is now more commonly used.

The WAIS-R was designed as a test of general intelligence, not for testing brain-injured patients. In fact it has been shown that IQ performance may remain intact after brain injury (Bennett, 1988). The entire battery or its various subtests are commonly used in neuropsychological assessment of brain damage, vocational counseling,

psychiatric assessment, and evaluations of mental retardation and genetic disorders (Goldstein, 1984).

The WAIS-R consists of verbal and performance scales. (See Table 20-1) The verbal scale includes six tests which measure verbal functioning and reasoning. The performance scale includes five speeded tests which measure psychomotor and perceptual integrative skills. It has been suggested that the verbal and performance subscales represent measures of crystallized and fluid intelligence, respectively (Sattler, 1982).

WAIS-R Verbal Scale. *The WAIS-R Information Test* consists of 29 questions measuring general knowledge. An example of the types of questions might be: "What was Marie Curie famous for?" This test is a measure of long-term semantic information.

The Vocabulary Test consists of 35 words to be defined. It taps long-term semantic knowledge. Vocabulary scores tend to be correlated with education.

The Comprehension Test includes 16 questions about practical situations. This test involves the ability to use proper judgment and integrate general knowledge.

The Similarities Test consists of 14 questions about the similarity between pairs of items, for example, "In what way are a button and zipper alike?" This test involves the ability to integrate semantic knowledge and to reason abstractly.

The Arithmetic Test consists of 14 mathematical word problems. This test involves the ability to reason abstractly and use stored knowledge of arithmetic rules.

The Digit Span Test requires the person to repeat strings of digits both forwards and backwards. The string of digits increases in length with each successive trial. This is a test of short-term memory and the ability to sustain attention. (See Table 20-2)

WAIS-R Performance Scale. *The Picture Completion Test* consists of 20 pictures with some crucial feature

Table 20-2
WAIS-R Verbal Scale
Example of a Digit Span Test

Trial 1	5 – 1	Score 2
Trial 2	4 – 8 – 6	Score 3
Trial 3	6 – 2 – 9 – 3	Score 4
Trial 4	7 – 4 – 9 – 1 – 5	Score 5
Trial 5	8 – 2 – 4 – 3 – 6 – 7	Score 6
Trial 6	3 – 8 – 1 – 9 – 7 – 4 – 6	Score 7
Trial 7	2 – 6 – 9 – 3 – 5 – 4 – 8 – 1	Score 8

missing. This test involves problem-solving skills and requires the ability to perceptually integrate information based on stored knowledge.

The Picture Arrangement Test includes 10 sets of pictures which tell a story. The subject is required to arrange the pictures in the proper sequence. This test involves the ability to conceptually sequence information to form a global story.

In the *Digit Symbol Test*, different symbols are associated with the numbers 1 through 9. The subject is given a paper filled with the symbols and the subject is required to write the corresponding number under the symbol. This test involves the ability to integrate new information and visual spatial abilities.

The *Object Assembly Test* requires the person to assemble four simple puzzles. This test involves the ability to integrate visual spatial information and psychomotor functioning.

The Block Design Test requires that red and white blocks be assembled into 9 different designs which are visually presented. This test involves visual spatial, psychomotor, and problem-solving abilities.

Psychometric Properties of the WAIS-R. A considerable amount of work has been conducted on the psychometric properties of the WAIS-R (Wechsler, 1981). Split-half and test-retest reliability studies have yielded very high reliability coefficients (Lindemann & Matarazzo, 1984). Studies of validity have examined the correlation of the WAIS scales to other tests of intelligence and studies of the factor analytic structure of the WAIS have supported the notion of verbal and performance scales (see Matarazzo, 1972 for a review). Wechsler (1967; 1974) has also developed the Wechsler Intelligence Scale for Children-Revised (WISC-R) and the Wechsler Preschool and Primary Scale of Intelligence (WPPSI) to assess the intelligence of children.

Summary and Comments. It can be seen from these brief descriptions that the WAIS-R is a comprehensive battery measuring many different components of cognition. The retrieval and integration of semantic information are involved in the verbal tests in addition to picture completion and picture arrangement. The retention of episodic information is necessary in both the digit span and digit symbol tests. Procedural memory could be tapped through the use of the block design and object assembly tests. Estimates of short-term memory capacity are often obtained from digit span. Furthermore, language comprehension and production, problem-solving skills, and the ability to sustain and focus attention are measured throughout these tests. The digit symbol test appears to be the most sensitive to brain injured patients.

The WAIS-R is considered a reliable and valid assessment tool for the measurement of intelligence. The subtests measure various components of cognitive functioning and can provide valuable information regarding specific deficits (e.g., short-term memory capacity) as well as more general deficits (e.g., visual spatial ability). Furthermore, the WAIS-R provides a global picture in which the pattern of deficits and assets can be assessed.

Halstead-Reitan Battery

The *Halstead-Reitan Battery* (HRB) is a widely used battery for general neuropsychological assessment. Halstead (1947) first developed a battery of tests based on his theory of biological intelligence which he felt could discriminate among levels of adaptive skills. He primarily developed the battery to answer research questions regarding brain-behavior relationships. His student, Reitan, later added more tests and was responsible for the empirical application of the battery as a neuropsychological assessment tool.

The HRB is standardized and needs to be administered with various equipment. It is a lengthy battery which takes approximately 6 to 8 hours to complete. However, each test is independent and can be administered at separate times. Although there are different versions of the HRB, the following tests are included in nearly all versions.

The Halstead Category Test is a test of concept formation. A series of trials are presented in which different visual forms or verbal material are presented on a screen. The patient's task is to identify the correct concept through feedback given after every trial. This test measures concept formation, problem-solving skills, and the ability to reason abstractly.

The Tactual Performance Test is a timed test in which the patient is asked to place various shaped blocks in their proper hole on a board. The patient is blindfolded and can only rely on sense of touch. The test is performed with the dominant hand, nondominant hand, and both hands. Then the patient is asked to draw from memory the board with the blocks in the correct position. This test involves the integration of tactual information with motor ability and memory for tactual information.

In *The Speech Perception Test* the patient is asked to listen to a taped recording of 60 non-words in which sounds are all similar and contain an "ee" sound in the middle (e.g., geend). Then the patient is given a multiple choice recognition test and asked to underline the correct response from among four alternatives. This test measures both the ability to discriminate speech sounds and memory for non-words.

The Finger-Tapping Test measures motor reaction time by requiring the patient to tap the index finger as rapidly as possible on a key which is attached to a mechanical counter for a period of 10 seconds. Several 10-second trials are performed with both the left and right hand.

The Seashore Rhythm Test measures the ability to discriminate rhythmic patterns and short-term memory. In this test, 30 pairs of rhythmic patterns are presented. The patient's task is to determine whether the two patterns in a pair are the same or different.

The following tests were added by Reitan:

The Reitan Aphasia Screening Test consists of a series of tasks related to language function including: repetition, spelling, reading, writing, naming, speech, and right-left orientation. This test also includes a copying task in which the patient is asked to copy a triangle, square, cross, and key. This test measures speech perception, comprehension, and production.

Trail-Making A and B includes Part A in which the patient's task is to connect a series of numbered circles on a sheet of paper in the correct order and Part B in which the patient must connect the correct numbers with letters (e.g., 1 to A, 2 to B). Both tests are timed and measure visual-spatial skills, sequencing skills, and motor skills. (See Figure 20-1)

The Perceptual Disorders Test consists of a series of tasks measuring perceptual discrimination skills, such as recognizing numbers traced on the fingertips and finger discrimination.

Often additional tests are administered with the HRB, such as some of the *Wechsler Intelligence Scales*, the Wechsler Memory Scale, the *Klove Grooved Pegboard test*, visual field examination, and the *Wide Range Achievement Test*.

The HRB is a comprehensive battery which taps many different components of cognition. The ability to sustain and focus attention is necessary throughout all of the tests. Higher order problem-solving skills and the ability to sequence are involved in the Category Test and the Trail Making tests. There is a substantial perceptual skills component associated with the HRB that is included in the Tactual Performance, Speech Perception, Seashore Rhythm, and Perceptual Disorders tests. Speech perception, comprehension, and production are tapped in the Speech Perception and Reitan Aphasia Screening tests. The HRB has been criticized for neglecting the area of memory (Goldstein, 1984), although memory is involved in the Tactual Performance, Speech Perception and Seashore Rhythm tests. This is the reason that the Wechsler Memory Scale is often used in conjunction with the HRB.

Psychometric Properties. Several studies on the validity of the HRB have been published (for a review see, Boll, 1981) with highly favorable findings. However, like the

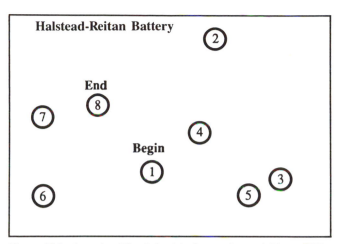

Figure 20-1. Assessing Visual Spatial, Sequencing and Motor Skills. Example of the Trail Making Test (Part A of the Halston-Reitan Battery).

WAIS-R, there has been relatively little work on the reliability of the HRB due to possible practice effects for the different tests and the spontaneous change often associated with brain-injured populations (Goldstein, 1984). Published norms for the HRB are available (Russell, Neuringer, & Goldstein, 1970), however, there is no published manual for the general administration and scoring of the battery.

Implications for Occupational Therapy. Rehabilitation programs have been developed on the basis of the HRB. The Reitan Evaluation of Hemispheric Abilities and Brain Improvement Training (REHABIT) was developed by Reitan as a program to rehabilitate different cognitive functions (Reitan & Wolfson, 1988). The REHABIT program involves both a neuropsychological evaluation with the HRB and specific training materials to remediate an individual's deficits as determined by performance on the HRB. There are five different tracks of training materials. Track A is designed to facilitate language and verbal skills related to academic ability. Track B includes training in language skills and more general problem-solving and reasoning skills. Track C emphasizes reasoning, abstraction, planning, and organizational skills. Track D emphasizes abstract reasoning skills with a focus on visual-spatial and tactile tasks. Track E is designed to develop more fundamental visual-spatial and manipulatory skills.

A particular patient may not need cognitive training on all five tracks. If the patient's deficits are relatively specific, then training on the related track materials would suffice. On the other hand, if the deficits are more general in nature, then cognitive training on all tracks would be employed. Unfortunately, little empirical work has been conducted on the efficacy of this program.

Goldstein and Ruthven (1983) have developed a vocational rehabilitation program based on the HRB with brain-injured patients. They found significant improvement on several tests following deficit-specific training, and many clients found jobs or resumed their educational activities upon completion of the program. Both the RE-HABIT and the Goldstein and Ruthven programs provide promising examples of the interface between standard neuropsychological assessment and rehabilitation planning. Clearly, more research is needed in this area.

Luria Nebraska
Neuropsychological Battery (LNNB)

The LNNB is a recently published battery (Golden, Hammeke, & Purisch, 1980) based on the work of the Russian neuropsychologist, Luria. Luria's test materials were first published by Christensen (1975) and later standardized and refined by Golden and his colleagues at Nebraska (Golden, Hammeke, and Purisch, 1978; Purisch, Golden, and Hammeke, 1978). The LNNB is a standardized battery including items that have been chosen based on substantial empirical work. It is now commonly used in clinical practice and is still undergoing revision.

The LNNB currently consists of 269 items representing the following 11 content areas:

The *motor scale* consists of a series of items to test voluntary motor skills, such as opening and closing a fist and performing motor actions based on verbal command. The *rhythm* scale primarily involves auditory perceptual skills such as pitch discrimination and repeating rhythm patterns. The *tactile* scale involves tactile recognition, such as identifying an item by touch or identifying a letter traced on the hand. The *visual* scale assesses basic perceptual and visual-spatial skills, such as mentally rotating objects and analyzing visual patterns. The *receptive speech* scale involves the ability to comprehend speech sounds, words, and more complex sentences and passages. The *expressive speech* scale involves the ability to produce speech sounds, words, and more complex narrative passages. The *writing* scale is an achievement scale which assesses basic writing skills such as spelling and writing sentences. The *reading* scale is an achievement scale which assesses basic reading skills. The *arithmetic* scale is an achievement scale which assesses fundamental mathematical skills, such as addition, subtraction, multiplication, and division. The *memory* scale assesses short-term memory and long-term memory for verbal and nonverbal information. The *intellectual* scale consists of items measuring problem-solving, verbal, and reasoning skills.

In addition, there are three derived scales: pathognomonic, left hemisphere, and right hemisphere. The pathognomonic scale consists of several items from various content scales which are primarily sensitive to discriminating between the presence and absence of brain damage. The left and right hemisphere scales consist of items from the motor and tactile content scales which are sensitive to left versus right sensory motor asymmetry.

Psychometric Properties. There have been several studies regarding both the reliability and validity of the battery (see Golden, 1981 for a review). The battery appears to have satisfactory discriminative validity in differentiating brain damage from normal controls, and results from the LNNB have been found to correlate with CT scan indices in various populations (Golden, Graber, Blose, Berg, Coffman, & Block, 1981; Golden, Moses, Zelazowski, Graber, Zatz, Horvath, & Berger, 1980). Reports of test-retest reliabilities for the content scales range from .78 to .96 (Golden et al., 1980). The published manual for the LNNB gives a detailed description of the testing procedures, scoring, norms, and validity and reliability studies.

Implications for Occupational Therapy. The LNNB has been criticized on both theoretical and methodological grounds (Stambrook, 1983). It has been argued that it does not reflect Luria's theory or methods (Goldstein, 1984) and does not provide a comprehensive assessment (Spiers, 1981). More specifically, it has been criticized for not providing an adequate classification of aphasia, and furthermore, because of the high verbal content of the battery, it would be very difficult to evaluate an aphasic patient's performance (Crosson & Warren, 1982). However, it is important to note that the LNNB is still being revised and reformulated.

At this time, there is no specific rehabilitation program associated with the LNNB, such as the REHABIT program for the HRB. However, there is a report of a case study utilizing the LNNB to guide a treatment plan and track the course of rehabilitation (Golden, 1984). It has been suggested that the LNNB may lend itself well to rehabilitation planning due to the specific nature of the items and content scales (Goldstein, 1987), however, such endeavors await empirical verification.

SPECIALIZED BATTERIES
TO ASSESS COGNITIVE DEFICITS

There are numerous **specialized batteries** for the assessment of specific cognitive deficits. Selected tests for each of the components of cognition (see Chapter 12) will be briefly discussed. For a more comprehensive presentation of the specialized batteries, the reader is referred to Lezak (1983).

```
M N K V E F H I L T W Y X F E T L I H F E V K N M W X
H M V E L W Y X K I F H E H T W V I H K X Y N E I L T
E K W X F T I H H W X T N V I H T L E M L T X E H I I
W M N V X E Y F H L T I N K K V X F I T E E I V M F F
T V M F I H N V W E E K M T V X F H T X M I F E F N Y
```

Figure 20-2. Example of a Letter Cancellation Task. The subject is instructed to cancel all of the "E's" by drawing a line through each.

Attention

Because attention guides most cognitive activity, aspects of attentional processing are included in many tests of cognitive dysfunction. For example, focused and sustained attention are crucial in the WAIS digit span test, the HRB speech perception and seashore rhythm tests, and the LNNB rhythm scale. The ability to shift attention is crucial in the Category test from the HRB. It is often difficult to measure attentional processes per se, because they interact with other components of cognition, such as short-term memory.

There are some tests used by neuropsychologists to primarily assess attentional deficits. Most attention tests require some form of perceptual tracking or scanning. Tracking tasks may involve simultaneously tracking more than one piece of information. The capacity to divide and rapidly shift attention often breaks down with brain damage (Lezak, 1983).

Vigilance tasks measure the patient's ability to sustain attention over an extended period and inhibit responding. Typically, a series of items (e.g., letters or numbers) are sequentially presented and the patient is asked to indicate every time a target item is presented (e.g., the letter "h"). The rate of presentation can be varied to make the task more complex. Also, the number of target items can be increased to assess the ability to shift attention.

Cancellation tasks are similar to vigilance tasks. Typically, rows of letters (or numbers) are interspersed on a sheet of paper and the patient's task is to cross off all the target letters on the sheet of paper within a certain period of time. (Figure 20-2). The complexity of the task can be varied by increasing the number of target items or decreasing the space between the letters. This task assesses the ability to sustain attention, visually scan information, inhibit responding, and shift attention (with more than one target). Diller and Weinberg (1977) found that performance on a cancellation task was associated with spatial neglect problems of patients with lesions of the right hemisphere.

The rehabilitation program for attentional deficits developed by Ben-Yishay and his colleagues (Ben-Yishay, Piasetsky, & Rattok, 1987; see Chapter 11 of this text for a description) is not based on neuropsychological evaluation, but does use performance on various neuropsychological tests

as pretest and posttest measures of the program's efficacy. In a case study report, they found that performance on the Visual Reaction Time, the Auditory Digits series and the WAIS Verbal IQ significantly improved after attentional training (Ben-Yishay, Piasetsky, & Rattok, 1987). Thus, neuropsychological tests can be used to assess the success of different rehabilitation programs.

Memory

Different aspects of memory functioning are involved in some tests in the comprehensive batteries since memory dysfunction is commonly seen in patients with brain damage and disease. For example, short-term memory is assessed in the WAIS digit span, the HRB seashore rhythm test, and the LNNB rhythm and memory scales. On the other hand, long-term semantic knowledge is assessed in all the verbal scale tests of the WAIS. There are also specialized batteries used to primarily assess memory function.

The *Wechsler Memory Scale* is a commonly used memory battery (Wechsler, 1945). The battery consists of six subscales:

The *personal and current information test* includes questions regarding age, birth date, and current affairs (e.g., "Who is the president of the U.S.?"). The *orientation test* consists of questions about time and place. The *mental control test* assesses the ability to recite well-learned information (e.g., the alphabet) and track conceptual information (e.g., count by threes from 1 to 50). The *logical memory test* assesses episodic memory of verbally presented paragraphs. The digit span is similar to the WAIS digit span test to assess short-term memory capacity. The *visual reproduction test* assesses visual memory for designs. The *associate learning test* assesses episodic memory of easy and difficult paired associates.

The *Wechsler Memory scale* has been criticized on the grounds that it is not a "comprehensive" memory test, or in other words, it is not representative of a variety of memory processes and therefore is not useful in differential diagnosis among neurologic conditions (Lezak, 1983).

The *Wisconsin Neuromemory Battery* includes a series of memory tests associated with different components of memory processes (Grafman, 1984). There are 14 tests including selective reminding, word recognition, face recognition, recurring figures, 7-24 test, visual sequential coding, word learning, sentence recall, Peterson and Peterson tri-word recall, paired associate, story recall, word fluency, token test, and famous events. This battery has been used in conjunction with a memory retraining program described below.

There are many other more specialized memory tests. For example, there are numerous tests for verbal retention including an auditory-verbal learning test (Rey, 1964) and the new word learning and retention test which requires patients to learn definitions for unfamiliar words (Meyer & Yates, 1955). Memory for sentences, paragraphs and stories can also be assessed.

Visual memory is tapped in several tests, including the *Benton Visual Retention Test* (BVRT) (Benton, 1974). This test consists of a number of geometric designs which are shown to the subject one at a time. After each design is viewed for a period of time, the patient is asked to reproduce the design on a sheet of paper. The BVRT is commonly used because it is easy to administer and score. It is considered to be very sensitive to brain damage and can differentiate between brain damage due to cerebral damage and brain damage due to psychiatric disorders (Benton, 1974; Marsh & Hirsch, 1982).

There are a few tests for memory of tactile information, such as the tactual performance test of the HRB. Lezak (1983) has argued that this test often yields redundant information, and the need to blindfold patients in this task has clinical disadvantages. Often patients become so uncomfortable being blindfolded that it impairs their performance on this test.

There is often a need to assess very long-term (or remote) memory in certain patient populations, such as in those with retrograde amnesia associated with Korsakoff's disease. Remote memory is not typically measured in standardized batteries such as the *Wechsler Memory Scale*. Tests have been developed to measure remote memory for public events (Squire, 1974), famous people (Albert, Butters, & Brandt, 1980), and even television titles (Squire & Slater, 1975).

A rehabilitation program based on the *Wisconsin Neuromemory Battery* has been developed by Grafman and Matthews (1978). Performance on the battery's tests were initially used as baseline measurements and to provide a "memory profile" for individual patients. The memory training program includes the PQRSTP strategy (a strategy used to organize text material for retrieval), visual imagery, verbal mediation, and note taking. They found that 40% of their sample of patients with head injury showed 50% improvement in memory test performance after completing

the program. Some patients reported applying the learned strategies in daily activities.

Language

Language dysfunction will affect performance on many of the **comprehensive** and **specialized batteries**. Language based deficits will be apparent on the verbal scales of the WAIS, the Reitan aphasia screening test of the HRB, and the receptive and expressive speech tests of the LNNB. If an aphasia seems to be present based on any of these tests, a specialized battery will typically be administered.

There are four batteries of basic language ability that are commonly used. All the batteries include items which assess speech comprehension, speech production, reading, writing, and gesturing abilities. The *Boston Diagnostic Aphasia Examination* (BDAE) provides information regarding the localization of lesions and discriminates among the different types of aphasia (Goodglass & Kaplan, 1972). The *Porch Index of Communicative Ability* (PICA) allows for discrimination among types of language deficits and also provides prognostic information of recovery of function (Porch, 1971). The *Minnesota Test for Differential Diagnosis of Aphasia* (MTDDA) provides differential diagnosis of language deficits in terms of the specificity and severity of dysfunction and prognostic information of recovery (Schuell, 1972). The *Neurosensory Center Comprehensive Examination for Aphasia* provides information regarding differential diagnosis (Spreen & Benton, 1977), but is highly subject to interpretation (Kent-Udolf, 1984).

Because all of these batteries require one to two hours to administer, shortened versions have been developed for the BDAE, the MTDDA, and the PICA (Kent-Udolf, 1984). For example, the *Western Aphasia Battery* (Kertesz & Poole, 1974) is a modified version of the BDAE. All of these batteries represent comprehensive tests of language dysfunction. In addition, there are more specialized language tests such as the Token Test and verbal fluency tests.

The *Token Test* (DeRenzi & Vignolo, 1962) is a test of speech comprehension in which the patient is given several tokens which vary in size, shape, and color and is expected to arrange them according to the examiner's command (e.g., "place the small blue square next to the green triangle"). The length of the command and number of elements included in the command can be varied to increase the complexity of the task. The *Token Test* is considered a highly sensitive test of auditory comprehension and is widely used with aphasic patients (Kent-Udolf, 1984).

The *Verbal Fluency Tests* (Wertz, 1979) are tests of speech production. The test consists of open-ended questions which often require a timed response from the patient. For example, the patient may be asked to produce as many words as possible that start with the letter "s" in one minute. Although there are many versions of this test, verbal fluency tests are used to assess word-finding difficulty and brain damage.

The standard batteries of aphasia include subtests of many aspects of language processes but do not necessarily reflect functional language skills. More recently, Holland (1980) has developed a test of functional language referred to as the *Communication Abilities of Daily Living* (CADL). The CADL utilizes some role playing to assess language skills in daily activities, such as shopping or visiting the doctor's office. Test items from various domains are included in the test, such as utilizing verbal and nonverbal context, social conventions, and humor. The use of the CADL could provide valuable information for planning functionally oriented rehabilitation programs.

Aphasia therapy is largely based on a patient's performance on aphasia batteries. The numerous approaches to language rehabilitation and their efficacy have been reviewed by Basso (1987), Goodglass (1987), and Kent-Udolf (1984).

Problem-Solving

Higher order problem-solving skills are involved in many of the tests found in standardized cognitive batteries. There are many subcomponents of problem-solving (see Chapter 12) such as planning, initiation, reasoning, and mental flexibility. Different aspects of problem-solving are measured in some of the specialized batteries. However, it is often difficult to assess problem-solving skills independent of more basic attentional, memory, or language deficits. Problem-solving skills are assessed in the Similarities, Picture Completion, Picture Arrangement, and Block Design tests of the WAIS, the Category Test of the HRB and the Intellectual Scale of the LNNB.

Planning is an important component of problem-solving activities which involves being able to identify some goal and the steps necessary to achieve that goal. The *Porteus Maze Test* (Porteus, 1965) is used as an assessment of planning and foresight (Lezak, 1983). The test consists of a set of visual mazes through which the patient must trace the correct path without going down any blind alley.

The *Tinker-toy Test* (TTT) (Lezak, 1983) is an "unconstrained" constructional test used to assess planning and initiation. The patient is simply given a set of tinkertoys and told to construct anything he/she wishes. The examiner then asks the patient what the construction represents and scores it for appropriateness according to specific standards.

Another important aspect of problem-solving is the ability to form abstract concepts and generalize those concepts

Table 20-3
Assessing Verbal Reasoning
Examples of Poisoned Foods Problems

Meals and their Consequences to Consumers. *From the information given, the subject is asked to determine the poisoned food in each set.*

1. Coffee Lamb Corn — Died
   Coffee Beef Corn — Lived

2. Milk Veal Corn — Died
   Milk Lamb Corn — Died
   Milk Veal Peas — Lived

3. Tea Lamb Peas — Died
   Coffee Lamb Rice — Lived
   Milk Beef Rice — Lived
   Tea Beef Peas — Died
   Coffee Veal Peas — Lived

beyond the present situation to other appropriate situations. Abstract conceptualization is assessed in the *Proverbs Test* (Gorham, 1956) in which the patient is read a proverb and asked to give an interpretation. Scoring is based on the abstractness/concreteness of the response.

Sorting tasks are commonly used to assess concept formation. These tasks typically involve an assortment of objects from which the patient is required to sort out the objects that go together. Sorting involves the ability to form concepts and shift concepts when necessary. Such tests provide a measure of response perseveration and inflexibility in thinking.

The *Wisconsin Card Sorting Test* (Grant & Berg, 1948) is a commonly used sorting task which includes 64 cards, each card containing from one to four identical symbols (triangle, cross, circle, star) of the same color (red, green, yellow, or blue). The patient's task is to sort the cards according to a principle which the patient must deduce from the examiner's responses of "correct" or "incorrect" after each trial. This test is considered to be sensitive to frontal lobe damage (Goodglass & Kaplan, 1979).

Reasoning involves the abilities to understand relationships and integrate information. The *Poisoned Foods Problems* (Arenberg, 1968) is an example of a verbal reasoning task which was originally developed to assess the effect of aging on reasoning skills. In this test, a series of meals (e.g., peas, coffee, veal) are visually presented with the subsequent consequences to the consumer (i.e., lived or died). The patient must deduce from the list of meals which one was the poisoned food. (See Table 20-3)

The Picture Absurdities test of the Stanford Binet

Table 20-4: Assessing Mental Status Example Questions from the Mini Mental State Examination

1. What is the (year) (season) (month) (day)?

2. Where are we? (state) (county) (town) (hospital) (floor)

3. Name 3 objects: 1 second to say each. Then ask the patient to repeat all three after you have said them. Then repeat them until he learns them.

4. Spell ''world'' backwards.

5. Ask for the objects above.

6. Repeat — no ifs, ands or buts.

7. Follow a stage 3 command: "Take the paper in your right hand, fold it in half, and put in on the floor."

Excerpted from Folstein, MF, Folstein, SE and McHugh, PR (1975). "Mini-Mental State." Journal of Psychiatric Research, 12, 189-198.

(Terman & Merrill, 1973) is another test of reasoning in which a picture of a logically incorrect situation is presented and the patient is asked to report what is wrong with the picture. There is also a Verbal Absurdities test of the Stanford Binet which presents illogical stories.

The *Raven's Progressive Matrices* test (Raven, 1960) was developed as a reasoning task which was freer from cultural bias than other tests. In this test, visual patterns are presented with one part removed, and the patient must choose the correct pattern to complete the pattern from a number of alternatives. Although the *Raven's Progressive Matrices* test is useful for assessing visual-spatial reasoning, it has not been as useful for screening for brain damage (Heaton, Baade, & Johnson, 1978).

Goldstein and Levin (1987) have argued that an initial comprehensive neuropsychological assessment can be useful for understanding problem-solving deficits in light of other cognitive deficits. If problem-solving deficits are indicated, then a more specialized assessment would be warranted and a rehabilitation program would be implemented based on this assessment. However, they also propose that both traditional and nontraditional assessments be utilized in this process. Certain higher order functions such as initiation and planning may not be adequately tapped due to the highly structured nature of many neuropsychological tests, and thus may require the use of more nonstructured tasks (e.g., the Tinker-toy Test).

Mental Status Examinations

Before ending the discussion of standardized tests of cognitive function, it should be noted that there are several tests for the evaluation of dementia. In general, these tests are relatively short and are used as screening tests for dementia. The actual diagnosis of dementia is made in conjunction with other sources of information, particularly in structured interviews with the patient and/or family member in which the areas of attention, memory, language, and problem-solving are assessed.

The *Mini Mental State* (Folstein, Folstein, & McHugh, 1975) (Table 20-4) is a commonly used screening test which includes items to assess orientation, attention, calculation, and language skills. The *Short Portable Mental Status Questionnaire* (SPMSQ) (Pfeiffer, 1975) consists of ten questions assessing orientation, general knowledge, and mental tracking. Other dementia scales include the *Dementia Rating Scale* (Mattis, 1976), the *Memory Loss Scale* (Markson & Levitz, 1973), and the *Blessed Dementia Scale* (Blessed, Tomlinson, & Roth, 1968). There are also more detailed structured interviews for the staging of dementia, such as the *Washington University Clinical Dementia Rating Scale* (Berg, 1984; Hughes, Berg, Danziger, Coben, & Martin, 1982).

COMPUTERIZED ASSESSMENT

Although it has been used successfully in personality assessment for several years (Butcher & Keller, 1984), **computerized assessment** is a relatively new phenomenon in the area of neuropsychology. In this approach, the administration, scoring and interpretation of test results are done by a sophisticated computer program. Ultimately, such an assessment could even recommend a rehabilitation plan. Because of the highly structured nature of standard neuropsychological batteries, they easily may lend themselves to automated administration and scoring procedures. A patient might be able to sit in front of a computer screen and respond to information presented on the screen by using the keyboard or some adapted procedure. The program would be set up to branch to different questions or tests depending upon the patient's prior responses. The scoring and interpretation of results would be based upon a vast amount of clinical information which easily could be stored in the computer.

There are several advantages for the use of computers in cognitive assessment: (1) Computers can hold and process a vast amount of information whereas it may be impossible for clinicians to mentally access this vast amount of information. Interactive computer systems are already available to physicians for diagnostic and treatment problem-solving (Goldstein, 1987). (2) Scoring can be done quickly and would be less subject to human error in a computerized system. (3) Computerized scoring and interpretation is not subject to human biases. Although one may be concerned about the impersonal nature of the computer for assessment, it has been reported in the area of personality assessment that patients enjoy the computer interaction and often reveal more sensitive information to the computer than a clinical interviewer (Griest & Klein, 1980, 1981; Johnson & Williams, 1980).

There are some disadvantages in using the computer in cognitive assessment: (1) The interpretation of test results often calls for decision-making and clinical judgments that might be difficult to precisely define and program into the computer. In addition, it could be very difficult to program in all the extraneous variables involved in any particular patient's situation. (2) There is the possibility that the ease of using computerized assessment might encourage nonprofessional use and interpretation of test results (Goldstein, 1987).

Regardless of these potential problems, it is apparent that computerized assessment is likely to be used to a greater extent in the future given the advantages. Computers already are used quite frequently in rehabilitation (e.g., Bracy, 1983). It is unlikely that computerized assessment will totally replace the human clinician. However, such systems can be used effectively for initial assessment and preliminary interpretation which will guide further testing and treatment planning.

BEHAVIORAL ASSESSMENT

Behavioral assessment is an alternative method for the evaluation of cognitive dysfunction. Behavioral assessment involves specific methods of observing and assessing behaviors similar to those used by occupational therapists. Although the technique is relatively new in the area of neuropsychology, there is a substantial body of literature on the topic (e.g., Haynes, 1978; 1984; Hersen & Bellack, 1981; Nelson & Hayes, 1984). It is important to note that behavioral assessment does not involve merely a casual description of behavior by any observer, but rather it involves a systematic and quantitative method of assessing behavior by a trained observer.

Behavioral assessment serves several interrelated functions (Haynes, 1984): (1) Specific target behaviors or areas of dysfunction must be identified in terms of their frequency, intensity, and relation to the patient's overall function. (2) Alternative behaviors or areas of intact functioning can be identified to possibly compensate for dysfunctional behaviors. (3) The cause of a deficit possibly

can be identified through the assessment of situational and environmental variables. (4) A treatment plan can be derived based upon a detailed behavioral assessment.

There are different methods used in behavioral assessment. Naturalistic observation involves the systematic observation of specific behaviors in the patient's natural environment by a trained observer, such as in the hospital or home. Usually a schedule is pre-determined, and the occurrence/nonoccurrence of the behaviors are sampled during this time. In analogue observation, behaviors similarly are observed, but in a controlled situation. Behaviors can also be recorded through interviews and questionnaires or the self-reports of the patients themselves.

Combined Approach

Behavioral assessment and standard neuropsychological tests represent two very different techniques for assessing cognitive dysfunction. However, it seems that the two approaches could be combined quite nicely (see, Goldstein, 1987 for a more detailed discussion). The function of the standard neuropsychological test is to identify specific cognitive deficits. These cognitive deficits often result in dysfunctional behavior. Through behavioral assessment, it would be possible to precisely identify these behaviors and treat them as an indirect way of remediating the cognitive deficit. For example, a patient may demonstrate a memory deficit on a neuropsychological test battery. This patient also may exhibit wandering behavior which could be assessed carefully and treated through behavioral assessment.

THE ROLE OF THE OCCUPATIONAL THERAPIST IN COGNITIVE ASSESSMENT

What is the role of the occupational therapist in the assessment of cognitive function? In practice, the occupational therapist must consider the cognitive capacity of the individual and develop a treatment plan for some form of cognitive dysfunction. This task requires the therapist to have an understanding of the nature of the dysfunction. It is not likely that the therapist would be involved in the administration and scoring of many of the standardized cognitive batteries unless the clinician has received specialized training. However, a therapist may use a particular test as a screening assessment (e.g., the Mini Mental State Exam).

There are some perceptual/cognitive evaluations which have been developed for occupational therapists, such as the *Lowenstein Occupational Therapy Cognitive Assessment* (LOTCA) (Katz, Itzkovich, Auerbach, & Elazar, 1989), the

Santa Clara Valley Medical Center Perceptual Motor Evaluation for Head Injured and Neurologically Impaired Adults (Jabri, Zoltan, Ryckman, & Panikoff, 1987), and the *Test of Orientation for Rehabilitation Patients* (TORP) (Deitz, Berman, & Thorn, 1986).

Therapists often use activity as a means of cognitive assessment. Cognitive processes can be assessed through the patient's performance of a relevant activity. The following two tasks provide examples of how the systematic observation of activity can be used for cognitive assessment and thus form the basis for treatment planning. In the *Allen Cognitive Level Test* (ACL) a leather-lacing test which varies in the complexity of the lacing stitch is used to assess the level of cognitive disability (Allen, 1985). *The Kitchen Task* (Baum & Edwards, 1990) is another activity-based assessment of cognition which has recently been developed in relation to senile dementia of the Alzheimer type (SDAT). Cognitive processes, such as initiation, sequencing, and organization are assessed by examining the patient's ability to perform a cooking activity. In both of these tasks, the assessment of cognition is based on the performance of an activity.

The occupational therapist must have a working knowledge of commonly used test batteries to assess cognitive function. The neuropsychological assessment can provide the therapist with a clearer understanding of the nature of the cognitive deficit and how the deficit impacts on ADL skills, and hence render important information regarding treatment. Fitting within the occupational therapy holistic approach to treatment, the neuropsychological assessment illustrates both areas of cognitive dysfunction and areas of intact cognitive function. Treatment should be guided by both the deficits and assets of a patient. By focusing on the intact cognitive skills, alternative approaches can be examined and integrated into the treatment plan.

Because occupational therapists typically work as part of an interdisciplinary treatment team, it is also important that they have an understanding of and are able to communicate with other members of the team regarding test evaluations. Occupational therapy is a crucial link between the assessment of cognitive deficits and their treatment.

SUMMARY

Although assessment of cognitive function is often associated with the field of neuropsychology, occupational therapists must understand the cognitive functioning of their patients in order to plan effective rehabilitation programs. Several standardized tests and batteries designed to assess cognitive function have been reviewed in this chapter. The *Wechsler Adult Intelligence Scale, the Halstead-Reitan*

Battery, and the *Luria-Nebraska Neuropsychological Battery* have been identified as useful comprehensive batteries. In addition, several specialized tests which assess attention, memory, language, problem-solving and mental status were reviewed.

In contrast to standardized approaches, behavioral assessment involves specific methods of determining cognitive function through observation of the patient. In addition to deriving information from standardized and behavioral assessment approaches from outside occupational therapy, therapists can make use of several instruments developed within the field, such as the *Allen Cognitive Level Test.* It has been emphasized that occupational therapists should use an interdisciplinary approach to gaining understanding of the nature of cognitive function in their patients.

Study Questions

1. What does it mean when a test is "standardized?"

2. What are the similarities and differences among the WAIS, Halstead-Reitan, and LNNB?

3. Give an example of a specialized test for each of the following: attention, memory, language, and problem-solving.

4. What are the advantages and disadvantages of computerized assessment?

5. How is behavioral assessment different from casual observation?

6. What is the role of the occupational therapist in the assessment of cognition?

References

Albert, M.L., Butters, N., & Brandt, J. (1980). Memory for remote events in alcoholics. *Journal of Studies on Alcohol, 41*, 1071-1081.

Allen, C.K. (1985). *Occupational therapy for psychiatric diseases: Measurement and management of cognitive disabilities*. Boston, MA: Little, Brown and Co.

Arenberg, D. (1968). Concept problem-solving in young and old adults. *Journal of Gerontology, 23*, 279-282.

Basso, A. (1987). Approaches to neuropsychological rehabilitation: Language disorders. In M.J. Meier, A.L. Benton, & L. Diller (Eds.). *Neuropsychological rehabilitation*, New York: Guilford Press.

Baum, C., & Edwards, D. (1990). A test of cognitive performance in Senile Dementia of the Alzheimer type: The Kitchen Task Assessment. Unpublished manuscript.

Ben-Yishay, Y., Piasetsky, E.B., & Rattok, J. (1987). A

systematic method for ameliorating disorders in basic attention. In M.J. Meier, A.L. Benton, & L. Diller (Eds.) *Neuropsychological rehabilitation*, New York: Guilford Press.

Bennett, T. (1988). Use of the Halstead-Reitan neuropsychological test battery in the assessment of head injury. *Cognitive Rehabilitation, 6*, 18-24.

Benton, A.L. (1974). *The revised visual retention test.* (4th ed.). New York: Psychological Corporation.

Berg, L. (1984). Clinical Dementia Rating. *British Journal of Psychiatry, 145*, 339.

Berg, L., Storandt, M.A., Miller, J.P., Duchek, J.M., Morris, J.C., Rubin, E.H., Burke, W.J., & Coben, A. (1988). Mild senile dementia of the Alzheimer type: 2. Longitudinal assessment. *Annals of Neurology, 23*, 477-484.

Blessed, G., Tomlinson, B.E., & Roth, M. (1968). The association between quantitative measures of dementia and of senile change in the cerebral grey matter of elderly subjects. *British Journal of Psychiatry, 114*, 797-811.

Boll, T.J. (1981). The Halstead-Reitan neuropsychology battery. In S.B. Filskov & T.J. Boll (Eds.). *Handbook of clinical neuropsychology.* New York: Wiley.

Bracy, O. (1983). Computer based cognitive rehabilitation. *Cognitive Rehabilitation, 1*, 7.

Butcher, J.N., & Keller, L.S. (1984). Objective personality assessment. In G. Goldstein & M. Hersen (Eds.). *Handbook of psychological assessment.* New York: Pergamon Press.

Christensen, A.L. (1975). *Luria's neuropsychological investigation: Manual.* New York: Spectrum.

Crosson, B., & Warren, R.L. (1982). Use of the Luria-Nebraska Neuropsychological Battery in aphasia: A conceptual critique. *Journal of Consulting and Clinical Psychology, 50*, 22-31.

Deitz, J., Berman, C., & Thorn, D.W. (1986). *Test of Orientation for Rehabilitation Patients (TORP).* Seattle, WA: University of Washington.

DeRenzi, E. & Vignolo, L.A. (1962). The token test. *Brain*, 85, 665-678.

Diller, L., & Weinberg, J. (1977). Hemi-attention in rehabilitation: the evolution of a rational remediation program. In E.A. Weinstein & R.P. Friedland (Eds.). *Advances in neurology.* New York: Raven Press.

Folstein, M.F., Folstein, S.E., & McHugh, P.R. (1975). "Mini-Mental State." *Journal of Psychiatric Research, 12*, 189-198.

Golden, C.J. (1981). A standardized version of Luria's neuropsychological tests: A quantitative and qualitative approach to neuropsychological evaluation. In S.B. Filskov & T.J. Boll (Eds.). *Handbook of clinical neuropsychology.* New York: Wiley.

Golden, C.J. (1984). Rehabilitation and the Luria-Nebraska Neuropsychological Battery: An introduction to theory and practice. In B.A. Edelstein & E.T. Couture (Eds.). *Behavioral assessment and rehabilitation of the traumatically brain-injured.* New York: Plenum Press.

Golden, C.J., Graber, B., Blose, I., Berg, R., Coffman, J., & Block, S. (1981). Difference in brain densities chronic alcoholic and normal control patients. *Science, 211*, 508-510.

Golden, C.J., Hammeke, T., & Purisch, A. (1978). Diagnostic validity of the Luria neuropsychological battery. *Journal of Consulting and Clinical Psychology, 46*, 1258-1265.

Golden, C.J., Hammeke, T., & Purisch, A. (1980). *The Luria-Nebraska battery manual.* Los Angeles: Western Psychological Services

Golden, C.J., Moses, J.A., Zelazowski, R., Graber, B., Zatz, L.M., Horvath, T.B., & Berger, P.A. (1980). Cerebral ventricular size and neuropsychological impairment in young chronic schizophrenics. *Archives of General Psychiatry, 37*, 619-623.

Goldstein, F.C., & Levin, H.S. (1987). Disorders of reasoning and problem-solving ability. In M.J. Meier, A.L. Benton, & L. Diller (Eds.). *Neuropsychological rehabilitation.* New York: Guilford Press.

Goldstein, G. (1984). Comprehensive neuropsychological assessment batteries. In G. Goldstein & M. Hersen (Eds.). *Handbook of psychological assessment.* New York: Pergamon Press.

Goldstein, G. (1987). Neuropsychological assessment for rehabilitation: fixed batteries, automated systems, and non-psychometric methods. In M.J. Meier, A.L. Benton, & L. Diller (Eds.). *Neuropsychological rehabilitation.* New York: Guilford Press.

Goldstein, G. & Ruthven, L. (1983). *Rehabilitation of the brain damaged adult.* New York: Plenum Press.

Goodglass, H. (1987). Neurolinguistic principles and aphasia therapy. In M.J. Meier, A.L. Benton, & L. Diller (Eds.). *Neuropsychological rehabilitation.* New York: Guilford Press.

Goodglass, H. & Kaplan, E. (1972). *The assessment of aphasia and related disorders.* Philadelphia, PA: Lee & Febiger.

Goodglass, H. & Kaplan, E. (1979). Assessment of cognitive deficit in the brain-injured patient. In M.S. Gazzaniga (Ed.). *Handbook of behavioral neurobiology: 2 Neuro-psychology.* New York: Plenum Press.

Gorham, D.R. (1956). A Proverbs Test for clinical and experimental use. *Psychological Reports, 1*, 1-12.

Grafman, J. (1984). Memory assessment and remediation in brain-injured patients: From theory to practice. In B.A. Edelstein & E.T. Couture (Eds.). *Behavioral assessment and rehabilitation of the traumatically brain-damaged.* New York: Plenum Press.

Grafman, J. & Matthews, C. (1978). Assessment and remediation of memory deficits in brain-injured patients. In M. Gruneberg, P. Morris, & R. Sykes, (Eds.). *Practical aspects of memory.* London: Academic Press.

Grant, D.A. & Berg, E.A. (1948). A behavioral analysis of degree of reinforcement and ease of shifting to new responses in a Weigh-type card-sorting problem. *Journal of Experimental Psychology, 38,* 404-411.

Griest, J.H. & Klein, M.H. (1980). Computer programs for patients, clinicians, and researchers in psychiatry. In J.B. Sidowski, J.H. Johnson, & T.A. Williams (Eds.). *Technology in mental health care delivery systems.* Norwood, NJ: Ablex Publishing Corp.

Griest, J.H. & Klein, M.H. (1981). Computers in psychiatry. In S. Arieti (Ed.). *American handbook of psychiatry.* (2nd ed., Vol 7). New York: Basic Books.

Halstead, W.C. (1947). *Brain and intelligence: A quantitative study of the frontal lobes.* Chicago: The University of Chicago Press.

Haynes, S.N. (1978). *Principles of behavioral assessment.* New York: Gardner Press.

Haynes, S.N. (1984). Behavioral assessment of adults. In G. Goldstein & M. Hersen (Eds.). *Handbook of psychological assessment.* New York: Pergamon Press.

Heaton, R.K., Baade, L.E., & Johnson, K.L. (1978). Neuropsychological test results associated with psychiatric disorders in adults. *Psychological Bulletin, 85,* 141-162.

Hersen, M. & Bellack, A.S. (1981). *Behavioral assessment: A practical handbook.* (2nd ed.). New York: Pergamon Press.

Holland, A. (1980). *Communication abilities in daily living (CADL).* Baltimore: University Park Press.

Hughes, C.P., Berg, L., Danziger, W.L., Coben, L.A., & Martin, R.L. (1982). A new clinical scale for the staging of dementia. *British Journal of Psychiatry, 140,* 566-572.

Jabri, J., Zoltan, B., Ryckman, D., & Panikoff, L. (1987). *Perceptual motor evaluation for head injured and other neurologically impaired adults.* San Jose, CA: Santa Clara County, Santa Clara Valley Medical Center.

Johnson, J.H. & Williams, T.A. (1980). Using on-line computer technology to improve service response and decision-making effectiveness in a mental health admitting system. In J.B. Sidowski, J.H. Johnson, & T.A. Williams (Eds.). *Technology in mental health care delivery systems.* Norwood, NJ: Ablex Publishing Corp.

Katz, N., Itzkovich, M., Auerbach, S., & Elazar, B. (1989). Lowenstein Occupational Therapy Cognitive Assessment (LOTCA) Battery for brain-injured patients: Reliability and validity. *American Journal of Occupational Therapy, 43,* 184-191.

Kent-Udolf, L. (1984). Communication disorders of traumatically brain-injured persons. In B.A. Edelstein & E.T. Couture (Eds.). *Behavioral assessment and rehabilitation of the traumatically brain-damaged.* New York: Plenum Press.

Kertesz, A. & Poole, E. (1974). The aphasia quotient: The taxonomic approach to measurement of aphasic disability. *Canadian Journal of Neurological Science, 1,* 7-16.

Lezak, M. (1983). *Neuropsychological assessment.* (2nd ed.). New York: Oxford University Press.

Lezak, M. (1987). Assessment for rehabilitation planning. In M. Meier, A. Benton, & L. Diller (Eds.). *Neuropsychological rehabilitation.* New York: Guilford Press.

Lindemann, J.E. & Matarazzo, J.D. (1984). Intellectual assessment of adults. In G. Goldstein & M. Hersen (Eds.). *Handbook of psychological assessment.* New York: Pergamon Press.

Markson, E.W. & Levitz, G.A. (1973). A Guttman scale to assess memory loss among the elderly. *The Gerontologist, 13,* 337-340.

Marsh, G.G. & Hirsch, S.H. (1982). Effectiveness of two tests of visual retention. *Journal of Clinical Psychology, 38,* 115-118.

Matarazzo, J.D. (1972). *Wechsler's measurement and appraisal of adult intelligence.* (5th ed.). Baltimore: Williams & Wilkins.

Mattis, S. (1976). Mental status examination for organic mental syndrome in the elderly patient. In L. Bellak & T.B. Karasu (Eds.). *Geriatric psychiatry.* New York: Grune & Stratton.

Meyer, V. & Yates, A.J. (1955). Intellectual changes following temporal lobectomy for psychomotor epilepsy. *Journal of Neurology, Neurosurgery, and Psychiatry, 18,* 44-52.

Nelson, R.O. & Hayes, S.C. (1984). *Conceptual foundations of behavioral assessment.* New York: Guilford Press.

Pfeiffer, E. (1975). SPMSQ: Short Portable Mental Status Questionnaire. *Journal of the American Geriatric Society, 23,* 433-441.

Porch, B.E. (1971). *Porch index of communicative ability.* Palo Alto, CA: Consulting Psychologists Press.

Porteus, S. (1965). *Porteus maze test.* Palo Alto: Pacific Books.

Purisch, A.D., Golden, C.J., & Hammeke, T.A. (1978). Discrimination of schizophrenic and brain-injured patients by a standardized version of Luria's neuropsychological tests. *Journal of Consulting and Clinical Psychology, 46,* 1266-1273.

Raven, J.C. (1960). *Guide to the standard progressive*

matrices. New York: Psychological Corporation.

Reitan, R.M. & Wolfson, D. (1988). The Halstead-Reitan Neuropsychological test battery and REHABIT: A model for integrating evaluation and remediation of cognitive impairment. *Cognitive Rehabilitation, 6,* 10-17.

Rey, A. (1964). *L'examen clinique en psychologie*. Paris: Universitaires de France.

Russell, E.W., Neuringer, C., & Goldstein, G. (1970). *Assessment of brain damage: A neuropsychological key approach*. New York: Wiley.

Sattler, J.M. (1982). Age effects on Wechsler Adult Intelligence Scale-Revised tests. *Journal of Consulting and Clinical Psychology, 50,* 785-786.

Schuell, H. (1972). *The Minnesota test for differential diagnosis of aphasia (MTDDA)*. Minneapolis: University of Minnesota Press.

Spiers, P.A. (1981). Have they come to praise Luria or bury him? The Luria-Nebraska battery controversy. *Journal of Consulting and Clinical Psychology, 49,* 331-341.

Spreen, O. & Benton, A.L. (1977). *Neurosensory center comprehensive examination for aphasia (NCCEA)*. Victoria, BC: University of Victoria Neuropsychology Laboratory.

Squire, L.R. (1974). Remote memory as affected by aging. *Neuropsychologia, 12,* 429-435.

Squire, L.R. & Slater, P.C. (1975). Forgetting in very long-term memory as assessed by an improved questionnaire taxonomy. *Journal of Experimental Psychology: Human Learning and Memory, 104,* 50-54.

Stambrook, M. (1983). The Luria-Nebraska Neuropsychological Battery: A promise that may be partly fulfilled. *Journal of Clinical Neuropsychology, 5,* 247-269.

Terman, L. & Merrill, M. (1973). Stanford Binet Intelligence Scale. Boston: Houghton Mifflin.

Wechsler, D. *(1939, 1945)*. *The measurement of adult intelligence*. Baltimore: Williams & Wilkins.

Wechsler, D. (1945). A standardized memory scale for clinical use. *Journal of Psychology, 19,* 87-95.

Wechsler, D. (1967). *Wechsler Preschool and Primary Scale of Intelligence*. New York: Psychological Corporation.

Wechsler, D. (1974). *Wechsler Intelligence Scale for Children—Revised*. New York: Psychological Corporation.

Wechsler, D. (1981). Wechsler Adult Intelligence Scale—Revised. New York: Psychological Corporation.

Wertz, R.T. (1979). Word fluency measure. In F. L. Darley (Ed.). *Evaluation of appraisal techniques in speech and language pathology*. Reading, Mass.: Addison-Wesley.

CHAPTER CONTENT OUTLINE

KEY TERMS

Biopsychological assessment

Evaluation

Frame of reference

Functional assessment

Mental status exam

Projective activities

Projective assessment

Psychological constructs

Psychosis

ABSTRACT

This chapter explores the interaction between psychological influences, performance skills, and the environment. The chapter includes a brief history of the development of psychological assessment and the basic components which have shaped its development, including the various psychological constructs, frames of reference, and points of view. Each type of assessment is described (self-report, self-monitoring, behavior observation scales, projective tests, psychometric techniques, and biopsychological assessment), and the patient interview and factors influencing it are reviewed as crucial elements necessary to any psychological assessment.

Assessing Psychological Performance Factors

Barbara Borg
Mary Ann Bruce

"In our endeavor to understand reality we are somewhat like a man trying to understand the mechanism of a closed watch. He sees the face and the moving hands, even hears it ticking, but has no way of opening the case. If he is ingenious he may form some picture of the mechanism which could be responsible for all things he observes, but he may never be quite sure his picture is the only one which could explain his observations. He will never be able to compare his picture with the real mechanism and he cannot even imagine the possibility of the meaning of such a comparison."

—Albert Einstein, (Quoted in Zukav, 1979)

OBJECTIVES

The information in this chapter is intended to help the reader—

1. explain the meaning of the term "psychological construct."

2. describe the influence of medical diagnosis in psychological assessment.

3. give examples of the practical and professional boundaries influencing and guiding the assessment process.

4. describe the advantages and disadvantages of subjective and objective assessment.

5. describe and give examples of the following types of assessment procedures: (1) behavior observation scale, (2) projective test, (3) psychometric technique, (4) interview, and (5) self-report.

6. distinguish between assessments that elicit samples of behavior and those that elicit signs.

7. discuss the influence of therapist and patient bias upon assessment results.

INTRODUCTION

In accordance with the holistic view endorsed by occupational therapy theory and practice, it is generally agreed that the mind and the body are connected, each influencing the other within the individual. While this reciprocal relationship is not fully understood, it is believed that in order to gain a full understanding of human performance, one must evaluate the psychological factors which impact the individual's performance and ability in everyday life.

In the therapy setting, the psychological factors include the patient's needs, values, attitudes, feelings, interests, self-image, goals and aspirations, esteem, sense of control, and style of coping. These factors are constructs with no universally agreed upon definition and there are diverse approaches to understanding them. Most often in occupational therapy the interaction of psychological influences, performance skills, and environment are evaluated to assess the person's accomplishment of life tasks and the adequacy of the individual's performance in the environment. The diverse approaches for understanding the dynamic interaction of psychological influences, performance skills and environment are explored in this chapter.

WHAT IS PSYCHOLOGICAL ASSESSMENT?

Psychological assessment is the process of gathering information about the person's mind or mental function, including the individual's thoughts, perceptions, conscious and unconscious processes, and sensations. Since we cannot really "get into another person's mind," psychological assessment has historically included an evaluation of the influence of the mind on a person's behavior. The information that is collected via psychological assessment enables knowledgeable and responsible decision-making on behalf of the individual (Frey, 1984, p. 14).

Because occupational therapy is concerned with both the ability of the individual to meet personal needs and responsibilities through activity and with the influence of activity on well-being, the link between mind and activity is integral to the profession's use of psychological assessment. Assessment of patients with identified psychological problems in occupational therapy has included a focus on the following factors: (1) the ability for self-care and daily maintenance, (2) the extent of skills related to work and avocational pursuits, (3) the presence of certain kinds of information or knowledge, (4) the existence of identified cognitive structures, sensorimotor and sensory-perceptual skills, and (5) information regarding self-image, interests, values, social relationships, personal concerns and personal goals.

While many of these foci are also addressed in other areas of occupational therapy assessment, psychological assessment strives to pay special attention to the relationship of mind (e.g., thoughts and feelings) to performance. An assessment of functional ability, such as a test of dressing skill, might prove to be within the scope of assessment of persons with emotional disabilities. However, many **functional assessments** cannot be conceived as psychological assessment, except perhaps by inference.

HISTORY OF PSYCHOLOGICAL ASSESSMENT

The history of psychological assessment in occupational therapy is less extensive than that of psychology. However, it reflects the historical developments which have occurred in mental health and psychological evaluation systems. Some of these developments will be reviewed in order to give a basis for understanding psychological assessment within occupational therapy.

Early History of Psychological Assessment

The art and science of psychological assessment tries to answer the question, "What is the very nature of human nature?" (Sundberg, 1977, p. 2). As discussed by Reisman (1976), psychological assessment can only be understood as a part and reflection of the history of humanity. For example, people in the earliest cultures would tend to see magical forces as responsible for the personal events and feelings they could not otherwise explain, and people in Biblical times might view sin (or redemption) to be at work when behavior took a turn for the worse or for the better.

During the mid to late 1800's, a more systematic study or scientific approach began to develop. Generally the scientific study of people was either conducted in a psychology laboratory or educational institution or within a medical environment.

Psychology was established as a professional specialty in 1892 when the American Psychological Association was founded by a group of pioneer psychologists that met at Clark University at the invitation of B. Stanley Hall. Psychology had three primary routes by which it would try to understand human feelings and behavior (Sundberg, 1977):

1. by attempting to determine what made the individual unique,
2. by studying the features and feelings all people appear to share, and
3. by studying the roles and interrelationships between people and between people and the non-human environment.

In the late 1800's and early 1900's, psychologists began to try to identify individual differences related to psychophysical attributes. For instance, tests were developed to measure reaction time; keenness of hearing and touch; perception of time, size, pitch, and color; and accuracy of motor performance (Sundberg, 1977; Reisman, 1976). Psychology then moved in the direction of measuring intelligence partly in order to assist the armed services screen prospective inductees during World War I. Intelligence testing would come to dominate psychological assessment during the first 40 years of the twentieth century. While early psychologists typically saw their role as trying to understand normal personality and behavior (in contrast to medicine's concern for the abnormal), this distinction quickly blurred. Much of the work of early, medically-oriented analysts such as Freud, Breuer, and Jung stirred interest in the non-medical community. The importance of individual personality and the impact of person to person relationships in health and illness became increasingly recognized. In response, psychology developed assessment tools related to personality typing and to the clarification of human interests, values, aptitudes, and emotions.

The 1920's through 1940's brought the refinement of a great many psycho-physical and intelligence tests and the standardization of many of the interest, aptitude, and personality instruments which are still in use today. Psychology gradually extended its domain beyond intelligence to trying to assess the conditions that fostered learning and to study the needs of special groups, such as children, criminals, or mentally ill persons. Psychologists also began to study the influence of social systems on the individual and society in general.

Today psychological assessment continues to be concerned with gathering information about how people learn and how the environment influences human thought and behavior and in understanding what is special about each of us and common among us. The 1990's finds us a psychologically sophisticated culture in which the jargon of assessment has become part of popular speech. All of the helping professions have become acutely aware of the need to appreciate and respond to the psychological needs of their clients, and psychological assessment is discussed across literature. Occupational therapy, along with other human services, often uses the information gathered by psychologists. In some cases, occupational therapists use assessments of their own that are quite similar to those identified with psychology, such as interest or value inventories. Industry, education, health systems, and the military have made psychological assessment an important criterion upon which decisions are made regarding all of us. This might cause us to wonder what ethics govern the use of psychological assessments.

Centralization of Test Material and Adoption of an Ethical Code

During the early history of psychological testing, each individual therapist or institution often assumed responsibility for designing **evaluation** tasks, tests, and protocol. Some standardized tools were available but most were not designed for the ill. The norms against which the patient's performance was judged were based upon the therapist's testing and treatment experiences with previous patients. Thus the basis of evaluation in treatment settings was subjective and the assessment process was decentralized. As the field of psychology expanded and clinicians sought to establish a more scientific foundation for evaluation, the assessment process became increasingly refined and centralized. Through the efforts of researchers and publishers of test materials, task protocol and tests were published and available for broad dissemination to mental health professionals. In addition, technology was used to systemize the process of compiling, scoring, reporting, and reviewing data. With a shared pool of assessment resources, it became more feasible for the development of a shared professional ethic in regard to the use of these materials.

Originally and through much of the 20th century, evaluators and publishers adhered to an unwritten ethical code in which publishers monitored the purchase and use of psychological tests. However, in 1967 the Federal Trade Commission protested this trade constraint. In 1974, the American Psychological Association (APA) suggested that the responsibility for ethical use of tests be shifted from the publisher to the test purchaser. Rather than issuing an explicit test purchase code, the APA provided a guide which suggests that test purchasers evaluate their knowledge, skills, and expertise and purchase only those tests for which the evaluator is qualified (APA, 1974, 1978). Currently, the publishers may ask test purchasers to sign an agreement based upon the APA guide. The agreement requests that the assessor maintain test security, adhere to the confidential aspects of the test, and administer the test as directed. The agreement also reminds the purchaser of the importance of

---

Basic Competencies in Assessment

A. Recognizes the importance of using standardized, reliable, and valid instruments wherever such are appropriate.

B. Distinguishes between subjective and objective data and uses each accordingly.

C. Distinguishes the critical differences between standardized and non-standardized instruments.

D. Recognizes the need to use standardized instruments according to the instructions given in the test administration manual.

E. Recognizes that using standardized instruments in an unstandardized (or adapted) manner may result in an invalid assessment.

F. Recognizes that specialized training may be necessary to administer certain instruments correctly and to interpret the data appropriately.

G. Uses assessment data to document work with client so as to provide a logical, continuous record of performance, therapeutic goals and media, and outcomes.

H. Follows ethical practices in the use of assessments: recognition of copyright, protection of the security of tests, protection of the confidentiality of test results, use of assessments for which one's education and experience is sufficient.

Figure 21-1. Basic Competencies in Assessment for the Occupational Therapist. *From: AOTA. (1984). Hierarchy of Competencies Relating to the Use of Standardized Instruments and Evaluation Techniques by Occupational Therapists. American Journal of Occupational Therapy, 38(12):803-804.*

current assessment knowledge and skill and the need for critical evaluation of test claims and research (Cronbach, 1984).

The ethical guidelines of the APA and those suggested by publishers of test materials are consistent with the basic competencies expected of occupational therapists as delineated in the Hierarchy of Assessment Competencies document approved by the American Occupational Therapy Association (1984). See Figure 21-1.

Regardless of what type of test is used, whether it was purchased from a psychological resource, originated within the occupational therapy profession, or originally designed, the therapist-assessor should strive to achieve the following:

1. to respect the dignity of patients,
2. to understand that psychological assessment can be experienced as intrusive by patients,
3. to realize that patients have the right of refusal, and
4. to realize that patients have the right, when possible, to understand the purpose and goal of the assessment.

The Development of a Classification System in Mental Health

While strides were being made in psychological assessment, more was being learned about the "inner person" by the medical community, including information related to the origin and treatment of psycho-social problems. This study continued within the domain of medicine, and psychiatry emerged as a powerful specialty.

Emil Kraepelin was a German psychiatrist (1855-1926) who separated mental disorders into those caused by exogenous factors (external), which he considered curable, and those caused by endogenous factors (inherent or constitutional), which he considered incurable (Reisman, 1976). Following this model, psychiatrists have tried to make distinctions between those individuals perceived as normal, mentally retarded, and mentally ill. Psychiatrists tried to organize information regarding mental illness by means of classifying abnormal states into medical diagnoses.

The work of psychoanalysts in the early 1900's gave us the landmark and most influential literature pertaining to the classification of psychiatric problems. Their work was colored by the fact that these psychoanalysts were originally schooled in medicine or the neurosciences, viewed personality and psychiatric problems in terms of the psychoanalytic concepts popularized by Freud, and used their own patient experiences or case studies as the basis for their conclusions. Not only were psychiatric diagnoses established, but much effort and study where directed toward trying to understand the nature of the conflicts and disturbances that were experienced subjectively by individuals with mental illness.

Kraepelin and Freud and other members of the psychoanalytic community were originally seeking an organic (or physical) basis for behavior and emotional disorder; more specifically they believed the origins of dysfunction to be in the matter of the brain or within micro-organisms (Sundberg, 1977; Reisman, 1976).

Although many of the early psychoanalysts continued to look for physical causes, they became increasingly convinced that a person's early experience and especially unconscious desires wielded a powerful influence over one's behavior and emotional well-being. (Freud himself never gave up his belief that the brain, as a physical organ, held the secrets of the psyche.) Projective tests such as *Jung's Word Association Test* (1905) and the *Rorschach Inkblot Test* (1912) were developed to reveal the contents of the unconscious, and Freudian concepts became the basis for establishing diagnoses. Because occupational therapy emerged from within medicine, it was the psychiatric system of giving atypical behavior a medical diagnosis and the goal of assessment to support such labeling that especially influenced our profession during the earlier years.

Diagnostic and Statistical Manual of Mental Disorders.
The first *Diagnostic and Statistic Manual of Mental Disorders* (DSM) was published by the APA in 1952 as an effort to standardize psychiatric terms because there were multiple classification systems prior to that time. Subsequent revisions occurred in DSM-II in 1968, DSM-III in 1980, and the DSM-III-R in 1987. Standardization was intended to minimize the confusion caused by multiple systems and to aid in the retrieval of information. The DSM systems describe the similarities and differences between persons with disorders and through the descriptions of etiology, prognosis, and differential responses serve as a link between classification and intervention. The DSM manuals are intended to enhance professional communication and to provide a foundation for theory through the consistent classification of disorders (Morey, Skinner, Blashfield, in Ciminero, et al., 1986).

DSM I and DSM II promulgated the concept that mental changes and accompanying behavioral disorders are illnesses. Both the DSM I and DSM II were used quite heavily as sources for establishing psychiatric diagnoses for third-party payers (insurance companies, the government, etc.). An important guiding premise in these two versions of the manual was the distinction made between ''neurotic'' versus ''psychotic'' disorders with a strong basis in traditional (Freudian) ego-psychology. The content of these manuals was based primarily on the clinical experience of its contributors, thus there was criticism regarding the subjectivity of the material and questions regarding reliability and validity. Even more criticism was generated because the manuals labeled individuals seeking psychiatric assistance as *ill* or *deviant* (Morey, et al., 1986).

The criticisms regarding the system of psychiatric diagnosis and treatment have been expressed by clinicians as well as by social scientists. Sociologists have criticized the medical model of diagnosis and treatment for the following reasons (Scheff, 1975, 1984):

1. The criteria for mental illness are ambiguous.
2. The terms used to define mental illness lack precision and are influenced by societal values and culture.
3. Signs and symptoms suggested in the diagnostic classifications are not uniform.
4. The cause, course, and site of pathology in mental illness have not been verified scientifically.
5. The choice of treatment is based upon clinical experiences and professional lore rather than scientific verification.
6. The diagnosis labels a person (temporarily, or more frequently permanently).
7. Diagnosis and treatment in mental health are used to maintain order in society.

Rather than accept the psychodynamic classification of mental illness as presented in the medical model of psychi-

atric diagnosis and treatment, sociologists have suggested that mental illness is a form of deviance. Labeling of patients using the *deviance theory* rather than psychodynamic principles is based upon the following premises (Scheff 1975, 1984):

1. Symptoms may be caused by disease (as suggested by the medical model), stress, psychological conditioning, or intentional deviant behavior, or they may represent artistic innovations;
2. Symptoms represent a violation of social norms and should not be viewed as entities confined to an individual but understood in the context of the individual within a social network (i.e., family, school, work, society at large);
3. There are many external contingencies which lead to labeling (i.e., how the behavior or symptom violates society's expectations, the age or race of the violator, or the nature of the community in which the patient lives and functions);
4. Labeling deviant behavior as mental illness frequently occurs during childhood and may inadvertently be positively reinforced during social interaction; and
5. Once a person is labeled deviant, it is difficult for that person to return to a conventional role.

These premises of labeling have influenced contemporary psychological theory, treatment approaches in mental health, and diagnostic classification. Although the medical model continues to serve as the basis for psychiatric diagnosis, the broad influence of labeling theory is evident in the DSM III and DSM III-R.

DSM III-R (1987) and its predecessor DSM III (1980) depart from previous manuals in that they attempt to be as atheoretical as possible. Psychiatric conditions are conceived as disorders rather than diseases. Psychiatric terms are not eliminated; however, the emphasis is on description of behavior and not on etiology (Dubovsky, 1988, p. xv). For example, an individual will not be labeled a ''schizophrenic'' or ''alcoholic'' but rather ''as having problems related to schizophrenia'' and as ''having problems with alcohol dependence.''

Another significant change in DSM III and DSM III-R is their use of a *multiaxial evaluation system*. The intent of the multiaxial system is to encourage clinicians to evaluate psychiatric disturbance on more than one level (Dubovsky, 1988, p. xv). This purpose is achieved through increased content organized within a five axis system (see Figure 21-2). Axes I, II, and III are provided as a basis for establishing diagnosis. Axes IV and V are intended to aid in the planning for treatment and predicting outcome. During assessment, the patient's primary therapist identifies the criteria from each axis that best describes the disorder that the patient is presently experiencing, the environmental context of the disorder, and the previous and present level of functioning.

The members of the Task Force who prepared DSM-III sought to produce a manual that would be compatible with the *International Classification of Diseases* (9th edition), and many changes in DSM-III and DSM-III-R are intended to clarify criteria for labeling. However, both these newer diagnostic manuals have been criticized by various authors (Jampala, et al., 1986; Kendell, 1980; Morey, et al., 1986; Spitzer, et al., 1983) for the following reasons: (1) neglecting psychodynamic approaches to diagnosis and unjustifiably eliminating the concept of neurosis, (2) too much content for a manual, yet not enough information for a text,

(3) lack of cited references, (4) lack of sound empirical base for some diagnostic criteria, and (5) the descriptive approach detracts from a deeper understanding of psychological problems.

The reader should review the manuals for more detailed information regarding these changes made in the newer editions. In addition to the modifications, other classification systems are being proposed that would be empirically-based and focus on behavioral analysis, psychological responses, and environmental circumstances (Morey, Skinner, et al., 1986).

Occupational Therapy Assessment History

Developments in occupational therapy psychological assessment have followed those in psychology and psychiatry. As with assessment in the mental health system generally, assessment in occupational therapy began with individual therapists creating assessment formats specific to their individual settings. However, today, the field recognizes the need for assessment instruments that are widely available and empirically sound.

During the early years of the profession, the occupational therapist relied heavily upon a referral from the physician to treat the patient and followed the physician's recommendations in the implementation of treatment. The occupational therapist may or may not have done an evaluation to elicit data to support the physician's psychiatric diagnosis and to guide treatment.

The more commonly used psychologically-oriented assessments were the Azima battery and the Fidler battery. Both of these batteries have a psychoanalytic basis and use **projective activities** to elicit data that suggest the patient's needs, thoughts, feelings, and concerns. During the 1950's, these data were interpreted by the physician and the occupational therapist and used to establish or confirm a diagnosis and to suggest treatment approaches. If these assessments are used today, the data are usually interpreted using the combined views of the patient and therapist.

The Effects of the Community Mental Health Movement. This physician-guided approach predominated in occupational therapy into the 1960's, at which time the community mental health movement gained momentum. With the creation of many community-based mental health centers, the broad treatment responsibility of the physician became shared with the entire treatment team and the patient. The physician maintained the primary role as diagnostician and shared the responsibility for intervention with nurses, occupational therapists, psychologists, recreation therapists, social workers, and mental health technicians. The occupational therapist, like other team members, continues to work cooperatively with the patient within the therapeutic milieu of a hospital or mental health setting to

Axis I —	**Clinical Syndromes and V Codes*** All of the mental disorders that are classified.
Axis II —	**Developmental Disorders and Personality Disorders** Disorders that begin in childhood or adolescence and persist throughout life. May indicate personality traits.
Axis III —	**Physical Disorders and Conditions** Conditions listed outside of the mental disorders section of ICD-9-CM.** The condition may relate to the etiology of the mental disorder or impact case management.
Axis IV —	**Severity of Psychosocial Stressors** Life events that cause an individual distress are rated to determine their relationship to the current mental disorder.
Axis V —	**Global Assessment of Function** The clinician uses The Global Assessment of Functioning Scale*** to judge the person's psychosocial and occupational performance (current level and the highest level during the past year).

* V Codes—"Conditions not attributable to a mental disorder that are a focus of attention or treatment." DSM III-R, (1987), p. 17.

** ICD-9 International Classification of Disease-9.

*** The Global Assessment Scale: A procedure for measuring overall severity of psychiatric disturbance. *Archives of General Psychiatry 33:*766-771, 1976.

Figure 21-2. DSM III-R Multiaxial System. (A five axes evaluation system for planning and predicting outcome of treatment). *Adapted from The American Psychiatric Association (1987). Diagnostic and Statistical Manual of Mental Disorders, 3rd ed, Revised. Washington, DC: American Psychiatric Association, pp. xvii-20.*

identify problems, evaluate the effect of symptoms upon performance, design intervention strategies within the confines of the available treatment resources, and determine the possible living environment after discharge.

With the community mental health center movement came the recognition that professionals, other than the physician, could serve effectively as primary therapist for a patient. Social workers, psychologists, psychiatric nurses, chaplains, educational counselors, licensed marriage and family counselors, and others moved into positions of greater authority and responsibility. While the tie of psychiatry to the medical model continued as did the tie of occupational therapy to medicine, the bonds were loosened in many areas.

In working with these varying disciplines in psychosocial care, the expectations and needs for assessment in occupational therapy frequently changed. Occupational therapy evaluation was no longer intended to establish or support a psychiatric diagnosis or reveal intra-psychic content, but rather was directed toward assessing function regarding the following: daily living; work and avocational skill level; the ability for independent self-care and social relatedness; cognitive function, problem solving, and coping skills; and specific skills needed in the expected (post-treatment) environment.

This change in assessment was also consistent with the move in mental health care to more problem-oriented treatment and documentation. Evaluation documentation was no longer limited to narrative formats, but included checklists, Likert scales, and more structured data communication, some of which is computerized today.

Expanded Assessment Boundaries. As occupational therapy developed alternative theoretical frameworks specific to psychosocial assessment and treatment, occupational therapy assessment and treatment broadened and a proliferation of assessment instruments followed, many of which were designed to meet the program needs of an individual department in a particular setting. The American Occupational Therapy Association (AOTA) established the *Uniform Terminology for Recording Occupational Therapy Services* (1979) and the *Occupational Therapy Uniform Evaluation Checklist* (1981) in order to provide broad boundaries for assessment and documentation within which multiple frameworks could be implemented. It was also hoped that the documents would define the boundaries of occupational therapy and its services for the consumer and for the third party payer. These documents have now been supplemented with the release of the Second Edition of Uniform Terminology for Occupational Therapy (AOTA, 1989; Dunn & McGourty, 1989). (See Appendix)

Occupational therapy literature reflected an interest from the members of the profession in establishing a guide for both the development of assessment instruments (Benson &

Clark, 1982) and for determining the reliability and validity of the instruments that are used in occupational therapy settings (Hemphill, 1982). The American Occupational Therapy Association sponsored an assessment institute in 1979 in Detroit, prior to the annual AOTA conference, during which assessments used in current practice were presented and evaluated for research design, potential standardization, and future development. It was during this institute that the *Bay Area Functional Performance Evaluation* (BaFPE) was selected as having potential for fulfilling these criteria. To date research and development has occurred and standardization is in process (See discussion of the BaFPE in Chapter 15).

Thus we see that through the evolution of the mental health system, the interests of practitioners, and the support of professional organizations, occupational therapy assessment in mental health has evolved from a physician-guided, primarily diagnostic focus to an autonomous data gathering process that contributes to team decisions of treatment. This data gathering process now has a uniform guide, multiple evaluation tools, goals of establishing reliability and validity standards, and a uniform data base.

CONTEMPORARY PSYCHOLOGICAL ASSESSMENT IN OCCUPATIONAL THERAPY

Since occupational therapists frequently function as members of the medical team, they seek to elicit information which will complement, rather than duplicate, information obtained by other professionals. Even if involved in home care and/or private practice, the occupational therapist will inevitably interface with other professionals. Hence, the therapist must be able to understand the assessments and subsequent reports made by other professions and know the unique contributions that occupational therapy assessment and treatment can offer.

Assessment Terminology in Occupational Therapy

The *Uniform Terminology for Occupational Therapy* (2nd Edition, AOTA, 1989), defines occupational therapy assessment as *"the planned process of obtaining, interpreting and documenting [information about] the functional status of the individual. The purpose of the assessment is to identify the individual's abilities and limitations, including deficits, delays or maladaptive behavior that can be addressed in occupational therapy intervention. Data can be gathered through a review of records, observation, interview, and the administration of test procedures. Such procedures include, but are not limited to, the use of standardized tests, questionnaires, performance checklists, activities, and tasks designed to evaluate specific performance abilities."* (p. 811).

Psychological performance abilities have also been defined within the current Uniform Terminology document. It identifies psychological skills and psychological components as one of three performance component areas (AOTA, 1989). This area has psychological, social and self-management divisions, each with identified attributes or skills. Psychological components and skills include roles, values, interests, initiation of activity, termination of activity, and self concept. Social components and skills include social conduct, conversation and self-expression; while self-management components include coping skills, time management and self-control. It is within these very broad areas that the therapist identifies and uses specific psychological assessment strategies to determine a patient or client's characteristics or levels of performance.

Domains for Assessment

Consistent with these general areas of psychological concern, the occupational therapist is interested in assessing the patient's ability to:

1. state his/her perceived needs, feelings, conflicts, values, beliefs, and goals and those of others;
2. identify knowledge and performance boundaries, including strengths and limitations;
3. acknowledge capabilities and accomplishments;
4. identify the need for change and the response which will allow optimum function and benefits;
5. identify role expectations and the means to fulfill role responsibilities; and
6. identify the performance necessary for successful participation in group and individual social situations.

Psychological Assessment of Persons with Physical Disability

Psychological assessment is not primarily the obligation of those who treat psychiatric problems. As discussed by Fike (1984), psychological assessment and restoration may be "deemphasized" in physical medicine because of occupational therapy's "stronger identification with physical care" and the need to document to third-party payers the physical changes that result from intervention (Fike, 1984; pp. 226-227). Both the theoretical and philosophical base of the occupational therapy profession "fully support involvement in intervention for the psychological needs of the physically disabled" (Fike, 1984, p. 228). It is also evident that what we think of

ourselves, our health, and our illnesses can greatly influence our personal well-being and our ability to participate in and profit from health care (Frey, 1984; Doneson, 1984; Barry, 1984; Watson, 1986; Bond, 1986). Moreover, as presented in Chapter 4, research suggests that emotional stress may be an important predisposing factor to certain kinds of illnesses and accidents (Holmes & Rahe, 1967; Jemmott & Locke, 1984; Ornstein & Sobel, 1984; Selye, 1976, 1979).

It is generally agreed that knowledge of psychological components is essential to having a picture of the whole person. There is far less agreement regarding the following issues of how to best achieve psychological assessment, what constitute domains of concern, and to what extent occupational therapists should hope to address all of their client's needs (Denton, 1986; Allen, 1985).

Purposes of Psychological Evaluation in Occupational Therapy

The assessment process is being more frequently used as a means to gather information regarding the patient's ability for problem-solving. It is less often used to support diagnoses. The occupational therapy literature establishes multiple purposes of psychosocial evaluation. Of these general assessment goals, those more frequently encountered in contemporary practice include: (1) determining what thoughts and feelings the patient has about self, others, and personal life experiences; (2) determining a patient's current level of performance in daily life and contrasting the present function with the highest level previously achieved; (3) providing a foundation for treatment planning; (4) determining the nature and quality of change which has occurred in response to treatment interventions, and (5) contributing to the master treatment plan.

ELEMENTS OF PSYCHOLOGICAL ASSESSMENT

Each therapist conducting a psychological assessment does so with goals specific to the treatment setting, his/her treatment philosophy, and the needs of his/her clients. However, there are several elements that can help the therapist select an appropriate assessment tool, make effective use of available instruments, and help in the interpretation of assessment data compiled by others. The following questions will help the therapist in focusing on these important elements:

1. How are **psychological constructs** conceived within the assessment?
2. Which practice **frame of reference** provides the assessment context?

3. Does the assessment tool gather data from the patient's perspective (insider/subjective) or the therapist's perspective (outsider/objective)?

4. Does the assessment process attempt to gather signs or samples of patient behavior?

5. What are the practical boundaries influencing the assessment process?

Psychological Constructs

Since we are unable to see thoughts and feelings, we must use psychological concepts or constructs when describing psychological phenomena. **Psychological constructs** are terms that are commonly used to describe mental states, but they have no universally agreed-upon dimensions. These phrases taken from the *Uniform Terminology of Reporting Occupational Therapy Services* (AOTA, 1979) describe skill components representing psychological constructs: ''self-concept;'' perceiving one's ''power;'' sensing one's ''competence;'' having a sense of ''psychological safety;'' handling ''stress;'' and ''understanding social norms.'' There are a great many more psychological constructs used in psychological dialogue, both within occupational therapy and across professions, as well as in everyday speech. Without such constructs, it would be difficult and perhaps impossible to talk about what people think or feel; we could only discuss what we do. Psychological constructs give us the language to discuss our feelings, to reflect upon what we have done, and to ponder where we are heading in our lives. However, the difficulty in using constructs is that there is no agreement on what the myriad of psychological constructs actually includes or excludes. Nor is there agreement regarding which constructs deserve priority and should be studied in relation to the inner-person, how internal states can be identified and measured, and how construct validity is best established for specific assessment instruments.* This problem does not pertain to psychological assessment alone but, rather, is part of a greater ''conceptual enigma'' that exists within and across all rehabilitation assessment (Frey, 1984).

Physical Changes as Indicators of Constructs. For a long time therapist-assessors have looked at the individual patient's physical appearance as a means to identify psychological state. The feelings conveyed by a person's face, dress, posture and demeanor, or in some instances one's non-verbal communication (the totality of which is often referred to as one's affect), might be summarized as ''sad,'' ''angry,'' ''guarded,'' ''optimistic,'' or ''cheerful.'' An

assessment of affect and judgments related to non-verbal communication is included in many assessment procedures and may also be a matter of course in the daily charting within a hospital or mental health setting. Yet, these judgments are often made at the discretion of the observer, without particular guidelines.

As previously discussed, psychological assessment has a history of assessing psychological states in terms of specific measurable physiologic changes. For instance, emotional depression has been related to decreased respiration, slowed response time, loss of appetite, and changes in REM sleep. Conversely, anxiety states may be associated with heightened arousal of the sympathetic nervous system, tremors, numbness, and palpitations. Psychosis may be associated with changed activity of the neurotransmitter dopamine.

Self Statements. Certainly the most common and straightforward means of identifying the existence of certain internal or feeling states has been to rely on what the individual says about oneself. For example, the person may say, ''I have no self-confidence,'' or ''I am worried about how I'll manage at home,'' thus suggesting anxiety or a lack of self-confidence.

Observation of Motor Performance. Psychological inferences of functional performance have also been made through the observation of motor performance or behavior in the everyday setting. For example, the assessor may conclude that an individual is confident in a particular setting if the person works independently on an activity, or the therapist may see social withdrawal as an indicator of the patient's depression. It should be noted that not all observations of performance are conducted to discover the client's mental state. In the behavioral frame of reference, the primary concern is the client's adequacy of performance as determined through use of a functional assessment.

In some instances observation of a patient's actions and affect may be combined in evaluative comments regarding personality, personality traits, or personality style (Allport, 1950, 1966; Allport & Odbert, 1936; Barry, 1984; Fidler & Fidler, 1963; Kahana & Bibring, 1964; Usdin and Lewis, 1978). Assessments might identify a patient's style as being ''controlled,'' ''demanding,'' ''sexualizing,'' or ''aloof.'' These, too, are constructs created to describe behavior. There is no one agreed upon scale for identifying such personality styles or traits.

Pfeiffer and Jones (1973) provide an enlightening group experiential exercise that illustrates the arbitrary nature of inferring personality traits from behavior. In the exercise , each group participant is given a large piece of paper and pencil and asked to make as many ''T's'' as he or she can, during a one-minute time period. When the minute has lapsed and each participant's score tallied, the assessor or

---

*''The end goal of validation is explanation and understanding, and many in the psychological profession are beginning to view all validation as construct validation'' (Cronbach, 1984, p. 126).

group leader asks, "What did this test measure?" The authors report that participants typically hypothesize that one or more of the following has been measured: eye-hand coordination, dexterity, ability to follow directions, creativity, competitiveness, T-making behavior, anxiety, quickness, achievement need, and compulsiveness. The point is made that any of these hypotheses may be correct since the traits inferred from the assessment process are identified and created by the scientist or test's architect in order to permit the "orderly description of behavior" (Pfeiffer & Jones, 1973, pp. 41-44).

Constructs as Defined by Frame of Reference. In addition to looking at affect, self-statements of feelings, and performance in the general manner that we have described, each of the theoretical frameworks imposes its own specialized set of psychological constructs and related assessment systems and measures. For example, a Freudian psychodynamically grounded framework may utilize such metaphorical concepts as the "id," "ego," "superego," "conscious," "unconscious," "defenses," and "drives." A related assessment might identify signs of adequate ego-function by noting the ability of the patient to realistically assess alternatives, to postpone a need for immediate gratification, or to follow a specified task procedure (Bellak, 1984; Fidler & Fidler, 1963; Prelinger & Zimet, 1964). Goldsmith (1984, p. 46) suggests that Freudian constructs can be operationalized as specific behaviors and clarity can be achieved if the parameters of assessment constructs are well-defined. But in her view, these psychological constructs lose their utility if one attempts to concretize images to the point where we talk about "the superego...[as] the little man in our head hitting us."

Mosey (1970) emphasizes the guiding role that a theoretical frame of reference provides in determining which constructs will be assessed and by what means. However, even when two assessment procedures or instruments are identified with the same frame of reference, psychological constructs may be conceived quite differently. For example, positive self-esteem might be judged in relation to patient independence in one assessment, by statements related to feelings of "attractiveness" in another, or by good grooming in a third.

Some authors point out that the lack of professional clarity and agreement regarding the various psychological constructs weakens the extent to which any profession (alone or in conjunction with other professions) can plan, implement, demonstrate, and scrutinize the treatment of those it serves (Anthony, 1979; Cohen & Anthony, 1984; Frey, 1984; Watts & Bennett, 1983). Because occupational therapists currently use a wide range of assessment instruments and often use an assessment process that is idiosyncratic to their institution, the therapist-assessor must know

with which theoretical framework a given assessment tool or process is aligned. The therapist must also understand the meaning of the identified psychological constructs in the context of specific assessment procedures, how related behaviors are recognized and documented, and along what axes and to what degree a desirable versus undesirable psychological status is conceived. In other words, in order to use an assessment tool effectively, the assessor must understand and be able to speak the language specific to that tool.

In some instances the assessment protocol, rationale, and constructs may be well described, such as when assessment batteries are introduced to the professional population within professional literature. However, the therapist may also encounter those without a clearly stated theoretical foundation, and thus will then need to further explore the theoretical assumptions and psychological constructs upon which the assessment is based.

Frames of Reference and the Evaluation Process

A frame of reference is the body of theoretical assumptions and related principles of practice that give unity and direction to practice and research. These frameworks determine the nature of the information sought in order to direct treatment and render a rationale for treatment. Therapists espouse a particular frame of reference; as do departments and institutions. Particular assessment tools and processes have been designed to gather information that is vital to certain theoretical frameworks and thus tend to become associated with a particular frame of reference. Sometimes an evaluation instrument will be clearly identified with a given framework, and other times, the relationship is less apparent. Therapists must take great care in selecting or using assessment instruments in accordance with specific theoretical and practice beliefs.

There are multiple frames of reference used in psychosocial occupational therapy which have been identified and classified in the literature with some variation (Bruce & Borg, 1987; Denton, 1986; Llorens, 1984; Mosey, 1970, 1986; Reed, 1984). In this chapter we will discuss the following frames of reference most frequently used in mental health and how they influence the assessment process: psychoanalytic, behavioral, developmental, acquisitional, neurodevelopmental, neurobehavioral, occupational behavior, and occupational performance.

There are several commonalities found among these multiple frames of reference in the occupational therapy literature. The first commonality is the emphasis on the partnership that exists between the occupational therapist and the patient during the assessment process. The partnership provides an opportunity for shared learning and interaction and provides a supportive structure from which therapist and patient can explore the patient's present situation and better understand the events that led to the need for treatment. As the patient and therapist explore in the present, they increase their understanding of each other and what each can contribute to the treatment process as trust grows. This element of humanism exists within all the theoretical approaches to assessment.

The second commonality is that all theoretical frameworks support the use of a combination of interview and task (structured and/or unstructured) which will accomplish the following: (1) help to identify the patient's discomfort or desire for change and/or growth, (2) enable the observation of behaviors and affect, (3) elicit verbalizations regarding the presenting concerns, (4) give information regarding the patient's strengths and capabilities, (5) help to identify resources (personal and environmental) which support the patient in the pursuit of growth and/or change.

The third and final commonality is that all the theoretical approaches identify the need for the initial and ongoing (continuous) assessment process. Throughout the treatment process the occupational therapist continues to observe the patient's participation in occupational therapy, to note and assess changes that occur during treatment, to revise intervention strategies as needed, and to plan for the eventual termination of treatment.

In any given theoretical viewpoint, there are distinguishing features of the assessment process. These distinguishing features can be categorized as: (1) the intended goal or outcome of the interview; (2) the activities chosen and the variations in particular activities used to elicit data; and (3) the manner in which the data are collected and interpreted. These three distinguishing features are discussed in each of the following frames of reference.

Psychoanalytic Frame of Reference

The psychoanalytic frame of reference is also referred to as the *object relations frame of reference*. This theoretical view acknowledges the role of the past or history as having a significant effect on the individual and constituting one important area of assessment. The goal of assessment is to identify the pressing needs, feelings, thoughts, and previous experiences which are influencing the person's behavior and presenting problems and/or symptoms. Goals may also include the identification of growth areas for the person and the resources which are capable of promoting that growth to enhance that person's quality of life.

The therapist uses insider-oriented projective tasks and the interview approach allows for open-ended responses. The interview is intended to determine the following from the patient's point of view: view of self concept of others, ego organization, conscious and possible unconscious conflicts, and other dynamics which influence the patient's behavior, personal development, and response to change.

During the assessment, the therapist discusses observations with the patient in order to increase his or her self awareness and involvement in the treatment process and to validate impressions of the patient's performance. The therapist observes the patient's approach to the evaluation activities and "listens" for feelings, needs, values, and interests and the manner in which these are communicated. The therapist focuses on the quality of the patient's interpersonal relationships, the patient's ability to invest energy in an adequate number and quality of need-satisfying activities, and the patient's ability to cope and defend against stress without a loss of personal integration.

In summary, the psychoanalytic approach uses an historical process to gain an understanding of the conflicting thoughts and feelings which cause discomfort and influence the coping styles the individual uses day-to-day. The therapist helps the person understand through a logical, at times inferential process, the psychological factors that are influencing the patient's behavior so that the individual can more effectively choose how he/she wishes to act.

Behavioral Frame of Reference

The behavioral frame of reference, also referred to as the acquisitional frame of reference, emphasizes learning theory and functional assessment. This theoretical view assumes that all behaviors are learned. Behavior may be adaptive or maladaptive and is represented by the repertoire of skills and habits that a person possesses. The primary goal of the behavioral evaluation is to determine the adequacy of the person's skills and habits for performance in a specific environment and the environmental forces that are influencing performance.

To determine adequacy of performance the occupational therapist observes the patient in the natural environment or in contrived situations (also referred to as *analogues*). When contrived situations are used, it is assumed there will be generalization of behavior, thus leading the patient to respond similar to what they would in similar natural circumstances. In recent literature, the term *functional assessment* is used to refer to the behaviors that are very specific to the environment in which the patient can be expected to function. For example, functional assessment of food preparation skills of a person who will be living in a halfway house would be minimal when compared to the assessment of those skills if that person plans to live at home alone.

The behavioral interview is more structured than that of the open-ended approach used in the object relations framework. Possible assessment tools may include questionnaires, behavioral observation scales, and self-report measures. The focus of the interview is to determine *how* the person behaves and not to establish reasons for this behavior.

Observations and interview data are used to form a behavioral baseline which *quantitatively* depicts the following information: (1) those skills and habits which are adaptive and/or those that interfere with daily function and adaptation, (2) the frequency of behavior, (3) the stimuli and reinforcers that influence behavior (their sources and frequency), and (4) the patient's ability to discriminate and respond effectively to the environment.

In summary, the emphasis of the behavioral evaluation is on what is observed and not on inferences, and the focus of assessment is on the skills necessary for function in specific post-treatment settings. Observation must be objective and is always considered within the context of the environment and its influence on learning.

Developmental Frame of Reference

The developmental frame of reference is founded on principles of normal growth and development throughout the life span. Assessment within the developmental framework strives to compare the person's physical and psychosocial performance to a normal developmental profile. The normal profile reflects physical patterns of growth and development, normative life tasks, and expected social roles.

The goal of the developmental assessment is to identify the person's level of physical and/or psychosocial skill performance and what is needed to master a specific developmental period within the life span. Some discussions do not identify specific assessment protocol for the developmental framework (Denton, 1986). Others suggest that performance be identified by using standardized tools, nonstandardized tests, and by observation of performance during activities, such as activities of daily living, pre-vocational activities and work (Reed, 1984).

During the interview, the therapist elicits historical information to determine if the patient has mastered life tasks and has the knowledge, skills, and attitudes for meeting social role responsibilities. The data elicited by the interview, tests, and activities are viewed holistically with the intent of identifying the uniqueness of each individual.

In summary, the developmental assessment summarizes the patient's physical and psychosocial performance within a specific life stage. The assessment also identifies the present stresses which the patient must confront in order to grow, change, and/or adapt to the present stage of development and identifies the available resources which can assist the patient to cope with life's changes.

Occupational Behavior Frame of Reference

The occupational behavior frame of reference has been further elaborated through a *model of human occupation*. In this model, the person is seen as an open system with three component subsystems: *volition* (motivation), *habituation*, and *performance*. During assessment, the occupational therapist seeks to identify the interrelationship of the subsystems and the adequacy of each system in maintaining order and facilitating the role performance of a person in the environment.

The occupational behaviorist uses interview, observation, history taking and tests (standardized and nonstandardized) to determine the level of occupational disorder and function. There are multiple assessment instruments suggested for this framework (Barris, Watts, Kielhofner, 1983; Kielhofner, 1985). Some have been developed by occupational therapists, others are available in unpublished masters theses, and others have been developed by non-occupational therapy members of the mental health community.

The data and performance observations that are elicited by the activity and interview strategy frequently are interpreted by using the *Occupational Case Analysis Interview and Rating Scale*. This system of case analysis was developed by Cubie and Kaplan (1982) and is used to identify the following: (1) personal causation (the sense of being effective and in control), (2) the person's goals, interests, and values, (3) the person's roles, habits and output, (4) the physical and social environment of the person, and (5) the feedback that the person receives. Cubie and Kaplan (1982, p. 649) also recommend that the therapist identify the dynamics of the (person) system, the compatibility of the system to the environment, and issues from the past, present or future that affect the system.

Neurodevelopmental Frame of Reference

The neurodevelopmental framework (also referred to as neuropsychiatric) in psychosocial occupational therapy is based upon the neurobehavioral theory developed by A. Jean Ayres for sensory integrative approaches for children with learning disorders. Ayres developed standardized tests for children ages four through eight. These tests required children to perform structured tasks that allow the therapist to observe the child's visual perception, figure-ground perception, position in space, design copying, motor accuracy, kinesthesia, manual form perception, finger identification, graphesthesia, localization of tactile stimuli (single and double), imitation of postures, crossing the midline of the body, bilateral motor coordination, and right-left discrimination (Ayres, 1973, p. 97).

Ayres' theory has been adapted by others (King, 1982; King, 1988; Ross and Burdick, 1981) for the evaluation and treatment of regressed psychiatric and geropsychiatric patients. Ross and Burdick suggest a sensorimotor-cognitive assessment for adults that is similar to that developed by Ayres. However, there are no standards of performance established for their instrument. The assessment requires the patient to perform structured tasks in order to identify the patient's sensorimotor functioning (range of motion, balance, posture, general strength, proprioception, crossing midline, finger identification, graphesthesia, stereognosis, unilateral neglect, and speed), and perceptual cognitive functioning (auditory, figure-ground perception, visual problems, fine motor coordination, bilateral coordination, body scheme, and image and linguistic output) (Ross & Burdick, 1981, pp. 45-47). This and other neuropsychiatric evaluations are used to give a general impression of the patient's general intelligence, attention span, perseveration, coping style, and skills that are needed to meet the required performance in self-care, work, and leisure pursuits.

Cognitive Frame of Reference

The cognitive developmental frame of reference is represented by the work of Claudia Allen. Allen's model focuses on cognitive disabilities associated with illnesses or injuries to the brain. Assessment is concerned with the patient's ability to process information. Cognitive processing is evaluated by observing sensorimotor operations, such as that of voluntary motor actions. Allen designed three assessment tools which are suggested for use in an acute setting to identify level of competence; the *Allen Cognitive Level Test* (ACL), the *Lower Cognitive Level Test* (LCL), and the *Routine Task Inventory* (RTI). These instruments are used in conjunction with a chart review and interview. The interview is used to obtain a routine task history and to identify the patient's functional abilities in past performance, during recent performance, *and* in present and possible future performance (Allen, 1985, 1988). During the evaluation, the therapist observes the patient's performance and tries to identify (1) the symptoms of illness, based on DSM-III information, (2) the patient's awareness of illness, based upon identification of strengths, limitations and assets, (3) the patient's cognitive level, based upon the level of behavioral responses during the ACL and the LCL, and (4) the patient's goals from those quoted by the patient (Allen, 1985). The occupational therapist then reviews the data to identify a specific cognitive level of function and then compares it to the highest level of function ever achieved by the patient, to that achieved during the past year, and to that which is chronologically expected (Allen, 1985).

Summary

Each of these frames of reference, plus others, are evident in occupational therapy practice. They are being used either as a singular guiding framework or within systematic, yet eclectic combinations, such as in Fidler's Life Style Performance (Fidler, 1982, 1988) and Mosey's Model of Role Acquisition (Mosey, 1986).

While a therapist's frame of reference bears directly on the substance and manner of the assessment process, there are several related dimensions of the assessment, including (1) the assessment point of view, (2) the conditions under which the assessment occurs, and (3) whether the assessment is designed to elicit signs of psychic conditions or samples of behavior. We turn now to a consideration of the interrelations between these dimensions.

ASSESSMENT POINT OF VIEW: SUBJECTIVE OR OBJECTIVE?

Assessment points of view can be broadly categorized as (1) the so-called insider or subjective point of view that takes the view of the patient, (2) the outsider stance or the view of an objective third person, and (3) a combination of both the insider and outsider perspectives.

Subjective Approach: The Insider Perspective

The insider approach to assessment raises three other influencing questions: (1) who chooses the feelings or behaviors that are to be assessed, (2) who monitors or reports on psychic states, and (3) who makes the judgment that feelings have changed or behaviors have been performed (Margolin & Jacobson, 1981).

The insider view may be taken within diverse assessment contexts including the initial interview, less structured media experiences, projective tests, activity configurations, patient questionnaires, self-rating scales and inventories, and patient journals. If the patient's point of view is the source relied upon, then the information given about himself/herself and the changes are genuine.

The *Body Parts Satisfaction Scale* (Noles, et al., 1985; Berscheid, et al. 1973) is an insider-oriented assessment that consists of a list of 24 body parts plus an overall-appearance item. The patient is asked to rate each body part on a six-point scale that ranges from "extremely dissatisfied" to "extremely satisfied." The *Body-Self Relations Questionnaire* (Noles, et al., 1985; Winston & Cash, 1984) consists of 140 items concerning the person's attitudes and actions regarding physical appearance, physical activity, and health items, to which the person must respond on a five-point scale ranging from "definitely disagree" to "definitely agree." These tools are very different from objective measures in which an outsider assessor-observer views an individual and rates physical appearance according to established criteria (Noles, et al., 1985).

BECK'S DEPRESSION INVENTORY
(selected items)

C. (Sense of Failure)

0   I do not feel like a failure

1   I feel I have failed more than the average person

2a   I feel I have accomplished very little that is worth-while or that means anything

2b   As I look back on my life all I can see is a lot of failures

3   I feel I am a complete failure as a person (parent, husband, wife)

L. (Social Withdrawal)

0   I have not lost interest in other people

1   I am less interested in other people now than I used to be

2   I have lost most of my interest in other people and have little feeling for them

3   I have lost all my interest in other people and don't care about them at all

O. (Work Retardation)

0   I can work about as well as before

1a   It takes extra effort to get started at doing something

1b   I don't work as well as I used to

2   I have to push myself very hard to do anything

3   I can't do any work at all

Figure 21-3. Sample Self-Inventory: Insider Perspective. *From: Beck, A.T. (1967). Depression: Clinical, Experimental and Theoretical Aspects. Harper and Row, NY, pp. 333-335.*

Phenomenology

The insider or subjective point of view brings into focus the *theory of phenomenology* or the belief that behavior is determined not by external but rather subjective reality. The therapist-assessor taking an insider or subjective perspective must consider that reality may depend on from what perspective it is viewed. For example, five people attending a concert or any event might each have a different description of the event because each one might notice and experience something different than the other four. Each person would organize and give meaning to what they experienced according to their personal viewpoint and in accordance with their life experiences. Not one of these five descriptions of the event would be any more correct than any of the others.

An insider-assessment philosophy holds that just as the patient will have a unique perspective on life, each treatment staff member encountering the patient cannot help but gain a unique assessment picture of this individual.

Collins describes it thus, "there is no real picture of . . .[the patient] . . . Just as there is no 'real recipe' for cure or restoration" (Collins, 1984, p. 185).

Examples of insider approaches that allow the patient to guide the content to be addressed are non-structured interviews in which the patient is asked to "tell about himself" with little direction given by the assessor, and draw-a-person procedures in which the patient is asked to "tell about" the drawing. These less-structured assessment experiences can be contrasted to the structured interview formats such as the *Adolescent Role Assessment* (Black, 1976) and the *Occupational Role History* (Moorehead, 1969) in which the therapist asks the patient to respond to specific questions identified by the assessor. The interview as an assessment tool is discussed in more detail later in this chapter.

A keenly subjective stance in assessment is also taken by humanistic existentially-oriented therapies, including those identified with client-centered, Gestalt, phenomenology, and field theories. Humanistically-oriented assessment procedures most often have an emphasis on feelings and are designed to

YOUNG'S LONELINESS INVENTORY
(selected items)

1. 0   I have someone nearby I can really depend on and who cares about me.

1   I'm not sure there's anyone nearby who I can really depend on and who cares about me.

2   There's no one anywhere I can really depend on and who cares about me right now.

3   For several years, I haven't had anyone I could really depend on and who cared about me.

7. 0   When I want to do something for enjoyment, I can usually find someone to join me.

1   Often I end up doing things alone even though I'd like to have someone join me.

2   There's no one right now I can go out and enjoy things with.

3   There hasn't been anyone I could go out and enjoy things with for several years.

8. 0   There are no groups I'd really like to belong to that won't accept me.

1   There is a group of people I know that I'd like to belong to but don't.

2   It bothers me that there is a group of people I know right now who don't like me.

3   For the past several years I've felt excluded by group(s) of people I've wanted to belong to.

Figure 21-4. Sample Self-Inventory: Insider Perspective. *From: Young, J.E. (1981). Cognitive Therapy and Loneliness. In Emery, G., Hollon, S., Bedrosian, R.C. (Eds.). New Directions in Cognitive Therapy: A Casebook. NY, Guilford Press, pp. 139-159.*

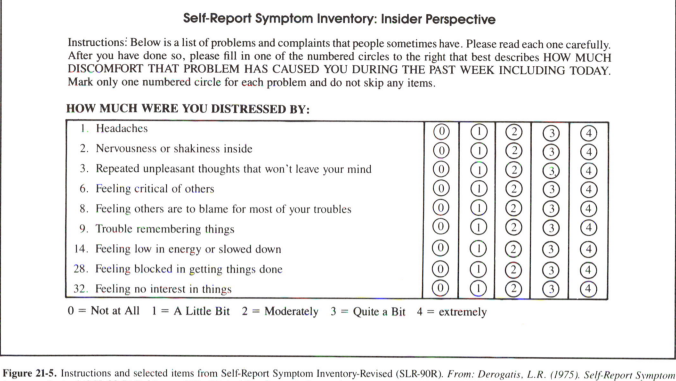

Self-Report Symptom Inventory: Insider Perspective

Instructions: Below is a list of problems and complaints that people sometimes have. Please read each one carefully. After you have done so, please fill in one of the numbered circles to the right that best describes HOW MUCH DISCOMFORT THAT PROBLEM HAS CAUSED YOU DURING THE PAST WEEK INCLUDING TODAY. Mark only one numbered circle for each problem and do not skip any items.

HOW MUCH WERE YOU DISTRESSED BY:

		0	1	2	3	4
1.	Headaches	⓪	①	②	③	④
2.	Nervousness or shakiness inside	⓪	①	②	③	④
3.	Repeated unpleasant thoughts that won't leave your mind	⓪	①	②	③	④
6.	Feeling critical of others	⓪	①	②	③	④
8.	Feeling others are to blame for most of your troubles	⓪	①	②	③	④
9.	Trouble remembering things	⓪	①	②	③	④
14.	Feeling low in energy or slowed down	⓪	①	②	③	④
28.	Feeling blocked in getting things done	⓪	①	②	③	④
32.	Feeling no interest in things	⓪	①	②	③	④

0 = Not at All   1 = A Little Bit   2 = Moderately   3 = Quite a Bit   4 = extremely

Figure 21-5. Instructions and selected items from Self-Report Symptom Inventory-Revised (SLR-90R). *From: Derogatis, L.R. (1975). Self-Report Symptom Inventory-Revised (SCL-90-R) Baltimore, MD: Clinical Psychometric Research.*

elicit patient thoughts and feelings through the use of expressive media and/or loosely structured formats. Humanism has influenced assessment across theoretical frameworks in occupational therapy. Evidence of the influence is seen by the profession's emphasis on individualization of patient care and therapists' attempts to view each patient's concerns from his or her own point of view (Bruce & Borg, 1987; Devereaux, 1984; Yerxa, 1978; Baum, 1980).

Behavioral and Cognitive Behavioral Assessment

The insider perspective in assessment has also been used frequently in behavioral and cognitive-behavioral assessment. Self-report procedures, self-inventory, and self-rating scales such as the *Body Parts Satisfaction Scale* (described previously), the *Beck Depression Inventory* (Beck, 1967), *Young's Loneliness Inventory* (Young, 1981), and the *Self-Report Symptom Inventory-Revised* (Derogatis, 1977) represent formats found frequently in behavioral and cognitive-behavioral literature (see examples in Figures 21-3, 21-4, and 21-5).

Other insider-oriented assessment instruments used in occupational therapy to ascertain the attitude of patients toward engagement include the *Role Checklist* (Oakley, et al., 1986) and the *Interest Checklist* (Matsutsuyu, 1969).

Figure 21-6 shows the categories assessed in a broad-based Self-Management survey and Figure 21-7 gives an example of the types of questions asked in the category of citizenship (Spiegler & Agigian, 1977, p. 359). These are typical of self-management surveys used for functional assessment in psychiatric rehabilitation.

The insider approach may be used as an initial or early stage assessment strategy, and may then be continued in monitoring therapy. For example, patients may be asked to keep a diary of daily events to log changes that occur in relation to their thoughts, feelings and/or actions or they may keep a time-log showing how they structure their time. They may also be asked to repeat an initial assessment inventory to demonstrate the changes in attitudes or behaviors that have occurred. The patient may also be involved in an interview or more formalized assessment batteries following a duration of therapy to determine readiness for the cessation of therapy.

It has been well documented that patients' appraisals of their own performance and attitudes correlate only moderately with the appraisals of those who assess them from the outsider (objective) perspective (Bem & Allen, 1974; Dellario, et al., 1984; Leff, 1978). Thus, the conclusions of others who judge patients' behaviors and/or interpret their feelings such as teachers, therapists,

Categories Assessed in Self-Management Survey

Basic Needs
 Food
 Clothing
 Shelter

Citizenship

Vocabulary and Reading Comprehension

Transportation

Money Management

Self-Medication

Communications
 Telephone usage
 Letter writing & postal service

Figure 21-6. Categories Assessed in Self-Management Survey. *Adapted from Spiegler, M. & Agigian, H. (1977). The Community Training Center. New York: Brunner Publishers. Appendix B, pp. 351-363.*

spouses, or parents, may differ from those of the patients themselves. One problem may result from different perceptions of terms and constructs used in describing their emotions.

Reactivity and Other Bias

Results of insider-oriented assessments can be skewed by reactivity—which is the tendency for individuals to rate themselves higher or demonstrate improved performance during the time they are being observed or evaluated (Nietzel & Bernstein, 1981). In direct contrast, there are also some individuals who may skew assessment outcomes by appearing less capable or having less internal strengths in the hope that this might minimize the amount of responsibility expected of them in therapy or at home.

Some patients are better able to reflect on their own feelings and behaviors than others. Some individuals can give seemingly insightful judgments regarding themselves, while others may respond simply that they ''never think much about themselves,'' and still others may resist the task of describing their feelings and behaviors.

This inner-oriented assessment may become much more difficult, when a patient's judgment is compromised by a status of confusion or disorientation. In severe cases of **psychosis**, the therapist may not understand the language of the patient, although it should be emphasized that such language is not without meaning or value. Insider assessment has been used in the treatment of psychoses, as for example in the self-assessment of hallucinations (Baker, 1975).

Summary of the Insider Perspective

An insider perspective espouses the philosophy that life is a uniquely subjective experience. Assessment from the insider (subjective) perspective is designed to gain an understanding of the patient's unique perspective of personal experience and to provide a means by which the patient takes responsibility for the therapy process. The insider approach is generally accepted as the most direct method of eliciting patient feelings and thoughts, and therefore requires the least inference from the assessor. The limitations of the insider approach are: (1) the risk that when

SAMPLE ITEMS FROM SELF-MANAGEMENT SURVEY: CITIZENSHIP

1. **How often do you read the newspaper?**
 a. Daily
 c. Hardly ever

2. **What are the names of the following public individuals:**
 a. President of the US?
 c. Governor of . . .?
 d. Two Senators from . . .?
 f. One city official where you live?

3. **Name three important current events that have happened during the past month.**

4. **Opinions**
 a. What is your opinion on the Vietnam War?
 b. Do you think there should be a death penalty? Why or why not?

5. **Personal Knowledge**
 b. When were you born?
 c. What is your address?
 d. What is your phone number?
 e. What is your social security number?
 f. What country do you live in?
 g. When were you in the military service?
 k. Do you have a guardian? If yes, give name.
 l. What is your highest level of education?

6. **VA Information**

7. **What should you do if:**
 a. you are the first to notice smoke and fire in a movie theater?
 c. you see someone breaking into the house next door to you?
 d. you are the first to come upon the scene of an accident?

8. **Jury Duty**

9. **Miscellaneous**

Note: Selected answers shown, not complete list

Figure 21-7. Functional Assessment: Insider Perspective. *Adapted from Spiegler, M. & Agigian, H. (1977). The Community Training Center. New York: Brunner Publishers, pp. 354-355.*

people are asked to assess themselves, they may try to anticipate the social desirability of responses; (2) the differences in interpreting constructs between patients and assessors; and (3) that patients' subjectivity may limit their ability to judge themselves as perceived by others, particularly if cognitively-impaired.

OBJECTIVE APPROACH: THE OUTSIDER PERSPECTIVE

The difference between an insider and outsider perspective is not identical to the difference between a ''feeling'' versus behavioral approach. In the outsider approach, the assessor may be concerned with patients' feelings, thoughts and/or behavior. In outsider assessment, the assessor determines what content areas will be assessed and makes judgments regarding the individual's efficacy (and progress) in these areas.

Some common outsider assessment formats include the structured interview, behavioral rating scales, structured task experiences, simulated setting observations (analogues) and natural setting observations. Outsider-oriented assessment procedures vary in relation to several key factors: (1) the nature of the setting in which the observation occurs, (2) the structure of the tasks in which the patients engaged, (3) the content and degree of inference which is drawn from the observation, and (4) the duration and schedule of observation.

Reducing Inference or Observer Bias

Outsider assessment can be used to assess patient feelings. Examples of this can be seen in the physician's narrative summary of the patient's mental status or in the occupational therapist's daily note in the patient's chart which might read as follows: ''Mrs. Jones is exhibiting motor agitation and appears to have difficulty with concentration. She speaks hesitantly and appears confused about the reasons for her hospitalization.'' The accuracy of this kind of interpretation depends largely on the therapist's judgment and skill and even at times intuitive ability. There is the risk when making such inferences that the observer's own (subjective) feelings may greatly influence the behaviors noticed within the assessment situation and thus bias the conclusions. Figure 21-8 lists the typical categories addressed in a **mental status exam**.

In order to reduce the role that assessor intuition plays in the assessment process, many outsider assessment tools provide behavioral criteria for making observations. These serve as a means to objectify the observation or reduce the role that observer bias will play. An outsider assessment with clear observation criteria should be capable of yielding

---

Categories Considered in a Mental Status Exam

1. *General description:* (a) appearance, (b) behavior and psychomotor activity, (c) speech, and (d) attitude toward the examiner.

2. *Mood, feelings and affect:* that which is pervasive; the amount and range; and the appropriateness to setting and culture.

3. *Perceptual disturbances:* existence of hallucinations and illusions and depersonalization.

4. *Thought process:* content, spontaneity, continuity, language impairment; preoccupations, thought disturbances (delusions, ideas of reference); abstract thinking; information and intelligence; concentration.

5. *Orientation:* time, place, and person

6. *Memory:* remote, recent, immediate retention and recall, coping mechanism for memory problem.

7. *Impulse control*

8. *Judgment:* social judgment and test judgment.

9. *Insight:* awareness and understanding of illness; intellectual insight; emotional insight; reliability (accurately report experiences).

Figure 21-8. Categories Considered in a Mental Status Exam. *From: MacKinnon, R.A. & Yudofsky, S.C. (1986). The Psychiatric Evaluation in Clinical Practice. Philadelphia: J.B. Lippincott Co.*

---

similar results for the same individual in a specified situation regardless of who the assessor might be. When outside assessment is focused on performance criteria, outsider assessment generally becomes consistent with the philosophy of behavioral treatment and with the mandates of those who call for functional assessment in psychiatry (Anthony, 1979; Dellario, et al., 1984; Spiegler & Agigian, 1977; Watts & Bennett, 1983).

Conditions of Outsider Assessment

Outsider, behavior-based assessment occurs on what Kazdin refers to as a continuum of the following ''conditions of assessment'' which can affect the outcome (Kazdin, 1981, p. 110):

1. *Naturalistic-contrived.* When naturalistic observation occurs, the assessment environment has not been structured for the patient by the assessor, for example when the home care therapist observes the patient at home during his normal routine. Such observation and assessment might also occur at the patient's place of employment or school. While such natural conditions may seem ideal, they may have problems as well, such as when the necessary behaviors do not occur in the natural setting or when unexpected

disruptions and alterations occur in routines.

In contrast, the therapist may assess the patient in a therapeutically structured environment (i.e., in the clinic) or may try to create a particular situation for the patient to respond within a treatment setting. In these situations, the therapist can typically guarantee that the patient will be exposed to the performance-demand that needs to be observed. For example, the patient may be assessed while engaging in a role-play simulating an employer-employee interaction, or he or she may be assessed while engaging in a battery of

---

Comprehensive Evaluation of Basic Living Skills (CEBLS)*

Rating: Observe the client performing the following skills. Place the number corresponding to the client's correct level of function in the blank preceding each skill.

4 Performs skill independently and correctly.

3 Requires some assistance to perform skill correctly.

2 Requires much assistance to perform skill correctly.

1 Cannot perform skill independently or correctly.
Indicate N/A if the item is not applicable.

Hair Care

____ shampoo hair

____ dry hair

____ set hair

____ comb & brush hair in organized way

Dressing

____ choose adequate clothing appropriate for physical/social situation

____ put on undergarments

____ put on shirts, blouses

Meal Planning

____ knowledge of basic four

____ menu planning

____ formation of grocery list

Meal Preparation

____ can follow recipe

____ get things from refrigerator

____ operate small appliances

____ prepare baked foods

*Note: only selected skills shown; not inclusive list

Figure 21-9. Sample Items from Comprehensive Evaluation of Basic Living Skills (CEBLS). *From: Casanova, J., Feber, J. (1976). Comprehensive Evaluation of Basic Living Skills. American Journal of Occupational Therapy 30(2):101-105.*

self-care tasks designed to represent the everyday tasks that must be completed at home. The *Comprehensive Evaluation of Basic Living Skills* (Casanova & Ferber, 1976) is an example of an outsider-oriented behaviorally-scaled assessment in which the patient is observed while engaged in what are judged to be typical self-care tasks (see Figure 21-9). By comparing this tool to the insider-oriented tool, the *Self-Management Survey* in Figure 21-10, it is easy to see two very different methods of assessing similar data regarding basic living skills.

The usefulness of assessment in a simulated setting or with therapist-structured tasks is generally related to the extent to which the behavior performed within the assessment actually compares to the real or home situation (Kazdin, 1981, pp. 116-117). Anyone creating an analogue must realize that just the presence of an observer can be expected to affect that performance. Even the most seemingly straightforward task such as buttoning a shirt or preparing a cup of coffee might be made easier or more difficult when one is in the presence of another person. The situation-specificity of virtually all human endeavor has become increasingly recognized by those concerned with psychiatric rehabilitation (Anthony, 1979; Cohen & Anthony, 1984; Frey, 1984; Spiegler & Agigian, 1977) and challenges the assumption performance in a simulated structure will be identical to the individual's performance in the natural environment.

2. *Unobtrusive vs. obtrusive observation.* A second element of the outsider observation condition that can affect the outcome is whether or not the patient is aware of being observed and/or has knowledge of the particular behaviors being observed. There are obviously degrees of obtrusiveness. The therapist-assessor can sit in front of the patient with a checklist in hand as the patient follows a task procedure, can mingle with several patients in a clinic and make more casual and intermittent observations, or can observe just one patient during the assessment situation. If the assessor chooses to be a non-participant observer, immediate recording of observations is possible, so that the therapist does not need to rely on memory for accurate recording of information. If the therapist chooses to be a participant-observer, the therapist must decide whether to use immediate recording or retrospective recording of information (Sundberg, 1977, p. 75). The therapist must weigh the risks of interrupting the assessment process to record observations which can disrupt the continuity of assessment and make the patient uncomfortable against the risk of relying on one's memory to accurately record information.

The varying degrees to which the patient is aware of what is being assessed can affect outcomes. The therapist may tell the patient specifically what is being observed in a task (e.g., ''I would like you to follow this mosaic design and I will be looking to see how adept you are at following diagrammatic directions.'') or the patient might be instructed to engage with other patients to prepare a meal and simply be told that social skills will be observed. As discussed previously, the reactivity factor comes into play when an individual is aware of being observed; thus, casual participant-observation may prove to be less of an influence. When patients are observed without their knowledge or consent (as through a one-way mirror), there are serious ethical considerations.

3. *Temporal conditions.* A third condition of outsider assessment relates to the time span in which assessment occurs. Most occupational therapy tools described in the literature provide assessment around a one-time task or series of tasks. *The Allen Cognitive Level Test* (Allen, 1985) provides observation criteria for observing and categorizing the skills for a patient engaged in leather lacing. *The Magazine Picture Collage* (Lerner & Ross, 1977; Lerner, 1979) provides criteria for judging both the process and end-product when a patient creates a collage. *The Milwaukee Evaluation of Daily Living Skills* consists of 21 subtests, each of which is designed to test in a brief time specific task behaviors (Leonardelli, 1988).

Data gathering over an extended period is another approach to outsider assessment. This type of assessment is referred to frequently in the psychological and educational literature, but less often in occupational therapy. Examples of this type of assessment include: (1) the *Child Behavior Checklist* (Achenbach 1978; Achenbach & Edelbrock, 1979) in which a child's behavior at home is documented on a behavioral scale by the parents of children ages 4 through 16, (2) the *Psychotic Inpatient Profile* (Lorr & Vestre, 1968) in which a patient's ward behavior over a three-day period is documented by a staff member, and (3) the *Bay Area Functional Performance Evaluation* (Bloomer & Williams, 1986). Examples of these extended assessments are provided in Figures 21-11, 21-12, and 21-13.

Assessments made over extended periods and made in multiple situations may be more time-consuming and therefore less cost-efficient. They have the advantage, however, of potential for yielding a more representative sampling of behavior. This can be especially significant when a patient's moods or ability to function are highly erratic.

SAMPLE ITEMS FROM THE SELF-MANAGEMENT SURVEY
BASIC NEEDS

A. Food

1. . . . what percent of your income do you need for food?
4. Are there particular foods that you should not eat because of a health problem?
5. Circle the staple food items (food you need not buy each time you grocery shop).
   a) salt
   b) meats
   c) corn meal
   d) rice
   e) ice cream
   f) milk
   g) coffee
   h) lettuce
   i) cheese
   j) eggs

B. Clothing

2. How many times should you wear a pair of socks before washing them?
22. Do you wash your own clothes at the present time: If yes, how often do you wash them?

Note: Only selected items presented from evaluation

Figure 21-10. Functional Assessment—Insider Perspective. *From: Spiegler, M. & Agigian, H. (1977). Self-Management Survey, Appendix B. The Community Training Center. New York: Brunner/Mazel Publishers, pp. 351-353.*

The Outsider Interview. Almost all occupational therapy assessment involves some degree of patient dialogue and interview. The outsider interview is characterized by both of the following: (1) the therapist-assessor has a predetermined agenda of questions or content items to be addressed and follows a set interview format and (2) the therapist-assessor observes the patient's affect and behavior and makes judgments regarding the patient's affect, style and/or performance during the interview.

The structured interview is recommended by Hemphill (1982, p. 6) for three reasons: (1) its ability to obtain ''objective'' information that can be compared to data gathered on another occasion and by another assessor (if needed) (2) it helps avoid the compilation of conflicting or incomplete information, and (3) it is time-efficient. With differing concerns, Barry (1984) suggests that a tightly structured interview (one highly outsider-oriented) may fail to deliver information in the areas of concern to the patient or may fail to allow the patient an opportunity to express feelings about specific content areas.

**Bay Area Functional Performance Evaluation
Task Oriented Assessment**

Tasks Used to Determine Function
Sorting shells
Bank deposit slip
House floor plan
Block design
Draw a person

Functional Abilities Assessed
Paraphrase (verbal or written instructions)
Decision-Making (productive)
Motivation
Organizaton (time and materials)
Mastery and Self-esteem
Evidence of Frustration
Attention Span
Ability to Abstract
Evidence of Thought or Mood Disorder
Correct Task Completion

Sample Functional Scale
Organization (of time and materials)
1. May manipulate materials but shows no orderly or logical progression in approach. Does not attempt task.
2. Deals with materials with disorderly or illogical progression. May or may not finish task in allotted time.
3. Deals with materials in orderly or logical progression but does not finish task in allotted time.
4. Deals with materials in orderly or logical progression and finishes task in allotted time.

Figure 21-11. Bay Area Functional Performance Evaluation Task Oriented Assessment. *Reproduced by special permission of the Publisher, Consulting Psychologists Press, Inc., Palo Alto, CA 94306, from Manual for the Bay Area Functional Performance Evaluation, 1st ed, by Susan Williams and Judith Bloomer © 1979. Further reproduction is prohibited without the Publisher's consent.*

Summary of Outsider Assessment. Outsider assessment provides a means by which the public self can be judged. In order to reduce the need for therapist-assessor inference regarding an individual's thoughts or feelings and provide objectivity, the outsider assessment frequently relies on observable, performance criteria. Such criteria increase the likelihood that two or more independent assessors will make similar conclusions. However, the varying conditions of the assessment process, including the nature of assessment environment and the degree of assessor involvement, can be expected to influence assessment outcomes.

Combining Objective and Subjective Views

Many assessments, regardless of the frame of reference, attempt to glean both the insider (subjective) viewpoint as well as the outsider (objective) view. In a combined approach, patients may be asked to describe themselves or

give a personal history allowing them the opportunity to define their own personal strengths, needs, limitations, and probable treatment expectations and they may also be observed engaging in a specific task and/or social behavior with the behavior and affect rated by a specified observer. In some instances, as with the *Schroeder-Block-Campbell Adult Psychiatric Evaluation* (Schroeder, et al., 1978), the areas in which patients describe themselves is complementary to but not intended to match the assessment of performance skills by the therapist.

There are assessments constructed so that the patient and assessor independently rate the patient on identical skills or constructs, such as in the *Multi-Function Needs Assessment* (Dellario, et al., 1984) which is a functional assessment designed for use with patients identified as schizophrenic (see Figures. 21-14 and 21-15).

**BAY AREA FUNCTIONAL PERFORMANCE
EVALUATION
SOCIAL INTERACTION SCALE**

Using direct observation and/or reported behavior observed by other staff member, the patient's functioning is rated on a five point continuum.

Verbal Communication
(Note if patient's primary language is not spoken in setting):

_____ 1. not able to assess due to degree of dysfunction _____, or language barrier _____.
_____ 2. avoids verbal interaction; withdraws or verbal interaction inappropriate
_____ 3. verbal interactions appropriate only when directly questioned
_____ 4. able to sustain a logical conversation with others some of the time
_____ 5. will initiate or sustain a logical conversation most of the time

Ability to Work With Peers
_____ 1. not able to assess due to degree of dysfunction
_____ 2. sets self apart in task or work oriented setting (may exclude self from peers through markedly irritating, inappropriate or isolative behavior)
_____ 3. some interaction with peers, but distances self (i.e., through isolative or irritating behavior)
_____ 4. usually works well with others, is generally cooperative
_____ 5. almost always works well with others (may encourage or stimulate others)

Figure 21-12. Sample Behavior Scale. *Reproduced by special permission of the Publisher, Consulting Psychologists Press, Inc., Palo Alto, CA 94306, from Manual for the Bay Area Functional Performance Evaluation, 1st ed, by Susan Williams and Judith Bloomer © 1979. Further reproduction is prohibited without the Publisher's consent.*

SELECTED PSYCHOTIC SYNDROMES IN THE PSYCHOTIC INPATIENT PROFILE

Excitement
Talks in a loud voice
Jokes, talks or laughs excitedly; seems "high"

Seclusiveness vs. Sociability
Mixes with other patients
Shows pleasure in recreation

Care Needed vs. Competence
Needs help in dressing
Needs help in going to the bathroom

Depressive Mood
Says he is a failure and a disappointment
Reports he cannot concentrate or remember things

Each of the items is rated on a frequency scale:
0 — Not at all
1 — Occasionally
2 — Fairly often
3 — Nearly always

Figure 21-13. Sample Behavior Scale: 3-Day Observation Period. *From: Lorr, M., Vestre, N. (1969). The psychotic inpatient profile: A nurse's observation scale. Journal of Clinical Psychology 25(2):137-140. Available from Western Psychological Services.*

Assessment processes may represent a mixture of insider and outsider perspectives in a variety of ways. The *Adolescent Role Assessment* (Black, 1976) elicits patient (insider) views, but then scores the responses according to outsider criteria. Many behavioral scales have an outside rater, but then assessment outcomes are shared with the patient (insider) who is asked to make judgments regarding the significance of the performance observed.

Because the sum of the assessment process in any setting may involve such variety in the mix of subjective and objective assessment procedures, it is not possible to specifically discuss the effectiveness of combining the two viewpoints. However, some combination of insider and outsider assessment is evident in virtually all programs allowing both the patient and the therapist-assessor to make judgments regarding the nature of the patient's skills, needs, feelings, strengths, deficits, and progress.

By eliciting both the patient and therapist perspective, one can conceive of a partnership in the assessment and treatment processes (Bruce and Borg, 1987). Both are seen as having unique and valuable insight regarding areas of concern to the patient. When judgments are in agreement,

then their essential veracity is strengthened. When there is disagreement or even a difference in emphasis, both the therapist-assessor and the patient are provided an opportunity to broaden their views and reconsider (or perhaps consider for the first time) options they might have otherwise failed to notice.

An assessment process that combines both the insider and outsider perspective must do so with clarity and towards a consistent goal. One of the most blatant and disheartening examples of inconsistency occurs when an assessment process or instrument seeks to elicit the patient's viewpoint but the resultant data are essentially disregarded in the conclusions drawn by the therapist-assessor. To avoid negating the patient's viewpoint, the therapist should ask the questions: "How can I best gain the necessary information?" and "From whose perspective is this information most sensibly approached?" Once these questions are answered, the therapist-assessor can identify and consistently use assessment tools capable of gaining the information.

SAMPLE ITEMS FROM MULTI-FUNCTION NEEDS ASSESSMENT

---

1 = No Assistance
2 = Prompting/Structuring
3 = Supervision
4 = Some Direct Assistance
5 = Total Assistance
Circle the appropriate response.

Self-Care:
With what type of assistance does this person currently:

1. perform toileting functions (i.e., maintain bladder & bowel continence, clean self, etc.)   1   2   3   4   5

2. perform feeding functions (i.e., drink liquids & eat, etc.)   1   2   3   4   5

3. perform bathing functions (i.e., laying out clothes, putting on clothes, etc.)   1   2   3   4   5

4. perform the functions of self-medication (i.e., prepare & administer all medications, etc.)   1   2   3   4   5

Figure 21-14. Combined Objective and Subjective Perspectives: Assessor's Portion of the Assessment. *From: Multi-Function Needs Assessment, Division of Human Resource Development, Rhode Island Department of Mental Health, Retardation & Hospitals. Cranston, RI. Excerpt adapted from Dellario, et al. (1984) p. 244. In Halpern, A. & Fuhrer, M. Functional Assessment in Rehabilitation, Baltimore, MD: Brookes Publishing Co.*

Items from the Multi-Function Needs Assessment

Practitioner Item

With what type of assistance does this person currently perform all aspects of the maintenance of his/her appearance including, but not limited to, cleanliness of hair, teeth, fingernails, and is able to maintain adequate and appropriate dress?

1. No assistance
2. Prompting/structuring
3. Supervision
4. Some direct assistance
5. Total assistance

Client Item

I can maintain a neat and appropriate personal appearance:

1. Without any assistance
2. With a little assistance
3. With a lot of assistance

Figure 21-15. Combining Objective and Subjective Perspectives: Sample items from practitioner assessment and client self report in the Multi-Function Needs Assessment. *Reprinted with permission. Dellario, D., Goldfield, E., Farkas, M., Cohen, M. (1984). Functional Assessment of Psychiatrically Disabled Adults. In Halpern, A., & Fuhrer, M. (Eds.), (1984). Functional Assessment in Rehabilitation, Baltimore, MD: Brookes Publishing Co. p. 248.*

SITUATION-SPECIFIC ASSESSMENT ITEMS: SIGNS OR SAMPLES?

Sign Approach

A *sign approach* is designed to give information about the patient's general style of performing, general mood, or manner. For instance, when the *Shoemyen Battery* (Hemphill, 1982) is used and the patient is asked to work with clay or create a tile trivet, the primary assessment concern is not the ability to use these media *per se,* but, rather, the patient's comfort with general classes of materials (unstructured versus structured) and processes (i.e., constructive versus destructive). The therapist may also be concerned with the patient's ability to follow instructions, sustain attention, and manage frustration.

Basic to this approach is the assumption that certain consistencies in feelings and behavior (i.e., traits) exist independently of situational variables (Goldfried and Kent, 1972, p. 410). For example, the patient who becomes angry and frustrated when unable to control the materials used in the assessment may be expected to become angry and frustrated in many life situations which are out of the patient's control. Similarly, the person who dislikes being "messy" with clay might be judged to be more globally uncomfortable with messy materials. In this assessment approach, the behaviors that an individual displays in the assessment and the feelings identified may be construed as signs of more pervasive psychological constructs. Such constructs are a way to conceive of and address personality variables. With the information that therapists gain from a sign-oriented assessment, they may proceed to work with the patient toward adapting styles or traits to specific situations.

One advantage of the sign-approach is that it helps the therapist identify patterns and informal relationships across multiple situations. It has been difficult to prove empirically the meaning of specific personality traits or styles, and their usefulness in documenting treatment outcomes has been questioned (Goldfried & Kent, 1972).

Sample Approach

The sample approach allows the therapist-assessor to select an assessment in which the patient is asked to address situation-specific tasks regarded as key to successful everyday function. For instance, in addition to completing the *Self-Management Survey* (Spiegler & Agigian, 1977), the patient may be asked to balance a personal or sample checkbook in order to assess skills specific to money management. In contrast to the sign-oriented approach that views patient responses as an "indirect manifestation" of underlying personality, the sample approach uses tests behaviors believed to "constitute a subset of the actual behaviors of interest" (Goldfried and Kent, 1972, p. 413). There is a need to establish that the sampled behaviors do in fact accurately represent the behavior in question.

When the sample approach is used, it has the advantage of reducing the requirement for therapist-assessor inference. When samples of behavior are elicited or addressed, no inferences need to be made about overall function nor personality (Goldfried & Kent, 1972 p. 419). The sample approach easily lends itself to establishing a database for comparison for re-testing.

Spiegler and Agigian (1977) emphasize the need for situation-specific behaviors in the everyday world. In discussing the Community Training Center, a treatment setting designed to meet the needs of a chronically limited population, they insist that for psychiatric rehabilitation to be successful, clients must demonstrate specific behaviors and definitive cognitive information (knowledge) if they are to succeed outside of the treatment setting. They advocate that it is situation-specific behaviors and not global styles that need to be assessed.

The trend within psychiatric and physical health care has

been toward this sample-orientation in assessment. Realizing that we all behave a little differently in various situations, we must ask the questions regarding the sample approach: Will the teaching of skills specific to a situation ultimately enhance or limit the patient's ability to generalize? Will the patient be able to use specific knowledge and skills in unexpected or novel situations in the future?

Other questions therapists will be trying to answer in the future relate to: (1) whether there are differences among individuals in terms of their ability to use assessment feedback related to sign or sample behaviors and (2) whether or not it is possible to use both the formal, sample outcomes that are most directly reflected in documentation and research and less formal sign indices that can help the assessor and patient put sample data into a conceptual context.

FACTORS THAT SHAPE AN ASSESSMENT

An assessment is shaped by the following factors: (1) the manner in which psychological constructs are conceived and expressed, (2) the theoretical framework for occupational therapy services, (3) the patient's ability to form a partnership and contribute to the psychological assessment process through subjective observation and interpretation of life experiences, and (4) the therapist's expertise.

When considering assessment in a particular practice setting, there are several additional factors that act as boundaries to the assessment process and should be considered:

1. The guidelines for assessment established by the occupational therapy profession;
2. The environment and mandates particular to the institution or setting in which the patient is being managed;
3. The characteristics of the patient population served;
4. The body of available assessment formats and procedures;
5. The nature of the information that is to be elicited; and
6. The interests, philosophies, and skills of the therapist-assessor(s).

Professional Mandates

Guidelines for assessment can be found in the Standards of Practice and the Uniform Occupational Therapy Evaluation Checklist (AOTA, 1979, 1986) which have been adopted by the American Occupational Therapy Association.

The Standards of Practice include both generic guidelines and those specific to mental health. The Standards of

Practice suggest that the occupational therapist use interviews, observations and tests to screen and evaluate clients to identify those persons with problems in occupational performance (work, self-care and play/leisure). The guides also indicate that the therapist has the responsibility for interpreting, summarizing, communicating with the treatment team and significant others, and documenting evaluation results (AOTA, 1986, p. V. 1-2).

The *Uniform Occupational Therapy Evaluation Checklist* is a general guide for gathering baseline data. During the evaluation of psychological/emotional performance, the checklist suggests that the occupational therapist seek information regarding the client's self-concept/identity, ability to cope, involvement in the community, ability for self-expression and self-control, and ability to interact in group and individual situations (AOTA, 1986 p. VIII. 22-23).

The Mental Health Standards of Practice reiterate the guides previously discussed. (AOTA, 1986, p. V. 8-9).

The Treatment Setting and Working as a Team Member

Once the broad professional boundaries have been established, the next step is to evaluate the mental health system in which the occupational therapy program exists. In the mental health system there are multiple factors to consider:

1. the system's environment—whether it is a private psychiatric hospital, community mental health center, etc.,
2. the mission statement—whether the focus is on patient care, education, and/or research,
3. the organizational structure—such as, who approves new programs or reviews quality of patient services,
4. the existing policies and procedures—such as, the referral and documentation requirements,
5. the nature of existing treatment programs—such as, crisis intervention, inpatient or outpatient, day care, etc.,
6. the theories and philosophies endorsed by the practitioners within the institution, such as psychoanalytic, behavioral, cognitive, etc.,
7. the members of the treatment team and their responsibilities in the assessment process—such as the social worker providing the patient's social history, the psychologist conducting personality testing, the recreation specialist providing the leisure history, etc.,
8. the predominant patient population including age, primary problems, length of stay, etc.,
9. the resources in the occupational therapy department—such as, theories endorsed, expertise of the therapist, the clinic environment, etc., and

10. the constraints that exist—such as, existing treatment schedule, patient case load, number of staff, etc.

After evaluating the ten system components, the therapist can determine if the department goals are compatible with the mission of the institution and whether his/her theoretical and philosophical views are synchronized with those of the treatment programs and the team of practitioners who implement them. Both the therapist and the institution will most likely have a predominant frame of reference that guides their treatment approach. In some mental health settings, different clinicians and physicians may operate from varying theoretical bases with their patients. The occupational therapist's theoretical and practice framework may or may not be identical to the frameworks favored by other treatment staff. However, it is important that the assessment and treatment provided by the therapist is complementary to that of other treatment staff and that information provided is pertinent and useful. For example, in a setting that is highly behavioral in orientation, non-specific feeling-oriented information might not be as pertinent, or in a setting that is highly feeling-oriented, information related to cognitive level might not be perceived as useful.

The arts of compromise and education can both be very useful in establishing a good working relationship with others on the treatment team. Occupational therapists can learn from what others profess, and they can choose to orient occupational therapy from a theoretical framework identical to or compatible with theirs. Other team members and the patient may learn from what the occupational therapist has to offer, and the unique vantage it may bring. This can only occur if the occupational therapist takes the time to explain to others the principles behind occupational therapy assessment information and the relationship of these data to the overall approach to the patient.

The occupational therapist must make the effort to understand and use the assessment data made available by others. Also knowing the contributions of other team members to patient assessment helps avoid duplication of services.

The system's structure and its policies and procedures, provide one set of guidelines for establishing the occupational therapy department's assessment protocol. These guides also establish institutional requirements necessary for approval of occupational therapy services.

General Considerations in Occupational Therapy Assessment

The occupational therapy department assessment program includes the following: (1) a referral system, (2) the time frame for completion of the evaluation interview, (e.g., within 48 hours of admission), (3) the system of documentation, (e.g., specific forms), and (4) the evaluation instruments used.

The Patient Population. The selection of a particular assessment process can be influenced by the type of individuals served in the treatment setting, such as the age of the patients, the type or nature of the dysfunction or presenting problem, the level of skill of the patient, and the general goal(s) in discharge planning.

Many assessment tools are designed specifically to be used with an identified age-range of individuals. The *Adolescent Role Assessment* (Black, 1976) is specifically designed for use with teens. *The Role Change Assessment* (Jackoway, et al., 1987) is identified for an older population (see Figure 21-16).

The Psychotic Inpatient Profile is designated for individuals with a given (or suspected) diagnostic problem. The authors are familiar with one mental health setting in which referral to occupational therapy is made only for patients who are believed to have a problem with body image and praxis. In this type of setting, a sensory motor assessment would be appropriate. In a setting in which occupational therapy evaluation is designated as a means to identify the likelihood that given patients will be able to function independently in a half-way house, then post-discharge assessment would focus on activities of daily living.

Assessment Modification. Some assessment procedures can be easily modified to meet an individual's special needs. For example, in an assessment interview, the therapist can choose a vocabulary and content focus to which the patient can relate. Some instruments require that patients have given skills and cognitive function, such as being able to read, to write, or do computation, or that they have a certain degree of attention and concentration. While it is certainly possible to adapt existing assessment tools to meet the special needs of a patient population, most tools with normative standards do not take into account such modifications. In general, it is better to avoid such adaptations. If such adaptations are made it must be recognized that the assessment was not used for its intended purpose, and thus the norms and validity data established for the standardized version do not apply.

Assessment Resources. There are multiple resources from which the occupational therapist can select an assessment instrument. These include resources in occupational therapy, nursing, education, sociology, vocational rehabilitation and psychology. There are numerous psychological evaluations documented in the mental health literature and numerous evaluations presented in the occupational therapy literature. However, in spite of extensive resources, the

ROLE CHANGE ASSESSMENT

Roles

Family and Social:

	Past	Present	Change	Value
Spouse				
Parent				
Visitor				
Pet Owner				

Organizational:

	Present	L/M	Past	L/M	Change	Value
Religious						
Civic						
Support/Self-help						
Special Interest						

Vocational:

	Present	Past	Change	Value
Worker for pay				
Caregiver				
Student				

Leisure:

	Present	Past	Change	Value	1	2	3	4
Hobbyist								
Walker								
Collector								
Observer								

Value—Positive Negative Neutral

L = Leader
M = Member

1 = done primarily at home
2 = done primarily away from home
3 = solitary activity
4 = social activity

Figure 21-16. Sample of Older Adult Evaluation: Insider Perspecstive. *From: Role Change Assessment. Jackoway, I., Rogers, J., Snow, T., (1987). The role change assessment: An interview tool for evaluating older adults. Occupational Therapy in Mental Health 7(1):17-37.*

choice for test adoption is complicated by the number of evaluation instruments. One must also consider the availability of the instrument and its psychometric qualities.

In her chapter on Assessment and Informed Decision-Making, Opacich suggests that task protocol, test descriptions and evaluation research are summarized in texts, references, and scholarly publications. Among the resources most familiar to educators and health professionals are:

Measurement Resources

Bearry, W.H. (Ed.) Improving educational assessment and an inventory of measures of affective behavior. Washington, DC: National Education Association, 1969.

Biesheuvel, S. (Ed.) Methods for the measurement of psychological performance. International Biological Program Handbook Number 10. Oxford: Blackwell, 1969.

Bolton, B. (Ed.) Handbook of measurement and evaluation in rehabilitation. Baltimore: University Park Press, 1976.

Boyer, E.G., Simon, A., & Karafin, G. (Eds.) Measures of maturation: An anthology of early childhood observation instruments. Philadelphia: Research for Better Schools, Inc., 1973.

Cattell, R.B., & Warburton, F.W. Objective personality and motivation tests. Urbana: University of Illinois Press, 1967.

Chun, K.T., Cobb, S., & French, J.R.P., Jr. Measures for psychological assessment. Ann Arbor, MI: Institute for Social Research, University of Michigan, 1975.

Comrey, A.L., Backer, T.E., and Glaser, E.M. A sourcebook for mental health measures. Los Angeles: Human Interaction Research Institute, 1973.

Hoepfner, R., et. al. CSE-RBS test evaluations: Tests of higher order cognitive, affective and interpersonal skills. Los Angeles: Center for the Study of Evaluation, University of California, 1972.

Johnson, O.G. (Ed.) Tests and measurements in child development: Handbook (2 vol.). San Francisco: Jossey-Bass, 1976.

Kapes, J.F. & Mastie, M.M. (Eds.) A counselor's guide to vocational guidance instruments. Falls Church, VA: American Personnel and Guidance Association, 1982.

Lake, D.G., Miles, M.B., & Earle, R.B., Jr. (Eds.) Measuring human behavior: Tools for the assessment of social functioning. New York: Teachers College Press, 1973.

Pfeiffer, J.W., & Heslin, R. Instrumentation in human relations training. La Jolla: University Associates Consultants, Inc., 1974.

Robinson, J.P. & Shaver, P.R. Measures of social psychological attitudes. Ann Arbor: Institute for Social Research, University of Michigan. 1973.

Rosen, P. (Ed.) Test collection bulletin. Issued quarterly by Educational Testing Service, Princeton, NJ.

Shaw, M.E., & Wright, J.M. Scales for measurement of attitudes. New York: McGraw-Hill, 1967.

Simon, A., & Boyer, E.G. (Eds.) Mirrors for Behavior: An anthology of observation instruments. (24 vol.). Wyncote, PA: Communications Materials Center, 1967-74.

Wylie, R.C. The self-concept. (2 vols.) Lincoln, NB: University of Nebraska Press, 1974; 1979.

Figure 21-17. Measurement Resources. *Sources are selected from Appendix A, Sources Listing Specialized Tests and Measurement Devices in Cronbach, L.J. (1984). Essentials of psychological testing, 4th Ed. New York: Harper & Row, Publishers.*

1. *The Mental Measurement Yearbook* (Buros, 1970, 1972),
2. *News on Tests* (Educational Testing Service),
3. *Tests on Microfiche* (Educational Testing Service),
4. *Tests: A Comprehensive Reference for Assessments in Psychology, Education and Business* (2nd Ed.) (Sweetland & Keyser, 1986),
5. *Test Critiques Vol. 1-5* (Sweetland & Keyser, 1984-85),
6. *Health Instrument File*—Behavioral Measurement Database Service (Box 110287, Pittsburgh, PA 15232).

Other resources are identified in Figures 21-17 and 21-18. In addition, libraries and universities may also have a file of technical manuals and specimen test sets which are available to professionals. However the file's availability may be limited in order to prevent improper use by possible test takers. In occupational therapy, there are two useful evaluation texts edited by Hemphill (1982, 1988). Also, recent occupational therapy texts summarize tests frequently used by the occupational therapist during psychological assessment (Denton, 1986; Kielhofner, 1985; Mosey, 1986; and Bruce & Borg, 1987). These tests have been developed by occupational therapists as well as by professionals from related fields, such as nursing and psychology.

Exploring the assessment literature in occupational therapy and related fields can help the therapist avoid the likelihood of trying to duplicate an assessment tool that already exists. It can also reveal just how difficult it is to design a useful and valid assessment tool. Designing an assessment tool takes a great deal of care and patience requiring a solid theoretical foundation. From the literature, one can see that numerous trials with an assessment process may not be adequate to gain a clear picture of its strengths and limitations. As occupational therapy undertakes to broaden and strengthen its professional base, the experiences of others may remind us of the need to take one judicious step at a time.

TYPES OF ASSESSMENT

Self-Report Formats

Self-report measures are a means by which individuals can describe and/or rate their thoughts, feelings, or behaviors, according to their experience. Self-report procedures can include those with a structured response format including checklists, true-false questionnaires, and performance scales. There are also formats with the option for less structured responses, such as asking open-ended questions such as "What would you do if I . . ?" or "How do you feel when I . . ?" Clients may be asked to depict a typical day in an activity configuration (Mosey, 1970, 1986) or asked to engage in a "pie-of-life" activity in which a drawing experience is used to depict the patient's

life activities (James & Jongward, 1971). Patients can be asked to report on thoughts or behaviors experienced in the past, their current thoughts or behaviors, or their plans for the future.

Self-report measures are generally easy to administer and inexpensive in terms of time and dollars. They have been used to establish information in a broad number of areas and can be adapted for use with a variety of patient populations. Self-report questionnaires generally possess face validity, that is they appear to address the issues and behaviors as subjectively understood by the patient and therapist (Jensen & Haynes, 1986, p. 151). One must be cautious in choosing a self-report instrument, as many self-report formats have been adopted without adequate attention to the relationship between their underlying assumptions or originally intended purposes and their actual use (Jensen & Haynes, 1986, p. 151).

Validity. The validity of the information gained by self-report formats is influenced by several variables, including: (1) the perceived social desirability of given responses or the role of reactivity, (2) the clarity of the language of the assessment and the respondent's ability to understand what is being asked, including one's ability to understand the vocabulary and constructs, (3) the respondent's cognitive skills related to recall and the ability to pick out the most salient features of a mental or physical event (Jensen & Haynes, 1986 p. 164) or the ability to put into

---

Assessment Publishers and Distributors

American Guidance Service: Circle Pines, MN, 55014.

CTB/McGraw-Hill: Del Monte Research Park, Monterey, CA, 93940.

Consulting Psychologists Press, Inc.: 577 College Ave., Palo Alto, CA, 94306.

Grune & Stratton, Inc.: 11 Fifth Ave.; New York, NY, 10003.

Institute for Personality and Ability Testing: 1602 Coronado Drive; Champaign, IL, 61820.

NFER—Nelson Publishing Co., Ltd.: 2 Oxford Road East; Windsor, Berks, SL4 1DF, England.

Psych Systems; 600 Reisertown Road: Baltimore, MD, 21208.

Psychological Corporation: 7500 Old Orchard Road, Cleveland, OH 44130.

Publishers Test Service: 2500 Garden Road; Monterey, CA, 93940.

Research Psychologists Press: P.O. Box 984; Port Huron, MI, 48060.

Riverside Publishing Co.: 1919 S. Highland Ave.; Lombard, IL, 60148.

Science Research Associates: 155 N. Wacker Drive; Chicago, IL, 60606.

Sheridan Psychological Services: P.O. Box 6101; Orange, CA, 92667.

Western Psychological Services: 1203I Wilshire Blvd.; Los Angeles, CA, 90025.

Figure 21-18. Assessment Publishers and Distributors. (This list is not all inclusive.) *These assessment sources are selected from Appendix B in Cronbach, L.J. (1984). Essentials of Psychological Testing, 4th Ed. New York: Harper & Row Publishers.*

words one's feelings or describe one's actions in less structured formats, and (4) the respondent's motivation and desire to provide accurate information.

As an insider-oriented approach, self-report has been questioned regarding the validity and accuracy of such data (Bellack & Hersen, 1977; Mischel, 1968; Nietzel & Bernstein, 1981). Whether one views self-report data as more or less accurate than data gathered by an objective observer depends on the philosophy of the assessor and the kind of information elicited. Self-report is one clearly identified method of obtaining the subjective perspective. Since the patient is the one providing the information, it is important that the therapist be certain that the patient understand exactly what is meant by assessment constructs and what response is desired.

Frame of Reference.   Self-report measures are not unique to any particular frame of reference. They can be used to gather information related to signs or samples of behavior and have been used to gain a measure related to patient feelings, cognitive content, interests, and task-behavior.

The following are examples of these types of self-reports:
Patient feelings — The *Young Loneliness Inventory,* (Young, 1981), *Depression Adjective Checklists* (Lubin, 1967);
Cognitive content — the *Daily Record of Dysfunctional Thoughts* (Coleman, 1981);
Interests — *Interest Checklist* (Matsutsuyu, 1969);
Task-behavior — the *Self Management Survey* (Spiegler & Agigian, 1977), *Activity Laboratory Questionnaire* (Fidler, 1982; Hemphill, 1982, p. 379), and *Survey of* **Heterosexual Interactions** (Twentyman & McFall, 1975).

Before selecting a self-report format for a particular individual, the following are important questions for the therapist-assessor to ask:
- What exactly am I trying to assess?
- Why am I trying to assess this construct?
- Is self-report the optimal (i.e., most direct) means to gather this information?
- Will I have confidence in the validity of the information gathered?
- Will my patient be able to understand the language and relevance of the assessment?
- Does the patient have the ability to report on the information the test seeks?
- Are there outsider-assessment formats which I will want to use to complement the information gathered?

Self-monitoring

Another type of insider-oriented assessment tool is that used for the self-monitoring of behavior or changes in thoughts and/or feelings. With self-monitoring, the patient-respondent records specified responses as they occur. This form of assessment has been used to establish goals prior to treatment, to gauge the effectiveness of treatment, and to help the patient become more aware of internal or external processes as they occur. The duration of the monitoring period can be as brief as a minute or two or can be extended for a period of weeks or months.

In order to help assure that the desired data are collected, the self-monitoring procedure needs to be carefully explained to the individual. A training period followed by a trial-run is useful. The immediate responses of self-monitoring offer the potential to yield greater accuracy than self-report information that often relies on longer periods of recollection. This is especially true when trying to record short-term thoughts or actions that are often forgotten by day's end.

Applications of Self-monitoring.   Self-monitoring as a means of assessment has been documented extensively in relation to cognitive-behavioral and behavioral treatment in the following applications: for headaches (Bootzin & Engle-Friedman, 1981), for smoking (Murray & Hobbs, 1981), for chronic pain (Zlutnick & Taylor, 1982), for health diaries (Verbrugge, 1980), and for monitoring the work performance of persons with developmental disability (Zohn & Bornstein, 1980). Self-monitoring can be carried out both within and outside of the treatment setting while the individual is at school, at work, or with peers at social functions. Figure 21-19 gives an example of a format for self-monitoring.

Self-monitoring can be a form of treatment within itself, for example, the act of pausing to observe or reflect upon one's own actions or thoughts as they occur may have a significant effect on that behavior. This effect on behavior can be viewed as another form of reactivity. An example would be the rather common process of recording one's own eating behaviors and caloric intake. Often such awareness of one's food intake can have a notable subduing effect on eating habits.

Recording Methods.   Self-monitoring may take the form of paper and pencil formats, including unstructured narratives, structured self-reports, checklists, and graphs. Some have incorporated the use of timing devices (tapes, timers, etc.) and video and audiotapes (Brantley & Bruce, 1986).

In order for self-monitoring to be accurate, thoughts, feelings and/or behaviors must be recorded upon their occurrence. This can be achieved by the use of frequency-related measures and time-related measures.

Frequency counts are used primarily when the behavior, thought or feeling of interest occurs as a "discrete event with an identifiable beginning and end" (Bornstein, et al., 1986, p. 178). It is often useful to classify the responses as

DAILY RECORD OF DYSFUNCTIONAL THOUGHTS

Date	Situation Describe:	Emotion(s)	Automatic Thought(s)	Rational Responses	Outcome
	1. Actual event leading to unpleasant emotion, or 2. Stream of thoughts, daydream or recollection, leading to unpleasant emotion.	1. Specify sad/ anxious/angry, etc. 2. Rate degree of emotion (1-100%).	1. Write automatic thought(s) that preceded emotion(s). 2. Rate belief in automatic thought(s) (0-100%).	1. Write rational response to automatic thought(s). 2. Rate belief in rational response (0-100%).	1. Rerate belief in automatic thought(s) 0-100%. 2. Specify and rate subsequent emotions (0-100%).
	Enter store.	Very anxious 100	Felt trapped. Knees feel weak, worried that I won't be able to stay. I feel I'm going to faint. Something may happen to me. No one will help me if I faint.	I will not faint. I haven't fainted in a store yet. If I faint people will help me. Someone will come to my aid.	

Figure 21-19. Sample of Self-Monitoring. When you experience an unpleasant emotion, note the situation that seemed to stimulate the emotion. (If the emotion occurred while you were thinking, daydreaming, etc., please note this.) Then note the automatic thought associated with the emotion. Record the degree to which you believe this thought: 0%=not at all; 100%=completely. In rating degree of emotion: 1=a trace; 100=the most intense possible. *From: Coleman, R.E. (1981). Cognitive-Behavioral Treatment of Agoraphobia. In Emery, G., Hollon, S., Bedrossian, R.C. (Eds.). New Directions in Cognitive Therapy. New York, Guilford Press.*

"performed or not performed," "appropriate or inappropriate," or "pleasant or not pleasant" (Kazdin, 1974, p. 104). For example, a patient in occupational therapy might be asked to check off the steps achieved each day on a list of items necessary to get the patient to therapy.

Time-related measures include time-sampling and duration measures. In time-sampling, a block of time or blocks of time throughout the day are designated and the patient is asked to record whether or not a given behavior or thought occurred during the specified interval(s). Duration measures can be added to time-sampling to record how long a given action or thought lasted. Occupational therapists may use daily journals or activity configurations to help their patients record their activities throughout the day as they occur (Mosey, 1976). In the most structured measures, the day can be subdivided into time intervals of 15 minutes, 30 minutes, or one hour, and patients are asked to record their activities and/or thoughts during each of these intervals.

Less Structured Self-monitoring. A less structured form of self-monitoring has been used by the authors on several occasions. In these instances, patients who were having difficulty while in the therapy setting were asked to discontinue the structured therapy task and record their thoughts in a notebook. This allowed them to record both their thoughts and feelings and the circumstances surrounding the therapy session. The inferences drawn from such an informal diary would be different, and certainly more subjective than the highly structured data organized according to duration or frequency measures.

Reactivity. Reactivity may significantly effect self-monitoring, as it does in self-report. Whether because the patient sees himself differently than others or because of a desire to please the therapist, a patient may not always record thoughts or behaviors with complete accuracy, particularly if accuracy is measured by objective means.

Effects of Self-monitoring. Some of the most potent effects of self-monitoring relate to the fact that recording one's own responses necessitates an interruption of activity, often an interruption of the very activity in question. For

COMPREHENSIVE OCCUPATIONAL THERAPY EVALUATION SCALE (COTE Scale)*

Date																
General Behavior	1	2	3	4	5	6	7	8	9	10	11	12	13	14	15	16
Appearance																
Non-productive behavior																
Activity level																
Interpersonal Behavior																
Independence																
Sociability																
Self-Assertion																
Task Behavior																
Engagement																
Coordination																
Follow Directions																
Sub-total																
Total																

Scale 0—Normal, 1—Minimal, 2—Mild, 3—Moderate, 4—Severe

Comments

_____

_____

_____

_____

_____

*Note: Sub-categories are not inclusive; refer to original source for complete listing.

Figure 21-20. Sample Behavior Observation Scale: Outsider Perspective. *From: COTE Scale. Brayman, S. & Kirby, T. (1982). The Comprehensive Occupational Therapy Evaluation. In Hemphill, B. (Ed.). The Evaluative Process in Psychiatric Occupational Therapy. Thorofare, NJ: Slack Inc.*

example, asking individuals to record every time they interrupt a conversation (a negative verbal behavior) or every time they ask for assistance in the clinic (a positive verbal behavior), stops the flow of the behavior itself. At times, as with the example of recording one's eating habits, stopping the flow of activity might be just what is desired in therapy. However, in other instances these interruptions of the natural sequence of thought or activity may not be so desirable, and hence are viewed as a drawback of self-monitoring.

Much has been written about the role that self-monitoring

can play as a vehicle of treatment beyond assessment (for reviews of the literature see Bornstein, et al., 1986; Ciminero, Karoly & Kanfer, 1981; Nelson & Lipinski, 1977; Stuart, 1977). Although we cannot explore these here, suffice it to say that self-monitoring has been successfully accomplished with both high and lower functioning individuals, both children and adults.

Nelson and colleagues (1978) used self-monitoring with retarded adults in a classroom, and Zohn & Bornstein (1980) used self-monitoring with retarded adults in a sheltered workshop setting. In both instances, the clients were first trained in how to conduct the self-monitoring with a subsequent high degree of accuracy. Summaries of the literature indicate that self-monitoring can be used effectively in behavioral and cognitive-behavioral treatment with a diverse patient population. However, as with all inner oriented assessments, there remains the question of whether the patients perceive themselves as others do.

Selecting a Self-monitoring Format. Before selecting a self-monitoring format, the therapist should ask the following questions:

- Is this patient capable of the diligence required for self-monitoring?
- Is the patient motivated to persist at this procedure?
- How can I ensure that the patient understands what is expected during the self-monitoring task?
- What effect might self-monitoring be expected to have on desirable/undesirable behavior or feelings?
- Can significant others in the patient's environment be expected to be supportive/nonsupportive of the self-monitoring process?
- What might I do to engage their support?
- Will I have confidence in the integrity of the data gathered?
- What would be a reasonable length of time for self-monitoring to take place? Would this process be a useful ongoing treatment tool?

Behavior Observation Scales

In contrast to the self-report tools, the behavior observation scales are outsider-oriented instruments designed to help organize the observations of the therapist-assessor and make them more objective. Behavioral observation is used to sample behavior viewed as necessary for adequate everyday function. Personality or inner conditions are not inferred. Behavior scales are particularly consonant with the behavioral frame of reference, but they may also be used within other frameworks when behavioral baselines are desired.

The most common assessment formats in which behavioral sampling is the primary goal are: (1) behaviorally-oriented interviews (also called interviewing for problem behavior), (2) observation in natural or analogue settings, (3) problem checklists filled out by the therapist-assessor, and not the patient, and (4) reinforcement or environment checklists (Sundberg, 1977, p. 171) *The Comprehensive Occupational Therapy Evaluation* (COTE) is an example of a behavior observation scale (Figures 21-20 and 21-21).

According to Sundberg (1977, pp. 163-164) regardless of whether the patient is being observed in a clinical or natural setting, behavior observation scales generally seek to document evidence of the following:

Samples From the Comprehensive Occupational Therapy Evaluation Scale Definitions

General Behavior

Appearance

The following 6 factors are involved: clean skin, clean hair, hair combed, clean clothes, clothes ironed and clothes suitable for the occasion.

0—No problems in any of the 6 areas
1—Problems in 1 area
2—Problems in 2 areas
3—Problems in 3 or 4 areas
4—Problems in 5 or 6 areas

Interpersonal

Sociability

0—Socializes with staff and patients
1—Socializes with staff and occasionally with other patients or vice versa
2—Socializes only with staff or with patients
3—Socializes only if approached
4—Does not join others in activities, unable to carry on casual conversation even if approached

Task Behavior

Follow Directions

0—Carries out directions without problems
1—Occasional trouble with more than 3 step directions
2—Carries out simple directions—has trouble with 2
3—Can carry out only very simple one step directions (demonstrated written, or oral)
4—Unable to carry out any directions

Figure 21-21. Samples from the Comprehensive Occupational Therapy Evaluation Scale Definitions. *Definitions are excerpted from Appendix X, Comprehensive Occupational Therapy. Evaluation Scale Definitions, in Hemphill, B. (1982). The Evaluative Process in Psychiatric Occupational Therapy, pp. 383-385, Thorofare, NJ: Slack Inc. Reprinted with permission.*

1. behavioral excesses (i.e., hyperactivity, overeating);
2. behavioral deficits (i.e., lack of social skills, lack of work-related skills);
3. behavioral inappropriateness (i.e., developmental delays, "bizarre" behavior);
4. behavioral assets (i.e., skills, knowledge, or achievements); or
5. environmental contingencies (i.e., persons, events, and/or objects in the patient's environment that are supportive or non-supportive of cited behaviors).

Selecting a Behavior Observation Scale. Behavior scales should possess criterion validity; that is, the test needs to contain samples of behavior that relate to actual performance standards and everyday success. As discussed, specific assessments of the behavioral observation type may vary according to several factors. The therapist trying to select the most appropriate format for a specific patient might consider the following questions:

1. Who will do the actual observation? What training and/or guidelines will be needed to help assure observer objectivity?
2. Will the patient be watched in isolation, or will several patients be observed at one time?
3. Will only specified events be sampled by the observer (e.g., only recording when the patient is conciliatory or finishes a task) or will the assessor record all behaviors that occur within a given time frame?
4. Will the assessment occur within the constraints of a specified test battery, or will the observation setting be minimally structured?
5. Will the observer record observations immediately or retrospectively?
6. What role will reactivity likely play in influencing the patient's performance?
7. Will insider-oriented procedures be used to complement the data that have been gathered by objective means?
8. To what extent might there be pre-conceived biases on the part of the therapist or observer that can color what is perceived during the observation?

Individual test formats may indicate whether the observer is to sit with or apart from the patient, how the observer is to handle questions that may be raised by the patient and to what extent assistance may be provided by the observer. When such guidelines are not provided by a specific test protocol, the therapist will have to consider the likely influence that therapist participation and/or obvious presence may have.

Observer Biases. While striving for objectivity, behavior observation scales cannot avoid being influenced to some extent by therapist-observer biases. Previous experiences with a given individual or with other patients color the therapist's expectations of what to see. Even for the most open-minded observer, observation is selective in nature and there is a tendency to see what we want to see and miss that which lies outside our expectations. Nevertheless, behavior-oriented, outsider scales provide a structure that helps the observer notice significant behaviors. These behavioral guides have been cited for their value in making the therapist and patient define clearly what is meant by their concerns and goals (Sundberg, 1977, p. 169). Observation formats may vary in terms of the duration of observation, the extent of training required of potential observers, the extent and scope of the behavior observed, and the structure of the observation setting. Thus, it would be difficult to draw any general conclusions regarding the time or expense involved in using such formats.

Projective Tests

The term "projective" was coined by Lawrence Frank (1939) who wanted "indirect methods for eliciting patterns of internal organization." Projective tests are based upon the Freudian belief that the most influential aspects of personality are not in the individual's conscious awareness, and therefore cannot be reported by the patient. According to Freudian thought, much of these significant data are held in the individual's unconscious by a censoring superego, or the practical ego. Projective tests are designed as a means to sidestep the constraints of the ego and superego and reveal data that represent the underlying personality or suggest themes in thought and behavior. They do not examine samples of behaviors. Behaviors are often viewed in terms of their symbolic function.

Types of Projective Tests. Projective tests are typically designed to provide a great deal of choice in patient response. Rather than using a true-false format or other structured response scale, they most often provide a stimulus to which the individual can respond freely by verbal or nonverbal means. As reported by Sundberg (1977, pp. 202-205), Lindzey (1959, 1961) categorized projective devices into five groups, based upon the nature of the response desired of the patient:

1. Association techniques ask the patient to react to a stimulus with the first word or image that comes to mind. Examples of such tests include the *Rorschach Ink Blot* (1921) and word-association tests.
2. Construction techniques require the subject to create something such as a drawing or story. Examples include Lerner's *Magazine Picture Collage* (Lerner & Ross, 1977, Lerner, 1979), the *Azima Battery* (Azima, 1959) and variations on Draw-a-Person. Two of the more commonly referenced Draw-A-Person tests are *Machover's Draw-A-Person* (Machover, 1949) and *Buck's House-Tree-Person* (Buck & Jolles, 1972).
3. Completion techniques require the individual to finish an incomplete task however he wishes, such as in sentence completion tests.
4. Choice or ordering techniques require the patient to select among alternatives and/or order according to preference.
5. Expressive techniques allow the patient to reveal personal style, as in unstructured drawing tasks, clay construction tasks, or puppet-play with children.

Therapist Inference. Of all the types of psychological assessment discussed, projective techniques require the most therapist inference. The therapist must be knowledgeable in Freudian theory and trained in the use of projective tests in order to note the patient's responses and interpret their meaning. This interpretation may or may not be shared with the patient. When signs of personality or themes in behavior are deduced, the therapist may attempt to determine with the aid of the patient, specific instances in behavior where this personality style becomes problematic. Construct validity is important in such projective devices because the therapist seeks to verify whether the assessment indicates a presumed personality construct. As discussed previously, it has not been possible to gain agreement regarding the myriad of psychological constructs employed in assessment.

Although occupational therapy assessment in the 1950's and early 1960's used these projective batteries, occupational therapists do not typically have the special training needed for psychoanalytic interpretation. Assessment in psychiatry, psychology, nursing, and occupational therapy all reflect movement away from psychoanalytic interpretation and towards more functional assessment. However, this should not suggest that expressive media do not have a place in occupational therapy assessment or treatment, but rather that interpretations of such expression should not be overextended and conclusions drawn should be understood as tentative. Formats such as those used in **projective assessments** also tend to encourage fantasy and may not be judged as suitable for individuals with a tenuous reality orientation.

Psychometric Techniques

Psychometric techniques is the term used by Sundberg (1977) to describe many of the personality, interest, and attitude inventories commonly associated with psychology. These are not the type of tests typically used by occupational therapists, but these tests may be discussed in the context of the patient's history. In psychometric tests, the patient's responses are treated as correlates of something else (not signs, nor samples). For example, the test may set out to define a human trait such as aggressiveness. A scale is then created to test behaviors that would be exhibited by an individual possessing this trait and the patient is asked to choose which behaviors he/she would use. Once the patient has completed the test, the responses can be directly tallied to produce a score for aggressiveness.

Personality inventories are often of this type. One of the best known personality inventories is the *Minnesota Multiphasic Personality Inventory*. Other popular personality inventories used by psychologists include the *California Psychological Inventory*, the *Eysenck Personality Inventory*, and the *Myers Briggs Type Indicator*.

Interest inventories are also often in this category. The *Strong Vocational Interest Blank* for Men, first published in 1927, selected items for occupational scales by comparing the responses made by the test-taker with those responses made by men who were successfully engaged in identified occupations (Sundberg, 1977, p. 187) For example, if a male test-taker's responses indicated responses that he enjoyed the same activities as did men already employed in an identified occupation, then his score would show a high correlation to that occupation. One assessment of this type referred to in the occupational therapy literature is the *Self-Directed Search* (Holland, 1982).

Attitude, value and opinion scales may also be psychometric techniques of this sort. A typical attitude scale will obtain a score on 10 or 20 items that is then correlated to positive or negative feelings toward an object or events (Sundberg, 1977, p. 192).

How Test Items are Chosen. Psychometric techniques are usually created by the initial identification of a pool of items that are believed to be indicative of an identified domain of interest. Frequently, psychological constructs are identified in terms of this item pool. Once the test-taker makes responses, the answers are translated into a numerical score and there is no therapist interpretation involved. Personality, interest, and attitude inventories are usually true-false or multiple-choice, paper and pencil tests. They are typically inexpensive and easy to administer. They do, however, necessitate certain cognitive skills of the test-taker and depend on truthful answers.

Use of Psychometric Tests. Although many tests have been created, there is no consensus on their utility or dependability. One common use of psychometric tests has been to help screen applicants for vocational, military, and educational programs. Test-takers can often determine what trait is being tested by the nature of the test items. Whether or not this knowledge will influence the outcome of the test and the validity of the results depends on both the test-taker and the test.

Biopsychological Assessment

Biopsychological assessment is designed to find out more about the relationship of bodily states to thoughts and emotions, or to determine how the central nervous system (CNS) affects behavior. Anyone who endorses the holistic premise that body and mind must be understood as a unit, could argue that all assessment is, in one way or another, biopsychological assessment. However, in the therapeutic context biopsychological assessment has been directed toward understanding the influence of the CNS damage on specific sensory-perceptual and motor functions, cognitive processing and feeling states, and on understanding the relationship between physiologic parameters and emotion (e.g., pulse rate, respiration, galvanic skin response). Biopsychological assessment has been used by psychologists and occupational therapists in relation to the special problems of brain and spinal cord injury, substance

---

ITEMS FROM THE SCHROEDER BLOCK CAMPBELL ADULT PSYCHIATRIC SENSORY INTEGRATION EVALUATION

1. Dominance (eye, hand, foot)
2. Posture (lordosis, kyphosis, etc.)
3. Neck Rotation (restricted, jerky range of motion)
4. Gait (shuffling, lack of restricted arm movements)
5. Hand Observation (ulnar deviation, thumb adduction, thenar atrophy)
6. Grip Strength (number of pounds)
7. Fine Motor Control (number of taps)
8. Diadochokinesis (deterioration, slowing of response, tremor, etc.)
9. Finger-Thumb Opposition (visual clues needed, variation, slowing of response)
10. Visual Pursuit (excessive blinking, strabismus, unable to track, unable to converge)
11. Bilateral Coordination (incorrect size, irregular shape, 2-3 trials to complete, etc.)
12. Crossing the Midline (slow, hesitant, hands switch, unable to complete)
13. Stability—UE (moves stance to maintain balance, offers no resistance, etc.)
14. Stability—Trunk (rigid muscle tone, excessively fluid, etc.)
15. Classical Romberg (performance awkward, balance lost once, twice, etc.)
16. Sharpened Romberg (can't hold position 30 seconds, 15 seconds, etc.)
17. Overflow movements (distal movements present, unable to hold position, etc.)
18. Neck Righting (arms move as head turns, arms align with head, etc.)
19. Rolling (moderate difficulty, unable to change direction, etc.)
20. Asymmetrical Tonic Neck Reflex (change in tone, tremor noted, contralateral limb flexion, etc.)
21. Symmetrical Tonic Neck Reflex (dorsiflexion, ventroflexion)
22. Tonic Labyrinthine Reflex (arm or leg tremors, unable to hold for 30 seconds, 15 seconds)
23. Protective Extension (slow or delayed response, absence of protective extension)
24. Seated Equilibrium (anxiety present, inflexible muscle tone, etc.)
25. Body image (size, anatomy indicators)
26. Abnormal Movements (hyperkinesia, hypokinesia, extrapyramidal)
27. Self-Reported Childhood History (general history, delayed development, neurologic soft signs, hyperactivity)

Figure 21-22. Sample Biopsychological Assessment. *Adapted from the Schroeder-Block-Campbell Adult Psychiatric Sensory Integration Evaluation (1981). Kailua, Hawaii: Schroeder Publishing and Consulting.*

abuse, anxiety, depression, schizophrenia, psychosomatic illness, cognitive dysfunction and developmental disability (retardation), and those problems globally referred to as "sensory-integrative" in nature.

Screening for Central Nervous System Damage. Some assessments have been used by clinicians from a variety of disciplines as a means to determine whether or not organic brain damage is present. The *Bender-Gestalt,* based upon the work of Lauretta Bender in the 1930's, uses nine geometric shapes, presented in order of maturational difficulty, which the subject is asked to duplicate (Hutt, 1969; Hutt & Briskin, 1961).

The *Draw-a-Person,* discussed previously as a projective device, is used also as an indicator of body-image, maturational, and/or neurological change. Research suggests that these instruments are valid only as rough screening tools and must be used in conjunction with other tests in order for differential diagnoses to be made (Buros, 1972; Cohn, 1960 and King, 1982). Some assessments may be particular to specific body systems, such as the auditory or visual systems, while others include many subtests and are designed to assess multiple CNS functions or the synthesis of functional systems.

The *Benton Neuropsychological Assessment* includes 12 tests intended to screen for and specify the nature of CNS impairment. Assessment in this battery includes temporal orientation, right-left orientation, form recognition, tactile recognition, serial-digit learning, phoneme recognition, and motor impersistence. (Benton, et al., 1983).

The *Schroeder-Block-Campbell Adult Psychiatric Sensory Integration Evaluation* was designed for screening sensory-integrative difficulties with an adult psychiatric population (See Figure 21-22) and the *Halstead-Reitan Neuropsychological Test Battery* (also referred to as the Halstead Reitan or the Halstead-Indiana Battery) are frequently referenced in the occupational therapy literature. Since there exists a wealth of assessments of the biopsychological type, one needs to investigate to determine which assessments would be most appropriate for a given patient population.

The Interview

The last type of assessment to be discussed is the interview. After reviewing the interview literature there are two conclusions that can be drawn: (1) interviewing is a crucial component of any assessment used to plan treatment interventions; and (2) there are multiple ways to conduct an interview and not any one method is correct. The literature has extensive recommendations for guiding the interview process, many of which are summarized here. The manner in which an interview is conducted is influenced by: (1) environmental factors (e.g., the institutional setting and the specific interview setting), (2) the interviewer's beliefs, biases, and theoretical orientation, (3) the characteristics of the patient, and (4) the dynamic interactions that occur while establishing the therapeutic relationship (e.g., time pressure, patient-therapist responses, etc.).

The Environmental Setting. The environment includes multiple professionals who contribute to each patient's treatment program. Each person may vary the interview style or type of interview to plan their segment of the intervention. Regardless of the type of interview, there are specific factors which can influence the interview outcome. The interview room should have adequate lighting, heat and air, and comfortable seating. Seating should allow the patient to be seen and heard easily. The atmosphere should convey a feeling of warmth and have minimal distractions. Any task or testing materials should be made available in advance and be easily accessible during the interview. The room should allow for privacy, thus telephone calls should be intercepted by a secretary (or answering machine) and a sign should be posted on the door to the interview room indicating that an interview is in progress.

Influence of the Therapist. The therapist's interview skills, personal values, beliefs, and theoretical orientation influence the interview style and strategies, and thus can possibly influence interview outcome. The therapist should make every effort to avoid influencing patient responses because the primary purpose of the interview is to elicit the patient's needs, concerns, problems, and capabilities.

Influence may be verbal or nonverbal. For example, the therapist's facial expression or head-nodding in affirmation may communicate criticism or acceptance of the patient's comments or feelings. The interviewer's self-knowledge also allows the therapists to listen and identify with the patient (frequently called empathy), while maintaining his or her own identity.

Theory guides interview behavior and the evaluation of behavior (Turkat, 1986). Thus the therapist's theoretical framework has a major influence upon the interview strategy. For example, in occupational therapy, the behavioral interview is structured, systematic, action-oriented, and focused. In contrast, the psychoanalytic interview provides a framework with open-ended questions in which multiple responses are possible, and the communication process and the interpretation of behavior are used to develop a patient profile.

Patient Influences. The individual being interviewed also has needs, values, beliefs, biases, and experiences which they bring to the interview setting, all of which can influence their responses and behavior during the interview and the outcomes. Patients may come to the interview with expectations. They may be fearful, wonder what is permissible to discuss, or may have a specific agenda they wish to share. Their previous therapy experiences may confirm their discomfort or support their investment in therapy. The therapist is encouraged to allow time during the interview to learn about influential patient factors.

Patient Symptoms and Interviewer Responses. Patient symptoms also may influence the type of interview strategy that is required. The literature suggests approaches for patients who are aggressive, demanding, paranoid, depressive, and seductive, etc. (Levinson, 1987; MacKinnon & Michels, 1971).

The aggressive patient may be verbally hostile and/or restless and hyperactive. These behaviors may suggest that the patient needs physical and/or psychological space because of feeling trapped or confined by the interview questions, personal problems, or the hospital experience. Aggression may also be a reaction to a loss of self-esteem and control. If possible, the therapist should try to determine the reason for the anger before reacting and give the patient physical and emotional space or bolster self-esteem as indicated (Levinson, 1987).

The demanding patient may be irritable, uncooperative, or verbally and physically demanding. When responding to this patient, the therapist should be sensitive to the deprived and neglected feelings that are usually the source of the demands. The therapist should try to minimize the stress of the interview and avoid questioning that could be perceived as interrogation by the patient (Levinson, 1987).

The patient with paranoia is suspicious and usually makes accusations. The individual will frequently refuse to be interviewed or may ask for justification of the information requested, for example asking: "Why do you need to know that?" They may also demand that the therapist identify the source of information by asking, "Who told you that?" It is best to recognize that the patient's thoughts are delusional and that the patient may not respond to reason. The therapist should not dispute the patient's false ideas and should, if possible, abandon the line of questioning that causes suspicion (Levinson, 1987).

The depressed person's symptoms represent the patient's loss of esteem, independence, and sense of wholeness. The symptoms may have a lifelong pattern of expression as feelings of worthlessness, hopelessness, apathy, guilt and loneliness. The patient's sadness is expressed by his tone of voice, posture, and speech. The therapist can respond to these behavioral expressions (i.e., "You look sad.") and usually must assume more responsibility for the direction of the interview by actively questioning the patient and periodically summarizing the interview information (Levinson, 1987).

A seductive response from the patient may take the therapist by surprise and initially may make the assessor (interviewer) feel flattered. However, it is important not to satisfy the romantic fantasies of the patient and to redirect the interview to the focus of patient treatment. If such seductive behavior should occur, the therapist should reevaluate the interview setting to guard against the patient's ability to make false charges regarding the interviewer's conduct. It may be necessary to use an assistant during the interview or change the interview setting (Levinson, 1987).

The patient who is resistive during an interview may be garrulous, may intellectualize, generalize, or remain silent. These behaviors may express a conscious or unconscious attitude that is opposed to treatment. In general, it is best not to directly tell the patient that he/she is resistant or say such things as, "I can't help you if you don't cooperate." When the therapist feels that the patient is at ease and ready to listen, then the therapist may identify possible feelings and solicit affirmation of the feeling and its possible sources. The therapist might choose to evaluate the silence by asking, "Are you at a loss for words?" or "Is it difficult for you to discuss what you're thinking? (MacKinnon & Yudofsky, 1986).

The previously described behaviors are only a few of the patient symptoms which continually challenge the therapist to individualize interview approaches—approaches which usually represent the collective efforts of experienced clinicians. Thus, it is recommended that the therapist consider consulting a colleague when difficult patients refuse intended assessment strategies.

Patient Age and Interview Response.   There are also age considerations when selecting interview strategies. Recent literature identifies interview approaches for children (Levinson, 1987; Simmons, 1987) and the older adult (Levinson, 1987).

Interviewing Children.   The therapist interviewing children should use a combination of verbal and play activities and structure the environment to minimize the child's anxiety and to maximize the opportunity to express feelings and concerns. Since children are usually seeking therapy at someone else's request (teacher, parent, physician), they may be fearful of what is to happen, naive about their problems, deny having problems, or be in therapy against their wills. Simmons suggests that the therapist state the reason for referral so that the child will not worry about what the therapist knows. The therapist should discuss confidentiality to minimize the child's suspicion that the therapist is an ally of the parents, teachers, or others. The therapist should use language that is appropriate to the child's vocabulary (Simmons, 1987). The interview environment should include both an area to talk and an area to play. The play area should have a variety of materials available from which the child chooses. Suggested materials include: (1) creative, drawing, and expressive media, (2) dolls, puppets, and stuffed animals for viewing personal interactions and which allow projective expression, (3) table games, and (4) toys which specifically promote expression of aggression (soldiers, guns), action (cars, trucks), etc. Other materials may include water and sand play, tools, building blocks, models for assembly, and other age related activities (Simmons, 1987).

Interviewing the Older Adult.   Usually the older adult who seeks treatment has complex problems that may be physical and psychosocial in nature, thus the therapist may be viewed as a resource for responding to multiple difficulties such as limited funds, isolation, unsatisfactory living condition, recreation needs, and transportation. In order to establish rapport with the older adult, therapists should convey respect, allow patients to discuss their accomplishments, allow them to maintain as much independence as possible, give them control over decisions about their own care, and assume that they are capable of scientific understanding and explanations of the treatment process (Levinson, 1987). When empathizing with the patient, the therapist should be sensitive to the "generation gap" (if one exists). If the therapist is much younger than the patient, rather than stating, "I know how you feel," it would be better to use comments such as, "My grandmother had a similar problem," (Levinson, 1987). The therapist should be careful in the phrasing of questions and avoid setting the patient up for failure, for example, rather than stating, "I'd like to ask you some simple questions," the therapist might phrase it as, "I'm going to ask questions that identify your ability to remember." If the patient feels they are unable to answer "simple questions," their sense of defeat may be greater (Levinson, 1987). It is best to begin questioning with open-ended questions and become more specific as the need arises. The therapist should speak clearly, but not loudly, and when speaking, the therapist should assume a position which will allow the patient to see him/her. Many older patients lip read and are unaware of doing so. If patients are slow to answer, the therapist should not fill in for them. Allow time for patients to remember and to respond (Levinson, 1987).

In addition to the interview environment, the therapist's expertise, the patient characteristics, and the nature of the therapeutic relationship, the outcome of the interview will be influenced by the interview's primary goal.

Types of Interviews

According to Turkat (1986) there are seven types of interviews identified by their primary goal: (1) diagnostic interview, (2) intake interview, (3) psychometric interview, (4) crisis interview, (5) history-taking interview, (6) patient management interview, and (7) informant interview. Of these seven, the occupational therapist more frequently uses crisis, history-taking, patient management, and informant interviews. However, all types of interview are briefly described here.

Diagnostic Interview. The diagnostic interview is conducted most frequently by a psychiatrist in order to classify the psychopathology that the patient presents. During the diagnostic interview, the psychiatrist uses the mental status exam and other questions pertinent to the patient's presenting problems. From the mental status questions, the interviewer notes the patient's appearance and behavior, sensorium, thought processes, thought content and intellect, perceptual disturbances, emotional regulation, volition, and somatic tendencies (Turkat, 1986).

Intake Interview. During the intake interview the therapist seeks to identify the patient's needs and determine if these needs can be met by the available treatment resources. In essence, the patient is screened for clinic suitability. This interview may lead to a referral to another setting or assignment of the primary therapist (Turkat, 1986).

Psychometric Interview. The psychometric interview is one which represents the traditional role of the psychologist. It occurs when the interviewer does formal psychological testing. In contemporary practice, the psychologist has an expansive role in which he may use multiple types of interview (Turkat, 1986).

Crisis Interview. When there is an emergency situation, such as when a person has attempted suicide, has lost contact with reality, or is unable to perform in one's job, there is a need for quick identification and conceptualization of the problem and a prompt intervening response. Such a brief, prompt, action-oriented response is a crisis interview (Turkat, 1986).

In acute short-term treatment settings, the occupational therapist is constrained by a limited time for evaluation and treatment and therefore may use an interview strategy which combines problem identification and intervention simultaneously. This has not been labeled crisis interviewing. Based upon a developmental frame of reference, Peloquin (1983) designed an *Occupational Therapy Interview/Therapy Set Procedure* which responds to a large case load and a short hospital stay (12 days). The interview gathers data for establishing the intervention plan and orients the patient to the occupational therapy process, including its opportunities and purpose. The procedure includes a letter to the patient, a guide to helpful activity, and an occupational therapy objective checklist (see Figure 21-23).

History-taking Interview. Turkat (1986) identifies the social worker as the professional responsible for the history-taking interview. This interview covers the patient's medical, family, marriage and sexual history, occupational data, history of mental illness, substance abuse, etc. There is usually a historical component to the occupational therapy interview. The occupational therapy history-taking interview focuses on the patient's abilities related to work, self-care, and leisure, and the skills for adequate performance in these areas.

Moorehead (1969) developed *The Occupational History* (OH) for reviewing occupational function in the context of social role theory. She assumed that each individual has family, sexual, and occupational roles and that these roles form one's identity. One's performance in these roles develops throughout life and early experiences influence adult role performance. To gain an understanding of adult role performance, the occupational history is used. The OH uses a semi-structured interview to gain an understanding of the conditions that influence performance and how the patient has learned to approach tasks and fulfill roles. Questions seek to identify the patient's level of competence and potential for improvement in role performance. Although the interview is structured the therapist is free to probe and clarify responses, and findings are discussed openly with the patient (Moorehead, 1969). The Occupational History is again referenced and used as a screening tool by Florey and Michelman (1982), who reiterate the value of history-taking as a means to establish a context for understanding presenting problems (Figure 21-24).

Patient Management Interview. The patient management interview is used to identify the type of therapy needed and is practiced by multiple professionals in outpatient or inpatient settings (Turkat, 1986). Most occupational therapy assessment interviews could be considered under this broad classification. Occupational therapists use the patient management interview to identify the following: (1) the patient's strengths which facilitate coping, (2) the current problems that the patient is experiencing, and (3) data which will increase the understanding of the patient's past and expected environments. During an interview, the occupational therapist learns about the patient's learning style and can then target approaches to tasks, the kind of supervision needed, and possible individual and group activities that could benefit the patient.

Informant Interview. The informant interview occurs when information is gathered from significant others, such as family members, teachers, etc. (Turkat, 1986). In general, the literature emphasizes that the informant interview should not be a substitute for interviewing the patient. Interviewing significant others can provide information about the patient and the interactions within the patient's social network. The therapist has the opportunity to gain an understanding of how significant psychosocial events produce symptoms and problems; and view the interactions between the patient and significant others. When opening the interview, the therapist should emphasize that this is a time for the significant others to express their views of the problems. The therapist should make it clear that everyone who wishes to speak will be given an opportunity. He/she should also point out that solutions will not be identified during this first session, but will evolve from problem-solving during family therapy sessions. During this interview discussion, the therapist should be careful not to place blame upon significant others, nor to take sides. The therapist acts as a discussion monitor and actively controls and directs the interview by asking specific questions to learn about problems. It is important to periodically summarize what has occurred, as this invites clarification or differing view-points, and allows the therapist to provide support as needed. The therapist also monitors the communication to prevent interruptions, retaliation, rambling, and "scapegoating" of individuals in the group. During the interview, the therapist can observe the significant others' ability to communicate, their stability and the closeness of their relationship with the patient. Additionally, it is possible to determine their capacity for cooperation during treatment, their status of health and how attuned they are to psychological processes, the cultural values that exist and their relationship to the community.

SUMMARY

Psychological assessment in occupational therapy is a mechanism for understanding the relationship between mind and body and how the mind-body connection influences human performance. As the occupational therapist-assessor gathers information about the patient's needs, values, attitudes, feelings, interests, goals, style of

---

Occupational Therapy—A Guide to Helpful Activity With Your Thinking

1. Have you been having any problems with your memory? _____
2. Has it been difficult for you to keep your attention on things? _____
3. Has making decisions become more difficult recently? _____
4. Do you find yourself thinking about your problems more than you'd like to? _____
5. When you leave the hospital, will you be returning to a responsible position or job (mother, worker, housewife)? _____

   The activity program can help you. When you become involved in activity, you are using important skills that are all part of the thinking process: choosing, deciding, problem-solving, remembering, and concentrating.

   Putting yourself back into a routine of activity will help smooth out any thinking problem you've had and keep you alert and ready to deal with returning to your responsibilities at home.

   Often people fail to realize how physical exercise helps their thinking. It does. Regular exercise helps regulate the nervous system, which in turn regulates a person's thinking. Daily exercise helps maintain and improve thinking abilities and it increases physical well-being.

Occupational Therapy Goals Toward Improved Functional Performance

Occupational Therapy will be working to help you in the following areas, hoping you will experience the benefit of activity that has purpose.

With Your Thinking Skills:

_____ improving your concentration by providing crafts, hobbies, and daily exercises that require you to concentrate

_____ reducing your confusion through activities that provide clear directions for you to follow

_____ building your problem-solving skills through activities and puzzles that encourage you to figure out problems

_____ keeping you alert and thinking in order to prepare you to return to your home and community

_____ helping you reduce racing thoughts through organized and calming projects

_____ providing you with opportunities to organize your thinking and behavior through structured tasks

---

Figure 21-23. A Structured Interview Format. *Peloquin, S. (1983). The Development of an Occupational Therapy Interview/Therapy Set Procedure. American Journal of Occupational Therapy 37(7):457-461.*

coping, sense of control, and self-image, the patient emerges as a unique individual who in his or her own way strives to accomplish life tasks and achieve a quality of life. To gather information, the therapist may use an interview, plus tests and activities. Psychological assessment strategies include projective tests, self-report and self-monitoring methods, subjective or objective approaches, sign and sample approaches, and behavior observation scales. Prior to selecting an assessment strategy, the occupational therapist may wish to review the assessment protocol of the department and consider characteristics of patient and environment. There is no single correct approach to assessment.

As therapist-assessors, occupational therapists need to recognize that the type of assessment chosen will determine what information is obtained. It is essential that an assessment tool is compatible with the treatment setting and theoretical frame of reference, is sensitive to the abilities and limitations of patients, and is suited to their assessment needs and the therapist's assessment goals. Ideally, patients should have ample opportunity to consider and communicate their treatment needs while the therapist is evaluating them. This shared responsibility for data gathering begins the partnership of patient and therapist in the process of assessment and intervention.

Study Questions

1. What is psychological assessment?

2. Is psychological assessment within the domain of occupational therapy?

3. If psychological assessment is within the domain of occupational therapy, then how is it different from a psychologist's report? How is it different from an intake report which is completed by the psychiatrist or primary therapist?

4. Do you think psychiatric labels are helpful in the treatment of patients? Support your answer.

5. How does a frame of reference influence psychological assessment?

6. Given the historical development of occupational therapy, how has psychological assessment changed?

7. What is (are) the difference(s) between an insider-oriented (subjective) and an outsider-oriented (objective) assessment?

8. Give an example of when insider-oriented assessment might be preferred. Identify specific setting, therapist, and patient conditions.

9. Give an example of when outsider orientation is

> **SAMPLE ITEMS FROM THE OCCUPATIONAL ROLE SCREENING INTERVIEW**
>
> **Worker/Homemaker**
>   1. What is your current occupation?
>   2. How/why did you choose this occupation?
>   3. What kind of tasks does it include?
>   4. How did you learn the daily routine?
> 10. Is there anyone you admire or want to be like, now and in the past?
> 14. How do you spend your leisure time?
> 20. What was the best period of your life?
> 22. What would you like to be doing a year from now?
> 23. How will you go about doing that?
>
> **School**
>   1. What school(s) did you go to?
>   2. How did you do in school?
>   3. What did you like about school?
>   8. Who did you admire during that period? Why?
>   9. Did you have any favorite teachers?

Figure 21-24. A Structured Interview Format. *From: Occupational Role Screening Interview. Florey, L. & Michelman, S. (1982). Occupational Role History: A Screening Tool for Psychiatric Occupational Therapy. Am J of Occup Ther 36(5):301-308.*

preferred. Identify specific setting, therapist, and patient conditions.

10. What is the function of psychological constructs in assessments? How might the occupational therapy profession come to an agreement on the meaning of these constructs? Is agreement necessary? Useful? Possible?

11. What are the differences between a functional assessment and a projective assessment?

12. How might the occupational therapist's bias influence the outcome of the assessment?

13. What factors will influence the nature of the assessment approach chosen by the occupational therapist for a particular patient?

14. Does the therapist's interpretation have a place in assessment?

References

Achenbach, T.M (1978). The child behavior profile I: Boys aged 6 through 11. *Journal of Consulting & Clinical Psychology, 46,* 478-488.

Summary of Selected Assessments

CATEGORY	TYPICAL FORMAT	PERSPECTIVE EMPHASIZED	CHARACTERISTICS	CLINICAL EXAMPLES (ASSESSMENTS)

1. Self Report	Questionnaire
	Checklists
	True-False
	Performance scales
	Narrative
	Activity configuration
		Subjective
		(Patient's view)
			Considered the most direct means to elicit patient views; can be influenced by reactivity; generally possesses face validity	*Activities Configuration* (several variations,
				  see Spahn, 1969; Mosey, 1973)
				Activity Laboratory Questionnaire (Fidler,
				  1982 in Hemphill, 1982)
				Beck Depression Inventory (Beck, 1967)
				Body-Self Relations Questionnaire (BSRQ)
				  (Noles et al, 1985)
				Depression Adjective Check List (Lubin,
				  1967)
				Interest Check List (Matsutsuyu, 1969)
				Role Checklist (Oakley et al, 1986)
				Self Management Survey (Spiegler & Agigian,
				  1977)
				Survey of Heterosexual Interactions
				  (Twentyman & McFall, 1975)
				Young's Loneliness Inventory (Young, 1981)

2. Self Monitoring	Frequency counts Time and duration sampling Narrative Activity configurations Checklists	Subjective (Patient's view)	A form of self-report used to determine changes in feelings or behavior; Can be used as a form of treatment; Often requires a training period (regarding methods)	*Daily Record of Dysfunctional Thoughts* (Coleman 1981)

3. Behavior Observation Scales	Problem-oriented interview
	Problem checklists
	Task experiences
	Reinforcement checklists
	Environment checklists
		Objective
		(Therapists view)
			Gathers samples of behavior; Used to objectify assessment process; Consistent with functional assessment; uses quantitative data	*Bay Area Functional Performance Evaluation*
				  (BaFPE) (Bloomer & Williams, 1978)
				Comprehensive Occupational Therapy Evaluation
				  (COTE) (Brayman & Kirby, 1982)
				Comprehensive Evaluation of Basic Living Skills
				  (Casanova & Ferber, 1976)
				Nurses' Observation Scale for Inpatient Evaluation (NOSIE)
				  Honigfield et al, 1966;
				  Behavior Arts Center, 90 Calla Ave., Floral Park, NY 11001
				Parachek Geriatric Rating Scale (Miller &
				  Parachek, 1974)
				Psychotic In-Patient Profile (Lorr & Vestre, 1986)

Figure 21-25. Summary of Selected Assessments.

Summary of Selected Assessments (continued)

CATEGORY	TYPICAL FORMAT	PERSPECTIVE EMPHASIZED	CHARACTERISTICS	CLINICAL EXAMPLES (ASSESSMENTS)
4. Projective Tests	Construction techniques Drawing Sentence completion Word association Play techniques Complete-a-story	Subjective/ Objective Patient's view/Assessor's interpret- ation	Relies on therapist inference; uses qualitative data Elicits signs of behavior and unconscious content	*Azima Battery* (Azima & Azima, 1959; Hemphill, 1982) *BH Battery* (Hemphill, 1982) *Draw-a-Person* (Available, Western Psychological Services) *House-Tree-Person* (Buck & Jolles, 1972) *Hutt Adaptation of Bender Gestalt Test* (Huff, 1969) *Lerner's Magazine Picture Collage* (Lernern & Ross, 1977; Lerner, 1979) *O'Kane Diagnostic Battery* (O'Kane, 1969) *Rorschach Ink Blot*
5. Psycho-metric Techniques	Paper & pencil test True-false Multiple choice Interest, value, opinion scales	Subjective/ Objective Patient's & Assessor's views	Most often used by psychologists, not occupational therapists; Patient responses treated as correlates of some attribute; Test items typically drawn from a pool of test items	*California Psychological Inventory* *Minnesota Multiphasic Personality Inventory* (MMPI) *Self-Directed Search* (Holland, 1982) *Strong-Campbell Interest Inventory* (Consulting Psychology Press)
6. Biopsycho-logical Assessment	Task experiences Dialogue/interview Cognitive problems Motor-performance tests	Subjective/ Objective Patient's & Assessor's views	Looks at CNS function, motor performance, cognitive processing, body image changes, etc.; Can include self report, behavior scales, interview, and other types of assessment	*Allen Cognitive Level Test* (ACL) (Allen, 1985) *Benton Neuropsychological Assessment* (Benton et al, 1983) *Draw-a-Person* (King, in Hemphill, 1982; Cohn, 1960) *Halstead Reitan Neuropsychological Test Battery* (Boll, 1981) *Hutt Adaptation of the Bender Gestalt Test* (Hutt, 1969) *Mental Status Exam* (Kaplan & Sadock, 1988)
7. Interview	Structured & loosely structured dialogue with patient Focus can be on intake, history, crisis- intervention, patient- management; Structured dialogue with significant others.	Subjective/ Objective Patient's and/ or assessor's views	Some form of interview is common to all frames of reference Can vary greatly according to the degree to which the assessor structures it	The following are structured interview formats: *Adolescent Role Assessment* (Black, 1976; Black in Hemphill, 1982) *Occupational Role Screening Interview* (Florey & Michelman, 1982) *Occupational Therapy Interview/ Therapy Set* (Peloquin, 1983)

Figure 21-25. Continued.

Achenbach, T.M. & Edelbrock, C.S. (1979). The child behavior profile II: Boys aged 12-16 and girls aged 6-11 and 12-16. *Journal of Consulting & Clinical Psychology, 47*, 223-233.

Allen, C. (1985). *Occupational therapy for psychiatric diseases: Measurement and management of cognitive disabilities.* Boston: Little, Brown & Co.

Allen, C. (1988). Cognitive disabilities. In Robertson, S. (Ed.). Mental health focus: Skills for assessment and treatment. (pp. 3-18 through 3-33). Rockville, Maryland: American Occupational Therapy Association.

Allport, G.W. (1950). *The nature of personality: Selected papers.* Cambridge, MA: Addison-Wesley.

Allport, G.W. (1966). Traits revisited. *American Psychologist, 21*, 1-10.

Allport, G.W. & Odbert, H.S. (1936). Trait names: A psycholexical study. *Psychological Monographs, 47*(211), 1-171.

American Occupational Therapy Association. (1979). *Uniform terminology for reporting occupational therapy services.* Rockville, MD: AOTA.

American Occupational Therapy Association. (1989). Uniform terminology for Occupational Therapy—2nd Ed. Rockville, MD: AOTA.

American Occupational Therapy Association. (1984). Hierarchy of competencies relating to the use of standardized instruments and evaluation techniques by occupational therapists. *American Journal of Occupational Therapy, 38*, 803-804.

American Personnel and Guidance Association. Responsibilities of users of standardized tests. *Guidepost,* Oct. 1978, 5-8.

American Psychiatric Association. (1952, 1968, 1974, 1978, 1981). *Diagnostic and statistical manual of mental disorders.* Washington, DC: APA.

American Psychiatric Association. (1987). *Diagnostic and statistical manual of mental disorders revised (DSM III-R).* Washington, DC: APA.

American Psychological Association, American Educational Research Association and National Council on Measurement in Education. (1974). *Standards for educational and psychological tests.* Washington, DC: American Psychological Association.

Anthony, W.A. (1979). *The principles of psychiatric rehabilitation.* Amherst, MA: Human Resource Development Press.

Arieti, S. (1967). *The intra-psychic self.* New York: Basic Books.

Ayres, A.J. (1973). *Sensory integration and learning disorders.* California: Western Psychological Services.

Azima, H. & Azima, F. (1959). Outline of a dynamic theory of occupational therapy. *American Journal of Occupational Therapy, 8*(5), 215.

Bahnson, C. (1980). Stress and cancer I: The state of the art. *Psychosomatics, 21*, 975.

Bahnson, C. (1981). Stress and cancer II: The state of the art. *Psychosomatics, 22*, 207.

Baker, R.D. (1975). Behavioral techniques in the treatment of schizophrenia. In Forrest, A.D. & Affleck, J.W. (Eds.). *Handbook of schizophrenia.* Edinburgh: Churchhill Livingstone.

Barris, R., Watts, J., & Kielhofner, G. (1983). *Psychosocial occupational therapy: Practice in a pluralistic arena.* Laurel, MD: Ramsco Publishing Co.

Barry, P.D. (1984). *Psychosocial nursing assessment and intervention.* Philadelphia: J.B. Lippincott Co.

Baum, C. (1980). Occupational therapists put care in the health system. *American Journal of Occupational Therapy, 34*(8), 505-516.

Beck, A.T. (1967). *Depression: Clinical, experimental and theoretical aspects.* New York: Harper and Row.

Beck, A.T., Rush, A.J., Shaw, B.F., & Emery, G. (1979). *Cognitive therapy of depression.* New York: Guilford Press.

Bellack, A.S. & Hersen, M. (1977). Self-report inventories in behavioral assessment. In Done, J.D., Hawkins, R.P. (Eds.). *Behavioral assessment: New direction in clinical psychology.* New York: Brunner/Mazel.

Bellak, L. (1984). Basic aspects of ego function assessment (pp. 6-19). In Bellak, L. Goldsmith, L.A. (Eds.). *The broad scope of ego function assessment.* New York: John Wiley & Sons.

Bem, D.J., & Allen, A. (1974). On predicting some of the people some of the time: The search for cross-situational consistencies in behavior. *Psychological Review, 81*, 506-520.

Benson, J. & Clark, F. (1982). A guide for instrument development and validation. *American Journal of Occupational Therapy, 36*(12), 789-800.

Benton, A., Hamsher, K., Varney, N., et al. (1983). *Contributions to neuropsychological assessment: A clinical manual.* New York: Oxford University Press Inc.

Berscheid, E., Walster, E. & Bohrnstedt, G. (1973). The happy American body: A survey report. *Psychology Today,* Nov: 119-131.

Black, M. (1976). The adolescent role assessment. *American Journal of Occupational Therapy, 30*(4), 73-79.

Bloomer, J. & Williams, S. (1986). *Bay area functional performance evaluation (BaFPE): Task oriented assessment and social interaction scale manual.* San Francisco: USCF.

Boll, T.J. (1981). The Halstead-Reitan neuropsychological battery. In Filskov, S.B., & Boll, T.J. (Eds.). *Handbook of clinical neuropsychology.* New York: John Wiley & Sons.

Bond, J.E. (1986). Increasing motivation in the practice of occupational therapy. *Occupational Therapy Forum,* II (32), 22-24.

Bootzin, R. & Engle-Friedman, M. (1981). The assessment of insomnia. *Behavioral Assessment, 3,* 107-126.

Bornstein, P., Hamilton, S. & Bornstein, M.T. (1986). Self-monitoring procedures. In Ciminero, A., Calhoun, K. & Adams, H. (Eds.). (1986). *Handbook of behavioral assessment.* New York: John Wiley and Sons.

Brantley, P., & Bruce, B. (1986). Assessment in behavioral medicine. In Ciminero, A., Calhoun, K. & Adams, H. (Eds.). (1986). *Handbook of behavioral assessment (2nd ed.).* New York: John Wiley & Sons.

Braun, P.R. & Reynolds, D.N. (1969). A factor analysis of a 100 item fear survey inventory. *Behavioral Research & Therapy, 7,* 399-402.

Brayman, S. & Kirby, T. (1982). The comprehensive occupational therapy evaluation. In Hemphill, B. (Ed.). (1982). *The evaluation process in psychiatric occupational therapy.* Thorofare, NJ: Slack Inc.

Brenner, C. (1980). Metapsychology and psychoanalytic theory. *Psychoanalytic Quarterly, 49,* 189-214.

Bruce, M.A. & Borg, B. (1987). *Frames of reference in psychosocial occupational therapy.* Thorofare, NJ: Slack Inc.

Buck, J. & Jolles, I. (1972). *House-tree-person projective technique.* California: Western Psychological Services.

Burdock, E., Sudilovsky, A. & Gershon, S. (1982). *The behavior of psychiatric patients.* New York: Marcel Dekker Inc.

Buros, O.K. (1970). *Personality tests and reviews.* Highland Park, NJ: Gryphon Press.

Buros, O.K. (1972). *The seventh mental measurements yearbook, vols. 1 & 2.* Highland Park, NJ: Gryphon Press.

Casanova, J.S. & Ferber, J. (1976). Comprehensive evaluation of basic living skills. *American Journal of Occupational Therapy, 30*(2), 101-105.

Churchman, C.W. (1979). *The systems approach.* New York: Dell Publishing.

Ciminero, A., Calhoun, K. & Adams, H. (1986). *Handbook of behavioral assessment.* New York: John Wiley & Sons.

Ciminero, A.R., Nelson, R.O. & Lipinski, D.P. (1977). Self-monitoring procedures. In Ciminero, A.R., Calhoun, K.S. & Adams, H.E. (Eds.). *(1986) Handbook of behavioral assessment.* New York: John Wiley & Sons.

Cohen, B. & Anthony, W.A. (1984). Functional assessment in psychiatric rehabilitation (pp. 79-100). In Halpern, A. & Fuhrer, M. (Eds.). Functional assessment in rehabilitation. Baltimore: Brookes Publishing Co.

Cohn, R. (1960). *The person symbol in clinical medicine.* Springfield, IL: Charles C. Thomas.

Coleman, R.E. (1981). Cognitive behavioral treatment of agoraphobia. In Emery, G., Hollon, S. & Bedrosian, R.C. (Eds.). *New directions in cognitive therapy: A casebook.* (pp. 101-119). New York: Guilford Press.

Collins, L.B. (1984). The role of the clinical social worker on the rehabilitation team. In *Rehabilitation psychology.* (pp. 183-192) Rockville, MD: Aspen Systems Corporation. ration.

Cone, J.D. (1981). Psychometric considerations (pp. 33-68). In Herson, M. & Bellack, A. (Eds.). *Behavioral assessment (2nd ed.).* New York: Pergamon Press.

Cormier, W.H. & Cormier, L.S. (1979). *Interviewing strategies for helpers: A guide to assessment, treatment and evaluation.* Monterey, CA: Brooks/Cole.

Coulton, C. (1984). Person-environment fit and rehabilitation. In *Rehabilitation psychology.* (pp. 119-129) Rockville, MD: Aspen Systems Corporation.

Cromwell, F.S. (1965). *Occupational therapists' manual for basic skill assessment: Primary prevocational evaluation.* Pasadena, CA: Fair Oaks Printing Co.

Cronbach, L.J. (1984). *Essentials of psychological testing (4th ed.).* New York: Harper & Row Publishers.

Cronbach, L.J., Gleser, G.C., Nanda, H. & Rajarathnam, N. (1972). *The dependability of behavioral measures.* New York: John Wiley & Sons.

Cronbach, L.J. (1980). Validity on parole: How can we go straight? *New Directions for Testing and Measurement, 5,* 99-108.

Cubie, S. & Kaplan, K. (1982). A case analysis method for the model of human occupation. *American Journal of Occupational Therapy, 36*(10), 645-652.

Cummings, E. & Henry, W.E. (1961). *Growing old: The process of disengagement.* New York: Basic Books.

Dellario, D., Goldfield, E., Farkas, M. & Cohen, M. (1984). Functional assessment of psychiatrically disabled adults. In Halpern, A. & Fuhrer, M. (Eds.). *Functional assessment in rehabilitation.* (pp. 239-252) Baltimore, MD: Brookes Publishing Co.

Denton, P. (1986). *Psychiatric occupational therapy: A workbook of practical skills.* Boston: Little, Brown.

Derogatis, L.R. (1977). *Manual for SCL-90: Administration, scoring and procedures manual II.* Baltimore, MD: Clinical Psychometric Research.

Devereaux, E. (1984). Occupational therapy's challenge: The caring relationship. *American Journal of Occupational Therapy, 38*(12), 791-798.

Doneson, I.R. (1984). The role of the physical therapist in emotional rehabilitation. In *Rehabilitation psychology.* (pp. 201-212) Rockville, MD: Aspen Systems Corporation.

Dubovsky, S. (1988). *Clinical psychiatry.* Washington, DC: American Psychiatric Press, Concise Guides Series.

Dundon, D.H. (1963). Psychiatric occupational therapy. In Williard, H. & Spackman, C. *Occupational therapy*. Philadelphia: J.B Lippincott Co.

Dunn, W. & McGourty (1989). Application of uniform terminology to practice. *American Journal of Occupational Therapy*, 43, 817-831.

Educational Testing Service (ETS). *News on tests*. Princeton, NJ: Author.

Educational Testing Service (ETS). *Tests on microfiche*. Princeton, NJ: Author.

Emery, G., Hollon, S. & Bedrosian, R. (Eds.). (1981). *New directions in cognitive therapy: A casebook*. New York: Guilford Press.

Fidler, G.S. (1982). The activity laboratory: A structure for observing and assessing perceptual, integrative and behavioral strategies. In Hemphill, B. *The evaluative process in psychiatric occupational therapy*. (pp. 195-207) Thorofare, NJ: Slack Inc.

Fidler, G. (1988). The life style performance profile. In Robertson, S. (Ed.). *Mental health focus: Skills for assessment and treatment*. Rockville, Maryland: American Occupational Therapy Association.

Fidler, G., & Fidler, J. (1963). *Occupational therapy: A communication process in psychiatry*. New York: Macmillan Co.

Fike, M.L. (1984). The role of occupational therapy in psychological rehabilitation of the physically disabled. In *Rehabilitation psychology*. (pp. 221-233) Rockville, MD: Aspen Systems Corporation.

Florey, L. & Michelman, S. (1982). Occupational role history: Screening tool for psychiatric occupational therapy. *American Journal of Occupational Therapy*, 36(5), 301-308.

Frank, L. (1939). Projective methods for the study of personality. *Journal of Psychology*, 8, 389-413.

Frey, W. (1984). Functional assessment in the 80's. In Halpern, A. & Fuhrer, M. (Eds.). *Functional assessment in rehabilitation*. (pp. 11-43) Baltimore: Brookes Publishing Co.

Gates, C. (1978). *A manual for cancer*. Boston: American Cancer Society.

Gillette, N. (1971). Occupational therapy and mental health. In Willard, H. & Spackman, C. (Eds.). *Occupational therapy*. Philadelphia: J.B. Lippincott Co.

Goldfried, M.E. & Kent, R.N. (1972). Traditional versus behavioral personality assessment: A comparison of methodological and theoretical assumptions. *Psychological Bulletin*, 77, 409-420.

Goldsmith, L.A. (1984). Ego function assessment considered in relation to current issues in psychoanalytic theory. In Bellak, L. & Goldsmith, L.A. (Eds.). *The broad scope of ego function assessment*. (pp. 31-68) New York: John Wiley & Sons.

Goleman, D. (1985). *Vital lies, simple truths: The psychology of self perception*. New York: Simon & Schuster.

Goleman, D. (1987). Who are you kidding? *Psychology Today*, 21(3), 24-30.

Goodenough, F.L. (1949). *Mental testing*. New York: Rinehart.

Greer, J.H. (1965). The development of a scale to measure fear. *Behavioral Research & Therapy*, 3, 45-53.

Grossman, W.I. (1967). Reflections on the relationship of introspection to psychoanalysis. *International Journal of Psychoanalysis*, 48, 16-31.

Halstead-Reitan neuropsychological test battery. Reitan Neuropsychology Laboratories, University of Arizona.

Harris, D.B. (1963). *Children's drawings as measures of intellectual maturity: A revision and extension of the Goodenough Draw-A-Man Test*. New York: Harcourt, Brace and World.

Hemphill, B.J. (Ed.). (1982). *The evaluative process in psychiatric occupational therapy*. Thorofare, NJ: Slack Inc.

Hemphill, B.J. (Ed.). (1988). *Mental health assessment in occupational therapy*. Thorofare, NJ: Slack Inc.

Henry, A.D., Delson, D. & Duncombe, L.W. (1984). Choice making in group and individual activity. *American Journal of Occupational Therapy*, 38(4), 245-251.

Holland, J.L. (1982). *The self directed search manual*. Palo Alto, CA: Consulting Psychologist Press.

Hollis, L.I. (1974). Skinnerian occupational therapy. *American Journal of Occupational Therapy*, 28(4), 203-213.

Hollon, S. (1981). Cognitive-behavioral treatment of drug induced pansituational anxiety states. In Emery, G., Hollon, S., Bedrosian, R.C. (Eds.). *New directions in cognitive therapy: A casebook*. (pp. 120-138) New York: Guilford Press.

Hollon, S.D. & Bemis, K.M. (1981). Self report and the assessment of cognitive functions. In Herson, M., Bellack, A. (Eds.). *Behavioral Assessment, (2nd Ed)*. (pp. 124-174) New York: Pergamon Press.

Holmes, R. & Rahe, R. (1967). The social readjustment rating scale. *Journal of Psychosomatic Research*, 11, 213.

Honigfield, G., Gillis, R.D., & Klett, G.J. (1966). NOSIE-3, a treatment-sensitive ward behavior scale. *Psychological Reports*, 19, 180-182.

Hopkins, H.L. (1978). An historical perspective on occupational therapy. In H.L. Hopkins, H.D. Smith (Eds.). In *Willard & Spackman's Occupational Therapy (5th Ed.)*, Philadelphia: J.B. Lippincott Co.

Hutt, M.L. (1969). *The Hutt adaptation of the Bender-Gestalt Test (2nd Ed.)*. New York: Grune and Stratton.

Hutt, M.L. & Briskin, G. (1961). *The clinical use of the revised Bender-Gestalt Test*. New York: Grune and Stratton.

Jackoway, I., Rogers, J. & Snow, T. (1987). The role change assessment: An interview tool for evaluating older adults. *Occupational Therapy in Mental Health, 7*(1), 17-38.

James, M., & Jongward, D. (1971). *Born to win: Transactional analysis with Gestalt experiments.* Reading, MA: Addison-Wesley Publishing Co.

Jampala, V.C., Frederick, S.S. & Michael, A.T. (1986). Consumers' views of DSM-III: Attitudes and practices of U.S. psychiatrists and 1984 graduating psychiatric residents. *American Journal of Psychiatry, 143*, 148-153.

Jemmott, J.B. & Locke, S.E. (1984). Psychosocial factors, immunologic mediation and human susceptibility to infectious disease: How much do we know? Psychological Bulletin, 95, 78-108.

Jensen, B.J., & Haynes, S.N. (1986). Self-report questionnaires and inventories. In Ciminero, A., Calhoun, K. & Adams, H. *Handbook of behavioral assessment.* (pp. 150-175) New York: John Wiley & Sons.

Kahana, R. & Bibring, G. (1964). Personality types in medical management. In Zinberg, N. (Ed.). *Psychiatry and medical practice in a general hospital.* New York: International Universities Press.

Kane, R. (1982). Lessons for social work from the medical model: A viewpoint for practice. *Social Work, 27*, 315-321.

Kaplan, H., & Sadock, B. (1988). *Modern Synopsis of Comprehensive Psychiatry V (5th ed.).* Baltimore, Williams & Wilkins.

Karoly, P. & Kanfer, F.H. (Eds.). (1981). *Self management and behavior change: From theory to practice.* New York: Pergamon Press Inc.

Kazdin, A.E. (1981). Behavioral observation . In Herson, M. & Bellack, A. (Eds.). *Behavioral assessment (2nd ed.).* (pp. 101-124) New York: Pergamon Press Inc.

Kazdin, A.E. (1974). Self-monitoring and behavior change. In Mahoney, M.J. & Thoresen, C.E. (Eds.). *Self-control: Power to the person.* Monterey, CA: Brooks/Cole.

Kendell, R.E. (1980). Book review, American Psychiatric Association, diagnostic and statistical manual of mental disorders (3rd ed.). *American Journal of Psychiatry, 137*, 1630-1631.

Kielhofner, G. (Ed.). (1985). *A model of human occupation: Theory and application.* Baltimore: Williams and Wilkins.

Kielhofner, G., & Burke, J.P. (1985). Components and determinants of human occupation. In Kielhofner (Ed.). *Model of human occupation: Theory and application.* (pp. 12-36) Baltimore: Williams and Wilkins.

King, L.J. (1982). The person symbol as an assessment tool. In Hemphill, B.J. (Ed.). *The evaluative process in psychiatric occupational therapy.* (pp. 169-194) Thorofare, NJ: Slack Inc.

King, L.J. (1988). Occupational therapy and neuropsychiatry. In Robertson, S. (Ed.). *Mental health focus: Skills for assessment and treatment.* (pp. 3-52, 3-59) Rockville, MD: American Occupational Therapy Association.

Kluckhohn, D., Murray, H.A., & Schneider, D.M. (Eds.). (1953). *Personality in Nature, Society and Culture.* New York: Knopf.

Lazarus, A.A. (1976). Multimodal Behavior Therapy: Treating the ''BASIC ID.'' *Journal of Nervous & Mental Disease, 156*, 404-411.

Lazarus, R. (1977). Cognitive and coping processes in emotion. In Monat, A., Lazarus, R. (Eds.). *Stress and Coping: An anthology,* New York: Columbia University Press.

Leff, J.P. (1978). Psychiatrists' versus patients' concepts of unpleasant emotions. *British Journal of Psychiatry, 133*, 306-313.

Leondardelli, C. (1988). The Milwaukee Evaluation of Daily Living Skills (MEDLS). In Hemphill, B. (Ed.). *Mental health assessment in occupational therapy.* (pp. 151-162) Thorofare, NJ: Slack Inc.

Lerner, C. (1979). The magazine picture collage: Its clinical use and validity as an assessment device. *American Journal of Occupational Therapy, 33*, 500-504.

Lerner, C., & Ross, G. (1977). The magazine picture collage: The development of an objective scoring system. *American Journal of Occupational Therapy, 31*, 156-161.

Lerner, E.A. (1972). *The projective use of the Bender-Gestalt.* Springfield, IL: Charles C. Thomas.

Levinson, D. (1987). *A guide to the clinical interview.* Philadelphia: W.B. Saunders Co.

Lindzey, G. (1959). On the classification of projective techniques. *Psychology Bulletin, 56*, 158-168.

Lindzey, G. (1961). *Projective techniques and cross-cultural research.* New York: Appleton-Century-Crofts.

Llorens, L. (1984). Theoretical conceptualizations of occupational therapy: 1960-1982. *Occupational Therapy in Mental Health, 4*, 1-14.

Lorr, M. & Vestre, N.D. (1968). *The psychotic in-patient profile manual.* Los Angeles: Western Psychological Services.

Lubin, B. (1967). *Manual for the depression adjective checklists.* San Diego: Educational and Industrial Testing Source.

Machover, K. (1949). *Personality projection in the drawing of the human figure.* Springfield, IL: Charles C. Thomas.

Mack, J.L. (1969). Behavior ratings of recidivist and nonrecidivist delinquent males. *Psychological Reports, 25*, 260.

MacKinnon, R.A. & Michels, R. (1971). *The psychiatric*

interview in clinical practice. Philadelphia: W.B. Saunders Co.

MacKinnon, R.A. & Yudofsky, S.A. (1986). *The evaluation in clinical practice*. Philadelphia: J.B. Lippincott Co.

Mahoney, M.J. (Ed.). (1980). *Psychotherapy Process: Current Issues and Future Directions,* New York: Plenum Press.

Margolin, G. & Jacobson, N.S. (1981). Assessment of marital dysfunction. In Herson, M. & Bellack, A. (Eds.). *Behavioral assessment.* (pp. 389-426) New York: Pergamon Press Inc.

Matsutsuyu, J. (1969). The interest checklist. *American Journal of Occupational Therapy, 23*(4), 323-328.

McCarthy, J.M., & Paraskevopoulos, J. (1969). Behavior patterns of learning disabled, emotionally disturbed and average children. *Exceptional Children, 36,* 69-74.

Melamed, B., & Siegel, L. (1975). Reduction of anxiety in children facing hospitalization and surgery by use of filmed modeling. *Journal of Consulting & Clinical Psychology, 43,* 511-521.

Melvin, J.L. (1977). *Rheumatic disease: Occupational therapy and rehabilitation*. Philadelphia: FA Davis Co.

Messick, S. (1975). The standard problem: Meaning and values in measurement and evaluation. *American Psychologist, 30,* 955-966.

Miller, E.R. & Paracheck, J.F. (1974). Validation and standardization of a goal-oriented, quick screening geriatric scale. *Journal of American Geriatric Sociology, 22,* 278-283.

Mischel, W. (1968). *Personality assessment*. New York: John Wiley & Sons.

Moorehead, L. (1969). The occupational history. *American Journal of Occupational Therapy, 23*(4), 329-336.

Moos, R.H. (1970). Differential effects of psychiatric ward settings on patient change. *Journal of Nervous & Mental Diseases, 151,* 316-322.

Morey, L.C., & Blashfield, R.K. (1981). A symptom analysis of the DSM-III definitions of schizophrenia. *Schizophrenia Bulletin, 7,* 258-268.

Morey, L.C., Skinner, H. & Blashfield, R.K. (1986). Trends in the classification of abnormal behavior. In Ciminero A., Calhoun, K. & Adams, H. *Handbook of behavioral assessment (2nd ed.)*. NY: John Wiley & Sons.

Morganstern, K.P. & Tevlin, H.E. (1981). Behavioral interviewing. In Herson, M., Bellack, A. (Eds.). *Behavioral assessment, (2nd ed.).* (pp. 3-37) New York: Pergamon Press.

Mosey, A.C. (1970). *Three frames of reference for mental health*. Thorofare, NJ: Slack Inc.

Mosey, A. (1973). *Activities therapy*. New York: Raven Press Publishers.

Mosey, A.C. (1981). *Occupational therapy: Configuration of a profession*. New York: Raven Press.

Mosey, A.C. (1986). *Psychosocial components of occupational therapy*. New York: Raven Press.

Murray, R.G. & Hobbs, S.A. (1981). Effects of self-reinforcement and self-punishment in smoking reduction: Implications for broad-spectrum behavioral approaches. *Addictive Behaviors, 6,* 63-67.

Nelson, R.O., & Hayes, S.C. (1981). Nature of behavioral assessment,. In Herson, M., & Bellack, A. (Eds.). *Behavioral assessment, (2nd ed.).* (p. 3-37) New York: Pergamon Press.

Nietzel, M.T. & Bernstein, D.A. (1981). Assessment of anxiety and fear. In Hersen, M. & Bellack; A. (Eds.). *Behavioral assessment.* (pp. 215-245) New York: Pergamon Press Inc.

Nelson, R.O., Lipinski, D.P. & Boykin, R.A. (1978). The effects of self recorder's training and the obtrusiveness of the self recording device on the accuracy and reactivity of self monitoring. *Behavior Therapy, 9,* 200-208.

Noles, S., Cash, T. & Winstead, B. (1985). Body image, physical attractiveness, and depression. *Journal of Consulting & Clinical Psychology, 53*(1), 88-94.

Noy, P. (1977). Metapsychology as a multimodel system. *International Review of Psychoanalysis, 4,* 1-12.

Oakley, F., Kielhofner, G., Barris, R. & Reichler, R. (1986). The role checklist: Development and empirical assessment of reliability. *Occupational Therapy Journal of Research, 6*(3), 157-170.

O'Kane, C.P. (1969). *The Development of a Projective Technique for Use in Psychiatric Occupational Therapy*. New York: University of New York at Buffalo.

Ornstein, R. & Sobel, D. (1984). *The healing brain: A new perspective on the brain and health*. New York: Simon & Schuster.

Peloquin, S. (1983). The development of an occupational therapy interview/therapy set procedure. *American Journal of Occupational Therapy, 37*(7), 457-461.

Peterson, D.R. (1968). *The clinical study of social behavior*. New York: Appleton-Century-Crofts.

Pfeiffer, J.W. & Jones, J.E. (Eds.). (1973). *A handbook of structured experiences for human relations training, (vol. IV)*. (pp. 41-44). La Jolla, CA: University Associates Publishers & Consultants.

Prelinger, E. & Zimet, C.N. (1964). *An ego-psychological approach to character assessment*. London: Free Press of Glencoe, Collier-MacMillan Ltd.

Proger, B.B., Mann, L., Green, P.A., Bayuk, R.J., & Burger, R.M. (1975). Discriminators of clinically defined emotional maladjustment: Predictive validity of the Behavior Problem Checklist and the Devereux scales. *Journal of Abnormal and Child Psychology, 3,* 71-82.

Quay, H.C. (1977). Measuring dimensions of deviant behavior: The behavior problem checklist. *Journal of*

Abnormal and Child Psychology, 5, 277-289.

Quay, H.C., & Peterson, D.R. (1967). *Manual for the Behavior Problem Checklist*, Champaign: University of Illinois Children's Research Center.

Reed, K. (1984). *Models of practice in occupational therapy*. Baltimore: Williams & Wilkins.

Rehm, L.P. (1981). Assessment of depression,. In Hersen, M. & Bellack, A. (Eds.). *Behavioral assessment,* (p. 246-295) New York: Pergamon Press.

Reiser, M. (1984). *Mind, brain, body: Toward a convergence of psychoanalysis and neurobiology*. New York: Basic Books.

Reisman, J.R. (1976). *Story of clinical psychology (enlarged edition)*. New York: Irvington Publishers Inc.

Reynolds, C.R. & Gutkin, T.B. (1982). *The handbook of school psychology*. New York: John Wiley & Sons.

Ross, M. & Burdick, D. (1981). *Sensory integration: A training manual for therapists and teachers for regressed, psychiatric and geriatric patient groups*. Thorofare, NJ: Slack Inc.

Scheff, T. (Ed.). (1975). *Labeling madness*. Englewood Cliffs, NJ: Prentice Hall.

Scheff, T. (1984). *Being mentally ill*. New York: Aldine Publishing Co.

Schroeder, C.V., Block, M.P., Campbell, I., Trottier, E. & Stowell, M.S. (1978). *Schroeder, Block, Campbell adult psychiatric sensory integration evaluation (2nd experimental edition)*. La Jolla, CA: "SBC" Research Associates, Psychiatric Occupational Therapy.

Selye, H. (1976). *Stress in health and disease*. Boston: Butterworth & Co.

Selye, H. (1979aa). Stress without distress. In Garfield, C. (Ed.). *Stress and survival: The emotional realities of life-threatening illness*. St. Louis: C.V. Mosby.

Shaw, C. (1982). The interview process,. In Hemphill, B.J. (Ed). *The evaluative process in psychiatric occupational therapy*. (p. 15-42) Thorofare, NJ: Slack Inc.

Simmons, J.E. (1987). *Psychiatric examination of children (4th ed)*. Philadelphia: Lea & Febiger.

Spahn, R. (1969). The patient gets busy: Change or Progress? In Evaluation Procedures in Occupational Therapy. Illinois Council on Practice, Region IV, American Occupational Therapy Association, May 1969.

Speer, D.C. (1971). The behavior problem checklist (Peterson-Quay): Baseline data from parents of child guidance and nonclinic children. *Journal of Consulting & Clinical Psychology, 36*, 221-228.

Spiegler, M. & Agigian, H. (1977). *The community training center: An educational behavioral social systems model for rehabilitating psychiatric patients*. New York: Brunner/Mazel.

Spitzer, R.L., Williams, J.B. & Skodol, A.E. (Eds.). (1983). *International perspectives on DSM-III*. Washington, D.C.: American Psychiatric Press Inc.

Stuart, R.B. (Ed.). (1977). *Behavioral self management: Strategies, techniques and outcomes*. New York: Brunner/Mazel.

Sundberg, N.D. (1977). *Assessment of persons*. Englewood Cliffs, NJ: Prentice Hall.

Sweetland, R.C. & Keyser, D.J. (1984-85). *Test critiques (vol. 1-5)*. Kansas City: Test Corporation of America.

Sweetland, R.C. & Keyser, D.J. (Eds.). (1986). *Tests — a comprehensive reference for assessments in psychology, education and business (2nd ed.)*. Kansas City: Test Corporation of America.

Turkat, I.D. (1986). The behavioral interview. In Ciminero, A., Calhoun, K. & Adams, H. (Eds.). *Handbook of behavioral assessment (2nd ed.)*. New York: John Wiley & Sons.

Twentyman, C.T. & McFall, R.M. (1975). Behavior training of social skills in shy males. *Journal of Consulting & Clinical Psychology, 43*, 384-395.

Usdin, G. & Lewis, (Eds.). (1978). *Psychiatry in general medicine practice*. New York: McGraw-Hill.

Verbrugge, L. (1980). Health diaries. *Medical Care, 18*, 73.

Watson, L.J. (1986). Psychiatric consultation — liaison in the acute physical disabilities setting. *American Journal of Occupational Therapy, 40*(5), 338-342.

Watts, F. & Bennett, D. (1983). Introduction: The concepts of rehabilitation. In Watts, F. & Bennett, D. (Eds.). *Theory and practice of psychiatric rehabilitation*. (pp. 3-14) New York: John Wiley & Sons.

Weiss, P. (1969). The living system: Determinism stratified. In Koestler, A., Smythies, J.R. (Eds.). *Beyond reductionism: New perspectives in the life sciences*. (pp. 3-55) Boston: Beacon Press

Wiggins, J.S. (1973). *Personality and prediction: Principles of personality assessment*. Reading, MA: Addison Wesley.

Willard, H., & Spackman, C. (1963). *Occupational Therapy*. Philadelphia: J.B. Lippincott Co.

Winston, B.A. & Cash, T.F. (1984). *Reliability and validity of the Body-Self Relations Questionnaire: A new measure of body image*. New Orleans, Louisiana: Paper presented at the Southeastern Psychological Association Convention.

Winston, J. (1985). *Brain and psyche: The biology of the unconscious*. Doubleday.

Wolpe, J. & Lang, P.J. (1964). A fear survey schedule for use in behavior therapy. *Behavior Research & Therapy, 2, 27-30.*

World Health Organization. (1979). *International Classification of Diseases,* (9th Ed.) Geneva: Author

Yerxa, E. (1978). The philosophical base of occupational therapy. In *Occupational Therapy: 2001 A.D.* Rockville, Maryland: American Occupational Therapy Association.

Young, J.E. (1981). Cognitive therapy and loneliness. In Emery, G., Hollon, S. & Bedrosian, R.C. (Eds.). *New directions in cognitive therapy: A casebook.* (pp.139-159) New York: Guilford Press.

Zlutnick, S. & Taylor, C. (1982). Chronic pain. In Doleys, D., Meredith, R. & Ciminero, A. (Eds.). *Behavioral medicine: assessment and treatment strategies.* New York: Plenum.

Zohn, J.C. & Bornstein, R.H. (1980). Self-monitoring of work performance with mentally retarded adults: Effects upon work productivity, work quality and on task behavior. *Mental Retardation, 18,* 19-25.

Zukav, G (1979). The Dancing Wuli Masters: An overview of the new physics. New York: Morrow.

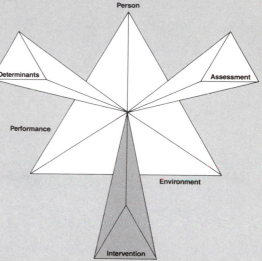

Section Four

Intervention Strategies

CHAPTER CONTENT OUTLINE

KEY TERMS

Bilateral integration

Equipment

Graded activity

Gratification

Proprioception

Self-care activities

Sex identification

Structured activities

Reality testing

Unstructured activities

ABSTRACT

This chapter focuses on the therapeutic use of activities, particularly the use of activities with meaning and added purpose (occupation) in helping to prevent or remediate dysfunction and maximize adaptation. The chapter explores how adaptation occurs, beginning with the use of activities of the performance hierarchy, progressing to the use of tasks, and lastly the performance of social roles. The chapter concludes with a discussion of the ways in which the components of performance and the therapeutic ''doing'' process are inextricably linked to the environment.

Occupation as a Therapeutic Medium
A Contextual Approach to Performance Intervention

22

Ruth E. Levine
Caroline R. Brayley

"Occupation is the very life of life."

—Harold Bell Wright, 1928

"The occupational therapy department constitutes a school of behavior in which patients, whose lives have become disorganized, are readjusted to their environment and set going again in normal channels."

—Horatio M. Pollack, 1927

OBJECTIVES

The information in this chapter is intended to help the reader—

1. appreciate the value of activities and tasks in remediating performance deficits and facilitating adaptation.

2. review historical antecedents to the use of occupation in promoting well-being.

3. appreciate how the use of occupation as therapy has changed during various periods during the profession's evolution.

4. identify important sociocultural dimensions of activity engagement.

5. list a range of factors which should be considered in activity analysis.

6. understand the rationale underlying the occupational therapist's choice of intervention in specific case descriptions.

7. review concepts related to occupational adaptation.

8. identify specific dimensions for classifying tasks.

INTRODUCTION

This chapter will focus on a fundamental process in occupational therapy— the therapeutic use of activities. It is useful to begin our exploration of this intervention strategy by considering a case study:

Case Study 22-1

Bruce Walker drove a truck for a major food company. Union wages and his overtime allowed him to command a high salary. Mr. Walker was a high school dropout and his reading and writing skills were poor, but he learned to cope with problems by being tenacious and by using his fists. His brother was a lawyer, and he took pride in the fact that he and his brother earned equally high incomes.

Mr. Walker's success came to a tragic end when he fell and fractured his scaphoid, underwent a bone graft, and suffered a subsequent non-union and then a successful graft. After the successful union, he continued to focus on the pain although there was no apparent reason for his discomfort. He was idle most of the day and began to lose contact with his family and job since he focused all his attention on his wrist (Kolman, 1987, p. 12).

Mr. Walker needed help. Although his wrist was medically cured and tests proved no inflammation was evident, he suffered from occupational dysfunction. His loss of role and deteriorated habits created a situation where he might never regain sufficient confidence to return to his previous work situation and lifestyle. Such a case of occupational dysfunction could benefit from the use of an intervention strategy involving the use of goal-directed activity.

The purpose of this chapter is to explain how occupational therapists use activities and tasks, to promote the highest degree of competence in an individual's life roles. We will start with an overview of the occupational therapy process, in which basic concepts and terms will be defined. A four-part conceptual hierarchy will be presented in which occupation and the environment are considered as an interdependent Gestalt, consistent with the general conceptual scheme of this text.

Occupational therapists use occupations in a highly specialized fashion so that people can attain improved functional performance. In short, occupational therapists are concerned with helping people to overcome performance deficits so they can achieve their life roles.

An effective activity program has both therapeutic and energizing power. The concept of occupation or goal-directed activity seems deceptively simple, yet it is profoundly complex. People, as doers, are so dependent on meaningful occupation that they often overlook just how important activities are to a satisfying and productive life. This importance seems to be tied to the perceived value of an activity, based on intrinsic and extrinsic factors that are related to the an individual's life roles (Christiansen, et al., 1988; Burke, 1977, 1983; Rotter, 1966; & Florey, 1969).

The doing process, which necessarily involves activity, has been the basis for occupational therapy practice since the profession emerged during the Progressive Era at the end of the 19th Century. Occupational therapy is based on the pragmatic philosophy of William James and John Dewey (Breines, 1987; Diasio-Serrett, 1985). From colonial times to the present, we maintain that individuals promote their own well-being by active participation in meaningful activity.

HISTORICAL OVERVIEW OF GOAL-DIRECTED BEHAVIOR

Occupation and the Arts and Crafts Movement

At the turn of the century, the term occupation was so commonplace that it was frequently mentioned in popular and scholarly literature. In fact, the word occupation was used so often that it was familiar to most educated people. This is much different from today, where few understand why the name occupational therapy reflects such a proud history. During this period, Americans were stressed and harassed; longing for a simpler life where they could return to basics and avoid the harried aspects of daily living. Essays appeared in newspapers, magazines, and books discussing the importance of occupation. Craft clubs, religious groups, and self-help groups implemented these ideas in an effort to promote health. Many people wove fabric, built furniture, created clay pots, hand-bound books, carved ornaments, and designed rooms and buildings in an effort to improve their lives (Lears, 1981; Beard, 1972; Boris, 1986; Kaplan, 1987).

These ideas were commonplace because of a lay health movement called the Arts and Crafts movement which swept across America from 1895 to 1920. The movement began in England during the 1850s and the movement's founder, John Ruskin and his follower William Morris, believed that industrialization compromised the human spirit because work was no longer completed in whole tasks but divided into meaningless, repetitive steps that were performed over and over again by the same person (Ruskin, 1884a, 1884b; Lears, 1981; Rodgers, 1974). In contrast, Ruskin and Morris believed that meaningful work was done by craftsmen who created Gothic cathedrals because they were involved in the product throughout their lives and could gain satisfaction from their accomplishments.

American dissatisfaction stemmed from the industrialization of the workplace, the influx of immigrants, the numerous financial panics of the 1890s, and changes in small town life and in the family (Burnham, 1972; Griffith, 1984; Wiebe, 1967; Wright, 1980). Thus, the ideals of the arts and crafts movement were adopted across America as a panacea for the stress of life. Prominent social reformers such as Jane Addams, Adolf Meyer, Clifford Beers, John Dewey, and Julia Lathrop applied the principles of the arts and crafts movement to their reform work. Crafts were used to teach immigrants good citizenship, a sense of self-worth and to prepare them for a worker role (Addams, 1920, 1935; Boris, 1986; Rodgers, 1974).

Americans, less opposed to industrialization than their British counterparts, interpreted the arts and crafts movement aesthetically. Instead of criticizing the social order and economic structure of society, many arts and crafts proponents focused on design, hand-made goods and their environment to improve daily life (Boris, 1986; Kaplan, 1987; Lears, 1981; Rodgers, 1974). According to the movement, a well-designed and beautifully executed project could help to center frenzied lives and cure poor habits. Environment could compromise or improve one's health, and an open, simply designed home or apartment could even improve moral character (Kaplan, 1987; Lears, 1981).

Occupation as Therapy

Occupational therapy founders applied the ideology of the arts and crafts movement to the treatment of individuals who were either mentally or physically disabled. Occupations were prescribed by progressive physicians and carried out with mental patients by nurses, social workers, or occupation or craft teachers.

Occupations were goal-directed, aesthetically designed activities that promoted the love of creation in every life task. Activities were presented so the child would learn to love active involvement in life. Mothers were responsible for making routine tasks interesting by using imagination "to rouse and excite his (or her) activity" (Washburne, 1915, p. 93). In addition to using household chores, other means such as toys, weaving, sewing, drawing, and painting were used to instill the appropriate attitude toward work, self-care, and leisure. Thus, the work ethic was a fundamental aspect of the arts and crafts movement. Values such as the following united the diverse individuals attracted to this movement:

1. Work could be made interesting by actively engaging the person's interest through the use of conversation and images related to the activity (Tracy, 1912).
2. Work must never bring on fatigue nor should individuals be allowed to "stop when they please" (Washburne, 1915, p. 94).
3. Role models must set an example of "willing industry" (ibid).
4. Monotony was detrimental and intellectual insights should constantly be offered (Ruskin, 1884a, 1884b; Dunton, 1918; Washburne, 1915; Slagle, 1922).
5. The child should learn the relationship between the larger world and daily routine (Washburne, 1915, p. 95).
6. Work was to be well-designed and attractive; the end product was important and must reflect the values of craftsmanship (Boris, 1986; Kaplan, 1987; Lears, 1981; Levine, 1987).
7. Nagging was counterproductive because it did not nurture the right attitude toward working (Washburne, 1915, p. 96).
8. Habits were the building blocks of the development of moral character (Slagle, 1922; Washburne, 1915).

Emergence of Occupational Therapy

The first occupational therapy text, written by Susan Tracy, a nurse; delineated the importance of understanding the patient's environment, lifestyle, values, interests, and roles (Tracy, 1912). Practice was directed toward motivating individuals by providing an occupation that stimulated interests and lead to an adjustment to their disability. During this time, scientists believed that people possessed a limited amount of energy. Once energy was used, it had to be replenished (Fuller, 1912; Dunton, 1928; Rosenberg, 1961). For the person who was preoccupied with "premorbid" or unhealthy thoughts, the prescription of a meaningful activity would restore a natural life balance. Thus, early occupational therapists felt that the mind influenced the body but this influence was based on the view of the person as a closed system. Environmental influences were viewed as providing opportunities for adaptation so that individuals could balance their inner lives (Meyer, 1922).

At first, practice was based solely on eliciting interest in an activity. Therapists thought that interest formed the foundation for adaptation to disability. The correct working environment and the personality of the therapist were important because the patient needed to learn improved habits and roles.

HISTORICAL OVERVIEW OF ACTIVITY ANALYSIS

Early Practice Focused on Generating Patient's Interest

The founders based their prescription of activities on the patient's interests. In the introduction to the first occupational therapy text, Fuller (1912) maintained that a dozen kinds of activities may be suggested but without an effective therapist, "daily expression of interest," and adequately graded occupations the "work is either never begun, or, if begun, is soon thrown aside" (Tracy, 1912, p. 5). Thus, the founders were truly committed to the therapeutic nature of the activity process, using the activity, the individual's role, the environment, and the therapist as elements of motivation.

Activity analysis was general at first, reflecting the ideology of the arts and crafts movement (Committee on Installations and Advise, 1928). Any art or craft activity could be used to increase interest, but good design and dedication to the entire production task was imperative. Therapists searched for novel tasks that would capture the patient's attention. Examples included bookbinding, leather-craft, wrought iron work, ceramics, weaving, basketry, square dancing, gardening, puppetry, toy making, print making, needlecrafts, hooking rugs, blacksmithing, chair caning, wood turning, papercraft, cement pot construction, games and play activities, and self-care skills. (Figure 22-1)

The Beginning of the Profession

The work-cure gained popularity during World War I along with the growing concern for the deleterious effects of idleness on large numbers of disabled veterans. Therapists were recruited to work on the war front, and they soon proved the importance of the occupation cure (Reed & Sanderson, 1983). The War ended before a great number of therapists were put to work. Instead, many searched for positions where they could apply their knowledge and skills.

In 1917, a group of dedicated occupationists met in Clifton Springs, New York and founded the profession of occupational therapy (Hopkins, 1988; Reed & Sanderson, 1983). It was no surprise, given the popularity and

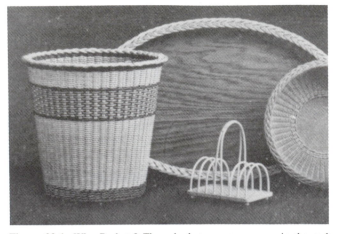

Figure 22-1. Why Baskets? These baskets were common in the early occupational therapy clinic. Basketry reflected the 'authentic' values of the arts and crafts movement. Using natural, high quality materials and good design, patients were encouraged to use their hands to center their lives. Occupational therapy was the amalgamation of this lay health movement and a medical process for helping the growing numbers of chronically impaired individuals.

widespread influence of the arts and crafts movement, that the founding group consisted of two architects, George Barton and William Kidner; an occupation teacher, Susan Johnson; a physician, William Rush Dunton; and a social worker, Eleanor Clarke Slagle. A nurse, Susan Tracy, was absent though invited to attend and was nevertheless given committee responsibilities

Early practice took place in mental hospitals, home health settings, manual training centers, schools for the handicapped child and hospitals. Early therapists were interested mostly in handicrafts and sought ways to prescribe occupations by medical diagnosis (Dunton, 1928; Haas, 1924; Sands, 1928). Modalities consisted of handicrafts, folk dancing, singing, gardening, bookbinding, games, sports, and plays. (Figure 22-2)

1930 to 1940: Crafts and Task Performance. As medical education shifted to a more scientific foundation, therapists tried even harder to match activity choices with the patient's medical diagnosis and functional problems. The activity analysis focused on the task, such as weaving, and the therapist's interpretation of what the patient could accomplish through this work. For example, metal hammering was prescribed for angry patients and not recommended for someone who was depressed.

Activity analysis became focused more narrowly as therapists searched for a prescription that could be dispensed like medication. The economic, social, and pragmatic pressures brought on by the Depression further obscured the importance of the motivational aspects of the activity process. Some therapists based activity assignments

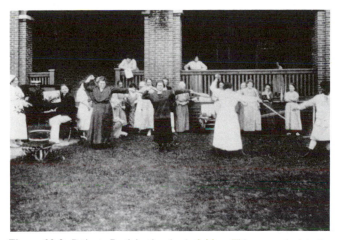

Figure 22-2. Patients Participating in Activities. This scene depicts the variety of activities that were used with patients. Here a piano is brought out of the ward and patients are encouraged to dance.

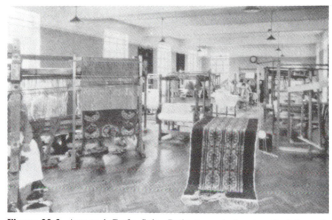

Figure 22-3. Arts and Crafts Sale. Patients made hand-crafted items in Occupational Therapy treatment and some of these items were sold to support the department. The sale of hand-made items was popular at the turn of the century since individuals were searching for activities or 'occupations' that centered their lives.

on their personal interests and skills. The patient's desire to pursue the task was considered, but since the arts and crafts ideology maintained that any well done occupation could bring satisfaction to the participant, the patient's values goals, motivation, and interests were not of central importance. This emphasis differed from the ideas offered by the founders of occupational therapy. Another seemingly contradictory idea was the sale of patient products to generate income for more patient supplies. Few therapists lost their jobs during the depression years, but they worked under pressure to deliver services to large numbers of patients, using projects that were developed from discarded or donated materials (scrap-craft). (Figure 22-3, 22-4)

In the thirty years since its formation, the profession had become an enigma to those who had not been part of the arts and crafts movement. Physicians whose medical education emphasized the inner workings of the mind, taught them to use sophisticated surgical techniques, and to develop scientific studies to prove the efficacy of their care, began to question whether weaving baskets could help their patients. One physician, who was familiar with the arts and crafts ideology, lamented that patients might participate more actively in therapy if they were more interested in the choice of occupation (Steckel, 1934). He recommended including the patient's roles, habits, and interests in the choice of activity.

Occupational therapists continued to focus on arts and crafts and on the products produced by patients because the joy of production was an important aspect of the arts and crafts ideology. This focus continued during World War II as occupational therapy expanded and physical dysfunction became more important. To help the physically disabled patient, therapists adopted a mechanical orientation toward movement and function. For example, weaving could reduce sensitivity in burned hands and hammering could strengthen weakened wrist muscles (McDonald, 1968; West, 1968). (Figure 22-5)

In psychiatry, therapists based their activity analysis on a Freudian interpretation of their patient's behavior. Working with clay could reveal a patient's inner fears and weaving could offer order and comfort to an anxious patient (Wade, 1947). Therapists working in pediatrics offered their services as surrogate mothers to normalize the child's experience during prolonged hospital stays while continuing to function within the constraints of the medical system. Play activities such as toys and games were prescribed with

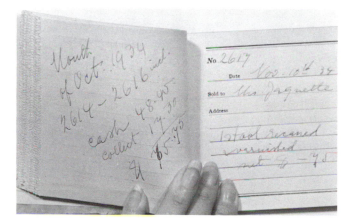

Figure 22-4. Receipt Book: Norristown State Hospital. This page demonstrates how early therapists kept track of their supply monies. The patients made projects that were sold for revenue for additional supplies. In some hospitals, patients had to buy their own supplies. Once a year the department would have a large sale to generate revenue.

consideration for appropriate developmental levels (Gleave, 1947).

During this period, the reasons for the arts and crafts activities became more unclear since students were taught basic science, liberal arts, and medical subjects during their education, but little information on why crafts were valued over other types of activities. The ideology of the once popular arts and crafts movement had long vanished from public interest. Therapists and patients began to question how craft activities could improve functional performance (Boris, 1986; Kaplan, 1987; Levine, 1987).

1940 to 1960s: Focus on Functional Performance and Rehabilitation. Rehabilitation medicine emerged during World War II and occupational therapists were considered valued members of the interdisciplinary team (Gritzer and Arluke, 1985; Licht, 1948). Therapists began to concentrate on activities of daily living, functional performance, household activities, and therapeutic exercise. Upper extremity prosthetic training was also important. Psychiatric specialists gathered and worked to develop theory that would improve the quality of clinical practice. Freudian theory was still widely used but therapists also began to consider social and psychological theories as a basis for practice. Medicine oriented toward acute care and most therapists worked in institutions.

The 1950s were a time of turmoil in the profession, partly because crafts were still the focus of treatment. The acute care orientation of medical training, which viewed patients as passive recipients of care; served to devalue the importance of activity; since patients in occupational therapy were expected to participate in their own healing process. Therapists began to question the value of certain treatment

approaches and leaders encouraged graduate education, research, and theory development.

In response, therapists tried to incorporate other activities into treatment and activity analysis forms reflected an in-depth analysis of the patient's interests. Most of the analysis was focused on either movement or interpretation of the patient's feelings; while little attention was directed toward the patient's values, goals, interests, roles, and habits. Therapists tried to concentrate on what the patient could do rather than on the healthful effect of occupations. The importance of motivation was deemphasized as therapists struggled to prescribe occupations from a functional perspective.

1960s to Present: Occupation and Goal-directed Activities. In the 1960s and 1970s, during a time of social dissent and activism in the United States, therapists began to question the activity basis of the profession. The health system was still oriented toward acute care, but the limitations of the health delivery system were discussed. Technology, once embraced as the answer to illness, now was viewed as a limited approach to promoting health. Self-care became popular as individuals slowly began to regard their health as a personal responsibility which could not be delegated to others without incurring a risk (Capra 1983; Ferguson, 1980; Illich, 1977; Laszlo, 1972; Mechanic 1979).

Medical practice continued to focus on technological advances and few practitioners offered restorative services. Reflecting society's interest in acute care, health care reimbursement was directly related to treatment that pro-

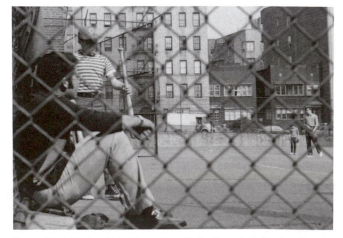

Figure 22-6. Playing Ball, Bronx New York: These individuals reflect the culture of urban living. The limitations of space are reflected in this ball field which is a school yard. Individuals must learn to share their space with many others. Games must be altered to deal with the many individuals who have the right to use the space. This is merely one aspect of the urban culture.

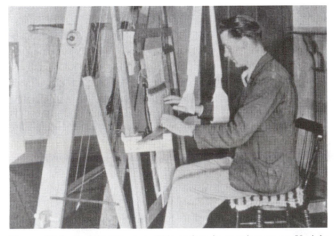

Figure 22-5. Upright Weaving. This patient is weaving on an Upright Loom. Note the similarity of this historical loom to those found in use today.

vided objective, measurable, physical changes with specific and narrow definitions of progress. These constraints splintered care for patients and healing was overlooked as a part of health delivery.

Occupational therapists, oriented to practice in an acute care focused delivery system, experienced conflict. On the one hand, they searched for specific modalities to promote independence and on the other hand, they valued a more holistic view of human performance. Therapists debated whether activities were important to patient care and how these activities should be used. Interest in the activity process was renewed and therapists began to explore the philosophy and beliefs of early practitioners (Diasio-Serrett, 1985; Kielhofner and Burke, 1977; Shannon, 1977).

Activity analysis became more complex as therapists began to move beyond a specific craft and functional orientation, to a multifaceted approach to dysfunction. Therapists began to consider the person's lifestyle and culture and the patient's motivation and capabilities. Research progressed and new ideas about the relationship between the nervous system and function began to influence practice (Ayres, 1966, 1969, 1979). Increasingly, therapists engaged in research and many earned graduate degrees (American Occupational Therapy Association, 1985). More specialty groups arose as therapists found that new information was available through continuing education workshops, graduate programs, publications, and research projects.

An increased number of therapists began to enter community settings such as workplaces, schools, community living centers, sheltered workshops, and geriatric facilities where they offered services for persons with chronic disabilities. Occupational therapists began to consider the person's lifestyle and culture and include the person receiving care in treatment planning. (Figures 22-6, 22-7, 22-8)

By 1980, work-related programming was becoming more important to the health care system, as the struggle began to contain escalating costs. Such programs were viewed as a cost-effective means to ease disabled persons into productive roles. At the same time, occupational therapists were gaining awareness of the impact of economics and politics on the profession and realized that their services needed to be promoted in an increasingly competitive health care marketplace. Product lines were developed and refined, and therapists participated in strategic planning activities to develop innovative approaches for meeting the emerging health needs of a changing society. Life skill training, work technology, leisure, driving, exercise, and fitness programs became more prevalent as therapists worked to secure their role in the rapidly changing, market-driven health care delivery system.

Today, the knowledge of occupation is based on research that links the physical, psychological, physiological, cognitive, and emotional factors of humans to performance of life roles. Occupation or goal-directed activity is a method to improve human performance in self-care, work, and play/leisure pursuits. As Reilly pointed out years ago, occupational therapy is one of the greatest ideas of the 20th century. (Reilly, 1962).

SYSTEMS THEORY

As introduced in Chapter 1, fundamental to an understanding of the use of activity as an intervention strategy in occupational therapy are concepts from general systems theory.

Systems theory or *general systems theory* (GST) (von

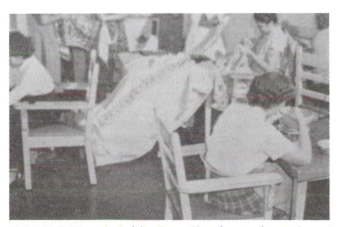

Figure 22-7. Women's Activity Group. Note the ceramic, weaving and sewing activities and compare these with the activities pictured in Figure 22-8.

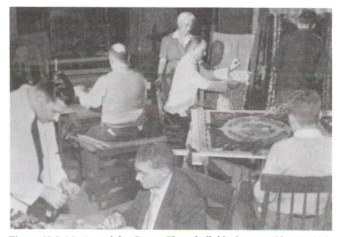

Figure 22-8. Men's Activity Group. These individuals are making Turkish knotted rugs, weaving and hooking rugs. Leatherwork, jewelry making and woodworking were also prescribed.

Bertalanffy, 1968; Boulding, 1961, 1968) is a conceptual framework that organizes knowledge in a manner that facilitates interdisciplinary communication. Mary Reilly, an educator and theorist, originally applied general systems theory to occupational therapy and suggested that occupation be viewed as a dynamic concept rather than a static and mechanistic idea (Reilly, 1962, 1974; Kielhofner, 1978, 1985).

According to theorists, a system may be either open or closed. A closed system is one that does not actively interact with the environment, thus, it cannot correct or maintain itself. The temperature control in an old stove is an example of a closed system. Once set, the control will maintain a certain level until the system malfunctions or until the setting is changed. Because the control does not interact with the environment, it does not realize when the cake is done and no further heat is needed.

In contrast, an open system interacts with the environment and is dynamic; that is, it changes as a result of its interaction. The function performed by the open system determines its future capacities. Compare the difference in musculoskeletal development between a weightlifter and a person who practices yoga. Both bodies share the same inherent arrangement of muscles, tendons and bones, but the different ways that these individuals use their bodies have changed the shape, structure, and performance capacities of the underlying components. All living things

are open systems because of their ability to adapt to conditions in the environment.

An open systems approach to humans favors a view that expresses a unity and interdependence among the individuals, their bodies and minds, and the world around them. An important value that emerges from an open systems perspective is the belief that humans can ''orchestrate their own health'' (Reilly, 1962). This requires the individual's active participation in the healing process. Illness is not viewed as a single germ that has attacked a person, but as a symptom of a total process that has influenced the person's mind and body (Johnson, 1983).

Occupational therapists rely on systems theory to explain why the occupational therapy process works. Meaningful occupations are used as means of promoting increased participation in daily life. Occupational therapy is not something that is done to a person but a process that is done with the individual (Kielhofner and Burke, 1985; Rogers, 1982, 1984; Yerxa, 1980).

A hierarchy is a group of ideas that are ranked or graded by complexity. In occupational therapy, a hierarchy allows therapists to organize occupational therapy knowledge and put concepts into practice. The ideas form a system in which interrelated parts are arranged in a deliberate order which creates an integrated whole. The structure for analyzing activities, tasks, and roles is an example of a hierarchy.

Table 22-1
Summary of the Development of the Therapeutic Use of Occupation

1890-1909	Group of dedicated individuals used occupation to teach work skills to immigrants, provide an outlet for mental patients and handicapped children and offer health services to chronically impaired individuals.
1910-1929	Group of physicians, nurses, craft teachers, architects and religious leaders combine ideals of lay health movement with medical care for chronically disabled. Used goal-directed activities or occupations to motivate individuals to overcome disability and illness. Therapists adapted supplies from environment to promote goals. Used bookbinding, weaving, basketry, ceramics, dance and gardening in an attempt to find a match between condition and media.
1930-1939	Depression years forced therapists to develop work strategies that offered maximum patient services despite limited resources. "Classes" were offered in variety of modalities such as sewing, weaving, drama, gardening, singing, and woodworking. The occupational therapist began changing from the "diversionist" who focused on arts and crafts to the "therapist" who promoted function through activity.
1940-1959	Casualties of World War II fighting required services of therapists who used activities to promote increased mechanical function. Therapists used crafts but focused on functional gains. Elaborate equipment set-ups were created to provide correct positioning during exercise so patient function was restored. Psychiatric practice became focused on the inner workings of the patient's mind and pediatric therapists became mother-surrogates. Play and human growth and development became integrated into treatment.
1960-1980	Mind/body unity was explored in research as therapists began to formulate advanced theories for improved care. Reimbursement focused on patient progress which must be completed within a prescribed time. Therapists used exercise and then realized the limitation of ignoring the patient's roles, values, interests, goals and interests. There was a renewed interest in activities that promoted intrinsic and extrinsic motivation. Research demonstrated the importance of activities to promote improved patient function. Treatment included non-medical problems as well as more traditional treatment.

Fiebleman (1954) described the laws which govern a hierarchy, as follows:

- higher components control or influence the lower components
- complexity of levels increases upward
- higher levels depend on the lower levels for continuation
- higher levels direct the lower levels
- both positive and negative forces reverberate throughout the hierarchy and all levels are affected
- higher levels require less time to make changes than the lower levels
- higher levels have broader categories than lower levels
- higher levels cannot be reduced to lower levels

In a hierarchy higher levels govern the lower levels, while at the same time, lower components constrain the higher levels. Because of these relationships, one cannot consider one level in isolation from the other levels. The Performance Hierarchy is presented in Figure 22-9. Note that activity is the bottom level or the foundation of the doing process. Activities constrain both task and role levels, and role and task levels depend on the activity level. Activity is governed by both task and role levels; however, benefits derived from one level affect the others. One can anticipate more rapid change in the role level than in the task or activity levels. One cannot reduce a higher level to a lower one.

Starting with the activity level (or foundation) of the performance hierarchy, each level will be explored with applicable concepts applied to a case study.

INTEGRATION OF EARLY CONCEPTS: MIND/BODY UNITY AND LIFESTYLE

Scholars in occupational therapy have recently attempted to integrate some of the field's earlier beliefs with current ideas and research. Two early concepts viewed as important to contemporary theory are those of mind/body unity and lifestyle.

Mind/Body Unity

The belief that a person's mind influences his/her body and vice versa appeared in medicine during the colonial period, disappeared before the Civil War, and resurfaced during the Progressive Era when Freud demonstrated the effect of the mind on the body. Today, this concept is once again gaining popularity as the public recognizes the limitations of scientific medicine (Ferguson, 1980; Capra, 1983). Contemporary literature (including print, tape, and film media) emphasize the phenomenon of mind and body

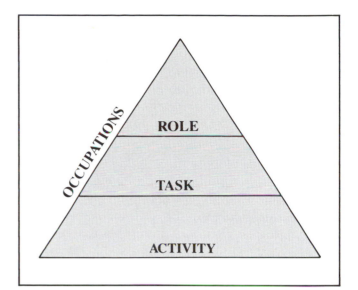

Figure 22-9. The Performance Hierarchy. Note that role is broader in conceptual scope than task or activity. Occupations cannot be prescribed without consideration of the task and activity components since the concepts are organized in a hierarchy where the higher levels dominate the lower levels but lower levels constrain the higher levels and each layer influences the others.

unity and that individuals can influence their health through behaviors and attitudes.

For example, the well-known author, Norman Cousins (1979), championed the interest in mind/body unity when he described his recovery from a life-threatening illness. In spite of dire predictions from his physicians and others around him, Cousins developed an ultimately lifesaving positive mental attitude by watching humorous movies, reading entertaining books, and taking vitamin C.

Oliver Sacks (1987) claimed that the separation between ''mechanism and life'' or mind and body can be explored through case histories which demonstrate the relationship between both. His humanistic descriptions of patients with neurological disorders offer insight into the suffering of people with sensory, perceptual, and physical disorders.

Clarissa Scott (1974) described the health beliefs of five ethnic groups in Miami and also the link between health and belief. In the study, one Bahamian woman came to the emergency room for treatment of a sore throat two days before her death. She never discussed her real problem (severe stomach and vaginal pain), which she believed was caused by witchcraft. Without understanding her beliefs and incorporating them into her healing process, the traditional medical system could not begin to help her.

Joan Borysenko (1987) described her recovery from severe migraines by use of relaxation techniques. She was impressed with a movie demonstrating acupuncture anesthesia. ''As assistants twirled a few needles, a surgeon incised a patient's chest, cracked the ribs, and removed a lobe of the lung—all while the patient, his head demurely hidden behind a sheet, talked and sipped tea.''

It is believed that the mind has the power to heal or to erode health through a complex pattern of interaction among body systems. External stress affects the internal body systems through hormones, neuropeptides, and the central nervous system. This can affect every part of the body. Thus, how a person feels about disease may be as important as the biological aspects of the disease process itself. While some researchers are exploring this issue, many questions concerning the influence of the mind on the body remain unanswered.

When a person suffers chronic pain from an injury, this pain literally can affect everything that the person does. If there is no cure for the pain, the person has two choices: to allow the pain to control his/her life or learn to focus on other things as a distraction.

One 54-year-old woman sustained a brachial plexus injury after a heavy carton fell off a shelf and hit her on the lower neck and shoulder. After four years of surgery, therapy, and counseling the woman still could not sleep because of her discomfort. In her desperation, she decided to find something to amuse herself during the hours of the early morning when her pain was overwhelming. She acquired an exotic snake that was nocturnal and observed the animal's behavior. Fascinated by the snake, she acquired more snakes and became an expert in snake behavior. She learned to change her sleep patterns and distract herself from her discomfort. Her interest expanded further and she began to lecture on the subject to students, collect data for research studies, and she eventually wrote several books on snakes.

Such an example demonstrates that an interesting task can promote adaptation and healing. Although the woman could never be free of pain, she used an interesting task to overcome her preoccupation. Anyone who has required extended bedrest for an illness appreciates how difficult the confinement becomes with the deprivation of stimulation and ensuing boredom. The mind and body cannot be separated when dealing with human beings. In occupational therapy, this concept is crucial to high quality intervention.

Lifestyle

Lifestyle is the belief that individuals must be considered in the context of their culture—their goals, values, interests, motivation, roles, habits and ability to perform tasks, and activities. As noted in the chapter by Krefting and Krefting, culture consists of thoughts and beliefs about the way life should be lived. As a template for living that is acquired very early in life, culture quickly influences our patterns of behavior and becomes a permanent imprint on our

existence. In considering the influence of culture, occupational therapists must become familiar with such things as an individual's patterns of roles and habits, their commitment to the work ethic, their compliance with taboos or myths, and their world view and relationship to other cultural groups. Beliefs about folk medicine and independence or health may also influence the success of intervention strategies (Leininger, 1978).

Successful occupational therapy programs reflect an individual's culture. Important considerations are values, motivation, goals, and interests. Participation in a meaningless activity quickly becomes an unpleasant burden. On the other hand, meaningful or relevant occupations promote optimal performance (Kielhofner and Burke, 1980; Mosey, 1981; Reilly, 1962; Rogers, 1982).

ACTIVITY

The most basic component of the performance hierarchy is activity. Since occupational therapy began as an organized discipline, the use of occupation (activity) as a means of providing treatment to patients has been an overriding premise of the profession. A philosophical base for occupational therapy, adopted by the Representative Assembly of the American Occupational Therapy Association in 1979, clearly states this premise as follows:

''Occupational therapy is based on the belief that purposeful activity (occupation), including its interpersonal and environmental components, may be used to prevent and remediate dysfunction, and to elicit maximum adaptation'' (American Occupational Therapy Association, 1981).

Activities are the foundation of the doing process (see Figure 22-10). An activity is any specific action or pursuit. These actions can be learned, involve a ''doing'' process, are specific in focus, and have a limited scope. Examples are brushing teeth, cooking a hot dog, weaving a paper mat, moving a skateboard back and forth on a table, swinging in a net, or riding a scooter board. An activity is the smallest conceptualization of the therapeutic ''doing'' process. The word *activity* was once used interchangeably with task, but for the purpose of this book activity will be considered the foundation of both doing and the performance hierarchy (Llorens, 1986).

Categories of Activities

An activity is something that is used therapeutically by occupational therapists, has a purpose for the individual patient/client and can be divided into various categories. Activities may be active or passive or involve individual or group participation. They can be categorized in numerous ways including characteristics, outcomes and meanings, or by the domains of self-care, work, and play/leisure. They may be defined in terms of the age-relatedness of an activity (developmental), orientation towards males or females (gender identification), by cultural factors, by the physical aspects, psychodynamic aspects, and social interaction. Occupational therapists may find other categories useful.

Functional and Diversional Activities. Occupational therapists use activities functionally, but at times the activity may be diversional. Functional activities are those used to improve function or prevent dysfunction and are utilized as such the majority of time by most occupational therapists. Diversional activities were used in early practice to divert attention from an unhealthy condition (Edgerton, 1947). Although therapists diverted attention from pain, hallucinations, and other unhealthy ideas, the term diversion implies a form of treatment which is solely based on amusement and recreation. For example, occupational therapists often provided craft activities, puzzles, games or hobbies to individuals in pain to displace their physical distress with some activity of interest. As we have already learned, some individuals find their own activity to displace their discomfort.

Today, therapists incorporate the diversional aspects of activities into their treatment but eschew the diversional label because it does not communicate the complexity of the activity process. For example, today's therapists involved in work hardening programs teach individuals how to participate in an activity safely while learning to live within the limits of pain.

Developmental Activities. Cynkin (1979, p. 25) stated that "activities have served as recognizable milestones that signal the progressive attainment of critical developmental steps toward physical, mental, and emotional maturity. Conversely, certain activities have become associated with specific age groups in terms of physical, mental, and emotional readiness for performance." Developmental theorists have determined performance expectations at various ages and stages. For example, we can expect that by age one year a child can feed him/herself with a spoon without spilling; by age three years a child is toilet-trained throughout the night; by age seven children know the value of the penny, nickel, dime, and quarter; and between the ages of 15 to 18 teenagers respond to hints or indirect cues in conversation. For these reasons, activity selection should be developmentally appropriate.

We also know that some activities are more relevant for one age grouping than another, while others may be appropriate for most ages. For example, playing with dolls may be more appropriate for young children, while playing

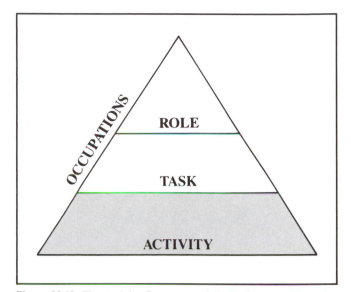

Figure 22-10. The Activity Component of the Performance Hierarchy Activity forms the basis of the occupational therapy process. Task and role levels of the hierarchy are constrained by the activity component but the higher levels rule the activity level.

checkers (draughts) is appropriate for children and adults alike. Thus occupational therapists must be conscious of the age-relatedness of an activity. For example, it is not appropriate to give an elderly person an activity which is associated with children, as it would degrade the elderly person and lower his/her self-image.

Activities Related to Gender. Even though many disagree, some individuals feel that particular activities are more appropriate for one sex or the other. For example, some men refuse to do household chores, while others willingly cook, dust, wash floors, vacuum, and shop for groceries. Some women enjoy doing woodworking activities, while others would not consider it believing it to be "man's work." The individual's sexual connotation of an activity must be considered when selecting it for therapeutic purposes, keeping in mind that this connotation is often culturally biased. By performing activity assessments, the occupational therapist can determine the interests, values, and capabilities of the individual and formulate a therapeutic plan that will meet specific individualized objectives.

Culture Influences Activities. Activities can represent cultural values and beliefs and thus influence the behavior or norms of individuals from a given culture. It is therefore important for the therapist to know what activities are culturally important and acceptable to their clients. For example, the daughter of an engineer might find it completely acceptable and interesting to restore antique cars as a hobby,

Table 22-2
Examples of Functional Activities in Occupational Domains

Self-Care	Work	Leisure
Grooming and hygiene	Homemaking	Hobbies
Feeding and eating	Child care/parenting	Sports
Dressing	Employment	Games
Functional mobility	School activities	Music/drama
Functional communication		

whereas the son of a lawyer might find working on cars either boring or confusing. An Italian-American patient might insist he will only allow his son to shave him or a Puerto Rican may identify his wife as his primary care-giver.

Culture "determines the relevance of activities to the world in which the individual is expected to function" (Cynkin, 1979, p. 27). Therapeutic activities should be selected in consideration of the patient's beliefs and values, not those of the therapist.

Functional Activities. Functional activities may be grouped as work-related, self-care, leisure, social and recreational (Cynkin, 1979; Pedretti, 1981). Work activities are typically those which are performed for remuneration or as a service to others and usually extend beyond the self and the immediate family. Work activities also include academic and homemaking activities. Home management includes those activities performed by any member(s) of a home and directed at maintaining the home, its furnishings and grounds as well as the skill and performance in homemaking and home management tasks. Such tasks may include meal planning, meal preparation and clean-up, laundry, cleaning, minor household repairs, shopping, and utilization of household safety principles. **Self-care activities** are those activities which individuals do to prepare themselves personally for a daily routine. Leisure activities are those activities which are performed to provide relaxation and enjoyment and include play activities of children which are conducted as part of normal development (American Occupational Therapy Association, 1978). This method of classification does not always result in pure categorization, since, for example, one person's perception of an activity as work may be perceived by another as leisure. An example of this concept is a person owning a business selling stamps and coins where sorting the products for sales may be the individual's vocation; conversely, a stamp or coin collector may consider the same activity to be leisure. Table 22-2 categories activities according to self-care, work, and leisure groupings.

Physical Characteristics of the Activity. Activities may be categorized by their physical characteristics including passive, active-assistive, active, and resistive. This classification is primarily related to physical functioning. *Passive activities* are those which require minimal or no physical exertion on the part of the individual. *Active-assistive activities* are those which require active motion from the individual, but mechanical assistance may be supplied from outside forces. In some instances the therapist is the external force. *Active activities* require active motion on the part of the individual without resistance. *Resistive activities* are those which utilize weight or tension and may be used to increase muscle strength. See Table 22-3.

Activities can also be classified on the basis of physical abilities necessary for competent performance. Such characteristics include gross or fine motor coordination, range of motion, dexterity, strength, endurance, prehension patterns, repetition, and posture. These are defined below.†

Gross motor coordination—skill and performance in gross motor activities using large groups of muscles to function together, usually the proximal muscles.

Fine motor coordination—requires small, discrete, specialized muscles to function together, usually the hand muscles, such as the opposing thumb-to-fingers position that is required to hold a pencil.

Eye-hand coordination—harmonious functioning of the eyes and the muscles required in grasping and manipulating objects.

Dexterity—skill in using one's hands or the required skill and performance for tasks using small muscle groups.

Endurance—the maximum amount of time an individual can perform one or more steps of an activity without fatigue.

Prehension patterns—the positions and grasp patterns of the human hand that allow an individual to perform various tasks or functions. Prehension patterns require minimal

---

†Note that these definitions differ from the ability categories identified in Chapter 1 (Figure 1-14). Those were derived from empirical research.

hand strength and flexibility (Pedretti, 1981). The various types of prehension patterns are described below.

Lateral prehension pattern—the thumb is adducted against the lateral side of the index finger (pad of thumb to side of index finger) as when opening a lock with a key.

Palmar prehension pattern—opposition of the pad of the thumb to the pad of the index finger. The Distal Interphalangeal (DIP) and Interphalangeal (IP) joint of the index finger and the DIP joints of the thumb may be fully extended or slightly flexed, as when holding a coin.

Tip-to-tip prehension pattern—a functional and precise opposition pattern requiring the pulp of the thumb to oppose the pulp of the index finger in an ulnar direction, as when using a needle to sew.

Spherical prehension pattern—similar to cylindrical grip except fingers are spread more to encompass object, as when holding a small ball.

Hook grasp—flexion of fingers around an object, usually sustained over a long period of time. The thumb is not usually involved, and when it is, the thumb is used primarily for stability, as when holding a suitcase or purse.

Cylindrical prehension—using flexors to place fingers around and maintain grasp on an object. The thumb is usually flexed and adducted around the object, as when holding a glass.

Sensory Characteristics. Sensory characteristics consist of the five basic senses of touch, visual, auditory, gustatory, and olfactory. Those terms which may be considered in relation to activities are defined below.

Touch—the sensation when the skin recognizes an object with which it comes in contact. Superficial sensation is concerned with touch, pain, temperature, and 2-point discrimination. Deep sensation is concerned with **proprioception,** deep muscle pain, and vibration.

Visual—the ability to see and identify by sight the components of size, color and shape.

Scanning—the ability to track or pursue an object or a series of visual stimuli such as a row of numbers.

Acuity—the relative ability of the visual organ to resolve detail, such as near (the ability to visually perceive objects in the near field of vision) or far (the ability to visually perceive objects in the distance.

Auditory—the differentiation and identification of sound, e.g., loud, soft, moderate or silent.

Auditory figure-ground—the ability to discriminate between the sound(s) made during or by the activity from the sounds in the environment.

Gustatory—the differentiation and identification of the tastes of sweet, salt, sour, and bitter.

Olfactory—the differentiation and identification of smell including pleasant, noxious, and familiar odors.

Perception. Perception is defined as the meaning the brain gives to sensory input. It is subjective while sensory is objective (Ayres, 1979). Appropriate terms are defined below.

Figure-ground perception—the ability to recognize forms and objects when presented in a configuration with competing stimuli.

Kinesthesia—the ability to consciously perceive muscular motion, weight, and position.

Spatial relationships—the ability to perceive the distances between relationships among objects in space.

Motor planning—the ability to plain and copy demonstrated acts or carry out movements commonly associated with tools and implements or action words (Pedretti, 1981).

Proprioception—the ability to identify the position of body parts in space.

Stereognosis—the ability to identify forms and objects through the sense of touch.

Bilateral integration—the ability to perform purposeful movement that requires interaction between both sides of the body in a smooth and refined manner.

Psychological Characteristics. The psychological aspects of activities can be used to provide individuals with insight into their abilities and limitations. "Often activities that involve manipulating objects, tools and materials, and which produce something finished at the end, provide concrete evidence which can be used to help the individual to test

Table 22-3
Physical Descriptors of Activities

Action	Examples
Passive	• reading a book • watching television • listening to a symphony
Active-assistive (therapist provides assistance)	• manually • with slings • with pulleys • with springs
Active	• using a telephone • brushing one's teeth • eating a meal
Resistive	• sanding a wooden board on an incline plane • cutting one's meat (depending on the texture and tenderness of the meat)

reality about himself or herself'' (Hopkins & Smith, 1983, p. 297). The psychological aspects of activities can be categorized in many ways including factors inherent in both the process and the product.

Self-concept. Self-concept can be categorized into sexual identification, body image, and self-esteem (Fidler, 1963). **Sexual identification** of an activity is the degree to which the activity has a traditional male or female connotation. Some activities are viewed as a strictly male oriented activity, such as woodworking, while other activities are viewed as female oriented, such as needlework. Other activities may be considered unisex, such as bicycling, dressing, and driving. Many activities provide the individual with the opportunity to symbolically express a sexual nature. ''Confusion about, distortion of, or lack of sexual identification is, of course, part of the patient's difficulties in self-concept'' (Fidler, 1963). We must always keep in mind that the connotation of sexual identification of activities is culturally and individually based.

Activities can provide the individual with the opportunity to become aware of his/her *body image*. Physical contact with others, participation in activities which require touching one's body parts, drawing a person, or creating a human figure from clay may reveal the individual's perception of his/her own body. For example, an obese person may perceive himself or herself to look like an elephant, and even when the individual has lost weight that perception may persist.

Self-esteem is confidence and satisfaction in self. Activities can enhance or diminish self-esteem. For example, teaching a male adolescent to budget his earned money appropriately could increase his self-esteem by providing a mechanism for him to be less dependent on his parents to provide for his needs. Conversely, asking an artist to paint by numbers would likely make that person feel as if he/she is no longer capable of performing previously mastered skills and thus lower self-esteem.

Psychodynamics. Activities can be categorized by the psychodynamics or defense mechanisms incorporated into the participation of the activity and the degree to which the activity encourages their expression. The therapist determines which defense mechanisms the individual manifests while manipulating the material used in the activity and the object itself, including those of regression, repression, projection, denial, avoidance, withdrawal, sublimation, and detachment. This is discussed in more detail in Chapter 12, Psychological Performance Factors.

Structured and Unstructured Activities. Activities can be structured or nonstructured. **Structured activities** have rules, can be broken down into manageable steps and can be preorganized or preplanned. **Unstructured activities** are not preplanned and not broken down into steps. There are various degrees of both structured and unstructured activities, and consideration of this category should be on a continuum, from highly structured to totally unstructured. For example, asking a patient to complete a woodworking kit with preset directions for putting the pieces together and steps for finishing the project is a structured activity. Giving the individual a piece of board with general directions to plan, cut, and complete their own woodworking project is more unstructured.

An example of a highly unstructured activity would be finger-painting because it does not require that any specific steps be followed once the paper is wet and the jars of paints are opened. It is a free-flowing and individualistic activity and can be performed with numerous objects, including the hand, fingers, fist, elbow, knuckles, or sponge. The technique used can be varied by overlapping the paints, smearing them, or using them in discrete isolation of each other. There are endless possibilities, making this a highly unstructured activity.

Social Interaction in Activities. Activities may be categorized by the degree of social interaction they produce or require. *Social interaction* relates to the amount of interaction necessary to effectively interrelate with other persons. Activities of social interaction which will be considered below are verbal, nonverbal, group, dyadic, and individual.

One method of categorizing the process involved in conducting activities is to separate the verbal from the nonverbal communication activities. An obvious example of a verbal communication activity would be a current events discussion group. This activity requires interaction between participants by discussing the local or world events of the day. It might not be as obvious to present the activity of cooking as a verbal communication activity; however, if the therapist planned the cooking activity in such a manner as to require the individual to respond to directions verbally, then the activity could be categorized as verbal. These two types of activities would also be considered group activities; thus, we can say that *verbal communication* requires interaction between two or more individuals.

A *nonverbal communication activity* is one that requires no verbal interaction between individuals, such as sitting at the computer and typing a manuscript. Nonverbal communication is a very important aspect of patient behavior that must also be observed by the therapist. We often use gestures, facial grimaces, and symbols to communicate nonverbally. For example, consider the various ways in which a smile can be used to convey one's thoughts. A certain type of smile can indicate pleasure, another can portray disapproval, and still another can indicate a smugness.

The process of conducting activities can include group and dyadic participation as well as individual participation. Group participation can be required through the action of doing the activity (sometimes called group activity, task-structured or project groups) or through a verbal group, which is "a group of people engaged in improving skills in communication through the use of discussion" (DeCado & Mann, 1985). A project group was defined by Nelson and associates (1988) as a group in which subjects worked together to make the same shared end product. A group activity may include making a collage from magazine pictures; playing sports or a game; planning, preparing, eating, and cleaning up after a meal; or preparing for a community trip. These types of activities can increase socialization, communication skills, self-concept, self-expression, self-confidence and independence.

Dyadic interaction refers to the degree of interaction required or possible with another individual and often can be regulated by the therapist as to the amount or structure of the activity. For example, the therapist either can provide an opportunity for the individual to ask questions and make comments during the process of the activity or the therapist can ask questions of the individual and promote conversation while the individual is participating in the activity.

Individual activities can include any activity which does not require the participation of another individual. In the psychosocial literature of occupational therapy this type of activity is frequently called a parallel group and is defined as individuals engaging "in the same types of activity to make individual products" (Nelson, Peterson, Smith, Boughton, & Whalen, 1988).

However, whether the activity has been designed to be conducted within a parallel group or individually, the activity is done by a single person. The card game, Solitaire, tells us by its name that it is a game to be played alone, but Gin Rummy must be played by more than one person. Pulling weeds from the garden, dressing oneself, reading a book, and doing needlepoint all can be individual activities. The occupational therapist must determine whether a group, dyadic, or individual interaction is in the best interest of the client when determining the therapeutic value of an activity. Occasionally, an activity must be adapted to achieve a desired type or level of social interaction.

Cognitive Abilities. Activities may be used to determine the individual's level of thinking and functioning in relation to objects and activity. Answering the following questions regarding cognitive abilities might assist the therapist to select an appropriate activity for the patient:

- *Does the activity require the individual to have long-term or short-term memory or short or long attention span to perform the activity?*
  Memory is the ability to retain and recall tasks or concepts from the past and can be categorized as short-term memory (1 hour to 2 days) or long-term memory (more than 2 days).

- *Does the activity require the individual to be oriented to time, place, and person?*
  Orientation is the ability to comprehend, define, and adjust oneself in an environment with regard to time, place, and person.

- *How much concentration is required to perform the activity?*
  Concentration is the skill and performance in focusing on a designated task or concept.

- *Can the directions for performing the activity be provided verbally, in writing, a combination of the two, or through demonstration, pictures, or diagrams?*

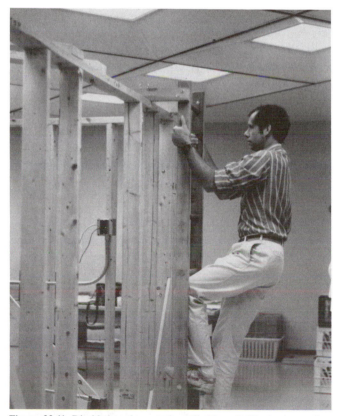

Figure 22-11. Disabled worker practices climbing a ladder in preparation for returning to work as a carpenter. The construction project allows the worker the opportunity to work on all aspects of building a room.

- *Are problem-solving skills required to be successful in completing the activity?*

    Problem-solving is the skill and performance in identifying and organizing solutions to difficulties.

- *Does the activity require concrete or abstract thinking?*

- *Is the activity a simple or complex activity? If it is a complex activity, can it be broken down into appropriate steps to make it more simple or is sequencing a requirement of the activity?*

    Sequencing is the ordering of steps of an activity in an organized, continuous manner.

- *Does the activity provide for symbolism and interpretation? Does the activity provide for cultural symbolism (e.g., flag, cross, Star of David) or individual (idiosyncratic) symbolism, such as when a picture of the ocean evokes pleasant feelings of home or summer vacations?*

    In relation to symbolic representation, the therapist should consider whether the patient's unconscious needs can be expressed or gratified through the activity. The symbolism involved in an activity can be either in a personal or a psychoanalytic framework. Symbols may be inherent in procedure, materials, equipment, or end product (Fidler & Fidler, 1963).

- *Does the activity provide for new learning or reinforce previous learning?*

- *Does the activity require the use of already known general information or does it provide an opportunity to learn experiences by trial and error, seriation, limitation, or casuality?*

- *Does the activity allow for **reality testing**?*

    Reality testing is the ability to know what is real and what is fantasy, usually accomplished through structured activity. Reality testing is important because often a patient's ''perceptual vagueness (sometimes) makes it difficult to be sure of what is real and what is not real, and such difficulties may be manifested in distortions about oneself and the external world and by confusion, impaired judgment, indecision, and even disorganization'' (Fidler & Fidler, 1963, p. 93). The act of performing activities and the finished product can help the patient determine what is real and what is fantasy.

Continuity. The activity must provide for various mental and physical abilities and must include continuity (Hamill & Oliver, 1980). *Continuity* in this context relates to the requirement of repetitive specific motions inherent in performing the activity; that is, an activity which provides for only one active motion lacks continuity and is ineffective if the remainder of the activity requires static positioning.

Activities must have a beginning, an ending, and a mechanism for judging the individual's performance and monitoring progress (Cynkin, 1979; Hamill & Oliver, 1980). Starting and ending activity provides a sense of achievement for the individual. Activities which can be stopped at a given point are more apt to be picked up again to be completed by the client; consequently, the components of the activity are more apt to be remembered. Conversely, those activities which can be completed in one sitting are more likely to be forgotten. This principle holds true when the activity has meaning for the individual and when the activity provides a means of checking progress (Cynkin, 1979). Individuals who feel that an activity is irrelevant lack the desire to complete the activity. The therapist's responsibility is to monitor progress with the activity and the level of continued interest and to provide feedback to the individual about the appropriateness of the methods employed to accomplish the activity. In this manner the therapist will encourage the individual to achieve the goals for which the activity was prescribed.

The range of activities used by occupational therapists is limited only by the creativity and imagination of the therapist. However the activity which is used therapeutically for a specific patient is determined by the psychological and physical capabilities of the individual. The goal is to increase the client's functioning and independence or prevent dysfunction. The activity selected must have relevance for the individual's needs if it is to enhance the development or restoration of function. Individuals can change and usually desire to change. Therefore, individuals are more likely to incorporate activities into their daily routines if they perceive them to have personal relevance.

Simulated Activities. Activities that artificially replicate endeavors the patient will perform in his or her own environment are termed simulated activities. Performing the actual activity is far better than a simulated activity, although simulated activities, if carefully designed, can be used as close approximations to the actual situation (Cynkin, 1979). Consider the activity of teaching an individual to dress. Is it more appropriate to practice at the time and place where the person usually dresses (i.e., in the morning upon arising) or later in the day in the occupational therapy clinic, at the convenience of the therapist? Similarly, will a person relearn the skill of cooking more quickly and efficiently in his/her own kitchen or in the occupational therapy setting? The answer seems obvious; tasks should be learned and practiced in the environment (and at the time of day) in which they typically will be performed. Unfortunately, this is not always possible.

For this reason, simulated activities have an important role in occupational therapy. When a more natural environmental setting places constraints on therapy, simulation is required. However, the setting, **equipment,** and materials should resemble the patient's actual environment as closely as possible. Simulations include both work and home activities and environments. Simulated activities are greatly used in work-oriented practice in occupational therapy. Simulations are particularly important in this area of practice because they provide an opportunity to assess the individual's ability to do meaningful work activities in a controlled environment and provide the individual with "a series of learning experiences that will enable him/her to make appropriate vocational decisions and develop work habits necessary for eventual employment" (Ad hoc Committee of the Commission on Practice, 1980).

One form of work simulation is the work simulator, a computerized apparatus that simulates the use of many tools and devices such as screwdrivers with various sized handles, a variety of knobs, steering wheels, different types of crank handles, a lifting tool that simulates rowing, bowling, a tennis racket, baseball bat, or ladder. Such devices are provided for the simulated activities one must perform in daily self-care and work life. It determines the amount of resistance desired and provides for the measurement and documentation of an individual's progress. One such device, manufactured by Baltimore Therapeutic Equipment, consists of two components: a shaft which protrudes from a controlled resistance assembly onto which the attachments are placed and a microprocessor and control panel from which one selects the desired amount of resistance and generates a print-out of the patient's time and performance data.

Other approaches to work simulations have been integrated into occupational therapy clinics. It is not possible to present all of the alternatives here; thus only a few examples are provided. A workstation that resembles construction of a section of a house assists in evaluation of the disabled worker's ability to return to work. By participating in the actual construction, the worker demonstrates the abilities of using a ladder, lifting, carrying, and holding heavy tools and materials, as well as working in a variety of positions such as stooping, crouching, upright standing, or overhead reaching. The workstation can also incorporate such activities as electrical wiring, plumbing, painting, siding, and tiling.

Another example of work simulation is a small appliance station where the individual works on repairing items such as toasters, tabletop ovens, mixers, radios, or televisions. Repairing such appliances indicates the individual's abilities with respect to such job requirements as manual dexterity, endurance, sitting or standing tolerance, adherence to safety regulations, attitude, and even reading and comprehending a manual. Figure 22-12 shows a working model of a pipe assembly project which was developed to provide practice with fitting various pipes together. It

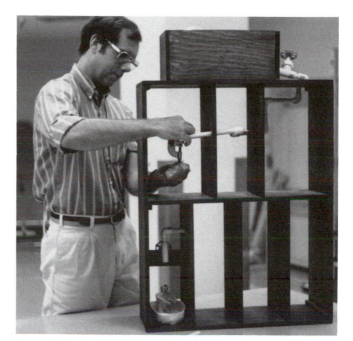

Figure 22-12. The Working Model of a Pipe Assembly Project. This is an example of simulated work activities designed by occupational therapist Norman Gustafson, St. Francis Hospital, Pittsburgh, PA.

enables the worker to fit together various shapes of joints and requires the client to assume numerous positions to accomplish the task. When assembled correctly, water that is poured in the receptacle at the top will run through the pipes and shower down on the miniature replica of a man in a bathtub.

Occupational therapists have designed numerous simulated activities for all types of work situations. Home situations are also simulated by the occupational therapists. For example, the occupational therapist may not have access to the person's home for teaching new cooking methods; therefore, the clinic should approximate the individual's kitchen and equipment as closely as possible. This requires direct communication with the patient and family members.

In some health care facilities an apartment is set up either in the facility or in an adjacent free-standing building to give an individual the opportunity to experience living in a home-like environment prior to discharge. In some instances, the individual may be in the apartment overnight while in other instances the individual may live there with a family member for a week. The dwelling may contain specialized equipment that the individual will require when discharged and provides the individual or family member with experience using the equipment and the opportunity to ask questions of the professional staff prior to being discharged.

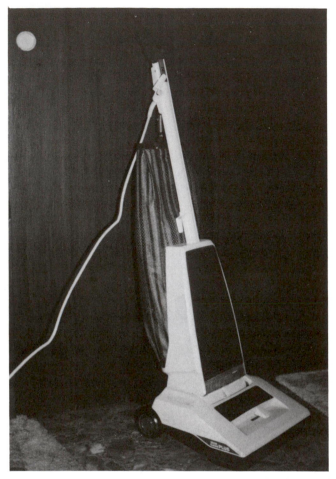

Figure 22-13. Upright Vacuum. This upright vacuum depicts the type of equipment used when completing the Activity Analysis. *Photo by David Murphy, Sr.*

To accomplish an appropriate simulation, the therapist must be versatile and adaptable. The simulated activities must be carefully selected and can be "justified by assuming that learning is transferrable from one situation to another" (Cynkin, 1979, p. 51).

Case Study 22-2

Intervention Strategies for Bruce Walker: The following is the intervention strategy planned for Bruce Walker, the truck driver who fractured his wrist in a fall (described in the beginning of the chapter).

While recovery from the fracture was successful, he continued to focus all of his attention on the pain in his wrist and withdrew from work. He was placed in a work-related program where the therapist first evaluated his condition. Mr. Walker's medical history was reviewed. Range of motion, sensation, strength and endurance, sitting and standing tolerance and edema were then assessed. It was

determined that sensation, sitting and standing tolerance were within normal limits. He had no edema. However, his range of motion, strength and endurance were slightly limited. Mr. Walker's self-care abilities were evaluated and found to be satisfactory. His pain was evaluated through the use of a pain chart on which he indicated where the pain was located when performing activities. This is a subjective evaluation which is done by the patient. Following this evaluation, short-term and long-term goals were established in collaboration with Mr. Walker and a treatment program established as follows:

Short-term goals
- To increase short-term range of motion
- To increase strength of the wrist

Long-term goals
- To adapt to pain
- To return to work as a truck driver
- To increase endurance

Treatment Program
- Therapeutic activities to increase range of motion and strength of affected wrist (e.g., woodworking, hammering, sawing, screwdriving)
- Increasing the amount of work time to increase endurance
- Continuation of completing pain chart on hourly basis to determine the severity and location of pain while completing activity
- Upper extremity exercise with and without resistance, using a computerized work simulator, particularly the steering wheel for trucks

Mr. Walker participated in the work-related program for two weeks, at first attending occupational therapy three times a day for about 45 minutes each session. Within three days the length of two treatment sessions per day increased to 2 hours. By the second week he was attending treatment five hours per day, and at the end of that week he was able to return to work as a truck driver. The physical limitations of his wrist had been alleviated. The amount of strength required to turn the steering wheel of the truck was determined by the therapist in collaboration with the company which employed him. The amount of resistance was then gradually simulated by the computerized work simulator. While he continued to report pain in the wrist, he determined that he "could live with it;" thus he had proven to himself that he could return to his former work by experiencing the actual demands of driving a truck.

Activity Analysis

Activities are selected for their potential to meet the goals of the therapeutic intervention. Activities are influenced by psychosocial, physical, cognitive, sensory, and perceptual functioning, as well as environmental factors. The psychosocial component is very important and includes motivation, upon which everything else is dependent. Activities must be analyzed by the therapist to determine the components inherent in the activity. The act of analyzing

Table 22-4a
Activity Analysis

ACTIVITY TO BE ANALYZED
Vacuuming with an upright vacuum

A. THE ACTIVITY PROCESS

1. **Activity of** Self-care _____✓_____
   Work/school _____
   Play/leisure _____

2. **Indicate appropriateness for**
   age range _Adolescent — adult_
   sex   F/M (Dependent on patient's sexual connotation)
   individual _✓_   group participation _____

3. **List sequence involved in the activity**
   (break activity down into logical steps, indicating natural pauses)
   Step 1: Unwind cord on vacuum
   Step 2: Plug cord in at waist height receptacle
   Step 3: Depress handle release button with right foot
   Step 4: Depress button to turn on vacuum
   Step 5: Push vacuum forward with one step forward
   Step 6: Pull vacuum backward

4. **Time factors**
   length of time for each step
      Unwind cord-30 seconds
      Plug in cord-15 seconds
      Step on release lever to use handle-2 seconds
      Step on button to start vacuum-1 second
      Push vacuum forward with one step forward-5 seconds
      Pull vacuum backward with one step backward-4 seconds
   delays inherent in the process: there can be a delay after each step;
   that is, the process can be stopped at any point.
   length of time for total completion: 55 seconds

5. **List materials required**
   None

6. **List tools and equipment required**
   Vacuum
   Floor/rug

7. **Indicate cost of materials**
   None.   Equipment approximately $250.00

8. **List safety precautions**
   Be careful when putting in and removing plug

B. ENVIRONMENTAL CONSIDERATIONS

1. **Indicate space required** (clinic, bedside, home, etc.)
   Clinic and/or home

2. **Indicate furniture/positioning devices** (chair, table, floor, lapboard, etc.)
   None

3. **Indicate external stimulation** (noise level, lighting, people, space, etc.)
   Noise level is dependent on the type of vacuum
   Lighting required—good

C. CHARACTERISTICS OF THE ACTIVITY

1. **Physical**
   a. Positioning of patient
      sitting _____   standing _✓_   side lying _____
      supine _____   prone _____
      other (indicate) _____
   b. Positioning of activity
      eye level _____   overhead _____   lap level _____
      floor _✓_
      other (indicate) Handle of vacuum at level of trochanter
   c. Physical requirements
      Upper extremities: Bilateral _____   Unilateral _✓_
                         right _____   left _____
      Lower extremities: Bilateral _✓_   Unilateral _____
                         right _____   left _____
      Coordination: Gross _✓_   Fine _____   Eye-hand _____
      Dexterity: Fine dexterity for using plug

Endurance: 15 minutes required
Repetitions: 10 repetitions to unwind cord from side of vacuum
   0 repetitions for putting plug in receptacle
   0 repetitions for vacuuming forward and backward
Prehension patterns: Lateral _____   Palmar _____
   Tip-to-tip _____   Spherical _____
   Hook _✓_   Cylindrical _✓_
Muscle and joint analysis: (Use Table 22-4b)

2. **Sensory Awareness**
   (Does the activity require discrimination of these aspects?)
   Touch
   sharp _____   dull _✓_
   deep pressure _✓_   pain _____
   light touch _____   vibration _✓_   texture _✓_
   hot _____   cold _____
   Visual
   size _____   color _✓_   shape _✓_   scanning _✓_
   acuity: near _____   far _✓_
   Auditory
   noisy _✓_   loud _____   soft _____   moderate _____
   figure-ground _____   none _____
   Gustatory
   salt _____   sour _____   bitter _____   none _✓_
   Olfactory
   pleasant _____   noxious _____
   familiar _____   none _✓_

3. **Perception** (Does the activity require these components?)
   body scheme _____   figure-ground _____   kinesthesia _✓_
   spatial relationships _✓_   motor planning _✓_
   proprioception _✓_   stereognosis _____
   bilateral integration _____

4. **Cognition** (Does the activity require these components?)
   orientation _____   concentration _____   generalization _✓_
   creativity _____   attention span (in terms of time) _____
   memory: short term _____   long term _____
   problem solving: trial and error _____   planning _____
      sequencing _____   cause and effect _✓_
      initiation _____   safety & judgment _✓_
   following instructions: written _____   verbal _____
      demonstration _✓_   interpretation of signs/symbols _____

5. **Psychosocial** (Check characteristics of activity)
   Structure _✓_   Non-structure _____
   Dependence _____   Independence _✓_
   Sex identification: Male _____   Female _____   Either _✓_
   Increase Self-image _____
   Affect: Quieting _____   Stimulating _____
      Monotonous _✓_   Varied _____
   Outlet for aggression _✓_
   Tests reality _____
   Symbolism involved _____
   Allows for controlling impulses _____
   Gratification: Immediate _✓_   Delayed _____
   Probability for success _✓_   failure _____

6. **Social Interaction** (Can the activity be performed as indicated?)
   Interaction
   Individual _✓_   Dyadic _____   Group _____
   Competitive _____   Cooperative _____
   Leadership potential _____   Follower _____

7. **How activity promotes goals, motivation and interest**
   (Describe briefly)
   This activity was selected for this male patient whose goals
   included being able to be independent at home upon discharge.
   Since he lives alone, he will have to clean his apartment using his
   upright vacuum cleaner.

activities is particularly important for the novice since it teaches the new occupational therapist to dissect each activity into its component parts and, thereby, understand the complexity of the components and characteristics inherent in each activity. After the process has been well integrated into practice, the experienced occupational therapist may not need to analyze each element in the activity with exacting detail.

Activity analysis can be found throughout the occupational therapy literature, at first emphasizing the prescriptive nature of activities and later encompassing the many and varied components of doing the process. In all forms of activity analysis, the activity is broken down into steps and component parts so that one may analyze the abilities required to complete each step. The activity analysis in Table 22-4a is presented to provide the student with a systematic way of considering the therapeutic aspects of activity. It should be noted that the activity is analyzed in a comprehensive manner, first considering the processes, materials, and equipment involved in the activity, and then the environmental considerations. The characteristics of the activity are then identified, including physical, sensory, perceptual, cognitive, and psychosocial aspects.

The example analysis was completed on the activity of vacuuming as a specific patient accomplished the activity. An upright vacuum was used by the individual who was tall enough to have the end of the handle approximately at the height of his trochanter. The individual was right-handed. The activity of vacuuming was performed once in the forward motion and once backward for this presentation, but it should be understood that the requirements of vacuuming a rug would require more repetitions. It should also be kept in mind that the amount of resistance would change with different types of carpeting. The analysis is based on this patient's individual method of vacuuming.

The activity analysis form should be used to consider all of the components and characteristics of any given activity. Items are relative to the activity and the person performing the activity. Students find it most beneficial to practice analyzing activities as they or their classmates perform them before involving a patient in the activity.

Grading Activities

Once skill has been obtained in analyzing activities, gradability and adaptation can be added to the process. These concepts are basic to the therapeutic use of activities. The activity must be capable of being graded if it is to be used therapeutically. Sometimes more than one activity is required to obtain the degree of grading desired to reach the client goals. Pedretti (1981) stated, "Gradation of activity means that the activity should be appropriately paced and modified to demand the client's maximum capacities at any point in his (or her) progress" (p. 103). **Grading activity** is always individualized to the patient's needs.

The gradability of the activity relates to the manner in which the physical and psychological characteristics of activities can be gradually modified to meet therapeutic requirements. Many aspects of activities may be graded, such as increasing range of motion, strength, coordination, muscle control, dexterity, speed, and endurance. That is, activities can be graded to increase the amount of distance joints must move to accomplish the activity, change the amount of resistance required to increase strength, increase the time and speed factor, reduce gross movement while increasing fine motion and increase the amount of time necessary to practice the activity. For example, if we wanted to grade the activity of vacuuming as previously presented in the Activity Analysis, we could increase the distance that the vacuum must be pushed or pulled to increase range of motion (providing that the full range was not incorporated initially), start with vacuuming a bare floor and progress to increasingly higher piles on the carpeting to intensify the degree of friction to increase strength and increase the number of repetitions for endurance.

Activities may be graded by increasing the number of steps as well as increasing the complexity of the steps, requiring more independence in planning and problem solving and changing the degree and kind of social interaction (Pedretti, 1981). Gradation in giving instructions may be accomplished by the therapist first demonstrating the activity to the individual, then giving verbal instructions, and finally providing written instructions. The therapist may also decrease the amount of cueing provided as the individual becomes more proficient in performing the activity. Problem solving ability may be increased from trial and error to planning, sequencing, and initiation. The amount of concentration and attention span required for the activity may be increased. This may be accomplished by increasing the number of repetitions required by the activity, the length of time spent performing the activity or the complexity of the steps within the activity. Structured activities can be graded to non-structured or vice versa or activities may be graded from immediate to delayed **gratification.**

Students frequently have difficulty knowing when to grade an activity in order to meet the needs of the client. As a general rule, an activity should be graded up when the patient is able to accomplish the task and further progress is desired or graded down when the patient is having difficulty with performance. The therapist must decide when change is indicated. Analyzing the activity will enable the therapist to determine the "qualitative differences in the complexity of the (activity) and suggest

Table 22-4b
Muscle and Joint Analysis

Steps required to perform activity	Joint motion (in degrees)	Muscle Groups Required	Type of Contraction	Strength Needed	Direction of Resistance
1. Unwind vacuum cord Person is seated*					
Scapula protraction		Serratus anterior	Concentric	Poor +	Parallel to floor opposite direction of protraction
elevation		Upper trapezius Levator scapulae	Concentric	Fair	➡ vertically downward
Shoulder flexion	80	Anterior deltoid	Concentric	Fair	➡
Elbow flexion	65	Brachialis	Concentric	Fair	➡ Movement is with gravity (no resistance)
extension	−30	Triceps (slight to initiate)	Concentric	Poor	
Forearm mid-position	0	Supinators/pronators to maintain position	Co-contraction	Poor +	➡
Wrist extension	30	Extensor carpi radialis longus and brevis; Extensor ulnaris	Isometric	Fair	➡
neutral for radial/ulnar deviation	0	Extensor carpi radialis longus Flexor carpi radialis	Isometric	Fair	➡
Hand Lateral pinch MP flexion	20	Flexor pollicis longus/brevis; adductor pollicis;	Isometric	Fair +	➡
IP flexion (digits curled lightly at cord)	40	First dorsal interossei			
MP flexion	30	Palmar dorsal interossei			
PIP flexion	90	Lumbricals		Fair +	
DIP flexion	45	Flexor digitorum profundus/superficialis	Isometric		
2. Unwind cord using a counter-clockwise motion					
a) Top bracket to bottom bracket*					
Scapula retraction; downward rotation		Serratus anterior upper/lower trapezius	Eccentric	Fair	Movement with gravity
Shoulder extends throughout	80 to 0 flexion	Anterior deltoid	Eccentric	Fair	Movement with gravity
horizontal adduction then abduction	0 to 45 to neutral	Pectoralis major Mid-deltoid; supraspinatus	Concentric Concentric	Fair Poor +	⇕ gravity eliminated plane
Internal rotation	0 to 65	Infraspinatus/teres minor to control	Eccentric	Fair	Motion is with gravity
then external rotation	65 to neutral	Teres minor—infraspinatous	Concentric	Poor +	Gravity eliminated (external rotation occurs at bottom)

Table 22-4b (continued)
Muscle and Joint Analysis

Steps required to perform activity	Joint motion (in degrees)	Muscle Groups Required	Type of Contraction	Strength Needed	Direction of Resistance
Elbow extension	+70 to −20 flexion/ extension	Brachialis	Eccentric	Fair	With gravity
Forearm mid-position to pronation	0 to 80	From mid-position to 80 pronation/supinators	Eccentric to control	Fair	Movement is with gravity
Wrist extension	30	Contraction of wrist extensors (depending on orientation of forearm)	Isometric	Fair	�
b) Bottom bracket to top bracket*					
Scapula protraction/upward rotation		Serratus	Concentric	Fair	Opposite protraction in gravity eliminated plane
		Upper/lower trapezius	Concentric	Fair	➤
Shoulder abduction (bottom)	0 to 45	Middle deltoid/ supraspinatus	Concentric	Fair	➤
then horizontal adduction (top)	45 to neutral horizontal abduction	Pectoralis major	Concentric	Fair	➤
external rotation (bottom)	0 to 30	Infraspinatus; teres minor	Concentric	Poor +	◊ gravity eliminated plane
then internal rotation (top)	30 to 30 external rotation/ internal rotation	Pectoralis major; subscapularis to initiate Internal rotation; then infraspinatus & teres minor to control	Concentric Eccentric	Fair Fair	gravity eliminated with gravity
The humerous flexes throughout	0 to 80	Anterior deltoid	Concentric	Fair +	➤
Elbow flexion	20 flexion to 80	Biceps; brachialis	Concentric	Fair +	➤
Forearm supination	0 to 50	Supinator; biceps (to initiate) then pronators to control	Eccentric	Fair	Movement is with gravity
then pronation	50 supina-tion to mid-position	Pronator teres, pronator quadratus	Concentric	Fair-Fair +	➤
Wrist maintained in slight extension	30	Flexor carpi radialis, ulnaris (depending on forearm position)	Isometric	Fair	➤
Hand (Same as in step 1)					

Table 22-4b (continued)
Muscle and Joint Analysis

Steps required to perform activity	Joint motion (in degrees)	Muscle Groups Required	Type of Contraction	Strength Needed	Direction of Resistance
3. Plug cord into waist high receptacle					
Scapula					
upward rotation protraction		Upper trapezius Serratus anterior	Concentric	Fair Good	➡ Parallel to floor against direction of protraction
flexion	45	Anterior deltoid	Concentric	Good-/ Good	➡
Elbow					
flexion	45	Brachialis	Concentric	Fair +	➡
Forearm					
mid-position	0	Pronator/supinators to give stability at mid-position	Co-contraction	Fair	
Wrist					
extension	30	Extensor carpi radialis, longus and brevis and Extensor carpiradialis	Isometric	Fair	➡ (Toward ulnar deviation)
neutral for radial/ulnar deviation	0	Extensor carpi radialis, longus and brevis; Flexor carpi radialis	Isometric	Fair	➡
Hand					
Lateral pinch (Same as step 1)					
4. Step on handle release with right foot, placing toe on button					
Hip					
flexion	30	Iliopsoas	Concentric	Fair	➡
abduction	15	Gluteus Medius	Concentric	Fair	➡
Knee					
flexion	30	Hamstrings	Concentric	Fair	➡
Ankle					
dorsiflexion (depress handle release using plantar flexion; knee and hip passively flex as a result of this action)	15	Tibialis anterior	Concentric	Fair	➡
Hip					
flexion	30-45	Passive	No additional contraction		
Knee					
flexion	30-40	Passive	No additional contraction		
Ankle					
dorsiflexion to plantar flexion	15 to 45	Gastrocnemius-soleas	Concentric	Good	⬆

NOTE: Stance leg: isometric contraction of hip/knee, and ankle musculature to maintain stability and additionally a contraction of gluteus medius to prevent lateral hip movement.

Table 22-4b (continued)
Muscle and Joint Analysis

Steps required to perform activity	Joint motion (in degrees)	Muscle Groups Required	Type of Contraction	Strength Needed	Direction of Resistance
5. Position foot to depress button					
Hip					
flexes	30	Iliopsoas	Concentric	Fair	←
Knee					
flexes	30	Hamstrings	Concentric	Fair	←
Ankle					
dorsiflexes	15	Tibialis anterior	Concentric	Fair	←
a) Depress button					
Hip					
extends	30 to 15 flexion	Iliopsoas Gluteus maximus	Eccentric Slight Concentric	Fair Good	← Movement is with gravity
Knee					
maintains itself in flexion	30	Hamstrings	Isometric	Fair	←
Ankle					
remains in dorsiflexion	0	Tibialis anterior	Isometric	Fair	←
b) Return foot to floor					
Hip					
flexion	30 to 40	Iliopsoas	Concentric	Fair	← Movement is with gravity
extension	neutral	Iliopsoas	Eccentric	Fair	
Knee					
extension	0	Hamstrings	Eccentric	Fair	← Movement is with gravity
Ankle					
remains at neutral	0	Tibialis anterior	Isometric	Fair	←
6. Push vacuum forward with one step forward*					
Scapula					
protraction		Serratus anterior	Concentric	Good	Gravity resists upward rotation; force of friction transmitted through handle resisting protraction
upward rotation		Upper Trapezius			
Shoulder					
flexion	40 to 40 extension/ flexion	Anterior deltoid	Concentric	Good	Parallel to floor; opposite direction of vacuum
Elbow					
extension	70 flexion full extension	Triceps	Concentric	Good	Parallel to floor; opposite direction of vacuum
Forearm					
mid-position	0	Pronators/supinators to maintain	Co-Contraction Isometric	Poor +	Essentially none
Wrist					
extension	30	Extensor carpi radialis, longus and brevis; extension carpi ulnaris	Isometric	Poor +	Essentially none

Table 22-4b (continued)
Muscle and Joint Analysis

Steps required to perform activity	Joint motion (in degrees)	Muscle Groups Required	Type of Contraction	Strength Needed	Direction of Resistance
Hand cylinder grip MCP flexion	60	Flexor digitorum profundus	Isometric	Good	Weight of handle gives resistance
PIP flexion	70	Flexor digitorum superficialis			
DIP flexion	45	Palmar/dorsal interossei Lumbricals			
Thumb abduction		Adductor pollicis	Isometric		on hand ➡
IP flexion	30	Flexor pollicis			
MCP flexion	20	longus and brevis			
7. Pull vacuum back					
Scapula retraction downward rotation		Middle trapezius and rhomboids	Concentric	Good	Opposite backward motion of vacuum. Parallel to floor
Humerus extension	40 to 40 flexion/ extension	Posterior deltoid; Latissimus dorsi; Teres major	Concentric	Good-	Opposite backward motion of vacuum. Parallel to floor
Elbow flexion	From full exten- sion to 70 flexion	Brachialis	Concentric	Good	Opposite backward motion of vacuum. Parallel to floor
Forearm mid-position	0	Slight contraction of pronators/supinators	Isometric	Poor	0
Wrist (Same as in step 6)					
Hand (Same as in step 6)					

* 1. Top of cord holder is just below shoulder height at arm's length; reach/grasp cord with right hand; slight movement in shoulder.

2a. Combined movements of horizontal adduction, internal rotation, then abduction, external rotation, with shoulder extension throughout the top to bottom movement.

2b. Using combined movements of abduction, external rotation, then internal rotation and horizontal adduction. The humerus flexes throughout.

6. To thoroughly analyze the lower extremity movements involved in the step forward requires gait analysis which essentially involves the coordinated movements of hip, knee and ankle, but would require more space than available to describe in detail. This activity differs from normal gait in that there is a more pronounced weight shift onto the support leg requiring eccentric contractions of the quadriceps and gastrocnemius and soleus. (Push vacuum forward; left leg is forward; right leg back; handle in right hand with cylindrical grasp.)

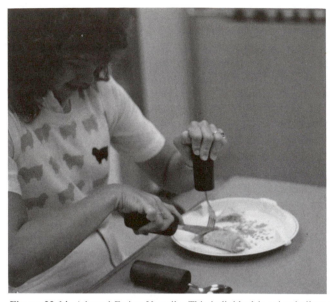

Figure 22-14. Adapted Eating Utensils. This individual is using built-up eating utensils and plate guard to attain independence in feeding. The individual has devised her own method of grip to hold the fork. (St. Francis Hospital, Pittsburgh, PA.)

changes in a typical procedure that will alter the (activity's) complexity'' (Allen, 1985, p. 101).

ADAPTATION

Adaptation is another concept basic to occupational therapy. Individuals use adaptation in response to the demands placed on them by their environments. Therapists may also modify or adapt environments to facilitate the therapeutic process. Such therapeutic adaptations are individualized.

Adaptation requires problem-solving by occupational therapists. Adapting to physical and environmental changes and to stress is of primary concern to the occupational therapist who, with the patient, problem solves a variety of ways of performing activities in order to achieve successful daily living.

When the individual accommodates to environmental demands, this may be called an *adaptive response*. King (1978) described four characteristics of the adaptive response:

1. *It requires a positive role for the individual*; that is, the individual is actively performing the activity; it is not being done to the individual. Consequently, through the individual's participation, the individual is actively adapting to the environment, the situation or the activity and, therefore, is actively involved in the occupational therapy process.

2. *The demands of the environment require adaptation;* that is, occupational therapy uses goal-directed activities ''in a specially structured environment to trigger the unfolding of a need adaptation'' (King, 1978, p. 432). The occupational therapist uniquely uses activities to provide the integration of adaptation into the daily life routine. If individuals want or need to do something and are obstructed by their own inabilities or changes in the environment, then individuals must learn to adapt themselves to the environment or adapt the environment to meet their needs.

3. *Adaptation is most efficient when it is organized on the subcortical level*. For example, when an individual is asked to do an activity, the individual is more successful in accomplishing it when the activity is performed on the subcortical level. Dr. Yerxa, in her Eleanor Clarke Slagle Lecture (1967), aptly described this adaptive response as follows:

   ''A year ago I helped evaluate a brain-damaged patient's function. She was asked to open her hand. No response occurred, except that she was obviously trying. Next she was moved passively into finger extension while the therapist demonstrated the desired movement. This time the patient responded with increased finger flexion. In frustration she cried, 'I know, I know.' Finally she was offered a cup of water. As the cup was perceived, her fingers opened almost miraculously to grasp it'' (p. 5).

   What better example could one use to demonstrate the value of purposeful activity on the subcortical level, rather than exercise. The focus is on the activity or the outcome, providing organization ''of sensory input and motor output to the subcortical centers where it is handled most efficiently and adaptively'' (King, 1978, p. 433).

4. *Adaptation is self-reinforcing*; each successful adaptation serves as a stimulus for attempting the next step. As the individual achieves success in performance, he/she is prompted to attempt more activity at a high level. King (1978, p. 433) states that: ''With purposeful activity, the activity itself is an end, as well as being a means to a larger end, therapy or adaptation. . .'' Consequently, there is motivation for the individual on two levels: (1) for participation in the activity itself, and (2) for establishing or maintaining health or preventing disability.

Adaptation of the therapeutically-used activity is fundamental to the occupational therapy process. When adapting activities, the therapist considers the components of the activity analysis. For example, one can adapt the process of the activity, devising methods of changing the simple performance of the activity through progressions of increasing complexity. The therapist can change the weight of tools to increase or decrease the strength required to progress the patient from hand tools to power tools to increase the complexity of the activity. The materials used in an activity can produce a variety of desired effects such as increased tactile stimulation, increased coordination, or decreased hostility.

Adapting Equipment. The therapeutic environment or the activity and/or tools can be adapted to meet the needs of the individual. Environmental adaptations are described in Chapter 26. Examples of adapting activities include the use of counterbalanced slings to facilitate the use of the upper extremity while performing an activity or utilizing a U-shaped neck support to increase head control of an individual in a wheelchair. Eating utensils can be adapted in numerous ways. For example, the handles of spoons, forks, and knives can be enlarged in size (built-up) to accommodate a weakened grasp; handles can be elongated to accommodate limited range of motion of the upper extremity; knives can be given a curved blade to allow for one-handed cutting; a plateguard may be attached to a plate or a plate designed with a built-in plateguard may assist an individual with incoordination to place food onto utensils (see Figure 22-14). The use of a triangular chair or the corner of a room may enhance a child's ability to support him/herself for an activity (Howison, 1983).

Many homemaking devices can be adapted such as cooking utensils, bowls, cutting boards, and mixer. Many of these adaptations allow for one-handed independence. Self-care devices can also be adapted to increase the individual's ability to be independent. The therapist must consider what adaptations are necessary for independent functioning (see Figure 22-15).

The adaptability of the characteristics of an activity should be considered carefully. An example which has been used by both Cynkin (1979) and Pedretti (1981) is playing board games such as checkers (draughts). The game can be played on a tabletop, on the floor, and vertically, and the playing pieces can be adapted by increasing their size and shape to promote varying degrees of coordination, grasp and release, finger function, and range of motion. It can be played on a floor grid to simulate proper lifting behaviors. The weight of the pieces can be changed to increase the amount of resistance offered to develop strength. Other forms of resistance can be provided, for instance, by adding Velcro to the pieces and the playing board. The texture of the pieces can range from rough to smooth to facilitate tactile sensation and graded prehension strength. These adaptations to the game of checkers are only a few of many that can be developed to adapt a relatively simple activity.

These and other adaptations can be applied to many activities; however, adaptations should not be considered until the normally acceptable methods of performing an activity are understood.

The adaptations to be used by occupational therapists are limited only by the creativity and imagination of the therapist and should be considered a challenge to the practice. It should be stated, however, that the most important criterion of the adaptations incorporated into the activity should be their relevance to the client. The adaptations should also be relatively simple and require only natural movements for their performance. The client should be willing to use the adaptation in performing the activity. If the patient does not value the adaptation, he/she will not achieve the goal of integrating the activity performance into the subcortical level as previously discussed and will not maintain interest in the activity.

The degree of interaction occurring during the activity may also be adapted. The therapist may increase or

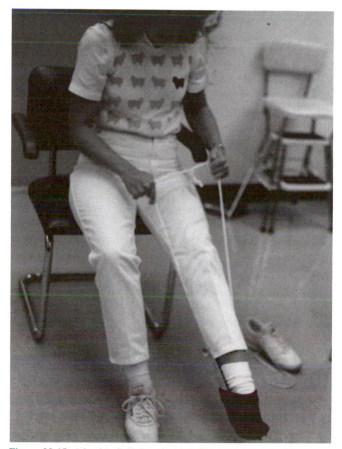

Figure 22-15. Adaptive Self-Care Device. This individual has learned to don her sock with a stocking aid. This assistive device enables her to complete the task inspite of her limited hip and knee flexion. (St. Francis Hospital, Pittsburgh, PA.)

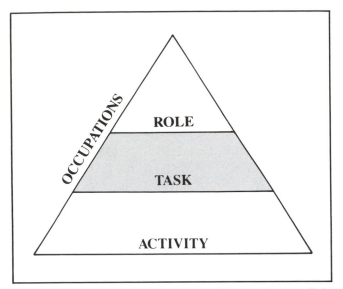

Figure 22-16. The Task Components of the Performance Hierarchy. Tasks require more motivation and commitment from the individual who is influenced by internal factors such as motivation, emotions, abilities and skills. Environmental influences include social system, culture, physical setting and the availability of necessary objects (such as tools and materials).

decrease the number of individuals involved in the activity, just as an activity which as been designed for involvement of one person may be adapted to include two or many more. The directions or rules of the activity may change accordingly. Competition may be added or subtracted. Cooperation of the members of a group may be enhanced by the way the activity is designed or the environment may be set up in such a way as to deter or promote other types of interaction.

One of the areas of primary concern for the occupational therapist is the patient's ability to perform those activities which are part of the individual's daily routine. Many times independence can be achieved with adaptations to those activities which the client performs every day. Occupational therapists may provide commercially available equipment or design individually adapted devices to those individuals who cannot or should not perform the activity in the usually accepted manner. For example, built-up handles on eating utensils or tools may be offered to individuals who have weakened grasp. (See Chapter 26). The number of available adapted devices is almost limitless. Numerous companies have developed and made available such adapted devices for sale. Often the commercial devices are more acceptable to clients because they are more cosmetically acceptable, more durable and less costly than devices fabricated by therapists. Therefore, the advantages of fabrication should be clearly identified before the therapist begins constructing an adapted device that is available commercially.

Avoiding Unnecessary Adaptation. The grading of activities and the adaptation of activities are two concepts that are vital to the therapeutic process. However, they should be considered only after the activity has been analyzed as it is usually performed and then in consideration of the individual's ability or inability to perform the activity. Gradations and adaptations must be incorporated into the treatment plan with careful consideration of the individual's psychosocial and physical needs. The patient should be fully informed and accepting of the activity and environmental adaptations being prescribed to promote his or her progress and independent functioning.

TASK

The next level of the hierarchy is the concept of a task. A task is a set of activities sharing some common purpose recognized by the task performer. This involves a **sequence of actions** involving some labor and difficulty. The work may be assigned or demanded from the person and may prove difficult or taxing. Individuals participate in these actions to satisfy "either societal requirements or internal motivations to explore, become competent or achieve goals in the environment" (Barris, et al., 1985, p. 49). Little (1983) maintains that these actions can be used as units to analyze personality research (p. 276).

Task is a broader concept than activity, and performance will involve either internal or external motivation. Compare the performance levels in Figure 22-16: note that task behavior is goal-directed, so that the environment will influence the individual's performance. Applying the rules of the hierarchy offered earlier, one notes that there are fewer instances of tasks when compared to activities because tasks rule the activity level. Activities are organized or grouped into tasks that have a clear purpose to the task performer. The doer must also have a commitment in the task. For example, getting into a bathtub is an activity but bathing is a task. Activities and tasks are compared in Table 22-5.

In each example, the task requires more concentration and focus than the activity because it is complex and demands attention. Tasks are comprised of activities that are integrated into a meaningful whole, creating a larger unit of doing. Based on the laws of the hierarchy, one cannot isolate a task from its activity components nor can one perform an activity without any regard for how task and role influence the activity components.

Returning again to Table 22-5, note that tasks are more complex than activities but less complex than roles. Thus, one can reason that engaging the patient in an activity affects his or her task and role behavior. Barris and her associates (1985) have maintained that tasks are goal-directed as well as governed by external or internal rules for satisfactory performance. The concept is divided into five dimensions: complexity, temporal boundaries, rules or structure, emotional dimensions, and social components. Each of these dimensions is described in further detail in the following sections.

Task Complexity

One can determine the complexity of a task by determining the "level of skill and the number of steps required to complete the task" (Barris, et al., 1985, p. 49). Skill level is determined by the individual's past and present abilities in sensory, cognitive, perceptual-motor, emotional, social, and cultural aspects of the task. Consider a spinal cord injured patient who has learned how to dress himself but prefers to hire a caregiver to perform this task so he can conserve his energy for other interests. The task of dressing is complex because of the inherent physical, emotional, and sensory components. For the spinal cord injured patient, the cognitive and perceptual aspects of dressing might not be difficult but motor and sensory dysfunction may pose overwhelming obstacles.

In comparison, what if the patient suffered from a cognitive disorder? The physical and sensory aspects of the task may be easy but the cognitive aspects might prove difficult. Thus the cognitively disabled person may chose inappropriate clothing, apply too much shaving lotion, or pull his belt too tight but could easily put on pants and a shirt if properly cued.

In many instances, the complexity of the task increases as the person becomes more accomplished. For example, consider a marathon runner who becomes interested in triathalon competition because this event is more challenging. Even so, one must consider how quickly accomplished individuals can lose interest in familiar tasks even if they are complex. The key issue is how to keep the person motivated and internally challenged. A therapist may create more complex and intricate hand splints after working as a hand therapist for five years but may find the task less interesting than it was initially. Thus, complexity may increase or decrease the person's interest and commitment to the task.

Temporal Boundaries

Tasks may be "time-limited and performed in a discrete unit of time, or they may be continuous, occurring over a long interval with no identifiable point of conclusion" (Barris, et al., 1985, p. 49). Tasks may be designed to be completed in a predetermined period or they may be carried out over an extended time frame. Some tasks have continuous responsibilities such as caring for a child while others may be discharged in a discrete time frame.

Temporal boundaries can make a task enjoyable or stressful. Individuals may find time limitations exciting as they race to meet a predetermined goal. On the other hand, some people may find that the anxiety arising from a time boundary may diminish their performance and compromise their ability to complete a task. For example, some students do well on examinations which have time limits, while others may become too anxious to be successful.

Task Rules

Rules are the standards by which one can judge the quality of a person's participation in a task. A rule is an established guide or regulation for an action, or a customary and familiar way to perform an action. Rules make performance criteria either flexible or rigid. Compare a friendly game of volleyball played with friends with the way that rules and standards are implemented during a tournament.

Emotional Aspects of Tasks

Tasks evoke positive or negative sensations or internalized reactions. Humans react to situations through their sensory organs and these sensations influence task performance. Sensory organs receive input from the environment and the perceptual-motor receptors organize the input so that an appropriate reaction is operationalized. Emotions are also influenced by social factors since tasks may require different degrees of communication and personal interaction. The task of refinishing a table may be enjoyable if an individual likes to work alone, but if she doesn't the assistance of a friend may make the task more acceptable.

Finally, tasks have cultural components which influence feelings. Cultural values are developed during childhood.

Table 22-5		
A Comparison of Selected Activities and Tasks		
ACTIVITY		**TASK**
Brushing teeth		Mouth care
Cooking a hot dog		Meal planning, preparation and clean-up
Weaving a paper mat		Making placemats
Swinging in a net		Play evoking vestibular system
Riding a scooter board		Play requiring balance and coordination
Vacuuming		Housecleaning

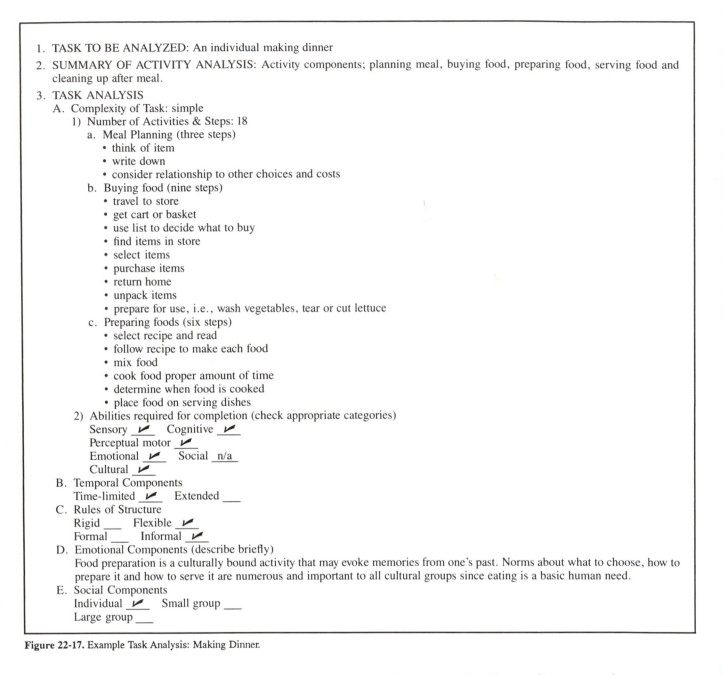

1. TASK TO BE ANALYZED: An individual making dinner
2. SUMMARY OF ACTIVITY ANALYSIS: Activity components; planning meal, buying food, preparing food, serving food and cleaning up after meal.
3. TASK ANALYSIS
   A. Complexity of Task: simple
      1) Number of Activities & Steps: 18
         a. Meal Planning (three steps)
            - think of item
            - write down
            - consider relationship to other choices and costs
         b. Buying food (nine steps)
            - travel to store
            - get cart or basket
            - use list to decide what to buy
            - find items in store
            - select items
            - purchase items
            - return home
            - unpack items
            - prepare for use, i.e., wash vegetables, tear or cut lettuce
         c. Preparing foods (six steps)
            - select recipe and read
            - follow recipe to make each food
            - mix food
            - cook food proper amount of time
            - determine when food is cooked
            - place food on serving dishes
      2) Abilities required for completion (check appropriate categories)
         Sensory ✔ Cognitive ✔
         Perceptual motor ✔
         Emotional ✔ Social n/a
         Cultural ✔
   B. Temporal Components
      Time-limited ✔ Extended ___
   C. Rules of Structure
      Rigid ___ Flexible ✔
      Formal ___ Informal ✔
   D. Emotional Components (describe briefly)
      Food preparation is a culturally bound activity that may evoke memories from one's past. Norms about what to choose, how to prepare it and how to serve it are numerous and important to all cultural groups since eating is a basic human need.
   E. Social Components
      Individual ✔ Small group ___
      Large group ___

Figure 22-17. Example Task Analysis: Making Dinner.

Ideas concerning lifestyle, likes and dislikes regarding choices of food, clothing, manners, time use, recreation, work, daily habits and family relations are established by family members and caregivers. Individuals develop a penchant for a given task because of their values and interests. Consider how some men would not know how to cook a meal where others prepare dinner every night and how some women make home repairs while others could not hold a hammer.

The desire to engage in a particular task depends on a number of factors which include both physical, mental, social, and emotional issues. Culture pervades every aspect of a task as individuals decide whether they find the task relevant or not worth the bother. These judgments are based on feelings about the match between the task and the person's lifestyle.

Another cultural aspect of task performance is the degree of task seriousness or playfulness. Barris, et al., (1985) maintained that this is determined by the "context in which it is performed and the consequences that are contingent upon successful performance" (p. 51). Tasks that evoke playfulness seem to promote more experimentation and exploration because there is less at stake if a failure occurs. Therapists often use the playfulness of a task to elicit different emotions from patients. Individual feelings about tasks are diverse so assumptions about a person's regard for a task must be corroborated.

Try to remember an event that really made you laugh and consider if all of your friends thought that the incident was as funny as you did. Usually there are some members of the group who do not view the event in the same way.

Social Dimensions of Tasks. The social dimensions of a task dictate the degree to which that task promotes interaction with others. A task with few social dimensions is done alone. One can even be alone while working in a group if the task does not promote interaction or if the feedback from others is not used to measure performance. These standards may become a source of motivation since interest can be generated from both internal or external sources for motivation (Burke, 1977, 1983; Rotter, 1966). Social factors create opportunities for communication, standard setting, and motivation.

Task Analysis. A task analysis should be used to organize activities into meaningful units. The analysis should consist of consideration of each of the five components of task: complexity, temporal boundaries, rules or structure, emotional dimensions, and social components. The results of activity analysis form the foundation of the task analysis, since the task level rules the activity level on the performance hierarchy. (Figure 22-17)

ROLE

As described in Chapter One, the highest level of the occupational performance hierarchy is the role. Recall that role is a concept relating to expectations or requirements for the performance of specific activities and tasks necessary to fulfill positions in society. According to Kielhofner, roles can be sexual, familial or occupational; informal or formal. However, virtually every role, regardless of classification, has an occupational component in that it requires the competent performance of specified activities and tasks.

Examine the performance hierarchy in Figure 22-18 and note that roles govern both the task and activity domains. It is important to note that while specific activities and tasks may be relevant to more than one role, it is the role that defines (and therefore governs) the tasks and activities necessary for competent performance. Having the abilities and skills to execute certain tasks may enhance performance in a variety of roles. An example can be provided from the occupational domain of self-care. The tasks of dressing and

grooming are important for success in virtually every role, ranging from that of spouse to employee or president of the local social organization.

Similarly, some work-related activities and tasks may be specific to performance of the worker role in a single vocation. From these examples it can be readily appreciated that role requirements are unique to the individual, and vary in complexity according to the number of roles a person may be occupying at any one time.

Role Function Evaluation

Using the concept of performance to determine appropriate boundaries for occupational therapy practice, one will find that treatment is based on what the person can do. Kielhofner (1985) developed a classification system based on the concept of adaptation which is useful because the individual's occupational function is evaluated in two ways: one satisfying external and the other satisfying internal needs.

External needs are determined by environmental forces. If someone can perform successfully then he/she is occupationally functional, but this is not the complete picture. One must also consider the person's internal needs. Thus, another important aspect of adaptation is whether individual skills, habits, roles, interests, values, motivation, and goals are satisfied. For example, if a genius is afraid to interact with other people, he may be considered as handicapped as a mentally deficient person. However, each has a different occupational dysfunction.

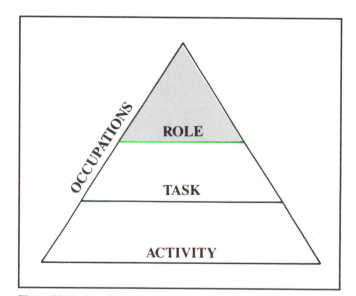

Figure 22-18. Role Component of the Performance Hierarchy. The role components must incorporate the individual's values, personal causation, goals, interests, and habits since role governs the task and activity levels of the Performance Hierarchy.

Individuals who meet both environmental demands and their own internal needs have no need for occupational intervention. An example is a person who has fractured his leg but is able to successfully attend classes and work without professional guidance (Rogers, 1982).

On the other hand, the occupationally dysfunctional person cannot meet societal demands and expectations for productive and playful behavior. Instead, behavior threatens to disrupt all of the other aspects of the person's life, leaving unfulfilled opportunities to explore and master the environment (Cubie and Kaplan, 1982; Kielhofner, 1985; Kielhofner and Burke, 1980).

OCCUPATION

In this text, occupation is used as a general term that refers to engagement in activities, tasks and roles for the purposes of meeting the requirements of living. While occupational domains of work, self-care and leisure are commonly identified, this is not meant to be restrictive. The perspective taken in this text is that all goal-oriented behavior related to daily living is occupational in nature.

The occupations in which one engages are defined by both form as well as performance (Nelson, 1988) and are therefore influenced by personal abilities as well as environmental factors. We have seen that in addition to physical demands, these various influences on occupational performance include values, goals, motivation, interests, roles, and cultural influences; as well as the setting in which occupation occurs. Before prescribing occupations for specific therapeutic goals, the therapist must attempt to understand as much as possible about the individual's lifestyle. By doing so, the promotion of occupational performance is more likely to be viewed in the context of specific role requirements and therefore more likely to be of greater relevance (and benefit) to the individual.

Systems Theory and Occupations

Matching the individual with an appropriate occupation requires knowledge of the individual, his/her lifestyle and occupations. To explain the complexity of the occupation level we return to the view of humans as open systems (Reilly, 1974, 1978; Kielhofner, 1978, 1985). Open systems are dynamic and influenced by function. The open system is part of the environment, which means that individuals perform actions and influence the world around them. This influence is not unidirectional; the environment influences the individual as much as the individual influences the environment. At times, the environment may either promote or retard adaptation to internal and external

demands. This concept is discussed at the beginning of this chapter and in Chapter One.

Occupational Adaptation

Adaptation is the process by which individuals make their behavior, attitudes, or values more suitable to meet external and internal demands. An adaptive being can accept the positive and negative opportunities, challenges, and expectations of the environment and can use these to "maintain and enhance personal integrity and potential" (Kielhofner, 1985, p. 63). The degree of success in changing or adapting performance to meet environmental demands indicates role function. Individuals have many roles and each demands different behaviors. In contrast to open systems, static systems do not respond to external demands. The open system uses information from the environment and creates responses based on this feedback. Occupational therapists use this concept and adapt ccupations by making specific alterations that enhance the individual's performance, such as using a built-up handle to make grasping easier or color-coding dials for the cognitively impaired.

Reilly (1974) originally described a person's function as a continuum of occupational performance. Her ideas were taken from systems theory, sociology, and psychology. Rogers (1982) developed the concept further and urged occupational therapists to focus on occupational dysfunction rather than on remediation of medical problems. Consideration of the individual's occupational abilities will promote care in neglected areas. For example, the truck driver mentioned in the introduction to this chapter suffered from occupational dysfunction. His medical needs were satisfied but he suffered from a loss of roles and habits.

Evaluating Occupational Performance

Before assigning activities, tasks or roles, the therapist must assess the level of occupational performance of the individual. Kielhofner's continuum is a useful tool to describe the varying degrees of occupational function or dysfunction (Kielhofner, 1985). The therapist will use observation and evaluation instruments to determine an appropriate level of performance. *The Occupational History* (Moorhead, 1969), the *Role Checklist* (Oakley, 1982), the *Role Assessment* (Jackoway, Rogers, and Snow, 1987) and *Occupational Role History* (Florey and Michelman, 1982) can be used to evaluate role performance.

Occupational performance can be categorized as:

1. *achievement*: demonstration of knowledge, skills and attitudes needed to perform an occupational role (Reilly, 1974, p. 146; Kielhofner, 1985, p. 64).
2. *competence*: adequate performance that can be im-

Table 22-6
Example Occupational Analysis: Caring for Wild Birds

VALUES

A. *What does the individual value?*

Mrs. Rose values her home and family. She enjoys watching game shows on television. She also seems to view independence as important since she dislikes asking for help.

B. *What objects, tasks, social organizations and cultural values are important?*

OBJECTS: Mrs. Rose values her home and garden. Her son-in-law cuts the grass but the flower beds are overgrown and she expresses concern about this. She takes care of african violets which are carefully tended. She also enjoys several other plants. TASKS: She enjoys looking out her breakfast room window and watching the animals that inhabit the field in back of her home. Mrs. Rose watches television most of the day. She was independent in self-care but now must rely on her daughter or grandsons to dress her. Her daughter supervises her bathing and dressing. She can prepare simple meals but frequently tells her daughter that she is not hungry. SOCIAL GROUPS AND ORGANIZATIONS: Mrs. Rose only relates to her family: a son and daughter-in-law, a daughter and son-in-law and two young adult grandsons. On holidays, she will call her sister who lives in Florida. CULTURE: Mrs. Rose is Episcopalian. She has not attended church services since her husband died twelve years ago. Her husband was a policeman for the local township. Mrs. Rose was a housewife who reared her family without any outside help. She did not often socialize with others. She liked animals and had three dogs and four cats until they each died of natural causes. She tended her garden with enthusiasm until her husband's death. She refuses to attend any senior citizen activities claiming that she would rather be left alone.

C. *How will the occupation be integrated into the individual's value system?*

The importance of animals and wildlife must be considered in proposing occupational enrichment for Mrs. Rose's life. Exercises for improving range of motion in the fractured arm should incorporate her interest in animals and plants.

GOALS

A. *Does the individual have any goals? What are they?*

Mrs. Rose has few goals. She does not want to be sick and dependent on her family. She says that she wants to die.

B. *How does the individual attain his or her goals?*

Mrs. Rose works on her self-care. She works to be independent, expressing anxiety about burdening her family.

C. *How will this occupation promote attainment of individual's goals?*

Mrs. Rose will use veachers to fill the bird feeders and place them on hooks on the back of the house. She will assume the role of a caregiver instead of a dependent role. She must also use her arm to fill the feeders and place them on hooks. The different types of seed will attract different species of birds and she will be able to see the birds up close as they feed on the seed.

PERSONAL CAUSATION

A. *Is the individual self-motivated or influenced by external sources?*

Mrs. Rose is motivated by external sources. She works to dress herself to save her family from bother. She will accept her son's advice because he is a man and she will comply with her physician's orders.

B. *Will the individual pursue occupation without external prompting?*

Mrs. Rose will require external motivation to pursue this occupation. The family members are prepared to encourage her in this role since a new housing development will eliminate the birds' present habitat and Mrs. Rose's feeding program will help the birds to adjust to the new limitations.

INTERESTS

A. *What aspect of the occupation does the individual enjoy?*

Mrs. Rose will enjoy seeing the birds up close since they will feed right at the window. She will enjoy seeing the different species and noting which birds like to eat certain types of feed. She also is interested in how the birds react to the changes in the weather.

B. *How does the occupation fit the individual's other interests?* (Occupational choice)

Mrs. Rose is interested in watching wildlife. She does not want to own another animal; yet, she can watch wild animals for hours at a time.

C. *How is this occupation linked to other interests?*

Occupation will encourage use of upper extremity and offer new interests and habits.

ROLES

A. *What role does this occupation fulfill?*

Mrs. Rose will fulfill caregiver role.

B. *Compare this role with the individual's other roles.*

She is frequently in role of care recipient.

C. *Does fulfillment of the role promote role balance?*

Mrs. Rose will be caregiver for animals and be able to see effect of her role. This is in contrast to other roles where she is a recipient of care. She can control when, where, what, how and how much to feed birds. She can practice making decisions.

HABITS

A. *Does the occupation promote habit patterns?*

Mrs. Rose must be dressed to go outside to replenish feeders. She must use her injured arm to steady feeder and fill it. She then can enjoy all of the birds who feed at her windows.

B. *Will these patterns be consistent with other daily habits?*

Yes, if a habit is established as a bird caregiver, Mrs. Rose will have a role with responsibility for the welfare of the animals.

PERFORMANCE SKILLS

A. *Does the occupation promote task and activity skills?*

Yes.

B. *Integrate task components of the occupation into the occupation.*

TASKS: Selecting and ordering seed from catalog. Filling bird feeders and water containers. Watching birds feed.

C. *Analyze the activity components and incorporate into the occupational analysis.*

ACTIVITIES:

Ordering seed; 4 steps—opening catalog, finding desired item, ordering item by telephone or order and paying for items.

Filling bird feeders; 4 steps—opening seed container, putting funnel into feeder, filling feeder by scooper, returning funnel and replacing lid of feed, replacing feeder in hook using reacher.

Watching birds; 4 steps—focus on particular bird, watch approach to feeder, focus on feeding behavior, watch bird fly away or interact with other birds.

From: Cubie, 1985; Kaplan and Cubie, 1982; Kolodner and Papougenis, 1982; Kielhofner and Burke, 1985; Kielhofner, 1985.

proved and organized into consistent habits and patterns (Reilly, 1974, p. 146; Kielhofner, 1985, p. 66).

3. *exploration*: manipulation of objects, skills, and communication tools that provides an opportunity for learning. Can be playful and entertaining with little serious commitment (Reilly, 1974, p. 47; Kielhofner, 1985, p. 67).

Note that the occupationally functional person begins by exploring the environment sometimes using playful behaviors. Consider your own behavior when you were learning a new occupation. Did you begin with little investment or with commitment and energy? Once invested, you may have gained competence but wanted to learn more about the occupation and improve your performance. Finally, you may have worked very hard to achieve a high degree of success so that your performance was expert.

In contrast, the three levels of occupational dysfunction indicate a diminishing ability to be engaged in the environment. Personal satisfaction may be minimal as the individual receives little positive reinforcement. This creates a spiral of negative feedback. Kielhofner described three dysfunctional levels: (1) *inefficacy* or when interference with performance is coupled with internal dissatisfaction, (2) *incompetence*, which is loss or limitation of skills, with limited satisfaction and inadequate performance, and (3) *helplessness*, when there is total disruption of performance combined with anxiety and feelings of inadequacy (Kielhofner, 1985, pp. 69, 71, 72).

Consider these three levels in a person who is not occupationally functional. At the first level, the person experiences little or no satisfaction from his/her role performance. Feedback is negative and performance is inadequate. The person may display poor work habits, disorganized personal hygiene, and minimal social relations. If the poor performance continues, the individual may deteriorate and performance will become more limited. Satisfaction decreases further as more and more negative feedback is received. Finally, the person may lose all sense of competence and feel anxious and useless (helplessness). Occupational therapists can analyze an individual's level of performance and determine the intervention required. Therapists design activities on an exploratory level, promoting feelings of efficacy and success. These opportunities should be playful and non-threatening, an attempt to capture the individual's interest. Once the patient indicates a degree of interest, the therapist upgrades the activity to keep the individual engaged. If unsuccessful, the therapist will select another activity, trying different experiences. When the individual shows interest the therapist expands the activity and upgrades the success until competence is achieved, using tasks and possibly occupations. At times, intervention will reach the achievement level.

Occupational Analysis

The occupational analysis will require the enlistment of the individual's values, goals, personal causation, interests, roles, and habits. One would call this the volitional and habituation subsystem, if using the model of human occupation (Kielhofner and Burke, 1980, 1985). The occupation level involves the person in a long-term commitment to a particular goal-directed process.

Case Study 22-3

Mrs. Rose, is an 81-year-old woman who sustained a Colles fracture of her dominant, right upper extremity when she fell down the stairs in her home. Although Mrs. Rose lives next door to her daughter, she rarely ventures out of her home. Confused and depressed, she does not like to participate in any activity. She was independent in her own self-care until she was injured. Even though the cast was taken off two weeks ago, she still requires assistance with fasteners, cooking, laundry, shopping, and ironing. She has no friends and talks to her daughter and grandsons once every few days. The therapist has initiated some upper extremity exercises (activities) and some cooking (tasks) which Mrs. Rose seems to enjoy. The occupational therapist would like Mrs. Rose to develop an occupation which will promote both physical and psychosocial function and offer opportunities for a new role and new habits. Table 22-6 is an example of an occupational analysis of Mrs. Rose.

ENVIRONMENTAL INFLUENCE ON PERFORMANCE

The environment is defined as a composite of all external forces and influences affecting the development and maintenance of an individual (Hopkins & Smith, 1983, p. 920). Occupational therapy uses the doing process to promote the highest degree of function in individuals who suffer from performance deficits. Understanding the doing components (role, task, and activity) is one aspect of the therapist's understanding of the individual's problems. The performance hierarchy is part of the individual's world since humans are viewed as open systems. What does this mean to the practicing therapist?

No one functions in a vacuum. Thus, it is important to consider the environment as a part of the performance hierarchy. Adjusting the original performance hierarchy, we now add the last level of environment (see Figure 22-19).

When considering how to use the doing process the therapist must consider the individual's environment. The environment consists of the conditions, circumstances and influences that effect the development of an organism. The environment has always been part of the occupational therapy process (Meyer, 1922; Dunning, 1972). Barris (1982, Barris, et al., 1985) analyzed the concept of environment in relation to occupational therapy practice. She depicted the environment as a series of concentric circles: objects, tasks, social groups and organizations, and culture (Barris, et al., 1985, p. 43).

The encompassing influence of the environment must be considered when developing roles, tasks, and activities for the individual. To assist with the evaluation of the environment, Cubie (1985) suggested consideration of the objects, tasks, social groups and organizations, and culture before prescribing a task, or activity. The importance of the environment has been described in greater detail in Chapter 5, The Physical Environment and Performance. The purpose here is to link environment to the performance hierarchy.

Occupational therapists have a unique perspective on individual performance. This perspective began with the founders of occupational therapy. Instead of focusing on the individual's diagnosis or pathology or what is medically wrong, occupational therapists consider the functional performance of the patient. This means that the medical diagnosis is merely one of many important considerations that include the person's goals, values, motivation, interests, roles, and habits. In fact, therapists are presently treating people who are considered medically sound but dysfunctional in selected roles and habits. The absence of a medical diagnosis does not preclude the possible value of occupational therapy intervention (Rogers, 1982). For example, consider a therapist's treatment of a learning disabled child. There is nothing medically wrong with the child, but he/she suffers from neurological problems which impair learning as well as some other aspects of performance. The occupational therapist will use activities and tasks to promote increased competence in the roles of student, sibling, and peer. (See Figure 22-20.)

Three important concepts are presented here: (1) the activity, task, and role levels of the performance hierarchy, (2) the importance of the environment, and (3) the function/dysfunction continuum. The application of these ideas is presented in the case study that follows. Every aspect of the individual's life had been adversely affected by his disability, and the therapist uses a holistic approach in motivating the patient to participate in his recovery.

Case Study 22-4

Ned Nitsky is a 26-year-old, robust, athletic man who was injured on the job when the scaffolding on which he was standing collapsed. Ned was initially rushed to a trauma

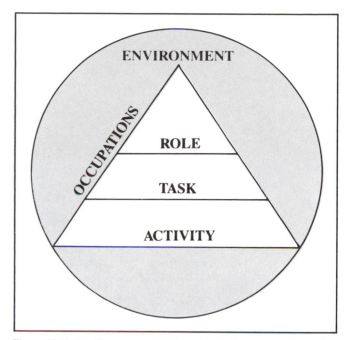

Figure 22-19. The Environmental Influence in the Performance Hierarchy. The pervasive influence of the environment affects every level of the performance hierarchy. Environmental considerations must be included in every aspect of treatment planning.

center where he was found to have a spinal cord injury at the C7 level. The injury left Ned quadriplegic with the loss of all voluntary motion below the level of the lesion. After four weeks in the hospital, his condition stabilized, and he was transferred to a rehabilitation center.

Ned was the middle child of three boys. A talented athlete in high school, he won a college scholarship by playing soccer and tennis, which gave him the financial resources to complete his course of study in philosophy in three years. Undecided about his future, Ned decided to work in a trade before settling into a chosen vocation. A friend asked him to work as an electrician and Ned discovered that he enjoyed the pragmatic balance between planning and application. He enrolled in a training program and completed his apprenticeship in four years. During this time he continued to work for a contractor and was soon supervising other apprentices.

Ned's social life revolved around his family and fiancee, Irene. Ned and Irene had dated since their college days together and they planned to marry in a short time. Ned lived in his own apartment a short distance away from his family. This was a familiar community since he had lived there as a child.

Ned worked diligently during the day but valued his freedom. He liked to return to his own apartment after work, relax, and have no constraints placed on his time. He would listen to music, care for his apartment, complete personal chores, or shop. Ned did his own cooking and made simple meals for himself and Irene at least three times a week. He

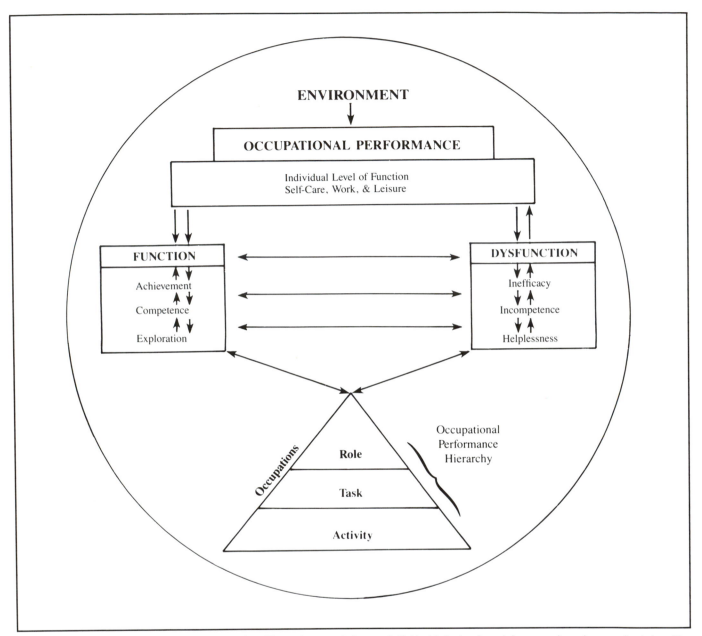

Figure 22-20. Promoting Function through Occupation. The environment influences individual behavior through human and non-human stimulation. The individual is an open system so that performance is affected by the environment and the environment is affected by the performance of the individual.

was also a frequent visitor to his parent's home and enjoyed the camaraderie of his parents and brothers. He also visited Irene's family several times a month.

Ned was a loner. Irene was his only close friend. He occasionally would meet some friends from work and share an evening with them but this was not a common occurrence. He especially enjoyed the company of his older brother and they would work on fixing and rehabilitating cars and vans. Ned loved to work on his own van as well. He would clean and wax it, creating his idea of a perfect form of transportation and luxury. His other interests included country and western

music and the outdoors. Ned was deeply committed to environmental issues. He enjoyed backpacking and hiking. He had tried mountain climbing but disliked all of the trappings and socialization that were required. Ned liked to be alone with Irene and come and go as he pleased.

Ned had no intention of participating in a rehabilitation program. In fact, his first words to the admitting nurse at the center were, "I am not going to therapy. No one can help me. This is all so useless since I am a cripple."

Angry and depressed, he refused to do anything. Ignoring social workers, psychologists, and family members, he withdrew further into himself. He would not even allow Irene to see him or talk to him. On the ward, he was angry and verbally abusive to the nursing staff. Soon his behavior deteriorated to the point that the nurses dreaded working with him. They reported that he was noncompliant and difficult.

After two weeks of this behavior the rehabilitation hospital director visited Ned and told him that he would have to attend therapy within 24 hours or else he would be discharged, since he was using space that could be better used by another person. Ned's response was to throw himself out of bed onto the floor. The commotion that resulted brought him a lot of attention but he asked to be left alone. Nurses on duty reported that he cried softly to himself for several hours. Feeling that he preferred to work these emotions through by himself, they gave him as much privacy as possible.

The next day he allowed the staff to wheel him into physical and occupational therapy but he refused treatment. He permitted the physical therapist to passively range his extremities but cut short all attempts to engage him in conversation.

The occupational therapist asked Ned what he liked to do. He responded negatively and the therapist then commented that the hospital had many recreational activities that he might find enjoyable. Ned stared at the therapist as if he was unsure whether she was teasing him or trying to involve him in some odious chore.

Suddenly, in a torrent of pent-up emotions he described the pleasures of his former life: how he loved to work with his hands, how he loved to fix mechanical things—vans, motorcycles, and cars, how he enjoyed electrical work because of the concentration, knowledge, and skill that were required to keep simple errors from resulting in dangerous mistakes. He spoke with longing about his own van and how he missed working on it. The van was something that he had created with Irene and they both traveled every weekend to open spaces experiencing a sense of freedom and abandon.

Suddenly, Ned stopped and looked at the therapist in anger. He said, "What does it matter now? A cripple can't drive a van, get married, or have kids." When the therapist tried to tell him that all of these goals were realistic and plausible, he became agitated and demanded the termination of the therapy session. For the next three days, he refused all therapy and acted as he had before.

The next incident demonstrates the motivating power of activities. The therapist decided to visit Ned on Saturday because she was working anyway. She brought a catalog of equipment used to modify cars and vans for people with disabilities. Ned was taken by surprise and he agreed to look at the catalog. While turning pages, the therapist pointed out several adaptations which might make Ned's van more serviceable for his interests and needs. Ned started to get excited; hooked, he was anxious to get more information. The therapist had prepared for this possibility and was equipped with a telephone book and some page-turning devices. She showed him how to look up the dealer who had adapted vans for some other patients. Ned learned how to dial the telephone and use the page turner by himself.

Ned thought that the adaptive devices were humorous but he telephoned the dealer and made an appointment for the following Monday. Using the initial activity of looking through a catalog, Ned began to engage in a task. The task became the renovation of his van. The next activity was looking up the telephone number of a dealer and next using the telephone. These three activities stimulated Ned's interest in the renovation and adaptation of his van. He could imagine himself in a competent role, using the vehicle to pursue his favorite occupation—travel outdoors.

Note the hierarchy of doing that bridged Ned's present and former lifestyles. The activity moved him from the level of helplessness to a level of incompetence because he realized that he had to learn a number of new skills. However, he also realized that although his life had drastically changed, there were still a number of opportunities that he could pursue to make his present life meaningful.

At discharge Ned was evaluated as having full strength in his shoulder muscles, with elbow extension, supination, and wrist extension, but weakened pronation and ulnar wrist flexion. His incomplete lesion left him with partial hand function, including limited grasp, release, and dexterity. The thumb had weakened function, but he was able to abduct and extend it. Ned demonstrated sensory loss along the ulnar nerve. He lacked trunk stability, but had bed mobility; that is, he could sit up in bed, roll over, and move about. He was confined to a wheelchair, but he was expected to gain full wheelchair independence and the ability to transfer from bed to wheelchair.

Everything did not fall magically into place for Ned after discharge. He could dress independently and feed himself without the aid of assistive devices. He could perform all hygiene activities and had independent bowel and bladder control; however, he could not change his catheter independently. Emotionally, he still experienced times of intense anger and sadness, but tried to work through these emotions and accept his life of daily challenges.

THERAPEUTIC EFFECTS OF OCCUPATION

The dramatic difference in Ned's performance demonstrates the therapeutic effect of the activity process. Success on a small scale made Ned feel better, and he was skillfully engaged in occupations that promoted his performance in self-care, work, and leisure pursuits. As he received more positive feedback from the environment, he was energized to try new activities and tasks. He ultimately developed new occupations which were compatible with his former lifestyle. The change in Ned was based on the concepts introduced throughout this chapter.

Occupational therapy problem-solving is based on systems theory. The environment influences role behavior, offering a myriad of life choices. After the overwhelming stress of Ned's accident, he had to reconsider his values, goals, interests, roles, habits, and skills. The interrelationships among all of these factors is presented in Figure 22-20. The performance hierarchy is expanded so that the individual can be considered in the context of the environment.

SUMMARY

The foundation of the occupational therapy process is based in commitment to the benefits of activities, tasks, and roles on individuals. Stimulating interests through activities can prove beneficial to individuals who are occupationally dysfunctional. Therapists work to keep the arousal high by expanding the activities offered into tasks that sustain the individual's interests and promote new roles and habits. Ultimately, therapists work to introduce occupations that can provide sustained, positive reinforcement from the environment.

Study Questions

1. What is the ideological basis of occupational therapy?

2. Explain the systems theory and its importance to occupational therapy practice.

3. Explain how activities can stimulate interests.

4. Compare an activity and a task.

5. Think of a patient who visited the occupational therapy clinic and then refused treatment. What factors may have contributed to this patient's negative attitude toward occupational therapy? Use the performance hierarchy to explain how occupational therapists could improve their services.

Acknowledgements

The authors wish to acknowledge the collaboration of Susan Cook Merrill, MA, OTR/L, who offered invaluable assistance with formulating initial ideas for this chapter and developing the case study 22-4. We also thank Gary Kielhofner, DrPH, OTR, FAOTA, for his careful review and feedback on this chapter, and David L. Nelson, PhD, OTR, FAOTA, for sharing his thought-provoking ideas on how to define occupation. Our appreciation is also extended to Norman Gustafson, OTR/L, Staff Therapist, St. Francis Hospital, Pittsburgh, PA, who collaborated in analyzing the vacuuming activity and developed the Working Model Pipe Assembly Project. We thank Kathleen Bakis, COTA, St. Francis Hospital, Pittsburgh, PA, who graciously gave her time and effort in providing the photos of self-care, and Doris Kaplan, former director of Norristown State Hospital, Norristown, PA for hospital photographs. We also thank the American Occupational Therapy Foundation and Williams and Wilkins Company for permission to use photographs.

References

Addams, J. (1920). *Democracy and social ethics*. New York: Macmillan Company

Addams, J. (1935). *My friend Julia Lathrop*. New York: Macmillan Company.

Ad hoc Committee of the Commission on Practice (1980). The role of occupational therapy in the vocational rehabilitation process: Official position paper. *American Journal of Occupational Therapy, 34*, 881.

Allen, C.K. (1985). *Occupational therapy for psychiatric diseases: Measurement and management of cognitive disabilities*. Boston: Little, Brown and Co.

American Occupational Therapy Association. (1978). *Occupational therapy product output reporting system and uniform terminology for reporting occupational therapy services*. Rockville, MD: American Occupational Therapy Association, Inc.

Anderson, R.S. (Ed.). (1968). *Army Specialist Corps*. Washington, D.C.: Office of the Surgeon General, Department of the Army, U.S. Government Printing Office.

Aquaviva, F. (Ed.). (1985). *Occupational therapy manpower: A plan for progress*. Rockville, Maryland: American Occupational Therapy Association.

Ayres, A.J. (1966). Interrelationships among perceptual-motor functions in children. *American Journal of Occupational Therapy, 20*, 68-71.

Ayres, A.J. (1969). Deficits in sensory integration in educationally handicapped children. *Journal of Learning Disabilities, 2*, 160-168.

Ayres, A.J. (1979). *Sensory integration and the child*. Los Angeles: Western Psychological Services.

Barris, R. (1982). Environmental interactions: An extension of the model of occupation. *American Journal of Occupational Therapy, 36*, 637-644.

Barris, R., Kielhofner, G., Levine, R., & Neville, A.M. (1985). Occupation as interaction with the environment (pp. 42-62). In Kielhofner, G., (Ed.). *A model of human occupation: Theory and application*. Baltimore: Williams and Wilkins.

Beard, G.M. (1972). *American nervousness: Its causes and consequences*. New York: Arno Press.

Boris, E. (1986). *Art and labor: Ruskin, Morris, and the craftsman ideal in America*. Philadelphia: Temple University Press.

Borysenko, J. (1987). *Minding the body: mending the mind*. Reading, MA: Addison-Wesley.

Boulding, K.E. (1961). *The image*. Ann Arbor, MI: University of Michigan Press.

Boulding, K.E. (1968). General systems theory—the skeleton of science (pp. 3-10). In Buckley, W., (Ed.). *Modern systems research for the behavioral scientist*. Chicago: Aldine.

Breines, E. (1987). Pragmatism as a foundation for occupational therapy curricula. *American Journal of Occupational Therapy, 41*, 522-525.

Burke, J.P. (1977). A clinical perspective on motivation: Pawn vs. origin. *American Journal of Occupational Therapy, 31*, 254-258.

Burke, J.P. (1983). Defining occupation: Importing and organizing interdisciplinary knowledge (pp. 125-138). In Kielhofner, G., (Ed.). *Health through occupation*. Philadelphia: F.A. Davis.

Burnham, S.C. (1972). Medical specialists and movements toward social control in the progressive era: Three examples. In J. Israel (Ed.). *Building the organizational society*. (pp. 19-30), New York: Free Press.

Capra, F. (1983). *The turning point: Science, society, and the rising culture*. New York: Bantam Books.

Christiansen, C.H., Schwartz, R.K., & Barnes, K.J. (1988). Self-care: Evaluation and management (pp. 95-115). In DeLisa, J., Curie, D.M., & Gans, B. (Eds.). *Principles of rehabilitation medicine*. Philadelphia: J.B. Lippincott.

Committee on Installations and Advise. (1928). Analysis of crafts. Continuation of the report of the Committee on Installations and Advise. *Occupational Therapy and Rehabilitation, 7*, 131-133.

Cousins, N. (1979). *Anatomy of an illness*. New York: W.W. Norton.

Cubie, S.H. (1985). Occupational analysis (pp. 147-155). In Kielhofner, G., (Ed.). *Model of human occupation: Theory and application*. Baltimore: Williams and Wilkins.

Cubie, S.H. & Kaplan, K.A. (1982). Case analysis method for the Model of Human Occupation. *American Journal of Occupational Therapy, 36*, 645-656.

Cynkin, S. (1979). *Occupational therapy: Toward health through activities*. Boston: Little, Brown and Company.

DeCarlo, J.J. & Mann, W.C. (1985). The effectiveness of verbal versus activity groups in improving self-perceptions of interpersonal communication skills. *American Journal of Occupational Therapy. 39*, 20-27.

Diasio-Serrett, K. (1985). Another look at occupational therapy's history: Paradigm or pair-of-hands? *Occupational Therapy in Mental Health, 5*, 1-31.

Dunning, H. (1972). Environmental occupational therapy. *American Journal of Occupational Therapy, 26*, 292-298.

Dunton, W.R. (1918). The principles of occupational therapy. *Public Health Nursing, 10*, 316-321.

Dunton, W.R. (1928). *Prescribing occupational therapy for nurses*. Springfield, IL: Charles C. Thomas.

Edgerton, W.M. (1947). Activities in Occupational Therapy (p. 41). In Willard, H.S. and Spackman, C.S., (Eds.). *Principles of occupational therapy*. Philadelphia: J.B. Lippincott.

Ferguson, M. (1980). *The Aquarian conspiracy: Personal and social transformation in the 1980's*. Los Angeles: J.P. Tarcher, Inc.

Fidler, G.S. & Fidler, J.W. (1963). *Occupational therapy*. New York: Macmillan Company.

Fiebleman, J.K. (1954). Theory of integrative levels. *British Journal for the Philosophy of Science, 5*, 59-66.

Florey, L. (1969). Intrinsic motivation: The dynamics of occupational therapy theory. *American Journal of Occupational Therapy, 23*, 319-322, 1969.

Florey, L. & Michelman, S.M. (1982). Occupational role history: A screening tool for psychiatric occupational therapy. *American Journal of Occupational Therapy, 36*, 301-308.

Fuller, D.H. (1912). Introduction: The need of instruction for nurses in occupations for the sick (Foreword). In Tracy, S.E. *Invalid occupations: A manual for nurses and attendants*. Boston: Whitcomb and Burrows.

Gleave, G.M. (1947). Occupational therapy in children's hospitals and pediatric services. (pp. 141-174). In Willard, H.S. and Spackman, C.S., (Eds.) *Principles of occupational therapy*. Philadelphia: J.B. Lippincott.

Griffith, E. (1984). *In her own right: The life of Elizabeth Cady Stanton*. New York: Oxford University Press.

Gritzer, G. & Arluke, A. (1985). *The making of rehabilitation: A political economy of medical specialization, 1890-1980*. Berkeley: University of California Press.

Haas, L.J. (1924). One hundred years of occupational therapy, a local history. *Archives of Occupational Therapy, 3*, 83-100.

Hamill, C.M. and Oliver, R.C. (1980). *Therapeutic activities for the handicapped elderly*. Rockville, MD: Aspen Systems Corporation.

Hopkins, H.L. (1988). A historical perspective on occupational therapy. In Hopkins, H.L. & Smith, H.D. (Eds.). (1988). *Willard and Spackman's occupational therapy*. Philadelphia: J.B. Lippincott.

Howison, M.V. (1983). Occupational therapy with children—cerebral palsy. In Hopkins, H.L. and Smith, H.D. (Eds.). (1983). *Willard and Spackman's occupational therapy*. (pp. 671-675). Philadelphia: J.B. Lippincott.

Illich, I. (1977). *Medical nemesis: The expropriation of*

health. New York: Bantam Books.

Jackoway, I.S., Rogers, J.C., & Snow, T. (1987). The role change assessment: An interview tool for evaluating older adults. *Occupational Therapy in Mental Health*, 7, 17-37.

Jacobs, K. (1985). *Occupational therapy: Work-related programs and assessments*. Boston: Little, Brown and Co.

Johnson, J.A. (1983). The changing medical marketplace as a context for the practice of occupational therapy (pp. 163-177). In Kielhofner, G. *(Ed.)*. *Health through occupation: Theory and practice in occupational therapy*. Philadelphia: F.A. Davis.

Kaplan, W. (1987). *The art that is life: The arts and crafts movement in America, 1875-1920*. Boston Museum of Fine Arts. Wilmington, MA: Acme Publishing Co.

Kielhofner, G. (1978). General system theory: Implications for the theory and action in occupational therapy. *American Journal of Occupational Therapy, 32*, 637-645.

Kielhofner, G. (1983). Occupation (pp. 31-41). In Hopkins, H.L. & Smith, H.D. (Eds.). *Willard and Spackman's occupational therapy*. Philadelphia: J.B. Lippincott.

Kielhofner, G. (1985). The human being as an open system (pp. 2-11). In Kielhofner, G. (Ed.). *The model of human occupation: Theory and application*. Baltimore: Williams and Wilkins.

Kielhofner, G. & Burke, J.P. (1977). Occupational therapy after 60 years: An account of changing identity of knowledge. *American Journal of Occupational Therapy, 31*, 675-689.

Kielhofner, G. & Burke, J.P. (1980). A model of human occupation, Part 1: Conceptual framework and content. *American Journal of Occupational Therapy, 34*, 572-581.

Kielhofner, G. & Burke, J.P. (1985). Components and determinants of human occupation (pp. 12-36). In Kielhofner, G. (Ed.). *A model of human occupation: Theory and application*. Baltimore: Williams and Wilkins.

King, L.J. (1978). Toward a science of adaptive responses. *American Journal of Occupational Therapy, 32(7)*, 429-437.

Kolman, C. (1987). Changing life roles after physical injury. *Occupational Therapy Forum. Atlantic Edition, 11(43)*, 12-13, 17.

Kolodner, E.K. & Papougenis, D.S. (1982). Occupational behavior evaluation outline (pp. 21-23). In Barris, R., Kaplan, K., Kielhofner, G., Kolodner, E., Levine, R., Neville, A., Papougenis, D., & Schaaf, R. *Occupational behavior: A clinical perspective: A workbook to demonstrate the application of the model of human occupation to occupational therapy practice*. Philadelphia: Department of Occupational Therapy, College of Allied Health Sciences, Thomas Jefferson University.

Laszlo, E. (1972). *The systems view of the world: The natural philosophy of the new developments in the sciences*. New York: George Braziller.

Lears, T.J.J. (1981). *No place of grace*. New York: Pantheon Books.

Leininger, M. (1978). *Transcultural nursing: Concepts, theories and practices*. New York: John Wiley & Sons.

Levine, R.E. (1987). Culture: A factor influencing the outcomes of occupational therapy. *Occupational Therapy in Health Care, 4*, 3-16.

Licht, S. (1948). *Occupational therapy sourcebook*. Baltimore: Williams and Wilkins.

Little, B.R. (1983). Personal projects. *Environmental Behavior, 15*, 273-309.

Llorens, L. (1986). Activity analysis: Agreement among factors in a sensory processing model. *American Journal of Occupational Therapy, 40(2)*, 103-110.

McDonald, M. (1968). *Occupational therapists before World War II*. In Army Medical Specialists Corps. H.S. Lee, H.S. and McDaniel M.L., (Eds.). Washington, D.C.: Office of the Surgeon General, Department of the Army, U.S. Government Printing Office.

Mechanic, D. (1979). *Future issues in health care*. New York: The Free Press.

Meyer, A. (1922). The philosophy of occupation therapy. *Archives of Occupational Therapy, 1*, 1-10.

Minutes of Representative Assembly (1979). Philosophical base of occupational therapy. *American Journal of Occupational Therapy. 33*, 785.

Moorhead, L. (1969). The occupational history. *American Journal of Occupational Therapy*, 23(4), 329-334.

Mosey, A.C. (1981). *Occupational therapy: Configuration of a profession*. New York: Raven Press.

Nelson, D.L. (1988). Occupation Form and Performance. *American Journal of Occupational Therapy, 42(10)*, 633-641.

Nelson, D.L., Peterson, C., Smith, D.A., Boughton, J.A., and Whalen, G.M. (1988). Effects of project versus parallel groups on social interaction and affective responses in senior citizens. *American Journal of Occupational Therapy, 42*, 23-29.

Oakley, F.M. (1982). *The role checklist*. College Park, Maryland.

Pedretti, L.W. (1981). *Occupational therapy: Practice skills for physical dysfunction*. St. Louis: C.V. Mosby.

Pollack, H.M. (1927). Educational principles in occupational therapy. *Occupational Therapy and Rehabilitation, 6*, 99-104.

Reed, K.L. & Sanderson, S.R. (1983). *Concepts of occupational therapy*. Baltimore: Williams and Wilkins.

Reilly, M. (1962). Occupational therapy can be one of the the great ideas of 20th century medicine. *American Journal of Occupational Therapy, 16,* 1-9.

Reilly, M. (1974). An explanation of play (pp. 117-149). In Reilly, M. (Ed.). *Play as exploratory learning: Studies of curiosity behavior.* Beverly Hills, CA: Sage Publications.

Reilly, M. (1978). *Curriculum planning in occupational therapy.* Workshop sponsored by Department of Occupational Therapy, Temple University, Philadelphia.

Rodgers, D.T. (1974). *The work ethic in industrial America 1850-1920.* Chicago: University of Chicago Press.

Rogers, J.C. (1982). The spirit of independence: The evolution of a philosophy. *American Journal of Occupational Therapy, 36,* 709-715.

Rogers, J.C. (1982). Order and disorder in medicine and occupational therapy. *American Journal of Occupational Therapy, 36,* 29-35.

Rosenberg, C.E. (1961). *No other gods: On science and American social thought.* Baltimore: The Johns Hopkins University Press.

Rotter, J.B. (1966). Generalized expectations for internal versus external control of reinforcement. *Psychological Monographs: General and Applied, 80,* whole number, 609.

Ruskin, J. (1884a). *Lectures on Architecture and Painting delivered at Edinburgh in November, 1853.* New York: John Wiley & Sons.

Ruskin, J. (1884b). *Pre-Raphaelitism.* New York: John Wiley & Sons.

Sacks, O. (1987). *The man who mistook his wife for a hat.* New York: Perennial Library.

Sands, I. (1928). When is occupation curative? *Occupational Therapy and Rehabilitation, 7,* 115-122.

Schmale, A.H. (1958). Relationship of separation and depression to disease: A report on a hospitalized medical population. *Psychosomatic Medicine, 20,* 259-277.

Scott, C.S. (1974). Health and healing practices among five ethnic groups in Miami, Florida. *Public Health Reports,* 89, 524-532.

Shannon, P.D. (1977). The derailment of occupational therapy. *American Journal of Occupational Therapy, 31,* 229-234.

Slagle, E.C. (1922). Training aids for mental patients. *Archives of Occupational Therapy, 1,* 11-17.

Steckel, H. (1934). Retrospective evaluation of therapy. *Psychiatric Quarterly, 8,* 489-498.

Tracy, S.E. (1912). *Studies in invalid occupation: A manual for nurses and attendants.* Boston: Whitcomb and Burrows.

von Bertalanffy, L. (1968). General system theory—A critical review. In Buckley, W. (Ed.). *Modern systems research for the behavioral scientist.* Chicago: Aldine.

Wade, B. (1947). Occupational therapy for patients with mental disease. In Willard, H.S. and Spackman, C.S. (Eds.). *Principles of occupational therapy.* Philadelphia: J.B. Lippincott.

Washburne, M.F. (1915). *Study of child life.* Chicago: American School of Home Economics.

West, W.L. (1968). *Professional services of occupational therapists, World War II.* In Army Medical Specialists Corps. Lee, H.S. and McDaniel, M.L., (Eds.). Washington, D.C.: Office of the Surgeon General, Department of the Army, U.S. Government Printing Office.

Wiebe, R.H. (1967). *The search for order, 1877-1920.* New York: Hill and Wang.

Wright, G. (1980). *Moralism and the model home: Domestic architecture and cultural conflict in Chicago 1873-1913.* Chicago: University of Chicago Press.

Yerxa, E.J. (1967). Authentic occupational therapy. *American Journal of Occupational Therapy, 21,* 1-9.

Yerxa, E.J. (1980). Occupational therapy's role in creating a future climate of caring. *American Journal of Occupational Therapy, 34,* 529-534.

Yerxa, E.J. and Sharrott, G. (1986). Liberal arts: The foundation for occupational therapy education. *American Journal of Occupational Therapy. 40,* 153-159.

CHAPTER CONTENT OUTLINE

KEY TERMS

Bilateral integration

Hypotonicity

Internal postural control

Motor planning

Neuromuscular re-education

Perceptual motor skill

Sensory integration

Spasticity

Visual neglect

Visual orientation

Visual perception

ABSTRACT

This chapter explores various treatment strategies to improve functional motor
performance following neurological insult to the brain. The factors affecting the
ability to move purposefully are examined in two major categories: those that
influence a person's ability to produce movement (neuromotor factors), such as
degree of voluntary movement, abnormal tone, orthopedic limitations and
endurance, and those which influence the person's ability to learn and organize
movement for adaptation, such as postural adaptation, motor planning and visual
awareness. General guidelines for treatment and for designing integrated
treatment programs are offered, including principles to guide task selection.

Strategies for Sensory and Neuromotor Remediation

Mary Warren

''Without movement there is no adaptation and without adaptation there is no life.''

—Elnora Gilfoyle, Ann Grady, and Josephine Moore, 1981

OBJECTIVES

The information in this chapter is intended to help the reader—

1. understand the components of motor learning ability and neuromotor control and how these components contribute to the person's ability to move.

2. understand the similarities and differences between the major neuromuscular treatment techniques.

3. understand how the spiral of spatiotemporal adaptation is applied to postural adaptation in the brain-injured adult, and appreciate the importance of postural adaptation to motor and perceptual learning.

4. identify motor planning deficits in adult brain-injured patients and design treatment strategies to facilitate motor planning skill.

5. identify visual scanning deficits in adult brain-injured patients, understand the neurological basis for these deficits, and design appropriate treatment interventions using therapeutic activities.

6. understand how to design treatment programs which facilitate integration of the patient's perceptual, cognitive, and motor function.

INTRODUCTION

This chapter explores various treatment strategies used to improve the efficiency of a patient's functional motor performance following neurological insult to the brain from a cerebral vascular accident (CVA) or head injury. Before one can understand how to apply treatment strategies, the purpose of movement and its intrinsic components must first be understood. Movement is the physical means by which man interacts with the environment, and therefore movement is integral to survival. When the ability to move is disrupted by injury or disease the central nervous system (CNS) automatically strives to compensate. Normal movement has a purpose or a goal; we work to accomplish a task. Purpose for movement is supplied by an environmental event and an innate desire to adapt to it; for example, a friend throws a book at you and you duck; you walk by a bakery, smell fresh donuts, and go inside; or your bus starts to leave without you and you run after it. As occupational therapists, we work with brain-injured patients to regain movement, not for its own sake, but for the accomplishment of a purposeful activity. We want a patient to gain sufficient sitting balance in order to bend down and

put on socks, or we want a patient to develop grasp in order to grip an orange and peel it.

Components that Enable a Person to Respond to the Environment

As previous chapters have shown, many intrinsic enablers contribute to human motor performance. Sensorimotor, cardiovascular, cognitive, and psychosocial factors each exert unique influence on the individual, and help shape response to the environment. Movement is the end product of the integration of these components. Each component must contribute its share to enable a person to respond purposefully to the environment. Basic physiological functions such as respiration, heart rate, and blood pressure must be sufficient to support life. Sensory information must be registered from the body and from the environment. The person must attend to this sensory information, categorize it, compare it to past events of a similar nature and decide whether it is important. (See Figure 23-1)

Consider the following scenario:

> You're on a playground. Suddenly your friend yells, "catch!" You look up and your visual system detects a ball coming towards you (the environmental event). You check your somatosensory system. It tells you that you're standing on two feet and that you have your hands in your pockets. You compare this new incoming, somatosensory and visual information with past experiences in catching balls, and you realize that in order to successfully catch the ball, you must take your hands out of your pockets and widen your stance. Then you ask yourself, "Do I care if I catch it?" You decide the answer is "yes," and you execute your plan. The ball lands in your hands, and hence, you succeed! You toss the ball back to your friend, and the process begins again.

This entire process occurs within seconds. A deficit in any one of the components affects the quality and quantity of the entire motor response. One must be able to see the ball to judge when to respond to it and to sense feeling in one's legs to determine whether one is standing on one or both. One must be able to compare the incoming sensory information with past experiences to determine a plan of action, the

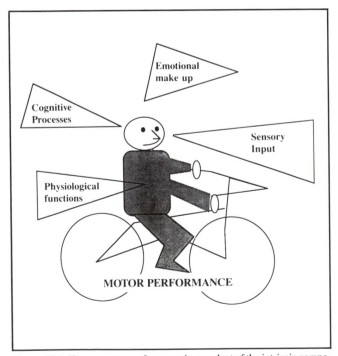

Figure 23-1. Human motor performance is a product of the intrinsic components of sensory input, physiological functions, cognitive processing and emotional make up.

importance of the event to motivate execution of the plan, and adequate physiological support needed to physically execute the plan.

Neurological insult to the brain from disease or injury can affect the integrity and functioning of one or all of these components. Therefore, successful treatment programs address the strengths and weaknesses of each component. Overlooking any component reduces the effectiveness of the treatment program and, ultimately, the patient's ability to re-adapt to the environment.

The ability to move purposefully involves the interaction of a number of neuromotor, cardiovascular, musculo-skeletal, sensory, and psychological factors. These factors can be categorized into two general groups: (1) those that influence the person's ability to produce movement and (2) those that influence the person's ability to learn and organize movement for adaptation. For the purposes of discussion, the first category can be labeled *neuromotor control* and includes such factors as the degree of voluntary movement present, the presence of abnormal tone, the presence of orthopedic limitations and pain, and limited endurance. The second category can be called *motor learning ability* and includes postural adaptation, motor planning, and visual awareness. Each factor in the two categories contributes equally to the person's ability to physically adapt to the environment. (See Figure 23-2)

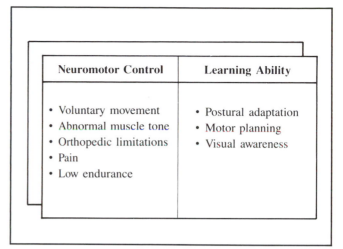

Neuromotor Control	Learning Ability
• Voluntary movement • Abnormal muscle tone • Orthopedic limitations • Pain • Low endurance	• Postural adaptation • Motor planning • Visual awareness

Figure 23-2. Two categories of factors which affect an individual's ability to move purposefully. *Neuromotor control* influences the ability to produce movement; *learning ability* affects the ability to organize movement.

NEUROMOTOR CONTROL DEFICITS AND STRATEGIES

Neuromotor Factors

The following discussion provides a more general overview of the influence of neuromotor factors on the quantity and quality of the movement regained following neural insult. These factors were discussed in detail in Chapters 9 and 10.

Degree of Voluntary Movement Present. One of the first determinations a therapist must make when assessing the movement potential of a patient is to establish how much voluntary movement the patient can produce. The diagnosis may provide some guidance. A patient with a complete lesion of the spinal cord below C6 should exhibit good strength in the deltoid, biceps, latissimus dorsi, serratus anterior, pectoralis, and radial wrist extensor muscles. Likewise a patient with occlusion of the middle cerebral artery will probably experience hemiplegia of the contra-lateral side. Diagnoses give the therapist a starting point for assessment and treatment, but one of the first lessons learned in the clinic is that few patients exhibit all of the

classical symptoms of a given diagnosis. Most patients exhibit individuality in movement ability, much the same as they exhibit individuality in personality. Because of this, a careful movement assessment must be completed on every patient.

The potential to regain voluntary motor control is also partially dictated by diagnosis. Patients with injuries or disease affecting the spinal cord and/or peripheral nervous system are limited in the ability to regain movement by the extent of the damage done to motor pathways. An individual with a complete lesion of the spinal cord at C6 will not regain movement of the lower extremities even with extensive and expert therapy. Individuals sustaining brain injuries have greater potential to regain voluntary control due to the greater plasticity of the central nervous system (Moore, 1986). However brain-injured individuals often have an overlay of sensory, cognitive, and emotional deficits which significantly limit the ability to realize this potential. A patient's ability to regain movement often depends on the therapist's ability to act as a facilitator and guide and perhaps even push the patient to achieve his or her maximum potential. The patient's diagnosis should guide, but not restrict, the goals set for a patient because tests cannot measure a person's desire to adapt.

Presence of Abnormal Tone. Damage to the brain and spinal cord nearly always results in an alteration of muscle tone in the affected extremities. Muscle tone can be defined as a continuous mild contraction of the muscle tissue in its resting state (Chusid & DeGroot, 1988). Normal muscle has a certain resilience which is felt when stretched. The level of tone in a muscle can be increased or decreased by damage

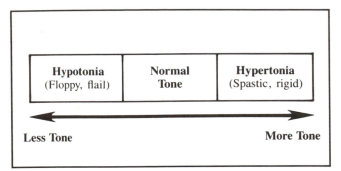

Figure 23-3. Muscle tone lies on a continuum with hypertonic and hypotonic tone on opposite sides. Normal muscle tone lies within the middle part of the continuum.

to the nervous system. As Figure 23-3 illustrates, muscle tone can be thought of as being placed on a continuum with severe **spasticity** and rigidity at one end and flaccidity on the other end. Normal muscle tone lies somewhere in the middle of the continuum. It is important that the therapist decide where the patient's muscle tone falls on the continuum before initiating a treatment program, because motor performance is affected differently depending on the amount of tone present.

When **spasticity** is present in a muscle, the level of tone in the muscle is higher causing increased responsiveness to stimulation. Spastic muscles are hyper-responsive to external sensory stimulation and to efferent commands from the brain. Unfortunately, it is the nature of spasticity to affect only certain muscle groups in the upper and lower extremities (Bobath 1978). The selective nature of spasticity results in a disruption of the synergy of the muscles during movement. When a person attempts to combine individual muscles to produce a certain movement pattern, the spastic muscles overreact and contract too strongly. This prevents the other muscles from completing their action and disrupts the synergy of the pattern. Figure 23-4 illustrates this problem. In this picture, a stroke patient with hemiparesis is attempting to reach out to grasp a cone. The normal muscle synergy for this act would involve combining elbow extension with shoulder flexion to extend the arm away from the body. But this stroke patient has spasticity in the elbow flexors, and when she attempts to reach for the cone, the elbow flexors are also stimulated and contract because of their elevated muscle tone, thus preventing the weaker elbow extensors from completing their action. Instead of movement of the hand away from the the body towards the cone, the stroke patient's hand moves towards the chin. Because spasticity increases with stress, the more the patient tries to move the arm away from the body, the stronger the elbow flexors contract and the more restricted the movement pattern becomes.

Spasticity results in decreased motor coordination and restricted movement. The person loses selectivity of movement, which results in decreased versatility and flexibility in adapting to the environment. In some cases, the level of spasticity can be reduced by drugs which relax the central nervous system. The effects can also be minimized by the therapist's approach to treatment (discussed later in this chapter). Some individuals can also learn to cortically relax their spasticity during movement through visualization. For example, they may picture their arm to be a "wet noodle" as it moves.

On the other end of the tone continuum is the person with *hypotonic muscle tone*. **Hypotonicity** can affect motor coordination and restrict movement as significantly as spasticity. Muscle tone provides the foundation for muscle movement. A certain amount of muscle tone must be present to generate an adequate muscle contraction. Hypotonic muscles are hypo-responsive to sensory stimulation and efferent commands from the brain. As a result, the patient must put much greater effort into contracting the hypotonic muscles. Most patients cannot sustain the mental effort needed to complete a purposeful activity using hypotonic muscles, so their nervous system looks for shortcuts. Shortcuts appear in the form of substitutions of stronger muscles and use of tonic reflexes such as the *asymmetrical tonic neck reflex* (ATNR). Research has shown that post-CVA patients purposefully will turn the head toward the involved side to elicit the ATNR to reinforce elbow extension when reaching for an object (Yamshon, Machek, Covalt, 1949).

Hypotonicity like spasticity affects movement by decreasing motor coordination and restricting motion. The person loses selectivity in movement and experiences decreased versatility and flexibility in adapting to the environment. However, the approach to treatment is very different. Instead of relaxing tone, the person must learn to increase it, and the therapist must apply techniques that facilitate rather than inhibit tone. The issue is made more complex by the fact that many patients exhibit mixed patterns of spasticity and hypotonicity in the same extremity, and both problems must be addressed simultaneously in treatment.

Presence of Orthopedic Limitations and Pain. In addition to muscle weakness, restrictions in the joint and ligamentous structures of the extremity significantly will affect the potential of the patient to regain purposeful movement. Restrictions may have been present before the injury/illness as a result of the person's lifestyle. For example, a truck driver is likely to have weak abdominals and shortened hamstrings as a result of prolonged sitting behind the wheel. This premorbid condition combined with hamstring spasticity may make it more difficult for a truck driver to relearn to ambulate following a stroke. The older the patient is, the more likely he/she is to have a preexisting orthopedic problem, such as chronic bursitis or arthritis.

Orthopedic limitations may also occur as a result of the sudden immobilization of the joints following paralysis. Adhesions may develop in the shoulder joint resulting in compromised circulation, restrictions in range of motion, and pain (Andersen, 1985). Edema may produce similar results in the hand. Subluxation of the humeral head is common following CVA due to weakness in the muscles surrounding the joint. Mishandling of the weakened extremity can result in tendonitis and bursitis (Caillet, 1981).

Most of these conditions result in pain. As Chapter 9 describes, pain is a complex neurophysiological event. However, it has a simple and nearly universal effect on a person's motivation to move: it destroys it. If a movement causes pain, that movement is avoided. Experiencing a stroke does not change the basic human nature to avoid unpleasant stimulation. In reducing motivation to move, pain also significantly reduces the patient's potential to regain movement. For that reason, the existence of pain is always addressed in treatment planning.

The most effective treatment approach to pain is a multidisciplinary approach involving physical therapy, nursing, the physician, and occupational therapy. The physician can prescribe drug therapy, the physical therapist can apply modalities to relieve the pain, the nurse can ensure that the patient is being properly positioned and moved, and the occupational therapist, by the use of activity, can elicit movement from the patient despite the pain. Each discipline must recognize its strengths and apply them. Physical therapists (PT's) are expertly trained in the application of modalities and exercise; most occupational therapists (OT's) are not. In contrast, occupational therapists are experts trained in the application of activity and activity analysis; physical therapists are not. While one discipline may gain expertise in the other's field, their basic approach to treatment is different. When the OT and PT team work together, this difference can enhance treatment rather than detract from it.

Endurance. As discussed in Chapter 8, cardiovascular and muscular endurance exert significant influence on motor performance. Limitations in endurance following brain injury may be either of the nature of physical fatigue, or fatigue from the mental exertion required to move weakened limbs.

Brodal, a neuroanatomist, described the influence of mental fatigue on motor performance in an article he wrote after sustaining a CVA resulting in weakness of his left extremities. In the article, he describes the deficits caused by his stroke, correlating them to the area of his brain which had been damaged (Brodal, 1973). At one point, he describes the great mental effort required to move his hemiparetic arm, stating, ''Subjectively this is experienced as a kind of mental force, a power of will. In the case of a muscle just capable of being actively moved, the mental effort needed was very great . . . it felt as if the muscle was unwilling to contract, and as if there was a resistance which could be overcome by very strong voluntary innervation.'' (p. 677). Brodal found that if the therapist passively moved his arm into the desired position several times before he attempted the movement, the effort required was lessened. The sensory input readied his nervous system to produce the movement and reduced the amount of mental exertion required. Passively moving a patient through a desired movement pattern several times before calling for active motion is a technique advocated by Bobath (1978) to facilitate movement.

One of the limitations imposed by reduced physical endurance is the patient's inability to participate in a full therapy program. Therapy sessions must be kept brief with frequent rest periods. If the patient has sustained an injury to the brain which affects his ability to learn new information in addition to decreased endurance, his potential to regain functional skills is even further reduced. The patient will require more time to process new information in order to learn a task and be physically unable to participate long enough for the processing to occur. Such patients can still relearn functional skills if activities in the therapy program

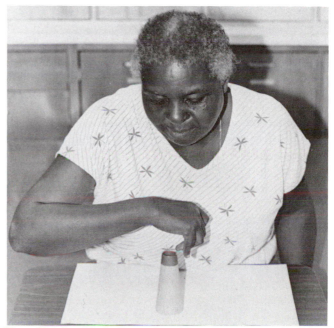

Figure 23-4. Spasticity in elbow, wrist and finger flexors prevents this patient from extending her elbow and fingers to grasp the cone.

are carefully graded to compensate for reduced endurance. Careful activity analysis must be applied, so that only the critical elements of task are taught and practiced. For example, in teaching an elderly stroke patient to put on a shirt, the first critical element of the task is to locate the sleeve and start the involved hand in the opening. The second critical element is to pull the sleeve onto the forearm, then to push it up the arm, then over the shoulder, and so on. To avoid fatigue, the therapist may require the patient only to initiate the critical elements of the task. That is, the patient starts the hand into the sleeve, and the therapist pushes the sleeve onto the hand. The patient starts pulling the sleeve onto the forearm, and the therapist completes it, and so on. As the patient's endurance improves, the therapist requires that he/she complete more and more of the task. Using a graded approach enables the patient to learn to organize and complete a task without becoming overly fatigued. *Grading activities so the task provides sufficient challenge to facilitate learning, but does not overwhelm the patient, is a crucial skill for clinicians treating patients with many types of deficits, including brain-injury.*

Neuromuscular Re-Education

Neuromuscular re-education is the term used to describe treatment to improve motor function in patients following brain and spinal cord injury. There are four major treatment approaches on neuromuscular re-education in current use by physical and occupational therapists. *Neurodevelopmental treatment* (NDT) is the approach espoused by Berta and Karl Bobath. *Proprioceptive neuromuscular facilitation* (PNF) is based on the work of Margaret Knott and Dorothy Voss. Margaret Rood developed an extensive and comprehensive body of knowledge on sensorimotor treatment known simply in clinics as *the Rood technique*. Signe Brunnstrom studied adult hemiplegia and developed an approach for movement integration following stroke known as *the Brunnstrom technique*. Several newer approaches gaining favor with therapists include the work of Carr and Shepard on motor relearning following brain injury and Margaret Johnstone on restoration of motor function in the stroke patient (See the recommended reading list at the end of this chapter for information on all of these techniques). Collectively, these frameworks comprise a shared body of knowledge between occupational and physical therapists. They are generally applied only to the treatment of motor dysfunction following brain injury, although some techniques such as PNF claim a more universal application. While some therapists ally themselves with one framework and strictly adhere to its principles, the majority of clinicians use an eclectic approach drawing from each.

The frameworks easily can be distinguished from each other in treatment emphasis and technique. But they share a common neurophysiological foundation based on two assumptions about central nervous system function:

1. *The central nervous system is capable of plasticity in response to damage.* That means that the CNS is able to change and modify its organization to compensate for damage. PNF theory refers to this as "human potential." If humans were not capable of CNS plasticity, then therapy would be limited strictly to teaching strategies to compensate for disability rather than remediation. As Chapter 9 discusses, research exists to support the capacity for CNS plasticity

2. *Motor output can be modified through application of sensory stimuli.* The organization and execution of movement can be modified by altering the type, amount, and timing of incoming sensory information. As discussed in Chapter 9, the motor system depends heavily on sensory processing to respond effectively to the environment. By controlling the sensory stimulation given, the therapist can either facilitate or inhibit movement in the patient.

The treatment approaches also share many principles based on a developmental perspective which holds that motor patterns develop in infancy and redevelop following brain injury in predictable patterns. For example, Brunnstrom identifies seven stages of motor return in adult hemiplegia. Bobath describes three stages of motor return and states that postural control precedes motor coordination. Rood identified the mobility/stability continuum, and Knott and Voss maintain that diagonal control develops in a supine to seated to standing progression.

Other treatment principles shared by the major approaches include:

1. *Motor control proceeds in a cephalocaudal fashion (head to foot) and proximal to distal.* The treatment emphasis in each theory is on developing trunk control first, then proceeding outward through the extremities.

2. *Movement should be relearned in purposeful patterns rather than specific muscle actions.* Motor learning is facilitated by the use of goal-directed and purposeful movement patterns. The goal of therapy is to enhance subcortical and automatic control, not cortical direction of movement. This differs markedly from approaches advocating the use of biofeedback and electrical neuromuscular stimulation in regaining motor control.

3. *Motor control is learned through repetition of purposeful movement patterns.* The patient will learn what he/she is required to practice.

All of the approaches share a common goal of the

reintegration of motor ability and the reorganization of a disorganized motor system. None promises normal movement, but each strives for the least stereotyped, most voluntary, and most flexible movement possible.

Where the approaches differ markedly is in treatment approach and technique. Treatment approach is determined by what each proponent sees as the major neuromotor problem following brain injury. While no approach arbitrarily advocates a single treatment technique, biases are readily apparent. Bobath (1978) identifies spasticity as the major obstacle to regaining motor control. According to Bobath, spasticity is the culprit responsible for both abnormal motor coordination and the disruption of body integration and the blending of posture and movement. Her treatment approach is directed towards inhibition and relaxation of spasticity. Gentle and light handling techniques are emphasized, which guide the patient away from patterns of spasticity into normal patterns of control. Bobath states that all movement must be performed effortlessly to avoid influence of the spastic pattern.

In contrast, Brunnstrom and PNF see the major obstacle to regaining motor control as weakness or a lack of voluntary control of movement. This lack of control disrupts body integration and the balance of flexor and extensor muscle groups and prevents normal movement patterns. Their approaches are directed toward facilitation and applying resistance and eliciting effort from the patient to gain movement. They emphasize patterns that promote strength and range of motion.

Rood takes the middle ground in advocating the use of either inhibition or facilitation depending on the patient's level of developmental control.

The treatment decision facing the clinician is whether to take an inhibitory or facilitory approach towards the patient. Each perspective tends to ignore the issue of the other. Brunnstrom and PNF never completely address the issue of spasticity and abnormal reflex patterning, and Bobath never completely addresses the issue of strength. This can create a dilemma for the therapist because patients usually present mixed problems of spasticity and weakness. Most therapists resolve the issue by matching the patient's major problem to the treatment approach best suited to remediate that problem and then execute that approach in such a way as to avoid exacerbating the other motor problems. That is, if the patient exhibits very little spasticity and a lot of weakness, a facilitory approach is used and emphasis is on applying resistance to elicit increased muscle contraction in such a way as to prevent a significant increase in spasticity. This is often accomplished by combining treatment techniques. For example, the therapist may use a resistive PNF technique such as *rhythmic stabilization* to elicit contraction of the proximal shoulder musculature. This may be applied with

the patient in a Rood reflex-inhibiting position of weight-bearing to prevent an increase in finger flexor spasticity. If the therapist understands the common treatment principles underlying the major approaches, he/she correctly can combine techniques for maximum treatment effectiveness.

SENSORY PROCESSING AND MOTOR PLANNING DEFICITS AND STRATEGIES

Factors Influencing Motor Learning Ability

Patients who have sustained injury to the spinal cord or peripheral nervous system primarily experience problems with neuromotor control as just described. Brain injuries however, usually result in more complex disruptions in movement.

Brain-injured patients not only experience problems with neuromotor control, but often their ability to learn new motor patterns and carry out motor sequences is impaired as well. They exhibit what is essentially a ''learning disability'' in the reorganization of movement, which reduces their ability to learn the compensatory motor strategies needed to increase their level of independence. Their disability stems from disorganization of **perceptual motor skill**. It is not a problem with motor strength, but a problem with motor organization and execution. **Perceptual motor skill** involves the ability to effectively organize and carry out movement to accomplish a goal-directed activity. The process involves sensory assimilation and integration (perception), and motor output (Kephart, 1971). *Sensory assimilation* involves the integration of two types of sensory information: sensory information coming from within the body through the somatosensory and vestibular systems and sensory information coming into the body from the environment through the visual and auditory senses. *Motor output* refers to motor planning or *praxis*, which is the ability to organize and execute complex voluntary movement. The assimilation of sensory information occurs both before and after the motor act in a sensory-motor-sensory sequence.

We can examine the sequence of events in this process by using the example given at the beginning of the chapter —that of a ball being thrown on a playground. The ball is thrown, the visual system registers the movement, the auditory system registers the shout of ''look out!,'' and the somatosensory and vestibular systems identify the body's position in space and readiness to catch the ball. The central nervous system integrates this sensory information, compares it to past sensory experiences, and issues a motor command. The person makes a motor accommodation by widening the stance and bringing the arms up to catch the ball. The motor accommodation creates sensory feedback which initiates the next motor response and so on. According to Gilfoyle, Grady and Moore (1981, p. 50), sensorimotor-**sensory integration** results in the maturation of sensory perception and skilled movement.

Injury to the brain can disrupt the organization of perceptual motor ability. When this occurs, the individual has difficulty learning new functional skills, often despite good physical ability. New skills, such as ambulating with a cane, writing with the non-dominant hand, or dressing one-handed are difficult to master. It is the learning disability and not the motor loss that limits potential for independence and leaves both therapist and patient frustrated in treatment. As stated previously, three ability areas support skilled movement: postural adaptation, motor planning, and visual awareness. Deficits may occur in one or more of the areas and contribute to disorganization of perceptual motor skill.

Postural Adaptation. Postural adaptation is the ability to remain steady and upright against gravity during changes in body position. It provides the foundation for controlled movement of the limbs. In adults, it is an internalized function whereby the body provides support for its own movement through midline stability and equilibrium reactions (Gilfoyle, Grady, & Moore, 1981). Infants must depend on external means of support from other people, the floor, the infant carrier and such, until they develop **internal postural control**.

While postural adaptation technically does not fall under the definition of perceptual motor ability, it can significantly affect the person's ability to relearn and execute purposeful movement and thereby contribute to the learning disability. Postural adaptation should occur automatically without conscious effort. We do not think about staying upright when we reach for a book on a shelf or put laundry in the dryer. We concentrate on the activity and let our bodies automatically program and execute the muscle contractions needed to keep us on our feet. When this ability is disrupted by brain injury, a person suddenly must concentrate all mental efforts on remaining upright against gravity. Little mental energy is left for relearning purposeful movement.

Mature Postural Strategies. Mature postural adaptation is characterized by a constant trade-off between the body sides for support and movement. For example, during ambulation, the lower extremities alternate between support and swing phases; when riding a bike, the upper trunk and extremities are held steady while the legs move; and when catching a ball, the legs and lower trunk stabilize while the arms reach out. Two methods are used to achieve the balance between stability and mobility: rotation-counter-

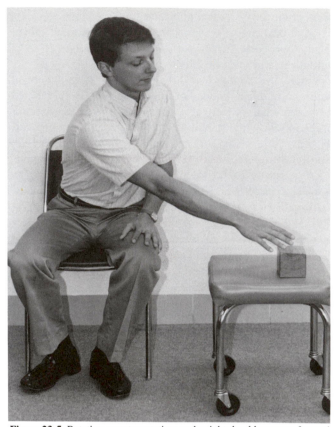

Figure 23-5. Rotation-counter-rotation: as the right shoulder rotates forward to extend the hand towards the block, the left shoulder rotates in the opposite direction to counter and control the pattern.

rotation and movement-countermovement (Gilfoyle, Grady, & Moore, 1981).

Rotation-counter-rotation occurs around the midline of the body. As one side or extremity rotates in one direction, the opposite side or extremity rotates in the opposite direction. For example, during ambulation, the pelvis and shoulder on the weight-bearing side rotate posteriorly as the pelvis and shoulder on the non-weight-bearing side rotate forward. In a mature segmental rolling pattern, movement of one half of the trunk (upper or lower) is countered by movement of the other half in the opposite direction. (See Figure 23-5)

Movement-countermovement occurs on a linear plane between the body sides or within the same extremity (Gilfoyle, Grady, & Moore, 1981). As the hand is projected forward to grasp an object, the shoulder moves backwards in a countermovement to add control to the pattern. (See Figure 23-6) If the person's center of gravity is shifted significantly forward as when the arm reaches for the object, the other arm will automatically counter the shift by extending backward.

Rotation-counter-rotation and movement-countermovement form the foundation for the equilibrium reactions and internal postural control (Gilfoyle, Grady, & Moore, 1981). They blend the two sides of the body together into a bilaterally integrated unit. **Bilateral integration** of the body sides is the hallmark of mature postural control.

Brain injuries typically cause paresis and spasticity in one half of the body. This is known as *hemiplegia* or *hemiparesis.* Motor accommodations are impaired on the affected side, preventing that half of the body from responding as efficiently as the other half. Subsequently, bilateral integration of the body sides is lost. Since internal postural control is dependent on bilateral integration, when bilateral integration is lost, mature postural control is also lost. However, the person's need to physically adapt to the environment remains unchanged following hemiplegia. This person still needs to dress, walk, roll over, and bathe. The motor system must adjust to the loss of mature postural strategies and find a way to compensate with its remaining motor abilities. Compensation is achieved through reenlistment of lower level patterns of posture and movement in accordance with the spatiotemporal adaptation framework developed by Elnora Gilfoyle and Ann Grady (Gilfoyle, Grady, & Moore, 1981).

Gilfoyle and Grady propose that the development of skilled movement proceeds along a spiraling continuum. (Figure 23-7) Early patterns of movement are integrated into higher level, skilled movement through a combination of environmental experiences and central nervous system maturation. These early patterns lose their original identity as they are absorbed into higher level patterns, but they continue to influence the individual's movement. Inherent

to this view is the principle that individuals never acquire totally new motor patterns. The ability to develop increasingly skilled movement is dependent on past acquired behaviors; for example, a child must learn to sit unsupported before learning to stand unsupported.

Spatiotemporal stress is the stimulus which organizes the motor system and provides the impetus for motor development. Spatiotemporal stress is defined by Gilfoyle and Grady as a "temporary state characterized by an inability to adapt one's highest level of posture and movement strategies to purposeful behaviors/activities" (p. 173). The motor system appears to have an established strategy for resolving stress. When first stressed, the individual attempts to adapt using the highest level posture and movement strategy. For adults, this is generally walking or standing. If this strategy fails, the individual slips down the spatiotemporal spiral and calls forth a lower level strategy to adapt to the situation. The person will continue to move down the spiral until a posture and movement strategy is found which meets the situation and resolves the stress. For example, an individual walks out onto an icy parking lot after the first winter storm of the year. Initially, one attempts to walk on the ice with arms at the sides using a mature reciprocal gait pattern. However, if one begins to slip (the stress), a lower level strategy is immediately enlisted. The arms are raised into a high guard position and legs are spread to widen the base of support. If this second strategy fails, one will slip automatically further down the spiral and call up cruising, grabbing onto a nearby railing or car. If that also fails, one will begin creeping on hands and knees, thus continuing to dip lower and lower down the spiral until the strategy is found which allows one to adapt and move on.

Patterns of Postural Dysfunction Following Brain Injury. Patients with paralysis and spasticity experience spatiotemporal stress with every postural adjustment and movement. Their motor system attempts to resolve this stress as genetically programmed by dipping down the spatiotemporal spiral until a successful posture and movement strategy is found. Many of the motor behaviors displayed by brain-injured adults are remnants of lower level behaviors integrated into the person's movement repertoire the first year of life. Following brain injury these more primitive patterns are reenlisted by the motor system to help stabilize and mobilize the body. They reappear as part of a normal stress reaction (Warren, 1984). How far the individual slips down the spiral depends on the severity of the motor loss. The slip may be barely noticeable, perhaps only a diminution of the equilibrium reactions, or it may be significant, leaving the person with the postural and movement strategies of a one-month-old child.

Persons who have sustained significant motor loss use several posture and movement strategies developed in the

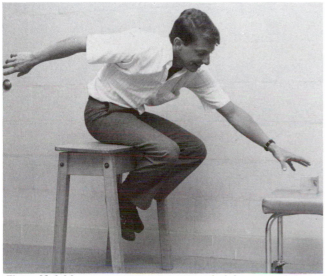

Figure 23-6. Movement-counter-movement: as the left arm extends forward to grasp the block, the right arm counters by moving backwards and the head and neck extend to prevent the person from falling forward.

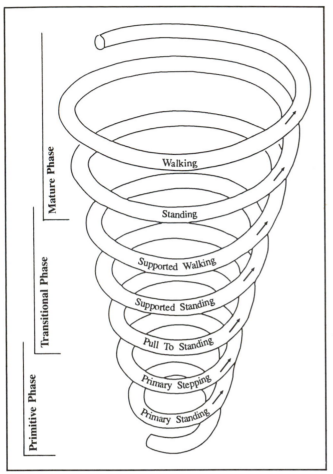

Figure 23-7. Key behaviors of standing/walking as illustrated through the spiraling continuum of spatiotemporal adaptation. *From Gilfoyle, Grady, & Moore: Children Adapt, 1981. (Courtesy of Slack, Inc.)*

first months of life to physically adapt to their environment. These strategies often can be observed readily as the patient moves about the clinic. They include the following patterns:

Upper Extremity Retraction-Fixation. This is a static pattern consisting of varying degrees of scapular depression and retraction, humeral abduction and internal rotation, elbow flexion, and pronation of the forearm. Wrist and finger flexion are also often present. The pattern is first observed in the pivot-prone posture assumed by infants and during early attempts to maintain a prone-on- elbows position. It reappears later as a high guard position when the child begins standing and walking (Figure 23-8). The pattern is purposefully used by the child to increase upper trunk stability and improve postural control (Gilfoyle, Grady, & Moore, 1981).

Following injury to the motor system, the pattern may be reenlisted to increase upper trunk stability when postural security is threatened. The pattern is typically observed on the involved side, when the adult patient is performing a

movement which is posturally stressful, such as walking or leaning forward to pick up an object. The pattern diminishes when the person is resting or is in a posturally secure and supported position.

Although the pattern is similar to the flexor synergy pattern identified by Brunnstrom, it is not the same. Brunnstrom's pattern occurs as the patient attempts to move the arm. The muscles involuntarily contract together as a synergy. The retraction-fixation pattern is a static response to postural stress and may appear in patients who have selective control of upper extremity movements, as is illustrated in Figures 23-9 and 23-10.

Undifferentiated Movements. These are mass movements of the trunk and/or extremities which occur through complete or nearly complete range of motion before antagonistic movement is initiated. They are observed in early infancy as movements of the extremities and trunk in bilateral reciprocal patterns of flexion and extension and are used to gain strength and control of movements against gravity (Gilfoyle, Grady, & Moore, 1981). The adult brain-injured patient may use undifferentiated movement

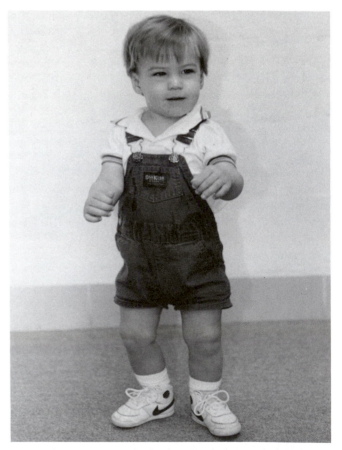

Figure 23-8. Upper extremity fixation-retraction pattern is observed as a high guard position in the child just beginning to stand unsupported.

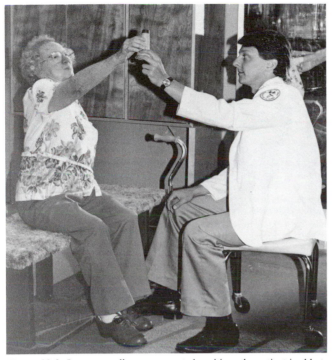

Figure 23-9. In a posturally secure, seated position, the patient is able to extend the affected upper extremity to reach out for a cone.

can be seen in art and sports. Hellebrandt (1956) among others has shown that they tend to reappear when the normal person's motor system is under stress and are used to reinforce postural control and direct movement.

With brain injury, remnants of these tonic reflexes are often apparent in the patient's movement. In some cases the reflexes reappear in a constant obligatory form, automatically triggered by external sensory input. The automatic grasp reflex associated with severe injury to the prefrontal motor area is such an example (Luria, 1980). However, most therapists report observing these reflexes only when the patient is posturally stressed. The positive support reaction is not observed until the patient attempts to walk, and the grasp reflex first becomes apparent during a transfer when the patient unconsciously clutches the wheelchair or the therapist's arm. Head turning is observed during ambulation as the patient attempts to use the asymmetrical tonic neck reflex to increase extensor tone in the weight-bearing leg. The reflexes may reappear in blatant or subtle

patterns to gain mobility. Such patterns are frequently observed when a patient rolls from supine to side-lying on the sound side. The patient uses undifferentiated flexion of the head and upper trunk to initiate the roll and inertia and push/pull of the sound extremities to complete the roll. The pattern is used because the patient lacks rotation-counter-rotation, a necessary component for mature segmental rolling. Similar patterns are seen when the patient moves from sitting to supine and vice versa. Instead of using movement-countermovement of the opposite limbs to control descent, the patient flexes the hips and "folds" in an undifferentiated pattern of trunk flexion and then swings into supine pivoting on the buttocks, as seen in Figure 23-11 and 23-12.

Tonic Reflexes. The tonic reflexes are used developmentally to increase postural tone and gain postural security (Gilfoyle, Grady, & Moore, 1981). They include the positive support reaction, grasp reflex, and the tonic neck reflexes. They are absorbed into higher level patterns and lose their obligatory nature as the individual matures; however their influence continues to be felt in mature adult movement. The tonic neck reflexes, in particular, have been shown to be easily elicited in normal adults and appear as a natural component of most of the postural patterns assumed by humans (Figure 23-13) (Hirt, 1967; Waterland & Munson, 1964; Fukuda, 1962). Examples of their influence

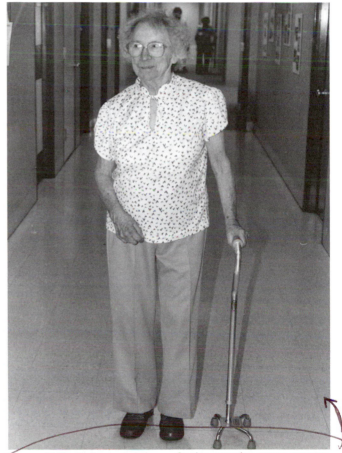

Figure 23-10. During ambulation, a fixation-retraction pattern automatically appears in the upper extremity on the affected side to increase postural tone in the upper trunk on that side. The patient would be unable to extend the arm to reach out for a cone in this less secure position.

forms, but they are used by brain-injured adults for the same purpose as they are used by infants, that is to increase postural stability and direct movement.

Use of the Upper Extremities for Support. The first combination posture and movement strategy learned by the infant is to use the upper extremities for support while mobilizing the lower extremities (Gilfoyle, Grady, & Moore, 1981). This is first observed in the prone-on-elbows position when the head, upper trunk, and arms are held firm as the legs kick away. The child returns to the strategy repeatedly as he or she moves upright against gravity. Pulling to stand, cruising, and supported sitting are examples of the strategy. It is not until the child gains lower extremity and lower trunk control against gravity that the arms can be freed from their support role and used for manipulation. Hence, a child is unable to reach out for an object in a prone-on-elbows position until co-contraction develops and anchors the pelvis to the support surface (Gilfoyle, Grady, & Moore, 1981).

Adult patients who lack internal postural control frequently resort to this strategy in their attempts to move. For example, during ambulation, the patient gains increased postural control by using his/her arms to hold onto the therapist, the walker, or the cane. Many patients require arm support in unassisted sitting. The need to use the upper extremities for support is due to inadequate co-contraction and control of the lower trunk and extremities. Unfortunately, if the upper extremities must be used for support, they cannot be used for manipulation, and many skilled movement patterns are lost.

Lower level patterns are used by adult patients when mature posture and movement strategies are no longer available. The motor system automatically employs these patterns through the spatiotemporal spiral to enable the individual to adapt to his or her environment. If reinforced through daily repetition, the patterns eventually will dominate the person's movement. This may be acceptable in the sense that the person is still able to move about the environment, but a great many of the activities that were an expression of the person as a individual become difficult, if not impossible. The individuals can no longer manipulate the environment. They cannot swing a golf club, ride a horse, play tennis, pick up a child, or hoe the garden. All of these activities require internal postural control and mature posture and movement strategies. It is very important that postural adaptation be addressed in the patient's treatment program and remediation provided whenever possible.

Prerequisite for Internal Postural Control. Failure to regain mature posture and movement strategies can be attributed in part to failure to establish the prerequisites necessary for internal postural control. Gilfoyle, Grady and Moore (1981) discuss the posture and movement capabili-

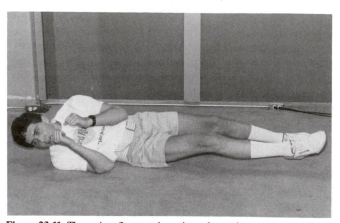

Figure 23-11. The patient flexes at the waist and uses the momentum gained in the upper trunk in an undifferentiated pattern to ring the legs over as he rolls from supine to sidelying. The patient's shoulder and hip on the left side move as a unit without rotation-counter-rotation.

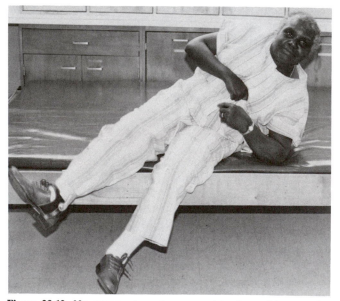

Figure 23-12. No movement-countermovement is observed between the patient's shoulders and hips as she comes into a seated position from supine. The patient flexes at the waist in an undifferentiated pattern and pushes herself into a seated position with the sound arm.

ties that children must develop in order to attain mature posture and movement strategies. These same capabilities or prerequisites apply to the brain-injured adult struggling to regain motor control: (1) The person must be able to produce movement through full range of motion in the trunk and extremities. The mature postural strategies of rotation-counter-rotation and movement-countermovement can be carried out effectively only if full range of motion is available. (2) In conjunction with full range of motion, the person must have the ability to differentiate body parts from one another, such as the ability to rotate the head independently of the shoulders. (3) The person must have the ability to stop and hold movement at mid-range of motion in order to stabilize against gravity. This ability is particularly critical for control of the body and/or body segments during changes in position, such as moving from a seated to standing position or during ambulation. (4) The person must have the ability to distribute normal postural tone in the body segments to support movement. This must be a fluid ability, and the individual must be capable of automatically increasing, decreasing, and redistributing postural tone with each change in position. (5) The person must possess symmetry. Symmetry used in this sense does not imply uniformity in posture or tone, but rather that both sides of the body are equally capable of motor response.

The degree of muscle tone present will influence the amount of range of motion, differentiation, and fixation that can be achieved. Patients with spasticity will have problems

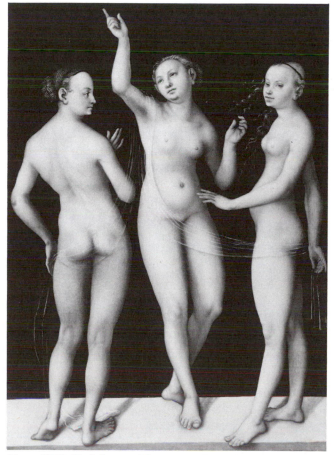

Figure 23-13. The influence of the asymmetrical tonic neck reflex (ATNR) can be observed in all three figures in this 15th century painting. The center picture is poised in a classic ATNR with extension of the limbs on the face side and flexion on the occiput side. More subtle influence of the reflex pattern is observed in the position of the upper and lower limbs of the other two figures. *"The Three Graces" by Lucas Cranach the Elder. Reprinted with permission from the Nelson-Atkins Museum of Art, Kansas City, Missouri, Nelson Fund.*

achieving sufficient range of motion and differentiation, while hypotonic patients will be unable to fix and hold patterns at mid-range. Orthopedic limitations and pain also can limit range of motion and differentiation significantly.

The ability to redistribute postural tone is critical for normal weight shift. Weight shift is the method the child uses to gain bilateral integration of the body sides. Children can be observed rocking, pushing, pulling, and twisting in each newly achieved position from the prone-on-elbows position to standing. Such movements cause weight shift to occur between the body sides and develop rotation-counter-rotation and movement-countermovement. Whenever a significant amount of paralysis or spasticity is present, the ability to redistribute postural tone is compromised. If too little postural tone is present, the individual lacks sufficient stability on the involved side. Too much postural tone severely restricts mobility on the involved side. In either case, weight shift diminishes and the person must rely on the sound side for control of all posture and movement.

Limited range of motion in a body part or alteration of muscle tone disrupts the symmetry of the body's response. This in turn reduces weight shift and prevents bilateral integration.

Treatment of postural dysfunction entails reestablishment of the prerequisites needed for internal postural control followed by practice of normal postural strategies. A variety of different techniques can be used including the bilateral asymmetrical patterns of proprioceptive neuromuscular facilitation and the Bobath prayer position. The technique used is not as critical as an understanding of what is needed (i.e., mobility or stability) to increase the patient's postural control.

The strategies employed by children as they come upright against gravity suggest the order of practice in therapy. Children gain internal postural control by imposing mobility on stability (weight shift) first with the hands and feet (distal ends) fixed and later with the hands and feet freed for skill. The arms are used for support first and later for manipulation after the lower trunk and extremities gain stability. Control proceeds proximally to distally with gross motor control of the midline developing before fine motor control of the extremities. Control also proceeds in a cephalocaudal manner with control of the head, neck, and upper trunk preceding control of the lower trunk and extremities. The value in approximating this developmental sequence as closely as possible is that it emulates the natural pattern of sensorimotor integration programmed by the nervous system. Because the pattern is familiar to the nervous system, less cortical effort is required to produce the movement.

Motor Planning. The second skill area affected by the learning disability is **motor planning**. The basis of motor planning skill is somatosensory integration. As Chapter 9 explains, somatosensory information is sensory information coming from within the body through tactile and proprioceptive senses. It provides information to the CNS on the state of the body and its readiness for action. The CNS uses this information with that coming in through vestibular, visual and auditory channels to plan and execute purposeful movement. How well movement is executed by the motor system depends partly on how much somatosensory information is available and the accuracy of this sensory information. The more complex the movement to be performed, the more complex the sensory information needed to execute it. Compare the act of tapping one finger with that of reciprocally tapping all of the fingers. In the first case, the CNS must monitor and coordinate the action of a single finger, and in the second, the CNS must monitor the actions of four fingers simultaneously and coordinate them so that the pattern progresses smoothly. *Motor-planned movements* are movements deliberately planned and executed by an individual to accomplish a purposeful task. Motor-planned movement is synonymous with skilled movement. Examples include writing, crocheting, opening jars, using tools, tap dancing, break dancing, and skiing. Motor-planned movements are the most voluntary, most complex movements in the CNS repertoire, and as such, they require the most complex sensory processing. Not only is the necessary sensory processing complex, but it must often be carried out very rapidly, such as a gymnast vaulting over a horse or a secretary typing 60 words per minute. Because of the complexity and speed of the sensory processing required to produce skilled movement, these movements must be centrally programmed and monitored within the nervous system by internal sensory feedback mechanisms (Taub & Berman, 1968; Melzack & Bridges, 1971).

Somatosensory Integration. As Chapter 9 discusses, the central nervous system relies on sensory input to organize, plan, and execute purposeful motor behaviors. To do this efficiently, the CNS must receive very precise sensory information about the state of the environment and the body. If the incoming sensory information is fuzzy or nebulous, the nervous system cannot anticipate and pre-plan its next move. If the sensory information comes in too slowly, the nervous system cannot anticipate its next move fast enough to be of use. Without the precise, rapid sensory information needed for motor planning, the motor system becomes reactive rather than proactive. The individual is able only to respond to the environment rather than actively manipulate it.

Animal research has shown that a number of motor planning deficits may be observed following disruption in somatosensory integration (Melzack & Bridges, 1971;

Melzack & Southmayd, 1974; Wall, 1970). These deficits include: (1) a failure to orient the head/body correctly to the task, (2) a failure to orient the hand correctly to objects, (3) poor use of tools, (4) a difficulty producing a sequence of movements, (5) a failure to initiate the first step of a sequence, (6) a failure to make anticipatory movement adjustments or to start and stop movements at an appropriate time, and (7) an ability to learn parts of a motor sequence, but inability to put the entire sequence together.

These deficits are most apparent during situations requiring new learning. A clinician familiar with brain-injured adults immediately will recognize these behaviors as examples of motor *apraxia*. As with animals, such deficits are typically seen when the patient is engaged in new learning such as wheelchair propulsion, one-handed dressing, using adaptive equipment, or changing hand dominance. Their presence often significantly impedes the patient's progress in acquiring functional daily living skills.

Treatment Principles for Remediation of Motor Planning Deficits. Because of the complexity of the sensory processing deficit, it is difficult to adequately remediate motor planning deficits within the time allotted for most rehabilitation programs. Therefore, the emphasis in treatment is often on compensation rather than remediation. Therapists attempt to circumvent the deficit when teaching patients independent life skills.

There are several principles that guide the teaching of compensatory skills to patients with motor planning problems:

1. *Use language to facilitate the motor planning process.* Research has shown that language serves a regulatory function in planning movement (Roy & Square, 1985). An internal linguistic reference system exists which acts as a voice inside one's head continuously identifying objects in the environment and their function. An example of this might be, if you see a tennis racket, the voice silently says, ''That is a tennis racket. — You use a tennis racket to hit tennis balls. — It looks sort of like a banjo, but you cannot play a tune on a tennis racket.'' By providing immediate information about the function of the object, the linguistic reference system assists the motor system in organizing its plan of action.

   Language allows us to put actions together in a sequence. A therapist can help patients use language to facilitate motor planning by requiring that they talk themselves through a task. The patient can be helped to understand the goal of an action by verbalizing what he/she is going to do, such as, ''I am going to put on my shirt.'' The plan of action can be facilitated when the patient verbalizes how he/she will complete the task, for example, ''I'm going to put my hand in the armhole of the sleeve, then I'm going to pull it up over my elbow . . ." The patient can evaluate the success of actions by describing what actions have just taken place. Talking through a task will also help to reduce perseveration and maintain concentration on the task.

2. *Teach in the style from which the patient best learns.* Individuals use three basic learning styles to acquire knowledge: visual learning, kinesthetic learning, and auditory learning (Bissell, White, & Zivin, 1971). Each of us prefers one or two styles to the others and attempt to structure our learning so that the favored style is employed. *Visual learners* like to look at graphic information such as found in pictures, graphs, illustrations, formulas. They are often good mimickers and are able to easily reproduce mirrored and non-mirrored movements. They like to read because reading requires visualization. They often have good memories for faces and previously known places. *Kinesthetic learners* learn by doing. They favor practica and lab sessions such as anatomy dissection. They reinforce learning by the manual act of writing, by taking and rewriting notes, or by drawing illustrations. They prefer to assemble kits without looking at the directions. *Auditory learners* concentrate on listening. They use tape recorders or read out loud. They often talk themselves through new or difficult activities. They are often good at games like ''name that tune'' and easily recognize voices on the telephone.

It is natural for us to present information the way we best learn it, for example, visual learners will cite landmarks to direct a lost traveler, auditory learners will give verbal instructions and street names, and kinesthetic learners will draw a map. However, the therapist's learning style may or may not match the patient's preferred style, or the patient may no longer be able to employ the favored style because of damage to that sensory system. Therefore, it is important that the therapist determine the patient's preferred and strongest style and employ that style during instruction in order to optimize learning. Careful observation of the patient as he/she attempts to learn a new skill or perform a test will give the therapist clues as to the preferred learning style.

3. *Approximate the natural context for the task as closely as possible.* All daily activities are performed within a certain context comprised of environmental surround and routine. For example, a person may dress every morning in the bedroom, sitting on the edge of the bed, first putting on the socks, then the pants, then the shirt, and finally the shoes. The context is so familiar that usually the person is not even aware of performing the task.

Hospital rooms and routines frequently destroy the context for self-care activities, thus making the new-old task of learning to dress oneself much more difficult for the apraxic patient. Dyspraxic patients often become more independent in their self-care when they return home than was thought possible based on their performance in the hospital. Approximating the patients routine for performing self-care will facilitate motor planning.

Visual Awareness. The third skill area affected by learning disability is visual awareness. The visual system is the most far reaching sensory receptor system for gathering information about the environment. It plays a dominant role in the integration of sensory information from the environment and in selective attention to the environment (Posner & Rafal, 1987). For example, you could be standing on a street corner having an animated conversation with the person of your dreams, but if you see out of the corner of your eye a bull charging towards you, you would forget the conversation and run. People will often believe what they see before they listen to their other senses.

Although vision often dominates the other senses, accurate visual interpretation of the environment is dependent on the integration of visual information with information from the other sensory systems. The visual and auditory systems are anatomically linked and function together (Cotman & McGaugh, 1980). When one hears a strange or unexpected sound, one automatically looks for the source; it is a natural uncontrolled reaction. The vestibular system contributes to accurate visual interpretation by providing information about the body's orientation to space. The somatosensory system gives definition and verification to what is seen. Just as there is a tendency to look toward the source of a sound, there is a natural tendency to touch what we see. The innate drive to verify visual information with somatosensory information is so strong that it literally must be trained out of children with their parent's monotonous chant of, ''Don't touch.''

All sensory systems are interdependent and work together to provide an accurate interpretation of the world (Cotman & McGaugh, 1980). We constantly use one sensory system to verify another system's perception. If you see a handbag in a store, and it looks like leather, you feel and smell it to make sure. Because of this interdependency, deficits in one system can adversely affect the interpretation of information by the other systems. Studies in perceptual discordance have shown that distorting visual input through the use of prism glasses causes misjudgments in the perception of somatosensory and auditory input (Freedman & Rekosh, 1968). But the reverse is

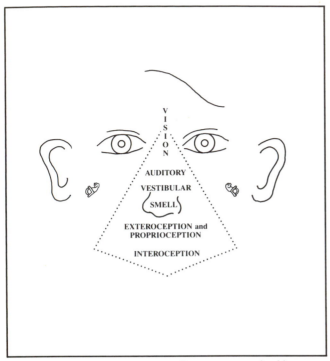

Figure 23-14. All sensory systems contribute to accurate visual interpretation of the environment. *Courtesy of Josephine C. Moore, PhD, OTR.*

also true. Intact sensory systems can compensate for individual senses that have been damaged; for example, persons with vestibular dysfunction can use vision to maintain balance, blind individuals compensate with auditory and somatosensory information, and deaf individuals compensate with visual information. When visual deficits occur, the person's ability to adapt to the environment physically, cognitively, and emotionally can be significantly limited. The severity of the limitation depends on the severity of the visual deficit and the integrity of the other sensory systems.

Following injury to the brain, two types of deficits may occur in the visual system.

1. Damage to the cranial nerves which innervate the extraocular muscles may result in *paralytic strabismus* in which the eyes do not align properly for conjugate vision, and the person experiences diplopia (double vision).

2. Damage can occur to the central neural structures that control the cranial nerves. Nearly every area of the brain is involved in the control of vision. Key areas include the frontal eye fields, parietal lobes, lateral geniculate, superior colliculus, cerebellum, and the occipital lobes. Damage to these structures or the pathways connecting them can create significant deficits in ocular control and perception (Leigh & Zee, 1983).

Modes of Visual Processing. Two modes of visual processing are believed to occur within the brain (Zihl & Von Cramon, 1979; Schneider, 1969). That is, two separate systems integrate visual information; operating simultaneously within the nervous system. While they are separate, their functions are intertwined so closely and are so equal in their contribution to vision that a deficit in one system affects the integrity of the other. The two systems are *focal vision* and *ambient vision* (Belleza, et al., 1979).

Focal Vision. Focal vision allows us to fix our attention and focus on a single object or a single aspect of an object to identify it and discriminate it from other objects in the environment. It is concerned with the identification of objects or **visual perception**. It relates to the ability to do puzzles, read, identify faces, etc. Focal vision allows us to distinguish the letter "b" from "d," or a tangerine from an orange (Gibson, 1976).

Focal vision is a learned response. The ability is refined over the lifespan through interaction with the environment. Individuals achieve different levels of this ability, for example, typesetters, artists, neurosurgeons, parts inspectors, and trackers all demonstrate refined levels of focal vision. Research has shown that this ability is partially shaped by culture and environment (Segal, Campbell, & Herskovits, 1966). Anthropologists have found that persons living in environments built by carpenters are more susceptible to certain types of visual illusions because of their constant exposure to right angles and straight lines than are individuals living in round huts on the plains of Africa where right angles are uncommon.

Ambient Vision. Ambient vision, often referred to as the second visual system, is concerned with the detection of events and their location in the environment (Zihl & Von Cramon, 1979). Ambient vision is involved in **visual orientation** or locating objects so they can be visually perceived. This system is more fundamental and holistic than focal vision. The capability for ambient vision is present at birth and is refined though experiences with the environment (Gibson, 1976).

Vision is actually only one component of this ability. Tactual, auditory, kinesthetic, and vestibular information are also required to accurately assess the relationship between the self and the environment. As Chapter 9 describes, information from all of the sensory systems is integrated together and used to supply the individual with an accurate environmental map. At the center of the map is the person's body, and the map changes as the person moves about in space. Because vision is a rapidly processed and far reaching sense, it contributes strongly to the shaping of the map and often dominates the other senses. This is why people can walk unsuspectingly into mirrors and plate glass windows or experience the sensation of falling or leaning in carnival fun houses.

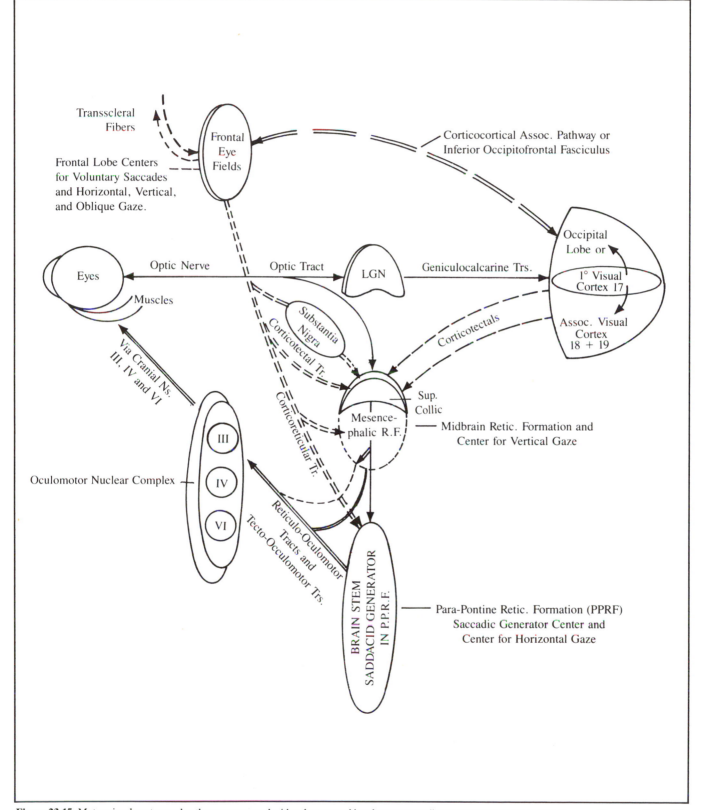

Figure 23-15. Motor visual centers and pathways concerned with voluntary and involuntary saccadic eye movements and conjugate gaze. *Courtesy of Josephine C. Moore, PhD, OTR.*

It is possible to maintain an accurate map and the subsequent accurate orientation to the environment without vision. Blind individuals, for example, are able to accurately navigate using other senses and some sighted individuals can successfully walk around at night without turning on a light.

To have a fully operational, efficient visual system, both systems of ambient and focal vision must work together. If you go to the store and buy a bag of Granny Smith apples, you would use ambient vision to locate the produce section and focal vision to distinguish the Granny Smith apples from the Golden Delicious. But, while both systems are necessary for efficient processing, ambient vision must be functioning properly for focal vision to be accurate. An individual must first notice the stimulus and attend to it before making an identification.

Visual Deficits Following Brain Injury.

Hemianopsia. Damage to the optic nerve, as it travels from the retina through the lateral geniculate body to the occipital lobe, can result in visual field cuts in which a portion of the visual field is lost (Chusid & DeGroot, 1988).

The most common visual field deficit following stroke is hemianopsia in which a person loses one half of the vision in each eye. If the lesion is on the right side of the brain, vision is lost in the left half of each eye. A lesion in the left hemisphere results in a visual loss of the right half of each eye. Persons with hemianopsia have difficulty initially

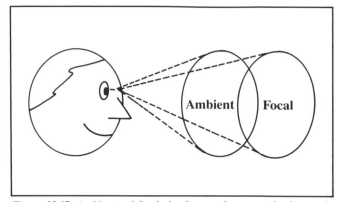

Figure 23-17. Ambient and focal visual processing occur simultaneously within the brain and overlap to provide an individual with functional visual skills.

readapting to the environment. They may exhibit such behaviors as eating food from only one half of the plate or bumping into objects on the blind side. However, most hemianoptic individuals learn to adjust to the loss of vision and develop effective compensation strategies within a few months of onset (Meienberg, Zangemeister, Rosenberg, et al., 1981; Zangemeister, Meienberg, Stark, et al., 1982). (Figure 23-18)

Hemispatial Neglect. A much more long-term and debilitating side-effect of stroke or head injury is a condition known as *hemispatial neglect* or *unilateral spatial neglect*. Hemispatial neglect is a condition where the person ignores visual stimuli occurring in the space on the involved side of the body. It may range from a mild form of extinction in which a person presented with two simultaneous visual stimuli will attend to the stimuli on the sound side and ignore (extinct) the stimuli on the involved side; to more severe forms in which the person acts as though vision is absent on the involved side. In some cases, hemianopsia may accompany neglect, but many brain-injured patients demonstrating neglect have intact visual fields (Albert, 1973).

Many theories have been proposed to explain the cause of neglect. The most widely accepted theory is that it occurs as a result of an attentional deficit in the brain (Mesulam, 1981) in which the brain no longer registers the visual information coming from the involved side as being important and does not attend to it or include it in its plans for adaptation. Somatosensory and auditory neglect often occur in conjunction with **visual neglect**. The person not only ignores visual stimuli, but also ignores the limbs on the involved side of the body and sounds coming from the involved side (Heilman, 1979). The person operates as though that half of the world does not exist.

There are a number of oculomotor deficits that accompany neglect, including:

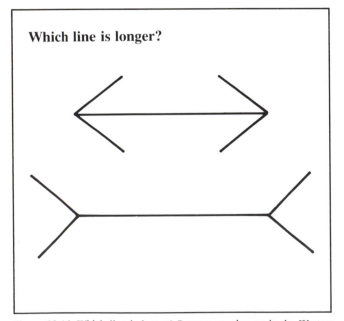

Which line is longer?

Figure 23-16. Which line is longer? Persons growing up in the Western Hemisphere are more susceptible to this type of optical illusion than persons growing up in environments in which they are not as exposed to right angles and straight lines. (The lines are the same length, despite the illusion that the lower line is longer.)

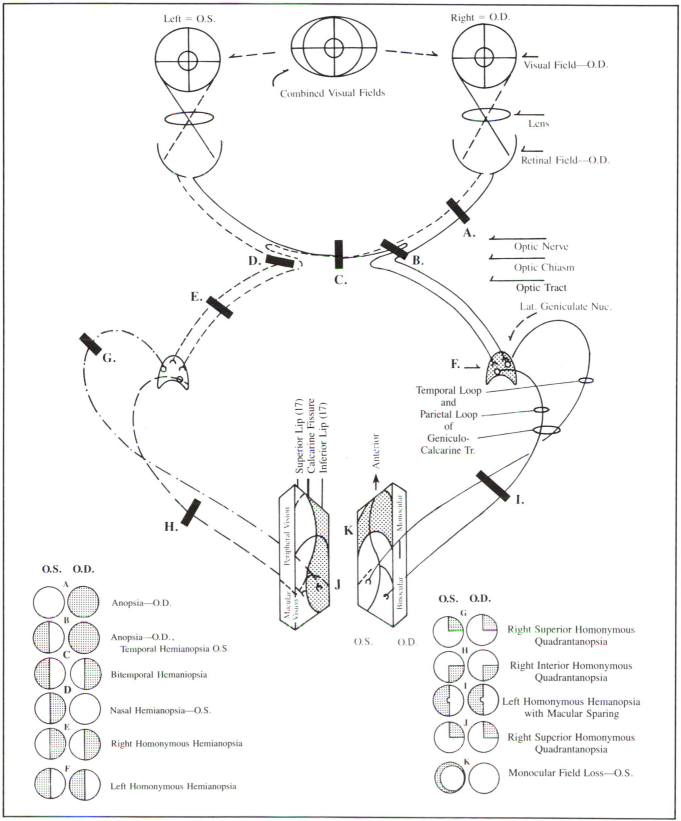

Figure 23-18. Visual field deficits resulting from various lesions in the optic nerve as it travels from the retina to the occipital lobe. *Courtesy of Josephine C. Moore, PhD, OTR.*

1. *An avoidance of shifting the eyes towards the involved side.* The eyes seem magnetized towards the intact side with a tendency to always fixate first on the most peripheral visual stimuli on the intact side. If a person is shown two objects in the intact right visual field, he/she will first attend to the object in the farthest right position even if both objects approximate midline (DeRenzi, 1982).

2. *The person may be unable to fixate his or her gaze in the involved space.* This is related to a condition known as *motor impersistence* in which a person is unable to carry out a sustained motor performance for more than a few seconds (Joynt, Benton, & Fogel, 1962).

3. *Eye movements towards the involved side are slower and take longer to initiate* (Ron, 1981).

These oculomotor deficits may result in use of an ineffective search pattern to explore the environment. Chedru and associates (1973) conducted a study of the scanning patterns of 36 normal and 115 brain-injured subjects. They found that normal subjects always used a logical scanning pattern to search for and locate a hidden object among other figures that were projected on a screen. Normal subjects scanned in a circular clockwise or counter-clockwise fashion, spending equal amounts of time exploring both halves of the visual field, until they found the designated figure. An equal amount of time was spent studying each figure until the desired one was located. In contrast, few brain-injured subjects demonstrated a systematic search pattern. Most began exploring visual space on the intact side. Those with right-sided lesions tended to spend a greater amount of time scanning the right half of the screen (the sound half), making only delayed and brief excursions towards the left half of the visual field. Brain-injured subjects were also slower at scanning, tended to fixate longer, and were less accurate identifying the designated form. Other studies have shown similar disruptions in scanning patterns (Belleza, et al., 1979; Diller & Weinberg, 1977; Tyler, 1969; Posner & Rafal, 1987).

Therapists often note that neglect seems to be more severe when it occurs in conjunction with right brain damage. The patient with left hemiplegia is typically known for inattention to events on the left side of the body and distractibility towards stimuli occurring on the right side. Heilman and Van Den Abell (1980) proposed a hypothesis to explain this clinical observation. Their research suggests that the right hemisphere has mechanisms for directing visual attention towards both sides of the visual field, whereas the left hemisphere only has mechanisms for directing attention towards the right side. A lesion in the left hemisphere may result in decreased attention to the right side, but the person is able to compensate for this decrease

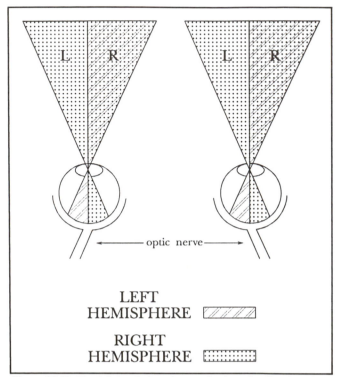

Figure 23-19. The left hemisphere has mechanisms for directing visual attention toward the right visual field only. The right hemisphere has mechanisms for directing visual attention toward both the left and right fields.

with the intact right hemisphere making the neglect less severe. There is no such compensatory mechanism with damage in the right hemisphere, thus resulting in much more severe neglect.

Neglect can create a variety of functional problems for the brain-injured patient. Patients with severe neglect frequently only dress one half of their body, shave or wash one half of their face, brush one half of their teeth, or eat food from only one side of the plate. They are often unable to turn toward the involved side and frequently run into objects on the involved side. They do not attend to environmental landmarks and frequently get lost in unfamiliar surroundings. They often have difficulty reading because they only scan one half of the page and difficulty with arithmetic problems because they only see half of the numbers on the page (Heilman, 1979).

Unlike patients with hemianopsia, they do not develop compensatory strategies for overcoming their visual deficits because their CNS is not aware that a problem exists. One group of researchers has linked impairments in scanning to accident prone behavior in post-CVA adults. Diller & Weinberg (1970) studied the accident reports of 270 post-CVA patients during a one year period. They found that hemiplegic patients comprised 24% of the patient population, but had 43.5% of the accidents reported. When they compared persons with left hemiplegia to those with right hemiplegia, they found that accident prone behavior correlated to speed and accuracy on a scanning task. The left hemiplegic individuals experiencing accidents tended to perform the scanning task very rapidly and with a large number of errors, reflecting inattention to the task. These patients tended to have accidents during wheelchair transfers and off hours when they were not in therapy. They would attempt to transfer without locking the brakes or removing the foot pedals and make other errors reflecting inattention to the task. In comparison, the accident prone behavior of right hemiplegics tended to be related to speed on a scanning task, but not accuracy. These patients tended to perform the scanning task slowly, but accurately. They were more likely to have an accident bedside when attempting to do something for themselves rather than ask for help. It was felt that this reflected difficulty with communication and language as many of these patients had some degree of aphasia.

Treatment Principles for Remediation of Hemispatial Neglect. While much literature exists on the identification and causes of unilateral neglect, very little has been published on the remediation of neglect. The limited research available suggests that patients must be made aware of the deficit and then systematically taught to compensate for it with an organized search pattern (Gianutsos & Matheson, 1987).

Weinberg, Diller, & Gordon, (1979) found anchoring techniques to be effective in improving the reading ability of 57 left hemiplegics exhibiting severe left side neglect. Patients were taught to locate the line they were reading by using the anchoring techniques (see Figure 23-20). An organized left to right scanning pattern, starting in the impaired space, was emphasized and reinforced in all activities. The patient was taught to consciously begin scanning on the involved side to compensate for the neglect and reorganize the scanning pattern.

Weinberg's study addressed scanning only as it pertained to an 8 and 1/2 by 11 inch sheet of paper. Successful performance of self-care and homemaking skills requires scanning of the broader visual space surrounding the body. Whether patients can be taught to scan their total environment more efficiently has not been proven. However, knowledge of the visual system and neglect suggests that if patients are taught to systematically scan a broader environment, similar to the way Weinberg taught them to scan a sheet of paper, improvement could be noted in scanning during ambulation, dressing and other self-care areas. Figures 23-20 and 23-21 demonstrate activities which require systematic scanning of a broad visual space.

Knowledge of how the brain processes or codes visual information also suggests that patients would be more likely to attend to visual information if required to use that information to physically adapt to the environment. Research has shown that visual and auditory information is coded more effectively if verified by somatosensory and vestibular information (Ayres, 1972). In other words, you

---

Table 23-1
Example of Anchoring Techniques Used to Improve Reading Skill in Patients with Left-side Neglect. A Patient Practices and Progresses Through Each Step Until Able to Read Without Clues.

Patient is asked to locate the vertical anchoring bar, then read the first line across using the numbers at the beginning and end of each line to avoid skipping lines.	**STEP 1**	1 - Humpty Dumpty sat - 1 2 - on a wall. Humpty - 2 3 - Dumpty had a great fall. - 3
Patient locates the anchoring bar and number of the line, then reads the line across.	**STEP 2**	1 - All the king's horses and 2 - all the king's men couldn't 3 - put Humpty together again.
Patient uses only the anchoring bar to locate the line.	**STEP 3**	Peter, Peter, pumpkin eater had a wife and couldn't keep her.
No cues are required to locate the line.	**STEP 4**	He put her in a pumpkin shell and there he kept her very well.

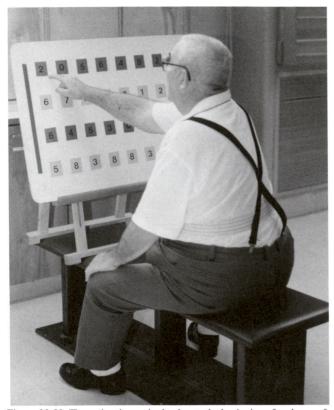

Figure 23-20. The patient is required to locate the beginning of each row of numbers by using the anchoring line on the left side and then reading the numbers across. Pointing to each number helps to pace the activity and ensure that the patient scans efficiently.

get a stronger, longer-lasting visual/auditory image if it is verified by a movement and/or tactual experience. For example, to teach the concept of "apple," a teacher can describe an apple as "An apple is hard, round, red, juicy, and delicious," and pupils, if they have good memories, will remember part of the description. If the teacher shows the pupil an apple, the pupil can associate the visual image of round and red with the spoken words and will develop a stronger concept of the apple. But, the optimum way to teach the concept of apple to ensure that the concept is retained would be to allow the pupil to explore the apple by feeling and tasting it. Through this exploration with hands and mouth, the pupil can verify the verbal and visual descriptions with somatosensory information. The pupil can feel that the apple is hard and round and juicy, see that it is red, and taste that it is delicious (Figure 23-22).

It is through this process of verification, integration, and feedback that children first develop concepts of space and form (Ayres, 1972). The implication to visual retraining in adults is that visual experiences can be more effectively integrated if verified by motor feedback. Visual activities should be structured so that the patient can physically

interact with the activity. Figures 23-23 and 23-24 provide examples of activities that require visual scanning and physical interaction.

In summary, three principles guide the selection of visual retraining activities for the patient with neglect: (1) draw attention to the impaired space first and teach the patient to systematically explore his surroundings starting in the impaired space, (2) broaden the visual space in which the patient is required to interact as much as possible, and (3) reinforce the visual experience with a sensorimotor experience by structuring activities so the patient is required to physically manipulate the activity.

INTEGRATING PRINCIPLES OF INTERVENTION

As stated in the introduction to this chapter, movement is the physical means by which we interact with the environment. Normal movement is goal directed, and the goal is supplied by an innate need to adapt to environmental events and manipulate them. According to Ayres (1972, p. 22), "The primary function of the brain is to translate sensory impulses into meaningful information and to organize an appropriate motor response." The brain receives isolated pieces of sensory information and filters, organizes, and integrates them to provide a complete and continuously updated picture of the environment. The person then uses this picture to make an adaptive response

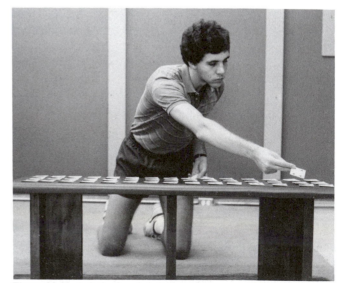

Figure 23-21. A deck of cards is laid out face up on a therapy bench. The patient holds another deck of cards in his hand and matches each card in this deck to one on the bench. He is required to search for the matching card by systematically scanning each row from left to right until the card is found.

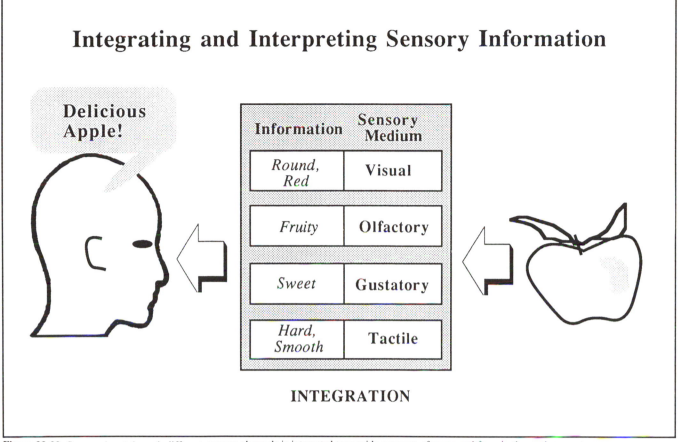

Figure 23-22. Sensory input through different sensory channels is integrated to provide concepts of space and form in the environment.

to the environment. Every movement is made within the context of this constantly changing picture.

Each sensory component of the picture must be there in order for an accurate response to be formulated. When one component is missing or garbled, the entire process is disorganized. If a component is damaged only slightly, one may not notice a change in the individual, but if significant damage occurs, the person will no longer be able to function productively. In treatment planning, the therapist must consider which sensory components are intact, which are missing or compromised, and the severity of the disruption to the overall system. Comprehensive evaluation is always the cornerstone to effective treatment.

As Chapter 9 discusses, the brain needs the "big picture" to operate efficiently and effectively. Our brain is structured to process sensory input most efficiently when it receives a variety of sensory information about an object or event in the environment. The example of teaching the concept of an apple illustrates this point. The brain needs and wants multiplicity of input, so it can use input from one sensory system to verify and enhance input from another system.

Importance of Activity Focus

Engaging in goal-directed activity is an optimum way to provide a patient with multisensory input in a controlled, focused manner. By carefully selecting an activity, the therapist can maximize sensory input and sensory integration. For example, to elicit visual scanning towards the neglecting side, the therapist may choose to engage the patient in the familiar game of tic-tac-toe using a large adapted board as illustrated in Figure 23-25. The width of the board requires the patient to scan past midline to see the columns on the involved side. Knowing that neglect is often a multisensory deficit, the therapist can structure the activity so that the patient is required to move and scan towards the involved side. This is accomplished by putting the game pieces on the patient's involved side so that he/she must reach into the involved space with each game move. If the patient is required to straddle a low therapy bench as shown in Figure 23-26, the game pieces can be placed near the floor, increasing the excursion into the involved space. With each game move, the patient simultaneously receives tactile and proprioceptive stimulation through the lower extremity on the involved side as she shifts her weight to reach the game piece, receives vestibular stimulation as her head accompanies the weight shift, and visual input as she scans for the piece. Auditory input may also be provided if the therapist provides verbal cues. Thus, by carefully structuring the activity, the therapist can provide sensory input simultaneously through four sensory modalities. Sensory integration occurs subconsciously as the patient seeks to adapt to the environment and play the game. Straddling the low, wide, bench has the added benefit of increasing the symmetry of the patient's sitting position and improving postural adaptation.

Principles Guiding Task Selection

As Chapter 9 states, registration of sensory information is the first step to adaptation. An individual must be aware of an object or change in the environment before he/she can formulate a response to it. Two types of stimuli activate sensory registration: *novel stimuli* and *important stimuli*. It is necessary to distinguish between the two because they do

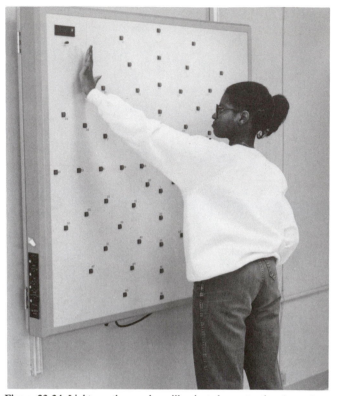

Figure 23-24. Lights on the panel are illuminated one at a time in random patterns. As each light comes on, the patient is required to locate it and press it to turn it off. As soon as the light is pressed, another light is illuminated. The patient tries to locate as many lights within a specified time period. *Eyespan 2064 by Performance Enterprises, Ontario, Canada.*

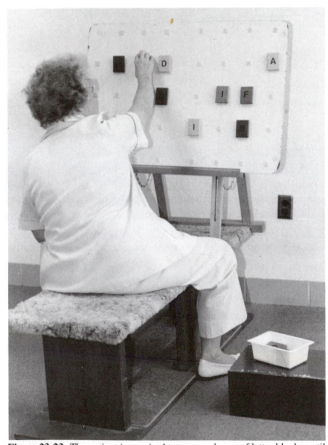

Figure 23-23. The patient is required to scan each row of letter blocks until she locates the one requested. When she finds the correct letter she removes the block and places it in the box on her right.

not ultimately produce the same level of adaptation. Novel stimuli such as a new voice or unusual sound is attended to initially but once categorized, is quickly forgotten. We may arouse a patient with a novel stimuli but we cannot always activate attention and elicit a response. The last step of the sensory registration process is effort which is activated most consistently by important stimuli. The most important stimuli are those which have survival value. The greater the survival value, the greater the inhibition of other sensory input so the person can concentrate on a specific stimulus. For example, food tastes best when one is really hungry.

The central nervous system also considers important, those stimuli which make a critical contribution to the person's ability to make an adaptive response to the environment at a given time. If one is playing a competitive game of checkers, the CNS will consider the visual information gained from scanning the board as important and focus concentration there. If one is walking a tightrope blindfolded, the CNS will consider information gained from the proprioceptors and tactile receptors in the feet as highly important. This is the justification for engaging patients in meaningful activity. Activity the patient perceives as meaningful will elicit sensory registration and in doing so develop sensory engrams for future learning.

The more meaningful the activity the more likely learning will occur. Task selection is very important. There are two rules of thumb which guide task selection:

1. *The activity should have some familiar qualities.* When the task is less familiar to the patient, it is less likely to be viewed as important by the patient. At the same time, if the task is too familiar, the patient may not make an effort to engage in it. The most effective activities have familiar qualities presented in a novel way, such as the enlarged tic-tac-toe board shown in Figure 23-26 and the scanning boards shown in Figures 23-20 and 23-23. These use numbers, letters, and a game concept familiar to most adults, but they are presented in an unusual way.

2. *The activity should be relevant to the person's age and lifestyle.* Computers are a familiar and relevant activity for young adults and teenagers, but older adults find them strange and threatening. Crafts, games, and activities of daily living have relevance to all age groups and lifestyles and thus are perhaps the most effective activities. A simple task such as

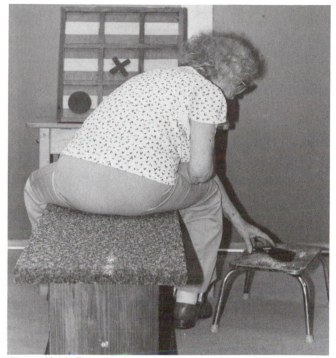

Figure 23-26. Example of an activity structured to provide multisensory input.

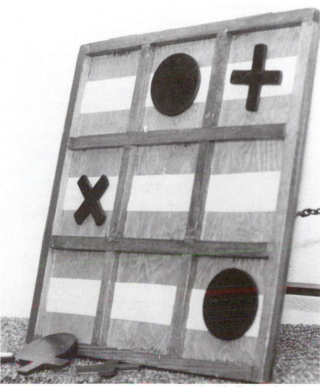

Figure 23-25. Tic-Tac-Toe board measuring 18 × 18. The board and game pieces have been adapted with velcro so the game can be placed in an upright position.

making a cup of coffee requires motor planning, concentration, and visual scanning and movement into the involved space, if structured to do so.

Designing Integrated Treatment Programs

One of the major frustrations of therapists today is the limited time available to work with a patient. A therapist may only work with a patient 30 to 60 minutes once or twice a day. The length of inpatient and outpatient programs are steadily decreasing as hospital costs rise. As stated earlier in this chapter, whereas a patient with spinal cord injury generally exhibits only two or three deficit areas (typically those of strength, endurance, and control), brain-injured patients can exhibit numerous neuromotor and learning deficits. Providing a cohesive, effective, and comprehensive treatment program in 60 minutes can be a difficult endeavor. The task is made easier when carefully selected activities are used as the focus of the treatment program. Activity acts as the glue that binds a treatment program together. Activities can be structured to provide multisensory input to the patient as previously described. They can also be designed to simultaneously address several deficit areas in an integrated fashion.

Before selecting and structuring an activity, evaluation must be completed to determine the patient's major deficit areas. The neuromotor components of voluntary movement,

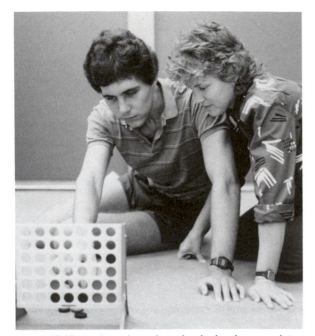

Figure 23-27. As the patient selects the checker, he moves into a side-sitting position bearing weight on the upper extremity to increase the proprioceptive and tactile input.

strength, muscle tone, orthopedic limitations, pain, and endurance must each be assessed. The patient's capacity for new learning must be determined in relationship to deficits in visual scanning, postural adaptation, motor planning, and motivation. Once deficit areas are identified, activities can be selected which simultaneously address two or more of the areas. The following are examples of how activities can be structured to provide an integrated treatment approach addressing several deficit areas at once.

Case Study 23-1

Patient Description: Jane is a 16-year-old woman who sustained a closed head injury resulting in ataxia in all four extremities, motor planning deficits particularly in sequencing motor actions, and poor concentration.

Suggested Activity: Playing a game of connect four on the floor, picking up the checker in a side-sitting position, and shifting into an all-fours position (on hand and knees) to place the checker in the board as illustrated in Figures 23-28 and 23-29.

How the Activity Increases Stability in the Extremities: Ataxia falls on the mobility side of the mobility-stability continuum; therefore the motor goal is to increase stability starting proximally at the shoulders and hips. The Rood neuromuscular reeducation approach dictates that weight bearing on the extremities facilitates co-contraction at proximal joints. Stability can be further facilitated by periodically applying the PNF technique of rhythmic stabilization during the activity or using the Rood technique of applying greater than body weight joint compression. Prolonged weight bearing and fatigue of the upper extremity is avoided by continuously changing positions between all-fours and sitting.

How the Activity Facilitates Motor Planning: Structuring the activity so that Jane picks up the checker in a side-sitting position and then shifts into an all-fours position to place the checker requires that she sequence four separate steps with each game move. To help carry out this sequence, the therapist can request that Jane verbalize the steps needed to complete the activity during each turn. Using language to direct the motor sequence will also help maintain Jane's concentration on the task. As Jane improves, the motor planning needed can be made more complex by requiring her to alternate side-sitting between the left and right sides as the game is played.

How the Activity Facilitates Concentration: The game requires that the player pay attention to the moves of her opponent as well her own moves to win. The game is familiar to Jane and one she enjoys. The therapist can increase Jane's concentration by having her analyze each move out loud before she makes it. Moving between the two postures provides continuous stimulation to Jane's vestibular system and increases her level of arousal which improves her concentration.

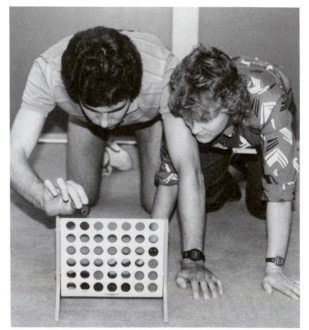

Figure 23-28. The patient shifts into a hands and knees position, continuing to bear weight on the left as he places the checker. The activity can be made more complex by requiring that the patient alternate side-sitting on the left and right sides.

Case Study 23-2

Patient Description: Jim is a 67-year-old man who sustained a right CVA resulting in left hemiplegia, sensory loss on the left side, neglect for the left visual field and body side, poor sitting balance, and poor attention span.

Suggested Activity: Placing shapes in a large formboard while straddling a low therapy bench as illustrated in Figure 23-29.

How the Activity Increases Sitting Balance: Straddling the therapy bench abducts the legs and places equal pressure on the buttocks which in turn elicits a support reaction in the trunk and increases postural control. Sitting balance can be challenged by placing the shapes for the formboard on a low stool to the side of the bench and asking Jim to reach down for the shapes. In the beginning, the therapist can sit behind Jim on the bench and guide his movement to ensure that he does not lose his balance and fall off of the bench. As his balance reactions improve, the shapes can be gradually placed on lower stools and eventually on the floor to require him to control balance reactions through greater and greater trunk range of motion.

How the Activity Increases Visual Awareness: The size of the board (34 × 24) requires that Jim scan past midline into the involved space to locate half of the openings. To reinforce an organized scanning pattern starting in the impaired space first, the therapist verbally cues Jim to start searching for the form in the upper left hand corner of the board and to point to each opening by moving from left to right until he locates the one which matches. This scanning pattern is repeated and reinforced with each form.

How the Activity Increases Awareness of the Left Extremities: By placing the forms on the left side, Jim is required to shift his weight onto the left lower extremity and move into the left space each time. Each weight shift increases proprioceptive and tactile stimulation to the left lower extremity. By placing the left elbow on his left thigh, the therapist can also guide weight shift onto the elbow to increase proprioceptive and tactile stimulation to the upper extremity. Jim also experiences increased vestibular input with the weight shift.

How the Activity Increases Concentration: The formboard is designed so that the forms must be matched by color and texture and shape, thus forcing Jim to closely observe the detail of each piece before it is placed. Concentration can be further increased by having Jim describe the opening for which he is looking as he scans the board and stating whether or not each opening matches the form. Pointing to each opening also will slow down his scanning speed and require that he attend to the activity more closely.

In designing programs for brain-injured patients, it is important to keep in mind that these individuals often have tenuous capabilities for registering, organizing and integrating sensory information. It does not take much sensory stimulation to overwhelm their integration processes and

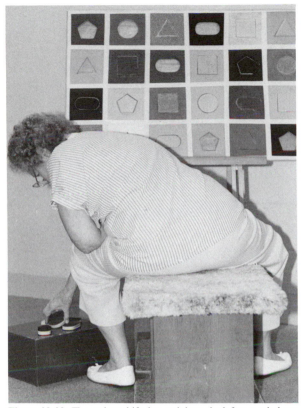

Figure 23-29. The patient shifts her weight to the left to reach down and pick up the form, then scans the board to locate the correct slot.

create distress within the system. Combining postural and perceptual activities is an optimum way to provide a multisensory experience, but activities must be balanced so that they provide challenge and not create distress. A simple rule to follow is to combine difficult perceptual and/or cognitive activities with less difficult motor activities and vice versa (Chapparo, 1980). For example, if the chosen activity has complex perceptual or cognitive qualities, the patient should be required to perform a relatively simple and posturally secure motor activity. Figure 23-30 illustrates this principle.

Gilfoyle, Grady and Moore (1981) list three basic stressors to postural control: *gravity, the complexity of the movement required,* and the *complexity of the activity to be performed.* If an activity is failing to produce the desired results, the therapist must consider whether the activity is too posturally threatening, too complex, or too strenuous for the patient. Chapparo (1980) suggests that a therapist should ask four questions in deciding whether to use an activity: activity:

- Is the activity relevant, meaningful, and goal-directed?
- Is it too high level or too low level for the patient?
- Does it provide multisensory input?
- Is the patient actively involved?

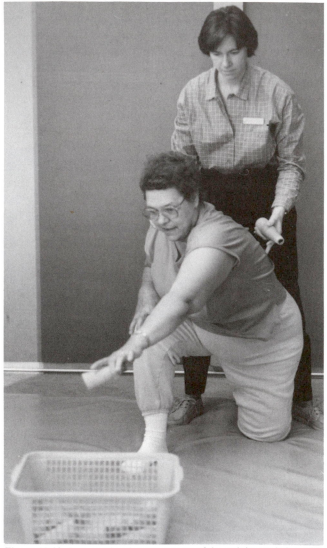

Figure 23-30. Perceptual and motor aspects of the activity are balanced to prevent stress by combining a simple perceptual activity (placing a cone in a basket) with a position that is posturally difficult for the patient to maintain (half-kneeling position).

If the activity meets these criteria it should achieve the desired results.

A final and important benefit of using an integrated activity based approach to treatment is its efficiency and cost effectiveness. By addressing two or three problems at once, the therapist can provide an intensive, comprehensive program in 30 minutes. In these days of streamlined hospital stays and limited outpatient coverage, efficient treatment that is also effective is clearly the most beneficial for the patient.

SUMMARY

Many of the activities and tasks required for competent role performance are dependent on purposeful movement. Coordinated, voluntary motion is synergistic, requiring the interaction of cardiovascular, neuromotor, sensory and psychological factors. In this chapter, attention has been given to approaches for remediating neuromotor and sensory deficits following damage to the central nervous system. The view has been taken that neuromotor control includes factors which influence the person's ability to produce movement, while sensory processing and motor planning are necessary to organize information and execute movement in accordance with environmental demands.

Neuromotor control is influenced by muscle tone, degree of voluntary movement, orthopedic limitations, pain, and endurance. Motor learning ability is influenced by postural adaptation, motor planning and visual awareness. Occupational therapists can draw from various approaches to provide intervention for deficits in each of the components underlying neuromotor control and motor learning ability. The general principles underlying intervention can be integrated in therapeutic activities carefully selected by the therapist. These tasks can be designed to provide engagement and challenge while simultaneously addressing areas of deficit.

Study Questions

1. How does spasticity influence motor control?

2. What affect does hypotonicity have on motor control?

3. How does mental endurance differ from physical endurance, and how do each impact on the patient's ability to participate in a treatment program?

4. What two neurophysiological premises underly the neuromuscular treatment approaches of Brunnstrom, Bobath, Rood and PNF?

5. What two methods are used by the adult to achieve balance between stability and mobility and gain internal postural control?

6. How does postural adaptation contribute to learning ability?

7. What strategy does the motor system automatically use to handle spatiotemporal stress?

8. What lower level patterns are used by adults to compensate for deficits in internal postural control?

9. What are the prerequisites for normal postural control?

10. What techniques can be used to circumvent motor planning problems in teaching a patient to dress?

11. How does visual neglect disrupt the normal visual search pattern used by adults? Why is visual neglect more often associated with right hemisphere damage?

12. What three principles guide the selection of activities for treatment of visual neglect?

Acknowledgment

The author would like to express her gratitude to the following dedicated persons who contributed their time and creative energy to the development of the treatment media shown in the pictures in this chapter: Wayne Benson, Jo Rinke, Linda Self, OTR; Diane Budic, OTR; and Jamie Mulder, OTR.

Recommended Readings

Ayres, A.J. (1972). Sensory integration and learning disorders. Los Angeles: *Western Psychological Services*, 190-206.

Bobath, B. (1978). *Adult hemiplegia: Evaluation and treatment.* (2nd Ed) London: William Heinemann Medical Books Limited.

Brunnstrom, S. (1970). *Movement therapy in hemiplegia.* New York: Harper and Row.

Carr, J.H. & Shepard, R.B. (1983). *A motor relearning programme for stroke.* Rockville, Maryland: Aspen Publication.

Gilfoyle, E.M., Grady, A.P., & Moore, J.C. (1981). *Children adapt.* Thorofare, New Jersey: Charles B. Slack, Inc.

Johnstone, M. (1978). *Restoration of motor function in the stroke patient.* New York: Churchill Livingstone.

Knott, M. & Voss, D.E. (1968). *Proprioceptive neuromuscular facilitation: patterns and techniques (2nd ed.).* Hagerstown, Maryland: Harper & Row.

Umphred, D.A. (Ed.). (1985). *Neurological rehabilitation.* St. Louis: C.V. Mosby Co.

References

Albert, M.L. (1973). A simple test of visual neglect. *Neurology, 23,* 658-664.

Andersen, L.T. (1985). Shoulder pain in hemiplegia. *American Journal of Occupational Therapy, 9,* 11-19.

Ayres, A.J. (1972). *Sensory integration and learning disorders* (pp. 190-206). Los Angeles: Western Psychological Services.

Belleza, T., Rappaport, M., Hopkins, H.K., & Hall, K. (1979). Visual scanning and matching dysfunction in brain damaged patients with drawing impairment. *Cortex, 15,* 19-36.

Bissell, J., White, S., & Zivin, G. (1971). Sensory modalities in children's learning. (pp. 130-155). In Lesser, G.S. (Ed.). *Psychology and educational practice.* Glenview, IL: Scott, Foresman and Company.

Bobath, B. (1978). *Adult hemiplegia: Evaluation and treatment (2nd ed.).* London: William Heinemann Medical Books Limited.

Brodal, A. (1973). Self observations and neuroanatomical considerations after a stroke. *Brain, 96,* 675-694.

Caillet, R. (1981). *The shoulder in hemiplegia.* Philadelphia: F.A. Davis.

Chapparo, C. (1980). Sensory integrative approach to the management of adult CVA and head trauma. Workshop sponsored by Professional Development Programs, Bloomington, Minnesota, November 7-9, 1980.

Chedru, F., Leblanc, M., & Lhermitte, F. (1973). Visual searching in normal and brain damaged subjects. *Cortex, 9,* 94-111.

Chusid, J.G. & DeGroot, J. (1988). *Correlative neuroanatomy (20th ed.).* East Norwalk, CT: Appleton & Lange.

Cotman, C.W. & McGaugh, J.L. (1980). *Behavioral neuroscience: An introduction.* New York: Academic Press Inc.

DeRenzi, E. (1982). *Disorders of space exploration and cognition* (pp. 57-125). New York: John Wiley & Sons.

Diller, L. & Weinberg, J. (1970). Evidence for accident prone behavior in patients. *Archives of Physical Medicine and Rehabilitation, 51,* 358-363.

Diller, L. & Weinberg, J. (1977). Hemi-inattention in rehabilitation: The evolution of a rationale remediation program (pp. 63-82). In Weinstein, E.A. & Friedland, R.P. (Eds.). *Advances in neurology.* New York: Raven Press.

Freedman, S.J. & Rekosh, J.H. (1968). The functional integrity of spatial behavior (pp. 153-163). In Freedman, S.J. (Ed.). *The neuropsychology of spatially-oriented behavior.* Homewood, IL: Dorsey Press.

Fukuda, T. (1962). Studies on human dynamic postures from the viewpoint of postural reflexes. *Acta Otolaryngologica, Supplement 161,* 1-52.

Gianutsos, R. & Matheson, P. (1987). The rehabilitation of visual perceptual disorders attributable to brain injury (pp. 202-241). In Meier, M.J., Benton, A.L., & Diller, L. (Eds.). *Neuropsychological Rehabilitation.* New York: Guilford Press.

Gibson, E.J. (1976). The development of perception as an adaptive process. *American Scientist, 235,* 98-107.

Gilfoyle, E.M., Grady, A.P., & Moore, J.C. (1981). *Children adapt.* Thorofare, NJ: Slack Inc.

Heilman, K. (1979). Neglect and related disorders (pp. 268-305). In Heilman, K. & Valenstein, E. (Eds.). *Clinical neuropsychology.* New York: Oxford University Press.

Heilman, K. & Van Den Abell, T. (1980). Right hemisphere dominance for attention: The mechanism underlying hemispheric asymmetries of inattention (Neglect). *Neurology, 30,* 327-330.

Hellebrandt, F.A., Houtz, S.J., Partridge, M.J., & Walters, C.E. (1956). Tonic neck reflexes in exercises of stress in man. *American Journal of Physical Medicine, 3,* 144-159.

Hirt, S. (1967). The tonic neck reflex mechanism in the normal human adult. *American Journal of Physical Medicine, 46,* 326-369.

Joynt, R.J., Benton, A.L., & Fogel, M.L. (1962). Behavioral and pathological correlates of motor impersistence. *Neurology, 12,* 876-881.

Kephart, N.C. (1971). *The slow learner in the classroom.* Columbus, OH: Charles E. Merrill Publishing Co.

Leigh, R.J. & Zee, D.S. (1983). *Neurology of eye movements.* Philadelphia: F.A. Davis Co.

Luria, A.R. (1980). *Higher cortical functions in man. (2nd ed.).* New York: Basic Books Inc.

Meienberg, O., Zangemeister, W.H., Rosenberg, M., Hoyt, W.F., & Stark, L. (1981). Saccadic eye movement strategies in patients with homonymous hemianopia. *Annals of Neurology, 9,* 537-544.

Melzack, R. & Bridges, J.A. (1971). Dorsal column contributions to motor behavior. *Experimental Neurology, 33,* 53-68.

Melzack, R. & Southmayd, S.E. (1974). Dorsal column contributions to anticipatory motor behavior. *Experimental Neurology, 42,* 274-281.

Moore, J.C. (1980). Neuroanatomical considerations relating to recovery of function following brain lesions. In Bach-y-Rita, P. (Ed.). *Recovery of function: Theoretical considerations for brain injury rehabilitation.* Baltimore: University Park Press.

Moore, J.C. (1986). Recovery potentials following CNS lesions: A brief historical perspective in relation to modern research data on neuroplasticity. *American Journal of Occupational Therapy, 40,* 459-463.

Posner, M.I. & Rafal, R.D. (1987). Cognitive theories of attention and the rehabilitation of attentional deficits (pp. 182-291). In Meier, M.J., Benton, A.L., & Diller, L. (Eds.). *Neuropsychological rehabilitation.* New York: Guilford Press.

Ron, S., (1981). Plastic changes in eye movements of patients with traumatic brain injury (pp. 233-240). In A.F. Fuchs & W. Becker (Eds.). *Progress in oculomotor research.* London: Elsevier North Holland Inc.

Roy, E.A. & Square, P.A. (1985). Common considerations in the study of limb, verbal, and oral apraxia (pp. 111-167). In Roy, E.A. (Ed.). *Neuropsychological studies of apraxia and related disorders.* Amsterdam: Elsevier.

Schneider, G.E. (1969). Two visual systems. *Science, 163,* 895-901.

Segal, M., Campbell, D., & Herskovits, M. (1966). *Influence of culture on visual perception.* Kansas City: Bobbs-Merrill.

Taub, E. & Berman, A.J. (1968). Movement and learning in the absence of sensory feedback (pp. 173-192). In Freedman, S.J. (Ed.). *Neuropsychology of spatially oriented behavior.* Homewood, IL: Dorsey Press.

Tyler, R. (1969). Defective stimulus exploration in aphasic patients. *Neurology, 19,* 105-112.

Vierck, C. (1978). Somatosensory system. In Masterton, R.B. (Ed.). *Handbook of behavioral neurobiology.* New York: Plenum Press. pp. 249-309.

Wall, P. (1970). The sensory and motor role of impulses traveling in the dorsal columns towards the cerebral cortex. *Brain, 93,* 505-524.

Warren, M.L. (1984). Comparative study of the presence of the ATNR in adult hemiplegia. *American Journal of Occupational Therapy, 38,* 386-392.

Waterland, J.C. & Munson, N. (1964). Reflex associations of head and shoulder girdle in nonstressful movements in man. *American Journal of Physical Medicine, 43,* 98-108.

Weinberg, J., Diller, L., & Gordon, W.A. (1979). Visual scanning training effect on reading-related tasks in acquired right brain damage. *Archives of Physical Medicine and Rehabilitation, 60,* 479-486.

Yamshon, L.J., Machek, O., & Covalt, D.A. (1949). The tonic neck reflex in the hemiplegic. *Archives of Physical Medicine and Rehabilitation, 30,* 706-711.

Zangemeister, W.H., Meienberg, O., Stark, L., & Hoyt, W.F. (1982). Eye-head coordination in homonymous hemianopia. *Journal of Neurology, 226,* 242-254.

Zihl, J. & Von Cramon, D. (1979). The contribution of the "second" visual system to directed visual attention in man. *Brain, 102,* 815-856.

CHAPTER CONTENT OUTLINE

Learning: A Mechanism for Social Control

The Adaptive Significance of Learning in Occupational Therapy

Behavioral Learning

Cognitive Strategies

Therapy as Learning

Learning Principles and Clinical Strategies

Cognitive Approaches and Strategies

Summary

KEY TERMS

Accommodation

Assimilation

Classical conditioning

Habituation

Learning

Operant conditioning

Schemata

Sensitization

Transfer appropriate processing

ABSTRACT

Therapy as learning is defined in this chapter as not only the means by which individuals acquire competent knowledge and skills; but also a mechanism for social control, whereby the rules, beliefs, and values of a society are transmitted from one generation to the next. Learning is explored as a crucial component in occupational therapy both from the perspective of the client to learn new behaviors and from the perspective of the therapist who must discover his/her own abilities to direct and control the behaviors of clients. The chapter explores the types of learning (both behavioral and cognitive processes) and clinical strategies associated with them.

Educational and Training Strategies
Therapy as Learning

Richard K. Schwartz

*" . . . but whatever we learn has a purpose and whatever we do affects
everything and every one else, if even only in the tiniest way. . . . And it's much
the same thing with knowledge, for whenever you learn something new, the
whole world is that much richer."*

—Norton Juster, 1961

OBJECTIVES

The information in this chapter is intended to help the reader—

1. describe the various types of behavioral and cognitive learning and explain
   their importance to occupational therapy.

2. discuss the role of the occupational therapist as a mediator of learning
   experiences.

3. suggest the types of assessment data which would be of value in determining
   the types of learning approaches to use with patients.

4. explain the concepts of ''criterial tasks'' and ''transfer appropriate
   processing'' in relation to the treatment of occupational therapy patients.

5. identify key learning issues and concepts for further study.

LEARNING: A MECHANISM FOR SOCIAL CONTROL

The ability of humans to learn is one of the most interesting and important of the biologically endowed behaviors which enable us to survive, reproduce, and be productive. Stop reading for a moment, and write down your own personal definition of **learning**. Each of us has an intuitive and personal appreciation of what is meant by the term *learning*. We have *learned* about anatomy in our studies to become occupational therapists and *learned* to fabricate splints and adaptive equipment. We have learned to handle difficult patients and stressful situations with tact and diplomacy. At first glance, it might appear that each of these learning experiences are examples of a similar process or skill, but this is not the case.

While one purpose of this chapter is to provide a general definition of learning, a far more important purpose is to define and describe different types of learning. Once differences among types of learning are appreciated, it will then be possible to provide principles and examples of how to improve therapeutic outcomes through the use of specific learning theories and principles.

Learning is not simply a mechanism by which individuals acquire knowledge and skills. Learning is also a mechanism for social control. The rules of any society or the beliefs and values of that society are transmitted from one generation to the next via learning. This distinction between personal learning and social learning is one that must be kept in mind when working with patients. Everything done to help others should capitalize, not only on the individual's innate abilities to learn and to change, but also on the therapist's abilities to direct and control the behaviors of others toward beneficial outcomes. Such social control functions, which may seem authoritarian at first glance, are best known under the general term of *teaching*.

Behavioral Approach versus Cognitive Approach

Learning is one of the most important functions of the human nervous system. All organisms which have a nervous system, from the lowly flatworm, planaria, to humans, have been found to be capable of learning. The capacity to learn seems to be genetically endowed and appears to permit the individual to benefit from prior experiences. Any definition of learning must take into account that learning is complex.

Current viewpoints on learning tend to fall into either the behavioral or cognitive categories.

Behavioral Approach. Definitions of learning have continued to evolve and focus attention on just those types of learning and learning issues of greatest interest at the time. Thus, from the early part of this century until the mid-1960s, most definitions of learning were strongly behavioral. This was due to the strong influence of Hull (1943), Thorndike (1898), Tolman (1932), Skinner (1938, 1968), Rescorla (1967), Garcia (1983) and others, who conceptualized learning as those processes which led to relatively long-lasting changes in observable behaviors. Schwartz's (1985) definition of learning is typical of this perspective:

> "Learning is the process whereby an individual modifies responsiveness to stimuli or acquires new patterns of behavior as a result of previous interactions with the environment, not including those changes due to growth, maturation, aging, trauma or disease, or those due to changes in motivation or awareness. Learning only occurs when such changes outlast the stimuli that cause them."

The behavioral school focuses on the ways in which the patterning of antecedent stimuli (S) influence behavioral responses (R). This stimulus-response approach has been especially useful for the study of perceptual-motor behaviors and the neurobiological bases of learning (Kandel, 1976).

The behavioral tradition endured for many years as the dominant view of learning among psychologists and educators. Then, as psychology and education began to surrender behavioral views of learning for more cognitively-oriented approaches, cellular neurobiology and the basic sciences concerned with the neural mechanisms of learning discovered and adopted the behavioral perspective on learning. Much of the current research on neural mechanisms of learning investigates observable behaviors with clear stimulus-response linkages. As we will see, there is still much that can be accomplished through clinical intervention that is based on a thorough knowledge of behavioral learning. Behavioral approaches alone do not provide an adequate basis for occupational therapy intervention. The shift from behavioral to cognitive perspectives should not be seen as negating the valuable applied principles of behavioral change which have evolved from behavior theories. Regardless of the inadequacies of such theories to explain complex human learning abilities, they do have an important role to play in understanding and modifying many aspects of human performance from sensory-motor skill development to the development of language and emotional behaviors.

Cognitive Approach to Learning. Most scientists currently interested in research on human learning have shifted their focus from behavior to cognition. It is no longer appropriate to claim that only observable behaviors constitute the domain of learning. Several important issues have been ignored by behavioral approaches, such as the development of knowledge; how individuals learn to learn; the role of thought, symbolic processes, and attention in human information processing; and especially how people come to understand and interpret their own experiences. These are all important influences and must be understood in order to fully comprehend the acquisition of competent human performance abilities. Cognitive theorists such as Piaget (1952, 1954, 1971), Ausubel and associates (1978), Miller and associates (1959), Gagne (1977), and Bransford (1979) have focused attention on constructs which cannot be directly observed, but which certainly influence observable behaviors.

Critics in the cognitive camp argue, with some justification, that the behavioral approach completely ignores important aspects of human mental activity such as attention, memory, thought, reasoning, and imagination. Weinstein and Mayer (1986) observe that the behavioral approach tends to focus on how the presentation of material or activity influences behavior. As such, it is particularly useful for the study of teaching and training methods, since there is an emphasis on controlling the experiences of the learner. Behavioral views usually see the learner as one who is passively driven by stimuli to respond to experiences. Cognitive learning theories seek to explain how information is processed and structured in memory by the learner. Cognitive views tend to see the learner as an active and important participant in the process. Thus, the behavioral viewpoint has been especially useful for investigating how teachers or therapists influence learners, whereas the cognitive viewpoint has emphasized the role of the learner in the processing and modification of information.

A perspective is needed that views behavioral learning and cognitive learning not as opposing theoretical perspectives, but as interdependent elements within the total set of learning processes. All forms of learning are apparently mediated by activity within the human nervous system. Thus, it may be useful to consider differences in the neural pathways and physiologic mechanisms which serve each type of learning. While the goal of reconciling these viewpoints is not likely to be accomplished in the near future, what should prove useful is a definition of learning which can be applied appropriately to either perspective. This is the definition which will be used throughout this chapter:

> **Learning** is a relatively enduring change in the ability of an individual to comprehend and/or competently respond to changes in information from the environment and/or from within the self. As one learns about the environment, the definition of the self and possible behaviors are altered.

This definition suggests that one's mental representations of the self and of the world help define the available behavioral repertoire of the person. Central to cognitive views of learning is the extensive body of research which demonstrates that mental representations of events often have priority over direct sensory experiences. An excellent example is provided by an experiment conducted by Johnson (1967) in which subjects were asked to perform a compensatory tracking task and led to believe that they were part of a two-person team, although there was no real partner. A two-person, group score was given. When told that they were performing below average, subjects tended to blame the poor scores on their fictitious partner. When told that they were performing above average, subjects accepted personal credit for the scores. When told that their performance was average, subjects tended to assume that their partner's poor performance cancelled out their own better-than-average performance. Clearly, the attribution of negative influences to a non-existent partner depended on a mental representation or model of a teammate. In spite of the fact that the only sensory evidence of the teammate came from the examiner, the subjects tended to assume that the teammate's inept performance accounted for undesirable outcomes. Even more indicative of this mental representation replacing sensory data is that the subject did not actually see or talk to the partner nor have any direct experience with the partner, yet was fully prepared to use the conceptual representation to avoid responsibility for failures on the experimental tasks. Although the tendency for mental representations to take the place of direct sensory experiences has been illustrated, the authors did not carefully explore whether or not such mental representations would be preferred over direct sensory data if both were available. This leaves an important issue unresolved for lack of appropriate evidence (Johnson, 1967).

Our everyday experiences tend to confirm the degree to which we rely upon mental representations of events. Consider the following scenario:

As I start my car each morning, I must decide among three possible routes to to arrive at my classes. As I drive the two miles out of the neighborhood onto the first main thoroughfare, I turn on the car radio and listen to a local traffic

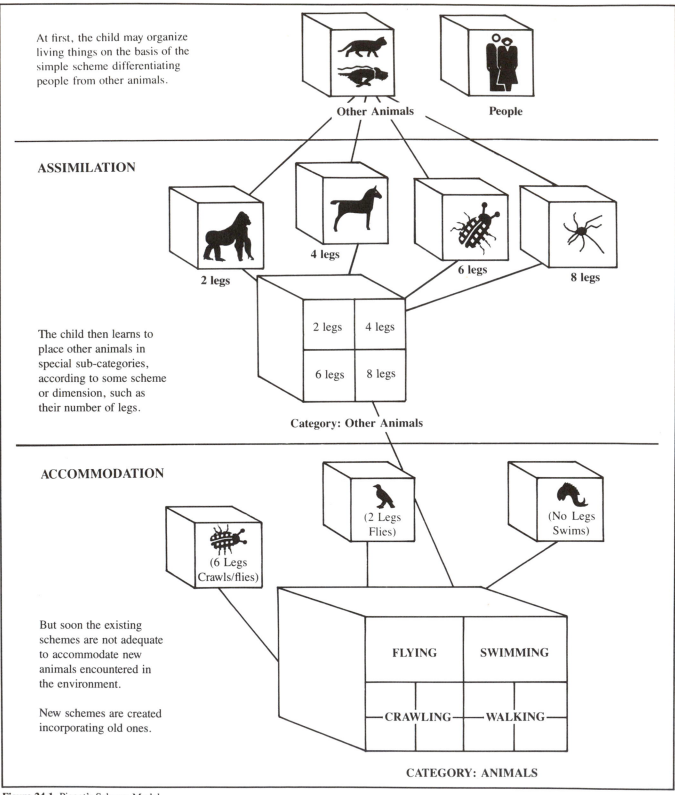

At first, the child may organize living things on the basis of the simple scheme differentiating people from other animals.

Other Animals

People

ASSIMILATION

2 legs

4 legs

6 legs

8 legs

The child then learns to place other animals in special sub-categories, according to some scheme or dimension, such as their number of legs.

2 legs	4 legs
6 legs	8 legs

Category: Other Animals

ACCOMMODATION

(6 Legs Crawls/flies)

(2 Legs Flies)

(No Legs Swims)

But soon the existing schemes are not adequate to accommodate new animals encountered in the environment.

New schemes are created incorporating old ones.

FLYING   SWIMMING

CRAWLING — WALKING

CATEGORY: ANIMALS

Figure 24-1. Piaget's Schema Model.

report. My decision of how to get to work is greatly influenced by mental representations. As I listen to the voice of the traffic announcer on the radio (my direct sensation), I immediately imagine the traffic announcer somewhere up above in the helicopter, alive and real, speaking into a microphone and sharing his direct sensory experiences of how the traffic looks on the highways of the city. As he describes an accident at a certain location, I conjure a mental image of cars backing up (image representation) and invoke my concepts of time, as I imagine how long it will take to get traffic flowing again after a serious accident. I decide to take an alternate route. My decision is confirmed when the traffic announcer says that traffic is moving well on that alternate route. Although I cannot physically see this alternate route, I do have mental representations of both the backed-up route and the free-flowing route and conceptual rules of how to spend the least time driving and get to my destination safely. Because the relevant traffic environment is so large that I could never directly gather all the data, I have chosen to use the mental model of the routes to make my decisions. The clear advantage of forming this representation rests in its predictive validity in helping me reduce delays and shorten the time of my commute.

Piaget's Schema Model. Cognitive scientists have proposed a number of models of mental representations ranging from those in which the human mind is thought of as a computer (*information processing models*) to those in which information in the various sensory registers of the brain may be interpreted in contrast to novel information (*Gestaltic models*). The model of mental representation which seems to hold the most promise for occupational therapy is Piaget's schema model. Piaget (1952, 1954) asserted that mental representations were organized constructions of human thought which begin with simple categories of sensorimotor experiences and eventually develop into complex and abstract categories of linguistic experiences. **Schemata** are considered to be the basic units of all knowledge. Each simple organization of experience and knowledge by the mind constitutes the original "schema" or framework, which represents our everyday experiences. Every experience, thought, and idea is a structural element in an organizational matrix that makes up a person's personal experiences and history. This matrix is comprised of a meaningful set of categories, each filled with data from one's memory of prior events (Schallert, 1982).

Schemata are dynamic mental structures. They undergo continual developmental modification each time an individual encounters novel information about any given category of experience. New knowledge and new information influence existing information via one of two fundamental learning or acquisition processes: **assimilation** and **accommodation** (Piaget, 1952, 1954). (See Figure 24-1)

All human actions and the contingent environmental responses to ourselves, provide new information which may be assimilated (added) into existing schemes or lead to the accommodation and revision of schemes. In this view, mental activity is not reduced to merely another form of behavior. Ideas and thoughts, beliefs and values, knowledge and memory comprise an information context or *map* of human possibilities which may both influence behavior and be modified by behavior.

The approach to learning suggested by the definition above is likely to frustrate those who prefer to see cognition and behavior as mutually exclusive processes. It will also disappoint those who would like to reduce cognition to behavior or behavior to the automatic and inevitable result of stimulus information processing.

Although there may be distinct anatomic and physiologic mechanisms serving each domain of learning, there is also a common set of neurobiological processes and constraints which apply to both cognitive and behavioral viewpoints. Both require incremental changes over time. In both, knowledge develops only through accretion. Both require an intact nervous system. Both lead to learning which can be stored in permanent memory. Both require a salient relationship among perceptions.

Piaget showed that the concept of schema could be applied to perceptual motor and developmental skills that are acquired through behavioral processes and cognitive knowledge. Once acquired these skills generalize to situations different from those present during the initial learning. It is this ability to generalize to other situations that enables patients in occupational therapy to greatly improve performance abilities when spending as little as two to three hours a week with a skilled occupational therapist.

One important difference between these viewpoints is that behavior theory deals only with relationships between stimuli and behaviors that can be directly observed and measured, whereas cognitive theories deal with abstract and/or *emergent properties* of the nervous system. These emergent properties are symbolic constructs which may only be inferred from observable phenomena. Another distinction, which is by no means absolute, is that behavioral learning most often focuses on the acquisition of perceptual-motor response skills, whereas cognitive learning most often deals with verbal, iconic and other symbolic processing skills. However, in the performance of occupational tasks, it is evident that both motor learning of performance skills and cognitive learning of how and when to use certain skills are simultaneously required for appropriate and competent performance.

THE ADAPTIVE SIGNIFICANCE OF LEARNING IN OCCUPATIONAL PERFORMANCE

Each one of us is biologically prepared to benefit from our experiences and interactions with the world. Granit (1977) has described the nervous system as "nature's greatest invention for enabling organisms to deal competently with their environment." All learning, whether behavioral or cognitive, enhances the individual's abilities to skillfully perform the occupations of life, those of self-maintenance, work and play, or leisure. As therapists, we are so often concerned with the specific content of the skills and ideas which we try to teach others, that we ignore the more general benefits of learning as an activity, yet this is where the adaptive significance of learning is best revealed and appreciated.

Learning is primarily a set of processes within the nervous system that enhance the survival and reproductive success of the individual. When we learn to avoid a hot stove or matches as a child, we decrease our chances of perishing from thermal injuries. When we learn to recognize the smell and sight of spoiled food, we decrease our likelihood of food poisoning. When we learn to read and write, we decrease our chances of being unemployed and of living in poverty. Learning alone does not guarantee that we will not be victims of accident, injury, or a hostile environment, but it does slant the odds in our favor. Biologically, such learning improves the chances that our individual genes will have a chance of being represented in the next and successive generations.

Learning also permits conservation of an individual's energy. Each new skill or ability decreases the likelihood of wasted time and effort from unsuccessful attempts to achieve a given goal. Learning enables us to act efficiently. From a biological perspective, it decreases the energy requirements for occupational performance. Less food and oxygen is needed to perform any given task at mastery than is required to accomplish the same task at any earlier point in the learning process. It may also mean that less time and energy are consumed performing essential survival tasks. This allows the individual more time for recreation, leisure, and creative activities.

Learning is also a way to prepare to deal with the unknown and unpredictable events in our lives. When we learn specific skills for each of our daily living tasks we also learn how to decide when to invoke such learning and when to invoke alternative means of reaching our goals. Inherent in the learning process is the process of making choices and decisions concerning our own actions. When we reflect on our learning experiences and think about our thinking ("metacognition"), we generate new knowledge concerning which learning approaches and strategies are successful in which types of situations. In essence, we learn about ourselves and the best methods of processing information. Thus, when we are confronted with the unexpected, we can make appropriate choices of how to act or how to learn more about the characteristics of the situation.

Learning also serves to prepare and enable us to live in social groupings with others. It enables us to structure the experiences of our children and to transmit the rules of acceptable behavior and interaction to improve social cohesiveness and minimize antisocial behaviors. When we learn to speak the language of our group, we gain a non-violent, non-physical means of conflict and conflict resolution. When we develop concrete and abstract reasoning abilities, we become better able to predict the consequences of our actions with respect to other persons and our environment.

Learning is a means of defining self. Learning establishes our identity to ourselves and others and partly determines the personality traits that we use to express our individuality. We learn to label our experiences and to use such labels to define ourselves.

One could not consider the specific applications of learning to the remediation of human problems, which is the major purpose of this chapter, without this larger context of what learning does for us. From a practical standpoint, we can use these personal benefits as additional criteria in assessing the effectiveness of therapeutic learning.

Table 24-1
Types of Behavioral Learning Important to Therapy

Type	Duration of Behavioral Change
Post-tetanic Potentiation (PTP)	Minutes to Hours
Post-tetanic Depression (PTD)	Minutes to Hours
Habituation	Hours to Weeks
Sensitization (Dishabituation)	Hours to Weeks
Classical Conditioning	Up to years
Operant Conditioning	Up to years

BEHAVIORAL LEARNING

There are six types of behavioral learning that are important for occupational therapy. Table 24-1 indicates the various types and the expected duration of behavioral changes. Each of these types of behavioral learning will be described below. The applications of the short-term learning approaches are described in great detail elsewhere (Schwartz, 1985), but both intermediate and long-term behavioral learning will be discussed in greater detail later in this chapter.

Post-Tetanic Potentiation and Post-tetanic Depression

Post-tetanic potentiation (facilitation) and post-tetanic depression are extremely ephemeral types of learning that last only seconds to minutes. They occur when there is a very rapid volley of afferent stimulation (sensory tetany) in a given neural pathway. Following such tetanic stimulation, it often is observed that there is a brief period in which post-synaptic neurons have either supernormal responses (in post-tetanic potentiation) or subnormal responses (in post-tetanic depression) to non-tetanizing presynaptic activity. Such learning is restricted only to the stimulated pathway and does not alter responses other than in the neurons immediately post-synaptic to those tetanized. It has been postulated that such learning is useful in explaining many of the results of neurorehabilitation (facilitation and inhibition) techniques (Schwartz, 1985).

Habituation

Habituation consists of reversible decreases in the amplitude (strength) of a response, when the response is repeatedly elicited through stimulation. A sudden or strong stimulus will immediately restore the habituated response to its original strength. This restoration is called ''dishabituation,'' and is actually a form of sensitization (the next learning paradigm to be considered).

Unlike the short-term paradigms just discussed, habituation is widely regarded as worthy of consideration as a type of behavioral learning (Kupferman, 1975). All animals, including humans, demonstrate this type of behavior modification (Kandel, 1979). Thorpe (1956) has defined habituation as ''. . . the relatively permanent waning of a response as a result of repeated stimulation which is not followed by any kind of reinforcement. It is specific to the stimulation and relatively enduring.''

The most distinguishing characteristic of habituation is the gradual recovery of habituated responses during periods of nonstimulation. In fact, the greater the period of nonstimulation, the more complete will be the recovery of the habituated response. This is a feature of habituation which is often overlooked by those who attempt habituation training. The most direct implication for intervention is that habituation trials must be provided in the context of frequent and repeated training sessions, because wide spacing of training over time totally reverses the learning results. It is generally accepted that the degree of recovery of a response during a fixed time interval is the most useful measure of the strength of habituation, i.e., the less the recovery per unit time, the stronger the habituation learning (Petrinovich and Patterson, 1979).

Bruner and Kennedy (1970) have suggested additional criteria to define habituation operationally. They argue that any change in the frequency of stimulation, regardless of direction, will restore some of the habituated response. Others (Petrinovich & Patterson, 1979) note that any novel stimulus or stimulus of significantly greater intensity (higher amplitude) than the habituation stimuli leads to some degree of recovery of habituated responses. It is argued that this requirement of habituation is essential to rule out such phenomena as receptor adaptation and fatigue. The reversal of habituation by other strong or novel stimuli is referred to as *dishabituation*.

The most comprehensive description of habituation is that of Thompson and Spencer (1966) who report that the greater the number of habituation trials, the more complete the response depression. If the habituation stimulus is presented in a series of trials, the briefer the time interval between trials, the greater (and more rapid) the response depression. In other words, for a fixed number of habituation trials, the more closely they are spaced in time, the more profound is the response decrement. There is also a relationship between stimulation intensity and rate of habituation. Using identical frequencies of stimulation but varying the intensity of the stimuli, the weaker of two habituation stimuli virtually always produces the more rapid, complete habituations. This is to be expected because the weaker the initial stimulus, the weaker the response it elicits. Weak responses naturally require less amplitude attenuation to reach a point of extinction. Finally, although habituated responses are capable of showing some degree of stimulus generalization (i.e., decreased responsiveness to stimuli similar to the habituation stimulus), for the most part, learning is restricted to the specific stimulus used to habituate that response.

Habituation is appropriately considered as having intermediate endurance effects. In many instances, the effects of repeated, non-noxious, and low intensity stimulation last from hours to days. It has been reported that habituation may last as long as three to four weeks following several sessions of ten stimuli each (Kandel, 1979).

Little debate or doubt exists regarding the adaptive significance of this type of learning. Habituation functions to screen out information which has little immediate significance to the organism. Environmental stimuli which occur repeatedly, yet offer no threat to an individual are usually ignored because they do not signal a need for an adaptive response. At least three distinct adaptive functions are performed by habituation:

1. *Habituation serves to limit defensive and escape behaviors to those stimuli most likely to signal true danger.* Any low intensity stimulus that poses little threat leads to rapid habituation of orienting and attending. Presumably, once free from the need to attend to each and every stimulus of the environment, only novel stimuli (be they dangerous or hedonistic), elicit orientation and attending behaviors. If this were not the case, every change in our environment would arouse and startle us.

2. *Habituation helps the individual to establish a territory.* When most features of an environment are familiar, habituation occurs and decreases the need for exploratory and/or defensive behaviors. This permits attention and energy to be focused on basic needs and drives, which enhance both individual and species survival.

3. *Habituation serves a social function.* Kinship bonds are maintained and strengthened by familiarity. Social behaviors which occur frequently and pose no particular threat are acceptable and demand no special responses since habituation has dampened such tendencies. Deviant behavior, which is unusual, potentially threatening, and occurs infrequently, is met by attention, defensive behaviors, and responses designed to restore the status quo and suppress deviant behavior.

This intermediate-term learning serves both longer lasting and more complex forms of learning by selectively focusing attention and sequentially structuring the individual's perception of the environment.

Sensitization

Sensitization consists of increases in the amplitude (strength) of a response to a given stimulus as a result of the presentation of another stimulus (often noxious or very strong), in which such enhancement does not depend on pairing of the stimuli. Sensitization learning is commonly regarded as the opposite of habituation learning. It is a process whereby stimuli that predict either danger or significant novelty in the environment act to increase pre-existing reflexive behaviors (Kupferman, 1975).

Sensitization often endures for minutes to weeks or longer after stimulation (Brunelli et al., 1976). The time course of sustained behavioral change is comparable to that of habituation and is the reason sensitization should be regarded as intermediate-term learning.

While habituation shows only a very modest stimulus generalization, sensitization is highly generalized to responses other than those previously habituated. Greenbaum (1979) has pointed out that sensitization may be a critical component of behavioral arousal. Sensitization is a process in which input activity modifies an output or response. It differs from classical conditioning in that the stimuli used to elicit a desired behavior need not have a temporal relationship. The most widely studied form of sensitization was termed dishabituation for many years until it was recognized to be a process separate and distinct from habituation. (Thompson & Spencer, 1966). Sensitization has been found to be a powerful restorative force with respect to both brief and long-standing habituated responses (Kandel, 1979).

The adaptive significance of sensitization can be considered by itself and with respect to habituation. Sensitization enables an individual to mobilize a range of responses to a single novel or threatening stimulus. Most of us have been startled by a foreign loud noise (such as a scream, explosion, or siren) that interrupts our daily activity. Our response is to become alert, with eyes open wide, ears attentive, and heart racing! This response differs from how we would respond to a friend or co-worker who might interrupt our activity without startling us. The familiarity of the voice, appearance, and other "stimuli" of a friend (learned via habituation and otherwise) tells us that this interruption poses no threat to us.

When sensitized by a scream or siren, it is unusual to be able to immediately return to one's previous occupation because of a heightened awareness and responsiveness to most other stimuli, even nonthreatening ones. Thus sensitization is not only significant in its own right as a form of arousal, but it also serves to restore habituated responses to nonthreatening and familiar stimuli, such as that experienced when one hears a strange sound during the night. We jump out of bed, turn on the lights, and immediately all of the familiar objects, furniture, doorways, and halls, elicit responses of attending and exploring even though no further sign of threat is present. For a period of time, we have heightened arousal to all features of our environment. When a threat is present, such dishabituation renders us cautious to all environmental features.

Sensitization, like habituation, serves to predict which responses will be most appropriate in a given environment at a given time. Habituation predicts that failure to attend or respond to a given stimulus will be of little or no consequence. Sensitization predicts that failure to respond to even seemingly trivial stimuli could have dire consequences.

Classical Conditioning

Classical conditioning is a process of repeatedly pairing a neutral stimulus with a stimulus that invariably elicits a response until the neutral stimulus alone is capable of eliciting the response (or one which closely resembles it). This type of learning is said to be *associative*. It is long-term learning and potentially can last indefinitely. The conditioned stimulus (CS) comes to be associated with or predicts the unconditioned stimulus (UCS). This is the result of the close temporal association of these two stimuli. The CS also becomes associated with certain aspects or components of the response elicited by the UCS. During the period of training, stimuli are repeatedly paired with one another in an invariant sequence in which the CS always precedes the UCS, and hence comes to predict that the UCS will follow whenever the CS is presented.

The most widely noted example of classical conditioning was provided by Pavlov (1906) who observed the response of dogs salivating when their attendants appeared. In a series of experiments he presented a CS (bell) immediately before a UCS (food) and found that salivation always occurred reflexively to food presentation as part of an unconditioned response (UCR) and would eventually occur as a conditioned response (CR) to the bell alone.

Modern View of Classical Conditioning. One interpretation of the classical conditioning process is that associative learning is critically dependent on the specific temporal ordering of training events. Such an interpretation implies that behavior changes because the individual is able to reliably predict that a neutral stimulus (CS) will be followed by a UCS. It is generally accepted that the optimal ordering of events for classical conditioning is to have the CS precede the UCS. Furthermore, the optimal interval between CS and UCS is generally accepted to be from one-half second to several seconds (Logue, 1979). One notable exception to the general principle that optimal conditioning requires very brief delays is *taste-aversion learning*. It has been shown that when food is consumed (CS) leading to gastric distress (UCS) and vomiting and/or nausea (R), there can be effective learned aversion even if the delay interval between stimuli is quite long (Logue, 1979).

Garcia (1983) and his colleagues at UCLA conducted a series of ingenious experiments designed to show that certain classically conditioned responses were more likely to be associated with stimuli naturally related to those responses than with other "neutral" or unrelated stimuli. In an initial experiment, water-deprived rats were simultaneously exposed to two conditioned stimuli (CS): saccharine taste added to the water and a flash of light with a clicking sound (audiovisual stimulus). These stimuli were both paired with radiation exposure to x-rays (UCS) leading to presumed nausea and other radiation sickness-induced responses (UCR). Following only three conditioning trials, these rats were offered sweetened water with no audiovisual

stimulus or plain water with the audiovisual stimulus on alternate days. Under these conditions, only the taste and not the audiovisual stimulus became aversive, such that the rats would avoid sweetened water when the audiovisual stimulus was absent, but not avoid the water when the audiovisual stimulus was presented. When another group of rats was trained using the same two CS (i.e., saccharine water and audiovisual stimuli) that were paired with electrical shock to the foot, the audiovisual stimulus became aversive and not the taste stimulus.

The series of experiments cited above are of significance in several respects since they tend to force a modification of the traditional views of classical conditioning. First, they force a revision of the widely held notion that classically conditioned learning depends on a close temporal association of CS and UCS. In conditioned taste-aversion learning, long delays between gustatory stimuli and the radiation (UCS), even from two to six hours, can lead to classically conditioned avoidance. Second, and perhaps of even greater significance, there appear to be certain "biologically prepared" tendencies to associate food-related stimuli with illness (i.e., gustatory stimuli with radiation induced illness) and to associate audiovisual stimuli with externally induced pain (i.e., light and sound with foot shock). This strongly suggests that it is the specific adaptive significance or information value of stimuli that determine their likelihood of becoming associated with specific UCS-UCR behaviors. An added note of interest is that such "prepared" associations seem to be species specific, such that Japanese quail, which lack taste buds, appear predisposed to associate visual cues related to food with subsequent illness rather than gustatory cues.

Classical conditioning can be classified into two broad categories based on the nature of the UCS. *Appetitive conditioning* occurs whenever the UCS is pleasurable or rewarding and consummatory or approach behavior is generally the response (R) to such stimulation. When the UCS is either noxious or punitive and the resulting response consists of either protective or escape (avoidance) behaviors, then the conditioned association of a neutral CS with such UCS is termed *defensive conditioning* (Kupferman, 1981). (Table 24-2)

Extinction. Reversal of learning or *extinction* is an important feature of classical conditioning. If a CR has been repeatedly elicited by a CS in the absence of any UCS presentations, then over time the intensity of the CR or the likelihood of its occurring after CS presentation will decrease. This is quite similar to the "forgetting" of habituated responses which follows a period of nonstimulation. In the case of classical conditioning, this phenomenon is known as extinction. Its adaptive significance seems to be that extinction eliminates those conditioned responses from an individual's repertoire that no longer predict an association between two stimuli. Kupferman (1985) has further observed that extinction is due most likely to active processes rather than to a passive reversal of changes serving the learned behavior.

Although classical conditioning can be extinguished, it is appropriately considered to be long-term learning. In some cases of both appetitive and defensive conditioning, a period of training may be sufficient to establish a CS-associated response that lasts the lifetime of the individual. Such learning is said to be relatively resistant to extinction. It is important to recognize that many forms of classical conditioning represent learning in relation to stimuli that are naturally paired. Where such natural pairing exists training is inherent in an individual's experience. Figure 24-2 illustrates that food preferences are an example of such naturally learned associations.

Adaptive Role of Classical Conditioning. The adaptive significance of classically conditioned learning has been discussed and explored by many learning theorists. Classical conditioning is established in human infants within three and four days after birth. Many have wondered about the value of such learning so early in life. Hence, the close relationship established between newborns and their mothers, known as *mother-infant bonding*, has received considerable attention in recent years. Some scientists have been interested in the degree to which common maternal-infant experiences influence such bonding. Freud suggested that infants sought close contact with their mothers because of the pleasurable (appetitive) association of the mother (CS) with the taste of her milk (UCS) and the visceral responses (UCR) elicited by the milk. Recent studies with infant rats, in which neutral olfactory stimuli (CS) were paired with milk (UCS) or no milk delivery while sucking a passive dam, showed that rat pups acquired a significantly greater preference for those odors paired with milk presentation over those paired with no milk (Brake, 1981). Although the generalization of results from rats to humans can be justifiably questioned, the study represents the first evidence that milk delivery in mammals may be responsible for developing learned associations between maternal behavior and infant responses.

Defensive classical conditioning appears to serve both adaptive and maladaptive behavioral learning. A form of learning called *rapid aversive conditioning*, takes advantage of innate defensive and/or escape responses. A neutral stimulus (CS) such as the visual image of a dog, if followed by a painful scratch or bite (UCS), may appropriately lead to avoiding other dogs by running away, screaming, or hiding (all UCRs and CRs). Such rapid learning is facilitated or prepared'' insofar as the conditioned responses, such as putting the hands in front of the face or freezing, are natural defensive reactions (Logue, 1979).

Many fears appear to be the result of classically associated stimuli. During the period of toilet training, a young child may come to associate the neutral stimulus of the bathroom with feelings of inadequacy or failure if the mother criticizes or scolds the child, and thus develops a conditional fear of bathrooms. The pervasiveness of such conditioning is attested to by Kushner (1981) when he questions, ''How many public and private superstitions are based upon something good or bad happening right after we did something, and our assuming that the same thing will follow the same pattern every time?''

Cognitive Processes can be Classical Conditioning. A dramatic example of classical conditioning is the association of neutral symbols, especially words, with emotional events. The word ''love'' connotes positive meaning only to the person who has been held (UCS), caressed (UCS), kissed (UCS), and smiled at (UCS). The expression, ''I love you,'' derives its power from previous paired associations of action-oriented stimuli with the utterance of the symbolic statement. The statement, ''I love you,'' would have no significance if said over the phone to someone who does not understand English. In such a case, the auditory stimulus is truly neutral. ''Love'' has different associations from person to person, because of the different events associated with it.

For most people, words eventually come to have a power of their own. A rational, mature mind would recognize that someone calling us ''no-good and stupid'' does not make that a reality. People can differentiate between what someone else says and what is, unless they have been consistently conditioned to think otherwise. Hence, we learn to respond to such words from prior learned associations.

Why do emotionally-laden terms seem especially susceptible to such associations? Perhaps because other more neutral descriptive terms such as ''brown-haired'' or ''carpenter'' are not likely to have occurred under conditions in which visceral or affective sensations (UCSs) were present and gave rise to

Table 24-2 Types of Classical Conditioning		
	Appetitive	**Defensive**
Nature of Unconditioned Stimulus (UCS)	UCS is pleasurable or rewarding	UCS is noxious or punative
Response (R) to Stimulation	Consummatory or approach behavior	Protective or avoidance behaviors

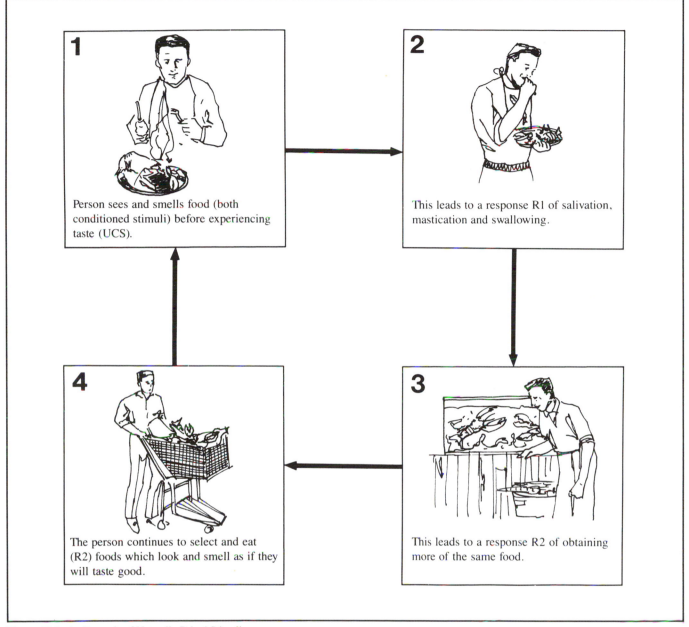

Figure 24-2. An Example of Naturally Paired Stimuli.

automatic or stereotyped responses (UCRs). Words that are rarely paired with situations having high affective content (good or bad) are unlikely to result in classically conditioned verbal associations. It is not only what we say, but how we say it that determines meaning. If one says ''I love you'' with a sarcastic or nasty tone, the message received will not be interpreted as an expression of genuine affection.

The examples cited thus far focus on some *autonomic* or *visceral responses*. By and large, there has been a tendency to identify classical conditioning with autonomic response learning, and *instrumental conditioning* with skeletal movement learning. Such a view may automatically reflect a general tendency, but ignores ever-increasing evidence that both types of conditioning have been employed to train autonomic and somatic learning (Hearst, 1975).

Instrumental or Operant Conditioning

Instrumental or **operant conditioning** consists of the presentation of a reinforcing stimulus after the occurrence of a given response so that repeated presentations of the reinforcing stimulus lead to an increase in the frequency and/or probability of the reinforced response. In operant conditioning, the close association is between the operants or emitted behaviors and any one of a number of positive reinforcers, negative reinforcers, or punishments which follow the behavior closely in time. In classical conditioning, this close temporal association is between the conditioned stimulus or neutral stimulus and the unconditioned stimulus, which elicits the unconditioned response.

Both classical and instrumental conditioning are said to be associative conditioning. Although the contiguity view of both classical and instrumental conditioning assumes that it is the close temporal association of events that is a necessary and sufficient condition for learning to occur, the *essential* element in all cases is the informative or predictive value of stimuli. Thus, in classical conditioning the CS must somehow be identified by the organism as predicting the arrival of the UCS, and in operant conditioning, the reinforcers or punishments must provide information that emitted behaviors are appropriate, serve adaptation, and/or will increase the future likelihood of pleasure or avoidance of pain.

Instrumental or operant conditioning procedures create an association not between two stimuli, but between a response and a stimulus that follows. Kupferman (1985, p. 808) notes that "Unlike classical conditioning, which is restricted to specific reflex responses that are evoked by specific, identifiable stimuli, operant conditioning involves behaviors (called operants) that apparently occur spontaneously or with no recognizable stimuli." (See Table 24-4)

Associative learning paradigms take great care to distinguish between classes of stimulus events. Two such classes have already been described: (1) eliciting stimuli, which call forth a reflexive response, and (2) reinforcing stimuli, which follow as consequences of voluntary or spontaneous behaviors. Stimuli act to set the stage or signal conditions that are ideal for behaviors reinforced previously. Instrumental conditioning may be used to modify behaviors by the presentation of reinforcing stimuli

Table 24-3
Classes of Reinforcing Stimuli

Class	Characteristic	Example
Positive	Reinforcer	Tokens
Negative	Removal or avoidance of aversive response	Loss of privilege
Punishments	Noxious stimuli	Electric shock

following the occurrence of the behavior. Since such behaviors often have no clear link to prior stimuli, they are most often considered voluntary behaviors.

Two distinct classes of behaviors also are influenced by associative learning paradigms: (1) reflexive responses or respondents, which usually occur after eliciting stimuli, and (2) operants or voluntary responses, whose frequency is modified by reinforcing stimuli. Instrumental conditioning was described first by Thorndike (1898) as the "*law of effect*," which proposed that rewards or reinforcing stimuli served to connect responses to stimuli and that large rewards produced stronger associations than small rewards. In other words, behaviors that produce the greatest pleasurable consequences are established more reliably than those which produce the least pleasurable consequences (Bitterman, 1975).

Just as Pavlov is most identified with classical conditioning, Skinner (1938, 1965) is most often associated with operant conditioning. Skinner's contribution was to focus on the modification of virtually any and all voluntary behaviors through the selective use of rewards and punishments.

Although there are many different "schedules" of reinforcement that may be effective, only the simplest example — that of continuous reinforcement — is described here. Repeated reinforcement of responses increases the frequency of the response during training and greater than the frequency recorded in the pretest. During the post-training periods, even if no reinforcement is provided, response frequency will increase over the pretest frequency. If reinforcement is totally ceased after training, a gradual decline in the frequency of the "learned" change will occur, and such non-reinforcement is said to lead to the extinction of the learned component of behavior.

Reinforcing stimuli fall into one of three primary classes: (1) *positive reinforcers*, which are rewards; (2) *negative reinforcers*, which consist of the removal or avoidance of aversive stimuli; and (3) *punishments*, which are noxious stimuli. A common misconception is that positive reinforcers increase the frequency of operants, and that punishments decrease the frequency of operants. Actually, under the right circumstances, rewards can be used to extinguish behaviors, and punishments can be used to increase the frequency of behavior. To understand this, it is necessary to consider the motivation of an individual to respond with a given behavior. White (1959) provides extensive evidence for at least three different types of motivation or "drives."

1. The *primary drives* are survival-oriented needs which represent conditions such as hunger and thirst and are associated with tissue deficits. They exist in a similar fashion for all members of a species. Behaviors such

as searching for food and/or water increase with non-reinforcement, but actually decrease with any positive reinforcement or reward that reduces the tissue deficit (e.g., food or water). Punishment of such behaviors only temporarily decreases frequency of searching behavior, and withdrawal of such punishment leads to increases in behaviors that seek to satisfy the need for food and water.

2. The *secondary drives* are thought of as hedonistic drives, in contrast to primary drives which are distinctly survival-oriented. Secondary drives include desires for recognition or approval, desires for money, and desires for certain material objects such as cars or televisions. These secondary drives are often called ''desires'' whereas primary drives are called ''needs.'' Behaviors such as working at a task to gain recognition increase in frequency when not reinforced or punished. For secondary drives, the association of positive reinforcement with increased operant frequency and punishment with decreased operant frequency is most appropriate.

3. The *competence drives* are drives that do not clearly fall into either of the above categories and include the need to manipulate objects, to explore one's environment, and to move one's body from place to place within one's environment. Although positive reinforcement tends to increase such behaviors and punishment to decrease them, there appear to be certain minimal needs for such activity. Thus, if all movement, manipulation, and exploration are not reinforced or even punished, the behaviors tend to increase in frequency—for example punishing a child for not sitting still or squirming in a chair is not likely to elicit a decrease in that activity. On the other hand, positive reinforcement most often increases behaviors that tend to fulfill competency needs.

To predict the effects of a given reinforcer, one must know something about the individual's motivation to perform an act and what has gone on previously with that individual and the environment. The misconception that rewards always increase frequency of behavior and negative reinforcement decreases frequency of behavior should be dispelled by a more accurate understanding of motivational influences.

Another issue centers on selection of the best operant or behavior to attempt to modify. For example, if the desired behavior is to have a rat jump over a metal strip dividing its cage, it is easier to obtain that behavior by punishing the rat for walking across the grid (i.e., by electrically shocking the rat for that behavior), than it is to positively reward the highly unlikely event of the rat jumping over the strip.

It should be noted that punishment suppresses, but does

Table 24-4
Comparison of Classical and Operant Conditioning

	Classical Conditioning	**Operant (Instrumental) Conditioning**
Neccessary Entering Behavior	Unconditioned reflex—an unlearned response to stimuli	Availability of a particular response
Nature of Reinforcement	Occurs on every trial	Occurs only when a correct response is made
Required External Learning Conditions	Contiguity (Pairing of UCS and CS) and Practice (repetition)	Reinforcement, contiguity and practice

not extinguish operants. Behaviors usually revert to pre-training levels once the punishment is removed. Furthermore, punishment has been found to usually elicit unpredictable responses from its victims (Woody, 1982). Only with intense punishment is undesirable behavior suppressed. *In general, non-reinforcement (ignoring) is a more effective means of extinguishing behaviors than is punishment.*

If instrumental conditioning only alters the frequency of an emitted response, one might wonder how the individual can learn new behaviors. The instrumental process whereby such complex learning occurs is known as *shaping* or *successive approximations.* Brady (1979, p. 26) provides an excellent description of this phenomenon:

''. . . it has been possible to make explicit the process called shaping, whereby a combination of operant conditioning and extinction (i.e., withholding reinforcers) can shape existing simple responses into new and more complex performances. Of critical importance for this shaping process is the observation that a reinforcing stimulus not only strengthens the particular response that precedes it, but also results in an increase in the frequency of many other bits of behavior (i.e., response generalization) and in effect raises the individual's general activity level.''

Thus, the shaping of behavior proceeds as reinforcers initially are presented following a response similar to or approximating the desired behavior. Since this tends to increase the strength of various other similar behaviors, the response still closer to the desired one is selected from this new array and followed by reinforcing stimuli. Shaping thus involves this progressive selection and refinement of the

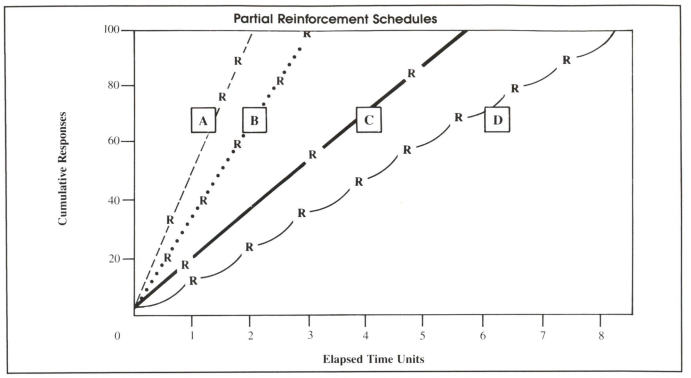

Figure 24-3: Each plot depicts actual performance according to a different reinforcement schedule. The vertical axis represents the cumulative number of times the subject demonstrates the target behavior. Each reinforcement is designated by a separate R. **Plot A:** *Variable ratio schedule* (reinforced according to varying number of responses). **Plot B:** *Fixed Ratio schedule* (reinforced according to a fixed number of responses). **Plot C:** *Variable interval schedule* reinforced according to varied interval) and **Plot D:** *Fixed interval schedule* (reinforced at fixed intervals).

desired response by reinforcement from among new arrays of available behavior. This shaping process is obviously of enormous clinical importance in behavioral medicine since many patients' performances can only be changed effectively in this way.

Toilet training of young children can be greatly enhanced by shaping or the rewarding of responses which successively approximate the desired response of urinating and/or defecating in the toilet. From personal experience with my own children, I have been able to experience the beneficial aspects of the progressive nature of shaping. We began by rewarding our daughter a penny each time she entered the bathroom before and after each meal, before naps, and before going to bed. We progressed to giving the penny only after sitting on her potty seat with clothes on, and then without pants, and finally the penny was given only when she actually urinated or defecated. This system worked extremely well, and she was toilet trained in much less time than her brother for whom we used the system of rewarding only when he actually used the toilet properly, an event that only rarely spontaneously occurred.

Schedules of reinforcement. Operant conditioning is long-term learning. It may endure months, years, or even the lifetime of an individual. The retention of such learning clearly depends on memory, which is a subject beyond the scope of this discussion, but *the single most important determinant of longevity of learning is the schedule of reinforcement used to establish and maintain operant learning.* A *reinforcement schedule* is a set of criteria or rules that govern exactly when reinforcement will be provided.

Longevity of learning cannot be directly assessed. It is impossible in most cases to know how much is being forgotten or lost and when such forgetting occurs. Instead, we measure the resistance to extinction or the degree to which operant conditioned behavior is maintained even when no reinforcement is given.

One quality of reinforcement schedules is the nature of the reinforcer, whether it is positive, negative, non-reinforcement, or punishment. Another key dimension is timing. Often a reinforcer must follow soon after the operant behavior or conditioning will be decreased (Kupferman, 1985). The extensive research on children generally shows that the best learning occurs when reinforcement is immediate.

When a reinforcement schedule requires every operant

response to be reinforced (positively or negatively), the schedule is termed *continuous reinforcement*. When only certain occasions of operant responding are reinforced, then the schedule is termed *partial reinforcement*. Resistance to extinction is greater using schedules of partial reinforcement rather than schedules of continuous reinforcement. For example, praising a patient for *every* small component of performance, will be less successful in altering behavior than praising only significant and/or new accomplishments. Continuous reinforcement may cause an individual to habituate to the reinforcing stimulus, therefore diminishing its effect. Since continuous reinforcement schedules are rarely appropriate, it is best to focus on partial reinforcement schedules.

Partial reinforcement schedules. The major categories are ratio and interval reinforcement and the subcategories of each are fixed or variable patterns of reinforcement (Brady, 1979). (see Figure 24-3)

Ratio reinforcement schedules are those that stipulate how many times an operant behavior must occur before it is reinforced. If reinforcements are provided at ratios that approach continuous reinforcement, the risk of decreased retention occurs. On the other hand, if an individual is rewarded too infrequently, there is a danger of extinction occurring during training because the desired behavior is not reinforced much of the time.

Interval reinforcement schedules provide for reinforcement at specified time intervals during performance independent of how many times the operant behavior has occurred. Interval schedules can also approach or even surpass continuous reinforcement if the intervals are too brief. Likewise, if intervals are too long, extinction will occur during training. But unlike ratio schedules, interval schedules have built-in reinforcement for persisting at a task, even if the target behavior occurs only rarely. Whereas a ratio schedule would discourage a slow learner or someone in the early stages of learning, an interval schedule rewards those trying to learn.

Ratio and interval schedules can be either fixed or variable. A *fixed schedule* is one in which the ratio or interval is constant; a *variable schedule* is one in which the ratio or intervals may change during training. With fixed schedules, the learner not only learns the operant behaviors desired, but also learns the schedule, and performance is altered by anticipation of those conditions that determine when reinforcement will occur. With variable schedules, learning about the schedule itself is difficult or impossible, and the seemingly random nature of reinforcement tends to minimize strategies that seek to perform at different levels during training.

Using these four descriptions of reinforcement schedules, virtually every complex schedule can be described. A compound schedule is one in which a given behavior may be reinforced only if it meets the requirements of two or more schedules. A concurrent schedule is one in which reinforcement is provided only if two or more behaviors (operants) meet the simultaneous demands of two or more reinforcement schedules. Other complex schedules fall into the categories of multiple schedules. In most natural learning situations, reinforcement typically follows compound, concurrent, or complex schedules (Brady, 1979).

In summarizing the importance of reinforcement schedules, we can clearly see that they are an extremely important determinant of the nature and extent of learning when carefully designed and implemented and when related to the underlying neural events that serve operant conditioning.

COGNITIVE STRATEGIES

Assimilation

Assimilation is the mental process which functions to increase the number of examples of objects, events, or processes represented by the larger schema concept. It expands the data or information within a given category or subcategory of a schema and helps to incorporate new information within the existing representational structure without requiring any reorganization or modification of prior knowledge. Assimilation may be thought of as an increase in the volume or amount of information in a given act or category.

Accommodation

Accommodation is the process whereby the organization of information within a schema must be revised or altered due to the inability to fit new information into any existing mental category. The most extreme instance of accommodation is the creation of a new schema. While this is a common occurrence for the young child who has not yet fully become aware of his or her own body and/or environment, it is rarely necessary for an adult to create an entirely novel mental representation. More often than not, a revised schematic organization is needed which permits data that cannot be readily classified and assimilated into a prior schema, to be subsumed under one or more of the revised schema categories.

Accommodation always alters the organizational structure or categories of schemata to permit inclusion of new information that could not fit into previously existing mental categories. An example of this can be seen within our own profession by the accommodation of electrical stimulation into occupational therapy treatment. Initially, it was thought of as a treatment based solely on the use of physical agents and thus within physiotherapy's domain. A middle ground was created with the advances in myoelectrically-controlled prostheses, robotic arms for functional assistance of disabled persons, biofeedback, and computer-assisted ambulation for those with spinal cord injuries. This middle ground between occupational and physical therapy treatment approaches was relatively ambiguous. Most occupational therapists who work in these areas had to accommodate a new category into the existing practice schema, that of *functional electrical stimulation*, which allows occupational therapists to use certain forms of electrical stimulation to control or use orthotics, but discourages the use of electrical current as direct treatment. Those who have made such an accommodation and modified their schema concerning occupational therapy practice view their professional role differently from those who adhere to the earlier schema.

As a learner is able to construct and elaborate upon a schema, there is an increase in familiarity with that schema and its elements. Assimilation or fitting new material into existing categories of knowledge requires considerably less mental attention and effort than accommodation of existing schemata. In short, assimilation is similar to filing information in existing slots or file folders, a process that is quick and relatively simple. Accommodation, on the other hand, requires that a new or revised organizational structure be created and tested to determine if it is appropriate for both our prior and our new knowledge. This is a considerably more challenging task than assimilation.

Verbal Learning

Verbal learning refers to the processes which lead to the acquisition of linguistic skills that enable an individual to express information through speech or writing and to receive information by means of listening or reading. One of the most useful views of such learning is provided by Roger Brown (1958). In the late 1950s, Roger Brown chose to address the debate (that is ongoing to the present day) of whether language learning in children proceeds from the general to the specific or from specific to general — for example whether a child first learns to think of all coins as "money" or whether they first learned to say, "penny," "dime," and "nickel" and then call them "money." In 1958, he set forth the radical proposition that neither directional hypothesis held, and that the discussion itself did not look at how children actually learned to name objects. Brown suggested that objects were named by adults for children in the way that the adult believed would be most useful or functional to the child in everyday usage, a concept that is now known as *functional labeling*. Brown showed that the acquisition of vocabulary could proceed either from general to specific or specific to general,

depending on which would be most useful for the child. Historically, this led to a significant shift from a polarized view of language acquisition to a more integrated, rational, and empirically verifiable approach.

THERAPY AS LEARNING

Therapy implies change. No therapeutic interaction with a patient is effective if the patient remains unaffected. The role of therapist as the agent who plans and structures the experiences of the patient in such a way as to effect beneficial changes is no longer satisfactory. Recently that there has been a willingness to shift perspectives and consider the role of the patient in this process.

The move towards synergy between behavioral and cognitive approaches highlights the need for such reciprocity in patient intervention. There are both intrinsic and environmental determinants of performance. In spite of paying lip-service to this distinction, many have focused their efforts almost entirely on the modification of environmental factors of performance. Even when attempting to alter the intrinsic factors (i.e., our patient's individual capabilities), we tend to manipulate and control environmental factors to make it easier for the person to change. In essence, our efforts have emphasized our own abilities to structure activities for our patients or to structure their external world through our own abilities to control and manipulate their sensory-motor experiences. It is crucial to realize that in addition to changing overt behavior via extrinsic performance factors, therapists can play a critical role in influencing intrinsic performance factors via cognitive intervention strategies.

Learning With and Without Mediators

Teachers and/or therapists, while capable of facilitating learning in many situations, are not essential for learning. You would quickly learn not to eat a certain new food, if eating that food subsequently made you sick (rapid aversive conditioning), even without the intervention of an instructor. Stroke patients might learn to use their unaffected arm to perform tasks that previously required the opposite paralyzed limb. Teachers or therapists can, of course, be helpful in facilitating learning by ensuring that the required stimulation occurs and that the learner is capable of responding. They must also ensure that the learner has the knowledge of how and when to use responses as they are learned.

Whenever formal instruction and supervised practice are provided by a teacher, therapist, parent, or other mediator, it may be said that the learning process involves education.

In fact, it is this dimension of formal and overt structuring of learning experiences by a mediator that distinguishes education from the general learning process. Consistency and adherence to fundamental learning principles during educational activities will induce desired changes in behavior and ensure teaching success.

Therapists must select and direct the experiences (i.e., the environmental stimulation) of their clients in ways that will change behaviors from maladaptive to adaptive. This is the educational component of therapy. Therapists must also motivate and educate patients to learn for themselves (i.e., learn to learn) if therapeutic activities are to be maximally effective.

If therapists could better analyze the sensations and motor responses associated with particular behaviors and determine the patterns of neural activity associated with such performance, it is plausible that they might be able to better modify the patterns of neural activity of a patient's nervous system. If therapists could better understand the biological predispositions of human performance in a developmental context, the selection of activities and reinforcers for those activities could be improved. If therapists were more aware of how individual patients represent knowledge concerning occupational tasks and skills and were cognizant of the role of attention and symbolic processing (language) in occupational performance, then the likelihood of successful habilitation or rehabilitation would be greatly increased.

Natural Learning

Learning that occurs without formal structuring (i.e., outside of educational processes) is considered *natural learning*. Humans are biologically prepared to learn basic perceptual and motor skills in this manner. No one has to *teach* the typical child how to smile, lift their head, sit upright, walk, or manipulate objects with the hand. It is only when there is pathology of either the CNS and learning mechanisms or of the biomechanical system, that a child may need specific intervention to learn such skills.

Most natural learning is behavioral. As the child repeatedly experiences a multitude of low level sensations, there is gradual habituation and lack of response to objects which pose no threat. On the other hand, when sudden intense stimulation occurs, the child is sensitized and all other responses are enhanced during this arousal period. Such a protective and defensive mechanism serves to mobilize the body and to focus attention on potentially threatening stimulus sources. Classical conditioning allows us to bring a number of visceral responses under voluntary control. For example, toilet training is enhanced by the predictive association of sensations of bowel fullness with defecation, thus permitting a voluntary effort to override the gastro-colic reflex. Operant conditioning principles account for almost all trial-and-error learning in humans. This is in fact a predominant mode of skill acquisition with respect to perceptual and motor learning (Cross, 1967).

Natural learning of this type may also serve the acquisition of attitudes and affective responses. The child who enjoys being cuddled by a parent will experiment with hugging and kissing others. When these behaviors are rewarded and encouraged, the child learns to demonstrate affection for others through such acts. Negative behaviors can also be learned in this manner. The shy teenage girl who accepts an invitation for a date, and then is embarrassed or teased about her own lack of social graces, will be negatively reinforced and will learn to avoid dating to minimize the risks of having such unpleasant feelings. The avoidance of the visceral sensations and terrible feelings serve as negative reinforcers of dating behavior. Initially this behavioral learning leads to a decreased frequency of action (dating), but natural cognitive learning sustains the avoidance. Cognitively, the teenager accommodates her scheme of self and begins to label herself as "inept," "awkward," or "undesirable." Once such an alteration in self-definition occurs, the problems are no longer amenable to behavioral modification alone.

For occupational therapists, there are two important points concerning natural learning which must be understood:

1. *Each therapist needs to learn how to decide whether their patients require a mediator's efforts to learn specific skills, tasks, and/or occupational behaviors.* Many patient behaviors acquired prior to needing therapy have been learned without mediators, and it is not certain that during therapy such learning will always be enhanced by the efforts of a mediator. For any specific patient the question of whether or not a mediator is needed for therapeutic changes to take place is a serious issue. This will be addressed in detail later in this chapter.

2. *When direct mediation is not needed for a specific learning goal, therapists may still play an important role as facilitators by helping patients to learn how to learn.* The teaching of cognitively-based strategies may be one of the most overlooked options for occupational therapy intervention in all areas, including physical disabilities, geriatrics and psychiatry.

Learning to Learn and Executive Control of Learning

The cognitive view of learning with its emphasis on the representations of experiences in the mind of the learner has focused considerable attention in recent years on the learner as an active participant in the teaching-learning process.

What a person remembers from prior experiences, what that person thinks about during learning, and the nature of active self-talk and cognitive processing by the learner have become important educational research issues (Anderson, Spiro and Montague, 1977; Weinstein and Underwood, 1985; Schuell, 1986).

Techniques which learners may be taught to use during learning experiences are termed learning strategies. These are defined as, " . . . behaviors and thoughts that a learner engages in during learning that are intended to influence the learner's encoding process" (Weinstein & Mayer, 1986). Learning strategies can influence successful acquisition of performance skills by teaching techniques that help the learner: (1) to use self-motivation and reinforcement to sustain interest in what is being learned, (2) to focus attention and concentrate on relevant and important information and ignore irrelevant and/or distracting information, (3) to acquire, organize, and interpret new information, (4) to enhance memory, including both retention and recall of information learned, and (5) to exercise *executive control* or use rational principles and problem-solving to make their own decisions about what to do to help themselves learn.

The cognitive approach to learning has effected a shift in how we think about the teaching-learning process. When we think of the individual and how information is encoded, organized, stored, and retrieved, it is clear that there is tremendous information processing potential available to each learner to use during skill and knowledge acquisition. The behaviorist tendency was to view environmental or extrinsic stimulation as the sole determinant of learning. The more modern and better substantiated position is that the learner actively processes and interprets information from extrinsic sources using intrinsic knowledge and strategies for organization and interpretation.

Learning strategies provide a powerful means of influencing learning abilities without depending on mediators/teachers. Teaching strategies, on the other hand, describe the ways in which individuals other than the learner may facilitate learning. These are also important in therapeutic intervention and must be considered.

Mediated Learning

When learning experiences are formally organized and feedback concerning performance is provided to the learner, the experience is termed *mediated learning*. Mediation always requires that some person other than the learner determine, in whole or in part, the nature of the learning materials, the learning activities, and the criterial tasks (i.e., evaluation methods) to be used with a given learner in a given situation (Bransford, 1979). Interestingly, this definition does not require direct human intervention during learning. Computer-assisted instruction, programmed texts with self-assessment workbooks, and interactive video are all forms of mediated learning in which a teacher/therapist need not be present. In such cases, it is assumed that the mediator such as the author(s) of the courseware have developed and tested the materials to ensure that structure, content, and feedback will be valid for all potential users.

The most common form of mediator is a person who acts as teacher to the learner. While this person may be a classroom teacher, a therapist, a parent, or any other person who instructs, there are common functions and behaviors shared by all mediators. (1) They transmit not only knowledge and/or skills, but are also responsible for motivating the learner to participate in learning activities. (2) They provide direction to the learner regarding what to do with which materials. (3) They detect and analyze systematic errors which the learner makes and help eliminate such errors by way of a variety of strategies. (4) They monitor the progress of the learner towards a goal(s) and give accurate assessments of that progress.

Mediation and Motivation. Therapists and other mediators can influence the amount of time, effort, and emotional investment which a patient or other learner makes when trying to acquire new knowledge and skills. Both behavioral and cognitive approaches can be effective in fulfilling this role. Behavioral approaches are especially effective in increasing the frequency and intensity of practice. Operant principles may be employed to maximize response rates through the use of rewards, punishments, and negative reinforcers such as avoidance of failure and/or pain. Sensitization may be used to focus attention on strong stimuli and enhance the ability of the learner to respond. Habituation may be used to teach patients to ignore trivial or irrelevant stimuli that act as distractors from the task at hand. Common to all such behavioral methods is the requirement that the therapist must actively control and structure the sensory experiences of the learner. For this reason, it is almost always necessary to use a clinic setting for therapeutic learning. The patient's home is too likely to present stimuli which cannot be controlled by the therapist or perhaps even by the patient. This means that the learning which is most capable of being motivated is not ideally occurring in the natural context to which it must later generalize. It is for this reason that cognitive approaches to motivation need also be considered. The therapist who wishes a patient to persist at a task, must minimize distractions. Cognitive theories of attention suggest that there is a limited amount of information processing capacity available to a person at any particular point in time.

Mediation and Structured Learning. Therapists or other mediators can enhance the success of learners by presenting materials and learning activities that have been proven effective in similar situations with persons of similar abilities and/or disabilities. For example, research has shown that young children are better able to use lighter and shorter tools accurately before gaining skill with longer and heavier tools (Schwartz and Reilly, 1981). An untrained parent or disabled child who attempts self-feeding with standard adult utensils can be expected to have many more failure experiences and to learn self-feeding more slowly than would be the case if special smaller utensils are used in therapy.

The organization of learning activities is also a responsibility of the therapist. Decisions such as whether to mass practice sessions with many repetitions or trials in a short period of time or whether to distribute practice such that trials are widely spaced over a long period of time, have a tremendous influence over the rate of learning and degree of retention (Cross, 1967). Even decisions of whether to give written or oral instructions to patients may affect learning. In each of these examples, the expertise of the mediator transcends the content of the learning and takes into account how, when, and where learning can best be fostered.

Mediation and Feedback. It is well established that the nature and extent of feedback which occurs during learning may influence how much is learned and retained. Two types of feedback which are especially important in occupational therapy are *ongoing feedback* and *after-the-fact feedback*. Ongoing feedback is that which occurs during learning and permits the learner to alter responses rapidly. After-the-fact feedback (sometimes called knowledge of results or KR) usually occurs only at the completion of a learning activity.

Both types of feedback depend on the ability of the learner to assess the degree to which a learning or performance goal is being accomplished and the nature and extent of errors in thought and/or behavior that account for deviations from the goal. Both types of feedback are important in natural learning as well as mediated learning. During natural learning, it is often the case that the individual knows that a goal is not yet being met, but is unable to identify specific errors or suggest specific remediations. This is the information which a trained mediator can provide to a learner that the learner might never appreciate if left unaided.

Occupational therapists play a critical role in recognizing, analyzing, and remedying these specific problems in habilitation, rehabilitation, or prevention of disability, particularly for those with impaired perception and/or judgment that makes it impossible for them to even recognize their own problems. For such patients it is essential to have a therapist provide performance feedback, since change is otherwise impossible.

Mediation and Monitoring of Progress. One of the most important roles of any mediator is to be able to organize and structure learning into a series of subgoals and sequenced activities designed to accomplish some larger goal. In order to do this effectively, the therapist needs to be able to establish an operational definition of the goal so that progress towards that goal can be measured. The selection of evaluation activities (*criterial tasks*) must be appropriate to the learning that is desired. Failure to recognize the importance of selecting the appropriate criterial task may lead a therapist to an inaccurate assessment of a patient's response to therapy. For example, it would be unwise to evaluate arthritic patients by asking them to verbalize what they have learned regarding training in joint protection and energy conservation techniques. The patient might understand fully and be able to verbalize their understanding of the training and techniques, but they may never change behavior or use it in any practical application. A more appropriate criterial task would be to either simulate ADL activities and observe the patient's performance or preferably to observe the patient at home doing actual tasks of daily living.

LEARNING PRINCIPLES AND CLINICAL STRATEGIES

The remainder of this chapter is devoted to exploring the application of both behavioral and cognitive learning principles to occupational therapy. A simple, but useful typology of intervention options is shown in Tables 24-5 and 24-6. It is possible and sometimes even desirable to use more than one of the four basic approaches of natural behavioral, natural cognitive, mediated behavioral, and mediated cognitive.

There are two types of decisions which need to be made concerning learning for any given patient and for any specific therapy goal: (1) Whether to use a behavioral approach, a cognitive approach, or some combination of behavioral and cognitive approaches, and (2) to decide if some form of mediated learning would be beneficial or if natural learning would be a more effective means of reaching the goal.

It would be unrealistic to attempt to include detailed practical guidelines for choosing among these options within this chapter. What follows describes some general principles that are useful in making such decisions and provides some illustrative examples of how such decisions may influence patient outcomes.

As a rule behavioral approaches are quite effective when dealing with the following kinds of individuals or situations:

1. *individuals whose cognitive abilities have been compromised or limited by disease, trauma or birth defects.* Severe mental retardation, head trauma, encephalopathies, and psychoses severely restrict symbolic processing abilities. In such cases where the formation of mental representations of events, such as schemata, is not possible or is severely limited, appropriate functional responses may be developed using controlling stimuli.

2. *individuals who are institutionalized and spend virtually all of their time in the same environment.* When there are few changes in extrinsic (environmental) performance factors, features of the environment may be used to predictably guide behavior. In such settings, it is possible to achieve a consistency of stimulation and reinforcement that is difficult to achieve in most outpatient or even home settings.

3. *individuals who need to learn specific perceptual-motor skills to enhance performance, such as eye-hand coordination, manual dexterity, or the use of tools, orthotics, or adaptive equipment.* When a task may be so highly structured and a goal so explicitly operationalized that a patient may not only monitor and correct errors but also monitor progress towards the goal(s) of therapy, then instrumental conditioning may be an ideal means of improving performance skills. If the individual does this without the assistance of a therapist, it is natural learning. If a therapist, computer program, or biofeedback device is used, it is mediated learning.

4. *individuals with normal attention span and normal memory abilities.* Where such skills are lacking, there is usually a need to employ cognitive learning approaches since an inability to attend to relevant task stimuli or to remember what is learned would otherwise render learning ineffective in the long run.

5. *individuals who are highly self-motivated to achieve operationally defined goals,* and

6. *in situations in which responses are invariant and little or no judgment is needed in determining what to do.* This includes tasks such as bringing a spoon to one's mouth or even most assembly tasks that are routine and require much repetition and only minimal judgment. On the other hand, if one were expected to inspect items as they came off of an assembly line, behavioral training alone would not suffice since a number of critical judgments would be required.

Cognitive approaches are especially effective in the following situations:

1. *when the individual must learn to solve a wide variety of problems as they arise.* In such situations, one must construct a schema of possible problem configurations and then utilize rules and logical processes to determine which would have the greatest likelihood of success.

2. *when the goal is to improve interactions and relationships with other persons.* Successful relationships depend on following accepted conversational conventions and the use of words in contexts and with meanings that can be readily understood by others.

3. *when there is impairment of attention span, memory, or other cognitive abilities that may affect performance of a wide array of tasks.* When memory and/or attention is deficient, but the individual still possesses basic representational schemes, it is possible to develop memory enhancement skills via taking notes and rehearsal of learned materials and to improve attention via cognitive strategies such as elaboration, and self-talk.

4. *when verbal mediation of behavior is essential to the performance of tasks* (i.e., operating a cash register or being a tour guide), and

5. *whenever the skills being learned need to be generalized to situations remote from those in which training occurs.* In such cases, the ability to identify and state abstract principles to guide action and the ability to apply such abstract principles to everyday activities may require cognitive approaches to learning.

Behavioral Approaches and Strategies

Common to all behavioral approaches, whether natural or mediated learning, is the notion of sensory/perceptual control. Because it is the pattern of stimuli that establishes the contingent associations essential to behavioral learning,

---

Table 24-5
Behavioral Learning Approaches

Natural Learning	Mediated Learning
Chaining of reflexes	Shaping techniques
Exploratory play	Behavior modification
Recalibration of body scheme	Computer assisted instruction
Conditioned aversions (phobias)	Biofeedback
Verbal-emotional associations	Rewarding to increase desirable behaviors
Habituation of familiar stimuli	Negative reinforcement or punishment to suppress undesirable behaviors
Sensitization to threatening stimuli	

the role of therapist is most often that of eliminating extraneous or distracting stimuli and organizing and controlling useful stimuli in appropriate doses at appropriate times. Environmental and temporal control are often described in occupational therapy research and texts, but rarely in the context of how this affects learning.

Control of Environmental and Temporal Conditions of Therapy

None of us would take a hyperactive child to Disneyland for a therapy session! We recognize that there would be too much to distract the child, or would overstimulate and arouse the child. Most of us would feel most comfortable treating this patient in a clinic setting in which we could take the patient to a small quiet room, free of clutter and distraction. While doing the proper thing for this child, it is actually learning theory that supports our rationale. In learning theory terms, Disneyland has a high sensitization potential. There are many strong and sudden, even potentially threatening stimuli. Such stimuli tend to enhance responsiveness to all stimuli rather than selective responses to specific stimuli. The ability to restrict stimulation to only those sensory experiences essential to learning will increase the rate and extent of learning.

In instrumental conditioning, it is important to control all reinforcers, both rewards and negative reinforcers, if one is to shape the behavior of another person. It would be ineffective for a therapist to praise a quadriplegic patient only when a sliding board transfer is safely and independently performed, if family members are offering praise when the patient waits for someone else to assist the transfer. Such inconsistent reinforcement of mutually exclusive behaviors would cause neither response to become firmly established. In fact this would be teaching the patient to learn to discriminate who is watching and then do what that particular person will reward. This situation would be most unfortunate for the patient whose goal in therapy is to achieve independence.

In many forms of neuromotor impairment, extraneous stimuli such as noise, cold, vibration, or other physical condition may serve to reflexively activate abnormal muscular responses such as spasticity, clonus, or tremor. Unless these stimuli can be controlled, there is the possibility that there will be classically conditioned associations of other neutral stimuli with these reflexes. Such conditioning would lead to inappropriate responses and the inability to inhibit undesirable movements.

Temporal control or timing of stimulation is as important as environmental control. For example, it would be ineffective for a severely depressed patient to express genuine and appropriate feelings and then have to wait until the next session with the psychiatrist or psychologist to be

Table 24-6 Cognitive Learning Approaches	
Natural Learning	**Mediated Learning**
Formation of perceptual-motor schemata	Teaching of learning strategies such as self-talk, elaboration, rehearsal, comprehension monitoring
Classification by quality, size, etc.	
Object permanence	Imagery techniques
Chunking of items in memory	Transfer appropriate processing
	Cognitive psychotherapies
	Conversational analysis and training

reinforced and rewarded. With so much time between reinforcement, the patient would miss the chance to increase the likelihood of other similar communications in the future.

Behavioral Suppression Strategies: Habituation and Extinction

Habituation is the decreased response caused by repeated stimulation. If you are working with a patient and another therapist begins a conversation nearby, you will glance that way to see what is going on. As the conversation continues, you will begin to forget or ignore those sounds which were initially a distraction and focus solely on your patient. This decrease in your glancing and listening (response) after repeated stimulation is *habituation*. In fact, if the same process occurs the next day, you will again show an initial orientation response to the distracting stimuli, but habituation will be rapid. The period of rest from one day to the next is all that is required to restore your initial sensitivity.

These examples of habituation appear to be both simple and direct, but there are also more complex functions of habituation, such as the role habituation may play in the neonatal and early cognitive development of the child (Jeffrey, 1968). The newborn child appears to orient toward and attend to virtually every stimulus in the environment. Because almost all stimuli are novel to the newborn and because most responses are initially reflexive, the infant appears to be driven by motor and perceptual responses to immediate surroundings. This does not mean that the infant is purely a stimulus-response organism whose behavior is wholly the result of environmental stimuli. As the newborn actively explores the environment, many novel stimuli will be encountered, some of which will have greater attraction and/or meaning for the infant than will others. Of course, even the newborn cannot attend to every stimulus. Certain more salient or powerful stimuli command attention, and other less salient cues are ignored. As those perceptual features of the environment that are initially most important (e.g., mother's face, odor, body heat) are gradually habituated, other cues that were initially less relevant (toys, mobiles, etc.) may become powerful in commanding orientation and exploratory responses. In this manner, habituation serves to establish a hierarchy of attending responses that structure the sequence of perceptual learning. This serial habituation allows the infant to respond progressively to more subtle and complex features of the environment. Presumably, habituation enables the individual to focus and attend to relevant cues long enough to respond with behaviors that maximize knowledge about the sources of these stimuli. Once these stimuli are familiar and demand no further exploratory responses (i.e., such responses have habituated), then other stimuli provoke exploration and attention.

A comparison between the behaviors of a two-year-old child and a 15-year-old will demonstrate the role habituation plays in development. If you give each child a large cardboard box without saying anything to them and observe their behavior, it is likely that the 15-year-old will look at the box, pick it up, look inside, and soon put it down. But for the two-year-old, the sequence of behavior will be highly variable and might include climbing onto or into the box, pulling and pushing it, banging on it, and perhaps tasting it. Because the 15-year-old has seen many other boxes like this one and has habituated effectively to the stimulus offered, the box does not really excite or motivate exploration. For the 2-year-old, this box may engage attention and behavior for a considerable period of time.

It does not seem unreasonable to suppose that childhood toys engage and fascinate because they teach the child about unfamiliar features of the physical and symbolic world. Likewise, the same toys, familiar to an adult, would offer little that had not been repeatedly habituated. Developmentally, serial habituation keeps us exploring and manipulating objects until they are thoroughly familiar in most, if not all, respects. It also permits new objects, persons, and places to command attention so that they too may be explored. In complex series, these events contribute to the formation of stores of information about the world that are increasingly complex and diversified.

For patients with head injuries or other brain damage, habituation offers a means to develop attention. Lack of cognitive mental abilities precludes cognitive approaches to developing attention for such patients. Such patients are often easily distracted and have severe attention deficits. By repeatedly presenting distracting stimuli and by avoiding any possible sensitizing stimuli, distraction responses can be extinguished. The selective aspect of attention can then be developed to permit the patient to learn to respond to stimuli related to occupational and/or therapeutic tasks.

In therapeutic applications, habituation has had its greatest impact on the extinguishing of phobic or avoidance behaviors. Such habituation is usually called *desensitization*. Sensitization often initiates phobias and usually sustains them; for example, if an elderly arthritic patient suffers a fall going from the shower to the bath mat and breaks a hip in the process, this creates such a strong sensitization that the patient is fearful of all transfers in therapy because of the association with the serious fall. Habituation or desensitization strategies suggest that frequent and repeated exposure to the stimuli which elicit such fearful conditions (when no real threat exists) will lead to a waning of the fearful responses.

The therapist may begin the desensitization strategies by showing the patient photographs or videos of other patients performing transfers. The next step might be for the therapist and patient to meet in the bathroom where the therapist would demonstrate and discuss safe transfer techniques, and finally the therapist would use a transfer belt and assist the patient to perform. For habituation to be effective stimuli must be repeated frequently. Most therapists spend 1/2 to 2 hours a day with each patient in periods of 1/2 hour to 1 hour. This necessarily leads to massed practice or the intensive grouping of habituation trials. Unfortunately, with long intervals between training sessions, the patient dishabituates and one must start all over again. True habituation would require that the patient spend 10 to 15 minutes at a time for 6 to 10 sessions a day for seven days a week to effect any lasting benefit that would lead to more rapid and complete habituation in later training sessions compared to earlier ones.

What has just been described for the fearful physically disabled person can be applied equally well to patients with phobic behaviors that lead to psychosocial impairment. Claustrophobia, agoraphobia, acrophobia (and related fear of flying), may all be approached effectively with habituation. It must be remembered that the goal is to extinguish the avoidance behaviors and fear behaviors which lead to dysfunction and not to actually teach the patient to perform the frightening act. This common error often leads therapists to attempt instrumental conditioning via shaping to establish the behaviors the patient fears. The problem is not that the patient is incapable of performing the act, but rather they are hampered in performing the act by the avoidance behaviors, such as closing the eyes, wringing the hands, pacing, and other nervous symptoms of phobias. Clearly, understanding the problem is crucial to effective configuration of the treatment approach.

Just as behavioral learning can lead us to naturally avoid certain stimuli, it is possible to use negative reinforcement to extinguish undesirable behaviors of patients in therapy. Certain biofeedback regimens create a contingent relationship between a behavior to be suppressed and a negative reinforcer. For example, to extinguish head drooping for an athetoid cerebral palsy patient, one might present an unpleasant loud tone whenever the head droops. The patient wears a simple headband with a mercury switch which completes a circuit only when the head tilts away from the horizontal. The avoidance of the unpleasant tone (negative reinforcer) may be paired with permitting the patient to listen to music whenever the head is erect (a reward). Not only is the drooping behavior (neck flexion or extension) quickly extinguished, but neck co-contraction is also established.

Behavioral Expression Strategies: Sensitization and Conditioning

Sensitization causes widespread arousal. This is in direct contrast to habituation which increases attentiveness and focus on relevant (nonhabituated) stimuli. Sensitization can be of value in therapy. The following is a case example of such.

Case Study 24-1

The case involved two 7-year-old boys who were learning-disabled and had minimal cerebral dysfunction. They were slightly overweight, physically undeveloped, and quite fearful. Both had been evaluated using the *Southern California Sensory Integration Tests* and found to have deficits of postural and bilateral integration which today might be termed postural-ocular and/or praxic deficits (Ayres, 1980). Both boys were extremely bright and verbal and tended to intellectualize and rationalize their fears concerning their bodies and movement. Most treatment sessions were a challenge as the boys were quite sensitive to failure and afraid to take risks. I was quite patient and proceeded cautiously for months to gain their confidence and to encourage and reinforce risk-taking and exploratory gross motor behavior.

One source of my frustration was that neither child could reciprocally climb stairs. The ''perceptual-motor room'' in the clinic was upstairs and for each session, they had to climb the flight of stairs. This was a time-consuming and obviously frightening experience for them. They accomplished it with a belabored ascent and descent holding on to the bannister with both hands.

After months of sensory integrative therapy, both boys began to make remarkable progress both during treatment and outside. One of the boys could now ride a two-wheeled bike and this quickly generalized to include stair climbing. But the other child still could not reciprocally climb the stairs even though he showed other marked improvements in therapy.

One day as the first child went up the stairs rapidly and reciprocally, the other still clung to the bannister. I became frustrated and raised my voice. This visibly upset him. I demanded that he ascend the stairs without the railing and reciprocally. For once, he did not intellectualize the situation or tell me I hurt his feelings, and without hesitation (and tearful), he climbed the stairs reciprocally without holding the railing. Then he turned around at the top, smiled tearfully, and climbed down reciprocally! Apparently, my anger posed a greater threat than that of falling. My young client was thrilled with himself and he rushed to get his mother and she watched while he ascended and descended the stairs perfectly. My sudden frustration had aroused skills (responses) in his repertoire that were never chained together successfully before that time. Since that experience, I have learned that such sensitization is not fortuitous, and have been known to mobilize other latent responses in clients by raising my voice.

A less dramatic example of sensitization is quick stretch, a facilitation technique of Rood and others (reported in Trombly, 1983; Farber, 1982). By shortening a muscle and then rapidly and moderately forcefully elongating it maximally (ideally just short of the painful range), subsequent responses of the muscle, especially voluntary, tend to be enhanced. Although stretch reflexes undoubtedly play a role in this augmentation, they are insufficient to explain the endurance of beneficial effect beyond the initial period of stimulation.

Voice modulation, especially a sudden and unexpected raising of the voice, is a method of coping with progressive habituation of attention. The telling of jokes and use of humor have similar arousal effect. Because such unexpected stimuli occur in situations where they are not predicted, they sensitize (arouse) responses and dishabituate orienting responses that have been habituated. For example, I have used exercise, such as jumping jacks followed by a joke to help maintain high arousal and alertness during exams for my students or used sensitization procedures to mobilize responses with comatose, stuporous, and traumatic head-injured clients.

Habituation and sensitization are complementary processes in that they strike a balance between focused concentration and generalized awareness. Both are nonassociative learning and both can last weeks, even months in some cases. Unfortunately neither alone is a basis for independent learning due to their impermanence. Only when followed by or used in conjunction with associative paradigms do these intermediate-term learning methods contribute effectively to therapeutic learning.

Classical conditioning. Evans (1980) has reported on the classical conditioning of movements in neonates. The unconditioned response of being picked up by the mother leads to a conditioned response of decreased excitability and inhibition of crying by the infant (via vestibular, tactile, and even olfactory pathways). When the infant's being picked up is paired with the sound of the mother's voice, it can lead to the voice alone becoming an effective calming agent. This illustrates how humans are prepared genetically to benefit from the natural associations of stimuli that exist in the world. Therapists can and should take advantage of such predispositions to learn naturally when working with infants at risk for developmental problems. The guided application of such naturally occurring stimuli may greatly enhance the infant's ability to develop self-regulatory mechanisms for behavioral control.

Classical conditioning can be used in occupational therapy when treating sleep impairment or insomnia that is often associated with many conditions such as back pain, arthritis, depression, and bipolar affective disorders. While it may be debated whether or not falling asleep is a true reflex, it appears that the classical conditioning paradigm holds here. To help patients go to sleep the therapist can instruct the patient or a family member to describe in detail the posture of the patient's body in the bed just before or just as the patient awakens. It is even better to identify the patient's positioning just as they actually fall asleep, but such information is more difficult to obtain. The patient is then instructed to assume this position (a presumed neutral stimulus set) when sleep is desired. The repeated pairings of the body position preceding sleep with the act of falling asleep is assumed to be a conditioning mechanism that the patient has already learned. Unfortunately, because one is losing consciousness just as one falls asleep, the positioning rarely is linked cognitively to induction of sleep. Thus, the patient starts each night experimenting with sleep positions until the appropriate one is once again discovered. This is especially true in chronic pain patients where CNS pathology of the reticular system is not a contributing factor.

Classical conditioning may also be useful to occupational therapists when dealing with bowel and bladder rehabilitation of spinal cord injured patients. Patients may be able to associate the stimuli of sitting on the commode (CS) with the application of a suppository (UCS) that leads to defecation. Eventually, this is further supported by the gastro-colic reflex, in which the bolus formed 15 to 20 minutes following a meal acts as a stimulus (UCS) for elimination, and the patient may be trained to defecate simply by sitting on the commode chair following the morning or evening meal.

Operant Conditioning Strategies. Operant conditioning is viewed as a valuable tool for therapeutic intervention. Individual differences greatly influence operant conditioning because one person may consider something a reward, but others may not. Drive level influences motivation and response to reinforcers along with age, social class, and previous exposure to reinforcers (Munsinger, 1975).

Any task for which we wish to shape or train behavior will have a hierarchy of positive and negative reinforcers. How rewards are selected and in what order makes a difference in outcome. Bitterman (1975) found that rats who initially were reinforced with a highly preferred reward performed significantly less well when less preferred rewards were used than did untrained controls only receiving the less preferred reward. North Americans have recently seen many manifestations of this phenomenon related to salaries during an economic slump with high inflation. Rather than accept their same jobs with reduced pay (a lesser reward), many chose to take their chances on being laid off (greatly reduced rewards) and not compromise salary demands during collective bargaining negotiations. One may think of a weekly or monthly salary as a fixed interval schedule of reinforcement. Presumably, we learn that although not every effort we put forth will be immediately rewarded, there will come a time when rewards will be received (Kupferman, 1985).

Of all the learning paradigms, operant conditioning has been explored most in relation to therapy. Trombly (1966) has described operant training of orthotic control for quadriplegics. Solomonow and associates (1979) have reported that two-point tactile discrimination thresholds can be reduced using operant conditioning resulting in decreased interelectrode distances on augmented or prosthetic sensory displays for the blind. This means patients can be taught finer discriminations for use with electronically controlled assistive devices. Shaperman (1979) has described the use of activity that would produce instrumental results in the early prosthetics training of child amputees. Murphy and Doughty (1977) report that contingent vibratory stimulation can be used with profoundly retarded students to improve control of arm movements. Burnside and associates (1982) have reported that a comparative study of biofeedback and simple exercise therapy shows that although equal levels of skill can be trained with either technique, biofeedback training is highly resistant to extinction, whereas simple exercise therapy is not.

Fiorentini and Berardi (1980) have demonstrated that practice at perceptual discrimination tasks which are rewarded leads to improvement in perceptual task skills. This supports a recent development in occupational therapy in which computer tasks and even commercial video games have been used in the treatment of perceptual-motor deficits. A careful analysis of one set of computer programs designed specifically for this purpose revealed that there was consistent and appropriate reinforcement which took full advantage of operant conditioning as part of the program design (Schwartz, 1987). Lucca and Recchiuti

(1983) have reported data showing that isometric strength training is more effective when biofeedback is used to increase performance feedback than when it is not used. Harris and associates (1974) have remediated postural deficits in children with cerebral palsy by giving them automatic reinforcement for using electronic signals to establish the location of their head and limbs in space. Hunt and associates (1979) have reported on the role of associative learning in habit formation and retention and suggest clinical methods of extinguishing undesirable behaviors. Even this brief sample of the literature related to operant conditioning and therapy demonstrates the expanding awareness of its role in clinical intervention.

Many of the operant techniques are considered to be behavior modification. Norman explains:

> "Behavior modification is an approach for changing behavior based on a preliminary study of the individual. Behavior change is attempted once the individual's learning characteristics and the identification of the optimal learning conditions for the learner have been analyzed. The ability to analyze systematically and to develop behavior-environment relationships also brings a responsibility to the user to understand and master the principles and procedures of behavior modification."

A number of the basic principles of operant learning were discussed earlier and are expanded here. Operant learning is based on a principle that individual differences in learners determine both their motivations and which reinforcers will be effective. Although reinforcement principles are the same for all learners with respect to schedules of reinforcement, it is always necessary for the therapist to know each individual client in order to determine potential positive and negative reinforcers.

Bandura (1969) has observed that the success of many reinforcement schedules can be enhanced whenever therapists share a knowledge of the process with clients:

> "In most real life circumstances the cues which designate probable consequences usually appear as part of a bewildering variety of irrelevant events. One must, therefore, abstract the critical feature common to a variety of situations. Behavior can be brought under the control of abstract stimulus properties, if responses to situations containing the critical element are reinforced, whereas responses to all other stimulus patterns lacking the essential element, go unreinforced. It should be noted here that the controlling function of various social and environmental stimuli is usually established simply by informing people about the conditions of reinforcement that are operative in different situations, rather than by leaving them to discover it for themselves through a tedious process of selective reinforcement. However, the existence of differential consequences is essential to maintain stimulus control produced through instructional means."

When behavioral contingencies cause certain behaviors to lead to predictable consequences, the learner's knowledge of this will lead to a more controlled response. This strongly supports the principal contention of this chapter that the interaction of cognitive and behavioral learning approaches is not impossible or undesirable and that they may mutually support one another in therapeutic learning.

In most, but not all cases, self-evaluation is of greater importance to a learner than the evaluation of a therapist. This may seem to contradict an earlier statement that mediated learning or guided learning may be more effective than "trial and error" approaches. Self-evaluations of specific tasks generally involve a determination after each task repetition of whether or not the task was performed successfully. Such a conscious evaluation of performance after the fact is termed *knowledge of results* (KR) feedback. Lucca and Recchiuti (1983) argue that biofeedback becomes a very special kind of KR in that it allows the learner to assess results, not only at the end of practice, but during practice as well. Reeve and Magill (1981) have shown that too much information in motor tasks may confuse the learner. They found that early in learning, information about the direction of motor errors was helpful to subjects as a form of KR, but that magnitude or distance of the errors was not useful KR information. Wallace and Hagler (1979) wanted to distinguish between final KR and intermediate KR (assessment of success during an activity rather that at the end). They continued to refer to final assessments as KR, but use the term, *knowledge of performance* (KP) for the intermediate assessment results. They compared the relative effectiveness of no feedback, KR, and KR plus KP on the learning and retention of a closed motor skill (shooting baskets). They found that KR plus KP was superior for both rate of learning and retention of learning over simple KR. Knowledge of performance involves a mediator of learning or facilitator since an individual often cannot stop an activity to assess how it is being performed. Knowledge of performance alone is insufficient information to direct learning without KR. Knowledge of results is thus superior to KP (i.e., self-assessment is superior to assessment by others), but KR plus KP leads to maximal learning and retention. This combination of KR and KP is the situation that prevails in therapy, hence leading us to the conclusion that such guided learning is superior to trial-and-error learning.

It is the role of the therapist to provide knowledge of performance feedback to clients in order to teach clients the response contingencies in operant conditioning and to allow clients to perform their own assessment of KR. Regardless of the type of learning, the therapist must analyze and prescribe a structure of intervention as well as methods or activities.

COGNITIVE APPROACHES AND STRATEGIES

Most therapists greatly underestimate the role of cognitive processes in everyday performance. We take for granted the tremendous amount of factual (declarative) knowledge and procedural knowledge which supports and guides even our simple actions. If we examine a simple "motor" act such as learning to use a hammer to nail two boards together, we can appreciate that most occupational skill development has both psychomotor and cognitive learning components. How does a skilled carpenter learn how hard or how fast to hit each nail? There are certainly cognitive rules which assist in this process. Often in the training of patients, we pay so much attention to the physical abilities and limitations of patients that we fail to assess to what degree cognitive abilities and skills may be used to compensate for lost physical function. This is especially true in *rehabilitation* as opposed to *habilitation*. The most ignored truth about individuals who have physical and/or perceptual impairments which severely compromise their functioning is that such persons will retain all of their cognitive abilities unless there is brain damage.

Attention Management Strategies

Attention is a set of processes in which a fluid or variable amount of available capacity must be allocated as a function of arousal to the particular set of activities present at a given time, to a person's enduring dispositions, and to a person's momentary intentions (Kahneman, 1973). In this conceptualization, attention is considered to be a limited resource. Determining the particular tasks or activities to which one will allocate some amount of attention is a function of the selective aspect of attention. The selective nature of attention helps explain why a person will process certain information present at any given time and ignore other information that is also readily available.

Any parent who has tried to get their child's attention to give them an instruction or request is familiar with this feature of attention. The child will often continue to play with a toy, a friend, or watch television even as the parent is talking. The momentary intentions of the child to enjoy the task at hand coupled with an enduring disposition to attend to the novelty of these activities leads the child to tune out the parent and selectively focus attention on the current task. Fortunately, most children also have an enduring disposition to attend to strong stimuli, such as the strong threats or the flailing arms and pacing back and forth of the irritated parent! As the child recognizes these particular patterns of environmental information, attention is shifted selectively to the parent, and a new set of tasks or activities can be presented for processing by the child.

The determination of what degree of conscious effort will be devoted to any particular task or activity is a function of the intensive aspect of attention. Tasks which are unfamiliar to a person demand a much greater allocation of one's total available capacity of attention (or mental energy) than those which are highly familiar. The degree to which a task or activity makes demands on one's total processing energies is the measure of the intensive aspect of attention. For example, when we read a story that we have read over and over to a child we assume that the spelling, punctuation, tense, and other formal/structural features of the text are accurate and appropriate and we attend only minimally to the story. Other stimuli, such as household noises, our recall of the events of the day, and the condition of the child's room may share our attention, and yet we easily can be successful in our reading task with only this minimal allowance of total available attention capacity. On the other hand, when one is proofreading a colleague's journal article on a new theory, one may lack familiarity with the format, the terminology, and the proposed relationships among constructs. In addition to this, there may be grammatical, spelling, and stylistic errors. Such a task requires an intensive allocation of attention resources. Even the slightest distraction will be highly irritating since the only available mental energy to attend, even briefly, to such distractions must come at the expense of our primary task at hand. In fact, our irritation with such minor interruptions is due to the fact that we perceive that it will not be possible to be successful at reading such text, unless we can fully allocate all attention to that task and that task alone.

As a learner is able to construct and elaborate upon a schemata, there is an increase in familiarity with that particular schemata and its elements. If one thinks of current or working knowledge as the content of schemata, then as a schemata is more richly and fully developed by prior experiences and learning, less attention is required. Novel material that fits an existing schema and simply represents an elaboration or extension of existing elements requires considerably less attention and mental effort than novel information that requires accommodation of existing schemata. Rather than simply fitting new information into existing mental structures, accommodation requires that we postulate and test a redesigned scheme to determine if it is equally appropriate to both prior knowledge and to the new information being processed.

When working with patients who have attention deficits, it is first important to determine if the problem affects the selective aspect of attention, the intensive aspect of attention, or both aspects. A learning disabled child may be hyperactive and distractible, yet have no deficit which affects intensive attention. To remedy this situation one would seek to free the environment from distracting stimuli, and at the same time to add novelty to activities requiring only assimilative processing (not accommodation). At the other extreme might be the patient with a closed head injury who is not particularly distractible, but who mentally fatigues very rapidly and cannot persist at tasks for very long periods. For this patient, tasks should be designed to allow the patient to alternate between activities rather than force the patient to sustain attention that is not available. This strategy is known as time sharing and allows for brief allocation of attention to one task after another over and over again, so that the patient will actually spend more total time on any given task as part of a group of activities than would be spent on any one task presented by itself.

Criterial Task Strategies. In the early 1970s, Craik and Lockhart (1972) proposed a concept known as "levels of processing" that postulated that inputs which were processed at deeper semantic levels would lead to better memory than would inputs that were processed at less semantic and more superficial levels of analysis. Morris, Bransford, and Franks (1977) conducted a series of experiments in which identical word lists were learned either in a sentence context (deeper semantic processing of meaning) or in a rhyming context (more superficial processing). Like Craik and Lockhart, they found that when tested for recognition with a list of the original target words and foils, deeper processing led to better recall. However, they also used a second experiment in which subjects were asked to determine whether or not words rhymed with the target words. Surprisingly, the more superficial processing was now associated with better recall.

To explain this observation, they postulated that it was the nature of the criterial task used to assess the learning rather than the levels of processing that determined whether deeper or more superficial processing led to better memory. They called this concept, **transfer appropriate processing** to emphasize that the type of processing used while learning determines the type of criterial task which will best elicit the information learned. Historically and theoretically this has led to a deemphasizing of the depth of processing model and to an exploration of the relationship of processing type to criterial task type.

One important area of application of these concepts to occupational therapy is that of patient education. Therapists teach energy conservation, work simplification, and joint protection techniques to arthritic clients. If patients are not trained and evaluated in their own homes or in simulated home environments, they quickly learn that the real criteria for success is being able to remember and articulate the biomechanical principles being taught, not to perform the tasks safely and appropriately. The patient's perception of the criterial task is the primary determinant of what will be learned. This has been quite apparent in work rehabilitation

in which the only techniques that have proven effective in returning workers to the job are those based on work-hardening or the actual performance of tasks for sustained periods of time by those undergoing rehabilitation. Even in psychosocial rehabilitation in which the criterial tasks of assessment do not directly and clearly predict how the patient will perform in actual life situations, patients learn to perform well in those areas they feel are directly related to evaluation.

Certain types of interventions, such as industrial accident and injury prevention programs, are a good example of how criterial task approaches may be used to improve patient learning. Traditional "back schools" have been used as both primary and tertiary prevention measures. Most primary programs work with small groups of 10 to 20 workers in one or two short sessions. Lectures, demonstrations, films, slides, models, and group practice in exercises and proper body mechanics are employed during the training sessions. Participants are usually trained in a classroom environment, taking notes as they are instructed and referring to manuals provided during the session. Tertiary prevention programs, often called *re-education programs,* are offered to those already having suffered back impairment of some kind. These differ from primary programs mainly in that they are often conducted either one-on-one or in small groups at a therapy or rehabilitation facility and emphasize the precautions related to each participant's particular injuries or condition.

The successes of such training programs in comparison with no intervention has been documented in most studies of "back school"(Schwartz, 1989). What is not obvious to those who have designed such programs are the intrinsic educational flaws in the rationale and methodology of these programs. For example, it might appear that the primary goal of such educational programs would be to teach proper methods of lifting, carrying, pushing, and pulling. Such a goal is totally unrealistic for at least the following reasons:

1. Most workers have established habits and patterns for performing work activities. Such habits cannot be altered easily simply by creating a new cognitive structure or scheme which describes the steps of safe lifting and material handling. What is needed is to strongly sensitize workers to the risks that they subject themselves to by not following safe and prudent body mechanics.

2. There is little reason to believe that knowing the ideal methods for performing tasks will guide workers towards making the proper decisions as to how to perform in most real life situations. Most importantly there is little reason to expect significant transfer of training or generalization of what is learned in back school to the actual work station. Classroom training

has very little relation to most hazardous work activities. While simulation activities might be of some benefit, workers should be trained in body mechanics by performing activities in the actual environments and under the actual work conditions in which they will be expected to use such learning.

3. The purpose of training should not be primarily to teach methods of performing, but rather to teach the worker how to employ general rules or principles of body use under less than ideal circumstances. In educational terms, this means teaching the worker cognitive skills to help plan and decide when to use the knowledge they have acquired. The learning can be made relevant to the unique worker and unique circumstances of each job by emphasizing methods of reducing the risk of injury even when circumstances are less than ideal and by training workers to make the best choices, rather than training them to perform ideal actions.

4. Most traditional programs do not have a formal set of evaluation activities (commonly known as criterial tasks) which are used to enhance worker attention to newly learned information and to assess the degree of understanding and retention of new learning. The relationship of cognitive processing type to criterial task is the most critical variable in the training situation. When workers are expected to practice proper body mechanics on the job, it makes little or no sense to have them take paper and pencil tasks to see how much they have learned. The importance of this conceptualization for back pain/back injury prevention was that it suggested that the use of lecture, reading and note-taking would only be justified if performance on paper and pencil tests were going to be used as the criterial tasks for programmatic success. Since this was not the case, the alternative was to recognize that any prevention program that was designed to change the body mechanics of workers should in fact emphasize practice and performance of work skills themselves.

Case Study 24-2

Development of an Accident/Injury Prevention Program: In my experience developing and implementing a comprehensive accident/injury prevention program for a major food distribution center, we decided that the program would consist of a series of small group education sessions conducted by a qualified medical expert and that workers would best learn by doing rather than by watching films or listening to lectures. This required that the program be conducted at the job site wherein each worker was trained at

his/her own work station. In attempting to educate the company management regarding safety measures, I emphasized that effective prevention must be directed at changing three types of contributing factors:

(1) the habits of workers, including poor body mechanics, improper pacing of rest/activity, and performing job responsibilities without thinking about them and carefully planning work actions, (2) the structure of tasks which may impose unnecessary demands for lifting, carrying, twisting, bending, which can often be altered at relatively low cost, sometimes by using special tools or procedures to decrease stresses and strains on the back; and (3) the unavoidable hazards within the physical environment of the work place that can often be reduced or eliminated through rearrangement/redesign of the work space.

The company was advised that there should be rewards to individual partners, whether management or worker, for participation and for making recommended changes in worker habits and the organization of work activities. For management, the benefits to be realized from a comprehensive program included: (1) the reduction of the incidence of reported back injuries, (2) the reduction in total time lost due to back injuries, (3) the reduction in worker's compensation insurance costs, (4) the reduction in employee turnover, and (5) the improvement in employer/employee relations.

For the individual worker, the benefits and rewards were less tangible but nonetheless beneficial, including: (1) the decreased likelihood of future back pain/back injuries, and (2) the decreased possibility of reduction or loss of future income resulting from back problems. Since management received most of the immediate and tangible rewards of a prevention program and not the workers, it was recommended that management consider the instituting of some incentive program (i.e., a behavioral learning strategy) with immediate and tangible rewards in order to motivate employee participation and compliance with the prevention program.

Linguistic and Other Symbolic Approaches. Because occupational therapy has emphasized occupation or the performance of purposive and meaningful occupational roles as important aspects of the profession, therapists have tended to be more aware and better trained in the psychomotor aspects of performance than in the cognitive processes which guide and sustain performance. Nowhere is this more apparent than in the treatment of psychosocial dysfunction. Therapists often minimize verbal interactions with patients, perhaps to avoid encroachment into the "talking therapy" realm of psychiatrists and psychologists. Occupational therapists are in an ideal position to provide cognitive therapies for such patients within the context of occupational performance.

Reviewing options for the treatment of a chronically

Role Playing as a Cognitive Strategy

The depressed or anxious patient who refuses to talk to members of the opposite sex, to date, or to socially interact with others, might be found to make the following statements: "I am no good at this" (probably a true statement), "No one likes me" (illogical and most likely untrue), and "I would just die if I were rejected one more time" (again, an undoubtedly false statement). In this situation, it is clearly the negative and self-defeating beliefs of the patient that lead to activity restrictions and depressive withdrawal.

Role playing in this situation would include someone playing the role of "the potential date" and the patient being asked to approach "the date" and ask him/her to go out for coffee or to a movie. The person playing the role of the date would be cued in advance to accept the invitation if and when the patient had the courage to articulate it, and the therapist would suggest what might be said to break the ice, how to ignore anxious feelings, and how to respond to "the date." At any point that the patient became frightened or frustrated saying, "I *can't* do this," the therapist would calmly countermand this irrationality by noting "You *can* do it, but right now you are frightened and upset and probably don't want to do it." The therapist must repeatedly identify all irrational statements and replace them with valid statements.

Some patients eventually learn what the therapist will say next and will be able to recognize the errors in their own thinking. However, there must also be behavioral learning (instrumental conditioning) to support the attack on inappropriate thinking and verbalization. The patient will be asked to do "homework" or "exercises" designed to test the irrational beliefs. If the person feels that they cannot get a date, they will be encouraged to try until they are successful.

The sad fact of depressive ideation is that it creates self-fulfilling prophesies. The patient who does not try cannot possibly succeed, and in fact, will remain the failure and fulfill that negative self-perception. Therapists might be surprised by the number of patients who can make the distinction between lack of success due to lack of effort and lack of success due to lack of ability.

Some of the most difficult patients to train successfully are those who are mentally subnormal. It is often assumed that complex tasks and sequences are beyond the scope of such patients and that the efforts involved in training are not adequately compensated by the benefits. Gold (1978) questioned this attitude and argued that the approaches to training and the activities of mediators were the impediment to high level skill acquisition. In his approach, the *try-another-way approach*, there are some simple cognitive rules that the trainer must follow. (1) Failures and non-reinforcement of even the simplest training responses are to be avoided at all costs. The patient can do no wrong when he or she is trying to succeed. (2) the patient is encouraged to do something different from the unsuccessful act and to independently determine what this is. This can be encouraged by the trainer always asking the patient, "Can you try another way?" (3) The trainer acts to coach the patient in options to reach the smaller subgoals during total task analysis when the task is broken down into the smallest chunks of procedural and declarative knowledge.

This approach assumes that the major block to skill acquisition is the trainer's inability to find appropriate directions or to give meaningful feedback. Gold suggests that the trainers deal with patient difficulties by asking, "Would some additional or alternative feedback work better?" or "Is there a different way to do the task or some part of the task?" or "Would another method of training work better?" Thus, the interference of cognitive processes (negative self-evaluations) with instrumental conditioning is eliminated by careful consideration of the verbal directions and verbal feedback used in training.

depressed patient is one way to explore the implications of cognitive-verbal approaches versus more traditional interventions. Seligman (1967, 1974) coined the term "learned helplessness" to describe what he believed was a major cause of depression in adults. *Learned helplessness* is the belief that one is without power to alter behavior or the events in one's own life. Many studies have supported the conclusion that repeated exposure to uncontrollable aversive stimuli can establish learned helplessness and the depressive behaviors that accompany those beliefs of helplessness.

The occupational therapist may see patients following episodes of depression, including the child who is abused by irrational parents, the child who repeatedly fails in school due to unrecognized perceptual-motor deficits, or the teenager who is unable to find employment due to lack of adequate education and lack of suitable role models. For such patients, it can be argued that natural (and unfortunately adverse) learning via instrumental conditioning has established the depressive pattern of patient withdrawal and depression, and this may, in fact, be true. This may lead therapists to the erroneous assumption that intervention should seek to reverse this learned helplessness via counter conditioning using a behavioral treatment approach that utilizes a high degree of therapist mediated learning.

The cognitive approach is a viable alternative to such behavioral intervention and has been proven successful. Beck (1976, 1979), Ellis (1984) and others have described the application of verbal/semantic interventions to psychotherapy in general, and Barris, Kielhofner, and Watts (1983) have directly applied the concepts of these cognitive psychotherapists to the practice of occupational therapy. The essential feature of these forms of intervention involves the identification of illogical or irrational beliefs of the patient regarding the self or the environment. Once the therapist identifies such ideas, the goal is to challenge and disprove them and force the patient to eliminate such untrue ideas from their belief schemata and to replace them with more accurate representations of reality (accommodation).

While most therapists would not be comfortable with the patient lying on a couch and engaging in an exclusively cognitive/verbal interaction, there are other alternatives. Role playing is one powerful cognitive technique which permits the direct attack on irrational beliefs of the patient.

Metacognitive Approaches to Learning

Imagery and Self-talk Strategies. The ability of patients to use their mental faculties to plan, rehearse, and evaluate performance without actually performing is a metacognitive skill which may be of great service in the course of occupational therapy interventions. The opportunity to discuss possible negative outcomes of each potential patient performance error and to determine how these can be avoided is a metacognitive approach. Teaching the patient how to think about the activity and how to plan for contingencies increases the likelihood of success.

Imagery techniques, or the imagining of possible difficulties, without actual physical practice is an important adjunct to such metacognitive preparation for performance. It is assumed that once the patient is willing to deal with the problems on the level of abstract imaging, that it is more likely that the patient will overcome fears and attempt to perform under safe and guarded conditions provided by the therapist. Such rehearsal also allows the patient to become very specific about fears related to performance and tells the therapist what specific aspects of action produce the most anxiety and need the most attention.

Conversational Learning. A final metacognitive approach to therapy concerns how patients are instructed and the role of conversation in therapy. Grice (1975), in his *conversational contract* or *cooperative principle*, has described a set of rules for human information exchange:

1. *Quantity*—The speaker should say only as much as the speaker believes the listener needs to hear, and no more!
2. *Quality*—The speaker must only say things which the speaker is confident are true, and the listener must assume that the speaker is telling the truth.
3. *Relation*—The speaker will always say something which is relevant to that which has already been said.
4. *Manner*— The speaker will be clear, concise, organized and to the point.

How many times in therapy are these rules ignored or violated? For example, this basic information exchange contract is violated whenever a therapist gives a family written instructions for a home program without adequate assessment of whether they comprehend the vocabulary and ideas, whenever a therapist uses lengthy discourse with an aphasic or other language-impaired patient, or whenever a therapist talks on and on without adequate opportunity to assess whether the patient has understood and assimilated.

Therapists must remember that regardless of how many stroke patients they have treated in the past, care must be taken to observe these basic rules with each one. We cannot expect patients to absorb too much information too quickly. We must always be direct and honest with patients and guard against our own anxieties that may cause us to offer unrealistic hopes of full recovery. Unless therapists follow these principles, there is little hope for being an effective mediator or therapist.

Learning Styles

Each individual learner acquires not only learning skills and learning strategies, but also learns to have specific preferences concerning the types of information and learning processes which are most comfortable. *Learning style* is the learner's preference regarding optimal conditions of learning.

One dimension of learning styles is that of *data modality* which is the sensory form of information presentation which is most conducive to learning and retention. For some people, visual presentation of information is essential; for others auditory is preferred (i.e., the person who would rather attend a lecture or hear a tape than read a book on a given subject), and still others prefer active kinesthetic/tactile experiences.

Another dimension of learning style is *cognitive processing preferences*. While one learner may prefer reflective and introspective consideration of information, another equally successful learner may tend to be intuitive and impulsive. The reflective, introspective types are often slow to process new information and do not feel comfortable in situations of high complexity. The intuitive, impulsive types tend to make many initial errors but handle information at a much faster rate. In Piagetian terms, the reflective learner accommodates well but assimilates relatively slowly, whereas the impulsive learner assimilates information rapidly but has difficulty with accommodations.

Dunn & Dunn (1978) and Dunn, Dunn & Price (1983) have developed a useful checklist of learning styles in which relevant factors have been grouped into one of four major categories. These are illustrated in Table 24-7.

While there is not an extensive literature to validate that an individual's preferred styles are actually optimal learning styles, the strong suggestion is that therapists should try to assess and accommodate to these learner characteristics whenever possible. Most, if not all, of these factors are potentially under the joint control of the therapist and the patient. There are no formal studies that show the importance of matching training conditions to learning styles of patients. However, from the standpoint of patient comfort and motivation, it should be apparent that the consideration of learning style may greatly enhance the patient's acceptability of therapy. In addition, an awareness of these options gives the therapist a basis for revising training strategies when results are not optimal.

SUMMARY

The issues of learning are complex. Every act may enhance or detract from the patient's learning and achieving the goals of therapy. To attend to the behavioral and cognitive dimensions of intervention is to recognize the essential fact that regardless of technique, diagnosis, or setting, all therapy is learning.

Study Questions

1. Why is a synthesis of behavioral and cognitive learning approaches more useful to occupational therapists than either approach by itself?

2. Why is the distinction between natural and mediated learning experiences an important one to make with reference to occupational therapy interventions?

3. What factors must one consider when planning therapeutic activities to ensure that changes in patient behaviors will be long-lasting?

4. What does one need to know about a patient in order to be effective in assisting the person to learn?

5. Why is learning the most critical consideration for occupational therapists who offer prevention services?

6. Given that learning is of vital importance to therapy outcomes, why do you think that there is so little formal emphasis on learning in occupational therapy treatment planning?

7. Do you believe the essential premise of this chapter—that therapy is learning? Why or why not?

Table 24-7
Checklist of Learning Styles

Environmental Conditions
1. Optimal noise level—from needs quiet to needs sound
2. Optimal lighting—from requires low illumination to requires high illumination
3. Optimal temperature—from needs cool to needs warm environment
4. Organization and structure—from needs highly organized room to needs chaos

Emotional-Motivational States of the Individual
1. From self-motivated to motivated by others to unmotivated
2. From highly persistent towards goals to not persistent towards goals
3. From very responsible to not responsible
4. From needs high task structure and specificity of assignments to needs little structure

Social Preferences of Learner
1. From likes to work alone to likes to work in groups
2. From likes to work with peers to likes to work with super- and/or subordinates
3. From likes to work in variety of settings to prefers single setting

Physical Characteristics and Needs of Learner
1. Sensory data preferences (auditory, visual, kinesthetic, tactile)
2. Prefers food and drink during learning to prefers no food or drink
3. Prefers mobility to prefers sedentary conditions
4. Temporal preferences—learns best in morning, afternoon, evening, night
5. Attention span—prefers short interval learning with breaks to prefers single long session

---

Source: Dunn, R., Dunn, K. & Price, G.E. (1983). Learning Style Inventory, P.O. Box 3271, Lawrence, Kansas.

References

Anderson, R.C., Spiro, R.J. & Montague, W.E. (1977). *Schooling and the acquisition of knowledge.* Hillsdale, NJ: Lawrence Earlbaum Associates.

Ausubel, D.P., Novack, J.D. & Hanesian, H. (1978). *Educational psychology: A cognitive view* (2nd ed.). New York: Holt, Reinhart and Winston.

Ayres, A.J. (1980). *Sensory integration and the child.* Los Angeles: Western Psychological Services.

Bandura, A. (1969). *Principles of behavior modification.* New York: Holt, Reinhart and Winston .

Barris, R., Kielhofner, G. & Watts, J.H. (1983). *Psychosocial occupational therapy: Practice in a pluralistic arena.* Laurel, MD: RAMSCO Publishing Co.

Beck, A.T. (1976). *Cognitive therapy and the emotional disorders.* New York: International Universities Press.

Beck, A.T., Rush, A.J., Shaw, B.F. & Emery, G. (1979). *Cognitive therapy of depression.* New York: Guilford Press.

Bitterman, M.E. (1975). The comparative analysis of learning: Are the laws of learning the same in all animals? *Science, 188*(16), 699-709.

Brady, J.V. (1979). Learning and conditioning. In Pomerleau, O.F. & Brady, J.V. (Eds.). *Behavioral medicine: Theory and practice.* Baltimore: Williams and Wilkins.

Brake, S.C. (1981). Sucking infant rats learn a preference for novel olfactory stimulus paired with milk delivery. *Science, 211,* 506-508.

Bransford, J.D. (1979). *Human cognition.* Belmont, CA: Wadsworth.

Brown, R. (1958). How shall a thing be called. *Psychological Review, 65,* 14-21.

Brunelli, M., Castellucci, V. & Kandel, E.R. (1976). Synaptic facilitation and behavioral sensitization in aplysia. *Science, 194,* 1178-1181.

Bruner, J. & Kennedy, D. (1970). Habituation: Occurance at a neuromuscular junction. *Science, 169,* 92-94.

Burnside, I.G., Tobias, H.S. & Bursill, D. (1982). Electromyographic feedback in the remobilization of stroke patients: A controlled trial. *Archives of Physical Medicine and Rehabiliation, 63,* 217-222.

Craik, F.I.M. & Lockhart, R.S. (1972). Levels of processing: A framework for memory research. *Journal of Verbal Learning and Verbal Behavior, 11,* 671-684.

Cross, K.D. (1967). The role of practice in perceptual-motor learning. *American Journal of Physical Medicine, 46,* 487-510.

Dunn, R. & Dunn, K. (1978). *Teaching students through their individual learning styles: A practical approach.* Reston, VA: Reston Publishing Co.

Dunn, R., Dunn, K. & Price, G.E. (1983). *Learning style inventory.* PO Box 3271, Lawrence, Kansas.

Ellis, A. (1984). Rational-emotive therapy. In Corsini, R.J. (Ed.). *Current psychotherapies* (3rd ed.). Itasca, IL: Peacock Press.

Evans, B. (1980). Learned responses to movement in neonates. *Developmental Psychobiology, 13,* 95-110.

Farber, S.D. (1982). *Neurorehabilitation: A multisensory approach.* Philadelphia: W.B. Saunders.

Fiorentini, A. & Berardi, M. (1980). Perceptual learning specific for orientation and spatial frequency. *Nature, 287,* 43-44.

Gagne, R.M. (1977). *The conditions of learning.* (3rd ed.). New York: Holt, Reinhart & Winston.

Garcia, J., et al. (1983). Taste aversions and the nurture of instinct. In McGaugh, J.L. & Thompson, R.F. (Eds.). *The neurobiology of learning and memory.* New York: Plenum Press.

Gold, M. (1978). *Try another way.* Champagne-Urbana, IL: Marc Gold Associates.

Granit, R. (1977). *The purposive brain.* Cambridge, MA: The MIT Press.

Greenbaum, H. (1979). The learning process in combined psychotherapy. *American Journal of Psychoanalysis, 39*(4), 303-310.

Grice, H.P. (1975). Logic in conversation. In Cole, T. & Morgan, J.L. *Syntax and semantics: Speech acts,* vol. 3. New York: Academic Press.

Harris, F.A., Spelman, F.A., Hymer, J.W. (1974). Electronic sensory aids as treatment for cerebral-palsied children. *Physical Therapy, 54*(4), 354-365.

Hearst, E. (1975). The classical-instrumental distinction: Reflexes, voluntary behavior and the categories of associative learning. In Estes, W.K. (Ed.). *Handbook of learning and cognitive processes, vol. 2, Conditioning and behavior theory.* Hillsdale, NJ: Lawrence Earlbaum Associates.

Hull, C.L. (1943). *Principles of behavior.* New York: Appleton.

Hunt, W.A., Matarazzo, J.D., Weiss, S.M. & Gentry, W.D. (1979). Associative learning, habit and health behavior. *Journal of Behavioral Medicine, 2*(2), 111-124.

Jeffrey, W.E. (1968). The orienting reflex and attention in cognitive development. *Psychological Review, 75,* 320-334.

Johnson, W.A. (1967). Individual performance and self-evaluation in a simulated team. *Organizational Behavior and Human Performance, 2,* 309-328.

Justin, N. (1961). *The phantom tollbooth.* New York. Random House.

Kahneman, D. (1973). *Attention and effort.* Englewood Cliffs, NJ: Prentice Hall.

Kandel, E.R. (1976). *Cellular basis of behavior: An introduction to behavioral neurobiology*. San Francisco: W.H. Freeman and Co.

Kandel, E.R. (1979). *Cellular insights into behavior and learning*. Harvey Lecture Series.

Klausmeier, H.J. (1985). *Educational psychology* (5th ed.). New York: Harper and Row.

Kupferman, I. (1975). Neurophysiology of learning. *Annual Review of Psychology, 26*, 367-391.

Kupferman, I. (1985). Learning. In Kandel, E.R. & Schwartz, J.H. (Eds.). *Principles of neuroscience* (2nd ed.). New York: Elsevier North-Holland.

Kushner, H.S. (1981). *When bad things happen to good people*. New York: Schocken Books.

Logue, A.W. (1979). Taste aversion and the generality of the laws of learning. *Psychological Bulletin, 86*(2), 276-296.

Lucca, J.A. & Recchiuti, S.J. (1983). Effect of electromyographic biofeedback on an isometric strengthening program. *Physical Therapy, 63*(2), 200-203.

Miller, G.A., Galanter, E. & Pribram, K.H. (1959). *Plans and the structure of behavior*. New York: Holt, Reinhart and Winston.

Morris, C.D., Bransford, J.D. & Franks, J.J. (1977) Levels of processing versus transfer appropriate processing. *Journal of Verbal Learning and Verbal Behavior, 16*, 519-533.

Munsinger, H. (1975). *Fundamentals of child development*. New York: Holt, Reinhart and Winston.

Murphy, R.J. & Doughty, N.R. (1977). Establishment of controlled arm movements in profoundly retarded students using response contingent vibratory stimulation. *American Journal of Mental Deficiency, 82*(2), 212-216.

Norman, C.W. (1967). Behavior modification: A perspective. *American Journal of Occupational Therapy, 30*(8), 491-497.

Pavlov, I.P. (1906). The scientific investigation of the psychical faculties of processes in higher animals. *Science, 24*, 613-619.

Petrinovich, L. & Patterson, T.L. (1979). Field studies of habituation. *Journal of Comparative Physiological Psychology, 93*(2), 337-350.

Piaget, J. (1952). *The origins of intelligence in children*. New York: W.W. Norton.

Piaget, J. (1954). *The construction of reality in the child*. New York: Basic Books.

Piaget, J. (1971). *Biology and knowledge*. Chicago: University of Chicago Press.

Reeve, T.G. & Magill, R.A. (1981). The role of the components of knowledge of results information in error correction. *Research Quarterly of Exercise and Sport, 52*(1), 80-85.

Rescorla, R.A. & Solomon, R.L. (1967). Two-process learning theory: Relationships between Pavlovian learning and instrumental learning. *Psychological Review, 74*, 151-182.

Schallert, D.L. (1982). The significance of knowledge: A synthesis of research related to schema theory (pp. 13-48). In Otto, W. & White, S. (Eds.). *Reading expository material*. New York: Academic Press.

Schuell, T.J. (1986). Cognitive conceptions of learning. *Review of Educational Research, 56*, 411-436.

Schwartz, R.K. (1985). *Therapy as learning*. Dubuque: Kendall-Hunt.

Schwartz, R.K. (1987). Evaluation of CAPTAIN Software for use by occupational therapists. *American Journal of Occupational Therapy, 41*(4), 265.

Schwartz, R.K. (1989). Cognition and learning in industrial accident injury prevention: An occupational therapy perspective. *Occupational Therapy in Health Care, 6*(1), 67-85.

Schwartz, R.K. & Reilly, M.A. (1981). Learning tool use: Visual-proprioceptive recalibration and the development of hand skills. *Occupational Therapy Journal of Research, 1*, 13-28.

Seligman, M.E.P. (1974). Depression and learned helplessness. In Freidman, R.J. & Katz, M.M. (Eds.). *The psychology of depression: Contemporary theory and research*. New York: Halsted Press.

Seligman, M.E.P. & Maier, S.F. (1967). Failure to escape traumatic shock. *Journal of Experimental Psychology, 74*, 1-9.

Shaperman, J. (1979). Learning patterns of young children with above-elbow prostheses. *American Journal of Occupational Therapy, 33*(5), 299-305.

Skinner, B.F. (1938). *The behavior of organisms*. New York: Appleton.

Skinner, B.F. (1965). *Science and human behavior*. New York: The Free Press.

Skinner, B.F. (1968). *The technology of teaching*. New York: Appleton.

Solomonow, M., Herskovitz, J.S. & Lyman, J. (1979). Learning in the tactile sense. *Annals of Biomedical Engineering, 7*, 127-13.

Thompson, R.F. & Spencer, W.A. (1966). Habituation: A model phenomenon for the study of neuronal substrates of behavior. *Psychological Review, 73*(1), 16-43.

Thorndike, E.L. (1898). Animal intelligence: An experimental study of the associative processes in animals. *Psychological Review Monograph Supplements*. No. 4, 2.

Thorpe, W.H. (1956). *Learning and instruction in animals*. London: Metheuen.

Tolman, E.C. (1932). *Purposive behavior in animals and men*. New York: Appleton.

Trombly, C.A. (1966). Principles of operant conditioning related to orthotic training of quadriplegic patients. *American Journal of Occupational Therapy, 20*(5), 217-220.

Trombly, C.A. (1983). *Occupational therapy for physical dysfunction* (2nd ed.). Baltimore: Williams and Wilkins.

Wallace, S.A. & Hagler, R.W. (1979). Knowledge of performance and the learning of a closed motor skill. *Research Quarterly, 50*(2), 265-271.

Weinstein, C.E. & Mayer, R.E. (1986). The teaching of learning strategies (pp. 315-327). In Whittrock, M.C. (Ed.). *Handbook of research on teaching.* (3rd ed.). New York: Macmillan.

Weinstein, C.E. & Underwood, V.L. (1985). Learning strategies: The how of learning. In Segal, S., Chipman, J. & Glaser, R. (Eds.). *Thinking and learning skills,* vol. 1. Hillsdale, NJ: Earlbaum.

White, R.R. (1959). Motivation reconsidered: The concept of competence. *Psychological Review, 56*, 297-333.

Woody, C.D. (1982). *Memory, learning and higher function: A cellular view.* New York: Springer-Verlag.

CHAPTER CONTENT OUTLINE

KEY TERMS

Accessibility

Architectural barrier

**American National Standards
  Institute (ANSI)**

Ergonomics

Workspace

ABSTRACT

Changes in the physical environment can greatly improve the level of
occupational performance for persons with disabilities. Change strategies can
include adding, rearranging or modifying environmental elements, or relocating
the client. This chapter examines several approaches for eliminating barriers that
prevent or interfere with the safe and optimal performance of activities and tasks
necessary for life's roles. Applicable standards and regulations for physical
accessibility are identified, and designs which enhance as well as enable
performance within home and work settings are described in detail. The need to
examine each client's situation and unique preferences and abilities before
modifications are made is emphasized.

Modification of the Physical Environment

Karin J. Barnes

"The task that faces us is to design truly responsive environments where all people have opportunities to develop competence. As we have seen, we cannot speak of competence as being a quality that lies exclusively within individual people. Rather, it is a relationship between each of us and the object that we are attempting to manipulate."

—Steinfeld, E., Duncan, J., & Cardell, P., 1977

OBJECTIVES

The information in this chapter is intended to help the reader—

1. become familiar with U.S. legislation and regulations pertaining to the elimination of architectural barriers.

2. identify factors in the physical environment which can interfere with optimal performance.

3. evaluate strategies for eliminating architectural barriers.

4. understand the relationships between occupational therapists and other experts concerned with the elimination of architectural barriers.

5. identify important considerations in adapting the home or work environment for individuals with reaching limitations.

INTRODUCTION

The physical environment influences the extent to which work, self-care, and leisure tasks are performed by all individuals. Unfortunately, customary designs of the physical environment can impede the performance of numerous activities for many individuals. For example, stairs in a restaurant can prevent an older person with depth perception problems from joining friends for a meal. Sling-type swing seats at a playground can prevent a child with neuromuscular disabilities from experiencing the pleasure of swinging. Meal preparation is impossible if the cook who uses a wheelchair does not have access to the refrigerator shelves.

The inability to optimally perform meaningful daily tasks due to conditions in the physical environment may influence an individual's psychosocial and economic well-being. This inability may also cause disruptions in family role delineation and daily routines (Christiansen, Schwartz, & Barnes, 1988; Slater, Sussman, & Stroud, 1970). Difficulty in performing meaningful tasks, and dependency on others for their completion, may lead to depression, diminished self-confidence, and lack of motivation (Aitken, 1982; Malick & Almasy, 1983).

Improvement in physical environmental conditions can improve the performance of daily tasks for individuals with disabilities (Colvin & Korn, 1984; Sandler, Thurman, Meddock, & DuCette, 1985; Steinfield, Schroeder, & Bishop, 1979). Colvin and Korn (1984) described a program in a major city in which **architectural barriers** were removed and environmental control devices were provided in the homes of people with disabilities. Participants in the project stated that the modifications made an improvement in their personal lives and their families' lives and that they felt safer and more independent as a result.

REGULATIONS CONCERNING ACCESSIBILITY TO PHYSICAL ENVIRONMENTS IN THE U.S.

In 1968 the Architectural Barriers Act was passed, making it the first federal legislation in the United States to require certain federal and federally-funded building projects to be readily accessible for individuals with physical disabilities (Federal Register, 1984; U.S. Department of Education, 1987). The federal Rehabilitation Act of 1973 further mandated that any institution receiving federal funds (such as a school) could not discriminate against persons with disabilities because of existing architectural barriers to the institution's facilities (Nugent, 1978). Moreover, the 1973 legislation created the Architectural & Transportation Barriers Compliance Board to enforce the provisions of the Rehabilitation Act. Compliance with the new regulations was inadequate, so in 1978 the Comprehensive Rehabilitation Services Amendment was passed, which increased the powers of the Architectural & Transportation Barriers Compliance Board (Hopf & Raeber, 1984; Ross, 1978). At this time the Architectural & Transportation Barriers Compliance Board was given the responsibility of issuing guidelines for standards of **accessibility** to buildings for persons with physical disabilities (Federal Register, 1984). The Uniform Federal Accessibility Standards were developed to meet these guidelines.

The Uniform Accessibility Standards were developed to be consistent with the standards of the **American National Standards Institute** (ANSI), a private organization (Federal Register, 1984). The ANSI standards are called, *"American National Standard for Buildings and Facilities— Providing Accessibility and Usability for Physically Handicapped People"* (ANSI, 1986). These standards were developed by an ANSI committee comprised of "organizational members representing disability groups, design professionals, rehabilitation specialties and services, building owners and management associations, building product manufacturers, building code developers and administrators, senior citizen organizations, and federal standard setting departments" (ANSI, 1986). The 1986 edition of this document states, "this edition of the standard (ANSI, 1986) reinforces the concept that a standard is basically a resource for design specifications and leaves to the adopting enforcing agency the application criteria such as where, when, and to what extent such specifications will apply" (ANSI, 1986).

Title VIII of the Civil Rights Act of 1968, which prohibited discrimination in the sale, rental, or financing of housing based on race, color, religion, sex, or national origin, was amended with the Fair Housing Amendment Act of 1988. The Fair Housing Amendment Act extended the coverage of Title VIII to prohibit discriminatory housing practices based on familial and disability status (Federal Register, 1988). This act "establishes an administrative enforcement mechanism for cases where discriminatory housing practices cannot be resolved informally, and provides for monetary penalties in cases where housing discrimination is found" (Federal Register, 1988).

ELIMINATION OF ENVIRONMENTAL BARRIERS

An environmental physical barrier is any element within the environment that impedes or prevents the safe and optimal performance of a desired task. This may occur in many sites including public parks, office buildings, schools, and homes. Barriers to access to and mobility within a structure can be created by such factors as stairs, door thresholds, width of a room, and height of a pushbutton. Other factors that may impede optimal function include furniture arrangement, **workspace** height, lighting, and floor surfaces. Problems that may occur as a result of these barriers range from total inaccessibility to an area, to inefficiency and inadequacy in task performance, fatigue, pain, and injury.

The improvement of environmental conditions and the elimination of environmental barriers is an area of interest in several fields. In industry, the study of workplace design in relation to the human worker has evolved into the multidisciplinary field called **ergonomics**. Ergonomics has been defined as "the science of workplace design; the designing and arranging of all architectural elements, furniture, equipment, and ambient factors in a manner compatible with human capabilities and limitations" (Raschko, 1982, p. x). Jobs are analyzed in order to:

"Improve worker productivity by eliminating unnecessary effort and designing tasks within the capabilities of most workers. Reduce opportunities for overexertion injuries. Curtail the development of fatigue over the shift. Utilize workers optimally, thereby increasing job satisfaction and individual fulfillment." (Eastman Kodak, vol. 2, 1986, p. 4).

The elimination of environmental obstructions frequently requires the expertise and planning of consumers, professional groups, and community agencies. Architects, engineers, computer experts, electricians, plumbers, and communication experts are among those involved in working with the occupational therapist to remove environmental barriers and design an optimal work and home environment. The occupational therapist should be familiar with these groups and be aware of the current governmental restrictions and regulations.

Using an understanding of the physical, perceptual, and psychosocial factors that affect occupational performance gives occupational therapists a unique role in eliminating environmental barriers. An awareness of the effects of disease processes on role performance enables appropriate intervention strategies.

DETERMINATION OF PERSONAL ROLE CHOICE

Each individual has a unique set of preferences and abilities which are independent of his/her age group or any medical diagnosis (Figure 25-1). Occupational therapy intervention involves understanding the attributes of the client and the environmental conditions so optimal independence in meaningful tasks can be assured. Intervention should aid the client in achieving active participation in home, work, and community settings.

The occupational therapist evaluates the specific tasks the client wishes to accomplish and the preferred manner of accomplishment before environmental modifications and/or other interventions are considered. This is crucial because intervention strategies developed from preconceived ideas about disability or age groups may result in an unsatisfactory intervention outcome. Additionally, client motivation to learn and maintain a skill is higher when the client, rather than others, determines goals and when he/she has control over the manner in which desired occupations are performed (Burke, 1977; Chiou & Burnett, 1985).

Factors Affecting Choice of Intervention Optics

As noted throughout this text, numerous factors affect the accomplishment of chosen tasks. Client characteristics, family and community situations, economic factors, and the physical conditions of a setting should be evaluated in relation to the improvement of environmental conditions. More detailed information concerning the assessment of the physical environment and personal and social behavior is presented in Chapter 16, Assessing Environmental Factors.

Personal Factors. Characteristics of the individual with a disability should be considered before planning the elimination of environmental barriers. While it is important to know the characteristics of various diagnostic groups, the occupational therapist should not categorize a client into a group as this impersonalized approach could jeopardize treatment results. It is important to plan the environment around the abilities, not the disabilities, of the client.

Physical impairment, including weakness, limb loss, paralysis, incoordination, pain, and orthopedic limitations, should be evaluated. These impairments may lead to difficulty in mobility, prehension, endurance, and balance,

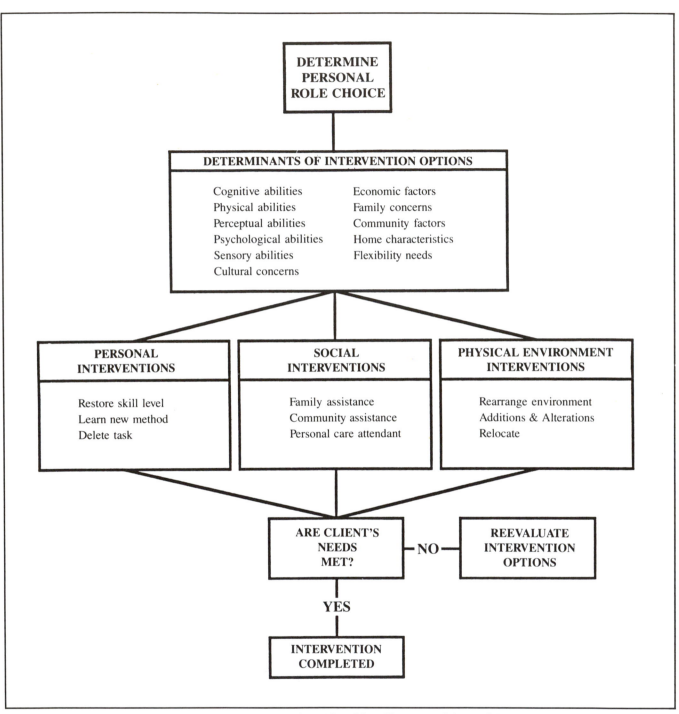

Figure 25-1. Decision-making in Elimination of Environmental Barriers. *Adapted from Christiansen, Schwartz & Barnes, 1988.*

thus impeding function and safety in role performance. The physical dimensions of the individual should also be evaluated. For example, height, width, weight, and arm and leg length are some of the physical characteristics that affect performance in the physical environment (Figures 25-2 through 25-5).

Sensory impairments, including hearing, vision, tactile, and kinesthetic losses and/or distortions, may cause communication and safety problems and jeopardize personal, social, and work role performance. Environmental modifications should be explored that will assist in overcoming these problems.

Perceptual, cognitive and psychosocial problems may be easily overlooked when determining intervention options related to environmental barriers. Yet, these problems contribute significantly to the manner in which an individual performs in the physical environment. For example, an individual with a visual form and space perception deficit may find it very difficult to select cooking utensils from a kitchen drawer in which many utensils of different sizes and shapes have been scattered. Appliances, such as a washing machine, which require several steps before operation may be difficult for those with sequencing problems, such as those found in apraxia or mental retardation.

Preferences in cultural and personal style should be considered in determining intervention because they influence the client's motivation and task choices. The habits, or styles of performance, that develop from these preferences are frequently the most comfortable style for the client and family members. The occupational therapist should be aware of these and provide intervention that allows tasks to be performed in the desired manner. Conversely, if the occupational therapist feels an intervention requiring habit changes may be useful, it should be offered as an alternative that the client may wish to explore.

Social Factors.

Another intervention determinant is the availability of assistance from other individuals. Assistance from others for the partial or total completion of desired tasks may negate the need for environmental modifications. This assistance may be from family, friends, community volunteer agencies, and/or contracted agencies, such as home health agencies, or from a private personal care attendant. Communication between the client, the individual assisting the client, and the occupational therapist, is needed to plan the best intervention strategies. Resources which address the use of health care attendants are available and may be of value to the client and his/her occupational therapist (Crystal, Flemming, Beck, & Smolka, 1987; Friedman, 1986; Fisher, & Gardner, 1987).

Economic Factors.

Economic considerations are very important in planning environmental changes. The cost range involved in modifying the environment is extremely wide. Inexpensive modifications include using small adaptive devices, retraining the client in the desired tasks, and rearranging the environment to minimize barriers. Moderately expensive interventions include additions to the environment such as special telephone receivers for the hearing impaired, hand-held showers, and lower storage shelves. Expensive interventions include major building renovations, computerized environmental control systems, and relocation to another building.

Individuals with disabilities may be able to obtain assistance for the elimination of physical barriers from their home and workplace through state and federal governmental agencies. *The Pocket Guide to Federal Help for Individuals with Disabilities* (1987) published by the U.S. Department of Education describes federal assistance programs available to eligible individuals with disabilities. It provides information concerning housing loans, rental assistance, and tax benefits related to the elimination of home physical barriers.

Physical Environment.

The physical environment is one determinant of the level of independence in occupational performance. The construction and site of a building influences the type of adaptations needed. Other factors include the building's age, the floor design, the type of materials used in construction, and ownership of the

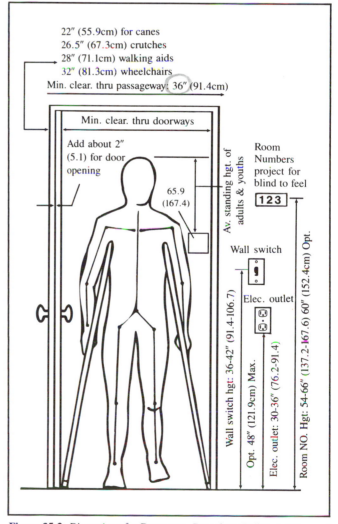

Figure 25-2. Dimensions for Doorways. *Data from Diffrient, Tilley and Bardagjy (1974). Humanscale 1/2/3. Cambridge, MA: MIT Press.*

| | DIMENSIONS | |
	Small Elderly Female	Large Elderly Male
	Inches (Cm)	Inches (Cm)
A. High Reach to Floor	63.0 (160.0)	77.9 (197.9)
B. Average standing height of persons over 65	57.4 (145.8)	71.5 (181.6)
C. Eye to floor distance	53.4 (135.6)	66.9 (169.9)
D. Shoulder to floor	46.4 (117.9)	58.7 (149.1)
E. Elbow to floor	34.5 (87.6)	43.4 (110.2)
F. High shelf	55.0 (139.7)	69.9 (177.5)
G. Low shelf	29.7 (75.4)	33.3 (89.7)
H. Low reach	21.7 (55.1)	27.3 (69.3)
I. Slump	1.0 (2.5)	1.3 (3.3)
J. Sitting ht. to seat	27.8 (70.6)	35.6 (90.4)
K. Eye to seat	23.6 (59.9)	30.9 (78.5)
L. High reach to table	19.7 (50.0)	26.7 (67.8)
M. Max forward reach	17.0 (43.2)	21.2 (53.8)
N. Shoulder to seat	17.1 (43.4)	22.8 (57.9)
O. Compressed st ht.	13.8 (35.1)	17.7 (45.0)
P. Max seat length	16.5 (41.9)	21.4 (54.4)
Q. Buttock to knee	19.8 (50.3)	24.4 (62.0)
R. Std. min foot room	19.0 (48.3)	23.0 (58.4)
S. Max. thigh hgt.	4.0 (10.2)	6.8 (17.3)
T. Table height	24.5 (62.2)	30.4 (77.2)

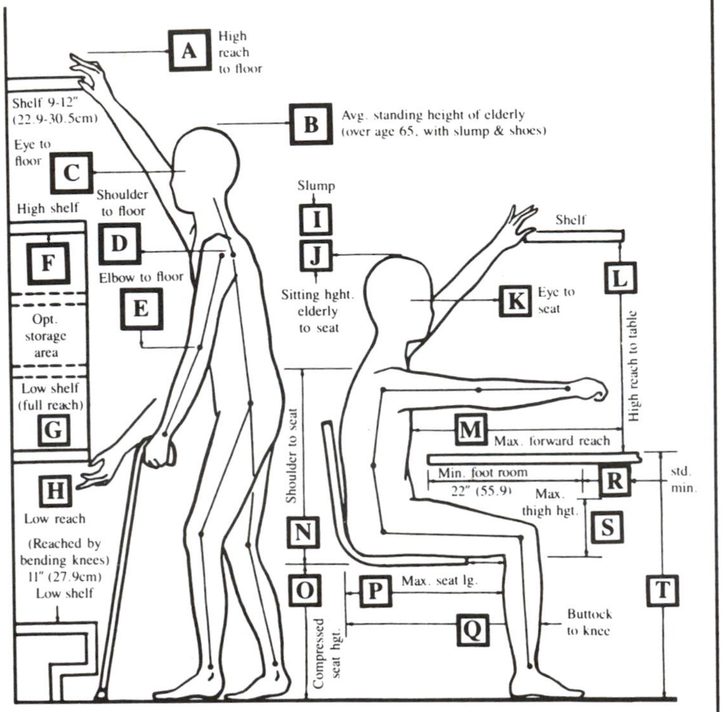

Figure 25-3. Reach Capabilities of Elderly Persons from Standing and Sitting Positions. *Adapted from Diffrient, Tilley and Bardagjy (1974). Humanscale 1/2/3: Cambridge, MA: MIT Press.*

building. Assessment of the house construction involves the teamwork of the client, an architect, and an occupational therapist (Orleans, 1981a). Thorough assessment helps to ensure ease in mobility, communication, work, dining, leisure, and self-care.

Strategies for Intervention

Once the factors that influence the accomplishment of desired tasks have been recognized, the occupational therapist can provide information about intervention options. The client can then make a successful choice concerning the manner in which environmental barriers are eliminated or the task performance is altered and/or improved. One of the therapist's highest priorities is to promote in the client a feeling of control and competency in daily tasks. There are different strategies for overcoming environmental barriers, ranging from simple to complex and from inexpensive to expensive. The factors mentioned above will help determine the choice. The following suggestions for overcoming environmental barriers are not exclusive of each other, and frequently an individual will use them in combination.

Personal Intervention Strategies. Sometimes the best way to overcome environmental barriers is to create new ways for the client to successfully complete a desired task. This may involve relearning the task or learning to perform the task using new procedures. For example, the therapist may retain a client with upper extremity weakness to cook a meal by using treatment that involves muscle strengthening. On the other hand, if strengthening is not feasible the client may be taught to cook with alternate movements and positions. These procedures are discussed in other chapters.

One may also explore the desirability of task performance. There may be self-care tasks which were accomplished before the injury or illness that the client now no longer chooses to perform. For example, an individual with hemiplegia who formerly baked bread may now choose to purchase it.

Social Intervention Strategies. Assistance from other individuals for the partial or total completion of a desired task is another option for the patient to consider. The assistance may be from spouses, friends, or from paid personal assistants. One of the occupational therapist's responsibilities is to instruct both the client and his/her helpers how to work together to complete the task (Christiansen, Schwartz, & Barnes, 1988). The use of social assistance may help a person with severe disability reside at home rather than in an institutional setting.

Physical Environment Intervention Strategies. Modifications to the living environment may be helpful in increasing the client's independence and functional capacity. Physical environment intervention options can be divided into three groups: (1) rearranging the living environment, (2) making additions to the environment and, (3) structurally modifying the environment. Within each group is a continuum of interventions that differ in expense, time consumption, labor and personnel requirements, and planning. These options may require the planning and assistance of electricians, architects, and carpenters.

Rearrangement of the physical environment can be an expeditious and inexpensive way to overcome physical barriers. In some instances, simply rearranging the physical setting may permit task performance. For example, moving dishes to lower kitchen shelves allows an individual sitting in a wheelchair to reach them. Furniture in the living room can be placed along traffic routes so the person who is blind will have contact points as he/she moves along (Dickman, 1983). A bed or extra sofa can be moved into the living room so the person who must lie down will be able to interact with others in an area other than the bedroom.

Additions to an existing environment can help to improve occupational performance. This includes the use of specially designed adaptive devices and other more commonly used equipment such as hooks, storage bins, and paint. These adaptations range from the very inexpensive to the very expensive. Painting a contrasting color on a wall around light fixtures for people with visual impairment is an example of a very inexpensive addition to the environment. For someone with a hearing impairment one might attach an electrical light to the doorbell. The occupational therapist should be acquainted with these devices, able to assist the client in determining whether they would be helpful, and capable of training clients in their use. There are numerous resources that discuss environmental adaptations. Several are included in the Reference and Recommended Readings sections at the end of this chapter.

Actual structural changes to the physical environment may also be made to allow the client to independently perform a task. These include the reconstruction of rooms to accommodate wheelchair movement or the addition of a ramp at the entrance to a building. Careful planning should go into changes in the structure of the home as these changes can be expensive. The planning and construction of structural changes requires teamwork among the client, occupational therapist and others assisting in the process. Major structural changes such as the installation of a wheel-in shower or wiring for a security system should be undertaken by licensed architects, builders, plumbers, or electricians as completion of such projects is outside the scope of occupational therapy.

A final alternative may be to move away from an environment that has physical barriers. Factors to consider in this change include the location of stores, transportation availability, proximity to family and friends, and expenses. Assistance from local agencies may be needed to direct the client to appropriate housing to meet his/her social, economic, and physical needs.

DESIGNS FOR MAXIMUM PERFORMANCE WITHIN THE ENVIRONMENT

The environmental design should aid function, maximize independence and efficiency, and prevent injury to people with and without disability. This should be done in the

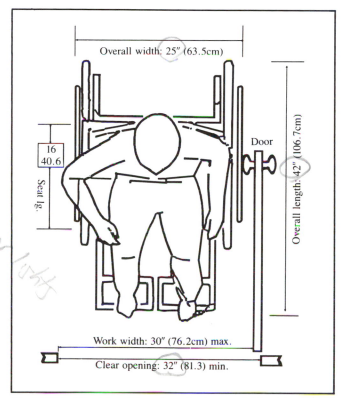

Figure 25-4. Wheelchair Dimensions for Average Adult. *Adapted from Diffrient, Tilley & Bardagjy (1974). Humanscale 1/2/3. Cambridge, MA: MIT Press.*

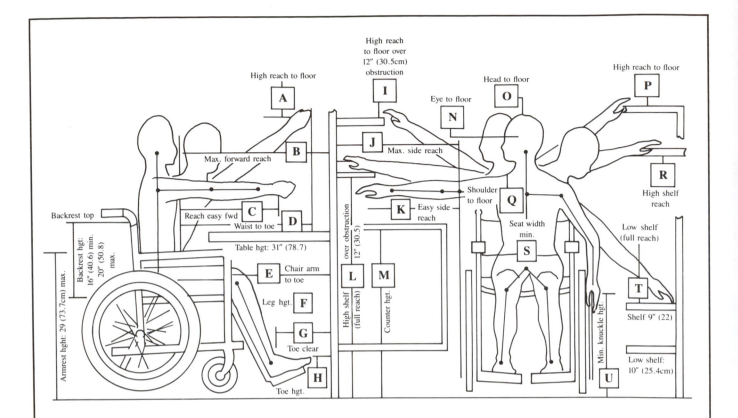

DIMENSIONS
Inches (Cm)

	Small Female	Average Adult	Large Male
A. High Reach to Floor	45.5 (115.6)	53.5 (135.9)	59.2 (150.4)
B. Maximum forward reach	31.3 (79.5)	35.3 (89.7)	38.3 (97.3)
C. Easy forward reach	18.5 (47.0)	20.8 (52.8)	22.3 (56.6)
D. Waist to toe	22.0 (55.9)	25.3 (64.3)	28.6 (72.6)
E. Chair arm to toe	12.5 (31.8)	15.5 (39.4)	18.5 (47.0)
F. Leg Height	23.5 (59.7)	25.0 (63.5)	26.5 (67.3)
G. Toe clear	4.5 (11.4)	6.6 (16.8)	8.8 (22.4)
H. Toe height	8.8 (22.4)	6.2 (15.7)	8.5 (21.6)
I. High reach to floor over obstruction	48.5 (123.2)	57.3 (145.5)	67.7 (172.0)
J. Maximum side reach	22.2 (56.4)	25.3 (64.3)	30.1 (76.5)
K. Easy side reach	16.2 (41.1)	18.6 (47.2)	22.5 (57.2)
L. High shelf over obstruction	38.0 (96.5)	50.5 (128.3)	60.0 (152.4)
M. Counter height	31.0 (78.7)	32.5 (82.6)	34.0 (86.4)
N. Eye to floor	42.8 (108.7)	47.7 (121.2)	51.1 (129.8)
O. Head to floor	46.8 (118.9)	51.8 (131.6)	55.8 (141.7)
P. High reach to floor	53.0 (134.6)	62.0 (157.5)	71.2 (180.8)
Q. Shoulder to floor	35.8 (90.9)	39.8 (101.1)	42.8 (108.7)
R. High shelf reach	43.6 (110.7)	53.1 (134.9)	62.7 (159.3)
S. Seat width minimum	16.0 (40.6)	18.0 (45.7)	18.0 (45.7)
T. Low shelf, full reach	18.7 (47.5)	15.3 (38.9)	10.0 (25.4)
U. Minimum knucle height	4.6 (37.1)	16.0 (40.6)	16.5 (41.9)

Figure 25-5. Anthropometric and Reach Data for Wheelchair Use by Small Females, Average Adult and Large Males. *Adapted from Diffrient, Tilley and Bardagjy (1974). Humanscale 1/2/3. Cambridge, MA: MIT Press.*

home, the workplace, and all other environments. The following general design goals and considerations for barrier elimination are adapted from Orleans (1981a):

1. Provide floor space for easy clearance, turning, and transferring for individuals with mobility disability, such as those using wheelchairs, canes, and crutches.
2. Arrange spaces to minimize unnecessary mobility, to simplify environmental control, and to facilitate ease of housekeeping.
3. Eliminate barriers which impede mobility and may cause injuries, such as door thresholds and throw rugs.
4. Provide sufficient, accessible storage.
5. Build usable work surfaces at appropriate countertop heights with sufficient knee space.
6. Locate mirrors, windows, light switches, electrical outlets, plumbing, and appliance controls at functional heights.
7. Provide as unobtrusive an access to the house as possible.
8. Survey the existing dwelling from a life safety standpoint.

The following sections describe components of the home and workplace which affect task performance. Environmental modifications designed to facilitate task performance are described, as well. An attempt has been made to include modifications and designs that are most frequently needed; thus, these suggested strategies should not be viewed as exhaustive.

Vertical Level Changes

Vertical level changes involve movement in which a person must travel up or down in relation to the surrounding structure, as with stairs, porches and door stoops. Vertical level changes pose one of the greatest threats to safe and independent movement for individuals with physical disabilities and are a potential safety hazard for all individuals. Even very small vertical level changes, such as door thresholds, can block passage for a person in a wheelchair or be a safety hazard for those with visual impairments.

No single vertical change adaptation will accommodate all disability groups due to the different biomechanical manifestations of the impairments. A ramp is often the best solution for individuals using wheelchairs, strollers and walkers as well as for those with limited ankle and knee mobility (Corlett, Hutcheson, DeLugan, and Rogozenski, 1972). Other individuals with walking disabilities, as seen in hemiplegia or lower extremity amputation, may find that stairs are preferable to ramps, particularly when descending, which requires considerable balance and muscular control (Goldsmith, 1976). Each client's abilities

must be carefully evaluated before determining the type of vertical level change that best meets his/her mobility and safety needs.

Ramps. Exterior ramps should not be placed in an isolated area away from the most accessible pathway into the building. People who need ramps for entrance to a house should not be required to travel long distances in secluded exterior areas to get to an accessible entrance. Ramps can be made so that they complement the exterior decor of the house by using matching or contrasting finishes and using plants and shrubs to enhance the landscape.

The following ramp dimension guidelines are from the American National Standards Institute (1986):

1. The slope of the ramp should be as small as possible. The maximum slope ratio should be 1:12, which means that for every inch of rise the ramp should be 12 inches long. Thus, for a 2 foot rise a 24 foot ramp is needed. Thirty inches is the maximum rise for any ramp.
2. For a ramp that has a slope of 1:12, the run (the horizontal projection) should be no more than 30 feet.
3. Ramp landings are the level surfaces at the bottom and top of each run. The landing should be as wide as the widest ramp run leading to it and have a length of at least 60 inches. If the ramp landing is adjacent to a door entrance, the landing should comply with American National Standards Institute (ANSI) regulations for door entrance space so the person will be able to open the door safely (See section on doors).
4. Ramps with a rise greater than six inches or a horizontal projection more than 72 inches should have handrails on both sides.
5. Ramps and landings with dropoffs should have edge protection to prevent people from falling off. This can be a curb, walls, railing, or projecting surface.

Further specifications concerning ramp dimensions may be found in the ANSI regulations (1986).

Ramps should be constructed so that the approach to the house is the most direct for those using it. Ramps can extend straight out from the house, be flush against the house, or at an angle from the house. In the cases in which the rise is very high, which would cause the ramp to be very long, the construction of a wrap-around ramp may be preferable (Figure 25-6). Wrap-around ramps are also helpful for clients with reduced endurance as this design allows them to rest at the middle landing.

Ramps may be constructed of concrete or wood. Wooden ramps are practical for the home ramp because they are relatively inexpensive and easier to construct than concrete ramps. The main drawback in the use of wooden ramps is the potential fire hazard. The wood used should be treated

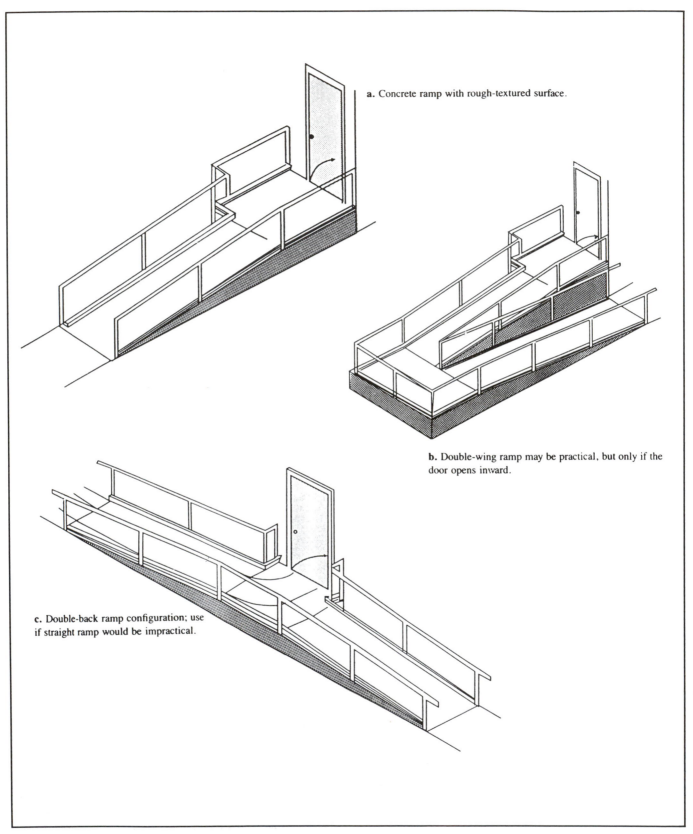

a. Concrete ramp with rough-textured surface.

b. Double-wing ramp may be practical, but only if the door opens inward.

c. Double-back ramp configuration; use if straight ramp would be impractical.

Figure 26-6a-c. Ramps.

to be resistant to decay and warping. The finish on the wood should be a weather resistive coating. Concrete ramps are fireproof and last longer than wooden ramps; however, concrete ramps are more expensive than wooden ramps and the margin for construction error is smaller because once the concrete has set it is difficult to alter. Employment of a professional concrete contractor may be advisable unless one is experienced in the use of concrete.

The ramp surfaces should be fireproof and made with a nonslip surface. The wooden surface can be made slip-proof by placing nonslip materials on it or painting it with skid-resistant paint (See Floor section). Concrete surfaces should not be smooth and should have a textured surface to prevent slips and falls. If the ramp is located so that it may became wet or slick due to ice, rain, or snow, it should be protected with a roof or enclosure.

Portable Ramps. There are portable ramps which may be transported in a car or van when going to buildings and houses that may not have ramps (Medical Equipment Distributors, Inc., 1987). They are also useful for getting into and out of vans. A disadvantage of portable ramps may be the size and weight of the ramp. Individuals with upper extremity weakness may not be able to lift and move them. Another disadvantage of some portable ramps is the time required to assemble and disassemble them.

Stairs. Stairs are potentially hazardous for any user and an attempt must be made to make them as safe as possible when they are a necessary part of a building. Each step on a stair should have a tread (or runner) depth of no less than 11 inches and a maximum riser height of no more than seven inches (ANSI, 1986). The nosing of each step should be rounded and extend no more than one and one half inches over the lower step (ANSI, 1986) (Figure 25-7). The surface of the steps should be made of a nonslip material. There should be no loose materials on the stairs, such as carpet edges, nails, or loosened wood. Open riser staircases should be avoided because people may catch their feet between the steps and the open view can make some individuals dizzy (Goldsmith, 1976). Doors should not be positioned directly at the top of the stairs and should not swing into the landing of the stairs. Stairs should not be exposed to any condition that may cause moisture on the steps. Handrails should be located on each side of the stairs and extend at least 12 inches beyond the top riser and at least 12 inches plus the tread width beyond the bottom riser (ANSI, 1986). Handrail height should be between 30 and 34 inches (ANSI, 1986). Additionally, the diameter of the gripping surface of handrails should be between 1.25 and 1.50 inches (ANSI, 1986).

Individuals with visual impairments, including some elderly people, may find stairs to be hazardous because it is difficult to differentiate one step from another as well as the top and bottom of the flight of stairs. Visual cues can make the stairs much safer. Dickman provides the following suggestions (1983):

1. The stairs should be well-lighted with a nonglare source of light. The top and bottom of the stairs should be accented with light, if possible.

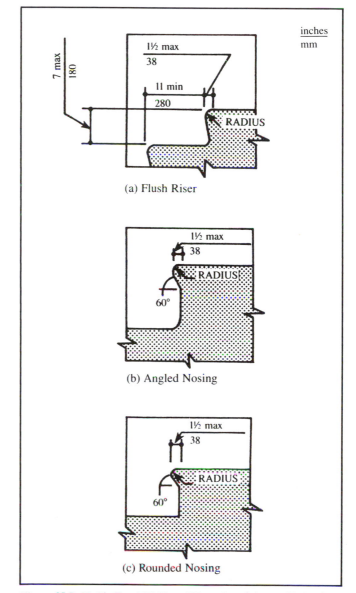

Figure 25-7. Usable Tread Width and Examples of Acceptable Nosings. *From American National Standard for buildings and facilities—providing accessibility and usability for physically handicapped people. ANSI-A117.1, copyright 1986 by The American National Standards Institute. Copies of this standard may be purchased from the American National Standards Institute at 1430 Broadway, New York, NY 10018.*

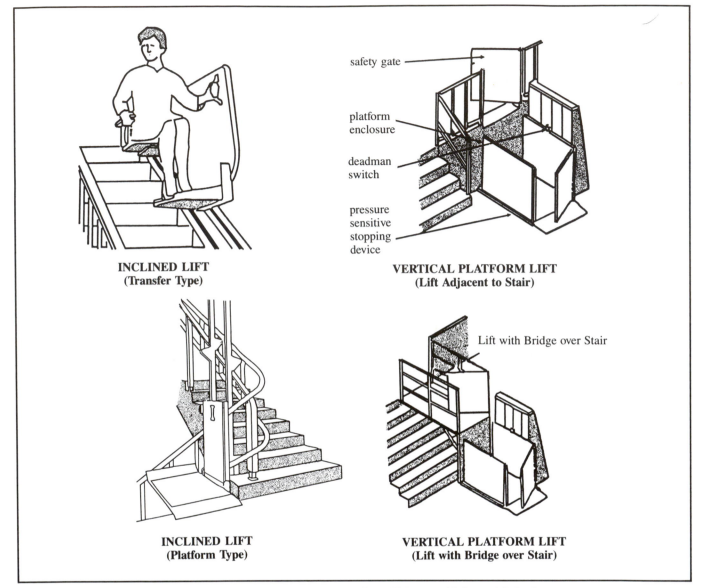

INCLINED LIFT
(Transfer Type)

safety gate

platform
enclosure

deadman
switch

pressure
sensitive
stopping
device

VERTICAL PLATFORM LIFT
(Lift Adjacent to Stair)

Lift with Bridge over Stair

INCLINED LIFT
(Platform Type)

VERTICAL PLATFORM LIFT
(Lift with Bridge over Stair)

Figure 25-8. Elevators & Lifts. *From Cotler, S. (1981). Access Information Bulletin: Elevators and Lifts. pp. 1-2. Washington, D.C. Paralyzed Veterans of America.*

2. Small, localized lights at each step, as used in darkened movie theaters, will help the user to see the location of each step.
3. The top and bottom landings should have a contrasting color to identify the end of the steps.
4. The hand rails should be a different, contrasting color from the supporting wall.
5. The leading edge of each step, on the runner, and the riser, can be marked with a contrasting paint or tape. This should run the entire width of the step and be two to three inches wide. Reflecting tape can be helpful. A textured material on the leading edge may also be helpful for feeling where the step is with one's foot.

Elevators and Lifts. Elevators and lifts are options for overcoming large vertical changes (Figure 25-8). These are available for use in private and public buildings for the exterior entrance as well as between interior floors. In the selection of elevators and lifts careful attention should be given to the size of the platform on which the individual will be carried. If the person will be sitting in a manual or electric wheelchair, there should be enough mobility space for getting on and off the platform and operating the control switches. The riding platform must be safely constructed so that the user will not fall or roll off. The control system must be within easy reach of the user and the control switches should be easily operated. Additionally, a backup electrical power source is needed in the event of fire or power outage.

An individual's needs must be carefully evaluated before purchasing an elevator or lift as they are expensive and require extensive construction time and labor. Architects, electricians, and construction contractors most likely will be needed for their planning and construction. Further information concerning the specifications of elevators and lifts for individuals with disabilities may be found in Cotler (1981) and ANSI (1986).

Doors

Doors are important environmental components of buildings and homes. They provide privacy, security, and protection from rain and snow. Doors also regulate temperature, air currents, and light. Additionally, doors and doorways are the indicators that role expectations may change upon entry into another room. For example, passage through a bathroom door cues the person of the social expectations for privacy and isolation while passage through a kitchen door provides cues for hospitality and activity.

While doors provide desired environmental restrictions, they can be a major restriction to movement for people with physical disabilities. Customary door designs can prevent passage for many individuals. The door weight, width, knob, threshold height, and location are features that may contribute to obstructed movement. Modifications to the door can be made to promote independent mobility.

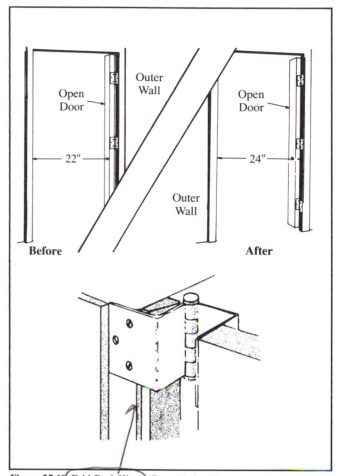

Figure 25-10. Fold-Back Hinge. *From Medical Equipment for the Rehabilitation, Treatment and Home Care of Children and Adults 1984/85 Catalogue. Forest Park, IL: AAMED, Inc. (1215 So Harlem Ave., Forest Park, IL 60130)*

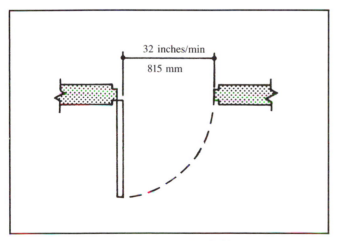

Figure 25-9. Interior Door Width. *Reproduced with permission from American National Standard for buildings and facilities—providing accessibility and usability for physically handicapped people (ANSI A117.1), copyright 1986 by the American National Standards Institute. Copies of the Standard may be purchased from the American National Standards Institute at 1430 Broadway, New York, NY 10018.*

Door Width. Exterior doors should be a minimum of 36 inches wide. This will provide a clear passage width of 34 inches between the face of the door and the doorstop. Interior doors should have a minimum width of 32 inches between the face and the stop (ANSI, 1986) (See Figure 25-9). The door should open to at least a 90 degree angle. This width allows wheelchair and walker users enough room to pass through the doorway.

The door width can be made larger in several ways. One way is to replace the entire door and frame with a wider door. This requires structural changes, time, and expense.

In some instances, the surrounding wall may not be wide enough to support a larger door frame. If a narrow interior doorway cannot be replaced with a wider door frame, the door can be removed from the frame, thereby adding one or two inches of width. Visual privacy may be provided by the use of a curtain hung from the door frame.

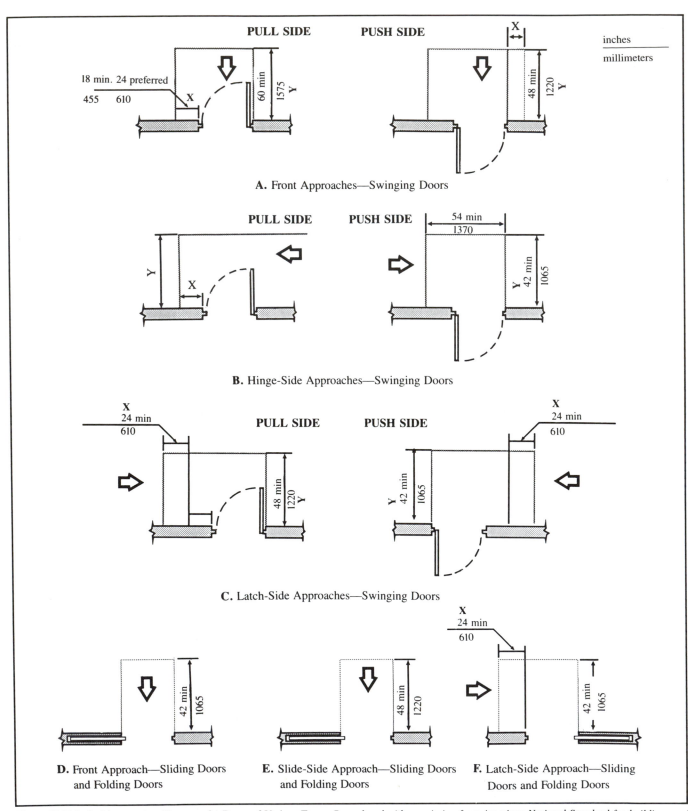

Figure 25-11 (a-f). Maneuvering Clearance for Doors of Various Types. *Reproduced with permission from American National Standard for buildings and facilities—providing accessibility and usability for physically handicapped people (ANSI A117.1), copyright 1986 by the American National Standards Institute. Copies of the Standard may be purchased from the American National Standards Institute at 1430 Broadway, New York, NY 10018.*

Sometimes if it does not open to 90 degrees or more, the open door will impede the passage through the doorway. Fold-back hinges are extended hinges that can replace regular hinges and allow the door to open flush with the wall. This increases the width because the door itself is out of the passageway (Figure 25-10).

If only one room or a closet has a doorway that is too narrow, the wheelchair or walker user may consider transferring onto a castor chair that will be used only in that room, and leaving the wheelchair or walker outside the doorway. This solution can only be used by individuals with adequate sitting balance and transfer abilities.

Maneuvering Space at the Door. Space around the door is needed to open the door, to back up while pulling the door open, and to pull the door closed once through the door. Space requirements to enter and close a door vary according to the type of door, the placement of the door, the approach to the door space, and the space needed to accommodate ambulatory devices or wheelchairs. Some individuals approach the door in a straight or perpendicular manner, while others may approach it parallel to the door from the hinge side or the handle side. The individual's abilities determine the best approach to be taken. Figure 25-11 shows the maneuvering space needed to open a door while sitting in a wheelchair. A space of 60 x 60 inches is needed for individuals in a wheelchair to be able to close a door (Raschko, 1982).

Door placement in the wall should be such that the door is able to swing completely open to at least 90 degrees without bumping into other structures. If the swing space of two doors intersects, the hinge side of one or both doors may be changed so there is no swing space intersection. Doors should open in a direction that allows maximum movement space. For example, a closet door should swing into the room or out of the closet so a person using a wheelchair or ambulatory device will be able to get close to the clothes rack.

Sliding doors allow maximum door width and eliminate door swing space requirements. Sliding doors do require installation into an adjacent wall that has an equal width to the door width and that is free of electrical wiring, etc. Sliding door tracks may be installed on the surface of the adjacent wall, which requires less construction but is not as attractive. Sliding door hardware may be difficult to grasp and operate for individuals with weak grasp, hand deformities or poor muscular coordination. A D-shaped handle can be mounted on the door front and back to ease operation. Folding doors must be placed in a door frame that is wide enough to allow a 32-inch passageway. Care must be taken in the choice of folding doors as some have operating controls that are difficult to manipulate.

Door Threshold. The door threshold height should be no greater than 1/2 inch for all doors except exterior sliding doors which should have a threshold height no greater than 3/4 inch (ANSI, 1986). Raised thresholds should be beveled, or sloped, so that the slope ratio is no greater than 1:2 (ANSI, 1986). Door thresholds that are greater than 1/2 inch (except for sliding doors) should be treated as vertical changes that require a ramped surface (see above). Door mats should be avoided because they can cause slipping and restrict mobility. The entrance floor surface should be of a nonskid material to prevent slipping due to moisture left from feet and ambulatory devices.

Door Opening Force. The maximum force needed to push or pull a door open is expressed in pound-force (lbf). The opening force should be no greater than 8.5 lbf for exterior doors and no greater than 5 lbf for interior doors (ANSI, 1986). The opening force for fire doors may vary depending on local fire safety authorities. The opening force is affected by the door weight, which varies depending on the type of construction and material. If there is a drag due to the door rubbing the door frame or the floor surface, the door side or bottom can be shaved down to decrease the drag. Door weather stripping should not be too thick, as it may increase the force needed to open the door.

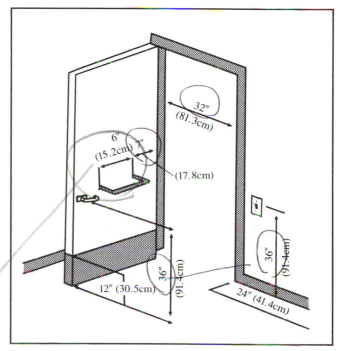

Figure 25-12. D-Shaped Pull-handle. *Source: Raschko, B. (1982). Housing interiors for the disabled and elderly. New York, NY: Van Nostrand Reinhold Company.*

Door Closing. Door closing can be difficult for users of wheelchairs, canes, and walkers because one must turn around and back up to push the door closed after passing through it. Following are several modification suggestions to make door closing easier:

1. A D-shaped pull handle can be placed on a door 7 to 8 inches from the hinge at the same level as the door knob. The person passing through can pull on it instead of backing up to grasp the door knob (Figure 25-12).

2. Tie a rope, approximately 2 feet long, to the door knob. The person passing through the door can grasp the end or secure it to a wheelchair or walker handle and pull the door closed while moving through the doorway.

3. Anderson (1981) describes a rope and pulley system that can be used to close a door (Figure 25-13). A sash cord, which runs through two pulleys, is mounted on the door and door molding. One pulley is located at the upper corner of the door near the hinge and the other is in the middle of the upper molding. The sash

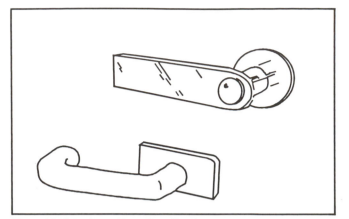

Figure 25-14. Horizontal Lever Door Handles. *From How to create interiors for the disabled: a guide for family and friends by Jane Rudolph Cary. Illustrated by Philip E. Farrell, Jr. Text copyright © 1978 by Jane Randolph Cary. Illustrations copyright © 1979 by Random House, Inc. Reprinted by permission of Pantheon Books, a Division of Random House, Inc.*

also runs through a screw eye at the side of molding. The end of the sash has a grasping ring. Once the person is through the door he/she can pull on the ring to close the door.

4. Mechanical door closers are also available. A consideration in choosing door closers is the fact that the door closer mechanism can make door opening more difficult. A door closer must not require more than 8 lbf for exterior door opening and 5 lbf for interior door opening (Barrier Free Environments, 1981). The most simple door closer is a spring attached to the door and the door frame, as frequently seen on wooden screen doors. Door closers which have a delay in the closing mechanism are desirable so that passage through the door can occur before it closes.

Electrically-Controlled Door Openers and Closers. Many types of electronically controlled door openers and closers are available, including electro-hydraulically operated and electro-mechanical pneumatic openers. A variety of operating switches are available including: floor sensing pads, wall switches, photoelectric beams, and radar and microwave devices (Barrier Free Environments, 1981). Doors are available that open out or slide open. Various features are available including variable speed settings, time delay for closing, and stopping for obstacles. Some require extensive structural modification while others may be installed on standard home doors with minimal installation requirements. Electrically operated door openers and closers should meet ANSI standards (1986). (See list of manufacturers at the end of this chapter.) Careful consideration should be given to selection as they may be expensive. An electrician or construc-

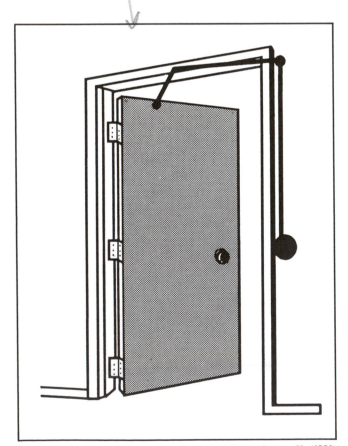

Figure 25-13. Rope and Pulley Door System. *From Anderson, H. (1981). The Disabled Homemaker. p. 252. Courtesy of Charles C. Thomas, Publisher, Springfield, Illinois.*

tion contractor should be consulted concerning the cost and feasibility of their use.

Door Handles and Locks.   A height of 36 to 38 inches is best for the door handles and locks (Anderson, 1981). The handle and locks should not require tight grasping or pinching or extensive forearm supination and pronation. Door handles and locks that require the use of only one hand are most accessible for persons with upper extremity impairments. The following suggestions are offered for making door handles and locks accessible:

1. Horizontal level door knobs can replace round door knobs for people with upper extremity weakness, limited range of motion (ROM) and hand dysfunction (Figure 25-14). These are available in hardware stores and through rehabilitation catalogues. Horizontal, closed end door levers can prevent the individual's clothing from being caught in the door handle while passing through (Cary, 1978).

2. A paddle type handle, which is pushed or pulled to work is another alternative to the conventional door knob (Figure 25-15). This can be useful for individuals with limited hand and forearm use.

3. Several devices are available that can be attached to round door knobs to make use easier. A rubber horizontal door knob attachment is easier to use because it has a surface which prevents slipping and because of its horizontal shape (Figure 25-16a). It is

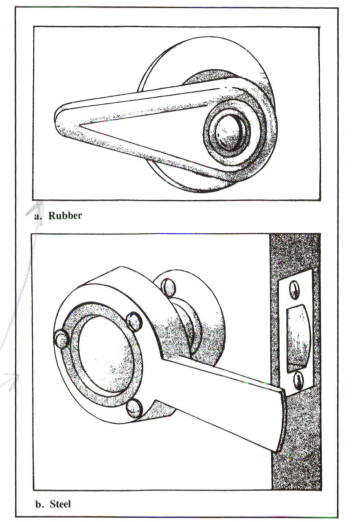

a. Rubber

b. Steel

Figure 25-16a, b. Door Knob Extensions. *From Fred Sammons 1989 Professional Healthcare Catalog (1989). Burr Ridge, IL: Fred Sammons, Inc.*

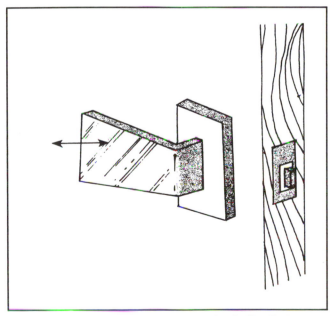

Figure 25-15. Paddle-Type Door Handle. *From Barrier Free Environments, Inc. (1981). Access Information Bulletin: Doors and Entrances. Raleigh, NC. Barrier Free Environments, Inc.*

placed over the door knob. Metal door knob extenders can convert door knobs into horizontal handles by screwing them on over the door knob (Figure 25-16b).

4. Portable door knob turners which slip over the door knob can also assist in door knob opening (Figure 25-17) and may be useful for individuals while they are away from home.

5. Deadbolt locks that are incorporated into the middle of the door handle make unlocking and opening easier as both are accomplished with one turn.

6. Individuals with visual impairments may have difficulty identifying, unlocking, and opening doors. To make things easier, doors can be painted a contrasting color to the wall and keys can be kept in order on a key

Lines on the floor

ring and coded by color or shape (Dickman, 1983). Individuals who live in apartments may have difficulty identifying which door is their own. Placing rubber-bands around the door knob or attaching felt decals to the door will facilitate that process (Dickman, 1983).

Door handles and other operating hardware which permit entrance to hazardous areas such as stairs, mechanical rooms, boiler rooms, and loading areas, should have a tactile surface that is textured as a warning to people with visual or mental impairments (Sorensen, 1979). This type of texturing can be achieved by roughing up the handle surface, knurling, or applying a rough surface paint or strips to the handle or hardware.

7. Electronic keys may be helpful for individuals with weakness and/or limited range of motion because they eliminate the need to turn the key in the lock, and may be activated by push-button or remote control systems.

8. Sliding doors should have easily operated handles and locks on both sides of the door that can be used when the door is fully open (Hopf and Raeber, 1984).

9. Holding packages while attempting to unlock and open an exterior door can be very difficult for any individual. Shelves or tables on which to place packages while opening or closing the door can be helpful in this situation. For an individual in a wheelchair the shelf or table height should be between 36 and 39 inches (Raschko, 1982). An individual who uses a cane or walker or who has back pain may want the shelf at a higher height to prevent stooping. The shelf or table should not interfere with the maneuverability space at the door.

outside room

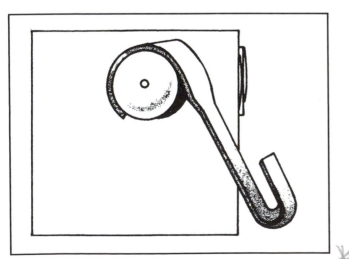

Figure 25-17. Portable Door Knob Turner. *From Fred Sammons 1989 Professional Healthcare Catalog (1989). Burr Ridge, IL: Fred Sammons, Inc.*

door bell on door

Door Communication.   Doorbells connected to lights, vibrators, or amplified sound systems are useful for the individual with a hearing problem, and intercom systems can provide safety.

Structural Protection.   Bumps and scrapes from ambulatory devices and wheelchairs can cause damage to the door and surrounding walls. Metal or plastic kickplates can be placed on the bottom of the door to prevent damage from wheelchair footrest or crutch tips being used to open the door. Carpet pieces can be fastened to door entrance ways to prevent injury from bumps and to prevent damage to the wall. Clear plastic molding strips can be placed on the wall corners and door frames to provide a smooth and softer edge and prevent damage.   *molding*

Outdoor Ground Surfaces

Outdoor surfaces on which travel will occur should be firm, stable, and slip-resistant (ANSI, 1986). Included in this category are sidewalks, porches, ramps, and stairs. These surfaces should be free of cracks, bumps, and loose gravel. Outside surfaces made of inlaid stone or rocks can be very hazardous if some edges stick up above others or if the pieces are unevenly spaced. Missing pieces of sidewalks can also be very hazardous. Concrete and other hard surfaces can be made slip-resistant by using nonskid finishes. Additionally, a mason can finish a new concrete surface with varying degrees of roughness.

Floors

A variety of floor surfaces are available for use within the home. Great differences exist in the usability, cost, and durability of each floor surface. The physical and economic needs of the resident will determine the types of floor modifications made. Changes of the floor surfaces may be extensive, such as carpeting over a vinyl floor, or simple, such as removing throw rugs in pathways. The following factors are considered in evaluating floor surfaces to promote mobility and safety:

Safety.   Floor surfaces greatly influence the safety of a home. Floors should be free of loose objects, frayed carpet, tacks, throw rugs, and furnishing which may cause falls. Gratings in the floor surface should have spaces no more than 1/2 inch wide (ANSI, 1986). Slippery surfaces, including highly waxed and polished wooden and vinyl floors, are hazardous for most people and are particularly hazardous for persons using walkers, canes, or crutches. Hard and resilient floors can be left unwaxed to decrease the slipperiness of the floor. Slippery areas can be made safer by using products such as Scotch Brand® Anti-Slip Tape (3M), which can be adhered directly to most surfaces including floors, steps, and bathtubs. Sorensen (1979) provides information on the friction of wet, dry, hard, and resilient floor surfaces as related to rubber and leather soled shoes, wheelchair tires, and crutch tips (Table 25-1).

Floor choices should be made with consideration to flammability. Manufacturers and retail stores can provide this information about floor coverings.

Cleaning.   Ease in cleaning is an important factor since dirt and grease may cause floors to be slick. Floors that require extensive maintenance should be avoided as cleaning may be difficult for the individual with a disability (Goldsmith, 1976). Considerations in carpet choice should include stain and moisture resistance.

Sound Quality.   Hard floors can be beneficial for individuals who are blind because they provide auditory feedback which allows them to hear the approach of others. However the noise from hard floors may be disorienting for people with hearing loss and/or auditory distortion problems. Carpet and resilient surfaces such as cork decrease floor noise.

Visual Quality.   Sunlight and indoor lighting on glossy floors can cause glaring reflections. This type of glare may impede the vision of individuals with poor visual acuity, visual accommodation, and dark adaptation (Levy, 1985). For individuals with visual acuity or depth perception problems, floor surfaces should have clearly defined visual edges in relation to the surrounding walls, doors, and other floor surfaces. Floor surfaces such as checkerboard tiles or large floral prints may be confusing to individuals with visual perception impairments.

Cost and Durability.   The cost of modifying floor surfaces may be very expensive for some clients. Inexpensive modifications can be explored for those with limited budgets, including the use of floor paints and finishings that alter the floor color, texture, and degree of friction. Any newly purchased floor covering should be chosen with durability in mind.

Comfort.   The type of floor covering chosen can influence the comfort of the residents. The resilience of floor surface influences the force on joints when standing and walking, an important consideration for people with arthritis. Increased padding under carpet and the use of resilient surfaces such as cork tiles, instead of hard surfaces such as ceramic tiles, may help improve comfort. The temperature of the floor surface also affects the comfort level of the people in the room. Carpet and linoleum with thick backing are usually warmer than hard surfaces in winter months.

Table 25-1
Friction of Surfaces

	RUBBER		LEATHER	
	Dry	Wet	Dry	Wet
Steel plate, phenolic resin/alundum grit surfaced	0.69	0.45	0.64	0.47
Concrete, carborundum grit	0.65	0.60	0.37	0.43
Smooth paving brick	0.68	0.38	0.27	0.27
Smooth terazzo	0.53	0.25	0.35	0.16
Terazzo, alundum grit	0.74	0.33	0.44	0.18
Smooth quarry tile	0.69	0.28	0.31	0.20
White oak, waxed and polished	0.49	0.19	0.24	0.17
Linoleum				
Clean	0.68	0.19	0.32	0.10
Solvent wax, polished	0.62	0.19	0.25	0.13
Water emulsion wax, polished	0.71	0.16	0.34	0.10
Rubber Tile				
Solvent wax, polished	0.61	0.17	0.29	0.16
Water emulsion wax, polished	0.80	0.32	0.42	0.20
Asphalt Tile				
Water emulsion wax, polished	0.72	0.22	0.37	0.15
Vinyl, smooth	0.47	0.22	0.25	0.21

For interior surfaces, dry rubber (shoes, heels, wheelchair tires, crutch tips) will be the usual condition

Coefficient of friction of less than 0.40 should be considered slippery and dangerous

Adapted from National Bureau of Standards, Research Paper RP 1879

From Sorensen, R. (1979). Design for Accessibility. NY, NY: McGraw-Hill Book Company.

Types of Floor Coverings.

Hard surfaces.   Hard surfaces include ceramic tile, concrete, wood, and marble. The individual using a wheelchair may find that hard surfaces are the easiest surface over which to maneuver a wheelchair (Sorensen, 1979; Wolfe, Waters, and Hislop, 1977). In a study of the influence of floor surfaces on energy requirements of individuals in wheelchairs, Wolfe, Waters, and Hislop (1977) found that a concrete floor surface required significantly less total energy to travel than did propulsion on indoor-outdoor carpet.

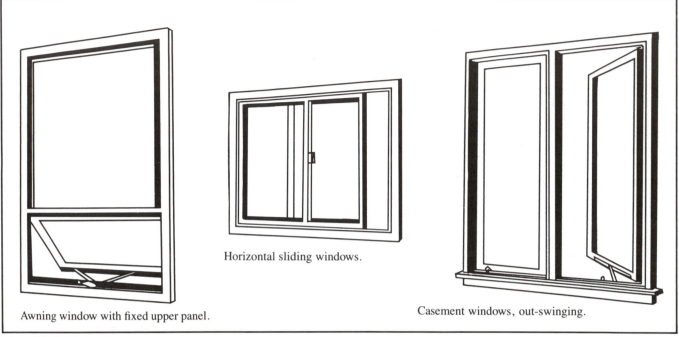

Awning window with fixed upper panel.

Horizontal sliding windows.

Casement windows, out-swinging.

Figure 25-18. Window Types.

Hard surfaces are more likely to be slippery than resilient or carpeted surfaces. Therefore, hard surfaces may not be the desired floor covering for individuals who may fall easily or who use ambulatory devices. If a hard surface is slippery, anti-skid compounds, such as Skid-Tex (Gamma Laboratories, Inc.) can be added to the floor finish to decrease slipperiness.

Resilient surfaces. A resilient floor surface such as cork or linoleum has a backing material that gives it the ability to spring back after being pressed down. This type of floor is better than a hard floor for ambulatory individuals who are prone to falls. Additionally, the resiliency of such a floor may be preferable for individuals with lower extremity joint or back pain.

Soft surfaces. Soft floor surfaces include carpeting and rugs. Rugs that have unsecured edges or are significantly higher than the surrounding floor should be removed as they make movement difficult in a wheelchair and may cause falls for ambulatory individuals. Deep carpet pile should be avoided as it makes wheelchair propulsion difficult and may cause tripping of individuals who are blind or who have ambulatory difficulty. ANSI guidelines state that carpet pile should be no higher than 1/2 inch. Other sources recommend even lower pile heights, between 0.15-0.25 inches (Kiewel, 1986; Raschko, 1982). The ANSI guidelines state that the carpet may have a "level loop, textured loop, level cut pile, or level cut/uncut pile texture" (ANSI, 1986). The carpet backing

or pad should be firm and dense since a backing material that is too soft will make wheelchair mobility difficult. Carpeting should be installed so the edges are securely fastened and the carpet is tightly stretched to prevent bunching or slipping under the wheels of a wheelchair (Anderson, 1981). Raschko (1982) provides a thorough analysis of carpeting including material types, construction methods, durability, flammability, and surface resistance to wheelchair travel.

Windows. Windows are important as they allow us to enjoy the outdoors while remaining sheltered inside and help to orient us to the time of day, weather conditions, and seasonal changes. Throughout the day, the ventilation and the temperature in a room can be altered by the opening and closing of windows. Windows also provide light for reading, growing plants, and other daily living tasks, and reduce the need for electrical lighting.

The ability to use windows is dependent upon their location and construction. An individual must be able to get close to the window and it must be at a height from which the person can view the outside. The opening mechanisms should be easy to reach and operate for the purposes of ventilation and temperature control. The curtains, drapes, or blinds should be easily manipulated in order to control lighting and privacy. Ease in cleaning also influences the use of the window. Additionally, ground level windows may be used as an alternate emergency exit in the case of fires, so it is essential that the person is able to get to the window, open it, and exit.

Dimensions. In order for people who are sitting or lying down to be able to see out of it, a window's lower edge must be no more than 15 to 20 inches above the floor (The American Institute of Architects, 1985). A clear space should be no more than 15 to 20 inches above the floor (The approach to the window, and low windows (such as floor-to-ceiling windows) should have guardrails or other means of protection to prevent accidents.

Mechanical features. Double-hung, vertically opening windows are usually difficult to operate for most individuals with physical disability due to the need for the use of both hands and the vertical movement range of the window. Awning and casement windows that open and close by the use of a crank handle located at the side or bottom of the windowsill may be the easiest to use for people with limited arm strength, low back pain, poor balance, or the use of only one hand (Figure 25-18). Horizontally sliding windows may be acceptable for individuals who are seated in wheelchairs as the vertical range of movement is eliminated. The mechanical features of any window should be well maintained so that it opens and closes with ease. No more than five pounds of force should be required to open or close windows (ANSI, 1986). Windows that are difficult to open may be sprayed with household lubricants. Controls for the window should be at a height that is convenient for the person using it; Raschko (1982) recommends that window controls be within the range of 28 to 42 inches.

Glass. Tempered, or "safety" glass, is a type of glass that breaks into small pieces instead of large sharp pieces, so that in the event of the accidental breaking of a window or glass door pane, tempered glass will be safer than regular glass.

Tinted glass can help control the glare that can impede the vision of elderly and visually impaired persons (Dickman, 1983). Decals or plastic strips can be placed on windows to make their presence more obvious for individuals with visual difficulties.

Coverings. Elderly people and people with visual impairments need a high level of illumination that is free of glare (Dickman, 1983). Blinds, drapes, curtains, and shades can help to control the amount of light that enters the room. The control mechanism of window coverings should be as easy to operate as possible. Extension handles, or wands, can be attached to the curtain or drape panel in order to pull it open or closed. Large circular rod rings attached to curtains or drapes make them move easily on the rod. Electrical drape openers are also available from drapery companies. If possible, windows should not be placed at the end of hallways and stairways as they may cause glare that can impede safe mobility (The American Institute of Archi-

tects, 1985). If there are windows in these locations, the window should be covered to prevent glare on the hallway or stairs.

Electrical Outlets and Switches

A clear approach area should surround outlets and switches so they are within easy reach and use for individuals using wheelchairs or walking devices (ANSI, 1986). The force needed to operate switches should be no more than 5 lbf and the switches should be operable with one hand (ANSI, 1986). Electrical outlets and switches should be mounted at a height not less than 15 inches above the floor for individuals using a forward reach (ANSI, 1986). When possible, it is advisable to locate switches and outlets at a comfortable reaching zone for the individual in a sitting or standing position (Figures 25-3 and 25-5). Raschko (1982) recommends that most electric outlets be installed between 27.3 and 36 inches above the floor. Additionally, the safety of all electrical switches and outlets is of utmost importance for all individuals and should be installed and inspected by a qualified electrician.

A variety of switches and outlets designed to make use of electrical devices easier and safer are available. Many of these are available in hardware and department stores or may be ordered through rehabilitation equipment companies. Following is a list of some adaptive devices:

1. Remote control switches that can be connected to control lights and other electrical devices from out-

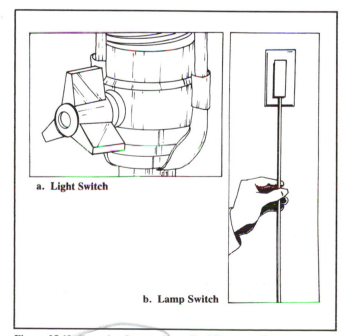

a. Light Switch

b. Lamp Switch

Figure 25-19. Extension Levers. *From Fred Sammons 1989 Professional Healthcare Catalog (1989). Burr Ridge, IL: Fred Sammons, Inc.*

side the home or from different rooms are available (Sears, Roebuck, and Company, 1987; Radio Shack, 1988).

2. Lamps which are activated by light touch to the lamp base eliminate the need to manipulate push-button or other on-off switches (Sears, Roebuck, and Company, 1987).

3. Wall light switches which have a rocker-type panel to activate lights can replace conventional wall switches for individuals with limited hand use (Sears, Roebuck, and Company, 1987).

4. Light switch extenders (a rod attachment that hangs down from the switch allowing the user to pull or push the rod) eliminate vertical reaching (Fred Sammons, 1988).

5. Lamp switch extension levers (Fred Sammons, 1988) and three spoke levers are available to replace standard lamp knob switches (Figure 25-19).

Lighting

The amount and quality of lighting is very important for task performance since it affects safety, task proficiency, and eye fatigue. Illumination "is a measure of the amount of light falling on, or incident to, a work surface or task from ambient and local light sources" (Eastman Kodak Company, 1983, p. 225). Illumination is measured with a lumination meter, which is placed directly on the work surface and measures the distance from the light source to the work surface. Eastman Kodak Company (1983) provides the recommendations of illumination levels for a range of tasks. The responsibility for the choice of the level of illumination in work settings should be left to the lighting engineer or supervisor at that work setting (Eastman Kodak Company, 1983).

Glare from light sources can decrease the contrast between work materials and the work surface, thus making task performance particularly difficult for those with limited visual capabilities. "Direct glare is caused when a source of light in the visual field is much brighter than the task materials at the workplace. Indirect glare, frequently called either veiling reflections or reflected glare, depending on its severity, is caused by light reflected from the work surface" (Eastman Kodak Company, 1983, p. 230). Grandjean (1971, p. 104) provides the following guidelines to avoid glare:

1. No light sources should appear in the visual field of the operator.

2. Unscreened illuminants should not be used in work rooms.

3. The angle between the horizontal line of sight and a line from the eye to the light source must be more than 30 degrees (Figure 25-20a).

4. If in large rooms an angle of less than 30 degrees cannot be avoided, the lights must be screened on the sides, and screened fluorescent tubes should lie across the line of sight.

5. To avoid glare from reflection, the workplace should be so positioned that the most frequently used lines of sight do not coincide with reflected light. No reflection area with contrast greater than 1:10 should lie within the visual field. (Figures 25-20b & 25-20c).

6. The use of polished surfaces or reflecting materials on machines, tabletops, switchboards, or other apparatus should be avoided.

Living Room Arrangement

A variety of activities take place in the living room. It may be used for conversation, leisure, or work tasks, depending upon the family customs. While construction of many living rooms is such that little structural modification is needed, the furniture arrangement should be such that all desired activities can occur with ease, independence, and safety for family members and friends.

The sofas and chairs can be placed closely together for individuals with hearing impairments so that it is easy to see the faces of other people as they talk (Levy, 1985). Individuals with movement disabilities should have the furniture arranged so that their approach to furniture is unobstructed. Wheelchair users need five feet of clear space for movement onto sofas and chairs. A clear pathway is also needed for individuals with movement disabilities, and it should be wide enough for the use of ambulatory devices or wheelchairs. For people with visual impairments, the living room should have a clearly established pathway, with certain pieces of furniture placed as guideposts along the way (Dickman, 1983). Items such as floor lamps, wastebaskets and magazine racks should be located outside of movement areas to prevent tripping.

The traditional low coffee tables placed in front of sofas restrict movement for people with mobility problems and cannot be used by those with poor sitting balance. Low coffee tables and other objects with horizontal projections can be a safety hazard for those with visual impairments (Dickman, 1983). Small, high tables at the side of a chair or sofa may be easier and safer to use than a low coffee table. Furniture is an intricate part of the environment which should not be overlooked when planning environmental modifications for individuals with disabilities. Chairs, tables, and shelves may impede task performance in the same manner that doors, walls, and steps do. When evaluating furniture for possible changes or modifications the following considerations should be kept in mind:

1. *Use of the furniture.* Determine who will be using the furniture and the purpose in which it will be used.

Evaluate the user's bodily dimensions, skills, and physical needs against the size, shape, and functional components of the furniture (See Figures 25-3 through 25-5).

2. *Ease in transfers*. The user should be able to move onto and off of the furniture with safety, ease, and comfort.

3. *Maintenance*. Evaluate the furniture's maintenance needs as well as the user's abilities and desire to perform maintenance.

4. *Flexibility*. Can the furniture be easily used for several tasks? Can it be used by more than one person?

5. *Safety*. The degree to which the furniture affects the user's and others' safety should be determined. Flammability is also an important safety consideration.

6. *Cost and durability*. The cost factor should be weighed against the durability of the furniture.

7. *Aesthetic and social appeal*. Furniture should be pleasant in appearance. Furniture that looks like it belongs in a hospital gives the appearance that the user is ill rather than having a disability, and may affect social interactions.

Kitchen Arrangement

Meal preparation is a task that involves many different activities including gathering and assembling food and tools, cooking, transporting food and utensils, serving, cleaning, and storage of food and utensils. The manner in which meal preparation is accomplished is greatly influenced by the kitchen's physical environment. Arrangement, workspace, appliances, and storage space all affect the ease, independence, and safety of meal preparation. It should be noted that a kitchen is a potentially dangerous location in any home. All modifications should be designed for optimal safety for all individuals within the household, including children.

Kitchen Floorplan. The amount and arrangement of space in the kitchen influences task organization and time and energy output. The number of movements one must make, the distance moved, and the amount of things to carry are all greatly affected by space and arrangement. This is an important consideration for individuals with weakness, incoordination, visual impairments, and those who are easily fatigued.

Kitchen design or layout should be determined by the needs of the individuals using the kitchens. The type of disability an individual has and the type of mealtime preparations he/she desires are important determinants. Obviously, in many situations it is impossible to change the

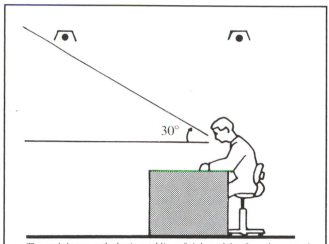

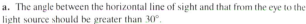

a. The angle between the horizontal line of sight and that from the eye to the light source should be greater than 30°.

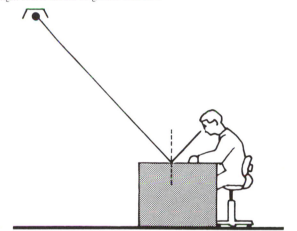

b. Unsuitable positioning of light source in relation to work place. Reflected light coincides with the line of sight, so that direct glare through reflection can occur.

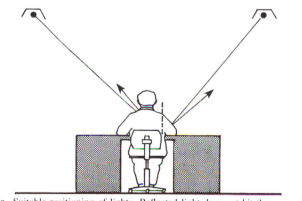

c. Suitable positioning of lights. Reflected light does not hit the eye and glare through reflection is avoided.

Figure 25-20a-c. Factors Effecting Glare. *From Grandjean, E. (1988). Fitting the task to the man—An ergonomic approach. 4th edition. New York, NY: Taylor and Francis, Inc.*

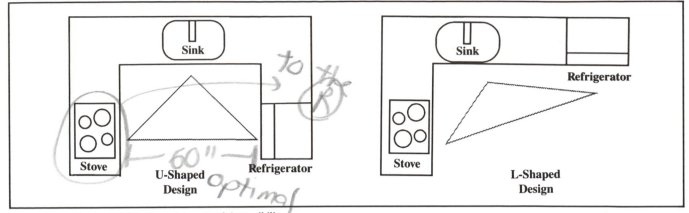

Figure 25-21. Kitchen Designs for Efficiency and Accessibility.

basic space design of the kitchen. In these instances, alternatives such as rearranging storage items, leaving items on the counter, and the use of movable carts for workspace may assist meal preparation.

The sink, range, workspace or preparation area, and refrigerator should be in easy access to each other to minimize movement during meal preparation (Sorensen, 1979; Wheeler, 1965). Ideally, the sink, refrigerator, and stove should be in a work triangle shape to minimize movement and concentrate work centers. There should be adequate work space on the sides of these stations for the placement and preparation of food and utensils. There should also be enough room so that the food and utensils can be moved by sliding rather than lifting and carrying.

An open area of at least five feet should be in front of each major appliance to allow for maneuverability of wheelchairs and ambulatory devices. Cabinet, refrigerator, or dishwasher doors should not be placed directly facing each other because when they are opened they will impede use. Following are several basic kitchen designs to consider for individuals with disabilities (Figure 25-21).

U-shaped and L-shaped designs. These two designs are generally considered the most desirable kitchen layouts. In a study to determine the most suitable arrangement for accessible kitchens, Steinfield, Schroeder, and Bishop (1979) found that the U-shaped and L-shaped kitchen designs were preferred by individuals in wheelchairs and that fewer bumps and accidents occurred in comparison to the one-wall and corridor kitchen layouts. These designs also reduce the distance traveled by an ambulatory individual. In these designs, it is preferable to place the sink in the middle, or corner, of the work triangle with a workspace on either side. Wheeler (1965) states that for ambulatory individuals, the stove should be placed at the right of the sink and within reaching distance of the sink so that minimal movement will be needed to reach between them.

The U-shaped design allows for continuous movement from one working space to another. Ideally, the sink and stove should be close to each other and separated by a working counterspace (Raschko, 1982). The distance between the two sides of the U-shape should be no less than 60 inches to allow for good turnaround space for people in wheelchairs and walkers (Anderson, 1981). However, the space should not be much larger than 60 inches to avoid fatigue due to long travel distances.

The L-Shaped design allows kitchen activity to be concentrated by placing working areas closer (Raschko, 1982). Movement between workcenters can be kept to a minimum in this design, reducing fatigue from lifting. Additionally, an L-shaped kitchen allows for the placement of a dining table in the corner, if desired (Goldsmith, 1976).

Corridor design. In this design the appliances and workspaces are on two facing walls and there is an opening at either end. This design can incorporate the basic triangle design between the sink, range, and refrigerator; however, utensils and food must be lifted and carried to different work areas instead of slid across the countertop, and frequent turning is needed. Another drawback of this design is that kitchen work may be interrupted by traffic through the room.

One-wall design. This design features all appliances and workspaces on one wall. This is the least efficient design as it requires moving across longer distance between work areas. It also requires turning in different directions which may be tiring for individuals using a wheelchair or walker.

Workspace. Workspace is needed for assembly, mixing and cleanup. The location and amount of work surfaces influences the organizational and time factors of mealtime activities. Work surface space should be designed so that minimal movement is required and so that a logical, efficient flow of tasks can be performed.

Workspace should be located near the stove, sink, and refrigerator. There should also be a place available to put dishes prior to serving meals. Orleans (1981) suggests a minimal counterspace of eighteen inches next to the opening side of the refrigerator door, twenty-four inches of heat-resistant surface to the left of the stove and thirty-six inches to the right, and twenty-four inches to the left of the sink. Work surfaces should be the same height for easy sliding of dishes and pans. Additional factors to consider when choosing the location of workspaces are any visual perceptual problems, such as hemianopsia.

Many kitchens lack an adequate amount of workspace. Extensions to the counter can be built to make additional space, or a table of a height suitable for the individual may be brought in to the kitchen. Fold-out tables or work surfaces can be installed on the wall and folded back up when not in use. Kitchen ''islands'' (free-standing cabinets) can also be installed to provide additional work surface. Counter extension boards, or bread boards, which slide back under the counter when not in use, are another alternative. Anderson (1981) suggests laying a piece of plywood over a drawer to make a pull out work area. Individuals using wheelchairs may want to use a tray on the wheelchair as a work surface.

A thirty-inch work surface should be available for food preparation (ANSI, 1986). Food preparation will be made easier if the workspace is adjacent to the sink. Stabilizing utensils and food while mixing, cutting, spreading, and rolling is difficult for many individuals with disabilities. Adaptations can be made to the work surface to provide stability during these activities. For instance, cutting boards can have holes cut into them for bowls to rest in while mixing; this will prevent the bowl from slipping (see figure 25-22). A plastic or wooden edge can be placed on the edge of the counter or cutting board so that bowls or food can be pressed against it as a means of stability. Another tactic for those with limited upper extremity use is to mount stainless steel nails in a cutting board so that vegetables can be stabilized by ''spearing'' them onto the nail. Numerous products are commercially available that can be used on the counter surface to aid in meal preparation (See Fred Sammons in list of manufacturers, Appendix B).

Counter Height and Depth. Figures 25-3 and 25-5 indicate the ideal height of counter surfaces for seated individuals. These measurements are for individuals without upper extremity dysfunction. Individuals with trunk or upper extremity limitations may not be able to reach as far and the counter will need to be adjusted to meet their needs.

Counter surfaces can be lowered by removing the baseboard of the counter (Garee, 1979). Wheeler (1965) suggests that for individuals in wheelchairs, a pull out board,

twenty-eight inches high, be used for heavy work tasks of stirring, chopping and slicing. This requires that the individual work parallel to the board because the wheelchair will not go under it. Knee and foot rest space under counters should be provided for individuals in wheelchairs (Figure 25-23). Opening or removing the counter doors beneath the work surface may provide the space needed for knees and footrests.

The work surface height will have to be adjusted for individuals who are ambulatory, so that they have an easy forward reach to the counter.

Storage Space. Storage spaces influence safety, task speed, amount of movement needed, and organization of meal preparation activities. Each work area should have storage space that is designed to facilitate the activities taking place there. Lowman and Klinger (1969) offer the following general guidelines for storage in the kitchen (p. 344):

1. Evaluate all utensils used. Keep only those necessary, replacing any nonessential ones with multipurpose tools.
2. Keep two sets of much used articles such as measuring spoons.
3. Store tools in such a way that they can be grasped easily.

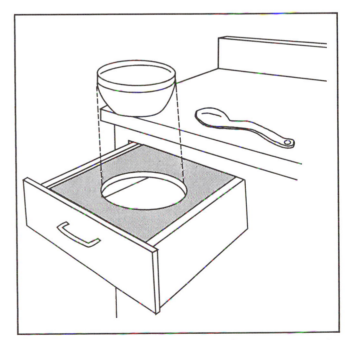

Figure 25-22. Kitchen Drawer Adaptation. *From How to create interiors for the disabled: a guide for family and friends by Jane Randolph Cary. Illustrations by Philip E. Farrell, Jr. Text copyright © 1978 by Jane Randolph Cary. Illustrations copyright © 1978 by Random House, Inc. Reprinted by permission of Pantheon Books, a Division of Random House, Inc.*

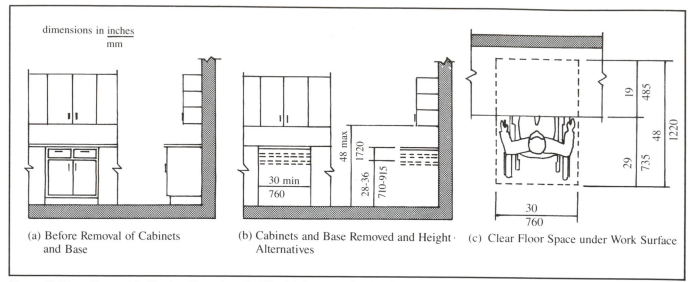

dimensions in <u>inches</u>
mm

(a) Before Removal of Cabinets and Base

(b) Cabinets and Base Removed and Height Alternatives

(c) Clear Floor Space under Work Surface

Figure 25-23a-c. Counter Modification Dimensions for Wheelchairs. *Reproduced with permission from American National Standard for buildings and facilities—providing accessibility and usability for physically handicapped people (ANSI A117.1), copyright 1986 by the American National Standards Institute. Copies of the Standard may be purchased from the American National Standards Institute at 1430 Broadway, New York, NY 10018.*

4. Group things by usage; for baking, keep ingredients, mixing bowls, rolling pin, cake, and pie plates in the same area.

5. Store items so that one may be removed without having to lift others.

6. Many utensils belong where first used; i.e., keep the coffee pot near the sink for water.

7. Have reaching device at hand.

8. Place heavy objects in such a way as to minimize or eliminate lifting. For instance, a countertop or pullout board can remain in place and simply be wiped off after use.

9. Keep food where there is adequate ventilation and even temperature.

Shelves.

1. Adjustable shelves allow placement at the optimal reaching zone for the user.

2. Shelves should be narrow in depth. A depth of four inches for shelves allows items such as cans and boxes to be stored without having other items in front of them (Rusk, Kristeller, Judson, Hunt, & Zimmerman, 1970). This allows items to be easily located and facilitates reaching.

3. A narrow wooden edge on the front of each shelf will help prevent objects from falling. This may be helpful for individuals with coordination or vision problems.

4. Corner areas in kitchens can be wasted areas. Shelves that are placed at a diagonal in the corner minimize reaching. Lazy Susans can also make corner space more usable.

5. Shelves with vertical partitions can be used to store

wide items such as pans and mixing bowls (Lowman & Klinger, 1969). This allows the cook to reach one item at a time without lifting or moving other items out of the way. Interval grooves allow the shelves to be placed at a desired width. This type of shelf is useful near the stove or mixing area.

6. Labels using words or pictures can be placed at each storage area to indicate the content. This may be helpful for those with cognitive disorders. Labels can be printed in braille for the blind.

Cabinets.

1. Individuals who use wheelchairs may wish to remove undercounter cabinets so that there is adequate footrest and knee space underneath the countertop. If it would be undesirable to remove the undercounter cabinets, a space next to the cabinet should be provided so that the person can reach into the cabinet from a side approach.

2. Some individuals may want to remove cabinet doors to aid in viewing and obtaining objects.

3. Items should be placed in the front part of the cabinet shelves. A narrow board can be attached to the shelf to prevent items from being pushed back out of reach. The location of the board on the shelf will depend upon the optimal reach zone of the users.

4. Cabinets with drawers that slide out can be very convenient because they reduce bending and reaching.

5. Vertical drawer partitions are helpful for storing items like cupcake pans, cookie sheets, and pan lids (Figure 25-24) (Lowman and Klinger, 1969).

6. Large D-shaped cabinet handles allow the hand to fit into the handle for easy opening. Handles should be placed at the bottom of the upper cabinets and at the top of below-counter doors. Pull strings may be attached to handles if they are difficult to reach.

7. Cabinet doors, drawers, and handles should be visually contrasted for those with visual impairments (Levy, 1985).

Pantries. Cary (1978) describes a roll-out pantry which is a free-standing, shallow storage unit that can be wheeled out from the wall so that the contents can be easily seen and reached (Figure 25-25). Each shelf has guard rails to prevent items from falling. A D-handle is used to pull each shelf out into the room. Laurie (1977) describes a series of pullout shelves which can be constructed as a storage and

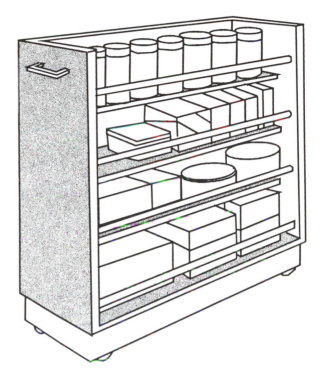

Figure 25-25. Roll-out Pantry. *From How to Create interiors for the disabled: a guide for family and friends by Jane Rudolph Cary. Illustrations by Philip E. Farrell, Jr. Text copyright © 1978 by Jane Randolph Cary. Illustrations copyright © 1978 by Random House, Inc. Reprinted by permission of Pantheon Books, a Division of Random House, Inc.*

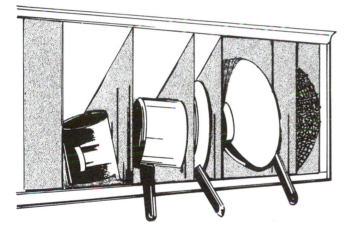

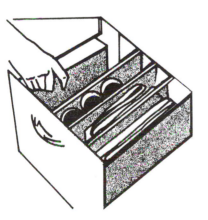

Figure 25-24. Vertical Storage. *From Lowman, E. & Klinger, J. (1969). Aids to independent living: Self help for the handicapped. New York, NY: McGraw-Hill.*

pantry area. Each shelf unit is mounted on wheels or a track which has a stop (Figure 25-26).

Additional storage options. Small adaptations that are inexpensive and require minimal construction can be made, and many of them may be purchased at hardware or department stores.

1. Storage bins on countertops may be used to provide additional storage that is within the user's reach zone.

2. Wall racks and hanging hooks can be placed in most locations in the kitchen for additional storage of pans and utensils.

3. Pegboard storage can be placed next to the stove, sink, and mixing areas, and on the inside of cabinet doors (Lowman and Klinger, 1969).

4. One- or two-tiered lazy Susans are convenient storage devices that help move small items closer to the user. They may be used on shelves or in cabinets, refrigerators, and bathrooms.

5. Utility carts may be used for storage as well as transportation.

6. Another alternative to storage problems is to leave

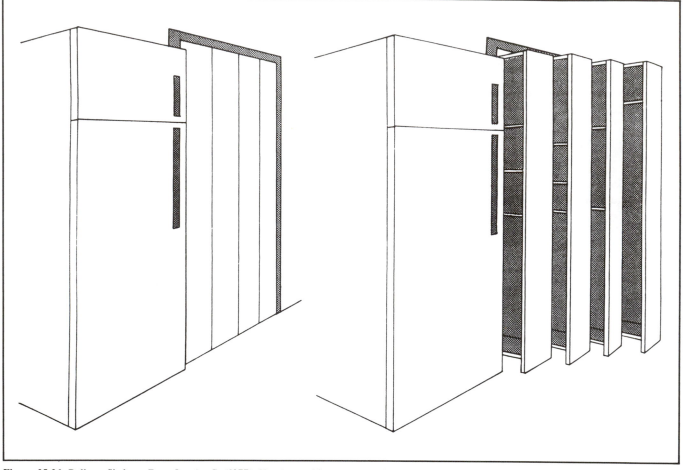

Figure 25-26. Roll-out Shelves. *From Laurie, G. (1977). Housing and home services for the disabled: Guidelines and experiences in independent living. Hagerstown, MD: Harper & Row.*

items in the place they are used rather than putting them away. For example, mixing bowls may be left on the counter and pans near the stove.

Refrigerator. The refrigerator may be a major physical barrier in the kitchen. Following is a list of some desirable features in a refrigerator:

1. A compact refrigerator may be more accessible for individuals with disability because the shelves and controls are easier to reach. Compact refrigerators should not be placed on the floor as this height is inconvenient for most individuals (Goldsmith, 1976). A compact refrigerator can be raised to an appropriate reaching level by mounting it on a stable base.

2. Refrigerator doors should open so that the door does not interfere with the pathway or movement of the users. The door should open away from the line of approach and, if possible, away from the the sink, stove, and work area. The door should open so that

the individual can remove objects from the refrigerator and easily place them on an adjacent counterspace. Refrigerators that have the option to hang the door from both the right and left side may be purchased.

3. A space next to the opening side of the refrigerator is desirable for wheelchair users so that a side approach is possible (Goldsmith, 1976). This may be a clear space under a countertop.

4. If the wheelchair user approaches the refrigerator from a side position the door should open 180 degrees (Goldsmith, 1976).

5. In many cases, the freezer should be at the top of the refrigerator with a door that opens in the same manner as the refrigerator door; however, very tall refrigerators may place the top freezer out of reach for many people. ANSI guidelines state that at least 50% of the freezer should be below 54 inches above the floor (1986). The freezer should not be below the refrigera-

tor, as the reach range is too great for many people who use wheelchairs or who have back injuries or weakness. Side-by-side refrigerator-freezers may be preferable for individuals who have a limited vertical reach; however, keep in mind that the doors open from the middle, which may cause approach and mobility difficulties.

6. Conveniences such as ice makers, self-defrosting freezers and external cold water spouts can be very helpful for individuals with upper extremity limitations. Units with these attachments require a plumbing hook-up and are more expensive than other refrigerators.

7. The door handle should be one which is easy for individuals with limited grasping abilities (for instance, a long D-shaped handle which allows the entire hand to be used in the opening). Magnetic door seals are helpful in the closing of the door (Raschko, 1982).

8. Refrigerator shelves should be vertically adjustable to meet the individual's reaching needs. Narrow shelf depth may be preferable for individuals with limited reaching capacities. Slide or swing out shelves may also be helpful features (Anderson, 1981).

9. Both the light and the temperature controls should be at the front of the refrigerator for easy access.

Sink. The sink dimensions affect all aspects of meal preparation including mixing, cooking, and cleaning and yet, the sink is frequently inaccessible for many individuals with disability. The faucet may be out of reach for a person sitting in a wheelchair. The sink may be too deep for the user's arms to reach the dishes. In some cases, the sink is totally inaccessible because the pipes underneath it are obstacles for the wheelchair user's legs and feet.

The sink's features should be evaluated in relation to the desired activities of the user and the user's skills. Modifications may range from simple additions to replacement with an accessible sink. The plumber should be made aware of the actual needs of the client so that appropriate modifications can be made.

ANSI (1986) provides the following guidelines for an accessible sink (page 70):

1. The sink and surrounding counter shall be adjustable or replaceable as a unit at variable heights between 28 and 36 inches (710 mm and 915 mm), measured from the finished floor to the top of the counter surface or sink rim, or shall be mounted at a fixed height no greater than 34 inches (865 mm), measured from the finished floor to the top of the counter surface or sink rim (Figure 25-27).

2. Where sinks are installed to be adjustable in height,

rough-in plumbing shall be located to accept connections of supply and drain pipes for sinks mounted at the height of 28 inches (710 mm).

3. The depth of a sink bowl shall be no greater than 6-1/2 inches (165 mm). Only one bowl of double-bowl or triple-bowl sinks need meet this requirement.

4. Base cabinets, if provided, shall be removable under the full 30-inch (760 mm) minimum frontage of the sink and surrounding counter. The finished flooring shall extend under the counter to the wall.

5. Counter thickness and supporting structure shall be 2 inches (50 mm) maximum over the required clear space.

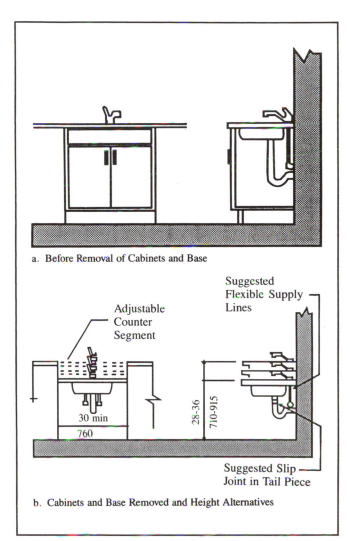

a. Before Removal of Cabinets and Base

b. Cabinets and Base Removed and Height Alternatives

Figure 25-27a, b. Adjustable Sink Specifications. *Reproduced with permission from American National Standard for buildings and facilities—providing accessibility and usability for physically handicapped people (ANSI A117.1), copyright 1986 by the American National Standards Institute. Copies of the Standard may be purchased from the American National Standards Institute at 1430 Broadway, New York, NY 10018.*

6. A clear floor space of 30″ by 48″ (760 mm by 1220 mm) shall allow forward approach to the sink. Nineteen inches (485 mm) maximum of clear floor space may extend underneath the sink. The knee space shall have a minimum clear width of 30″ (760 mm).

7. There shall be no sharp or abrasive surfaces under sinks. Hot water pipes and drain pipes under sinks shall be insulated or otherwise covered.

Many kitchen sinks are too deep for individuals in wheelchairs or with limited range of motion in the arms. If the sink cannot be replaced by a more shallow sink, drainage racks may be placed in the sink bottom to raise the height. If bumping and dropping cause problems, rubber mats can be used to line the sink to prevent breakage of dishes. To facilitate washing and scrubbing of dishes and pans, suction cup stabilizers or vertical scrub brushes with suction cup bottoms can be placed in the sink.

Frequently, sink drainage pipes come down from the middle of the sink and interfere with the wheelchair user's ability to get knees and feet under the sink. Additionally, exposed pipes may become very hot and be a hazard for those who have poor sensation in their legs. Sinks which have drainpipes in the back can be a good solution for this problem. Pipes should be insulated to prevent burns.

The faucet control levers should be easily operated with one hand and the force needed to activate them should not exceed 5 lbf (ANSI, 1986). Orleans (1981) recommends the use of faucets with single operation lever-type handles that control the water volume and temperature. Long-handled faucets which extend forward can be helpful for people with limited reach and limited strength. The faucet may be located at the side of the sink for individuals with severe strength and reach limitations. A tall gooseneck spigot can make tasks such as filling pans and washing large objects easier. The installation of retractable hose with a faucet end can be helpful for filling pans away from the sink or rinsing large objects in the sink.

Dishwasher. A dishwasher may be a helpful appliance for an individual who has difficulty washing and drying dishes. However, dishwashers may be difficult for many individuals to open, load, and empty as considerable bending and good balance are required. Orleans (1981) recommends that dishwashers have independent loading racks. The controls should be at the front of the dishwasher and require as little force as possible to start the machine. A side or front approach space of thirty to forty-eight inches is needed (Orleans, 1981).

Garbage Disposal and Trash Compacter. Garbage disposals and trash compacters can be very helpful for individuals with a disability because they reduce the amount of time and energy needed to package, carry, and dispose of trash. Consideration must be given to their cost, installation, maintenance, and space requirements.

Stove and Oven. Stoves and ovens should be evaluated carefully as these appliances greatly affect safety, speed of preparation, quality of food, and amount of cleanup needed. Conventional stoves may be barriers to cooking for individuals with disabilities, since the controls are frequently out of reach for users in wheelchairs or may be difficult for those with visual impairments to read. Reaching into the oven can be a safety hazard for individuals with poor balance or weakness.

Clear floor space of at least thirty by forty-eight inches should be in front of the stove and oven to allow for a forward or parallel approach. Countertop stoves which have knee space underneath are the most accessible for individuals who sit while cooking. The height of the stove should be the same as the adjacent counterspace and at an accessible height for the cook with a disability.

It is generally considered safer to have an electric stove rather than a gas stove because of the open flames of the gas stove (Goldsmith, 1976). The controls of the stove should be easily reached at the front or side and have lights to indicate whether the burners are on or off. The controls should be easily manipulated by individuals with poor grasp. Raised marks may be placed on the controls for individuals with vision impairments, and knob extenders are available for individuals with limited reach (Fred Sammons). The burners should be arranged to avoid

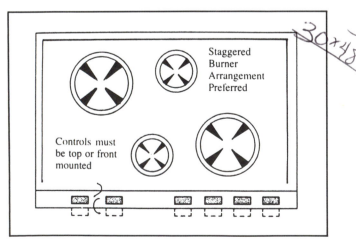

Figure 25-28. Recommended Stovetop Burner Arrangement. *From Garee, B. (1979). Ideas for making your home accessible, p. 59. Bloomington, IL: Cheever Publishing.*

[handwritten: 30×48]

*[handwritten: * Electric better than gas Don't get burner]*

reaching over hot surfaces to access rear heating elements, as seen in Figure 25-28. Metal guardrails around the side and front of the stove may prevent objects from getting knocked off the stove top. A mirror may be mounted at a 30-40 degree angle above the stovetop so that the seated individual will be able to see the contents of the pans more easily.

Steinfeld, Schroeder and Bishop (1979) studied oven types to see which type was easiest for individuals in wheelchairs to use. The results of their study indicated that individuals in wheelchairs could best use countertop ovens with side-hinged doors for cooking and oven cleaning. The conventional below-counter, drop door oven, without side space provided, was less satisfactory for individuals in wheelchairs as it was difficult to get close enough to transfer weighted pans into and out of the oven. It was also more difficult to clean this type of oven.

The height of the oven should be adjusted for the easiest reach into the oven. Goldsmith (1976) suggests that the height of the oven be adjusted so that the oven's middle shelf would be about the same height as the adjacent work surface. The shelves should move freely on the racks and should not tip. A stop on the shelves prevents accidentally pulling the shelves off the racks. Accessible space beside the oven is needed for placing pans as they are pulled out of the oven. Self-cleaning ovens are recommended. Oven controls should be on the front of the oven.

Small Cooking Appliances. When the use of an oven or stove is impractical or unsafe, one may consider the use of small electrical devices, such as microwave ovens, crockpots, or toaster ovens for meal preparation. Possible advantages include versatility in location and height, portability, cost, and ease in use. Klinger (1978) makes suggestions for choosing this type of cooking device:

1. Be sure that electrical outlets are powerful enough for the device to be used. If there are any doubts about the electricity, an electrician should be consulted.
2. Make sure that you can physically handle the appliance. Check out the type of handles and base it has. One should be able to safely move the appliance.
3. The appliance should have built-in safety features as well as switches and controls that adjust quickly. The appliance should be approved by Underwriters' Laboratories, a firm that tests products for manufacturers.
4. The appliance should be easy to clean.
5. The controls should be easy to read or understand and easy to manipulate.

Mealtime Transportation. Mealtime activities involve movement for preparation, serving, and cleanup. The distance traveled and number of repeated trips affects the endurance and efficiency of the involved individual. The kitchen environment should be arranged to decrease the amount of movement needed, as mentioned above.

Utility carts may be used to transport many items, reducing the number of trips, and requiring less energy to push than carrying heavy objects. Large castor wheels on utility carts make movement over carpet edges and bumps easier. The cart should be made of a heavy material so that it will not tip easily.

Dining Area

The psychosocial importance of eating should not be overlooked when planning the physical environment of the dining area. Meals represent more than the act of satisfying hunger. Meals provide the opportunity for social needs to be met. A disruption of this process due to environmental barriers can mean that an important chance to participate in social interaction is lost. The environment of mealtimes should be peaceful, easily accessible, and conducive to conversation. Attention should be given to the lighting, wall colors, acoustics, and spacing of tables and chairs.

Laundry

Laundry is a task that involves many activities. Washing activities include storage of dirty laundry, transportation of dirty laundry, sorting, placing laundry into the washing machine or sink, adding soap, and selecting the correct water setting. Once the clothes are washed, they are dried, folded, ironed, transported to storage areas, and placed in drawers or closets.

This lengthy chore requires skill in many performance areas. Cognitive and perceptual abilities are needed to plan and perform the task sequences and operate the machines. Necessary physical abilities include mobility, balance, grasp, and manipulation of the involved objects and machines. The manner in which the individual with a disability will perform laundry tasks will depend upon the client's preferences and an evaluation of his/her abilities as related to the tasks and the physical environment. The task can be accomplished by changing the activities of laundry or changing the physical environment. Modifying both may prove to be an effective solution.

Alternate procedures and shortcuts can reduce or eliminate laundry activities. For example, laundry duties can be assumed by other family members or the laundry may be done professionally, depending on the client's financial status. Some activities may be eliminated or changed. For example, if the dirty clothes are stored next to the washing machine instead of in a closet, laundry transportation is reduced. Anderson (1981) suggests placing different colored dirty clothes into separate sorting bins instead of placing them all into a large laundry basket, thus eliminating the requirement of sorting them from the large basket. Clothes removed from the dryer soon after they are dried may not need ironing if they are immediately hung up to dry. Sheet folding can be eliminated if the sheets are placed back on the bed soon after they become dry. Premeasured laundry soap packets that may be directly placed into the washing machine eliminate the need to measure and pour laundry soap.

Space around washers and dryers is needed to transport laundry and load and unload the machines. This space should be large enough for a person, any mobility device used, and the opened door of the machines. Individuals in wheelchairs need clear space to load the machines from a front, side, or parallel approach (Figure 25-29).

Front-loading washers and dryers are the best for individuals in wheelchairs as the bottom of the tub of top-loading machines is difficult to reach. The dryer lint trap should be in the front of the machine or in the door and the controls should be on the front of the machines, also. If the controls or lint trap are on the top side of the machine, a clear space at the side of the machine will allow closer contact to them. Reach extenders are available that may help the person reach the machine controls. If the person has a weak grasp, knob enlargers designed to aid in turning are available through rehabilitation equipment companies. Some washers and dryers have push-button controls that require very little strength.

A work table may ease some laundry activities, such as

spot removal and folding. The height should be between 28 and 36 inches, depending on the needs of the involved individual. The table depth should be no wider than a comfortable reaching distance. Anderson (1981) suggests attaching large snap clips on the wall above a laundry table so the corners of sheets and other laundry can be secured while the person with limited arm use folds over the other end.

The use of laundry or utility carts can ease laundry transportation difficulties. Bags with drawstrings or handles can also by used to transport laundry. Installing laundry chutes in two story houses can considerably reduce laundry transportation.

Individuals sitting in wheelchairs or with reduced standing tolerance may need to iron clothes while sitting. Small portable ironing boards are available that can be placed on table or counter tops. Ironing boards with wooden legs can be cut down to the desired height for ironing and ironing boards which are mounted to the wall or inside a closet or cabinet may be more sturdy than conventional ironing boards and can be moved out of the way when not in use. Lightweight irons and steamers may make ironing easier for people with weak upper extremities. Irons are available that automatically switch off if they fall or are left unattended which may be helpful for individuals with incoordination, weakness or forgetfulness.

Bedroom Arrangement

The bedroom should be designed so that sleeping, dressing and sexual activities may occur with as much ease, privacy, and independence as possible. The bedroom may also be used for other activities such as reading, conversing and watching television. The bedroom's environmental modifications will be determined by the activities to be performed and by the client's abilities.

The bedroom design should allow ease in bed transfers, access to dressers and closets, and convenient use of the telephone, light switches, and other necessary equipment. Sorensen (1979) recommends that there be five feet on one side of the bed for easy wheelchair transfers and three feet two inches on the other side of the bed. A free space five feet in diameter should be in front of the closet and dresser for forward and sideways wheelchair approaches and clear turnaround space. Individuals using crutches and walkers will need additional space to accommodate their assistive devices while using the closet and drawers. There must be enough space in front of the windows for opening and closing. Individuals who cannot get out of the bed may wish to have their bed moved to another room. In this case, Sorensen (1979) recommends that the bedroom door have a clearance of 44 inches to accommodate free access of a single bed.

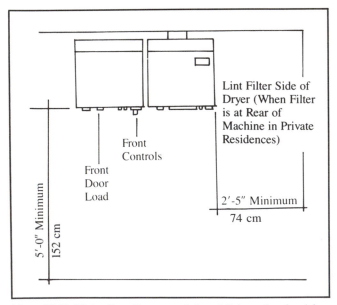

Figure 25-29. Washer/Dryer Recommendations. Minimum 1 washer, 1 dryer in each group to be wheelchair accessible (front controls, front load). Prefer front loading washer/dryer combination for wheelchair use where possible. *From Sorensen, R. (1979). Design for accessibility. New York, NY. McGraw-Hill Book Company.*

Bed. The bed choice depends upon the individual's disability and the physicians' recommendations. Those who eat, work, and spend leisure time in a bed may prefer an adjustable bed (so that, for instance, the head end could be raised). Lunt (1982) describes many types of adaptable beds including electrical hospital, manual hospital, and electrical nonhospital beds. She also describes bed equipment used to prevent skin breakdown, transferring devices, and positioning equipment.

The bed height affects transfers and visibility in the room and out of windows. The ideal height is determined by the individual's preferences and physical needs. An individual in a wheelchair usually needs the bed at the same height as the wheelchair seat to make transfers easier. Garee (1979) suggests that the bed height be no higher than 19 inches for wheelchair transfers and that there be 10-13 inches of clear space under the bed for the footrests.

An individual using a walker or cane may prefer the height of the bed to be equal to the distance between the floor and the back of the knee, while sitting with the hips, knees, and ankles at 90 degree angles. This height provides a stable base of support from which the individual can push off the floor with his/her feet. The bed height should not be lower than this, as pushing up from a lower height would require more strength and energy.

Individuals with arthritis, hip, or knee arthroplasty may have difficulty bending down to a typical bed height. In this case the bed height may be raised so that minimal hip and knee flexion are necessary. Sturdy side and head bed rails may be used to pull onto the bed and to prevent the individual from sliding off the bed.

Several options are available for bed height changes. The height can be lowered by cutting down the length of the legs or removing the bed castors. A large wooden platform placed at the side of the bed can be used as a step for beds that are too high. Bed legs can be made longer by using large wooden blocks with holes drilled in the middle in which to place the leg end. Commercially made, molded leg extenders are available that raise the bed leg three to five inches (Figure 25-30a, b). Another way to make the bed higher is to place the entire bed on a sturdy platform, thus raising it to the desired height. Commercially available adjustable beds allow the bed to be at the correct height during transfers and then changed for activities in the bed as needed.

Bed Work Surfaces. Bed work surfaces can be designed to allow many activities to be performed by individuals who lie or sit for long periods of time. These areas must be designed so that all items are within an easy forward and side reaching distance. A rim around the sides and back of the work area and bed tables prevents items from falling.

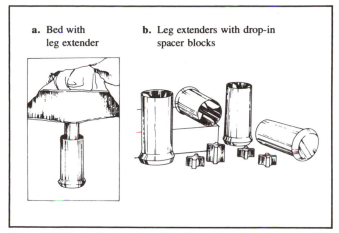

Figure 25-30a, b. Furniture Leg Extenders. *From Fred Sammons 1989 Professional Healthcare Catalog (1989). Burr Ridge, IL: Fred Sammons, Inc.*

Hospital tables, which are adjustable in height and angle, may be useful for home use. They are available through hospital supply companies. The "U" Modular Twin Turntable Desk (manufactured by Extensions for Independence) has an adjustable height work surface and built-in turntables on which items may be stored and easily retrieved while working in a bed, chair, or wheelchair (Figure 25-31).

Bedstands and Shelves. Bedstands and shelves placed at the side of the bed can increase the access to items needed for dressing, hygiene, work, hobbies, and eating. Telephones, emergency signals, and controls for the television, temperature and lights can be placed within easy reach on bedside tables or shelves. The height of bedstands and shelves should be no lower than the level of the bed mattress because reaching down while in the bed is an unsafe movement. The depth of tables and shelves should be no more than the distance the person can reach without loosing his/her balance. This furniture should be very stable to prevent it from being pushed over. Items placed on tables and shelves can be prevented from being pushed off by placing rims on the sides and backs.

Closets. The clothes rod should be at a height that is easy for the individual to reach. Raschko (1982) suggests that the clothes rod be mounted at a maximum height of 60 inches for ambulatory individuals. Individuals using ambulatory devices, or who have shoulder range of motion limitations will need the rod placed at lower ranges. Figure 25-32 shows the ANSI suggested maximum height for clothes rods for wheelchair users.

The clothes rod height can be adjusted by moving the hanging brackets. Another method to provide a lower clothes rod is to suspend a large dowel rod from the regular rod. This is accomplished by drilling holes in the ends of the dowel rod, placing a nylon cord through each end and tying the other ends to the rod. The length of the cords can be adjusted to suspend the dowel rod at the desired height.

Shelves in closets or in the room can be used for the storage of clothing and shoes. The height of shelves should be such that the farthest ranges, high and low, do not jeopardize balance or cause pain. Figure 25-32 shows the ANSI suggested shelf range for persons in wheelchairs. Many individuals with physical disabilities have difficulty reaching the floor. Shoes and other items can be stored on shelves instead of the floor. Also, hanging shoe and sweater racks, which are suspended from the closet rod, can be used inside closets. Wire racks mounted on the inside of closet doors can increase accessible storage space for shoes and folded clothing.

Drawers. Drawers should be placed at a height that is easily reached by the disabled individual. The drawers should be easy to push and pull. Narrow and shallow drawers are preferable because clothes removal is difficult from wide and deep drawers. A single, horizontally positioned, D-shaped pull handle, placed in the middle of the drawer, is the easiest for most individuals to use. Additionally, drawers should be equipped with stops to prevent the entire drawer from being pulled out of the dresser.

Bathroom

Customarily designed bathrooms pose one of the greatest architectural barriers for individuals with disabilities. The bathroom entrance, the floor plan, and the type of fixtures are frequently inaccessible for users of wheelchairs, canes, walkers, and those with weaknesses and incoordination. Glare from shiny porcelain, mirrors, and metal make

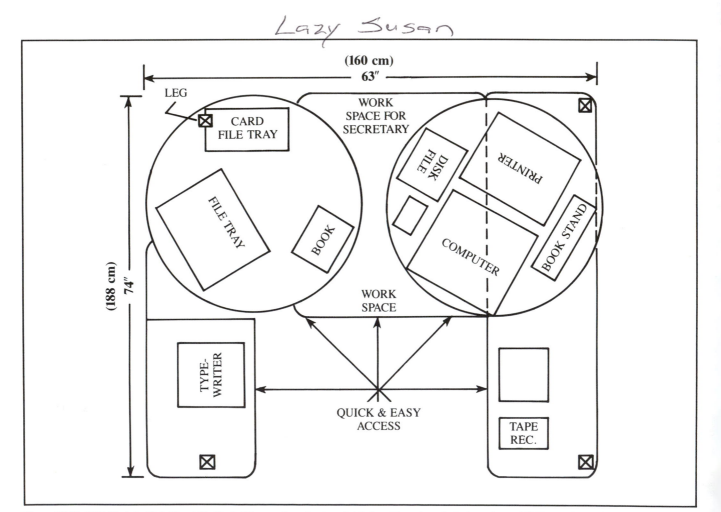

Figure 25-31. "U" Modular Twin Turntable Desk. *The creation of and available from Extensions for Independence, 757 Emory Street #514, Imperial Beach, CA 92032.*

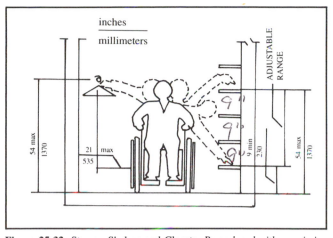

Figure 25-32. Storage Shelves and Closets. *Reproduced with permission from American National Standard for buildings and facilities—providing accessibility and usability for physically handicapped people (ANSI A117.1), copyright 1986 by the American National Standards Institute. Copies of the Standard may be purchased from the American National Standards Institute at 1430 Broadway, New York, NY 10018.*

activity difficult for those with visual impairment. The usual placement of cabinets, towel racks, toilet paper dispensers, and mirrors makes them hard for people with reaching problems to use. Additionally, the hard, slick, and wet surfaces of the bathroom are potentially hazardous for most individuals.

Floorplan. The bathroom floor space should be large enough for ease in entrance and exit through the door, approach to the sink, toilet, and bathtub or shower. Transfers at the bathtub and toilet and the use of additional equipment such as a wheelchair or a hoist also require sufficient floor space. A free space five feet in diameter allows for unobstructed maneuverability within the bathroom for wheelchair users. A minimum of four feet of clear area is needed in front of the sink, toilet, and tub or shower (Figure 25-33).

Toilet.

Toilet height. Toilet height affects the muscular angle of pull at the hips, knees, and ankles during transfer. Individuals with lower extremity joint pain, weakness, and limited range of motion may benefit from a raised toilet because less movement is required during transfer. Those transferring between a wheelchair and a toilet need a toilet height that is close to the height of the wheelchair seat. Cochran (1981) suggests a height of 19 inches at the top of the toilet seat. However, the best height must be calculated according to the person's size and abilities.

In the home, toilet height can be adjusted several ways. Commodes of differing heights are manufactured and can

be purchased for home use. A less expensive adaptation is the use of a raised toilet seat. A variety of raised toilet seats are available which, when attached to the toilet, add 2-6 inches in height to the seat. The seat should be stable during transfers and weight shifting while on the toilet. For individuals (particularly children) who need a lower toilet seat height, platforms can be constructed to facilitate standing transfers.

The posture of the individual on the toilet is affected by the toilet seat height. Standard toilet seats may be too high for children or small adults, causing their feet to dangle and placing the entire body in an abnormal, uncomfortable position. The height should be one in which the feet are stable and the angle of the hips, knees, and ankles are 90 degrees. This position places most people in a more relaxed and safe position. Foot platforms can be added at the base of the toilet to raise the feet and place the hips, knees, and ankles in a correct position. These platforms may be removed during assisted transfers, if necessary.

Grab bars and trunk support. Grab bars on reinforced walls are needed for stability on the toilet and during transfers. Some individuals who need help lowering and raising from the toilet may benefit from side and back grab bars (Figure 25-34). Toilet back supports, seat belts, and

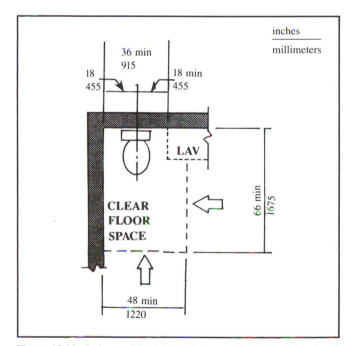

Figure 25-33. Bathroom Wheelchair Maneuverability. *Reproduced with permission from American National Standard for buildings and facilities—providing accessibility and usability for physically handicapped people (ANSI A117.1), copyright 1986 by the American National Standards Institute. Copies of the Standard may be purchased from the American National Standards Institute at 1430 Broadway, New York, NY 10018.*

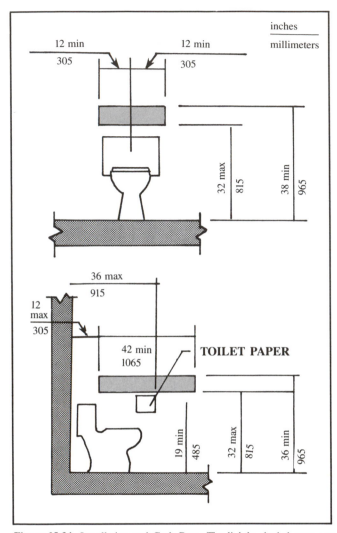

Figure 25-34. Installation and Grab Bars. The lightly shaded areas are reinforced to receive grab bars. *Reproduced with permission from American National Standard for buildings and facilities—providing accessibility and usability for physically handicapped people (ANSI A117.1), copyright 1986 by the American National Standards Institute. Copies of the Standard may be purchased from the American National Standards Institute at 1430 Broadway, New York, NY 10018.*

harnesses can be attached to the toilet for individuals who have poor sitting balance. These are available through rehabilitation equipment companies.

Flush control. Flushing the toilet can be difficult for persons with poor balance, weakness, or limited reach. The location and shape of the handle can make this activity more difficult, and various alternate flush controls are available, including light activated, weight activated, and push-button controls. Flush controls are standardly mounted on the left of the toilet tank. Toilet tanks with flush control on the right can be obtained for individuals with limited use of one side of the body. Flush control adaptations can be added to the

handle to make it longer and bigger for easier pushing (Fred Sammons, 1988).

Portable toilets. Some individuals may need a toilet in a location outside the bathroom. These are available through medical supply companies. The portable toilet must be stable for transfers and while sitting. Privacy considerations are important in the use of portable toilets and room partitions or curtains may provide some privacy.

Sinks. Conventionally installed bathroom sinks are inaccessible for many individuals with physical disabilities. The sink depth should be no greater than 6-1/2 inches (ANSI, 1986). The drainpipes should be in the back and should be wrapped or protected so that hot pipes or sharp edges will not harm legs (Figure 25-35). Faucets should be within easy reaching distance for the person using the sink and the controls should be easily operated. Wristblade faucet han-

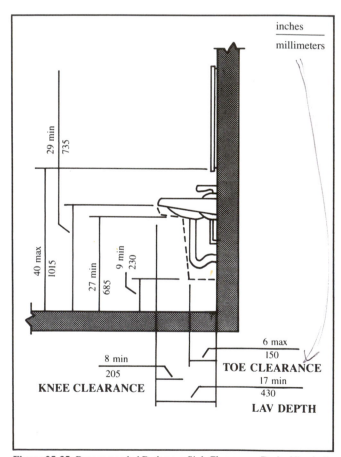

Figure 25-35. Recommended Bathroom Sink Clearances. Dashed line indicates dimensional clearance of optional underlavatory enclosure. *Reproduced with permission from American National Standard for buildings and facilities—providing accessibility and usability for physically handicapped people (ANSI A117.1), copyright 1986 by the American National Standards Institute. Copies of the Standard may be purchased from the American National Standards Institute at 1430 Broadway, New York, NY 10018.*

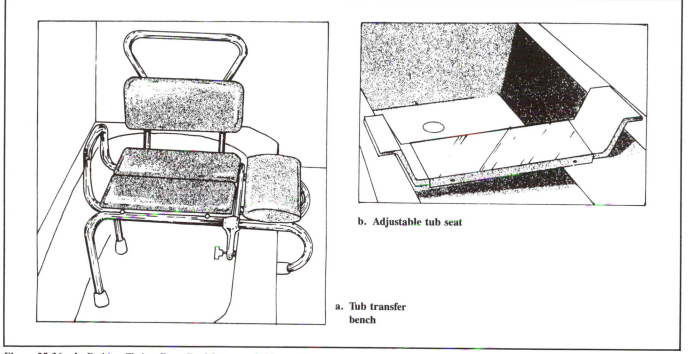

b. Adjustable tub seat

a. Tub transfer bench

Figure 25-36a, b. Bathing Chairs. *From Fred Sammons 1989 Professional Healthcare Catalog (1989). Burr Ridge, IL: Fred Sammons, Inc.*

dles, which are flat handles that extend forward toward the sink, are easily operated by the push of the hand, wrist, or elbow (Cary, 1978). Another faucet option is a lever action, single control faucet which can be mounted at knee level (Raschko, 1982).

The height of the bottom edge of the sink should be no more than 34 inches (ANSI, 1986). The top edge of the mirror can be tilted away from the wall for better visibility. Full length mirrors can be placed in the restroom at other locations if the area in front of the sink is inaccessible. Also, mirrors mounted on movable extension rods can be mounted near the sink.

Medicine Cabinet. Medicine cabinets in bathrooms are frequently placed too high for use by individuals with limited reaching range. New cabinets can be installed so that the bottom edge of the cabinet is only two inches above the sink height (Raschko, 1982). D-shaped handles can be mounted on the door to make opening and closing it easier.

The use of shelves, pegboards and hooks mounted to the wall near the sink can be an alternative to medicine cabinets. Storage bins placed in accessible locations can be used for the storage of hair dryers, large bottles of shampoo, and other large items. These open storage adaptations will be unacceptable for storage of medicines and potentially harmful items in households with family members who do not understand the danger of these products.

Towel and Clothing Racks. Towel racks should be securely mounted at an easy forward reach height for each person. The rack can be of contrasting color to the surrounding wall for individuals with visual impairments. Towel racks are not constructed sturdily enough to be used as grab bars. Plastic or wooden hooks and pegs are easily mounted alternatives to towel racks and may be used for towels or clothing. If hooks are used, they should be securely attached to the wall and should be big enough to hold large articles of clothing. Hooks should not have sharp, pointed edges.

Bathtub and Shower. The use of traditional bathtubs and showers is difficult for many individuals. Bathtub sides are too high and the bottoms are too low for some individuals to get out of once they are sitting. Shower stalls may be too narrow, the ledge may be difficult or impossible to step over, and the controls may be too high and too difficult to use. The surfaces of tubs and showers are hard and slippery and as such, are dangerous.

Structural changes to the bathtub or shower should be made with the advice of an architect, carpenter, electrician, and plumber as these changes are expensive and require the knowledge of structural support, electricity, and plumbing. Following are suggestions to make mobility easier and safer in the bathtub and shower:

1. Numerous types of bathtub and shower chairs are

Color contrast items for visually impaired individuals

available to be used while bathing (Figure 25-36a, b).

2. Flexible shower attachments which can be mounted on the wall at a desired height or held in the hand while sitting allow better control over water flow than traditional showers or bathtub faucets.

3. Nonskid mats or friction tape help prevent slipping in tub or shower and provide a color contrast for the visually impaired person.

4. Wide, contrasting color friction tape on the edge of the tub or shower helps people with visual impairment during transfers while bathing (Dickman, 1983).

5. Grab bars are needed on the side, front, and back tub and shower walls. Many people need a grab bar on the edge of the tub rim, as well (Figure 25-37a, b).

6. Faucets should have single mixing control and be easy to use. The temperature of the water should not exceed 115 degrees F (Raschko, 1982).

7. Sliding shower doors should be removed as they block transfers into the tub and, since they are not very sturdy, may present a safety risk.

8. Shower stalls may be safer and easier for transfers than bathtubs. However, they usually have an outside rim which makes wheelchair transfers difficult.

Shower chairs are helpful for individuals with poor standing abilities and endurance.

9. Wheelchair or ''roll-in'' showers allow the user in an ambulatory device or wheelchair to move into the shower without having to navigate ledges at the front of the shower stall. These are available in custom made or premade fiberglass units through manufacturers of bathroom facilities.

Workplace

Concern for the design of the workplace in relation to human function has gained considerable attention in many areas of industry (Eastman Kodak, 1983; Grandjean, 1971; MacLeod, 1982). As a result of this attention, two important factors have been recognized: (1) All people do not have the same bodily dimensions in weight, size, height, and strength, and (2) The work environment should be adjusted to ''fit'' the abilities and limitations of the human worker, not the reverse. This is important for all individuals, regardless of age, sex, or physical or psychosocial impairment.

Considerable research concerning worker and workplace fit has gone on in the field of ergonomics. Occupational therapists should be acquainted with this research as it

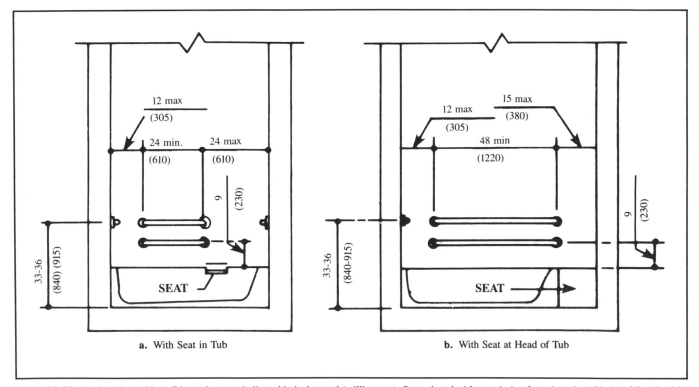

a. With Seat in Tub **b.** With Seat at Head of Tub

Figure 25-37a, b. Grab Bars. Note: Dimensions are indicated in inches and (millimeters). *Reproduced with permission from American National Standard for buildings and facilities—providing accessibility and usability for physically handicapped people (ANSI A117.1), copyright 1986 by the American National Standards Institute. Copies of the Standard may be purchased from the American National Standards Institute at 1430 Broadway, New York, NY 10018.*

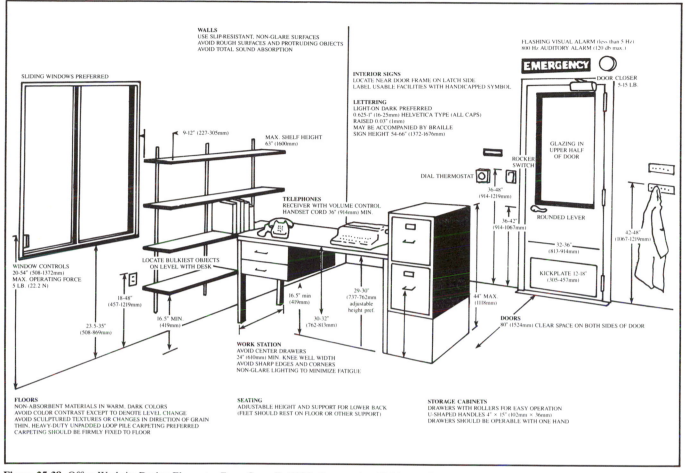

Figure 25-38. Office Worksite Design Elements. *From Gray, K. (1986). Ergonomics: Making products and places fit people. Illustration by James Mueller. Hillsdale, NJ: Enslow Publishers, Inc.*

directly relates to performance in work, school, and home settings. The Recommended Readings and Reference sections of this chapter list several excellent resources concerning ergonomics in the work and home settings.

Careful consideration should be given to the physical setting of the work environment. Figures 25-38 and 25-39 are examples of ergonomically designed office and industrial worksites. The following section addresses sitting and standing workstations. Niemeyer (1988) states that one purpose of workplace modification is to keep workers with pain in correct alignment to allow function and to allow frequent small postural adjustments as needed while working.

Seated Workplace. Seated work usually involves work on a surface in front of the body, as with such tasks as reading, typing, writing, and small assembly. Tasks that are best performed in seated positions are those in which (1) all needed items are within easy reach, (2) the hands will not

need to work above a six inch level above the table, and (3) no large forces are needed (no greater than ten pounds) (Eastman Kodak, 1983).

The chair is very important because it is the base of support for all tasks. The manner in which a person is seated greatly influences muscle tone, movement patterns, and skeletal integrity, which are needed for occupational performance involving the head and use of the arms and hands. Poorly seated individuals may not have the proximal hip, trunk, and shoulder mobility and stability to perform tasks, and thus are at risk to fatigue easily and develop contractures, pain, and pressure sores. For example, if a chair seat is too high, the posture assumed may be one of too much ankle plantarflexion, hip flexion, spinal kyphosis, cervical neck hyperextension, and elevated and protracted scapulae. This type of posture may contribute to back and neck pain, poor circulation in the legs and shoulder pain (Figure 25-40).

No one seating system, including wheelchairs, can meet

the needs of all workers. Further in-depth information concerning seating system design can be found in resources in the Recommended Readings section (Diffrient, Tilley, & Bardagjy, 1974; Eastman Kodak Company, 1983; Grandjean, 1971). In general, a good chair should maintain the hips, knees, and ankle joints at 90 degree angles. The natural lordosis of the lumbar spine should be maintained. Seating should be accessible for the users, with ease in approach and transferring onto and off of the chair.

The table height should be such that the seated individual has clearance for his/her knees. ANSI (1986) recommends a minimum of 27 inches for knee clearance for individuals sitting in wheelchairs. The angle of the elbows should be approximately 90 degrees when the upper arm is at the side of the body (MacLeod, 1982). Objects should not be placed outside the person's optimal reach zone (Figures 25-3 and 25-41). This means that the person should not have to bend at the spine in a forward or sideward manner, or lift up his/her hips to manipulate work materials.

Standing Work. Standing workplaces are generally used when objects to be handled weigh more than ten pounds, when reaching is required, when downward force is exerted and/or when movement around the workstation is needed (Eastman Kodak, 1983). Objects to be manipulated on the table should be within an easy reach.

The height of the work table depends upon the type of work being done. Precise, fine manipulation should be performed with the table height at approximately elbow height (MacLeod, 1982; Eastman Kodak, 1983; ANSI, 1986). However, some fine work will require higher tables due to visual requirements with small objects. Heavy and large work requiring strength is best performed with a lower table (Figure 25-42). ANSI (1986) suggests a height of approximately ten inches below the elbow height for heavy work for a standing person. However, it should not be so low as to require forward bending of the spine.

Footrests or rails can be used on which to place a foot

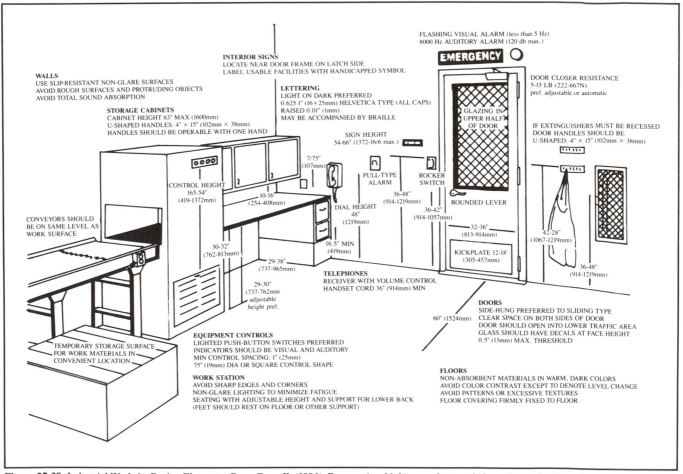

Figure 25-39. Industrial Worksite Design Elements. *From Gray, K. (1986). Ergonomics: Making products and places fit people. Illustration by James Mueller. Hillsdale, NJ: Enslow Publishers, Inc.*

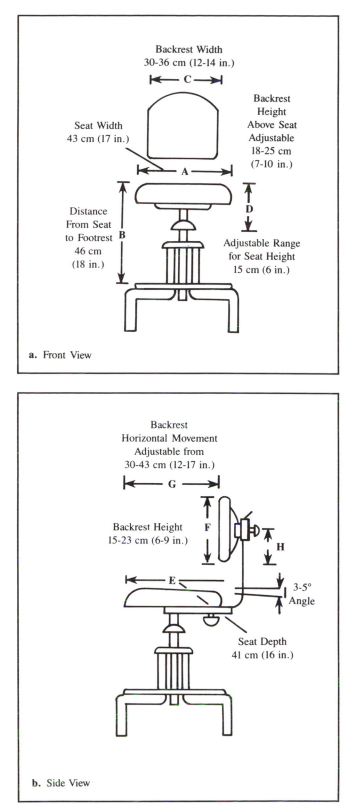

a. Front View

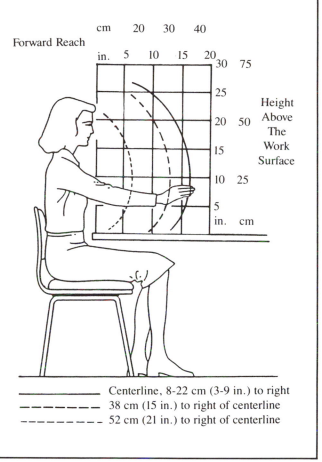

Figure 25-41. Forward Reach Capability of a Small Operator, Seated. Three curves describe the seated reach workspace for a 5th percentile female's right hand. The forward reach capability (horizontal axis) is affected by the height of the hands above the work surface (vertical axis) and by the arm's distance to the right of the body's centerline, as indicated by the three curves defined at the bottom of the figure. At 25 cm (10 in.) above the work surface, for example, the forward reach is 41 cm (16 in.) if the arm is within 23 cm (9 in.) of the centerline; if it is moved 53 cm (21 in.) to the right, forward reach falls to 18 cm (7 in.). *From Eastman Kodak. Ergonomic Design for People at Work, Volumes 1 and 2. Rochester, NY: Eastman Kodak Company.*

b. Side View

Figure 25-40 a, b. Recommended Chair Characteristics. *From Eastman Kodak (1983). Ergonomic Design for People at Work, Volumes 1 and 2. Rochester, NY: Eastman Kodak Company.*

while working in a standing position. This may relieve stress to the lower back while standing. Additionally, a high stool which has a footrest should be available if the worker chooses to sit while working.

Work Storage and Shelf Areas. Shelves and work storage should be within the optimal reach zone of the worker (Figures 25-3 and 25-41). Shelves and storage furniture should be very stable to prevent them from falling over onto the users. Clear space should be allowed in front of shelves for approach and reaching. If a forward approach

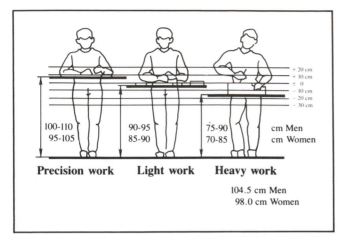

Figure 25-42. Optimal Counter Heights for Standing Workers. The horizontal zero line indicates the height of the elbow above the floor: on average this is 104.5 cm for men and 98 cm for women. When adjusting the height of the work for an individual it is necessary to start with the elbow height. *From Granjean, E. (1988). Fitting the task to the man—An Ergonomic approach. 4th edition. New York, NY: Taylor and Francis, Inc.*

is needed there should be space under the shelf to allow room for wheelchair arms and footrests.

The back of the shelf should not be deeper than the optimal reach zone, as items may slide back beyond the user's reach. If a shelf is too deep an edge may be placed on the surface at the limit of the reach zone so that items can not be pushed backwards. Edges may be painted a contrasting color for individuals with visual impairments.

SUMMARY

The physical barriers of the typical home and work environment are numerous and greatly influence the manner in which individuals are able to perform chosen occupations. These barriers may impede the performance of work, leisure, and self-care tasks. Task performance difficulty may result in loss of competency and feelings of low self-esteem. Additionally, inability to perform these tasks may result in dependence upon others and in changes in residency from one's home to a care facility.

Occupational therapists are instrumental in helping individuals to overcome physical barriers by discussing modification options and assisting in the implementation of their use. These options include personal, social, and physical intervention strategies. This chapter focused on intervention strategies to modify the physical environment. These intervention options vary greatly in cost, time consumption, and need for professional assistance.

The physical, cognitive, and perceptual characteristics of

the client are important factors in determining the manner in which barriers will be eliminated. However, the most important factors in the selection of intervention strategies are the desires and choices of the individual who will be using them. These must form the basis of the intervention used to overcome environmental barriers. The intervention goal should be to assist each person to live as independently as he/she chooses and to develop competencies in all valued roles. These are basic needs of all individuals, with or without disability.

Study Questions

1. Describe the purpose of the Architectural & Transportation Barriers Compliance Board.

2. List those factors, or determinants, which affect the intervention options in the development of an accessible environment.

3. Define the term "ergonomics."

4. Describe ways in which to eliminate barriers caused by traditionally-used doors within a facility.

5. Describe ways in which to enhance function and minimize hazards within a building for individuals with limited vision.

6. Discuss the benefits of the U-shaped or L-shaped kitchen designs over that of the corridor or one-wall kitchen designs.

7. Describe ways in which to adapt storage areas for individuals with reaching limitations.

8. Describe the important physical characteristics of an office workplace environment which may affect the efficiency of the worker.

Recommended Readings

American National Standards Institute, Inc. (1986). *American National Standard for buildings and facilities—Providing accessibility and usability for physically handicapped people.* New York.

Bednar, M.J. (1982). *Barrier-free environments.* New York: Van Nostrand Rheinhold

Cary, J.R. (1978). *How to create interiors for the disabled.* New York: Pantheon Books.

Dickman, I.R. (1983). *Making life more livable: Simple adaptations for the homes of blind and visually impaired older people.* New York: American Foundation for the Blind.

Diffrient, N., Tilley, A., & Bardagjy, J. (1974). *Human scale, 1/2/3*. Cambridge, MA: MIT Press.

Diffrient, N., Tilley, A., & Harman, D. (1974). *Human scale, 4/5/6*. Cambridge, MA: MIT Press.

Diffrient, N., Tilley, A., & Harman, D. (1974). *Human scale, 7/8/9*. Cambridge, MA: MIT Press.

Eastman Kodak Company. (1983). *Ergonomic design for people at work, vol 1*. New York: Van Nostrand Reinhold Company.

Eastman Kodak Company. (1986). *Ergonomic design for people at work, vol 2*. New York: Van Nostrand Reinhold Company.

Gay, K. (1986). *Ergonomics: Making products and places fit people*. Hillside, NJ.: Enslow Publishers.

Leibrock, C. & Rowe, L. (1981). Interior furnishings and space planning. *Access information bulletin*. Washington, DC: National Center for a Barrier Free Environment.

Lunt, S. (1982). *A handbook for the disabled: Ideas & inventions for easier living*. New York: Charles Scribners' Sons.

Raschko, B. (1982). *Housing interiors for the disabled and elderly*. New York: Van Nostrand Reinhold Company.

Sorensen, R. (1979). *Design for accessibility*. New York: McGraw-Hill Book Company.

Steinfeld, E., Duncan, J., & Cardell, P. (1977). Toward a responsive environment: The psychosocial effects of inaccessibility. In Bednar, M. (Ed.). *Barrier-free environments*. Stroudsburg, PA: Dowden, Hutchinson & Ross, Inc.

Steinfeld, E., Schroeder, S., & Bishop, M. (1979). *Accessible buildings for people with walking and reaching limitations*. Washington, DC: U.S. Government Printing Office.

Tichauer, E. (1978). *The biomechanical basis of ergonomics: Anatomy applied to the design of work situations*. New York: John Wiley & Sons.

U.S. Consumer Product Safety Commission. (1986). *Safety for older consumers*. Washington, DC: U.S. Consumer Product Safety Commission.

Wheeler, V.H. (1965). *Planning kitchens for handicapped homemakers*. New York: Institute of Rehabilitation Medicine.

References

Adaptive Environments Center. (1981). *Environments for all children*. Washington, DC: National Center for a Barrier Free Environment.

Aitken, M.J. (1982). Self-concept and functional independence in the hospitalized elderly. *American Journal of Occupational Therapy, 36,* 243-250.

American Institute of Architects Foundation. (1985). *Design for aging: An architect's guide*. Washington, DC: The AIA Press.

American National Standards Institute, Inc. (1986). *American National Standard for buildings and facilities—providing accessibility and usability for physically handicapped people*. New York: American National Standards Institute.

Anderson, H. (1981). *The disabled homemaker*. Springfield, IL: Charles C. Thomas.

Barrier Free Environments, Inc. (1981). Doors and entrances. Access Information Bulletin, Raleigh, NC: National Center for a Barrier Free Environment.

Burke, J.P. (1977). A clinical perspective on motivation: Pawn versus origin. *American Journal of Occupational Therapy, 31,* 254-258.

Cary, J.R. (1978). *How to create interiors for the disabled*. New York: Pantheon Books.

Chiou, I.L. & Burnett, C.N. (1985). Values of activities of daily living: A survey of stroke patients and their home therapists. Physical Therapy, 65*(6), 901-906*.

Christiansen, C., Schwartz, R., & Barnes, K. (1988). Self-care: Evaluation and management. (pp. 95-115). In DeLisa (Ed.). *Rehabilitation medicine: Principles and practice*. Philadelphia: J.B. Lippincott.

Cochran, W. (1981). Restrooms. *Access information bulletin*. Washington, DC: National Center for a Barrier Free Environment.

Colvin, M. & Korn, T. (1984). Eliminating barriers to the disabled. *American Journal of Occupational Therapy, 38*(11), 748-753.

Corlett, E., Hutcheson, C., DeLugan, M., & Rogozenski, J. (1972). Ramps or stairs: The choice using physiological and biomechanic criteria. *Applied Ergonomics*, December, 195-201.

Cotler, S. (1981). Elevator & lifts. *Access information bulletin*. Washington, DC: National Center for a Barrier Free Environment.

Crystal, S., Flemming, C., Beck, P., & Smolka, G. (1987). *The management of home care services*. New York: Springer Publishing Company.

Dickman, I.R. (1983). *Making life more livable: Simple adaptations for the homes of blind and visually impaired older people*. New York: American Foundation for the Blind.

Diffrient, N., Tilley, A., & Bardagjy, J. (1974). *Human scale, 1/2/3*. Cambridge, MA: MIT Press.

Eastman Kodak Company. (1983). *Ergonomic design for people at work, vol. 1*. New York: Van Nostrand Reinhold Company.

Eastman Kodak Company. (1986). *Ergonomic design for people at work, vol. 2*. New York: Van Nostrand Reinhold Company.

Federal Register. (1984). Volume 49, Number 153. Washington, DC: General Services Administration, Department of Defense, Department of Housing and Urban Development, U.S. Postal Service and the Architectural and Transportation Barriers Compliance Board.

Federal Register. (1988). Volume 53, Number 215. Washington, DC: Department of Housing and Urban Development.

Fisher, K. & Gardner, K. (Eds.). (1987). *Quality and home health care: Redefining the tradition*. Chicago: Joint Commission of Accreditation of Healthcare Organizations.

Friedman, J. (1986). *Home health care*. New York: W.W. Norton & Company.

Garee, B.E. (1979). *Ideas for making your home accessible*. Bloomington, IL: Cheever Publishing.

Gay, K. (1986). *Ergonomics: Making products and places fit people*. Hillside, N.J.: Enslow Publishers.

Goldsmith, S. (1976). *Designing for the disabled (3rd ed.)*. London: RIBA Publications Limited.

Grandjean, E. (1971). *Fitting the task to the man—An ergonomic approach*. London: RIBA Publications Limited.

Hopf, P. & Raeber, J. (1984). *Access for the handicapped: The barrier-free regulations for design and construction in all 50 states*. New York: Van Nostrand Reinhold Company.

Kielhofner, G. (1983). Occupation. In Hopkins, H. & Smith, H. *Willard and Spackman's occupational therapy*. Philadelphia, Pennsylvania: JB Lippincott Company.

Kiewel, H. (1986). Ramps, Stairs and Floor Treatments. *Access information bulletin*. Washington, DC: Paralyzed Veterans of America.

Klinger, J. (1978). *Mealtime manual for people with disabilities and the aging (2nd ed.)*. Camden, NJ: Campbell Soup Company.

Laurie, G. (1977). *Housing and home services for the disabled: Guidelines and experiences in independent living*. Hagerstown, MD: Harper & Row.

Leibrock, C. & Rowe, L. (1981). Interior furnishings and space planning. *Access information bulletin*. Washing-

ton, DC: National Center for a Barrier Free Environment.

Levy, L. (1985). Sensory changes and compensations. In *Role of occupational therapy with the elderly (ROTE)*. American Occupational Therapy Association, Inc.

Lowman, E. & Klinger, J. (1969). *Aids to independent living: Self-help for the handicapped*. New York: McGraw-Hill.

Lunt, S. (1982). *A handbook for the disabled: Ideas & inventions for easier living*. New York: Charles Scribners' Sons.

MacLeod, D. (1982). *Strains & sprains: A worker's guide to job design*. Detroit: United Automobile Workers Health and Safety Department.

Malick, M.H. & Almasy, B.S. (1983). Assessment and evaluation: Life work tasks (pp. 189-205). In Hopkins, H.L. & Smith, H.D. *Willard and Spackman's Occupational Therapy (6th ed.)*. Philadelphia: J.B. Lippincott Company.

Meredith Corp. (1981). *The Accessible Home: Remodeling Concerns for the Disabled*. Better Homes and Gardens Remodeling Ideas, July, 65-79.

Niemeyer, L. (1988). Job modifications for injured workers in sedentary jobs. *Work Programs Special Interest Section Newsletter, 2*(2), Published by The American Occupational Therapy Association, Inc.

Nugent, T. (1978). *The problem of access to buildings for the physically handicapped*. Farmington, CT: The Stanley Works.

Orleans, P. (1981). Kitchens. *Access information bulletin*. Washington, DC: National Center for a Barrier Free Environment.

Orleans, P. (1981a). Single family housing retrofit. *Access information bulletin*. Washington, DC: National Center for a Barrier Free Environment.

Raschko, B. (1982). *Housing interiors for the disabled and elderly*. New York: Van Nostrand Reinhold Company.

Ross, E.C. (1978). New rehabilitation law. *Accent of Living*, Winter, p. 23.

Rusk, H., Kristeller, E., Judson, J., Hunt, G. & Zimmerman, M. (1970). *A manual for training the disabled homemaker. (4th ed.)*. New York: The Institute of Rehabilitation Medicine.

Sandler, A., Thurman, S., Meddock, T., & DuCette, J. (1985). Effects of environmental modification on the behavior of persons with severe handicaps. *Journal of the Association for Persons with Severe Handicaps, 10*(3), 157-163.

Slater, S., Sussman, M., Stroud, M. (1970). Participation in household activities as a prognostic factor for rehabilitation. *Archives of Physical Medicine*, 605-610.

Sorensen, R. (1979). *Design for accessibility*. New York: McGraw-Hill.

Steinfeld, E., Duncan, J., & Cardell, P. (1977). Toward a responsive environment: The psychosocial effects of inaccessibility. In Bednar, M. (Ed.). *Barrier-free environments*. Stroudsburg, PA: Dowden, Hutchinson & Ross, Inc.

Steinfield, E., Schroeder, S., & Bishop, M. (1979). *Accessible buildings for people with walking and reaching limitations*. Washington, DC: U.S. Government Printing Office.

U.S. Department of Education: Clearinghouse on the Handicapped (1987). *Pocket guide to federal help for individuals with disabilities*. Washington, DC: U.S. Department of Education.

Wheeler, V.H. (1965). *Planning kitchens for handicapped homemakers*. New York: Institute of Rehabilitation Medicine.

Wolfe, G., Waters, R., & Hislop, H. (1977). Influence of floor surface on energy cost of wheelchair propulsion. *Physical Therapy, 57*(9), 1022-1027.

CHAPTER CONTENT OUTLINE

Introduction

Definitions of Technology

History of Technology

Competencies Required by
Occupational Therapists

Information Sources for Technology

Matching Technology to Individual
Human Needs

Technological Applications

Service Delivery Models

Societal and Professional Issues
Regarding Technology Service
Delivery

Mandate to the Occupational Therapy
Profession

Mandate to Therapists

The Future of Technology and
Occupational Therapy

Summary

KEY TERMS

Biofeedback

Cognitive Rehabilitation

Databases

**Functional Electrical
    Stimulation (FES)**

Hardware

Headstick

**Human-Environment/Technology
    Interface Model (HETI)**

Light Pointers

Microchip

Mobility

Motor Training Software

Mouthwand

Optical Pointers

Positioning

Robots

Seating

Selection Techniques

Single Switch

Software

ABSTRACT

This chapter identifies the competencies needed by therapists to understand and
use technology effectively. Current technologies for direct intervention and
client support are reviewed, along with models for technological service
delivery. Emphasis is placed on the importance of matching technology to
individual human needs. U.S. legislation that governs the delivery of technology
for improving functional performance is identified, along with information and
funding sources. Societal and professional issues affecting the use of technology
in rehabilitation are discussed, and the need for occupational therapists to
increase their awareness of the potential of technology for improving
independence is argued.

Technological Approaches to Performance Enhancement

Roger O. Smith

"Any sufficiently advanced technology is indistinguishable from magic."
—Arthur C. Clarke, 1962

"Tell a man that there are 300 billion stars in the universe and he'll believe you. Tell him that a bench has wet paint on it and he'll have to touch it to be sure."
—M-19 Murphy's Laws on Technology, 1981

OBJECTIVES

The information in this chapter is intended to help the reader—

1. describe the types of rehabilitation and assistive technologies relevant to occupational therapy.

2. explain the importance of having technology-expert therapists on rehabilitation and educational teams.

3. discuss the role of occupational therapists in applying technology in practice.

4. describe methods for obtaining additional information about technology.

5. list the sequence of steps required to appropriately apply technology.

6. describe the implications of the Parallel Interventions and Human-Environment/Technology Interface Models on technology application.

INTRODUCTION

For many people, technology is appealing—it has pizazz. Technology is often viewed as holding the magical new solution to every problem, including those related to disability. Television has fostered this image, creating the illusion that lost limbs and organs can be replaced by "bionic" substitutes. In fact, many people believe that bionic is a medical term, rather than one created by the media. These are the people who accept on blind faith that there are 300 billion stars in the universe. In contrast, there are skeptics who must touch the freshly painted bench to verify that the "wet paint" sign is valid. These people (including some human service and health care providers) believe that technology is a wasteful fad that will soon disappear.

In occupational therapy, technology is in a critical period, a time of transition. While technology is not the panacea for occupational therapy practice, it can certainly no longer be ignored or even viewed as a specialty for a selected few. Occupational therapy is pervasively integrating technology into practice.

Technology is not a new phenomenon to occupational therapy. Historically, occupational therapy and technology have had a close relationship, evolving from a low technological base in the 1950s to today's high technology which includes computers, robotics, adapted vehicles, electrical stimulation, and very sophisticated integrated electronic circuitry. Although occupational therapists need not become engineers or computer programmers, they do need to understand the increasing role of technology in all areas of occupational therapy practice.

This chapter has three goals:

1. To summarize the current issues and applications relevant to occupational therapists today,
2. To integrate technology related information that is presented in other chapters, for example, how technology affects cognitive rehabilitation, mobility, and activities of daily living, and
3. To provide a framework for using technology within occupational therapy practice.

DEFINITIONS OF TECHNOLOGY

Technology means different things to different people, therefore it helps to understand the varied perspectives from which technology is defined. Some definitions are based on the composition of the hardware; others are based on what it does; and still others focus on the newness or innovation of the technique or device. Many definitions are best described as dichotomies, as reflected in the following section.

High Technology versus Low Technology

Low technology usually refers to assistive devices such as button hooks, dressing sticks, long-handled sponges, rocker knifes, forks, Dycem™, Velcro™, and wash mitts. Many others round out an entire menagerie of low technological devices. Special devices for writing, splints, mouth-wands, head sticks, special seating systems, and even more common devices such as eyeglasses fall within this category.

High technology usually is differentiated from low technology by the use of electronics. Any device which requires electricity frequently is considered to be high technology, particularly those devices which use integrated microchips for electronic processing. The definitions of low and high technology change over time. The more familiar and common a technological device becomes, the more likely it is to be termed low technology. For example, the telephone was once considered high technology but today would be considered low technology. Calculators, radios, televisions, bank teller machines, and dishwashers have been perceived as less "high tech" as they have become more prolific in everyday use. One way of viewing this distinction would be to consider low technology as commonplace and high technology as having exotic features or devices.

Custom versus Commercial Technology

An important distinction among the types of technology is how they are made and whether they are available commercially. In the past, most devices were custom-made since few devices were available commercially. But within the last decade, this situation has changed drastically, and therapists use commercial products which cost much less.

Cost-effectiveness is a very important issue in the current health care and educational environment. A product made on an assembly line is much less expensive than a product which takes one to six hours to individually fabricate in the occupational therapy clinic. Commercial devices such as splints have become more available in a variety of sizes and styles which can be fitted quickly and modified to the client, thus avoiding the high cost of custom-made splints. The use of custom-made technologies is greatly shrinking as more commercially-available technologies are used.

This trend has critical implications for occupational therapy practice. Occupational therapists are doing less of this custom fabrication and more selection of the appropriate commercial products. Because of this, one of the new skills required by occupational therapists is the ability to review, analyze, and evaluate countless product descriptions in the extensive technology literature and databases to determine the best commercial product for their patient/client.

Minimal versus Maximal Technology

Technological applications to enhance human performance are used across a wide range of human ability levels. Technological devices once were implemented primarily to assist and support human performance; today they are being used to substitute for performance deficits. For example, in the past, technology intervention was limited to using a wash mitt or a long-handled sponge to assist individuals with washing and bathing activities. These devices provided some minimal assistance to improve an individual's independence. Although this minimal technology continues to be used, there are maximal technologies available for the person with severe motor deficits (e.g., high level quadriplegia) such as robots that can grab a sponge, dip the sponge into water, and wash the face.

Appliance versus Tool

Technology can be applied as an appliance or as a tool (Rodgers, 1985). The distinction between tools and appliances is crucial for proper technology application. An appliance operates independently; for example, a refrigerator serves its technological function by operating by itself once it is plugged in. Other appliance technologies include hearing aids, eyeglasses, and certain splints. They do not require the development of particular skills in order to be used.

In contrast, a tool requires certain skills and/or manipulation to serve a useful function. People think of some tools or higher technologies as appliances that require very little effort. This misunderstanding can have serious consequences. For example, communication aids are often thought to be a simple type of technology that helps an individual speak or write. However, communication aids cannot operate on their own and require many hours of both the user's time to learn their operation and the therapist's time to teach the user. Such tools of higher technology should not be perceived as an easy answer, but rather as implements that require skill and time in order to help individuals improve their performance and become more independent. When potentially valuable tools are treated as

appliances and training is not provided, the devices frequently end up being discarded or not used because the client does not know how to use them correctly. Just as a cook must learn to use a stove to make savory meals, one who wears a flexor hinge (tenodesis) splint must learn to manipulate the splint for grasp and pinch, and those who use a communication aid must develop the language skills and mechanical operations of the device to be able to functionally converse. Without user training, these tools may only exhibit a fraction of their potential.

Adaptive/Assistive Technology versus Rehabilitative/Educational Technology

Technology serves two major roles: helping and teaching. Those technologies that help an individual support their functional independence by enhancing or assisting performance in a functional activity are referred to as *assistive* or *adaptive technologies*. A device that helps support a person (orthosis) and a device that replaces a function (prosthesis) are both considered adaptive/assistive technologies. Other adaptive or assistive technologies include such products as an automatic page-turner, a one-handed denture brush, a laptop computer with accelerated writing system software, or a robotic device.

The second type are *rehabilitative* or *educational technologies*. Examples of this type of technology include cognitive rehabilitation software, **biofeedback** and **functional electrical stimulation** when applied for training muscle groups.

The distinction between these types of technologies is critical to understand. Although adaptive/assistive types of technologies can be extremely helpful in maximizing the independence of those with a disability, occupational therapists should avoid prescribing these devices too quickly and assuming that the person might never gain the skills necessary for independence. These assistive/adaptive technologies should be viewed as temporary measures, helping to maximize the person's performance within the context of their current deficits. Occupational therapists should always assume that the person's current deficits could change. Hence they should recognize that the individual's need for therapeutic intervention (rehabilitation and educational skill development and periodic re-evaluation) is likely to continue.

The other extreme is when therapists assume that their exclusive role is to provide therapeutic intervention in order to rehabilitate or educate an individual. Those who believe assistive and adaptive technologies only provide a crutch that prevents progressive skill development completely avoid the use of assistive/adaptive technology in hopes that the person will be motivated to reach his/her highest level of independence.

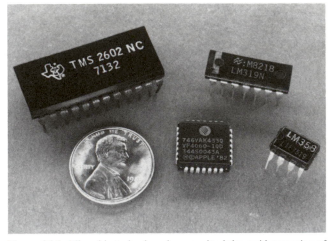

Figure 26-1. Microchip technology has permitted the rapid expansion of high technology into clinical practice.

The best approach is neither adaptive/assistive technologies nor rehabilitation/educational technologies alone. Effective occupational therapy should utilize both concurrently. For example, when a person uses an assistive technology, it is important to evaluate that person's skill levels over time to determine if and when more or less powerful technologies are required. Likewise, when rehabilitative or educational therapeutic intervention is provided, assistive and adaptive technologies must be considered as a way of maximizing an individual's functional performance—even as a temporary measure.

The traditional use of a crutch is an excellent example of integrating both adaptive/assistive technologies and rehabilitation/educational intervention. When the knee has been traumatized, therapeutic intervention is required to maintain and improve range of motion to normalize the joint motion as rapidly as possible. A continuous passive range of motion (robotic type of technology) might be used. At the same time, low technology is also incorporated into the therapy plan by prescribing the use of a crutch as a temporary assistive device. The individual is monitored continually as to the need for the crutch (adaptive/assistive) while concurrently receiving therapy (rehabilitative/educational). As the condition improves, the need for the crutch no longer exists.

This Chapter's Definition of Technology

As discussed, technology can be viewed and categorized in several different ways. A universal definition of technology taken from U.S. federal legislation defines the technology focus of this chapter. The Technology-Related Assistance for Individuals with Disabilities Act of 1988 (PL 100-407) defines *assistive technology device* as "any item, piece of equipment, or product system, whether acquired commercially, off-the-shelf, modified or customized, that

is used to increase, maintain or improve functional capabilities of individuals with disabilities" (Federal Register, 1988). While keeping all of these types of technology in mind, this chapter will focus on the newer and more exotic technologies.

HISTORY OF TECHNOLOGY

Technology and Occupational Therapy

Occupational therapists have been experts in the application of low technology for decades. Before the current age of computers, therapists applied handmade technology which was often constructed in their own clinic workshops. Early in this century, adaptation of equipment was used frequently as the approach was fundamental to occupational therapy philosophy. Whereas the public associates computer programmers, engineers, scientists, and commercial industry with technology, the occupational therapy profession has extensive experience in applying technology. The focus of technology in occupational therapy has always been targeted to helping facilitate the functional living skills of persons with disabilities.

The occupational therapy literature as early as the 1940s and 50s displayed low technological applications including such articles as, Adaptation of Media (Brokaw, 1948), Adaptations and Apparatus (Parlin, 1948), Toys for Children with Cerebral Palsy (Craig & Hendin, 1950), Two Feeding Appliances (Hall, 1951), Special Equipment Adaptable for Kitchen Use (Svensson & Brennan, 1953), Self-Care Board for Hemiplegics (Lepley, 1955), Adjustable Reading Rack for the Visually Handicapped (Moore, 1956), and Adaptation for Resistance to the Beater of the Floor Loom (Myers, et al., 1956).

In the late 1950s, Fred Sammons began work which led to his becoming a leading and significant figure in technology in occupational therapy, both nationally and internationally. He is cited as one of the first occupational therapists who seriously considered technology development. He expanded on innovative ideas from a foundation in orthotics and prosthetics at Northwestern University and created the first widely disseminated commercial button hook in 1958 (Sammons, 1988). His business was one of the first of today's many commercial manufacturers and distributors of technology devices used in occupational therapy. Occupational therapists have been experts in the application of technology for a long time and their expertise has been applied in a variety of clinical and educational environments such as long-term health care facilities, acute care hospitals, school districts, mental health facilities, and in community-based practices (e.g., independent living centers).

Computers

Technology is frequently equated with computers. While it is true that many technology applications are not computer applications, computers do provide a base for virtually all high technology applications, including functional electrical stimulation, biofeedback, robotics, powered mobility controls, environmental control systems, and electronic augmentative communication systems. The trend for the computer to be the platform for technology implementation is increasing, particularly as the costs of such components continue to decrease.

The increased use of computers and other electronic devices for use in rehabilitation largely is the result of the development of the **microchip**. Current microchips are small black squares (about the size of a thumbnail) with numerous protruding metallic pins. In engineering, they are known as IC's (integrated circuits), a label which conveys the fact that electronic impulses are routed through the complex microscopic circuitry contained in the microchip. Microchips are now so sophisticated and efficient that they have become entire computer processing units. Figure 26-1 shows internal and external views of an integrated circuits.

Integrated circuits have revolutionized the use of computers. Not only have they substantially reduced the cost of computers by over 95 percent, they have enabled the size of computers to shrink from apparatus which filled large rooms to much smaller pieces of equipment that fit easily on desktops. Thus, we have seen computer technology change from large mainframe computers to less costly, more lightweight and more powerful microcomputers, some laptop varieties of which now conveniently fit into briefcases. These dramatic reductions in size and cost have led to a significant development—the widespread availability of computers for individual use (See Figure 26-2). Their affordable cost and availability has made the use of computers in occupational therapy more feasible.

Occupational Therapy and Computers

Lau (1986) and Angelo and Smith (1989a) have reviewed the occupational therapy literature regarding the application of computers and identified several shifts in computer applications in the profession. They found that in the 1970s, many of the articles discussed computer use in the future tense, while articles written in the 1980s began discussing computer use in the present tense. There was also a substantial increase in the number of articles with only five articles appearing from 1971 to 1981. Figure 26-3 indicates the rapid increase in computer articles in occupational therapy literature from 1982 through 1988. These studies also found that the literature in the 70s focused on administrative uses, professional education, and research applications of computers while the more recent literature

began to highlight therapeutic applications. While these articles on application tend to be descriptive case study discussions, experimental research investigating the efficacy of using computers as therapeutic intervention is emerging. As occupational therapists increase computer use in clinical settings, it becomes important to clarify the appropriateness of when and how to best use this new technology.

Who are the Technologists?

Although society continues to be highly dependent upon engineers, scientists and computer programmers for developing and refining technology, a host of other disciplines have become involved with applying it to everyday problems. Since the 1970's, human factors engineers, rehabilitation engineers, bioengineers, speech and language pathologists, psychologists, and physical therapists, as well as occupational therapists, have become better acquainted with technology and its potential in clinical application.

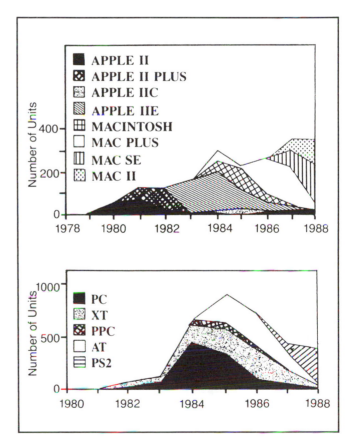

Figure 26-2. The Recency of Computer Technology. *The advent of personal computers: computer acquisition and obsolescence as inventoried at the University of Wisconsin-Madison. 1989. Madison, WI: University of Wisconsin-Madison.*

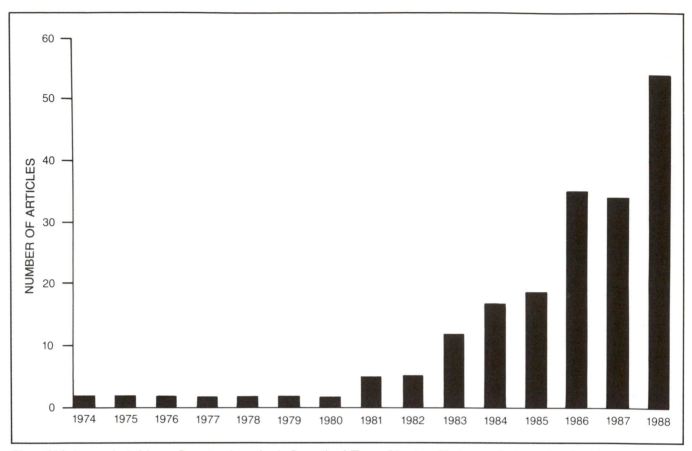

Figure 26-3. Increase in Articles on Computers Appearing in Occupational Therapy Literature. *The increase in the number of articles on computers in occupational therapy literature since 1974 is a dramatic indication of the increasing relevance of technology to OT practice. From Angelo, J. and Smith, R.O. (1989a). Indications of Computer Use: A Literature Review of Thirteen Occupational Therapy Periodicals.*

Technology cannot be applied in isolation; the process demands a team approach. Occupational therapists should become comfortable with technology and develop an awareness of the particular contributions they can make in applying it to clinical problems as part of a technology team. This requires the ability to be able to relate to colleagues in other disciplines that use technology, such as engineers.

Augmentative communication provides one example of the critical need for occupational therapy participation in a technology team (Angelo & Smith, 1989b; Finkley, 1988). Augmentative communication is primarily seen as the domain of speech and language pathology. Speech and language pathologists specializing in augmentative communication are experts in language, symbolic structuring, identifying appropriate vocabularies, and vocabulary arrangement. They are also familiar with the types of technological systems that permit appropriate language displays which optimize the conversational interaction between individuals. An individual's ability to use an augmentative communication system is, however, depend-

ent on his/her sensory-perceptual, cognitive, and motor skills. They must be able to perceive and comprehend the messages being expressed and control the system effectively in order for it to become a practical communication method, hence the role of the occupational therapist emerges.

Occupational therapists with backgrounds in physical disabilities or psychosocial disabilities, and those who are familiar with augmentative communication devices are particularly equipped to function as experts in interfacing the technologies. It is occupational therapists who can best help identify which control and display methods are best matched to an individual's sensorimotor and cognitive-perceptual deficits and potentials. Although occupational therapists usually are suited best for this task, the function of choosing the most appropriate augmentative communication system unfortunately often has been assumed by speech and language pathologists or others because occupational therapists have not been available for participation on the team.

COMPETENCIES REQUIRED BY OCCUPATIONAL THERAPISTS

The evolution of many of the newer technologies has made it difficult to know just how much background and experience a therapist needs in order to be competent in applying it. Competency levels range from the basic skills of a general practitioner, to the advanced skills of a technology-generalist, to those who specialize in an area such as seating/mobility or drivers' assessment and training. While advanced competencies are required for those who practice in these specialized areas, certain fundamental competencies are needed by all occupational therapists. These competencies fall into three learning domains, as follows:

1. an affective domain in which an adequate level of comfort with technology is necessary,
2. a knowledge domain that includes technology information which occupational therapists must understand, and
3. a psychomotor learning domain in which therapists must demonstrate skills in order to appropriately apply the technology.

Comfort Level for Therapists

It is essential that occupational therapists feel comfortable with technology. In the past, therapists' attitudes toward technology greatly varied. Some were relatively apathetic, some had an extreme aversion or fear of technology, others believed technology to be irrelevant to their practice, and still others had a fear that learning and mastering the necessary information and skills for competency would be frustrating. Because the use of technology is a relatively new phenomenon, the need to become comfortable with technologies is extremely high today. Over the next few years, however, increasing numbers of therapists will become comfortable with technology during their basic professional education or even during their pre-college education. Integrating technology education into curricula will help increase the number of therapists who feel comfortable with computers and other technologies (See Figure 26-4a).

Basic Literacy

Occupational therapists must have a working knowledge of technical vocabulary such as megabyte, digital, analog, sub-ASIS bar, transparent access, and augmentative communication. As occupational therapists apply this technology more, the need for basic technology literacy will increase. Over time this need will decrease as literacy education is integrated into basic, primary, secondary, and professional education and as manufacturers continue to develop more user-friendly systems which require less skill and literacy. Figure 26-4b displays the relationship of literacy need to the increase in education and user-friendly technology.

Potentials and Limitations of Technology

In order to apply technology appropriately, therapists must be familiar with its capabilities and limitations. This requires four areas of knowledge for the occupational therapist:

1. Occupational therapists should be familiar with the majority of commercially available products in order to know how technology might assist persons with disabilities.
2. Therapists should know when and what modifications of commercial products might be appropriate and when original fabrication of a device is needed.
3. Therapists must know how technological products are applied including the purpose of a product, the product function, how well it functions in various environments, and what type of training the user needs for the appropriate application.
4. Therapists must recognize when technology is not a desirable option. Some technology is often contraindicated either because it is more difficult to maintain or simply because a lower technology is more functional. Figure 26-4c depicts the steady and continuous increase in the need for therapists to become more familiar with technological products and their applications.

Matching Technology to Individual Human Needs

In order to select a technology, the therapist must also be able to match the technology to the particular client's deficits and skills and to the environment in which they will be used. For therapists to appropriately apply technology, they must assure that they have followed these four steps:

1. *assess the individual,*
2. *consider the living and working environments of the individual,*
3. *assess potential technologies,*
4. *match technological features to the specific needs of the individual.*

Each of these steps contributes to the successful matching of the individual and technology. As many more technology applications become available as options, it becomes more imperative for therapists to learn how to match technology to individual needs. Figure 26-4d shows the steady and continuous need for the occupational therapists to know how to match technology to individual needs as the use of technology expands. Critical concepts in this process are discussed in a later section of this chapter.

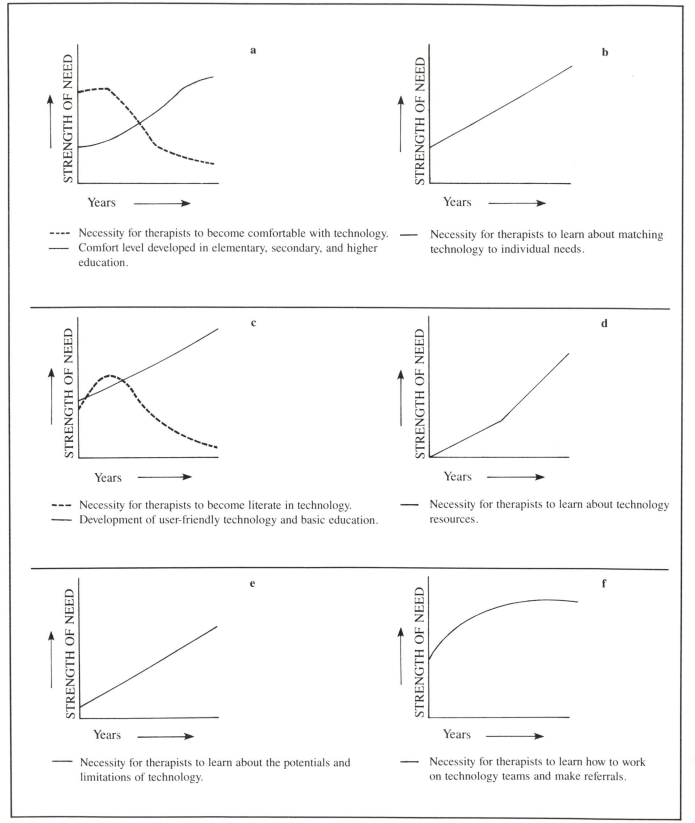

Figure 26-4a-f. Projected Technology Trends in Occupational Therapy.

Information Resources

As Naisbitt pointed out in his popular book, *Megatrends,* we are in an era of an information society. There is so much information available today that we cannot possibly keep all the information in our own brain banks. Occupational therapists need to be able to access key information and use supplemental information sources to support their own bank of knowledge. (See Figure 26-4e)

Team Work and Referrals

There is so much information and expertise today in various specialized areas that occupational therapists realize they cannot know everything about technology application in rehabilitation. Technology implementation requires the expertise from various clinical, physical, and social perspectives. Consequently, the most effective technology service delivery model is one where knowledge is cooperatively integrated by a team.

Perhaps the most important skill in technology application is using sound clinical judgment that leads to the appropriate referral. A therapist may need to refer to another specialist on the technology team or to an individual in an outside specialty evaluation center. Because local clinics often cannot afford all the costly equipment, local clinics often must refer clients to specialty evaluation centers for demonstration and hands-on trials on the range of potential devices and systems. Specialty evaluation centers are better equipped for hands-on assessment with the technology itself. Not every occupational therapy clinic will be able to comprehensively evaluate all patients for technology, but therapists in local clinics can evaluate the basic skills of the client and refer clients to a center where a complete technological assessment can be accomplished. Figure 26-4f illustrates that occupational therapists will continue to need to learn to work within technology teams and make referrals.

INFORMATION SOURCES FOR TECHNOLOGY

Technology information is pervasive. It is fortunate that so many resources are available, but this requires therapists to learn how to use an increasing number of resources. There are many types of resources available and each has advantages and disadvantages. While books, periodicals and databases are excellent sources for obtaining specific information, the application of technology is best learned in workshops, conferences and educational courses.

Books and Periodicals

Books and periodicals are the first line of information for therapists. A variety of textbooks, professional periodicals, and consumer newsletters are available, as listed below:

General Technology Text References
- *Assistive Technology Sourcebook* (1990), by Alexandra Enders. This is a comprehensive guide to technology resources.
- Veterans Administration Research and Development Progress Reports
- *Rehabilitation Technology Service Delivery: A Practical Guide* (1987a). Washington, D.C.: RESNA.
- *The Trace Resource Book* (1989), by Berliss, J.B., Borden, P.A., & Vanderheiden, G.C. Madison: University of Wisconsin, Time R & D Center Reprint Service. This book lists rehabilitation technology products with descriptions and photographs; biannually updated; and focuses on computer access, augmentative communication, and environmental control systems.

Texts Directed to Occupational Therapists
The following textbooks provide general descriptions and many case studies of a variety of technology applications particular to computers.
- *Computer Applications in Occupational Therapy* (1986), by Cromwell, F.S. (Ed.). New York: Haworth Press.
- *Microcomputers: Clinical Applications* (1986), by Clark, E.N. (Ed.). Thorofare, N.J.: Slack.

Proceedings of National Conferences
- Proceedings of RESNA (published annually)
- American Occupational Therapy Association (technology proceedings published annually)

Professional Periodicals and Newsletters
- *The American Journal of Occupational Therapy*
- *Assistive Technology*
- *Exceptional Parent*
- *The Journal of Rehabilitation Research and Development*
- *Augmentative and Alternative Communication*
- *Cognitive Rehabilitation*
- *The American Occupational Therapy Special Interest Section Newsletters*
- *RESNA Newsletter*

Consumer and Care-provider Publications and Newsletters
These publications are published by manufacturers of rehabilitation equipment or specialty centers.
- *Accent on Living*
- *Breaking New Ground*
- *Paraplegia News*

<table>
<tr><td>

Technology-Related Conferences

Abilities Expo
1106 2nd Street, Suite 118
Encinitas, CA 92024

American Occupational Therapy Association (AOTA)
1383 Piccard Drive
Rockville, MD 20850
(301) 948-9626

Association of Drivers Education for the Disabled (ADED)
c/o David Harden
33736 LaCrosse
Westland, MI 48185

Closing the Gap (CTG)
P.O. Box 68
Henderson, MN 56044

Compute-Able Conference on Adaptive Technology
Compute Able Network
P.O. Box 1706
Portland, OR 97207

Computer Technology/Special Education/Rehabilitation Conference
California State University, Northridge
18111 Nordhoff Street
Northridge, CA 91330

Human Factors Society
P.O. Box 1369
Santa Monica, CA 90406

International Seating Symposium
University of Tennessee Rehabilitation Education Program
682 Court Avenue
Memphis, TN 38163

International Society of Augmentative and Alternative Communication (ISAAC)
P.O. Box 1762
Station R
Toronto, ON M4G 4A3 CANADA

RESNA
1101 Connecticut Avenue NW
Suite 700
Washington, D.C. 20036

United States Society of Augmentative and Alternative Communication (USSAAC)
c/o Barkley Memorial Center
University of Nebraska
Lincoln, NE 68588

</td></tr>
</table>

Figure 26-5. Technology-related Conferences.

- *Closing the Gap*
- *Prentke Romich Expressions*
- *Positively Speaking* (newsletter of PRAB Command, Inc.)

Technology Databases

Databases are newer sources of information and several are available to help the clinician identify appropriate technology and applications (Hall, 1987). (See Appendix C for a list of various databases with information on technology and disability.) Two important ones are described below:

- ABLEDATA (1989) describes over 15,000 commercially available rehabilitation products from over 1900 companies. Each product listing gives a description of the equipment, the manufacturer's name, address, cost of the product, and other comments. This database is available through BRS, or in a desktop version as one of the distributed databases of Co-Net (See Appendix C, Manufacturers and Information Centers). Co-Net is a consortium of agencies invested in rehabilitation technology information and serves as a prime dissemination group for technology desktop databases.

- REHABDATA is a bibliographical database supplied by the National Rehabilitation Information Center, which includes commercial publications, government reports, journals, and unpublished documents on the general topic of rehabilitation. Technology entries are one area of focus within that database (see NARIC in Appendix C).

Networks

The technology revolution has seen the advent of networks and electronic bulletin board systems which provide on-line information. These networks can be accessed by a computer, modem, and telephone line. A variety of on-line networks provide computer bulletin boards which specialize in providing current answers to questions regarding disability and technology, such as Developmental Disabilities Connection, the Veterans Administration Bulletin Board on Compuserve, and the Bulletin Board on SpecialNet. In 1989, two more electronic bulletin board systems devoted specifically to occupational therapy were initiated, one out of Creighton University in Omaha, Nebraska and a second called OT Source from the American Occupational Therapy Association. Appendix C provides a listing of on-line bulletin boards and databases that provide information on technology and disability.

Conferences

Professional conferences are a rich source of technology product information since this is where developers and manufacturers frequently introduce their newest systems and products. Meetings and special interest group sessions also help clinicians to improve their knowledge base in technology and keep experienced technologists aware of the latest technology information. Figure 26-5 is a list of technology-related conferences. Some of the conferences focus entirely on technology while others are more general but include a special technology component.

Training Programs

Training programs are essential to the clinician. Occupational therapists who wish to either become more familiar with technology or expert in one or more specialty areas can enroll in technology training programs. There are three general types of training programs: (1) pre-service education programs, (2) graduate school programs, and (3) continuing education training programs.

Pre-service education programs are ones which offer technology training prior to entering the field. Most universities and colleges with professional OT programs now include one or more courses in computer and technology clinical applications. Formal technology programs for pre-service technology training are also emerging. In 1989, several of such programs were supported by federal funds including ones located at the University of Washington in Seattle; University of Wisconsin-Madison; Rancho Los Amigos Hospital; University of Southern California; and New York University. The technology program at the University of Washington was designed as a required part of the entry-level program for all professional OT students. Some programs award a certificate following an elective set of courses, such as the one at the University of Wisconsin at Madison.

The second type of program is offered at the graduate school level. Some programs are oriented specifically to occupational therapists (Gilkeson & Krouskop, 1987) and others are more broadly targeted. A few programs provide graduate degrees with an orientation in rehabilitation engineering, such as those at Louisiana Tech and San Francisco State University (for addresses, see listings under Manufacturers and Information Centers, Appendix C).

The third type of program is continuing education training. These programs usually take place in the form of workshops, seminars, and institutes offered at national conferences. There are also many national and regional workshop series sponsored by state organizations, specialty technology centers, local clinics, and school-based programs. Becoming a member of a professional technology organization usually automatically places one on related mailing lists for announcements of scheduled continuing education activities.

Videotapes

Many centers are producing videotapes about technology applications, and manufacturers are also using videotapes to introduce and demonstrate their products. Information regarding videotapes can be obtained from contacting manufacturers or by attending video sessions that are scheduled at most professional conferences.

Professional Organizations

Some organizations are professional and trade-oriented, while others are more focused on advocacy. The occupational therapist who wishes to become an expert in technology and remain current should be an active member of several professional associations. *RESNA* is an association for the advancement of rehabilitation and assistive technologies and is now the primary interdisciplinary professional association that addresses the full range of rehabilitation technology (RESNA was formerly an acronym for Rehabilitation Engineering Society of North America which changed its emphasis from engineering to rehabilitation technology during the past decade). The organization hosts an annual conference and publishes proceedings of research and practice activities in the field. RESNA oversees a set of special interest groups (SIG's) ranging from service delivery, to robotics, to gerontology. Figure 26-6 provides a complete list of RESNA special interest groups.

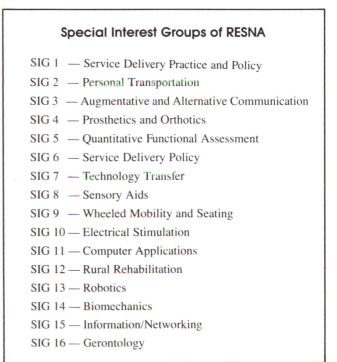

Special Interest Groups of RESNA

SIG 1 — Service Delivery Practice and Policy
SIG 2 — Personal Transportation
SIG 3 — Augmentative and Alternative Communication
SIG 4 — Prosthetics and Orthotics
SIG 5 — Quantitative Functional Assessment
SIG 6 — Service Delivery Policy
SIG 7 — Technology Transfer
SIG 8 — Sensory Aids
SIG 9 — Wheeled Mobility and Seating
SIG 10 — Electrical Stimulation
SIG 11 — Computer Applications
SIG 12 — Rural Rehabilitation
SIG 13 — Robotics
SIG 14 — Biomechanics
SIG 15 — Information/Networking
SIG 16 — Gerontology

Figure 26-6. Special Interest Groups of RESNA.

In the past few years, the American Occupational Therapy Association has sponsored a variety of technology-oriented institutes and technical sessions at its annual conferences. In the mid 1980s, the activities of a computer club sparked interest in what is now a technology special interest section that provides supportive technology update for clinicians. In 1989, in Baltimore, the American Occupational Therapy Association held its first technology forum as part of the annual conference and produced its first proceedings.

Other important organizations related to technology in occupational therapy are USAAC and ISAAC (the United States and International Societies for Augmentative and Alternative Communication). These memberships are primarily comprised of speech and language pathologists and educators. However, conferences and memberships aim to be interdisciplinary, and occupational therapists are beginning to play a more significant role.

The Association of Driver Educators for the Disabled (ADED) is an organization of professionals who work with adapted driving and drivers' education for persons with disabilities. ADED hosts a national annual conference and provides support materials for persons active in this area of technology.

The Human Factors Society has a more generic interest in technology and how it interfaces with people. Its orientation is from an engineering perspective, but its publications and conferences have substantial implications for occupational therapy and technology. Human Factors is the branch of engineering which focuses on the interface between humans and machines. The interests of this society focus on the limitations and potentials of human perception, motor control, and other areas of functional performance and their influence on the design characteristics of control systems, displays, and other aspects of machinery.

Disability organizations in the U.S., such as the Association for Retarded Citizens (ARC), Easter Seals, and United Cerebral Palsy (UCP) increasingly are involved in assistive technology application. These organizations function as local community-oriented chapters with a national coordinating office. They assist technologists to work closely with and be responsive to the needs of the users of technology, their families, and community support systems.

Rehabilitation Engineering Centers (RECs) conduct technology research and serve as information centers. There are about 16 REC's distributed throughout the country and each center performs technology research activities in a specialized area ranging from sensory aids for blind and deaf individuals to augmentative communication, prosthetics and orthotics, and modifications to worksites and educational settings (See Appendix C for a listing of RECs). These REC's are funded by the National Institute on Disability and Rehabilitation Research within the Office of Special Education and Rehabilitation of the U.S. Department of Education.

Specialty Clinical and Research Centers

These centers offer training, evaluation, and specialty service delivery in a particular area of technology expertise. Many are based in universities, but some are also affiliated

---

Elements of Technology Application

1. Locating people who can make use of the technology and giving them an awareness of the possible uses of technology.
2. Establishing their needs, capabilities, and the potential benefits of the technology.
3. Selecting and acquiring appropriate technology components including special market hardware and software and general market hardware and software.
4. Assembling the technology system.
6. Mounting the technology system on the user's wheelchair, shoulder bag, bed, office workstation, etc.
7. Fitting the system to the user, including adjustments, modifications, and initial customization.
8. Selecting the most effective training, such as manuals, video tapes, demonstration programs, etc.
9. Initially training the user in the basics of the technology and how to optimize it for their own use.
10. Training the people in the user's environment who will need to help the user maintain the technology.
11. Providing ongoing training to make sure users get all possible benefit from the technology.
12. Being on call to answer subsequent questions about the technology as it is being used.
13. Providing ongoing preventive maintenance and replacing worn parts.
14. Providing repairs.
15. Updating the system when significant improvements make it desirable.
16. Periodically re-evaluating the success of the technology in the user's life and providing suggestions or further training as necessary.
17. Using helpful information gained from users to help refine and improve the technology.
18. Providing different and more appropriate technology when the user's needs or capabilities change.
19. Providing different and more appropriate technology when significant advances in technological design render more useful systems available.

Figure 26-7. Nineteen Elements of Technology Application.

with rehabilitation hospitals and other facilities that have specialty technology centers. These centers frequently provide intense interdisciplinary evaluations and can provide substantial information to clinicians who encounter questions regarding their particular specialty area. These specialty centers are located throughout the country and vary widely in their emphasis in specific rehabilitation and education technology areas. A directory of such services is available from the RESNA office (RESNA, 1989b). Many Rehabilitation Engineering Centers also can supply listings of service delivery programs and specialty evaluation programs related to their particular focus area of research (Appendix C).

MATCHING TECHNOLOGY TO INDIVIDUAL HUMAN NEEDS

The Process of Providing Technology

With the rapid developments in this field and sufficient technology literature available, theorists have begun to describe the process of providing technology. Rodgers (1985) identified 19 steps for appropriate technology application (Figure 26-7). He points out that technology service delivery cannot focus just on the technology, but must direct substantial attention to providing service. Only Step 3 specifically focuses on the **hardware** or **software** itself. The others relate to the various services that support the user of the system over time. This is a very vital concept in the application of technology—emphasis should be focused on the procedures for applying the technology devices to real-life use (i.e., ongoing training) rather than on the technology itself.

Smith (1988a) reduces Rodger's 19 steps to seven discrete functions which must be performed in order for a clinician to appropriately match a technological system with an individual:

1. Understand the potential technology has for persons with disabilities. This understanding is a pre-requisite and fundamental to the clinician's knowledge-base.
2. Assess the person with the disability and the environments in which he/she must function to ascertain inherent abilities and functional areas of deficit. This evaluation must investigate the individual's ability to perform in a variety of functional activities from basic self-care skills to community integration activities. The evaluation must also look at specific components, skills, and abilities such as range of motion and visual perception. The individual's abilities must be evaluated in the context of the environment in which he/she will be functioning, and the environment itself

---

Matching Technology to Individual Needs

Although it is obvious that advanced technology can help many people, it does not follow that the more advanced or higher technology always provides a better solution. In some cases, electronic devices are inappropriately applied simply because nothing else has worked. In other cases, devices are selected based on the mistaken belief that any technology is better than no technology, or that advanced technology is always better than fundamental devices or techniques. People are often given communication aids which they do not need, simply because these aids are more technologically advanced than the one they currently use. Consider, for example, the following true story:

A therapist, after successfully interfacing a young girl with a switch, decided that an electronic scanning communication should be purchased for the girl. Because the therapist was unable to locate funding for the aid, a local television station became involved and ran a special fund drive. Each night on the evening news, the television station showed a thermometer demonstrating the amount of donations and how much was needed to reach the goal. The station received enough donations and the aid was obtained. On the day the girl was to receive the aid, the TV station ran live coverage from the rehabilitation center. With all eyes trained on her, the young girl hit the switch and the lights began to move slowly down the display, row by row, then across item by item, until it finally reached a square with a prominent, "Thank You" written on it. The light behind the "Thank You" began to flash and this was greeted by applause from the audience. The TV stations of course reported the wonders of modern technology. But with the camera still on her, the young girl took her finger off the switch and proceeded to point, rapidly and accurately, to each of the 100 squares on the communication screen. It turned out that the young woman was perfectly able to point and already had a communication board with 280 squares, which she used on a daily basis.

What the wonders of modern technology had given her was a $1,000 switch and 8,000 transistors which allowed her to communicate 10 times more slowly and with a vocabulary only a third as large as the one she had used previously with the communication board.

Once the aid was brought into the classroom, it became instantly apparent that it would be of no use to her. It took several weeks before she could get rid of the aid and return to her communication board because of all the publicity and media attention surrounding its acquisition.

Figure 26-8. Matching Technology to Individual Needs. *From Vanderheiden (1987b).*

must be assessed for its inherent abilities and areas of deficit.

3. Evaluate technology intervention alternatives. An appropriate match of technology to the person's

disabilities cannot occur if the therapist is not familiar with the capabilities and limitations of the technology. Vanderheiden (1987b) provides a clear example of an inappropriate person-technology match in the case study described in Figure 26-8.

4. After complete evaluation of the individual, the environment, and available technological systems, select the appropriate system.

5. Acquired the technology and make it available. This involves the therapist locating the funds to purchase the device. This can often be a very complicated, arduous, and delayed process. The therapist must work with funding agencies and give the agencies written justification for the need for the equipment to assist the funding agency in making a rational decision. This is described in more detail in a later section of this chapter.

6. When the equipment or device arrives, the person who will be using the system must be trained in the appropriate techniques for properly applying the system in their day-to-day environment. This will sometimes require many months of training.

7. The technological system which is implemented must be monitored and revised as ongoing evaluation and revised implementation is imperative.

The Parallel Interventions Model

In 1989, the cost of a technological system ranged from $2,000 to $50,000. With more expensive systems, the financial impact of the wrong choice of technology can be catastrophic. The policies of many funding agencies allow the funding of only one technological system every several years for each individual. For example, Medicare reimbursement policies in the U.S. consider a wheelchair in the category of durable medical supplies and assume a wheelchair will last a few years. Thus, Medicare generally will not fund another replacement, regardless of added technological advancements, immediately following a purchase.

The role of the occupational therapist is not simply to identify the correct technology at any given point in time, but to predict what the individual may need in the immediate future. To do this, the therapist must determine the performance level which an individual may be able to achieve within a reasonable length of therapy intervention. For example, during an evaluation, an individual with significant motor deficits may exhibit minimal control of a device. Consistent and reliable technology access may be limited to the activation of a single switch. However, after a month of graded motor training with a head light-pointer aimed toward enabling direct selection techniques, the same individual might be able to gain sufficient function to access

a much more powerful technological system. (A head light-pointer is a flashlight-type of pointer that is worn on the head to enable individuals who have little control over other parts of their bodies to use head and neck control for pointing at targets.) In this case, it could be unwise for a therapist to prescribe a single-switch device as an optimal long-term access system. Single-switch access would be appropriate as a temporary control, but light-pointing training should also be implemented to occur concurrently, as a parallel intervention.

This is an example of a *parallel interventions model* (DePape & Smith, 1987; Angelo & Smith 1989b) which maximizes functional abilities with technology by simultaneously incorporating intervention in parallel tracks. The first track temporarily adapts the environment to the individual needs of the client, while the second track improves the client's skills and abilities to minimize the degree of dependency on an adaptive environment.

The parallel intervention philosophy holds that this process cannot occur in a sequential fashion. Human disability rarely progresses rapidly enough to warrant a serial method of intervention when dealing with technology. The environment should be modified as a temporary measure, while at the same time skill acquisition, rehabilitation, and training are implemented as the focus of therapy. This implies that the individual's environment should be re-evaluated and modified as necessary while skill level improves. This iterative technique is based on the belief that a person's skill level and his/her environment are dynamic and inter-related. Figure 26-9 illustrates the parallel interventions model.

The Human-Environment/Technology Model

A method of evaluating a person and the person's environment is to view both as a *unified interactive system*. This systemic view aids the therapist's assessment of the potential of the technology and improves the process of matching appropriate technology to an individual's needs. Conceptually, there are six primary functions technology can serve; three of them address human deficits and the other three address the technological environment. This model is based on the human-machine interaction model discussed in human factors literature (Meister, 1971; Chapanis, 1976).

In this chapter, the **Human-Environment/Technology Interface Model** (HETI) is the framework for understanding these functional relationships (see Figure 26-10). HETI proposes that a person must first receive information in order to interact with the environment. The person must then process the information to make meaningful judgments and proper decisions. Finally, the person must respond motorically to the information. This is

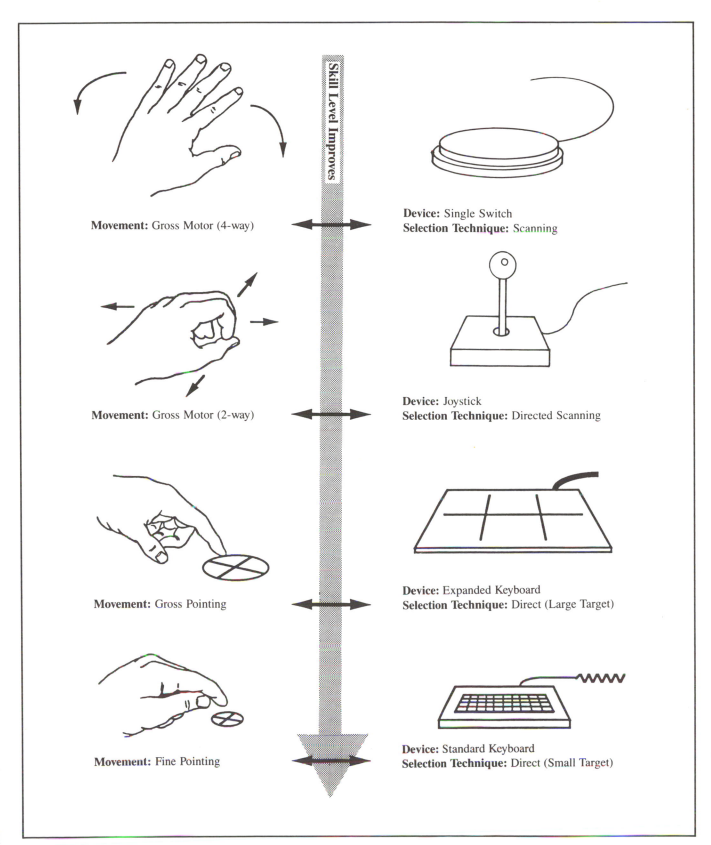

Movement: Gross Motor (4-way)   **Device:** Single Switch
Selection Technique: Scanning

Movement: Gross Motor (2-way)   **Device:** Joystick
Selection Technique: Directed Scanning

Movement: Gross Pointing   **Device:** Expanded Keyboard
Selection Technique: Direct (Large Target)

Movement: Fine Pointing   **Device:** Standard Keyboard
Selection Technique: Direct (Small Target)

Skill Level Improves

Figure 26-9. Parallel Intervention System.

consistent with sensory input, cognitive throughput, and motor output, which is the base of much occupational therapy theory and practice. In this conceptual model, these three functional capacities are labeled *human input (HI), human processing (HP), and human output (HO)*. All sensory dimensions fall under human input including perceptions that are tactile, proprioceptive, visual, vestibular, auditory, olfactory, and gustatory. Human processing is made up of all cognitive dimensions including memory, orientation, attention span, recognition, thought-processing, problem-solving, generalization, sequencing, concept formation, categorization, and other intellectual operation. Human output includes the neuromotor dimensions such as fine motor coordination, gross motor coordination, muscle tone, reflexes, range of motion, strength, endurance, soft tissue integrity, skeletal integrity, postural control, and activity tolerance.

In this conceptual approach, adequate sensation, cognitive skills, and motor skills are generic in their interaction with the environment and not specific to a given activity. For example, visual sensation allows an individual to visually perceive all of the environment. Deficits in visual perception do not affect one specific activity, but tend to encompass many activities. Therefore, both visual skills and visual deficits tend to be fundamental.

The second half of the HETI Model is the machine or technological environment. The components mirror the human side of the model. Any type of dynamic and functional machine has some type of method to sense or receive information, hence the *environment/technology input (EI)*. These types of technologies also have a specific function and purpose which are termed *environment/ technology applications (EA)*. Functional machines and technology are not useful unless there is a way to demonstrate their capabilities by way of some motor or display presentation, which is the *environment/ technology output (EO)*. The technology half of the model tends to be fairly specific to one or a few activities; thus, they are more limited in application, as opposed to the more generic capabilities and functions of the human half of the model.

To illustrate this model, consider the example of a person interacting with a computer. When people first encounter a computer, they must see the computer, the keyboard or mouse, and visually perceive the display on the computer monitor (human input). As they use the computer, they must integrate information (words, pictures) that they read or see from the monitor and convert that information into appropriate motor responses. When the computer beeps to indicate an error, they must decide what the beep signifies (human processing). Motor output is then aimed back to the computer (human output). This

human-machine interaction, however, would be absolutely useless if the computer did not have some method of acknowledging and acting on the person's motor output. The person presses a key or moves a mouse to tell the computer what to do next (environment/technology input). But the computer must have a program which reads, interprets, and analyzes what the key and mouse movements mean. The particular computer program becomes the computer's processing side of the human's cognitive processing (environment/technology application). The computer then must convert the new information it has calculated into a presentation which is perceivable by a human being. It takes its imperceptible (below human threshold) electronic impulses and converts them into auditory signals and visual displays (environment/ technology output). This completes the human machine cycle.

These six components are essential for the functioning of this human-technology model. If an individual needed to use a computer, but had any disability in sensory perception, cognitive processing, or motor output, the person would have difficulty using the computer. Likewise, this would be a non-functional interaction if the computer had a disability. A disabled computer would either fail to accept information the way the person was providing it, fail to process information in appropriate applications, or fail to output information so the person could perceive it. This model operates in a cycle and, as in most chains, is only as strong as its weakest link. Consequently, if an individual were blind, the cycle would be broken and the person could not use a computer unless one of two things were to occur: (1) either the person's input system (blindness) was somehow remediated or (2) the computer expressed some additional type of output which could be perceived by somebody who could not see the monitor.

This computer example provides a realistic example of human-machine interaction. It applies to technology application in general, and the role of occupational therapy in applying technology. Another example can be seen in a person driving a power wheelchair, in which the person needs to see where he/she is going (human input), decide where to go (human processing), and control the joystick (human output). The wheelchair requires a method of control, which is the joystick (environment/technology input), must process the information for directing the chair movement (environment/technology application), and actually move the chair in that direction (environment/ technology output). The model assists the therapist by identifying potential breakdown sites in therapeutic interventions and provides a framework for discussing the potentials and limitations of technology.

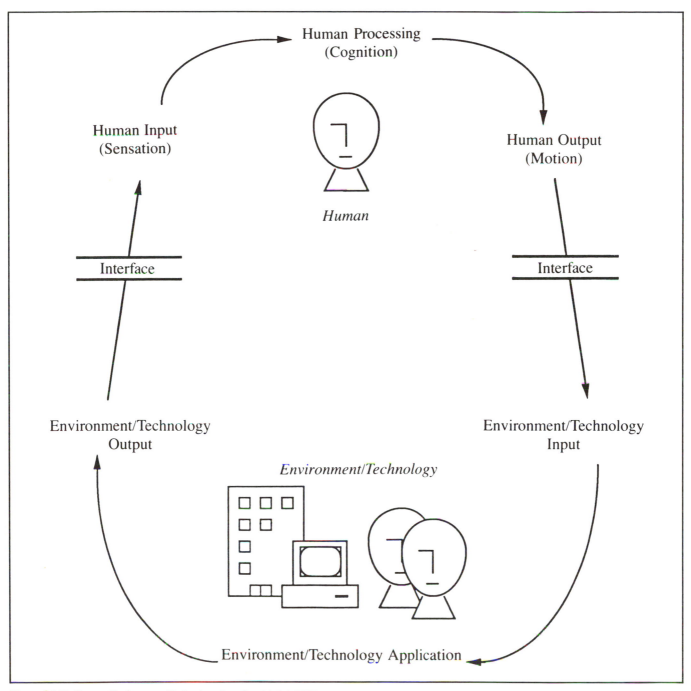

Figure 26-10. Human-Environment/Technology Interface Model (HETI).

TECHNOLOGICAL APPLICATIONS

There are two primary classes of technological applications in occupational therapy practice: (1) *direct intervention technology* which is used in direct patient care, and *supportive technology* which is used in nondirect patient care. Direct intervention technology includes two major categories (1) assistive/adaptive technologies and (2) rehabilitation/education technologies. Whereas, support technology commonly includes the following four areas: (1) administration, (2) documentation, (3) research, and (4) professional education (Figure 26-11).

Direct Intervention Technologies: Patient Care

In direct patient care, occupational therapists use a wide spectrum of intervention technologies including both assistive/adaptive techniques and rehabilitative/educational technologies.

Intervention Technology for Human Input. For the person with a human input deficit, an assortment of assistive/adaptive technologies are available to magnify his/her remaining perception or to substitute for his/her nonexisting perception. The types of assistive/adaptive technologies addressing human input are applied by specialized medical practitioners and are usually outside the domain of occupational therapy clinical practice. Examples of this type of technology include eyeglasses, hearing aids, or other more specialized devices such as tactile sensing gloves. The occupational therapist may serve a critical role in screening sensory deficits and helping individuals with sensory deficits accommodate their disability, but occupational therapists commonly do not evaluate and select eyeglasses, hearing aids, or tactile sensing gloves.

Occupational therapists do, however, frequently treat individuals with sensory impairments and apply specific training technologies to improve human sensation, such as sensory desensitization techniques. Also biofeedback is used in many applications with sensory and motor training (Abildness, 1982; Basmajian, 1989). Biofeedback can be used effectively in stress and pain reduction techniques to train an individual to sense their own muscle tension, heart rate, and other physiological responses. In this way, biofeedback expands human sensory awareness.

Furthermore, occupational therapists frequently apply assistive and adaptive devices which aid those with sensory/perceptual deficits, but implement them for very specific tasks for use in a particular environment, thus placing them more in the category of environment/technology output.

Intervention Technology for Human Processing. Persons with cognitive deficits such as individuals who have had strokes, head injuries, mental retardation, Alzheimer's disease, or schizophrenia can benefit from some assistive/adaptive technologies (both high and low technologies). Low technologies have been available for many years. Examples of this low technology used for people with memory or cognitive vigilance include such things as making grocery shopping lists or a list of steps on how to take the bus from home to a sheltered workshop, or using a watch that has an alarm set to sound to remind one of appointments, or to take medication.

The high technological systems are only beginning to be used by persons with cognitive disabilities. Examples of high technology in the assistive/adaptive category designed for persons with human processing deficits include the VIC system (Steele, Weinrick, Kleczewska, et al., 1988) and the COGORTH programming and application projects (Jaros, et al., 1987; Kirsch, Levine, & Jaros, 1987). The VIC system (developed at the Palo Alto Veterans Administration Hospital/Medical Center) uses a Macintosh computer to interface between a person with a specific aphasic (language deficit) and those with whom they communicate. VIC incorporates a pictorial/symbolic vocabulary on the Macintosh screen and the person who has left brain damage with oral apraxia can use the intact right hemisphere capabilities of spatial-orientation and cognition to help communicate by way of the computer (Figure 26-12).

The COGORTH system (University of Michigan) is a programmed language that is oriented towards helping individuals who have memory and problem-solving difficulties such as those who have suffered traumatic brain injuries. As a high-level programmed language, it helps set up a computer to assist an individual to follow through on a set of activities in any task. Both the VIC and COGORTH systems began experimental applications in the late 1980s. In the area of human cognitive processing, it is critical for occupational therapists to be aware of the types of technologies available. A large proportion of patients whom occupational therapists see have these deficits. The occupational therapist who is knowledgeable about the evaluation of cognitive deficits is a vital member of the treatment team for recommending appropriate low or high cognitive, orthotic, or prosthetic technologies.

Occupational Therapy Applications of Technology

Therapeutic Interventions (Direct Patient Care)	Support of Therapy (Non-Direct Patient Care)
1. Assistive/Adaptive Technologies	1. Administration/Management
2. Rehabilitative/Educational Technologies	2. Documentation
	3. Research
	4. Professional Education

Figure 26-11. Types of Technology Applications.

In addition to these adaptive/assistive technologies, the occupational therapist is also called upon to select and use a variety of software products which facilitate rehabilitation or education to remediate deficits in human cognitive processing. This technology group is usually classified as **cognitive rehabilitation** in the health science literature and thinking or problem-solving skills in educational research (Sidler, 1986). More than 25 cognitive rehabilitation and visual/perceptual integration programs are cataloged (see Trace R & D Center in Manufacturers and Information Centers listing). Software format and content range from highly structured game-like programs that isolate only one stimulus-response action (e.g., attention and discrimination) to multi-level, flexible branching programs that teach problem-solving strategies through everyday life simulations. Designers of cognitive software study the human input (e.g., sensory and motor limitations) of different groups of cognitive disabilities and attempt to improve human processing deficits or provide compensatory techniques (Sidler & Hutchins, 1987). A list of software titles and their manufacturers is presented in Appendix D. Cognitive rehabilitation software applications have substantial potentials, but some scholars continue to be skeptical and feel that much research is needed to empirically document and clarify the clinical efficacy of this type of technology.

Intervention Technology for Human Output. Occupational therapists work intensively with persons having human output deficits. Many patients whom occupational therapists treat have motor deficits that can benefit from low or high technology assistive/adaptive devices. Those with severe human output deficits benefit greatly from seating systems, positioning systems, and mobility systems (Taylor, 1987; Trefler, Kozole & Snell, 1986; Jaffe, 1987). These systems are crucial if functional motor skills are affected by activity intolerance, poor balance, or abnormal tone. An individual without proper trunk support or body positioning may be unable to effectively use their arms or hands. With proper positioning, however, their functional motor control can be improved considerably.

It is not uncommon to see children or young adults in technology evaluation centers who have never been able to voluntarily manipulate objects in their environment. They seem amazed to find their functional skills greatly improved with the introduction of fundamental seating and positioning components, such as a firm seat, firm back, lateral trunk support, head/neck support, and a lap tray that optimally positions objects in front of them. Sometimes the implementation of proper seating and positioning can have remarkable results. With correct seating and positioning devices, a child who could never play with toys while sitting can immediately manipulate a

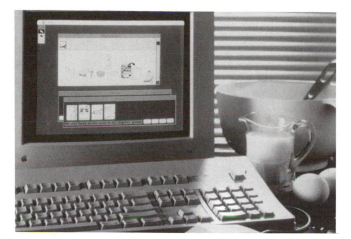

Figure 26-12. The VIC Communication Program.

toy voluntarily. Even more important is that these seating, positioning, and mobility technologies allow individuals to access new locations and educational environments in which they once could not go without the technology. Many more opportunities become available, such as sitting to watch a television or a puppet show or even visiting a park, a zoo, or museum.

Seating and **positioning** and **mobility** represent an important aspect of rehabilitation technology. This is evidenced by a special interest group in RESNA and major category heading in the ABLEDATA product listings.

Human output technology applications can also assist with fine motor tasks in helping people who have paralysis due to spinal cord injury, cerebral palsy, multiple sclerosis, or amyotrophic lateral sclerosis. When someone is unable to use their arms and legs, technology can extend their motor functioning by capitalizing on head and neck or mouth control with the use of **mouthwands** or **headsticks** (Figure 26-13a, b). **Light pointers** and **optical pointers** (commonly used in augmentative communication systems) and **single switch** activations can be the primary method of output for someone who has severe physical limitations (Figure 26-14a, b). In Brandenburg and Vanderheiden (1987a,b,c) and Borden and Vanderheiden (1988), these types of technologies were categorized as Pointing and Typing Aids.

Individuals with functional deficits resulting from less severe or isolated orthopedic or neuromuscular trauma or disease also benefit from a range of technology. For example, a person with C-5 quadriplegia due to spinal cord injury may have no intrinsic hand function, but by using a tenodesis splint, they can gain the fine motor capabilities to manage most tasks requiring basic hand function. An individual with a Colles wrist fracture who is being treated in a hand rehabilitation clinic may benefit from a wrist splint

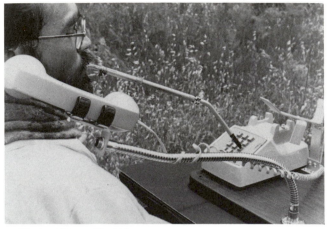

a. Person using mouthwand.

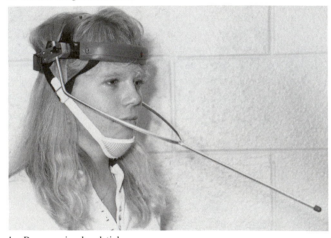

b. Person using headstick.

Figure 26-13a, b. Mouthwands and Headsticks.

which improves the person's ability to maintain hand function.

As a recently developed technology, functional electrical stimulation (FES) is being used as an orthotic approach to substitute for inadequate functioning of specific muscle groups (Benton, Baker, Bewman, & Walters, 1981). Appendix C highlights the types of FES research and development projects as presented at the International Conference of the Association for the Advancement of Rehabilitation and Technology in Montreal (ICAART, 1988). A Functional Electrical Stimulation Information Center is now available for responding to clinical and research questions (see Manufacturers and Information Centers listing, Appendix C).

Robots are yet another example of high technology which provides support primarily to persons with human output deficits (Figure 26-15a, b). Robots are found in a variety of settings, including homes and workplaces. PRAB Command, Inc. and Rehabilitation R & D Center—Palo Alto Veterans Administration are two centers developing

such systems (see Manufacturers and Information Centers listing). Figure 26-16 is a listing of the robotics research and development projects.

In occupational therapy, there is much interest in the technology available for motor training. The goals of technologies in this area range from increasing endurance and strength to range of motion. Developing technologies that address motor training include motor training software, functional electrical stimulation, biofeedback, robotics, and work hardening systems. Some motor training software such as reaction-time exercises are packaged with programs for cognitive rehabilitation. Individuals with apraxia, exhibited by some persons who have brain injury, may benefit from cognitive rehabilitation programs which have included praxis exercises within cognitive software.

Other **motor training software** programs are designed specifically for developing motor skills in order to gain access to the technology. Switch training programs are examples (see Figure 26-17). Functional electrical stimula-

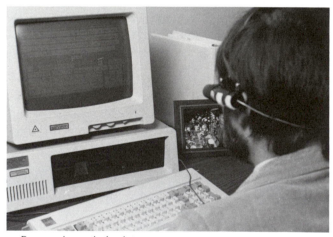

a. Person using optical pointer.

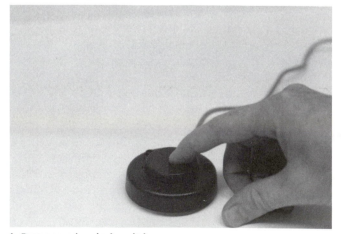

b. Person pressing single switch.

Figure 26-14a, b. Optical Pointer and Single Switch.

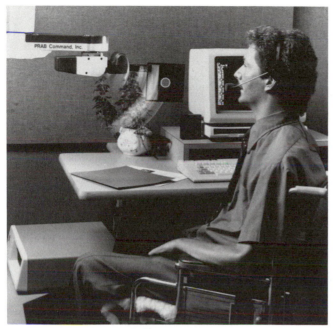

a. Robot workstation (PRAB Command).

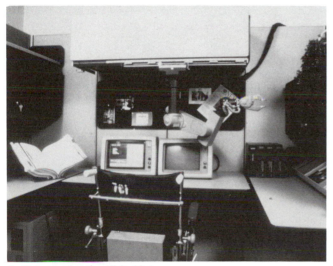

b. Robot workstation (Palo Alto).

Figure 26-15a, b. Robots as Assistive Technology Systems.

tion, biofeedback, and the integrated use of functional electrical stimulation and biofeedback have been implemented actively as motor training technologies and are discussed at length in other chapters. In the past, biofeedback systems commonly used simple meters, scales, and auditory signals for the biofeedback mechanism, but today, powerful biofeedback systems tend to be computer-based and incorporate two-dimensional and three-dimensional visual feedback on a computer monitor (Figure 26-18).

Robots are beginning to find their way into a variety of unexpected applications, including facilitating social inter-

action of autistic children (Durie, 1988; Howell & Campbell, 1988) and using robots as an automated motion-training assistant (Kristy, 1988). Passive range of motion machines are a focused and single-function type of robot which have been on the market for several years.

Intervention Technology for Environment/Technology Input. Frequently, the design of machines, furniture, architecture, and even technology does not accommodate able-bodied persons, much less persons with disabilities. Such poor design can frustrate or even further antagonize those with disabilities. *Human factors engineering* is an entire field which addresses the specific issues of human limitations and capabilities and their influence on machine technology or environmental design. Although human factors engineers investigate and refine the design of technology for persons without disabilities, they have found that a design that accommodates persons with disabilities usually also makes it easier or more efficient for able-bodied persons. For example, a poorly-engineered heavy entrance

---

Robotics Research and Development

Design And Evaluation Of A Vocational Desktop Robot

Education And Research Issues In Designing Robotically-Aided Science Education Environments

The UT/HMMC Robotic Aid

Hardware And Software Considerations In The Design Of A Prototype Educational Robotic Manipulator

Developing Specifications Of A Robot For Health Care Use; Step 1: Data Collection

Design Of A Human-Machine Interface Of A Voice Controlled Vocational Robotic Work Station

Sensory Feedback And Automated Grasping For A Vocational Robotic Work Station

Mobile Robot System For Rehabilitation Applications

Development Of Automated Grasping And End-Effector For Robotic Aid Using Multiplexed Infrared Sensors

Todus: An English Interface With Rehabilitation Potential

Integrated Robotic Assisted Environment

Applications Of The Curl Programming Environment

Development Of A Programming Environment For Rehabilitation Robotics

MOUSETRAP

User Selection Criteria For A Voice Activated Robotic Work Cell

Figure 26-16. Robotics Research and Development Project Titles.

door to a building will not only prevent persons with disabilities from entering, but also restricts many individuals considered normal or able-bodied (i.e., those who are short in stature, those that lack good grip-strength, or those susceptible to back injury). In contrast, a lighter door that is well-designed will allow access to persons with disabilities as well as most able-bodied persons. Figure 26-19 describes another example of how making adaptations for persons with disability improves the environment for everyone.

Unfortunately, not every device or environment satisfactorily meets ideal human factors requirements. This is quite evident when an occupational therapist helps a person with a disability confront a hostile environment. Adaptive and assistive technologies are often needed to permit the person with a disability to input or access a machine or environment. Occupational therapists should be among the first to identify and recommend appropriate modifications.

Other examples of environment/technology input adapta-

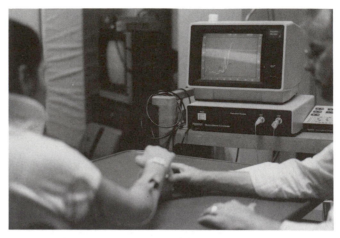

Figure 26-18. Biofeedback System for Muscle Re-Education.

tions are alternative and expanded keyboards for computer or typewriter access, voice recognition control systems for power wheelchairs, and environmental control systems (Figure 26-20a-f). An example of low technology in this category would include an adaptation of a regular knife for a person who has the use of only one hand (called a rocker knife).

These assistive/adaptive technologies have become so numerous that they require a classification system of their own. Borden and Vanderheiden (1988) use 30 different codes for describing input systems (Figure 26-21).

A key role of occupational therapy in technology service delivery is identifying the optimal input techniques for accommodating individual disabilities. Many different techniques are used to control technological devices. While these methods have been described in augmentative communication literature, the concepts can apply as well to access to computers, power wheelchairs, environmental control, and robotics. An occupational therapy technologist needs to be familiar with the breadth of these input techniques.

Vanderheiden and Lloyd (1986) carefully delineate many of the key components of access technologies. Five terms are briefly described here: direct selection, directed scanning, scanning, encoding, and acceleration methods. The first three are basic selection techniques.

Direct selection is how able-bodied people dial a telephone or type on a keyboard and is a very fast method. The individual simply identifies a target key and moves straight toward it (Figure 26-22). Similarly, picking a box of cereal off the shelf at the grocery store is direct selection. Unfortunately, even though this is frequently the method of choice because it is cognitively simple and rapid, direct selection also requires refined motor patterns. Thus, for people with severe motor deficits (HO) to use this method requires adapted methods of technology input (EI).

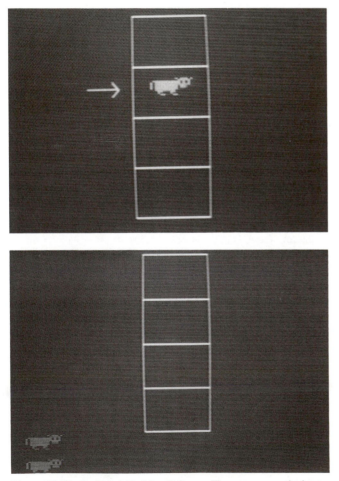

Figure 26-17a, b. Switch Training Software. The arrow scans the boxes. To catch the cow, the user hits the switch when the arrow is pointing at the cow.

Directed scanning is an alternate input method which requires less motor skill, but is a slower method when compared to an agile person using direct selection. For example, persons with limited motion might not be able to directly indicate a target. They may, however, be able to use a directed scanning input device such as a joystick or five switches to drive a cursor around a display to select a target which, in turn, might control the environment (Figure 26-22).

Scanning is another input method which requires even less motor function to access a large quantity of targets. Scanning is a start-stop technique in which the user starts the scanning and once the target is identified, the user stops the scan. Using binoculars to find a bird in a tree is an analogous process. The bird watcher scans the area in the tree until the bird is seen through the binoculars and then stops. In terms of motor control, one method of scanning can be operated simply by hitting a switch to start the scan and again to stop the scan (Figure 26-22).

These three generic selection methods can be implemented using many different techniques which are not discussed here. For example, scanning can be uni- dimensional or multi-dimensional or visual or auditory. When choosing the best method to use, the motor skill requirement is only one aspect of input skills to consider. For instance, the cognitive requirement usually increases as the motor requirement decreases, hence one must consider the cognitive capacity of the individual. Scanning is cognitively more difficult to use than direct selection.

Encoding is another dimension of selection methods. Encoding simply means that some input symbols represent other output symbols. There are a variety of coding methods available to persons with motor disabilities, such as Morse code, which is frequently used. (See Figure 26-23.)

Acceleration is another selection method which helps to speed up the input-output process. Acceleration techniques are elaborate coding structures or computerized algorithms which take a minimal number of input symbols and return them as expanded output. For example, with an abbreviation-expansion technique, an entire name and address might be represented by only two initials. Keying those two initials into the computer could generate information for a mail label. (See Figure 26-23.) Another example of an acceleration is word prediction, in which the computer tries to guess the next word after a cue word is typed. If the word "good" is input, then the computer might offer the following choice of words: "morning," "afternoon," "night," "bye," "riddance," or "grief."

Input techniques are not simple. There are many varieties and combinations of varieties. Occupational therapy technologists need to carefully examine the options to select the most appropriate adapted input method for an individual to access their particular environment.

Intervention Technology for Environment/Technology Application. Assistive/adaptive devices and systems all have the purpose of improving the functional performance of a person with a disability. Some of these devices or systems do not provide access, but actually perform the functional activity or directly assist in it.

Personal care activities: cleanliness, hygiene, and appearance. Assistive/adaptive technologies are currently allowing more independence and privacy in personal care activities for those who have disabilities. These include many adaptive and assistive devices now taken for granted by occupational therapists, including bathing aids such as bath mitts, bath benches, long-handled sponges; toilet hygiene aids such as elevated toilet seats, grab bars, special wiping and suppository devices; grooming aids such as denture brushes, special dental floss holders for oral hygiene, cosmetic holders, brushes and combs with

---

"Curb-cut Logic"

Curb cuts for city streets and sidewalks were intended to help individuals with mobility disabilities who did not have equal access to streets and sidewalks and for whom downtown areas, shops, and businesses were not accessible from a wheelchair. Because many cities are progressive and feel the responsibility to provide equal access to everyone, curbs are being broken apart and curb cuts are being laid into sidewalks for persons with wheelchairs. The result of this environmental adaptation for persons with disabilities, however, is better access between streets and sidewalks for many more individuals than just persons with disabilities. In fact, it is estimated that for every person in a wheelchair who uses a curb cut, ten able-bodied individuals use the curb cut for shopping carts, roller skates, strollers, high heels, hand trucks, etc. Today, much less expense is incurred when curb cuts are first being laid instead of the more costly approach of tearing old curbs up and replacing them.

This design concept is being extended beyond curbs. Vanderheiden (1983a,b), proposed that all the newer models of computers be designed to avoid retrofitting electronic systems at a later date when it is more difficult. The logic is that not only will more accessible computers enable persons with disabilities to function in a computer environment, but many of the design parameters required for persons with disabilities make computer use much more efficient for persons *without* disabilities. One of the first examples of computer "curb-cut logic" was the off/on switch of many computers which at one time was always located on the back of every computer but is now being located within easy reach for any computer user.

Figure 26-19. Making Environments Accessible for Persons with Disabilities Makes Environments Accessible for Everybody.

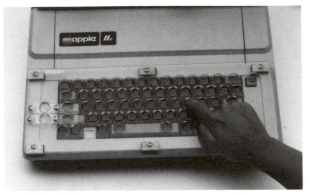

a. Keyguard.

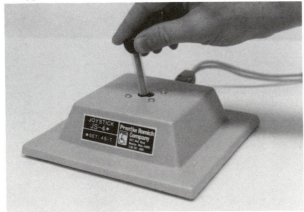

b. Joystick.

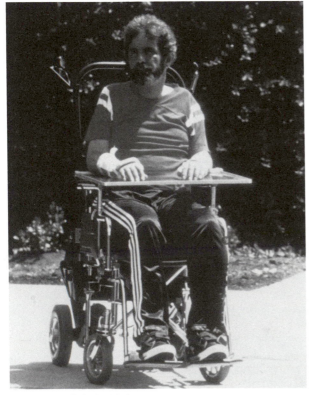

c. Head-controlled wheelchair.

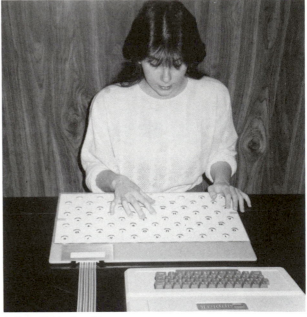

d. Expanded keyboard.

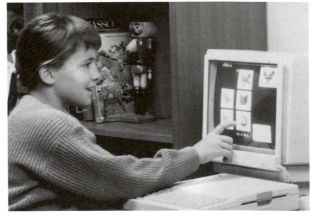

e. Touchscreen.

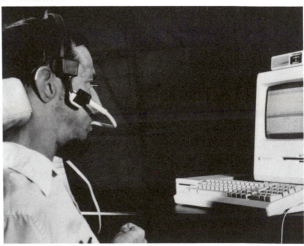

f. Ultrasonic mouse.

Figure 26-20 a-f. Input Technologies.

extended handles, holders for electric shavers, and dressing aids such as sticks, sock aids, apron hoops. Such low technology devices can be ordered from manufacturers such as Sammons, Preston, Maddak, or Cleo (See Appendix C at the end of the book). There are several thousand assistive and adaptive devices cataloged by ABLEDATA in the categories of cleanliness, hygiene, and appearance.

Extremely sophisticated high technologies are now being applied to personal care tasks. One system being used at the Palo Alto Veterans Administration Hospital and Medical Center includes a voice-activated robot which assists severely physically impaired individuals to brush their teeth, shave, and wash their faces (Figure 26-24).

Medical and health management. Technology offering cognitive support systems can help individuals to independently take the correct medications at the appropriate times. Such devices that help promote independent medication routines include: 7-day pill holders, special adaptive holders for self-administration of intra-muscular injections, medication pumps, special scoops for persons who have swallowing disorders, and adaptive medication bottle caps. Computer-based cognitive support systems are available which help individuals remember their medication routine and keep them apprised of current dangerous side-effects (Bagneski, 1985; Jaros, Levine & Kirsch, 1987).

Home exercise programs use assistive and adaptive devices such as checklists and videotapes in order to help individuals remember the therapeutic sequences for their physical and psychological health benefit.

To aid individuals in calling for help in emergencies, memory-dial telephones enable individuals with cognitive, motor, or sensory disabilities to quickly dial emergency telephone numbers. The advent of the 911 Emergency Hotline and Smart 911 systems in North America not only provides a number that is easy to remember, but also immediately identifies the origin of a telephone call if the caller is unable to specify their location.

Not only is this high technology available in acute care hospitals, but much of it can now be used in the home. Cardiac and EMG monitors are being sent home with clients in order to monitor their daily activity over a 24-hour period. In this way, clients can be monitored as they go about their daily routines and engage in exercise programs at home as if a therapist were present. They also provide feedback to clients and their family members.

Kitchen and nutrition activities. In this category, low technology vendors provide adaptive cooking devices including one-handed utensils, cutting boards, kitchen and tableware utensils, and adaptive dishwashing aids such as one-handed bottle brushes, can openers, and jar openers. High technology computers offer pre-planned menus, computer-assisted prompting systems, powered feeders, and independent simple meal preparation and feeding through the use of robotics.

Mobility activities. Products for basic mobility include the full range of bed mobility devices, transferring devices and systems, manual wheelchairs and the spectrum of wheelchair accessories, powered wheelchairs, and special control systems. Adaptive devices to aid driving include devices that accommodate the use of one hand, the use of only upper extremity, the use of only lower extremity, and extremely limited motor control driving. Adaptive devices

---

Assistive/Adaptive Technologies

Input Expand/Accel
Abbreviation expansion
Encoding (chart or memory based)
Levels or pages
Morse
Predictive

Input Method
Directed scanning
Scanning

Input symbol system
Auditory presentation (e.g., Auditory Scanning)
Bliss symbols
Photos/pictures/line drawings
User selectable symbols
Whole words

Input Type
Air (sip/puff)
Contact (zero pressure)
Eye movement and eye gaze
Head controlled
Input Jack—accepts any switch
Joystick/wobblestick
Light sensitive (optical)
Movement activated
Noise (sound or vocalization)
OCR (optical character recognition)
Pressure sensitive
Speech recognition
Wireless

Switch Inputs
Analog control
Dual switch
Joystick (4 or 5 switches)
Multiple switches (3 to 16 switches)
Single switch

Figure 26-21. Thirty Input Classifications.

Direct Selection

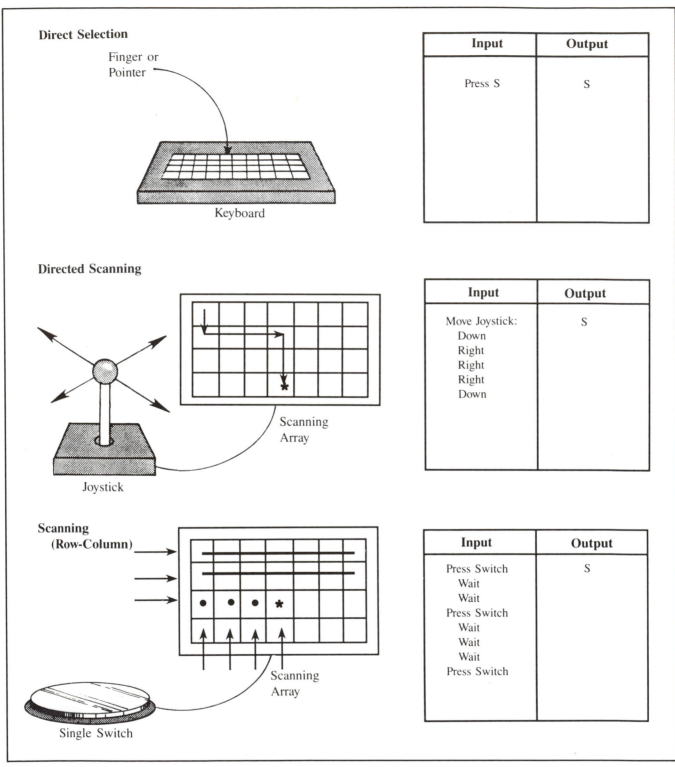

Finger or Pointer

Keyboard

Input	Output
Press S	S

Directed Scanning

Joystick

Scanning Array

Input	Output
Move Joystick: Down Right Right Right Down	S

Scanning (Row-Column)

Scanning Array

Single Switch

Input	Output
Press Switch Wait Wait Press Switch Wait Wait Wait Press Switch	S

Figure 26-22. Selection Techniques.

used in public transportation include low technology systems for cognitive-prompting such as special maps and pictures of the proper change required for a fare.

Communication activities. These activities include communication, writing, reading, and telephone use. Augmentative and alternative communication interventions fall under the assistive/adaptive technologies for communication activities. A number of textbooks describe the overall application of augmentative/alternative communication systems; some are more generic and introductory (Blackstone, 1986) and others more specific to high technology (Fishman 1987). Conversation technologies range from manual pointing boards and eye-pointing charts to elaborate systems which incorporate electronic voice output such as the Light Talker, Touch Talker, Intro Talker (Prentke Romich, 1989), Real Voice (Adaptive Communication Systems, 1989), Easy Talker and Equalizer (Words+, 1989), VOIS (Phonic Ear, 1989). Figure 26-25a-d shows samples of these systems.

Low technology writing devices include special pencil/pen holders, writing template guides, letter templates, electric typewriters, and word processors. Also higher technology writing systems with acceleration and special interactive software are being based on laptop computers. A noticeable difference between writing systems and conversation systems is that writing systems have printed output and the ability to manipulate text. Conversation systems tend to be used more as a temporary means usually with only auditory output which is serially delivered. As discussed earlier, abbreviation expansion, semantic compaction, and word prediction are computerized vocabulary-selection acceleration techniques used in both speaking and writing systems.

There are a number of devices available to aid in reading. Low technology adaptations for a person with a severe motor restriction include mouth-wand page-turners with an eraser tip and book clips; those of higher technology include electronic page-turners. Adaptations for individuals with visual impairments include systems with large print, talking books, and optical character recognition units such as the Kursweil (See Appendix C).

Telephone access can be provided through a variety of methods, including gooseneck receivers with mechanical flip-levers to depress the receiver switch. One product called the Directel (AT&T) allows *sip and puff* switch access to the operator, who then provides free dialing assistance (See Appendix C). Telephone technologies can also be integrated into more comprehensive environmental control systems.

Vocational role-related activities. Most of the technological applications in this area occur in the work site and tend to be specific to the individual's particular job duties and responsibilities. Technologies include robotics, environmental control systems, work modification devices, and rural rehabilitation technology. Robots have been effectively working in assembly lines for industry for many years. Acceptance of robots by occupational therapists seems to be growing (Glass & Hall, 1987). The specific applications of robots in the workplace for people with disabilities, however, is relatively new. In the past, robots required sophisticated and time-intensive programming, but newer robots are much easier to use. Since robots have been most beneficial for persons with severe physical disability such as high spinal cord injury, robotic workstations tend to be activated by voice. These robot stations are usually of industrial quality and consequently cost between $20,000 and $50,000 for the total workstation. Two organizations marketing early robotic workstations in the U.S. include: PRAB Command Inc. and Rehabilitation R & D Center in Palo Alto (See Appendix C). Smaller capacity robots, often defined as personal robots or toy robots (Campbell, 1986) are also being investigated for application in more workstations. However these smaller robots tend to be less durable, much less refined in their motor control, and more difficult to set up.

Although most of us take for granted simple movements such as turning on the lights, switching TV channels, answering the doorbell, or adjusting the heating device, not one of these tasks is easy for people with severe disabilities. Environmental controls such as those pictured in Figure 26-26a-d can help accomplish these tasks for those who have limited human movement (Dickey & Shealey, 1987).

Environmental control systems (sometimes called "ECU's" for Environmental Control Units) can be fundamentally electronic. Others mechanically control specific devices such as systems that draw curtains, open doors, and

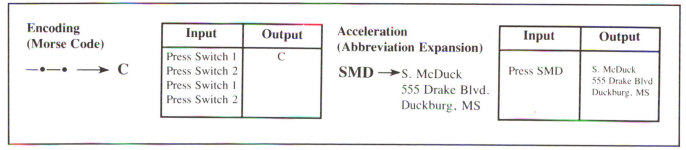

Encoding (Morse Code)	Input	Output
— • — • ⟶ C	Press Switch 1	C
	Press Switch 2	
	Press Switch 1	
	Press Switch 2	

Acceleration (Abbreviation Expansion)	Input	Output
SMD ⟶ S. McDuck 555 Drake Blvd. Duckburg, MS	Press SMD	S. McDuck 555 Drake Blvd. Duckburg, MS

Figure 26-23. Encoding and Acceleration Techniques.

open locks. Methods of controlling these systems include human voice frequency or sound stimulation such as whistling, ultrasound impulses, infrared controls such as the light waves used in remote TV controls, radio signals, and direct wiring. Most environmental control units are used within an individual's home for controlling the home environment, but there is an increase in environmental control systems being used at the worksite. Occasionally, they are linked to the newer robotic workstations and permit individuals to work outside of the home. Unfortunately, third-party reimbursement agencies often do not consider environmental control systems as being medically necessary, so reimbursement for such systems is difficult to obtain. The costs of such systems range from under $100 to several thousands of dollars for a complete, complex system.

Worksite modifications are another important area of assistive/adaptive technology. Some basic technologies simply apply known ergonomic principles such as in chairs with adjustable seat heights and backs, in the proper heights of keyboards, and the placement of monitors for technology workstations. Basic accessibility issues are also important in the worksite such as providing tables which permit wheelchair accessibility. Other commonly used assistive/ adaptive technologies include shop workbenches that have rotating, sliding or tilting table-tops, adjustable heights and specific equipment modifications that permit one-handed use of tools, and special jigs for placements of work pieces.

The National Institute of Disability and Rehabilitation Research in the U.S. recognizes the rural setting as a vital work setting and has highlighted rural technology as worthy of particular attention. Rural rehabilitation has many unique features, such as special equipment needed for mounting and dismounting from tractors. A Research and Training Center based in Montana was begun in 1988 to focus on rural rehabilitation (See Rural Rehabilitation R & T Center in Appendix C). Other centers have specialized in rural technology for many years, including those at North Dakota University and Purdue University. Purdue University also runs an intervention information service which provides key resources on rural technology applications (See Appendix C).

Technology as applied to assist in vocational role-related activities cannot be viewed as easy to select and implement. Identifying the right technologies and learning proper use is more time consuming than it appears. For example, learning how to use the "Butler in a Box" environmental control system, can be extremely difficult for a novice computer user or a person who has very little technological background. Consequently, training manuals and tutorials are vital to these technologies. Computer-based training systems increasingly are being developed for use to train technology use. Many computer software companies are incorporating more elaborate on-screen tutorials and help manuals that are context sensitive. Other companies, like the Free Wheel developers (Pointer Systems), determined that their computer access and writing systems required specific training and thus developed both a tutorial module to assist the new user in understanding the system and a trainer module to develop motor skills to optimize use of the pointing system.

Intervention Technology for Environment Technology Output. The last functional category of assistive/adaptive technologies is in the output area. Individuals with sensory impairments cannot perceive information presented by many machines and machine environments. For example, an individual who is blind cannot read text from a computer screen. Therefore, specific modification or peripherals are necessary to permit blind individuals to read computer information. Some methods of computer output for blind individuals include voice synthesis programs which read the text on the computer screen and print it from Braille printers. Other examples for sensory impaired individuals include phone receiver amplifiers, large print books, and large print software programs which provide magnifying capabilities on a computer system. Figure 26-27 lists the seven categories of output/display systems.

Low technologies in the area of adapted output include the analysis and modification of visual displays. Simplifying displays, instructions, and visually organized material can improve the presentation and output of machine environments for persons who have limited cognitive-perceptual abilities. Methods of optimizing visual displays include color coding of communication boards, rearranging point

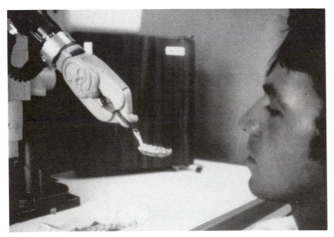

Figure 26-24. Robots in Personal Care. *Palo Alto robot - hygiene or grooming.*

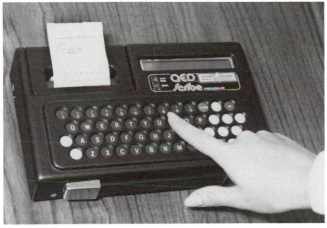

a. Red Scribe (Zygo).

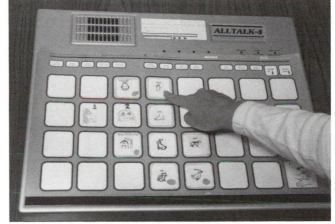

c. All Talk (Adaptive Communication Systems, Inc.).

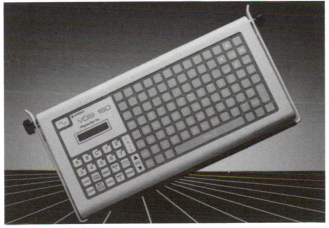

b. VOIS (Phonic Ear).

Figure 26-25a-d. Augmentive Communication Devices.

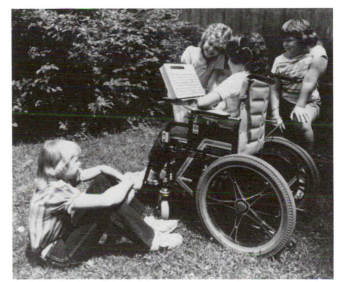

d. Light Talker (Prentke-Romich).

cells on communication boards, or using pictures instead of verbal models of information.

Some types of technologies are not used in direct patient care or therapeutic intervention, but rather assist therapists in performing clinical tasks, such as the numerous clerical tasks of administration, documenting/reporting, research, and professional education.

Administration. From the management perspective, technology provides a much faster and more comprehensive analysis of numbers and information. For therapists, this efficiency should be viewed as cost-effective management practice. Consequently, traditional computer applications used by businesses are being implemented in occupational therapy administrative practice in the form of word processors, spreadsheets, and databases (Smith, 1986; Sidler, 1986). Five general types of computer applications are

being used by occupational therapy managers and are important to review.

First, many managers are now billing charges by computers. Billing software programs are usually written for the particular setting and primarily have been governed by the organization in which the occupational therapy clinic resides, such as a hospital administration. However, now independent practitioners can set up their own computerized billing systems.

A second area of administrative technology application is the analysis of occupational therapy activity which includes examining the fiscal and work unit statistics to identify expenses, revenues, units of occupational therapy activity, and overall productivity of the occupational therapy clinic. In the larger organizations this information frequently is provided to the occupational therapy manager by management information services or data processing. In smaller

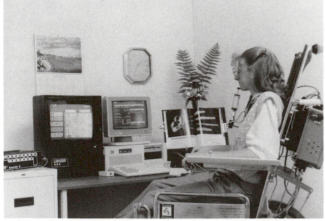

a. An environmental control system run with a joystick. DU-IT environmental control unit.

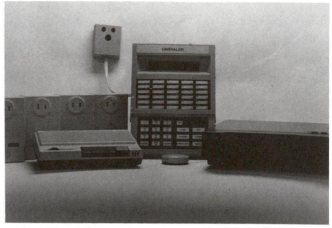

c. A modular environmental control system. Unidialer by TASH, Inc.

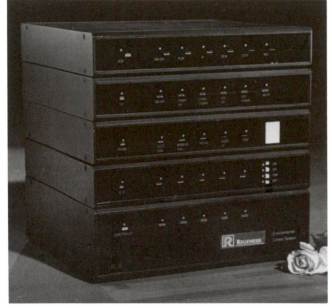

b. A system which includes dialing and managing telephone calls. Environmental control unit by Regenesis.

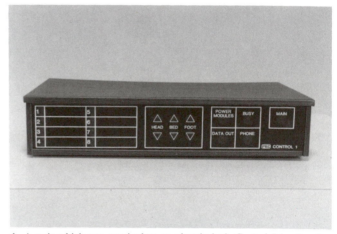

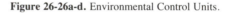

d. A unit which can manipulate an electric bed. Control I by Prentke-Romich Company.

Figure 26-26a-d. Environmental Control Units.

independent settings, the occupational therapy administrator is responsible for selecting their own particular analytical software package.

A third area of application is resource management in which computer applications are used in scheduling therapists, scheduling patients, scheduling therapy rooms and facilities, ordering equipment, and maintaining equipment inventories and vendor supply inventories.

A fourth area of application is personal management. Personal management software is evolving and these packages typically include methods of storing phone numbers, addresses and names of contact people, and "tickler" memory files. They can be connected to a modem for automatic telephone dialing. Examples of this are Apple Macintosh Hypercard (Apple, 1987), Agenda (Lotus, 1988),

as well as programs called desk accessory programs like Sidekick Plus (Borland, 1988). Lists of work tasks and work priorities are frequently included. Scratch pads, note pads, outliners, calculators, calendars, and clocks are common desktop applications.

The fifth type of administrative application is more clinically-oriented. Occupational therapists benefit from having computerized information systems. For example, a clinician needing to know if a certain rehabilitation product is available or desiring the cost and source of a given device can easily locate that information in Hyper-ABLEDATA (See Figure 26-28). Special information databases can also catalog the most commonly used activities and treatment modalities in a clinic so the therapist can type "visual perceptual" into the computer and receive a list of suggested visual perceptual training activities. These information databases may also catalog attendance records for continuing education courses for easy access when required by the Joint Commission on Accreditation of Health Organizations or the Commission for Accreditation of Rehabilitation Facilities. The RESNA Technology Service Delivery Guide is also available in an electronic database designed so that a clinician visually can view a map, point to the location where services are desired, and obtain service delivery listings. This is helpful for making referrals and identifying services in unfamiliar locations (Figure 26-29).

Documenting/Reporting. Computerized "Boilerplates" or standardized information are commonly used in occupational therapy clinics when the same information is required repeatedly for letters such as patient advocacy requests to funding agencies. These boilerplates are also being used in occupational therapy evaluation and progress note documentation. These tasks usually are performed with word processor or specific documentation programs. For example, there are several such programs available today to help in writing Individual Educational Plans required for students in certain school settings in the U.S.. (Trace R & D, 1989).

Computers are also enabling more efficient documentation systems for therapists. The computer can generate forms with blanks to be filled in by the therapist. One example is a system that helps customized home programs where the therapist writes the number of repetitions of a certain exercise and adds or deletes exercises. (Create, 1989).

Computer-assisted evaluation is becoming quite common within occupational therapy practice. These reporting systems frequently are linked directly into word processors so that a written summary of the evaluation is generated which can be included in the chart or used as a base for a narrative note in the medical or educational record. Some programs also compare information between admission and discharge and indicate the results on a graph. Appendix C lists titles and sources of computerized evaluations.

Research. Research applications of computers have been around longer than any others. Many occupational therapy researchers received their initial professional training on large mainframe computer systems which required using computer cards and keypunching. Today, research and statistical applications are much more user-friendly.

In research, computers are viewed typically as the mechanism for the statistical analysis of data. T-test, ANOVA, factor analysis, and tabulations are becoming easier to perform with increased availability of software and computers. In the 1970s, only mainframes in universities

would permit these functions. Today, compatible statistical analysis packages can be used by researchers on personal computers. Clinicians/researchers can now perform statistical analyses in the clinic and no longer require mainframe equipment. Additionally, the advent of laptop and hand-held computers permits actual on-site clinical data collection in an efficient manner (Schneider, Champoux & Beinert, 1987).

Professional Education. Early discussions of computer applications in occupational therapy literature addressed the use of computers for educating professional students. Such programs are commonly referred to with the following acronyms: "CAT" for Computer Assisted Training, "CAE" for Computer Assisted Education, and "CAI" for Computer Assisted Instruction. One of the newest technologies now being implemented in computer-assisted instruction is the video laser disk which permits fast interactive video systems (Dudley & D'Agati, 1989).

SERVICE DELIVERY MODELS

Service delivery in rehabilitation/education technology needs to be viewed from two perspectives: one which looks at the national service delivery scene and the other from the pragmatic occupational therapy perspective.

The occupational therapist is involved in delivering rehabilitation technology services in a variety of settings. Seven service delivery models have been identified by RESNA (Figure 26-30). Occupational therapists should understand that different areas of technology can be delivered using different models even with the same setting. For example, power mobility, seating, and positioning may be performed from within an occupational therapy department; whereas environmental control or augmentative communication systems may use a durable medical equipment

---

Output/Display

Braille Printer
Deaf Baudot (for TDDs)
Ideographic/Pictographic Symbols
Large Print
Modem (ASCII)
Speech Output
Tactile/Braille Display (Dynamic)

Figure 26-27. Seven Output Classifications.

supplier as the primary service delivery mechanism. For children in the same vicinity, the school district may provide the augmentative communication technology services, and drivers' training, and adaptive equipment modifications for community mobility may be provided by a private rehabilitation technology firm in the community. Such a dissociated delivery system involving many programs can be high quality, but requires careful coordination by the therapist. Occupational therapists must be cognizant of all of these delivery mechanisms to be able to appropri-

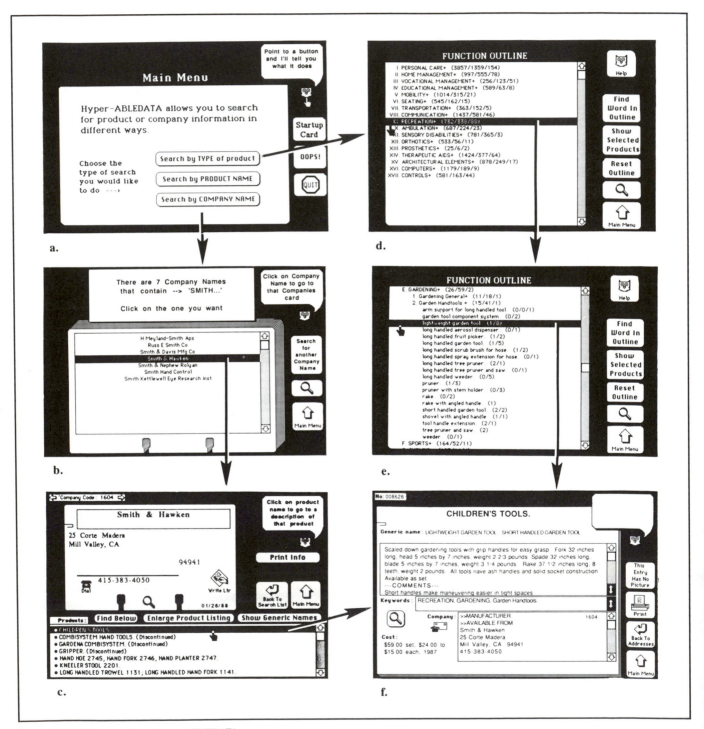

Figure 26-28a-f. Screens from Hyper-ABLEDATA.

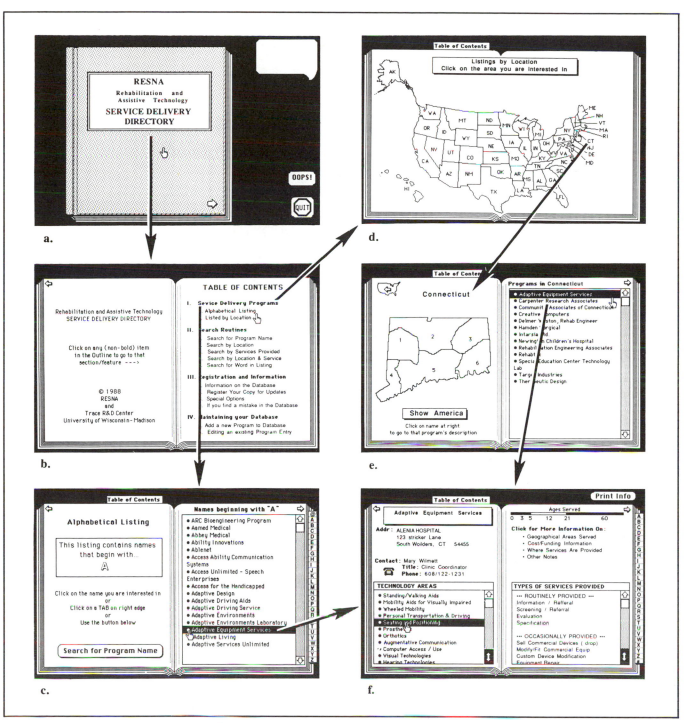

Figure 26-29a-f. Screens from Service Delivery Directory Database.

ately refer and to tap the necessary resources. One method of assuring coordination of resources is to list all the functional needs for the respective patient population and identify each mechanism being implemented to provide technology service.

Technology service delivery is also moving toward a system built upon regional expert centers (Vanderheiden, 1987a,b). There is a trend in rehabilitation and assistive technology to develop centers of excellence, such as the regional centers for powered mobility and seating and

Service Delivery Models	
Model 1:	The Durable Medical Equipment (DME) distributor
Model 2:	The department within a comprehensive rehabilitation program
Model 3:	The technology service delivery center in a university
Model 4:	The state agency-based program
Model 5:	The private rehabilitation engineering/ technology firm
Model 6:	The local affiliate of a national nonprofit disability organization
Model 7:	Miscellaneous types of programs, including the volunteer agency

Figure 26-30. The seven models of service delivery in rehabilitation technology.

positioning. Occupational therapy community clinics should know where the nearest centers are located and maintain fundamental knowledge about seating, positioning, and mobility in order to refer to the regional center as indicated. Ideally, each occupational therapy clinician should have information about the regional center and visit the site to see exactly what they do.

Technology service delivery poses a special problem for occupational therapy managers. Because of the technological advantages of the past decade, it has become impossible for any one individual to be an expert in all technology applications. It is increasingly evident that in current practice, larger occupational therapy clinics need to divide technology application areas between a group of therapists and/or hire technology experts. For example, a comprehensive rehabilitation occupational therapy clinic might identify a therapist with expertise in seating, positioning, and mobility, a second therapist with expertise in cognitive rehabilitation, a third with expertise in interfacing input and output systems with computers and communication systems, a fourth therapist with expertise in robotics and environmental control units, and a fifth with expertise in biofeedback and functional electrical stimulation. Depending on the size of the clinic, therapists or technologists might be assigned other technology application areas such as ADL's, driving, recreation, or job site. Obviously, all therapists must have a fundamental knowledge across all of the technological areas for general application. The individual resource person serves as the primary service provider and the resource expert for particularly difficult cases. These therapists must remain up-to-date on the current

changes in the technological area and provide staff training. Therapists need to consider themselves technologists in specialty areas but have basic fundamental knowledge in other areas of technology.

SOCIAL AND PROFESSIONAL ISSUES REGARDING TECHNOLOGY SERVICE DELIVERY

Legislative

Just as Public Law 94-142 was a major force in providing comprehensive multidisciplinary special education services for children with disabilities, other federal legislation in the U.S. is having an impact on technology service delivery. In the 1980s, two significant legislative decisions were enacted.

In 1986, amendments were made to the Rehabilitation Act of 1973 that defined and integrated rehabilitation engineering and technology services into the Rehabilitation Act. This recognized technology services as a part of rehabilitation and required that rehabilitation engineering services should be available in vocational rehabilitation departments throughout the country.

A second important feature of the 1986 Amendments to the Rehabilitation Act of 1973 was the mandate to make electronic systems used by government employees accessible to persons with disabilities. In other words, the federal government was required to purchase electronic equipment which meets accessibility criteria. This meant that corporations which sold electronic equipment and provided services to the federal government and other related agencies were required to provide electronic equipment that reasonably could be accessed by blind persons, deaf persons, motor impaired persons, and cognitively impaired persons. The significance of these revisions in the Rehabilitation Act is that the federal government was acknowledging the need for products designed for persons with disabilities. Perhaps even more significant was that these regulations suggested to the commercial sector that they should consider persons with disabilities when designing equipment. Procurement officers in the federal government now have criteria and recommendations for obtaining electronic equipment. These guidelines focus on personal computers but will include typewriters, copiers, and calculators. (Gray, LeClair, Traub, et al., 1987; Vanderheiden, Lee, & Scadden, 1988).

A second legislative act of major significance to technology and occupational therapy in the U.S. was Public Law 100-407, the Technology Related Assistance for Individuals with Disabilities Act, which became law in the summer of 1988. This Act made funds available to help state governors' offices coordinate technology service delivery in their respective states. The Act was extremely general and recommended that each state have a comprehensive plan to incorporate direct service delivery, and provide for equipment, education of professionals, awareness, public research, and information services. Services to persons of all ages are provided under the act, which did not focus on special populations of school-aged children, adults, or older people. The long-term impact of this Act will not be in financing services or technology, but rather in generating increased interest by state and local governments in technology service delivery. Over time, this will result in better technology service delivery.

Funding

A variety of resources are available to help therapists obtain better third party funding for technology, including case study examples of letters successfully requesting funding and how funding agencies view particular types of equipment. Many agencies are funding positioning and mobility aids, but it is still difficult to locate funds for other types of technology. Augmentative and alternative communication systems are also frequently viewed as non-essential. A list of resources for funding technology systems is found in Appendix C.

To facilitate the funding process, organizations and commercial vendors are more frequently working together as coalitions. One of the results of a coalition from the mid-80s is the Specialized Product/Equipment Council (SPEC). SPEC was aimed specifically toward improving use of and payment for specialized rehabilitation equipment. SPEC formulated documents to facilitate technology funding including several forms and standardized procedures to optimize communication with third-party payers.

Other Disciplines/Professions

As mentioned early in this chapter, technology is highly visible and glamorous because it appears to magically solve the problems of independence for persons with disabilities. Legislative efforts have been successful and very interesting programs on functional electrical stimulation and robotic applications have appeared on television. Because of the visibility and funding available, a variety of professions are becoming involved as providers of rehabilitation and assistive technology. However, this has created many problems. Many individuals have become involved in practicing technology without the necessary education and experience. Inappropriate recommendations may be made by clinicians who simply do not have the appropriate information available or who lack the experience to know which technologies are successful over time. With inappropriate recommendations, limited funding may be wasted and the individual may not receive optimal services. Consequently, a variety of agencies and professions are beginning to look at the quality assurance aspects of technology service delivery.

Assuring Quality

RESNA, the international association which addresses rehabilitation and assistive technologies, is in the process of clarifying quality assurance in the field. There is a pressing need for certification/accreditation of individual therapy teams and educational facilities that either apply technology or teach students. This is a very difficult and complicated process due to the number of disciplines involved in providing service delivery. It appears that quality assurance in technology cannot focus on a single profession, but must address the various types and functions of technology implementation across many professions. Because it has become increasingly difficult for one therapist to provide appropriate technology service delivery, the certification of technology teams may be more appropriate.

In the late 1980's, a variety of educational programs were beginning to improve the quality of technology service delivery through training. Occupational therapy professional programs were beginning to require computer courses and other courses oriented toward technology. Others were setting up elective programs for students to maximize their exposure and abilities in technology. No formal policy or certification procedure is supported by occupational therapy associations in North America.

Beyond professional qualifications, other aspects of quality assurance include the concern about product quality. A consumer of a commercial technology device should be able to assume that the product is not only delivered by a competent professional, but is a safe product.

MANDATE TO THE OCCUPATIONAL THERAPY PROFESSION

It has been emphasized throughout this chapter that occupational therapists have been providing technology service delivery for decades and that occupational therapy is one of the professions in the vanguard of technology service delivery. Occupational therapists need to continue updating their skills since technology is rapidly changing. While occupational therapists have been traditionally proficient in some areas of low technology, the profession must move to increase competency in both low and high technology.

There are three major directions in which the profession must move: (1) Practicing therapists must continue to be supported by administrators in order to participate in continuing education opportunities such as workshops, conferences, and opportunities for hands-on access to appropriate equipment to learn the technology. (2) Occupational therapy educators must seriously consider technology in undergraduate education programs. Occupational therapists must leave the university setting with increased familiarity and comfort with technology. Low and high technology must be better integrated into current curricula. (3) The occupational therapy profession must seriously consider technology as a legitimate research domain. Technology is a subject that has great impact on the ability of occupational therapists to provide appropriate therapeutic intervention. Research is needed in the clinic to determine which methodologies are most appropriate for clinicians. Occupational therapy publications on the topic of technology have multiplied rapidly over the past decade, but the frequency of research-oriented publication in technology has not increased as rapidly (Angelo & Smith, 1989a). Case studies continue to be needed, but other research approaches are important to guide future use of technology intervention.

MANDATE TO THERAPISTS

In order to appropriately enhance the performance of individuals with disabilities and maximize their independence, it is obvious that occupational therapists must be aware of the potentials of technology. Six simple tasks are mandates to all therapists:

Every occupational therapist should use his/her fundamental knowledge to become a technology problem-solver in striving to remove the limitations of persons with disabilities using the available technology.

Occupational therapists must begin to see themselves as human-technology/environment experts. They must obtain substantial interfacing skills in technology which are the natural extension of fundamental occupational therapy skills.

Every occupational therapist must gain a basic comfort level with low and high technology.

Occupational therapists must gain a basic literacy in technology-related areas. For example, every occupational therapist should be aware of the variety of seating and positioning systems available and why the standard manual wheelchair should become obsolete. Therapists should also become literate with computers and know the different types of floppy disks, how to boot up computers, how to load programs, and have a basic understanding of the types of programs available.

Occupational therapists must understand the limits of their knowledge in technology and their limits in evaluating and providing of technology. They must be able to refer to specialty centers as needed and understand and use technology resources for the successful application of technology.

Occupational therapists must be aware of their ethical responsibility to know what technology benefits individuals and to assure that appropriate technology is obtained and successfully implemented for persons requiring it.

THE FUTURE OF TECHNOLOGY AND OCCUPATIONAL THERAPY

The only two absolute facts known about the future of occupational therapy and technology are: 1) Technology is here to stay and occupational therapists must continue to integrate technology into practice and professional training. 2) Technology will change and occupational therapy will need to change along with the technology. No computer system has been able to sustain its application for more than five years without being superseded by a better system which is much more effective. It is certain that virtually every technology (both high and low) we use today will be modified and improved over the next five years.

The role of occupational therapy and technology service delivery will evolve over time. Our role on the technology team will continue to be clarified. Much of this will depend on the roles occupational therapists play in current technology service delivery and in educating themselves for the future. The involvement of occupational therapy in technology service delivery could either blossom or fade. Certainly other professions are viewing various areas of technology as their specialty, and there is potential for a new professional in this area, designated as a Rehabilitation/Educational Technologist. The relationship between occupational therapy and any new technology profession is being defined currently by occupational therapists throughout North America. The amount of occupational therapy involvement in technology for tomorrow will depend upon how much technology expertise is developed today.

SUMMARY

This chapter has attempted to provide an overview of the use of technology in occupational therapy. It has been shown that, for several decades, technology has been used to enhance the functional performance of individuals with disability. However, the advent of microcomputers and integrated circuits, along with other technological advances, has created vast new potentials for meeting mobility, communication, work, leisure and self-care requirements of persons with limited ability.

The application of technology in occupational therapy use can take the form of direct intervention, through assistive/adaptive and rehabilitative/educational technologies; or through supportive means, as used in management, documentation, research or professional education. One convenient method of viewing the application of technology in direct intervention is known as the HETI model, for Human Environment Technology Interface. The six components of this model are based on the input-throughput-output open system model described elsewhere in this text. There are many resources available to therapists which can facilitate the selection of suitable technologies, provide current information on state-of-the-art developments, or assist in professional education. It has been emphasized that the application of technology in rehabilitation is such a vast and complex area that interdisciplinary teams are necessary to provide intervention services of broad scope and high quality. However, with appropriate basic and continuing education in technology, occupational therapists can establish themselves as vital members of technology teams in rehabilitation.

Study Questions

1. What are the dichotomies presented in the various definitions of technology?

2. How new is the application of technology in the occupational therapy profession?

3. What is in the role of computers in occupational therapy today and for the future?

4. How does the parallel systems concept affect how an occupational therapist should go about applying technology in practice?

5. What are the components in the HETI Model? Why is it helpful for an occupational therapist to understand this model when applying technology?

6. What are the types of information resources available to occupational therapists in technology?

7. How can a database such as ABLEDATA be helpful to an occupational therapist in a practice?

8. What is the role of appropriate seating and positioning in any assistive/adaptive technology application?

9. What are the six competencies required by occupational therapists in order to apply technology appropriately? Why are they important?

10. What are the seven critical steps in providing technology for an individual?

11. Using the HETI Model, describe six different technology devices and their functions.

12. How is technology used by occupational therapists in nondirect patient care applications?

Acknowledgment

This work has been supported in part by grants H029F80083 and H133E80021 from the U.S. Department of Education, Office of Special Education Programs and National Institute on Disabilities and Rehabilitation Research.

The author would also like to thank the following individuals for their expert assistance, review, and comments: Jennifer Angelo, Denis Anson, Peter Borden, Bob Christiaansen, Alexandra Enders, Sharon Esser, Carol Gwin, Elizabeth Kanny, Bill Mann, Marilyn Sidler, Elaine Trefler, and Gregg Vanderheiden.

References

Abildness, H. (1982). *Biofeedback strategies*. Rockville, MD: The American Occupational Therapy Association.

American Occupational Therapy Association (1989). *Technology Review '89: Perspectives on Occupational Therapy Practice*. Rockville, MD: The American Occupational Therapy Association, Inc.

Angelo, J. & Smith, R.O. (1989a). Indications of computer use: A literature review of 13 occupational therapy periodicals. Unpublished Manuscript.

Angelo, J. & Smith, R.O. (1989b). The critical role of occupational therapy augmentative communication services. In American Occupational Therapy Association (Eds.). *Technology Review '89: Perspectives on Occupational Therapy Practice*, (pp. 49-53). Rockville, MD: The American Occupational Therapy Association, Inc.

Bagneski, L.K. (1985). *Computer system for geriatric memory maintenance* (GEMM). Madison, WI: Rehabilitation Care Consultants, Inc.

Basmajian, J.V. (Ed.). (1989). *Biofeedback, principles and practice for clinicians*. Baltimore: Williams and Wilkins.

Benton, L.A., Baker, L.L., Bewman, B.R., & Walters, R.L. (Eds.). (1981). *Functional electrical stimulation: A practical clinical guide,* 2nd ed. Downey, CA: Rancho Los Amigos Rehabilitation Engineering Center, Rancho Los Amigos Hospital.

Berliss, J.B., Borden, P.A., & Vanderheiden, G.C. (1989). Trace Resource Book. Madison: University of Wisconsin, Trace R & D Center Reprint Service.

Blackstone, S.W. (1986). *Augmentative communication: An introduction.* Rockville, MD: American Speech-Language-Hearing Association.

Borden, P.A. & Vanderheiden, G.C. (Eds.). (1988). *Rehab/education resourcebook series update.* Madison: University of Wisconsin, Trace R & D Center Reprint Service.

Brandenburg, S.A. & Vanderheiden, G.C. (Eds.). (1987a). *Rehab/education resourcebook series: Resource Book 1 -Communication Aids.* Boston: Little, Brown, and Company.

Brandenburg, S.A. & Vanderheiden, G.C. (Eds.). (1987b). *Rehab/education resourcebook series: Resource Book 2 -Switches, training, and environmental control.* Boston: Little, Brown, and Company.

Brandenburg, S.A. & Vanderheiden, G.C. (Eds.). (1987c). *Rehab/education resourcebook series: Resource Book 3 -Software and hardware.* Boston: Little, Brown, and Company.

Brokaw, E.H. (1948). Adaptation of media. *The American Journal of Occupational Therapy, 2*(2), 77.

Campbell, C.L. (1986). Introduction: Robotics and the disabled. In F.L. Cromwell (Ed.). *Computer applications in occupational therapy,* (pp. 93-98). New York: The Haworth Press.

Chapanis, A. (1976). Engineering psychology. In Dunette, Marvin D. (Ed.). *Handbook of industrial and organizational psychology,* p. 701. Rand McNally College Publishing Company.

Clark, E.N. (Ed.). (1986). *Microcomputers: Clinical applications,* Vol. 1, No. 2, Thorofare, NJ: Slack.

Clarke, A.C. (1962). *Profiles of the future: An inquiry into the limits of the possible.* New York: Harper & Row.

Craig, H.L., Hendin, J.S. (1950). Toys for children with cerebral palsy. *The American Journal of Occupational Therapy, 5*(2), 50.

Cromwell, F.S. (Ed.). (1986). *Computer applications in occupational therapy.* New York: The Haworth Press.

DePape, D. & Smith, R.O. (1987). Parallel interventions for congenital motor impairments. Presented at Working Together...American Speech & Hearing Foundation, International Society on Alternative and Augmentative Communication, Communication Aids Manufacturer Association Conference, October 1987.

Dickey, R. & Shealey, S.H. (1987). Using technology to control the environment. *The American Journal of Occupational Therapy, 41*(11), 722-725.

Dudley, S. & D'Agati, S. (1989). Interactive video: The Basics of Development. In The American Occupational Therapy Association (Eds.). *Technology Review '89: Perspectives on Occupational Therapy Practice,* (pp. 45-48). Rockville, MD: The American Occupational Therapy Association, Inc.

Durie, N.D. (1988). A robot for use with autistic children. *PRADNET.* Neil Square Foundation, 4381 Gallent Avenue, N., Vancouver, BC, Canada.

Enders, A. (1989). Assistive Technology Sourcebook. Bethesda, MD: RESNA Press. In press.

Federal Register. (1988). Technology Related Assistance for Individuals with Disabilities Act of 1988, PL 100-407.

Finkley, E. (1988). Occupational therapy in augmentative communication. *Occupational Therapy News, 42*(5), 14-15.

Fishman, I. (1987). *Electronic communication aids.* Boston: College-Hill Press.

Gilkeson, G.E. & Krouskop, T.A. (1987). A Master's degree program in occupational therapy with a rehabilitation technology focus. *The American Journal of Occupational Therapy, 41*(11), 22.

Glass, K. & Hall, K. (1987). Occupational therapists' views about the use of robotic aids for people with disabilities. *The American Journal of Occupational Therapy, 41*(11), 745-747.

Gray, D.B., LeClair, R.R., Traub, J.E., Brummel, S.A., Maday, D.E., McDonough, F.A., Patton, P.R., & Yonkler, L. (Eds.). (1987). *Access to information technology by users with disabilities: Initial guidelines.* Washington, DC: Department of Education, National Institute on Disabilities and Rehabilitation Research and General Services Administration, Information Resources Management Services.

Hall, M.E. (1951). Two feeding appliances. *The American Journal of Occupational Therapy, 5*(2), 52.

Hall, M. (1987). Unlocking information technology. *The American Journal of Occupational Therapy, 41*(11), 722-725.

Howell, R.D. & Campbell, K. (1988). Robotic devices as cognitive and physical prosthetic aids. Paper presented at the 68th Annual Conference of the American Occupational Therapy Association, Phoenix, AZ:

ICAART. (1988). *Proceedings of the 3rd International Conference of the Association for the Advancement of Rehabilitation Technology.* Washington, DC: RESNA: Association for the Advancement of Rehabilitation Therapy.

Jaffe, K.M. (Ed.). (1987). Childhood powered mobility: Developmental, technical, and clinical perspective. *Proceedings from the 1st RESNA: Association for the Advancement of Rehabilitation Technology Northwest Regional Conference.*

Jaros, L.L., Levine, S.P., & Kirsch, N.L. (1987). COGORTH: Cognition orthosis programming language. In *Rehabilitation R&D Progress Reports.* Baltimore: Veterans Administration.

Kirsch, N.L., Levine, S.P., & Jaros, B.S. (1987). Computerized task guidance for cognitively impaired people. In *Rehabilitation R&D Progress Reports*, (pp. 116-167). Baltimore: Veterans Administration.

Kristy, K.A. (1988). Use of robotic arm as a rehabilitation exercise partner: A therapeutic enhancement. *Proceedings of the 3rd International Conference of the Association for the Advancement of Rehabilitation Technology* (ICAART), 3, 452-453.

Lau, A. (1986). Computer applications in occupational therapy: A journal review. In Cromwell, F.S. (Ed.). *Computer Applications in Occupational Therapy*, (pp. 93-98). New York: The Haworth Press.

Lepley, M.G. (1955). Self-care board for hemiplegics. *The American Journal of Occupational Therapy, 9*(2-1), 68.

M-19 Murphy's Laws on Technology. (1981). New York: Harvey Hutter & Co.

Meister, D. (1971). *Human factors theory and practice.* New York: Wiley.

Moore, J.C. (1956). Adjustable reading rack for the visually impaired. *The American Journal of Occupational Therapy, 10*(2), 82.

Myers, C., et al. (1956). Adaptation for resistance to the beater of the floor loom. *The American Journal of Occupational Therapy, 10*(1), 13.

Naisbitt, J. (1982). *Megatrends: Ten new directions transforming our lives.* New York: Warner Books.

Parlin, F.W. (1948). Adaptation and apparatus. *The American Journal of Occupational Therapy, 2*(4), 206.

Rehabilitation R & D Center-Palo Alto, CA. (1989). *1988 progress reports.* Palo Alto, CA: Veterans Administration Medical Center.

RESNA. (1987a). *Rehabilitation technology service delivery: A practical guide.* Washington, DC: RESNA.

RESNA. (1987b). *Proceedings of the 11th Annual Conference on Rehabilitation and Assistive Technology.* Washington, DC: RESNA

RESNA. (1988). *Proceedings of the national planners conference on assistive device service delivery*, Carolyn Coston (Ed.). Washington, DC: RESNA.

RESNA. (1989b). *Rehabilitation technology service delivery directory.* Washington, DC: RESNA.

RESNA. (1989, June). Technology for the next decade.

Proceedings of the 12th Annual Conference on Rehabilitation and Assistive Technology. Washington, DC: RESNA Press.

Rodgers, B.L. (1985). *A future perspective on the holistic use of technology for people with disabilities.* Madison: University of Wisconsin, Trace R & D Center Reprint Service. Based on a paper presented at the Discovery '84: Technology for Disabled Persons Conference, Chicago, IL.

Sammons, F. (1988). Self-help innovation for the handicapped. *NEWS for Release.* Brookfield, IL: Fred Sammons, Inc., Box 32, Brookfield, IL 60513.

Schneider, M.L., Champoux, M., & Beinert, R.H. (1987). The use of computer-assisted behavior observation in sensory integrated practice and research. *Occupational Therapy in Health Care, IV.* 2. New York: The Haworth Press.

Sidler, M. (1986). Impact of technology on rehabilitation. In Cromwell, F.S. (Ed.). *Computer Applications in Occupational Therapy*, (pp. 55-84). New York: The Haworth Press.

Sidler, M. & Hutchines, S.E. (1987). Software testing: Potentials and problems in head injury, speech therapy, and sign language. *Proceedings of the Computer Technology/Special Education/Rehabilitation Conference at California State University at Northridge.*

Smith, R.O. (1986). Computers and the occupational therapy administration. 1985. In Cromwell, F.S. (Ed.). *Computer Applications in Occupational Therapy*, (pp. 99-115). New York: The Haworth Press.

Smith, R.O. (1987). Models of service delivery in rehabilitation technology. In *Rehabilitation Technology Service Delivery: A Practical Guide.* Washington, DC: RESNA.

Smith, R.O. (1988a). Service delivery and related issues at the Trace Research and Development Center. Paper invited for presentation at the National Planners Conference on Assisted Device Service Delivery. Chicago, IL. Published in *Planning and Implementing Augmentative Communication Service Delivery,* selected from conference presentations and published by RESNA, Association for the Advancement of Rehabilitation Technology.

Steele, R.D., Weinrick, M., Kleczewska, M.L., Carlson, G.S., & Hennies, D. (1988). Targeted applications for aphasia rehabilitation: Computer aided visual communication in aphasia. *Proceedings of the 3rd International Conference of the Association for the Advancement of Rehabilitation Technology* (ICAART), 3, 48-49.

Svennson, V.W. & Brennan, M.C. (1953). Special equipment adaptable for kitchen use. *The American Journal of Occupational Therapy, 7*(4), 190.

Taylor, J. (1987). Evaluating the client with physical

disabilities for wheelchair seating. *The American Journal of Occupational Therapy, 41*(11), 711-716.

Trefler, E., Kozole, K., & Snell, E. (Eds.). (1986). *Selected readings on powered mobility for children and adults with severe physical disabilities.* Washington, DC: RESNA: Association for the Advancement of Rehabilitation Technology.

Vanderheiden, G.C. (1983a). Computers: The greatest single handicapping condition of the future? Keynote address, Annual Governor's Conference for the Handicapped, Indianapolis.

Vanderheiden, G.C. (1983b). Curbcuts and Computers: Guaranteeing Access to Computers and Information Systems. *Proceedings of the Discovery '83 Computers for the Disabled Conference,* Minneapolis, MN. Madison: University of Wisconsin, Trace R & D Center Reprint Service.

Vanderheiden, G.C. (1987a). Issues in planning a statewide technology service delivery program for special education. Paper invited for presentation at the National Planners Conference on Assistive Device Service Delivery. Chicago, IL. Published in *Planning and Implementing Augmentative Communication Service Delivery,* selected from conference presentations and published by RESNA, Association for the Advancement of Rehabilitation Technology.

Vanderheiden, G.C. (1987b). Service delivery mechanisms in rehabilitation technology. *The American Journal of Occupational Therapy, 41*(11), 703-710.

Vanderheiden, G.C. & Lloyd, L.L. (1986). Communication systems and their components. In *Augmentative Communication: An Introduction.* S.W. Blackstone (Ed.). Rockville, MD: American Speech-Language-Hearing Association.

Vanderheiden, G.C., Lee, C.C. & Scadden, L. (Eds.). (1988). *Considerations in the design of computers and operating systems to increase their accessibility to persons with disabilities, Version 4.2.* Madison: University of Wisconsin, Trace R & D Center Reprint Service.

Veterans Administration. (1989). *Rehabilitation R & D Progress Reports*, 1988. Washington, DC: Veterans Administration, Office of Technology Transfer.

CHAPTER CONTENT OUTLINE

Introduction

Definition of Independence

Rehabilitation from the Consumer's Point of View

Proposed Programs (Products) and Referral Patterns of Occupational Therapy Services

Preparation for Discharge into the Community

Networking: An Organizational and Professional Tool

Achieving Occupational Performance

Summary

KEY TERMS

Caregiver

Excess disability

Independence

Long-term support system

Networking

Product line

Re-entry rehabilitation programs

ABSTRACT

In order for individuals with performance dysfunction to achieve independence, they must be given access to professionals who can help them obtain necessary services, programs, and resources. The occupational therapist's goal is to facilitate the client's independence and to design and implement systems of care to ensure the client has access to those needed services. This chapter describes the services available in the hospitals, as outpatient services, as home health services, and community programs. It also reviews methods of identifying and locating the needed community resources and services and emphasizes the importance of networking to give the therapist access to a referral and problem-solving system.

Identification and Use of Environmental Resources

Carolyn Baum

"Our role consists in giving opportunities rather than prescriptions. There must be opportunities to work, opportunities to do and to plan and create . . . It takes, above all, resourcefulness and ability to respect at the same time the native capacities and interests of the patient . . . We may well be able to shape for ourselves and our patients an outlook of sound idealism, furnished in a setting in which many otherwise apparently insurmountable difficulties will be conquered . . ."

—Adolph Meyer, 1922

OBJECTIVES

The information in this chapter is intended to help the reader—

1. appreciate the importance of resources in achieving independence.

2. recognize the difference between the approaches of the medical and rehabilitation models and how each influences a person's potential for living independently.

3. understand the product line approach to organizing and marketing occupational therapy services.

4. identify strategies for linking services between facilities and programs.

5. understand how consumer groups serve as valuable resources in assisting persons to achieve independence.

6. understand the concept of professional networking.

INTRODUCTION

Occupational therapists are guided by the principles of occupational therapy ethics. The preamble of the Code of Ethics states that occupational therapists should be dedicated ''to furthering peoples' ability to function fully within their total environment'' (AOTA, 1988). To further peoples' ability to function, occupational therapists must provide the intervention strategies to help individuals overcome disabling conditions, and help them learn to identify and use resources. In some cases, the needed resources do not exist, making it necessary to develop new resources.

The goal of this chapter is to help occupational therapists understand that they treat patients within a system; and that system has many resources to help individuals function. This chapter will also serve as a guide for learning how to access community resources.

Paul J. Corcoran, M.D., states in his monograph, *The Health Care Dilemma*, that physicians are not taught to operationalize health according to the definition established by the World Health Organization in 1946 (Corcoran, 1984, p. 1). This definition states that health is ''a state of well-being and not merely the absence of disease or infirmity.'' Corcoran perceives that medicine is practiced with the goal of trying to medically cure individuals, hence individuals remain ''patients'' until they become ''normal'' or cured. This medical approach views the patient in terms of the pathology (what is medically wrong). The patient who does not recover is considered ''a failure.'' Corcoran also states that it is a misnomer to categorize medicine as a health science because medicine continues to focus primarily on the issue of sickness, often excluding rehabilitation services and care for chronically impaired persons.

As medical technology has improved, we have seen a dramatic increase in the number of patients who survive sickness or injuries. This has greatly increased the demand for rehabilitation services. It is very important that rehabilitation services expand in a rehabilitation model of service rather than in the medical model. A rehabilitation model of service helps individuals overcome human performance deficits and assures that they have access to the services needed to shift from a ''patient-oriented'' status to one of functional independence.

Of course, the initial rehabilitation approach to patients must be oriented toward helping an individual achieve medical stability, but it is then important to view the person not as a patient, but as an individual who fills social roles —as worker, parent, student, homemaker, or volunteer (as examples). We have seen in earlier chapters that these roles define behavioral expectations and serve the important function of providing self-definition. The nature of practice advanced in this book is one of viewing clients as individuals with role-related performance problems that need to be solved. To overcome these problems and achieve maximum independence, clients require access to resources.

DEFINITION OF INDEPENDENCE

What is the real meaning of independence? If we consider independence as having adequate resources to accomplish everyday tasks, we must consider the individual with a disability as independent when they, too, have the resources to accomplish their everyday tasks. Corcoran reminds us that the term ''normal'' is relative. There are many variables that allow individuals to achieve different levels of performance, such as culture, education, physique, life demands and skills; but we are all dependent on environmental factors and countless other individuals in order to achieve our objectives on a daily basis. As Corcoran (1984) describes it: ''We may feel that we have bathed, dressed, and eaten our breakfast without any assistance or special adaptations. Further reflection would show an infrastructure of thousands of persons who grow, process, deliver and even prepare our food, others manufacture and clean our clothes, and yet others create the products we use to groom.''

It is inappropriate to define persons with disabilities as those who require special adaptations or human assistance to perform their daily life tasks, since we all require assistance of various types (Corcoran, 1984). Rather independence means having access to and using the necessary devices and human helpers in order to perform the tasks of daily living.

REHABILITATION FROM THE CONSUMERS POINT OF VIEW

Irving Kenneth Zola, Ph.D., (1982) in his commentary, *Social and Cultural Disincentives to Independent Living,''* challenges all rehabilitation professionals to treat patients as consumers; hence as partners in their own rehabilitation. Dr. Zola is a sociologist at Brandeis University who developed considerable right-sided weakness as a result of having polio in 1950 and an accident in 1954. He wears a long leg brace, a back support and walks with a cane. In his own words, Dr. Zola addresses some very important issues regarding the traditional U.S. approach to rehabilitation:

- *. . . many programs not only give up too early in the rehabilitation process but also have no systematic way of assessing our long-term progress and capability. In fact, most of us with disabilities are never given the chance to learn about new devices. I have never, in 25 years since my rehabilitation was completed, been called in by any of my orthopedists or prosthetists for a checkup or to discuss new ways I could do things or new devices I could use. I do not mean, of course, that I have not seen these people, but rather that I only did so when something was wrong and then we all focused on the trouble.*

- *Anything new that I do or use today I learned from friends or journals. Some might argue that that is the American way. I would argue that it is haphazard rehabilitation, a consigning of me and many like me to the ''we have done all we could category.'' I am not claiming callousness. I am claiming that there exists a system built on certain assumptions that prevents the rehabilitation world from ever really knowing if they have done all they can.*

- *We must expand the notion of independence from physical achievements to sociopsychologic decision-making. Independent living must include not only the quality of physical tasks . . . but the quality of life they (the disabled person) can lead. The notion of human integrity must take into account the notion of taking risks. Rehabilitation personnel must change the model of service from doing something to someone to planning and creating services with someone* [emphasis added].

The health care system has increased the demand for medical care that can measurably improve the patients' functional status and help them live independently. With this demand has come an increased use of occupational therapy. In order to achieve independence, an individual with performance dysfunction must be given access to those who can help obtain the necessary services, programs, and resources. The occupational therapist's goal is to facilitate the client's independence and to design and implement systems of care to ensure access to those services. By addressing services toward the goal of independence, occupational therapists play a critical role in health care.

Alvin Tarlov (1983) is a physician and a health care futurist who predicts that future health care will become

---

An Occupational Therapy Product Line

- Adapted sports and recreation programs
- Caregiver training programs
- Community education programs
- Exercise and fitness programs for elderly persons
- An independence center for selection of tools and techniques to support independent living
- Injury prevention at the work site
- School or vocational readiness
- Technology center to assess the need for computers and offer training
- Driving program for the assessment of driving capacity, recommendation of driving aids, and training in driving skills
- Return-to-work programs including work assessments, conditioning, and work hardening
- Training in the skills of living
- Wheelchair and mobility program

Figure 27-1. An Occupational Therapy Product Line.

---

more effective in terms of restoring the person's ability to function in activities of daily living and in their social and economic roles.

PROPOSED PROGRAMS (PRODUCTS) AND REFERRAL PATTERNS OF OCCUPATIONAL THERAPY SERVICES

Consumers of the health care system are taking a more active role by exercising their rights and demanding access to services that they believe are necessary for themselves and their families. Occupational therapists should develop product lines for this new type of health care consumer. A product line is a series of services offered to help individuals with their specific problems. Examples might include driving programs for older adults or wheelchair clinics. Presenting occupational therapy to the public as a product does not prevent the therapist from employing the full range of occupational therapy services; rather, it ensures that those with specific problems will recognize that occupational therapy is a service that can assist them. Figure 27-1 presents an example of an occupational therapy department's **product lines** (not meant to be inclusive).

Once occupational therapy services or programs (products) are defined, they must be put into operation in a variety of clinical settings to reach the people who need them. It is important to remember that people needing to

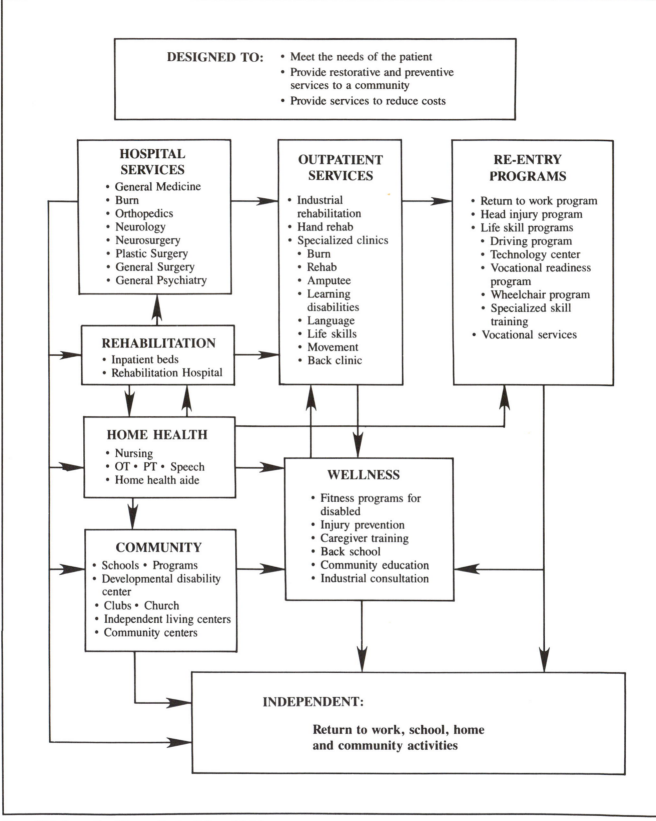

Figure 27-2. Occupational Therapy Service Delivery Model.

resolve performance deficits will need access to many services that will resolve their problems. Some of those services are totally within the domain of occupational therapy practice, while others are interdisciplinary.

The current structure of the United States health system does not allow a patient to stay in one level of care for the duration of the rehabilitation process. Many patients are discharged from the hospital to either a rehabilitation facility or to their home with home health services. Later in the rehabilitation process, they may use outpatient services or community services. To ensure that these individuals have access to the services needed to achieve independence, occupational therapists must design a system of care in their own facility or refer patients to other occupational therapists or programs in the community. It is the occupational therapist's responsibility to identify potential services and resources for the individual. A service delivery model for occupational therapy is presented in Figure 27-2, and the components of the model are described in the sections which follow.

Hospital Services

Patients are usually in the hospital for a very short period of time. The average length of stay is less than eight days. Table 27-1 lists the average lengths of stay in acute care for several illnesses or injuries.

During hospitalization, patients are usually medically unstable. Occupational therapy services are very important at this time to help patients learn basic skills that give them a sense of control over their environment and prevent further disabling conditions. Occupational therapy services in the hospital also help families solve basic problems such

Table 27-1
Average Length of Hospital Stay in Acute Care (U.S.A.)

AVERAGE LENGTH OF STAY	DIAGNOSIS
7.6 days	Heart failure and shock
8.9 days	Multiple sclerosis
9.9 days	Cerebral vascular disorder
17.0 days	Other disorders of nervous system
14.3 days	Amputations
11.9 days	Fractured hip/pelvis
8.6 days	Connective tissue disease

From: Background Paper (No. 531) by U.S. Department of Health and Human Services, Health Care Financing Administration, December 24, 1984, Baltimore, MD.

Table 27-2
Length of Stay and Cost for Selected Diagnostic Categories (U.S.A.)

DIAGNOSTIC CATEGORY	LENGTH OF STAY (DAYS)	CHARGE PER PATIENT ($)
Stroke	13 to 55	4,418 to 24,384
Spinal Cord Injury	7 to 89	2,911 to 38,625
Brain Injury	12 to 80	3,760 to 38,520
Neurological Disorders	8 to 54	2,972 to 22,116
Fracture of the Femur	8 to 46	0 to 34,146
Polyarthritis	11 to 41	3,389 to 14,803
Amputation	14 to 44	4,710 to 20,422
Congenital Deformities	9 to 43	2,424 to 17,758
Burn	12 to 38	4,935 to 13,739
Major Multiple Trauma	6 to 58	3,108 to 20,308
Other	2 to 66	0 to 32,243

From: The National Association of Rehabilitation Facilities, Position Paper on Prospective Payment System for Inpatient Medical Rehabilitation Services, 1985.

as how to get the patient home, how to manage after getting there, and how to find resources to help the patient become more independent in taking care of himself/herself. Patients who have experienced a disabling condition and their families should leave the hospital with a specific plan of how they are going to obtain these additional services.

Rehabilitation Hospital

Patients requiring rehabilitation services are transferred to rehabilitation hospitals (or to rehabilitation beds in general hospitals) as soon as they are medically stable. The average length of stay in a rehabilitation hospital is less than 34.1 days. Table 27-2 shows ranges for the length of stay and costs for patients in several diagnostic categories in medical rehabilitation facilities.

During this time, the rehabilitation process begins. An individual must become aware of his/her responsibility to work toward achieving the long-term goal of independence and moving away from the role of patient. Independence can rarely be achieved in this short period of time. Thus, before leaving the rehabilitation setting, individuals and their families should help develop a specific plan of how to obtain additional needed services to achieve independence. Figure 27-3 is a sample of a discharge assessment and

```
┌─────────────────────────────────────────┐
│      Discharge Assessment and Long-Term Plan      │
│                                                   │
│   Client Name _____         │
│   Address _____         │
│   _____           │
│   Phone # _____         │
│   Caregiver _____         │
│   Address _____         │
│   Phone # _____         │
│   DESCRIPTION OF LIVING ARRANGEMENTS              │
│   (accessibility, safety, distance from caregiver):│
│                                                   │
│                                                   │
│                                                   │
│                                                   │
│   DESCRIPTION OF TRAINING PROGRAM FOR             │
│   CAREGIVER                                        │
│   (Describe skills taught, amount of time caregiver was trained│
│   with patient. If other training is required state how this is to be│
│   accomplished):                                  │
│                                                   │
│                                                   │
│                                                   │
│                                                   │
│   FUTURE REHABILITATION PROGRAMS TO               │
│   CONSIDER                                         │
│   (Including method of contacting the program):   │
│   _____           │
│   Occupational Therapist              Date        │
└─────────────────────────────────────────┘
```

Figure 27-3. Discharge Assessment and Long-Term Plan.

long-term plan which should be completed with the patient and family.

Outpatient Services

Outpatient services traditionally have been associated with the hospital setting. This trend is changing, and many hospitals have developed satellite clinics that offer services in locations that are more easily accessible for individuals. Other locations where outpatient rehabilitation services are available include the physician's or therapist's office, health maintenance organizations, one-stop health care clinics, industrial sites, skilled nursing facilities, and rehabilitation clinics. In many outpatient settings, people

with disabilities are still perceived to be "patients" who need "curing," although many will not be cured. They should be viewed and addressed as individuals who are asking for assistance. The occupational therapist is responsible for planning with the individual and the family how to obtain additional services to help the client achieve independence, if returning to work and community activities is a goal.

Home Health Services

Home health services play a very important role in helping an individual achieve independence, because being in the person's home affords the opportunity to determine the environmental modifications (i.e., accessibility and use of adaptive equipment) that are necessary to achieve independence in home activities. Home health services are very limited and do not include activities that prepare an individual for work or community activities. For this reason, home health therapists should develop mechanisms for referring their clients to other rehabilitation services.

Community Programs

Agencies, schools, and day facilities also provide services to the disabled individual. Occupational therapists work in these settings either as staff or as consultants and apply a wide variety of services to help students or clients gain skills to achieve independence. Sometimes the services that are necessary to help an individual attain the highest level of independence are not provided in the community setting. In such cases, the occupational therapist should work with the staff of the agency, the individual, and the family, to develop a plan of how to obtain additional services needed to achieve a higher level of independence, such as driver training, instruction in the use of computers, and work hardening programs.

Re-entry Programs

Re-entry rehabilitation programs help provide individuals with the skills, the physical endurance, the emotional support, and family support needed to function independently at a community level. The timing of re-entry programs is a clinical judgment. Some individuals need to go through the total rehabilitation program immediately after an illness or injury, while others may need extended time to make adjustments and accept the lifestyle changes that can accompany a major injury or illness. This intervention should result in improved function for the individual and the family members who have undergone lifestyle changes during the period when the individual was greatly dependent on their assistance.

PREPARATION FOR DISCHARGE INTO THE COMMUNITY

Some individuals with disabilities will never be able to live totally independently or be employed. The goal for each individual is to live in the least restrictive environment and to attain the highest possible level of independence in order to express himself/herself as an individual.

Occupational therapists should help the client determine the level of services needed before discharge to the community. The relationship between occupational therapists and their clients and families should not terminate when they return to the community; rather the relationship should be ongoing. It is important to develop a long-term relationship with the individual to keep them informed of new advanced technology and equipment that could help them become more functional. During the last five years, we have seen the whole range of technological supports become affordable for most clients. For example, new affordable wheelchairs and seating devices have greatly enhanced the independence and activities of disabled people.

The client's functional status changes either by progress or, in the case of a progressive disease, by deterioration. As their status changes, these individuals and their families will continue to need access to occupational therapists who can help them solve their performance-related problems with the aid of all the new technologies and advances.

The process of occupational therapists keeping in touch with the health care consumer need not be complicated. Those in need of service should be responsible for making requests for service, but the therapist can facilitate this communication by providing a business card with the name of his/her facility and phone number. Some occupational therapy departments establish ''independence'' follow-up clinics that help provide a routine visit to determine if other services could be helpful. Clients returning to such clinics may need additional medical attention. In such cases, the occupational therapist can refer the individual to the physician for medical management.

A service profile should be completed prior to initial discharge from any level of care, to ensure that adequate resources are available to support the individual at the community level (see Table 27-3). The service profile is valuable in helping the family make decisions and giving the social workers information about the individuals' needs based upon their actual ability to perform life tasks. It is crucial that the evaluation be based on careful assessment of the individual's performance capabilities and not just inferred from communication.

Identification of Community Resources for Long-term Support

In order for occupational therapists to utilize community resources, they first must be familiar with the existing services available in the community where the individual lives. Some communities have extensive resources, while others do not; and some resources are more obvious than others. Occupational therapists must seek out the resources to support community placement of their clients. The search for resources can stimulate the need for additional services and establish an important link with the community. Table 27-4 is an example of a community resource assessment that can be used as a guide in identifying resources.

Federal and state governments have funded the development and maintenance of many services that are helpful to people with special needs, such as day care programs, senior citizen centers, or the Meals-on-Wheels program. The occupational therapist should be acquainted with these resources and collaborate with the social worker to assist the family in acquiring the services necessary to maintain the client's highest functional level. The goal in choosing services is to match the individual's capabilities and needs with the services to be provided. Table 27-5 presents the **long-term support system** as described by Brody and Masciocchi (1980).

The Importance of Caregiver Training

Support services can be provided in the home, in the community, and in hospitals. In order for a community support system to work and provide the necessary support for an individual, it is critical that those who give care on an ongoing basis be trained to understand the capabilities as well as the dysfunction of the individual.

To function as a **caregiver** may require new skills. Occupational therapists often assume responsibility for assisting caregivers to acquire the skills, attitudes, and confidence necessary to function in their helping role. One faced with providing ongoing care and support to a dysfunctional person has to assume many functions that are new to their daily activities. The following are important discharge planning considerations related to caregiver needs:

1. The caregiver needs sufficient understanding of the characteristics of the disease or disability in order to report changes in the person's status to the physician.
2. The caregiver needs to learn the techniques to solve problems on a daily basis. They must also acquire specific and unique skills that are required by the individual with a performance dysfunction.
3. The caregiver is responsible for knowing what services are available in the community and determining what is of benefit to the person and the family.

Table 27-3
Checklist of Services Necessary to Support Community Living

ACTIVITY	INDEPENDENT	FAMILY SUPPORT	NEIGHBOR	COMMUNITY
Adequate Housing				
Working Utilities				
Money for Food				
Safe Transfers				
Self Care				
Manage Medications				
Manage Hygiene				
Meal Planning				
Meal Preparation				
Grocery Shopping				
Light Housework				
Heavy Housework				
Yard Work				
Pay Bills				
Manage Finances				
Getting Mail				
Telephone				
Emergency Assistance				
Security				
Transportation				
Socialization				
Legal Assistance				
Medical Care				
Leisure Activities				
Physical Activities				
Church Activities				
Work				

4. The caregiver must be prepared for new situations and unexpected problems that are likely to arise.
5. The caregiver must provide the motivation and support for the client to continue making progress.

Teaching caregivers these responsibilities requires more than just giving them printed instructions and a few telephone discussions with the occupational therapist. Caregivers should be trained in all areas in which the individual continues to experience dysfunction including mobility, use of time, safety and emergency procedures, meal planning, and self care skills (particularly if the individual requires gestural or verbal cues to perform an activity). Caregivers must have strategies to deal with their own social isolation, frustrations, and the demands of their new role. The caregiver is not always a family member, but can include home health aids, volunteers, or neighbors who assist in the care of the individual. The occupational therapist should arrange for training for all those involved in the care of the individual. This training is critical to prevent the development of **excess disability** which is the disability that the individual sustains when not allowed to maintain the skills that he/ she possesses (Brody, 1974).

Table 27-4
Assessing Community Resources to Support Independent Living

RESOURCE REQUIRED AND POSSIBILITIES	AGENCY	ADDRESS AND PHONE NUMBER	FUNCTION/ SERVICE	FUNDING SOURCE	ROLE OF OCCUPATIONAL THERAPY PERSONNEL
Transportation Regional planning council (required to develop a transportation plan for each region—a helpful report)					
Driving program Driver evaluation program (usually associated with a rehabilitation facility)					
Advocacy Independent living center Voter registration council					
Aids and appliances, including technological aids, computers, and communication devices Occupational therapy department at a rehabilitation facility Medical equipment dealers					
Social and personal development Agencies, groups Peer counselor Independent living center Professional counselor (social worker) Hairdresser Makeup artist Clothing consultant Sexuality groups Discussion groups					
Financial guidance or assistance Social worker or caseworker to steer individual toward resources					

Authored by Carolyn Manville Baum, MA, OTR, FAOTA, and Aimee J. Luebben, OTR.

Consumer Groups

The 1970's and 80's brought voluntary health organizations into the mainstream of American medicine. Caregivers banded together to form support groups — initially to gain support and answers. Today these voluntary health organizations are major sponsors of research.

Voluntary Health Organizations are invaluable resources to help individuals achieve their long-term goals of independence. There are several resources available to guide occupational therapists in planning services for a disabled individual and the family. These books are comprehensive resource guides that will give the

Table 27-5

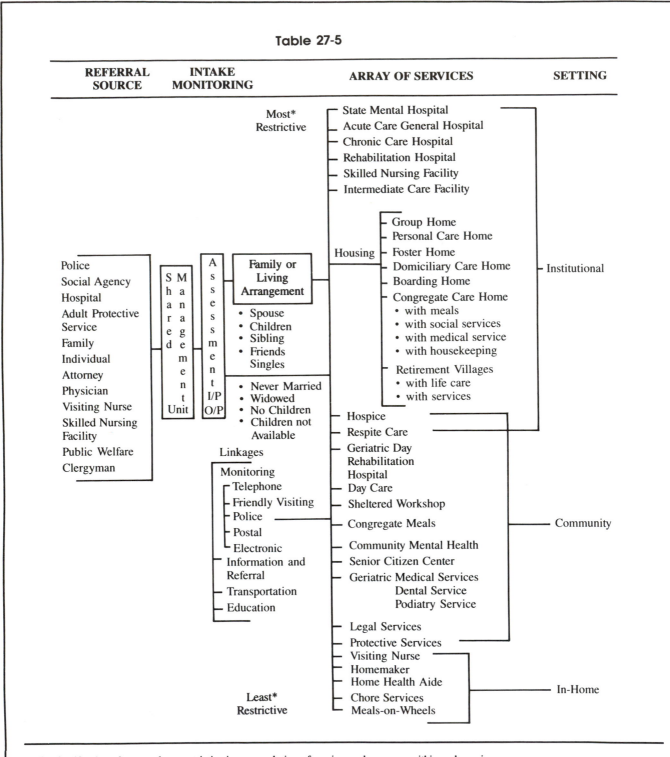

REFERRAL SOURCE	INTAKE MONITORING	ARRAY OF SERVICES	SETTING

* The classification of most to least restrictive is a general view of services and may vary within each service.
Long-term support system from Brody and Masciocchi: American Journal of Public Health 70:1194-1198, 1980.

occupational therapist information useful for long-term planning. These resources are also of value to caregivers, providing them with the information necessary to give them options in making very complex decisions.

- *Directory of National Information Sources on Handicapping Conditions and Related Services*, U.S. Department of Education, Publication No. E-82-22007, U.S. Government Printing Office.
- *Health Care U.S.A.* by Jean Carper, Prentice Hall Press, New York, 1987.
- *Information U.S.A.* (Revised Edition) by Matthew Lesco, Viking Press, New York, 1986.
- *Voluntary Health Organizations: A Guide to Patient Services*, L. Scheinberg and D. Schneider, Demos Publications: New York, 1987.

Resource Organizations for Disability Groups

The resources provided by organizations for disability groups vary; therefore it is necessary to check with each one to determine the scope of its services and its local resources. Some of the more common services available are: counseling, distribution of educational materials and newsletters, assistance with purchase or loan of equipment, patient clinics, research funds, seminars, support groups, and transportation services. At the end of this book (Appendix D) is a list of organizations that should assist the occupational therapy student or clinician in obtaining resources to help their clients. This list provides addresses and phone numbers of national organizations in North America, but many have local or regional organizations as well.

NETWORKING: AN ORGANIZATIONAL AND PROFESSIONAL TOOL

''Germinated in the uproar of the 1960's and born in the self-reflection of the 1970's, networks appear to be coalescing everywhere in the 1980's, an appropriate sociological response to bureaucratic logjams'' (Lipnack and Stamps, 1986).

Keeping current in an evolving field such as occupational therapy with all the changes in rehabilitation, new techniques, and new products requires therapists to develop strategies that link them with other colleagues. Professional networks serve the purpose of connecting people who share common goals. By developing a resource bank of people in one's own and related fields, one gains access to a referral and problem-solving system. Networks are something that must be developed and nutured, they do not just happen.

John Naisbitt (1982, p. 192) in *Megatrends*, cites the

Building and Maintaining a Network

- Carry a business card that gives your position at your facility, your business address, and your phone number
- Keep a professional address book
- Collect business cards and write reminders on the back of them regarding future opportunities
- Keep in touch with your contacts by telephone and occasional lunch dates
- Contact with periodic notes (holidays are a good time to re-establish contact)
- Make it a challenge to add one or two new contacts each month
- Increase contacts by being active in your professional organization (both locally and nationally)
- Shape resources with colleagues and peers
- Thank people who help you and help them as often as possible

Figure 27-4. Building and Maintaining a Network.

shift from hierarchy to networks as one of ten major trends shaping contemporary society.

Simply stated, networks are people talking to each other, sharing ideas, information, and resources. The point is often made that networking is a verb, not a noun. The important part is not the network, the finished product, but the process of getting there—the communication that creates the linkages between people and clusters of people. Networks exist to foster self-help, to exchange information, to change society, to improve productivity and work life, and to share resources. Networks are structured to transmit information in a way that is quicker, more high touch and more energy efficient than any other process we know.

Building and Maintaining a Network

The professional society or association is a ready-made network for the occupational therapist. Such organizations serve as resources to help their members solve clinical problems and issues. They also help to resolve problems faced in the delivery of occupational therapy services, such as problems relating to reimbursement, changes in policies or regulations, or access to services. Most problems faced by the occupational therapist have occurred with other therapists, and professional organizations help members take advantage of their colleagues' experiences.

It is important for occupational therapists to identify the people who will serve in their network. A network needs nurturing, hence it is beneficial to keep in contact with people who help you on a regular basis. Figure 27-4

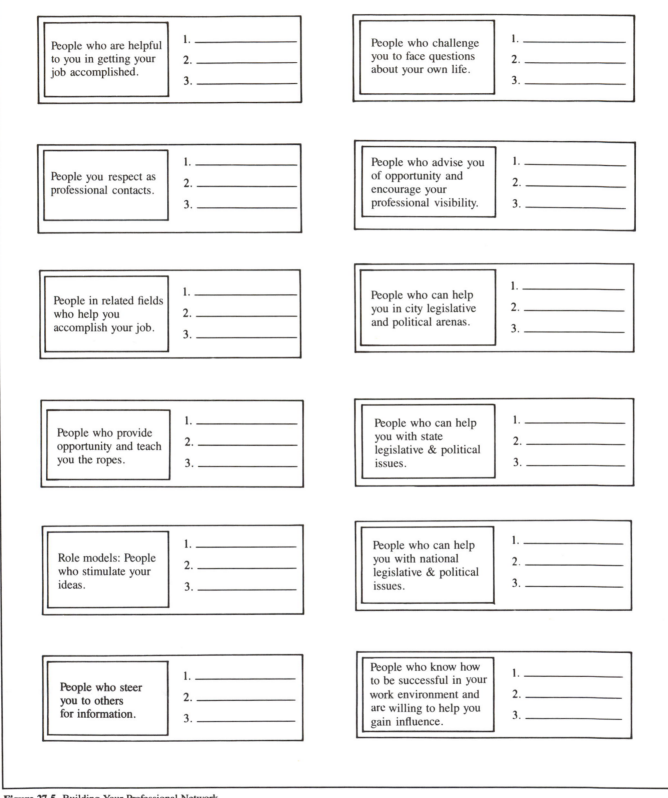

Figure 27-5. Building Your Professional Network.

presents a list of practical tips for helping one establish a network.

The type of people in a network include: experts in one's area of practice, local people who can help access services for persons with disability, colleagues to whom you can refer patients in their own geographic location, role models, mentors, individuals who can provide sources of information (i.e., a librarian), those who can offer professional challenge, and people who can give you political advice on health-related personal issues. Figure 27-5 is a guide to help the reader identify individuals for their own professional network.

Electronic Networking

The 1980's has opened a new dimension for networking with the new communications medium created by the merger of computer and telecommunication technologies. Electronic networking enhances an individual's ability to connect with other people. Within five years, we should see many expanded opportunities for professional growth through on-line conferences, electronic meetings, electronic publications, and on-line education. The technology already exists to tap into national resource databases to help the people we serve. Because of this rapidly-changing technology, it would be futile to describe the specific programs currently available since they would quickly become out-of-date. This is a perfect example of how a network could be used to remain current in the new technology.

ACHIEVING OCCUPATIONAL PERFORMANCE

The process occupational therapists use to help a person achieve community independence in their occupational role is a very complicated one. The process requires the therapist to integrate scientific knowledge with environmental determinants and employ clinical judgment on a case-by-case basis. Independence is not gained by merely allowing a piece of equipment to perform a task for the client, but rather by giving the individual the tools to engage in occupation. The total process of occupational therapy includes all of the following:

1. assessing a person's capabilities,
2. enhancing the individual's performance to the highest possible level,
3. determining the capacity of the caregiver to support performance,
4. being familiar with the resources that will provide the environmental support,
5. integrating all this information to support change in the person.

SUMMARY

The dynamic nature of health care services in the United States, greatly influenced by changes in consumer attitudes, has made it necessary for occupational therapy to reconsider its position in the marketplace. By emphasizing services that address areas of traditional strength within the field, occupational therapists can play an instrumental role in promoting independence for persons with disabling conditions. A more competitive posture in this area can be facilitated in several ways. Recommended strategies include understanding effective methods for organizaing and marketing services, (such as the product line approach), increasing awareness of community resources, developing more effective networking skills, and appreciating the value of professional organizations in supporting these efforts.

Study Questions

1. Why do some physicians have such a narrow concept of rehabilitation? What can you do to change this?

2. How can occupational therapists change rehabilitation services away from a focus on"doing to the client" and toward a focus for "planning and creating services with the client'?

3. Identify at least three additional occupational therapy products to add to the occupational therapy product line.

4. How can occupational therapists tap into the long-term support system network described by Brody and Masciocchi?

5. Contact one of the consumer organizations to obtain information about a problem of interest. What types of resources does the organization make available?

References

American Occupational Therapy Assocation. (1988). Guide to Official Documents, Rockville, Maryland.

Baum, C.M. & Luebben, A.J. (1985). Assessing Community Resources to Support Independent Living, in *Pivot, Planning and Implementing Vocational Readiness in Occupational Therapy*, Rockville, MD: The American Occupational Therapy Association, 95-98.

Brody, E.M. (1974). A longitudinal look at excess disability in the mentally impaired aged. *Journal of Gerontology, 29,* 79-84.

Brody, J.S. & Masciocchi. (1980). Data for long-term planning by health care systems agencies. *American Journal of Public Health 70,* 1194-1198.

Corcoran, P.J. (1984). *The health care dilemma*, RTC/IL Monograph, The Research and Training Center on Independent Living, The University of Kansas. 1.

Lipnack, J. & Stamps, J. (1986). *The networking book: People connecting with people.* New York: Routledge and Kegan Paul.

Meyer, A. (1922), The philosophy of occupational therapy. *Archives of Occupational Therapy, 1*, 1-10.

Naisbitt, J. (1982). *Megatrends: Ten new directions for transforming our lives.* (p. 192). New York: Warner Books.

National Association of Rehabilitation Facilities. (1985). *Position Paper on A Prospective Payment System for Inpatient Medical Rehabilitation Services.* Washington, D.C.: Author.

Tarlov, A. (1983). Shattuck Lecture: The increasing supply of physicians, the changing structure of the health-service system, and the future practice of medicine. *New England Journal of Medicine 308*(20), 1235-1244.

U.S. Department of Health and Human Services, Background Paper, (No. 531). Health Care Administration, Dec. 24, 1984, Baltimore, MD.

Zola, K.I. (1982). Social and cultural disincentives to independent living. *Archives of Physical Medicine Rehabilitation 63*, 394-397.

CHAPTER CONTENT OUTLINE

KEY TERMS

Compensatory power

Competition

Condign power

Conditioned power

Cost benefit analysis

Federal register

Legislative review

Bill mark-up

Medicare

Policy

Power

Representative assembly

Technology transfer

ABSTRACT

The health care system today is heavily governed by economics and cost containment, thus it is imperative that the public and the health care industry are aware of the benefits of occupational therapy in helping to reduce overall health care costs by helping to return disabled individuals to independent living. This chapter challenges and encourages occupational therapists to become active in developing professional policy, to influence public policy through the legislative process and through regulations, to challenge insurance denials, and to become involved in consumer groups and advocacy-oriented organizations that share the same concerns for persons with disabilities.

Professional Issues in a Changing Environment

Carolyn Baum

"The last twenty-five years have witnessed a great change in the prevailing conception of citizenship and citizenship training. Looked upon formerly as limited to the study of constitutions and government machinery, civics is now regarded as including also governmental functions and needs, and embracing, in addition, such relationships and problems as appear in everyday living."

—Howard Copeland Hill, 1928

OBJECTIVES

The information in this chapter is intended to help the reader—

1. appreciate the importance of educating policy makers about occupational therapy and its contribution to health care.

2. identify the different arenas in which policies are established.

3. recognize, define, and distinguish among different types of power.

4. identify strategies for influencing policy decisions that will ensure that occupational therapy is a viable service in the future.

INTRODUCTION

The United States health policy at this time is one of finance. Economics drives the system, and those who can pay are the ''haves,'' while those without financial resources are the ''have nots.'' As we near the end of the twentieth century, America is still without a national health policy that serves the American people. In spite of having one of the most sophisticated health care systems in the world today, there are still some very startling statistics about health care in the U.S. There are 37 million people without health insurance (an increase of 14 million from just 3 years ago) and another 15 million who are underinsured. Fifty percent of children living in families with incomes below the poverty level are without a system to pay for their basic health needs (Boyle, 1987).

In such an atmosphere of cost consciousness and cost containment in health care, occupational therapists must ensure that the public and industry are aware of the benefits of occupational therapy. The following questions should be answered in the affirmative:

- Do those involved in developing programs and policies for elderly persons know the potential contribution of occupational therapy?
- Are legislators who are debating new health finance laws aware of occupational therapy's contribution to health care?
- Do people in industry understand occupational therapy's potential to reduce their costs by returning disabled individuals to work?
- Do insurance companies realize that providing coverage for occupational therapy services can translate into a cost benefit?
- Do hospital administrators understand how occupational therapists can expand their markets?
- Do those involved in developing technology understand occupational therapy's contribution to linking human potential with technology?
- Do physicians who are using bioreplacement technology recognize the impact of occupational therapy on returning their patients to productive living?

WHY INFLUENCE POLICY?

It is through public **policy** that support is garnered for community living, that disabled children gain access to services, that the mentally ill have access to programs that give them the skills for living, and that disabled individuals gain access to the services that will help them learn to live and work as productive individuals. Governments in the United States provide funding for all of these programs.

Funding of rehabilitation programs has traditionally been carried out jointly by the state and federal governments. The Rehabilitation Act of 1973, a major piece of human rights legislation which has had subsequent revisions, serves as the guiding legislation for programming and research for the disabled persons. Table 28-1 presents an overview of the programs currently operating under the Rehabilitation Act.

Because occupational therapy is so closely linked to the legislative process, it is important for therapists to be informed and involved. Therapists' responsibilities go beyond their relationship with their clients and beyond their role as health care professionals. As citizens in a democracy, they also have a responsibility to propose policy and raise the issues that effect necessary legislation. To become vitally involved in the political system, each therapist must take the responsibility of gaining the skills necessary to influence policy. Such skills are acquired by mobilizing resources and learning the workings of the system in which the policy will be changed.

The goal of this chapter is to introduce the occupational therapist to the trends of the future, to define the therapist's right and responsibility to influence change, and to explore the skills needed to enhance the future of the profession.

HEALTH CARE: A CHANGING SYSTEM

Health care is in a turbulent period of change. The futurists, Johnson and Johnson (1986) call it a revolution. The U.S. health care system has developed within an environment and culture that are constantly adapting to new situations and being modified by new economics. Capra (1982) tells us that

Table 28-1
An Overview of Vocational Rehabilitation Programs in the U.S.

PROGRAM	DESCRIPTION
Basic State Grants	The law provides for a program of matching funds, eighty percent federal, twenty percent state. As mandated by law, funds are distributed on a formula basis and provided to individuals with the most severe handicaps. This is the major program under the Act.
Services to the Blind and Visually Handicapped	Services are geared to the development of specific salable job skills to expand suitable employment opportunities.
Client Assistance Projects	Grants go only to state vocational rehabilitation agencies. Projects provide an advocate for patients/clients to identify undecided complaints or problems with the system and seek solutions. Seventeen projects were funded in 1982.
Training	Grants go to universities for vocational rehabilitation training. Occupational therapy programs have traditionally received funding.
Special Projects for Severely Disabled Individuals	An example of such projects is the seventeen spinal cord centers funded in 1982.
Handicapped Migratory and Seasonal Farm Workers	Projects expand services to this highly mobile and rural population.
Special Recreation Programs	Recreational projects contribute to patients'/clients' overall vocational goals.
Projects with Industry	The private sector accepts a senior responsibility for each partnership job-training project.
Independent Living Centers	Services are geared to independent living or more effective community living. In 1982, 156 centers were supported. Services vary according to local needs.
National Institute of Disability and Rehabilitation Research (NIDRR)	The institute provides a comprehensive and coordinated approach to research for disabled persons, and facilitates and increases distribution of scientific and technical information.
Rehabilitation Research and Training Centers (RTCs)	Projects combine service, research, and training. Twenty-six centers were funded in 1982.
Rehabilitation Engineering Centers	Similar to RTCs in purpose, the centers provide information on durable medical equipment, prosthetics, and orthotics.
National Council on the Handicapped	The fifteen-member council appointed by the President advises the Commissioner of Rehabilitation Services Administration on policy.

we must think differently not only about health in general, but about how and where health care is delivered.

The interplay between physical and mental processes has been recognized throughout the ages and is the foundation upon which occupational therapy's originators based their concepts. Presently, in the changing health system, the understanding of mind/body interaction is re-emerging and rapidly gaining acceptance, especially with the growing public awareness of the relevance of stress.

Capra (1982) explains how this concept will continue to change the nature of health institutions and health care in general. The future will require that we develop psychological techniques that will facilitate the healing process. More serious illness will require greater efforts of regaining one's balance, generally with the help of a doctor or therapist, and the outcome will depend crucially on the patient's mental attitudes and expectations. Severe illness will require a therapeutic approach, dealing not only with the physical and psychological aspects of the disorder, but also with the changes in the patient's lifestyle and world view that will be an integral part of the healing process.

The basic aim of any therapy will be to restore the patient's balance, and since the underlying model of health acknowledges the organism's innate tendency to heal itself, the therapist will try to intrude only minimally and keep the treatments as mild as possible. The healing will always be done by the mind/body system itself; the therapist will merely reduce the excessive stress, strengthen the body, encourage the patient to develop self-confidence and a positive mental attitude, and generally create the environment most conducive to the healing. To do this hospitals will gradually transform themselves into humane institutions, with more comfortable and therapeutic environments modeled after hotels, and family members will be involved in the care. *"This process will require a considerable broadening of their scientific basis and much greater emphasis on the behavioral sciences and on human ecology.''* (Capra, 1982, p. 337).

The transition to this new approach is in progress, but it will occur slowly and carefully because of the great symbolic power of the biomedical system in western society.

Change Is Now

The Association of American Medical Colleges' report, *Physician for the Twenty-First Century* (1984), outlined the changing role of the physician and highlighted several major trends occurring in U.S. health care that are of major importance:

- '' . . . an increasing recognition that many factors determining health and illness are not directly influenced by interventions of the health care system, but are the consequences of lifestyle, environmental factors and poverty.''

- ''Environmental factors and lifestyle are increasingly targeted as more important determinants of health and illness than are medical interventions.''

- ''Medical faculties have thought it imperative that medical education keep pace with biomedical science and have expanded the base of factual knowledge that students must commit to memory. By this concentration on the transmittal of factual information faculties, they have neglected to help them (students) acquire the skill, values, and attitudes that are the foundation of a helping profession.''

The interdisciplinary approach to health care has also become a necessity, as reflected in this statement from the Health Policy Agenda for the American People (1987): ''Those persons engaged in programs of education for the health professions should learn to work effectively with health professionals in other disciplines. Interdisciplinary learning experiences are an important means to an end.''

The health community is becoming more receptive to occupational therapy's concepts and interventions, but it still requires a political effort on the part of all occupational therapists to influence the development of the new health system and to secure their places in that system. Although great strides have been made in developing new therapies to help the disabled person function independently, they will have been made in vain if therapists are denied access to the clients who need their services.

In the 1962 Eleanor Clarke Slagle Lecture, Mary Reilly (1962) proposed that occupational therapy could be one of the great ideas of twentieth century medicine. Today, our responsibility as occupational therapists is to take her message to the public and to the legislature.

The Impact of Public Policy on the Profession

In the United States, several laws have been enacted which have has substantial influence on the development of occupational therapy. For example, the 1965 Medicare law (P. L. 89-97) limited payment to occupational therapists by placing occupational therapy in **Medicare** Part A, the acute medical service of hospital and skilled nursing home care. From 1965 to 1983, while speech and physical therapists were building community-based practices, occupational therapists were limited to working in hospital-based positions. When Medicare was initiated, the significance of this limitation was not immediately clear, but as private insurers and Blue Cross and Blue Shield adopted the Medicare guidelines as a basis of payment over the years, it became clear that this severely limited occupational therapy's payment patterns in outpatient services. The changes in the Medicare laws in the early 1980's gave a boost to occupational therapy by opening access to outpatient payment.

Another example of legislation which limited access to occupational therapy is evident in the Medicaid program. Under Medicaid, states have the right to select the services they wish to provide from among those identified in the legislation. While occupational therapy is a covered medical expense in the federal law, not all states allow it as a covered outpatient service. This prevents many poor people (who rely on Medicaid for health care) from receiving occupational therapy services. Most health policy critics agree that the Medicaid system is in need of major reform.

Until two legislative initiatives changed the focus and availability of education for handicapped persons, therapists had a difficult time accessing children with developmental disabilities. The Education for All Handicapped Children Act of 1975 (P. L. 94-142) and Section 504 of the Rehabilitation Act of 1973 gave occupational therapists access to children who experience performance dysfunction. Presently, nearly 20% of all occupational therapists in the U.S. practice in a school setting. This statistic clearly exemplifies how professional involvement in the legislation process can greatly impact the parameters of the populations we seek to serve.

A LOOK AT THE FUTURE

Russell Coil (1986) in his book, *The New Hospital*, identifies megatrends that may shape the future of health care. Those of aging, **competition**, shifting health care dollars, technological advancements, and the rising costs of health care, will greatly affect occupational therapy practice and are addressed in the following.

The Growing and Changing Elderly Population

The demographics of our nation's population are greatly

changing. In 1980, one out of every nine Americans was over the age of 85 and by the year 2010, one out of five will be over that age. Clearly, elderly persons will comprise a large segment of our population, and this group places heavy demands on the health care system.

The elderly persons of the future, particularly those aged 50 to 70, will be in better physical condition, more educated, more affluent and better informed about their health. It is clear that occupational therapists will become more involved with both healthy and chronically ill elderly persons and the subsequent influences on their families and society.

Competition

The deregulation of health care will stimulate even greater competition than exists today. Industry has already taken on a greater role in determining the health benefits of its employees. Many have chosen to become members of Preferred Provider Organizations (PPOs) and Health Maintenance Organizations (HMOs) in order to hold down health care costs via competitive bidding. Such approaches to health care delivery do not always offer comprehensive services.

Therapists must demonstrate that the addition of occupational therapy services will result in a cost benefit to the payor. This can be accomplished through documented studies that are designed to measure the outcome of care through **cost benefit analysis**. It is also possible (and necessary) for occupational therapists to collect information about the patients that are being served in a program. It is important to know the average length of stay in a program, in addition to the average cost and discharge status of people who have been served. The insurers want to know that the services rendered have been effective in reducing costs. It is important for the occupational therapist to point out to insurers the number of people who are being returned to gainful employment as well as the number being discharged to community living instead of institutions.

Shifting Health Care Dollars

Health care dollars are being shifted from inpatient to outpatient services. The health care facilities of the future will need to establish an effective case management system to ensure that patients receive the services necessary to keep costs down. An internal referral process, along with the effective use of community resources, serves as a case management mechanism. Insurance companies hire case managers to manage complicated medical and vocational problems. The insurance company's goal is to reduce expenditures. If the rehabilitation team provides the coordinated level of care that prepares an individual for community living, the insurance company's cost will be reduced.

Hospitals must submit low cost bids to be selected as preferred providers by industry. Occupational therapy managers will have to design intervention strategies that keep costs lower. Some examples are: (1) the use of certified occupational therapy assistants and on-the-job-trained technicians, (2) the institution of group treatment, and (3) family involvement in the treatment process.

Technological Advancements

Coil identifies six technological advances as driving forces in health care: (1) computerization, (2) artificial intelligence, (3) office automation, (4) genetic engineering, (5) super drugs, and (6) bioreplacement technology. Four of these advances have direct application to occupational therapy and will be discussed below.

Computerization. Occupational therapists can expect computers to provide many more employment opportunities for their clients. Those who were previously unemployable because of age or disability will be in demand in the work force for two reasons: (1) they will be able to perform work in the "information society" with voice-activated and electronic controls and (2) the retirement of the "baby boomers" will create a tremendous vacancy in jobs that disabled persons can fill. We can already see evidence of this in the fast food industry, in which jobs previously held by teenagers are being filled by individuals who are elderly or mentally retarded.

Office Automation. Occupational therapists must actively design programs to incorporate technology to document the clinical progress of the people they serve. Database systems offer opportunities for computer-generated reports as well as program evaluation models.

Artificial Intelligence. Artificial intelligence could have major applications for occupational therapy practice. Mechanisms are being developed that could give verbal cues to individuals with cognitive loss. This advance could make treatment much more successful, particularly for those disabled by head trauma and stroke. The robot will also have an impact on the life-skill patterns of people requiring attendants.

Bioreplacement Technology. Bioreplacement technology could also have a major impact on the performance capabilities of occupational therapy clients. Advances in myoelectric limbs, as well as electronic stimulation to muscles in individuals with spinal cord injuries, will most certainly alter our practice strategies.

Significant advances in transplant technology are also

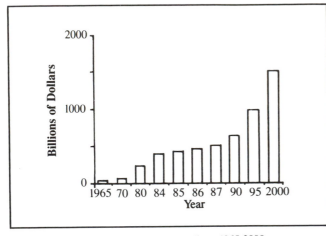

Figure 28-1. U.S. National Health Expenditure 1965-2000.

being made. Donor knee transplants are being performed, and in the next decade lung transplants, extremity transplants, and perhaps even brain transplants will be performed. All of these advances create new opportunities for the occupational therapist to help clients achieve independence.

The Rising Cost of Health Care

Rising medical costs not only threaten Americans' health, but the very economic strength of the U.S. Fein (1986) states that "Labor-management contracts, household budgets, corporate stability, and federal and state expenditures are held hostage to ever rising health expenditures." Figure 28-1 presents the U.S. health expenditures since 1965 and those projected to the year 2000. The following are some of the foreboding signs of this threat to our economy and to each of us individually:

- Medicare, the United States' largest health insurance program, provides diminishing protection to its beneficiaries.
- Medicare will have to be reformed or it will face bankruptcy (Annual Report of The Board of Trustees of the Federal Hospital Insurance Trust Fund, 1985).
- Health benefit plans have been reduced. In 1982, 30 percent of all health insurance plans required a deductible for hospital inpatient services, but by 1984, 60 percent required deductibles (Environmental Analysis, 1985).
- "Cost controls are being imposed without systematic assessment of their impact on the availability and quality of medical care. Efforts to shift costs divert increasing proportions of funds, energy, and ingenuity into administrative activities that do not save lives or alleviate suffering" (Fein, 1986).

The central policy issues are whether the U.S. can afford the kind of health system it has created and whether existing financial mechanisms will be adequate. The answers to these questions will come, not from physicians, not from the American Medical Association, not from scientists, not from professional associations in occupational therapy, but from politicians.

This next phase of development in health care will be different from the current system. In short, there will be major system reform. Advanced technology will continue to save more lives and more people will survive to live with disabilities. The system will begin to rely on more outpatient preventive measures, but they will be delivered at the work site, not at the hospital. Insurers will not pay for tests and procedures that are not shown to be necessary. The predicted overabundance of physicians will bring costs down, and doctors will become interested in using many of the same interventions that occupational therapists now employ. Competition will be further stimulated to control costs, and competition is a self regulating model in which only responsive and efficient producers are assured of survival (Fein, 1986).

ACHIEVING INFLUENCE AND ATTAINING POWER

Given the above scenario of the changing health care system in the U.S., we must ask what occupational therapists can do to influence the future changes. The occupational therapist must understand and gain skills in the use of **power** to influence change that will ensure that patients have access to occupational therapy services. *"Power is the possibility of imposing one's will upon the behavior of other persons"* (Weber, 1954).

Instruments for Using Power

Kenneth Galbraith (1983) identifies three instruments for wielding power and three traits that accord an individual the right to use it.

Condign power achieves control by imposing an alternative to the unpleasant or painful preferences of the individual or group so that such preferences are abandoned. An example of this would occur if a particular physician was prone to embarrassing the clinical staff, a therapist avoided talking to that physician. In such a case, the therapist would be controlled by condign power.

Compensatory power is exercised by giving something of value to the person submitting to that power. Praise is an example of compensatory power. In the modern economy, payment for services rendered is an important expression of compensatory power. That payment represents a submission to the economic or personal purposes of others. Occupational therapists wield considerable compensatory power by providing a service that both accomplishes the purposes of agencies and institutions and produces an income.

Conditioned power is exercised by changing the belief of an individual. Education, persuasion, or social commitment causes the individual to submit to the will of others. This type of power is central to the occupational therapist's role in helping insurers, payors, administrators, physicians, legislators, industry, and the public know and understand the occupational therapist's potential contribution to health care.

Galbraith further states that there are three sources of power behind the three instruments for exercising power:

Personality. An individual's personality and how he/she is perceived by others has a direct impact on the individual's ability to persuade or create a belief. It therefore is important for the occupational therapist to be known by the individuals he/she hopes to educate. By demonstrating leadership, the effective personality will be more persuasive. When it is impossible to form a relationship, the therapist must learn about the individual to be educated so that the interaction can be meaningful. The therapist's approach must be precise, cogent, and honest. To influence others the therapist must be confident in his/her knowledge and committed to the cause. In this manner, the therapist's personality functions through conditioned power.

Property. The therapist who generates income, brings in grants and/or attracts donations, or contributes by managing a department, is a valuable asset to the organization. By the same token, it is virtually impossible for an occupational therapist to wield power in an organization if he/she is not making the financial contribution that is expected. Property invites conditioned power, but primarily helps to exercise compensatory power.

Organization. Organization plays a very important role in influencing policy and is the most important source of power in modern society. It is taken for granted when power is sought or needed that an organization is required. An organized group's power is often measured in direct relation to the property that the group possesses. The American Occupational Therapy Association, the Canadian Association of Occupational Therapists, and the state and provincial occupational therapy associations are organizations whose primary purpose is to help the profession achieve influence through its collective membership. Organization as described here is most closely related to conditioned power.

INFLUENCING POLICY

Influencing Professional Policy

The policies of professional organizations guides its actions and positions as it represents the profession in the public arena. In North America, each state in the United States and each province in Canada has a professional association or society representing occupational therapy. While the sizes and organizational structures of these groups vary, each has a mechanism through which individual members can raise issues for official consideration by the entire organization. Frequently, these opportunities occur during annual meetings.

In Canada and the United States, the national organizations representing occupational therapists publish policies, standards and guidelines, and position statements. These documents can be requested by contacting the respective organizations, as follows:

American Occupation Therapy Association, Inc.
1383 Piccard Drive
Rockville, Maryland 20850-4375
U.S.A.
(301) 948-9626

Canadian Association of Occupational Therapists
110 Eglinton Avenue West
3rd Floor
Toronto, Ontario M4R 1A3
CANADA
(416) 487-5404

Influencing Policy through the Legislative Process

The process of achieving a policy or changing a policy that is made by government through its legislative bodies is as follows: an individual identifies his/her needs and garners the support of an organization. That organization convinces a legislator to introduce a bill that addresses those needs. The bill is then expounded before legislatures and political parties, enacted into law, and administered by the administrative departments of the government. How much the government can do depends on how much it is called on to do by the public.

Figure 28-2 demonstrates the process by which a bill becomes law in the United States Congress. The process is similar in most state legislatures. However, there are some differences from state to state that must be understood if one is to be effective in influencing the bill as it is being developed into law.

In order to influence the outcome of a bill, either positively or negatively, one must track the bill's progress through the system and lobby. Lobbying is one method organizations can use to communicate their concerns to public officials. Lobbying is a good example of applying conditioned power.

The following description of the lobbying process is adapted from the book, *Lobbying for Health Care* (1985), written by Susan Scott, OTR, and Jane Acquaviva, OTR. This is an excellent source for occupational therapists to learn the workings of the lobbying process.

Introduction of a Bill. Lobbying must begin before a bill is introduced into the legislature. The group that wants to create a change in the law must first find a legislator to sponsor the bill. Generally, the more respected a sponsor is in that area of concern, the more attention the bill will receive. Also, the more sponsors the bill has, the greater its chances for success.

Assignment of the Bill to Committee. Once a bill has been introduced, it is assigned to a committee. It is possible to lobby the leadership of the house and the senate for the best committee assignment, if there appears to be flexibility in the assignments. However, most bills are assigned according to their jurisdiction; for example health bills go to the health committee and education bills go to the education committee. There is some flexibility when the jurisdiction overlaps, as in the case of a bill requiring budget review. When there is overlap, the bills frequently go to more than one committee. In the United States Congress, the House of Representatives has 19 standing committees and the Senate has 15 standing committees that can receive bills. Bills may then be referred to a subcommittee.

Public Hearings. Federal law and most state laws require the legislature to hold public hearings. This is the time to

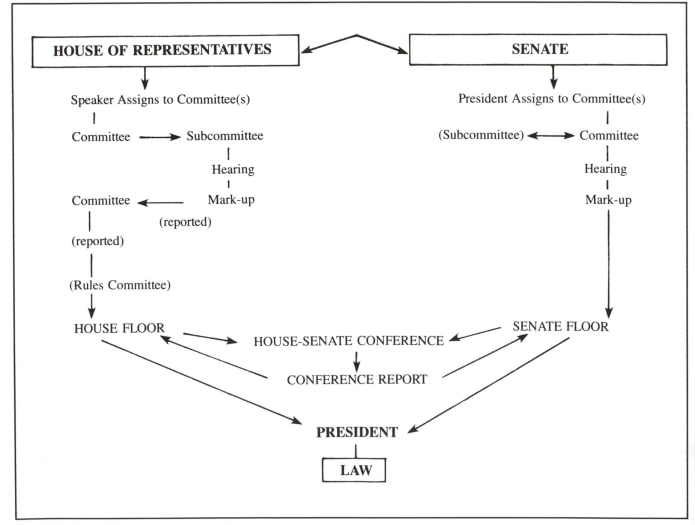

Figure 28-2. How a Bill Becomes a Law (United States Congress).

present prepared information both verbally and in writing. Prior to the hearing, it is important to educate the legislator with a letter or a phone call. Perhaps the most important strategy is to visit the representative's office. All representatives have local offices and local staff that keep them informed, so actual visits can make an impact.

Bill Mark-up. After the committee or the subcommittee has met, the committee members actually **mark up** the bill, amending it by either deleting, modifying, or adding to it according to their own inclinations and the wishes of their constituents and lobbyists. At this time, the lobbyist can and should make specific requests regarding the actual language of the bill, such as asking to delete offensive words or paragraphs or to insert special wording.

In the United States Congress the mark-up process may not begin for weeks or months after the hearing, but in the state legislatures mark up often begins as soon as the hearing ends.

Reporting the Bill to Committee. After the bill is marked up, the subcommittee reports the bill to the full committee. The report describes the bill's content and explains any amendments that have been made. This report helps to establish legislative intent and is frequently consulted when the agency later writes the regulations for the law. It is also used by lawyers and judges when interpreting the law, so it is important to lobby for the inclusion of explanations about important concerns (e.g., the qualifications of professionals providing services), so that there is no possibility of misinterpretation of the intent at a later time.

Voting on House or Senate Floor. A bill can be amended at any reading by a legislator on the floor. Once the bill has passed both chambers, it is referred to a *conference committee*, if there are differences in the bills, this committee works out such differences through compromise to arrive at a version to be reported.

Conference Committee Report. Select members of the Senate and the House of Representatives work together to reach compromises. If there are different versions of the bill, it is important to lobby for the version that most satisfies the original intent. When all of the differences have been resolved, the conference committee report is prepared and identifies and explains the compromises that have been reached.

Approval by the House and Senate. The report of the conference committee must be approved by both chambers and usually is. If the report is not approved, it is either recommitted to conference or the bill dies. If approved, it is forwarded to the chief executive, either the president or the governor.

Signature of the Chief Executive. The chief executive usually signs bills that have been passed by both chambers. If the chief executive vetoes the bill, it is sent back to both chambers with the objections noted. The legislature can override a veto with a two-thirds majority. An automatic veto of a bill occurs if the chief executive does not sign or veto a bill within ten days of receiving it — as long as the legislature is not in session (pocket veto). If the legislature convenes during that period, the bill automatically becomes law. A pocket veto cannot be overridden by the legislature, although it can be introduced at the next legislative session.

Influencing Policy through Regulations

Regulations are generated by federal and state agencies to implement the law. They translate the broad language of legislation into specific policies and procedures. Additionally, agencies can develop new regulations for matters on which the legislature is silent. They can also develop regulations that bring new programs into conformance with existing programs. Examples of state agencies affecting occupational therapy are: the State Office of Medical Assistance (Medicaid), the State Health Department, State Department of Education, Vocational Rehabilitation, and Worker's Compensation. State and federal agencies responsible for administering programs directly related to occupational therapy must be monitored to avoid surprises that could seriously affect the delivery of occupational therapy and other health care services. Figure 28-3 is a diagram of the federal regulation-making process. Variations on this process occur at the state level.

Formulation of Proposed Rules. The rule-making process begins within the agency. The agency writes the rules which interpret legislative intent.

Publication of Proposed Rules. Federal agencies publish proposed rules in the **Federal Register**, which is issued daily. Some states have registers that are published on a less frequent schedule. States that do not publish registers publish proposed rules in local newspapers (usually two to four of the major papers in the state). Some of the states that publish registers occasionally publish the rules in the newspaper as well when they are proposing changes in a popular or controversial program.

Invitation for Public Comment and Public Hearings. When the rules are published, they are accompanied by an invitation for public comment. The time limit for comment is detailed in the notice. It is very important for professional organizations and/or individuals to propose any changes at this time.

Sometimes public hearings are held. The location and the time of the hearings are published with the proposed rule. Usually the hearings are held in several locations around the state. Again, this is an important opportunity for the public to comment on changes they wish to have proposed in the rules.

Inter-agency Review and Comment. Usually the agency proposing the rule sends the rules to other agencies for their comments. It is a good idea to have contacts in all of the agencies that relate to occupational therapy interests. Particularly in non-licensed states, it is helpful if the state agencies can help the organization watch-dog legislation and regulations that could govern and define the practice of occupational therapy. The organization can also call upon these contacts to incorporate therapists' concerns into any comments they make to the requesting agency on the proposed rule.

Governor's Approval. The governor is the chief executive officer of the state and is ultimately responsible for the administration of all of the state agencies, and as such it is the governor's responsibility to accept or reject the rules. If the governor does not approve the proposed rules, they are sent to the agency for revision. Another alternative in attempting to change a proposed rule is to contact the governor's office and express your concern and ask for the changes. You may also request that the governor return the rule to the agency for further work.

Legislative Review. A **legislative review** of the rules occurs when the legislature perceives that an agency has misinterpreted its intent or excessively revised existing regulations. If a citizen or an organization believes that the agency has misinterpreted or changed the intent of the law in revising the regulations, it is possible to enlist the support of legislators who are friendly to the cause to ask for a legislative review.

Legislative Intervention. Legislative intervention involves considerable effort. It usually takes the form of an amendment to a bill that is currently being considered before the legislature. The purpose of the amendment is to more clearly define the intent of the law. This legal clarification makes it more difficult for the agency to ignore the actual intent of the law in the regulation.

Not all policy decisions are performed with such public scrutiny. Every day insurers, people in business, and administrators create policies regarding access to and payment for services. The occupational therapist in the clinic or in the community can be very influential in helping shape policy by demonstrating that occupational therapy services represent a cost-effective alternative to dependency.

Influencing Policy by Challenging Insurance Denials

The therapist should routinely challenge *insurance denials*, not to criticize the payment policies of the insurer, but to educate the insurer as to the value of occupational therapy in helping the insurance company achieve its objectives. Experience shows that many insurance companies know little about occupational therapy, but they will never know of its potential to help their subscribers unless therapists tell them. The best strategy is to educate them with actual cases by appealing their denial decisions. Physicians are usually willing to write a letter in support of the services they have ordered for their patients. If the company denies the appeal, the therapist should continue up the corporate ladder, from supervisor to manager, educating as he/she goes. If services are appropriately delivered and well documented, it is well worth the effort to challenge insurance denials. The results should be financially successful and professionally satisfying.

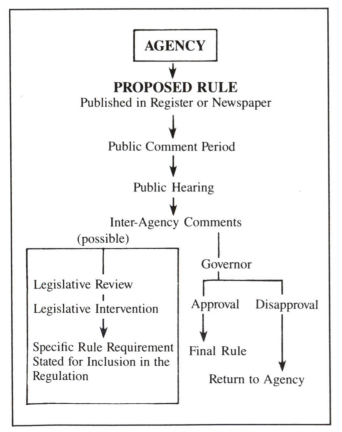

Figure 28-3. How Regulations Are Made.

Influencing Policy through Broad Community Involvement

When consumer groups and community organizations know that occupational therapy is valuable in helping disabled persons achieve independence, the profession will command support for its financial and legislative issues. With the backing of consumer groups, occupational therapy will be in a much stronger position to achieve its professional goals.

Occupational therapists should be involved with the consumer organizations identified in Chapter 7. Additionally, the highlighted advocacy-oriented groups share common concerns with occupational therapy. It is important to associate with these organizations to achieve important objectives for disabled persons.

ADVOCACY-ORIENTED GROUPS

The American Coalition of Citizens With Disabilities, Inc. is a group of organizations and individuals working toward improving conditions for the disabled in housing, employment, transportation, the media, and civil rights.
Address: American Coalition of Citizens With
Disabilities, Inc.
1012 14th Street N.W.,Washington, DC 20005
Telephone: (202) 628-3470 (voice and TTD)

The Center on Human Policy is an advocacy and research organization committed to the rights of people with disabilities to integrate educational, vocational, rehabilitative and residential services.
Address: Center on Human Policy
Syracuse University, 216 Ostrom Avenue,
Syracuse, NY 13210
Telephone: (315) 423-3851

Congress of Organizations of the Physically Handicapped (COPH) publishes the COPH Bulletin, a quarterly newspaper which provides information on developments in rehabilitation research and on state legislation affecting the physically handicapped.
Address: Congress of Organizations of the Physically
Handicapped (COPH)
16630 Beverly Avenue, Tinley Park, IL 60477
Telephone: (312) 532-3566

The Disability Rights Center was established in 1976 to advocate for the rights of all disabled persons. The Center monitors and seeks ways to strengthen the federal agencies' affirmative action programs for the employment of disabled persons.
Address: Disability Rights Center
1346 Connecticut Avenue, N. W.,
Washington, D.C.
Telephone: (202) 223-3304

The Foundation For Dignity promotes the dignity, civil rights, independence, and personal development of individuals with physical or mental handicaps.
Address: Foundation For Dignity
37 South 20th Street, Philadelphia, PA 19103
Telephone: (215) 567-2828

The Gray Panthers work to eliminate age discrimination and promote policies and attitudes that enable people to reach their full potential, regardless of age.
Address: Gray Panthers
311 South Juniper Street, Philadelphia, PA 19107
Telephone: (215) 545-6555

Consumer Organization for the Hearing Impaired (COHI)
Address: P.O. Box 8188, Silver Springs, MD 20907

OCCUPATIONAL THERAPY: ABILITY TO SHAPE THE FUTURE

Technology Transfer

The profession of occupational therapy continues to grow not only by generating knowledge about occupation and its effect on performance, but also by demonstrating how important it is for people with performance dysfunction to have access to occupational therapy services. The process of sharing scientific information about occupational therapy is called **technology transfer**. Occupational therapy is an applied science and its application must be known to the individuals who can benefit from it. The results of our research will give credence to our profession's image as a necessary health service if the people who influence the evolving health care system have access to those results. It is every occupational therapist's responsibility to transfer information about occupational therapy's technology to consumers, to providers, and to the public policy makers.

Results of Occupational Therapy Intervention

Nothing makes a stronger statement than results. Satisfied consumers are the profession's greatest asset. When people return to work and/or are successful in their daily life activities, when caregivers understand their tasks and when physicians and insurers see the effect of occupational therapy interventions, we are building a perception of the profession's importance in the health care marketplace. Business literature tells us how important a satisfied customer is in building a business. The business of occupational therapy is helping individuals overcome human performance deficits. Satisfied ''customers'' present occupational therapy to the policy makers.

Behaviors of the Professional Occupational Therapist

Occupational therapists are challenged to create an environment in which the people they serve can achieve an independent level of function. This continues to be a political process, one that each therapist is challenged to perform in the daily routine.

The United States only incorporated *guaranteed access* for disabled persons into law in 1973 (subsequently modified in 1990), and we are just beginning to see more liberal attitudes toward persons with disabilities. Accessibility standards assure that those disabled people who wish to pursue degrees can attend a university and be assured of physical access to that environment. Educational standards guarantee all handicapped children the right to an education. Non-discrimination clauses forbid employers to discriminate against the disabled worker. Although all of these rights are stated in laws and regulations, the average citizen is slow to accept the disabled person as a worker, a student, or a community member. Occupational therapists can and must continue working to break down the attitudinal barriers that limit the handicapped in our society. By accepting a role in changing attitudes, therapists will gain influence as health professionals who have the knowledge, skill, and ability to help people achieve occupational performance.

"He (man) has a set of gifts which make him unique among the animals: so that, unlike them, he is not a figure in the landscape—he is a shaper of the landscape" (Bronowski, 1973).

SUMMARY

In order to influence decision by policy makers which affect health care and the lives of their patients and clients, occupational therapists must have an understanding of how policy is shaped. This chapter has reviewed various public policy decisions in the United States which have influenced occupational therapy practice, both positively and negatively. Since power influences change, an understanding of how power is acquired and used is vital. Toward this end, various instruments for exercising power, including condign, compensatory and conditioned power, have been identified. Additionally, personality, property and organization were identified as important sources of power.

Since an understanding of the legislative and regulation making processes is necessary for influencing public policy decisions, these were summarized. Community involvement, the use of professional organizations, the practice of

challenging insurance denials, and the process of technology transfer were all described as useful mechanisms for influencing change.

Study Questions

1. Review Mary Reilly's 1962 Eleanor Clarke Slagle Lecture in light of Capra's comments regarding the therapist's role and the healing process.

2. What can an individual occupational therapist do about the federal laws that limit a patient's access to services?

3. What can the therapist do to ensure that administrators, physicians, insurers and legislators are aware of occupational therapy's role in health care?

4. Develop a justification for an insurance denial. Ask a clinical therapist to help you review a record on a claim that has been denied and find out whom you would approach about changing the decision.

References

U.S. House Document #99-47. (1986). *The 1985 Annual report of the board of trustees of the Federal Hospital Insurance Trust Fund*, (pp. 1-73). Washington, DC: U.S. Government Printing Office.

Boyle, J.F. (1987). *An agenda for the future. The health policy agenda for the American people: Status report* (p. v.). Chicago: American Medical Association.

Bronowski, J. (1973). *The ascent of man* (p. 19). Boston: Little, Brown and Company.

Capra, F. (1982). *The turning point: Science, society and the rising culture* (pp. 305-327). New York: Simon and Schuster.

Coil, R. (1986). *The new hospital: Future strategies for a changing industry* (pp. 6-9). Rockville, MD: Aspen Publications.

Fein, R. (1986). *Medical care, medical costs: The search for a health insurance policy* (pp. 1-2). Cambridge, MA: Harvard University Press.

Galbraith, J. K. (1983). *The anatomy of power* (pp. 2-13). Boston: Houghton Mifflin Company.

The health policy agenda for the American people (principle 2-2k) (1987). Chicago: American Medical Association.

Environmental analysis (1985). Hewitt Associates survey (pp. 18-19). Chicago: Blue Cross and Blue Shield Association.

Hill, H.C. (1928). *Community and vocational civics* (p. iii). Boston: The Atheneum Press

Johnson, E.A. & Johnson, R.L. (1986). *Hospitals under fire:*

Strategies for survival (pp. 437-443). Rockville, MD: Aspen.

Physician for the twenty-first century (pp. xiii-3) (1984). The report of the Panel on the Professional Education of the Physician and College Preparation for Medicine. Washington, DC: Association of American Medical Colleges.

Principles of occupational therapy ethics (1987). Ethic VII, Reference manual of the official documents of The American Occupational Therapy Association. Rockville, MD: *The American Occupational Therapy Association.*

Reilly, M. (1962). Occupational therapy can be one of the great ideas of 20th century medicine. *American Journal of Occupational Therapy, 16,* 300-308.

Rheinstein, M. (Ed.). (1954). *Max Weber on law in economy and society* Cambridge, MA: Harvard University Press.

Scott, S.J. & Acquaviva, J.D. (1985). *Lobbying for health care* (pp. 2-7). Rockville, MD: The American Occupational Therapy Association.

Uniform Terminology for Occupational Therapy—Second Edition (American Occupational Therapy Association)

Uniform Terminology for Occupational Therapy— Second Edition delineates and defines Occupational Performance Areas and Occupational Performance Components that are addressed in occupational therapy direct service. These definitions are provided to facilitate the uniform use of terminology and definitions throughout the profession. The original document, *Occupational Therapy Product Output Reporting System and Uniform Terminology for Reporting Occupational Therapy Services*, which was published in 1979, helped create a base of consistent terminology that was used in many of the official documents of The American Occupational Therapy Association, Inc. (AOTA), in occupational therapy education curricula, and in a variety of occupational therapy practice settings. In order to remain current with practice, the first document was revised over a period of several years with extensive feedback from the profession. The revisions were completed in 1988. It is recognized and recommended that a document of this nature be updated periodically so that occupational therapy is defined in accordance with current theory and practice.

Guidelines for Use

Uniform Terminology—Second Edition may be used in a variety of ways. It defines occupational therapy practice, which includes occupational performance areas and occupational performance components. In addition, it will be useful to occupational therapists for (a) documentation, (b) charge systems, (c) education, (d) program development, (e) marketing, and (f) research. Examples of how occupational performance areas and occupational performance Components translate into practice are provided below. It is not the intent of this document to define specific occupational therapy programs nor specific occupational therapy

interventions. Some examples of the differences between occupational performance areas and occupational performance components and programs and interventions are

1. An individual who is injured on the job may be able to return to work, which is an occupational performance area. In order to achieve the outcome of returning to work, the individual may need to address specific performance components such as strength, endurance, and time management. The occupational therapist, in cooperation with the vocational team, utilizes planned interventions to achieve the desired outcome. These interventions may include activities such as an exercise program, body mechanics instruction, and job modification, and may be provided in a work-hardening program.

2. An individual with severe physical limitations may need and desire the opportunity to live within a community-integrated setting, which represents the occupational performance areas of activities of daily living and work. In order to achieve the outcome of community living, the individual may need to address specific performance components, such as normalizing muscle tone, gross motor coordination, postural control, and self-management. The occupational therapist, in cooperation with the team, utilizes planned interventions to achieve the desired outcome. Interventions may include neuromuscular facilitation, object manipulation, instruction in use of adaptive equipment, use of environmental control systems, and functional positioning for eating. These interventions may be provided in a community-based independent living program.

3. A child with learning disabilities may need to perform educational activities within a public school setting. Since learning is a student's work, this

educational activity would be considered the occupational performance Area for this individual. In order to achieve the educational outcome of efficient and effective completion of written classroom work, the child may need to address specific occupational performance components, including sensory processing, perceptual skills, postural control, and motor skills. The occupational therapist, in cooperation with the team, utilizes planned interventions to achieve the desired outcome. Interventions may include activities such as adapting the student's seating to improve postural control and stability and practicing motor control and coordination. This program could be provided by school district personnel or through contract services.

4. An infant with cerebral palsy may need to participate in developmental activities to engage in the occupational performance areas of activities of daily living and play. The developmental outcomes may be achieved by addressing specific performance components such as sensory awareness and neuromuscular control. The occupational therapist, in cooperation with the team, utilizes planned interventions to achieve the desired outcomes. Interventions may include activities such as seating and positioning for play, neuromuscular facilitation techniques to enable eating, and parent training. These interventions may be provided in a home-based occupational therapy program.

5. An adult with schizophrenia may need and desire to live independently in the community, which represents the occupational performance areas of activities of daily living, work activities, and play or leisure activities. The specific occupational performance areas may be medication routine, functional mobility, home management, vocational exploration, play or leisure performance, and social skills. In order to achieve the outcome of living alone, the individual may need to address specific performance components such as topographical orientation, memory, categorization, problem solving, interests, social conduct, and time management. The occupational therapist, in cooperation with the team, utilizes planned interventions to achieve the desired outcome. Interventions may include activities such as training in the use of public transportation, instruction in budgeting skills, selection of and participation in social activities, and instruction in social conduct. These interventions may be provided in a community-based mental health program.

6. An individual who abuses substances may need to reestablish family roles and responsibilities, which represents the occupational performance areas of activities of daily living and work. In order to achieve the outcome of family participation, the individual may need to address the performance components of roles, values, social conduct, self-expression, coping skills, and self-control. The occupational therapist, in cooperation with the team, utilizes planned intervention to achieve the desired outcomes. Interventions may include role and value clarification exercises, role-playing, instruction in stress management techniques, and parenting skills. These interventions may be provided in an inpatient acute care unit.

Because of the extensive use of the original document (*Uniform Terminology for Reporting Occupational Therapy Services*, 1979) in official documents, this revision is a second edition and does not completely replace the 1979 version. This follows the practice that other professions, such as medicine, pursue with their documents. Examples are the *Physician's Current Procedural Terminology First-Fourth Editions (CPT 1-4)* and the *Diagnostic and statistical Manual First-Third Editions (DSM-I—III-R)*. Therefore, this document is presented as *Uniform Terminology for Occupational Therapy—Second Edition*.

Background

Task Force Charge. In 1983, the Representative Assembly of the American Occupational Therapy Association charged the Commission on Practice to form a task force to revise the *Occupational Therapy Product Output Reporting System and Uniform Terminology for Reporting Occupational Therapy Services*. The document had been approved by the Representative Assembly in 1979 and needed to be updated to reflect current practice.

Background Information

The *Occupational Therapy Product Output Reporting System and Uniform Terminology for Reporting Occupational Therapy Services* (hereafter to be referred to as *Product Output Reporting System* or *Uniform Terminology*) document was originally developed in response to the Medicare-Medicaid Anti-Fraud and Abuse Amendments of 1977 (Public Law 95–142), which required the Secretary of the Department of Health and Human Services to establish regulations for uniform reporting systems for all departments in hospitals. The AOTA developed the documents to create a uniform reporting system for occupational therapy departments. Although the Department of Health and Human Services never adopted the system because of antitrust concerns relating to price fixing, occupational therapists have used the documents extensively in the profession.

Three states, Maryland, California, and Washington, have used the *Product Output Reporting System* as a basis for statewide reporting systems. AOTA's official documents have relied on the definitions to create uniformity. Many occupational therapy schools and departments have used the definitions to guide education and documentation. Although the initial need was for reimbursement reporting systems, the profession has used the documents primarily to facilitate uniformity in definitions.

Task Force Formation

In 1983, Linda Kohlman McGourty, a member of the AOTA Commission on Practice, was appointed by the commission's chair, John Farace, to chair the Uniform Terminology Task Force. Initially, a notice was placed in the *Occupational Therapy Newspaper* for people to submit feedback for the revisions. Many responses were received. Before the task force was appointed in 1984, Maryland, California, and Washington adopted reimbursement systems based on the *Product Output Reporting System.* Therefore, to increase the quantity and quality of input for the revisions, it was decided to postpone the formation of the task force until these states had had an opportunity to use the systems.

In 1985, a second notice was placed in the *Occupational Therapy News* requesting feedback, and a task force was appointed. The following people were selected to serve on the task force:

Linda Kohlman McGourty, MOT OTR, Washington (Chair)

Roger Smith, MOT, OTR, Wisconsin

Jane Marvin, OTC, California

Nancy Mahon Smith, MBA, OTR, Maryland and Arkansas

Mary Foto, OTR, California

These people were selected based on the following criteria:
1. Geographical representation
2. Professional expertise
3. Participation in other current AOTA projects
4. Knowledge of reimbursement systems
5. Interest in serving on the task force

Development of the Uniform Terminology—Second Edition. The task force met in 1986 and 1987 to develop drafts of the revisions. A draft from the task force was submitted to the Commission on Practice in May of 1987. Listed below are several decisions that were made in the revision process by the task force and the Commission on Practice.

1. To not replace the original document (*Uniform Terminology for Reporting Occupational Therapy Services,* 1979) because of the number of official documents based on it and the need to retain a *Product Output Reporting System* as an official document of the AOTA.
2. To limit the revised document to defining occupational performance areas and occupational performance components for occupational therapy intervention (i.e., indirect services were deleted and the *Product Output Reporting System* was not revised) to make the project manageable.
3. To coordinate the revision process with other current AOTA projects such as the Professional and Technical Role Analysis (PATRA) and the Occupational Therapy Comprehensive Functional Assessment of the American Occupational Therapy Foundation (AOTF).
4. To develop a document that reflects current areas of practice and facilitates uniformity of definitions in the profession.
5. To recommend that the AOTA develop a companion document to define techniques, modalities, and activities used in occupational therapy intervention and a document to define specific programs that are offered by occupational therapy departments. The Commission on Practice subsequently developed educational materials to assist in the application of uniform terminology to practice.

Several drafts of the revised *Uniform Terminology— Second Edition* document were reviewed by appropriate AOTA commissions and committees and by a selected review network based on geographical representation, professional expertise, and demonstrated leadership in the field. Excellent responses were received, and the feedback was incorporated into the final document by the Commission on Practice.

OCCUPATIONAL THERAPY ASSESSMENT

Occupational Therapy Intervention

I. Occupational Therapy Performance Areas
  A. Activities of Daily Living
    1. Grooming
    2. Oral Hygiene
    3. Bathing
    4. Toilet Hygiene
    5. Dressing

6. Feeding and Eating
7. Medication Routine
8. Socialization
9. Functional Communication
10. Functional Mobility
11. Sexual Expression
B. Work Activities
   1. Home Management
      a. Clothing Care
      b. Cleaning
      c. Meal Preparation and Cleanup
      d. Shopping
      e. Money Management
      f. Household Maintenance
      g. Safety Procedures
   2. Care of Others
   3. Educational Activities
   4. Vocational Activities
      a. Vocational Exploration
      b. Job Acquisition
      c. Work or Job Performance
      d. Retirement Planning
C. Play or Leisure Activities
   1. Play or Leisure Exploration
   2. Play or Leisure Performance

II. Performance Components
A. Sensory Motor Component
   1. Sensory Integration
      a. Sensory Awareness
      b. Sensory Processing
         (1) Tactile
         (2) Proprioceptive
         (3) Vestibular
         (4) Visual
         (5) Auditory
         (6) Gustatory
         (7) Olfactory
      c. Perceptual Skills
         (1) Stereognosis
         (2) Kinesthesia
         (3) Body Scheme
         (4) Right-Left Discrimination
         (5) Form Constancy
         (6) Position in Space
         (7) Visual Closure
         (8) Figure-Ground
         (9) Depth Perception
         (10) Topographical Orientation
   2. Neuromuscular
      a. Reflex
      b. Range of Motion
      c. Muscle Tone

      d. Strength
      e. Endurance
      f. Postural Control
      g. Soft Tissue Integrity
   3. Motor
      a. Activity Tolerance
      b. Gross Motor Coordination
      c. Crossing the Midline
      d. Laterality
      e. Bilateral Integration
      f. Praxis
      g. Fine Motor Coordination/Dexterity
      h. Visual-Motor Integration
      i. Oral-Motor Control
B. Cognitive Integration and Cognitive Components
   1. Level of Arousal
   2. Orientation
   3. Recognition
   4. Attention Span
   5. Memory
      a. Short-Term
      b. Long-Term
      c. Remote
      d. Recent
   6. Sequencing
   7. Categorization
   8. Concept Formation
   9. Intellectual Operations in Space
  10. Problem Solving
  11. Generalization of Learning
  12. Integration of Learning
  13. Synthesis of Learning
C. Psychosocial Skills and Psychological Components
   1. Psychological
      a. Roles
      b. Values
      c. Interests
      d. Initiation of Activity
      e. Termination of Activity
      f. Self-Concept
   2. Social
      a. Social Conduct
      b. Conversation
      c. Self-Expression
   3. Self-Management
      a. Coping Skills
      b. Time Management
      c. Self-Control

Occupational Therapy Assessment

Assessment is the planned process of obtaining, interpreting, and documenting the functional status of the individual. The purpose of the assessment is to identify the individual's abilities and limitations, including deficits, delays, or maladaptive behavior that can be addressed in occupational therapy intervention. Data can be gathered through a review of records, observation, interview, and the administration of test procedures. Such procedures include, but are not limited to, the use of standardized tests, questionnaires, performance checklists, activities, and tasks designed to evaluate specific performance abilities.

Occupational Therapy Intervention

Occupational therapy addresses function and uses specific procedures and activities to (a) develop, maintain, improve, and/or restore the performance of necessary functions; (b) compensate for dysfunction; (c) minimize or prevent debilitation; and/or (d) promote health and wellness. Categories of function are defined as occupational performance areas and performance components. Occupational performance areas include activities of daily living, work activities, and play/leisure activities. Performance components refer to the functional abilities required for occupational performance, including sensory motor, cognitive, and psychological components. Deficits or delays in these occupational performance areas may be addressed by occupational therapy intervention.

I. Occupational Performance Areas
  A. Activities of Daily Living
    1. *Grooming*—Obtain and use supplies to shave; apply and remove cosmetics; wash, comb, style, and brush hair; care for nails; care for skin; and apply deodorant.
    2. *Oral Hygiene*—Obtain and use supplies; clean mouth and teeth; remove, clean and reinsert dentures.
    3. *Bathing*—Obtain and use supplies; soap, rinse, and dry all body parts; maintain bathing position; transfer to and from bathing position.
    4. *Toilet Hygiene*—Obtain and use supplies; clean self; transfer to and from, and maintain toileting position on, bedpan, toilet, or commode.
    5. *Dressing*—Select appropriate clothing; obtain clothing from storage area; dress and undress in a sequential fashion; and fasten and adjust clothing and shoes. Don and doff assistive or adaptive equipment, prostheses, or orthoses.
    6. *Feeding and Eating*—Set up food; use appropriate utensils and tableware; bring food

or drink to mouth; suck, masticate, cough, and swallow.
    7. *Medication Routine*—Obtain medication; open and close containers; and take prescribed quantities as scheduled.
    8. *Socialization*—Interact in appropriate contextual and cultural ways.
    9. *Functional Communication*—Use equipment or systems to enhance or provide communication, such as writing equipment, telephones, typewriters, communication boards, call lights, emergency systems, braille writers, augmentative communication systems, and computers.
    10. *Functional Mobility*—Move from one position or place to another, such as in bed mobility, wheelchair mobility, transfers (bed, car, tub, toilet, chair), and functional ambulation, with or without adaptive aids, driving, and use of public transportation.
    11. *Sexual Expression*—Recognize, communicate, and perform desired sexual activities.
  B. Work Activities
    1. *Home Management*
      a. *Clothing Care*—Obtain and use supplies, launder, iron, store, and mend.
      b. *Cleaning*—Obtain and use supplies, pick up, vacuum, sweep, dust, scrub, mop, make bed, and remove trash.
      c. *Meal Preparation and Cleanup*—Plan nutritious meals and prepare food; open and close containers, cabinets, and drawers; use kitchen utensils and appliances; and clean up and store food.
      d. *Shopping*—Select and purchase items and perform money transactions.
      e. *Money Management*—Budget, pay bills, and use bank systems.
      f. *Household Maintenance*—Maintain home, yard, garden appliances, and household items, and/or obtain appropriate assistance.
      g. *Safety Procedures*—Know and perform prevention and emergency procedures to maintain a safe environment and prevent injuries.
    2. *Care of Others*—Provide for children, spouse, parents, or others, such as the physical care, nurturance, communication, and use of age-appropriate activities.
    3. *Educational Activities*—Participate in a school environment and school-sponsored activities (such as field trips, work-study, and

extracurricular activities).

4. *Vocational Activities*

   a. *Vocational Exploration*—Determine aptitudes, interests, skills, and appropriate vocational pursuits.

   b. *Job Acquisition*—Identify and select work opportunities and complete application and interview processes.

   c. *Work or Job Performance*—Perform job tasks in a timely and effective manner, incorporating necessary work behaviors such as grooming, interpersonal skills, punctuality, and adherence to safety procedures.

   d. *Retirement Planning*—Determine aptitudes, interests, skills, and identify appropriate avocational pursuits.

C. *Play or Leisure Activities*

1. Play or Leisure Exploration—Identify interests, skills, opportunities, and appropriate play or leisure activities.

2. *Play or Leisure Performance*—Participate in play or leisure activities, using physical and psychosocial skills.

   a. Maintain a balance of play or leisure activities with work and activities of daily living.

   b. Obtain, utilize, and maintain equipment and supplies.

II. Performance Components

A. Sensory Motor Component

1. *Sensory Integration*

   a. *Sensory Awareness*—Receive and differentiate sensory stimuli.

   b. *Sensory Processing*—Interpret sensory stimuli.

     (1) *Tactile*—Interpret light touch, pressure, temperature, pain, vibration, and two-point stimuli through skin contact/receptors.

     (2) *Proprioceptive*—Interpret stimuli originating in muscles, joints, and other internal tissues to give information about the position of one body part in relationship to another.

     (3) *Vestibular*—Interpret stimuli from the inner ear receptors regarding head position and movement.

     (4) *Visual*—Interpret stimuli through the eyes, including peripheral vision and acuity, awareness of color, depth, and figure-ground.

     (5) *Auditory*—Interpret sounds, localize sounds, and discriminate background sounds.

     (6) *Gustatory*—Interpret tastes.

     (7) *Olfactory*—Interpret odors.

c. *Perceptual Skills*

     (1) *Stereognosis*—Identify objects through the sense of touch.

     (2) *Kinesthesia*—Identify the excursion and direction of joint movement.

     (3) *Body Scheme*—Acquire an internal awareness of the body and the relationship of body parts to each other.

     (4) *Right-Left Discrimination*—Differentiate one side of the body from the other.

     (5) *Form Constancy*—Recognize forms and objects as the same in various environments, positions, and sizes.

     (6) *Position in Space*—Determine the spatial relationship of figures and objects to self or other forms and objects.

     (7) *Visual Closure*—Identify forms or objects from incomplete presentations.

     (8) *Figure-Ground*—Differentiate between foreground and background forms and objects.

     (9) *Depth Perception*—Determine the relative distance between objects, figures, or landmarks and the observer.

    (10) *Topographical Orientation*—Determine the location of objects and settings and the route to the location.

2. *Neuromuscular*

   a. *Reflex*—Present an involuntary muscle response elected by sensory input.

   b. *Range of Motion*—Move body parts through an arc.

   c. *Muscle Tone*—Demonstrate a degree of tension or resistance in a muscle.

   d. *Strength*—Demonstrate a degree of muscle power when movement is resisted as with weight or gravity.

   e. *Endurance*—Sustain cardiac, pulmonary, and musculoskeletal exertion over time.

   f. *Postural Control*—Position and maintain head, neck, trunk, and limb alignment with appropriate weight shifting, midline orientation, and righting reactions for function.

g. *Soft Tissue Integrity*—Maintain anatomical and physiological condition of interstitial tissue and skin.

3. *Motor*
   a. *Activity Tolerance*—Sustain a purposeful activity over time.
   b. *Gross Motor Coordination*—Use large muscle groups for controlled movements.
   c. *Crossing the Midline*—Move limbs and eyes across the sagittal plane of the body.
   d. *Laterality*—Use a preferred unilateral body part for activities requiring a high level of skill.
   e. *Bilateral Integration*—Interact with both body sides in a coordinated manner during activity.
   f. *Praxis*—Conceive and plan a new motor act in response to an environmental demand.
   g. *Fine Motor Coordination/Dexterity*—Use small muscle groups for controlled movements, particularly in object manipulation.
   h. *Visual-Motor Integration*—Coordinate the interaction of visual information with body movement during activity.
   i. *Oral-Motor Control*—Coordinate oropharyngeal musculature for controlled movements.

B. Cognitive Integration and Cognitive Components
   1. *Level of Arousal*—Demonstrate alertness and responsiveness to environmental stimuli
   2. *Orientation*—Identify person, place, time, and situation.
   3. *Recognition*—Identify familiar faces, objects, and other previously presented materials.
   4. *Attention Span*—Focus on a task over time.
   5. *Memory*
      a. *Short-Term*—Recall information for brief periods of time.
      b. *Long-Term*—Recall information for long periods of time.
      c. *Remote*—Recall events from distant past.
      d. *Recent*—Recall events from immediate past.
   6. *Sequencing*—Place information, concepts, and actions in order.
   7. *Categorization*—Identify similarities of and differences between environmental information.
   8. *Concept Formation*—Organize a variety of information to form thoughts and ideas.
   9. *Intellectual Operations in Space*—Mentally manipulate spatial relationships.
   10. *Problem Solving*—Recognize a problem, define a problem, identify alternative plans, select a plan, organize steps in a plan, implement a plan, and evaluate the outcome.
   11. *Generalization of Learning*—Apply previously learned concepts and behaviors to similar situations.
   12. *Integration of Learning*—Incorporate previously acquired concepts and behavior into a variety of new situations.
   13. *Synthesis of Learning*—Restructure previously learned concepts and behaviors into new patterns.

C. Psychosocial Skills and Psychological Components
   1. *Psychological*
      a. *Roles*—Identify functions one assumes or acquires in society (e.g., worker, student, parent, church member).
      b. *Values*—Identify ideas or beliefs that are intrinsically important.
      c. *Interests*—Identify mental or physical activities that create pleasure and maintain attention.
      d. *Initiation of Activity*—Engage in a physical or mental activity.
      e. *Termination of Activity*—Stop an activity at an appropriate time.
      f. *Self-Concept*—Develop value of physical and emotional self.
   2. *Social*
      a. *Social Conduct*—Interact using manners, personal space, eye contact, gestures, active listening, and self-expression appropriate to one's environment.
      b. *Conversation*—Use verbal and non-verbal communication to interact in a variety of settings.
      c. *Self-Expression*—Use a variety of styles and skills to express thoughts, feelings, and needs.
   3. *Self-Management*
      a. *Coping Skills*—Identify and manage stress and related reactors.
      b. *Time Management*—Plan and participate in a balance of self-care, work, leisure, and rest activities to promote satisfaction and health.
      c. *Self-Control*—Modulate and modify one's own behavior in response to environmental needs, demands, and constraints.

References

American Medical Association. (1966–1988). *Physicians' current procedural terminology first-fourth editions (CPT 1–4).* Chicago: Author.

American Occupational Therapy Association. (1979). *Occupational therapy output reporting system and uniform terminology for reporting occupational therapy services.* Rockville, MD: Author.

American Psychiatric Association. (1952–1987). *Diagnostic and statistical manual of mental disorders first-third editions (DSM-I–III-R).* Washington, DC: Author.

Medicare–Medicaid Anti-Fraud and Abuse Amendments (Public Law 95–142). (1977), 42 U.S.C. §1305.

Prepared by the Uniform Terminology Task Force (Linda Kohlman McGourty, MOT OTR, Chair, and Mary Foto, OTR, Jane K. Marvin, MA, OTC, CIRS, Nancy Mahan Smith, MBA, OTR, and Roger O. Smith, MOT, OTR, task force members) and members of the Commission on Practice, with contributions from Susan Kronsnoble, OTR, for the Commission on Practice (L. Randy Strickland, EdD, OTR, FAOTA, Chair).

Approved by the Representative Assembly April 1989.

Appendix B
MANUFACTURERS AND VENDORS

Adaptive Equipment and Devices
USA and CANADA
(Please refer to product category code key at end of listing)

AAMED, Inc.
1215 South Harlem Avenue
Forest Park, IL 60130
(708) 771-2000
GEN

Ablenet
1081 Tenth Avenue SE
Minneapolis, MN 55414
(800) 322-0956
ECU/S

Adaptability
Norwich Avenue
Colchester, Ct 06415
(203) 537-3451
GEN

Alimed, Inc.
297 High Street
Dedham, MA 02026
(617) 329-2900
GEN

ARIS Isotoner, Inc.
417 Fifth Avenue
New York, NY 10016
(800) 223-2218
CL

Baltimore Therapeutic Equipment Company
7455-L New Ridge Road
Hanover, MD 21076-3105
(301) 850-0333
WAS

Canadian Wheelchair Manufacturing, Ltd.
3232 Autoroute Laval Quest
Laval, Quebec H7T 2H6
CANADA
(514) 687-0780
SS/M

Consumer Care Products, Inc.
P.O. Box 684
Sheboygan, WI 53082
(414) 459-8353
SS/M

DeWill Chairs
696 Alanbrook Street
London, Ontario N6J 3B4
CANADA
(519) 685-6599
SS/M

Dorma Door Control, Inc.
Dorma Drive
Reamstown, PA 17567
(215) 267-3881
ECU/S

Easy Street Environments
6908 E. Thomas Road, Suite 201
Scottsdale, AZ 85821
(602) 947-8078
FAS/E

Everest & Jennings Canadian Ltd.
111 Snidercroft Road
Concord, Ontario L4K 2J8
CANADA
(416) 669-2381
SS/M

Extensions for Independence
757 Emory Street, # 514
Imperial Beach, CA 92032
(619) 423-1478

E & J Avenues
3233 East Mission Oaks
Camarillo, CA 93010
(805) 388-7668
CL

Flaghouse, Inc.
150 North Macquesten Parkway
Mt. Vernon, NY
(800) 221-5185
GEN

Fred Sammons, Inc.
P.O. Box 32
Grand Rapids, MI 49501-3697
(800) 323-5547
GEN

Fred Sammons-Canada
1224 Dundas Street East,
Mississauga, Ontario L4Y 4A2
CANADA
(416) 566-9203
GEN

Forward Motions, Inc
214 Valley Street
Dayton, OH 45404
(513) 222-5001
VAN

Garaventa
P.O. Box L-1
Blaine, WA 98230
(800) 663-6556
L/R

G.E. Miller, Inc.
540 Nepperhan Avenue
Yonkers, NY 10701
(914) 969-4036
GEN

Gottfried Medical, Inc.
3350 Laskey Road
P.O. Box 8966
Toledo, OH 43623
(800) 537-1968
GPG

Hen's Nest
P.O. Box 531
Colby, KS 67701
(913) 462-3104
CL

Horton Automatics
4242 Baldwin Blvd.
Corpus Christi, TX 78405
(512) 888-5591
ECU/S

J.A. Preston, Corporation
60 Page Road
Clifton, NJ 07012
(800) 631-7277
GEN

J.A. Preston of Canada, Ltd
1224 Dundas Street East, Unit 5
Mississauga, Ontario L4Y 4A2
CANADA
(416) 566-9200
GEN

Jobst Division of Zimmer Canada
2323 Argentia Road
Mississauga, Ontario L5N 5N3
CANADA
(416) 858-8625
GPG

LCN Closers
P.O. Box 100
Princeton, IL 61356
(815) 875-3311
ECU/S

LMB Hand ReHab Products Inc
P.O. Box 1181
San Luis Obispo, CA 93406
(800) 541-3992
ORT

Lumex, Inc.
100 Spence Street
Bay Shore, NY 11706-2290
(800) 645-5272
GEN

Maddack, Inc.
P.O. Box 152
Pequannock, NJ 07440
(201) 694-0500
GEN

MED/WEST
702 S. 3rd Ave.
P.O. Box 130
Marshalltown, IA 50158
(515) 752-5446
L/R

Nor Am Patient Care Products, Ltd
2410 Speers Road
Oakville, Ontario L6L 5M2
CANADA
(416) 825-0094
GEN

Otto Bock Orthopedic Industry of Canada
251 Saulteaux Crescent
Winnipeg, Manitoba R3J 3C7
CANADA
(204) 885-1990
SS/M

Self Regulation Systems, Inc.
14770 NE 95th Street
Redmond, WA 98052
(800) 345-5642

Southpaw Enterprises, Inc.
800 West Third Street
Dayton, OH 45407-2805
(800) 228-1698
DTE

Smith and Nephew Richards, Inc.
1450 Brooks Road
Memphis, TN 38116
(800) 238-7538
(Kinetic continuous passive motion devices)

Smith and Nephew, Inc.
2100 52nd Avenue
Lachine, Quebec H8T 2Y5
CANADA
(514) 636-0772
ORT

Stanley Magic Door
Division of The Stanley Works
Farmington, CT 06032
(302) 677-2861
ECU/S

Ted Hoyer & Co., Inc
2222 Minnesota Street
P.O. Box 2744
Oshkosh, WI 54903
(414) 231-7970
L/R

Theradapt Products, Inc.
17 W 163 Oak Lane
Bensenville, IL 60106
(708) 834-2461
A/F

3M Household and Hardware Products Division
223-4S, 3M Center
St. Paul, MN 55144
(612) 733-1110
GEN

Touch Turner Company
443 View Ridge Drive
Everett, WA 98203
(206) 252-1541
GEN

WFR Aquaplast Corp
P.O. Box 635
Wyckoff, NJ 07481
(800) 526-5247
ORT

Winsford Products, Inc
179 Pennington-Harbourton Road
Pennington, NJ 08534
(609) 737-03297
E/F/D

Work Stations, Inc.
165 Front Street
Chicopee, MA 02023
(413) 398-8394
A/F

Product Category Codes

SS/M   = Seating Systems/Mobility
A/C   = Arts and Crafts Materials
A/F   = Adapted Furniture
CL   = Clothing
DTE   = Developmental Therapy Equipment
ECU/S   = Environmental Control Units, Switches
E/F/D   = Eating and feeding aids

FAS/E   = Functional Assessment Systems/Environments
GEN   = General
GPG   = Gradient Pressure Garments
ORT   = Orthotic and Orthopedic Materials and Equipment
L/R   = Lifts, ramps
VAN   = Van Conversions

*This listing is not considered to be an endorsement or recommendation of these manufacturers, vendors or their products. No responsibility can be assumed for errors or omissions.

Appendix C
TECHNOLOGICAL RESOURCES

List of Electronic Devices, Manufacturers and Information Centers

The following list of manufacturers and information centers is not intended to be exhaustive. Inclusion here does not constitute an endorsement of the manufacturers and centers or their products.

ABLEDATA. (1989). Newington, CT: Newington Children's Hospital. 181 East Cedar Street, Newington, CT 06111.

Adaptive Communication Systems, Inc. (1989). 354 Hookstown Grade Road, Clinton, PA 15026.

American Occupational Therapy Association. (1989a). OT Source. Rockville, MD: The American Occupational Therapy Association.

Apple Computer. (1987). Office of Special Education, 20525 Mariani Avenue, Cupertino, CA 95014.

AT&T. (1989). 2001 Route 46, Parsippany, NJ 07054.

Borland. (1988). 4585 Scotts Valley Drive, Scotts Valley, CA 95066.

Butler-in-a-Box. Mastervoice. 10523 Humbolt Street, Los Alamitos, CA 90720. 312/594-6581.

Christiaansen, R. (1989). Project TROCHOS video disc. Madison: University of Wisconsin, School of Allied Health Profession.

Closing the Gap. (1989). Route 2, Box 39, Henderson, MN 56044.

Co-Net. (1989). Trace R&D Center Reprint Service. Madison: University of Wisconsin. Trace Center, S-151 Waisman Center, 1500 Highland Avenue, Madison, WI 53705.

CREATE. (1989). Physical Dysfunction Home Programs and Physical Dysfunction Evaluations. P. O. Box 28, Hales Corner, WI 53130.

Functional Electrical Stimulation Information Center. (1989). 25100 Euclid Avenue, Suite 105, Cleveland, OH 44117.

Hyper-ABLEDATA. (1987). Co-Net Beta test version. Trace R&D Center. Madison: University of Wisconsin.

Kurzweil Computer Products, Inc. (1989). 185 Albany Street, Cambridge, MA 02139.

Lotus. (1988). 55 Cambridge Parkway, Cambridge, MA 02142.

Louisiana Tech. (1989). Rehabilitation Engineering Program, P. O. Box 10426, Ruston, LA 71272.

NARIC. (1988). 8455 Colesville Road, Suite 935, Silver Spring, MD 20910-3319.

Phonic Ear. (1989). 250 Camino Alto, Mill Valley, CA 94941

Pointer Systems. (1989). 1 Mill Street, Burlington, VT 05401, 802/658-3260.

PRAB Command, Inc. (1988). 4100 East Milham Road, PO Box 2121, Kalamazoo, MI 49003, 616/329-1096.

Prentke Romich. (1989). 1022 Heyl Road, Wooster, OH 44691.

Preston Corporation. (1988). 60 Page Road, Clifton, NJ 07012.

Purdue University. (1989). Breaking New Ground Resource Center. Department of Agricultural Engineering. West Lafayette, IN 47907.

Rehabilitation R & D Center - Palo Alto Veterans Administration, 3801 Miranda, Palo Alto, CA 94304.

Rural Rehabilitation R & T Center. (1988). University of Montana, Missoula, MT 59812.

San Francisco State University. (1989). Rehabilitation Engineering Technology, 1600 Holloway Avenue, San Francisco, CA 94132.

Tomlin, George. (1989). Interactive Video: "Help: Tutorial on Biomechanics" for Occupational Therapy Students. School of Occupational Therapy and Physical Therapy, Tacoma, WA.

Trace R & D Center. (1989). Quicksheets and TraceBase Search. Reprint Service, S-151 Waisman Center, 1500 Highland Avenue, Madison, WI 53705.

Words+. (1989). 1125 Stewart Court, Suite D, Sunnyvale, CA 94086.

On-Line Bulletin Boards and Databases with Information on Technology and Disability

4 Sights Network

National Information System for Visually Impaired

Teleconferencing, bulletin board, and database for blind persons and those working with them. Information available includes rehabilitation resources, public policy, calendar of events, software descriptions and reviews, etc.

ABLEDATA

Adaptive Equipment Center

Computerized listing of commercially available products for rehabilitation and independent living. Currently available on-line or on disk. Searches performed for a nominal fee.

Accent on Information

Computerized product database organized by categories of equipment and by disability function.

Blissymbolics Communication Institute

Computer conferencing network that enables users to establish and participate in technology-related forums and conferences regarding individuals with disabilities.

(BRS)

Robotics Information

EIC/Intelligence, Inc.

Database with journals, books, technical reports, and conference proceedings dealing with robotics.

C-CAD Online

Center for Computer Assistance to the Disabled

Bulletin board for the elderly and handicapped.

CompuHelp

National Association of Blind and Visually Impaired Computer Users

Menu-driven database and bulletin board for blind and visually impaired computer users. Information on hardware, software, publications in braille or tape, self-help groups, blind computer user groups, etc.

CompuServe

A nationwide network with bulletin boards that provide information on handicapped persons, issues, technology, and statistics, etc.

CTG Solutions

Closing the Gap

Information on computer technology for persons with disabilities, including information on hardware, software, publications, organizations, and practices/procedures.

ECER

(Educational Resources Information Center)

Council for Exceptional Children

ECER is the ERIC database. It has educational materials (including special education), reports, bibliographic information, available via computer, microfiche, or paper copy.

EQUAL BBS

Michael Bowen

Offers 20 databases, generally catagorized by disability type. Focus is on hardware, software, aids and adaptations to help persons with disabilities live more independently.

OT Source

American Occupational Therapy Association

AOTA member bibliographic and member database with practice bulletin board, employment listings.

Occupational Therapy Bulletin Board Service

Department of Occupational Therapy

School of Pharmacy and Allied Health Professions

Creighton University

Bulletin board, message, and software exchange system for occupational therapists.

REHABDATA

National Rehabilitation Information Centers

A database of rehabilitation-related literature.

SCAN (Shared Communication and Assistance Network)

Electronic mail, bulletin boards for persons with developmental disabilities.

SpecialNet

National Association of State Directors of Special Education

This network features telephone access, electronic mail, bulletin and data collection in the area of special education.

Rehabilitation Engineering Centers

Rehabilitation Technology Transfer
Professional Staff Association of Rancho Los Amigos
Medical Center, Inc.
P.O. Box 3500
Downey, CA 90242

Development and Evaluation of Sensory Aids for Blind and Deaf Individuals
Smith-Kettlewell Institute of Visual Sciences
2232 Webster Street
San Francisco, CA 94115
(415) 561-1630

Technology Resources
Institute for Human Resource Development
78 Eastern Boulevard
Glastonbury, CT 06033
(203) 659-1166

Augmentive Communication
University of Delaware
Department of Computer & Information Science
Newark, DE 19711
(302) 451-2712

Rehabilitation Technology Transfer
Electronic Industries Foundation
1901 Pennsylvania Avenue, NW #700
Washington, DC 20006
(202) 732-1115

Evaluation of Rehabilitation Technology
National Rehabilitation Hospital
102 Irving Street, NW
Washington, DC 20010
(202) 877-1932

Prosthetics and Orthotics
Northwestern University
633 Clark Street
Evanston, IL 60208
(312) 908-8560

Modifications to Worksites and Educational Settings
Cerebral Palsy Research Foundation of Kansas
2021 North Old Manor—Box 8217
Wichita, KS 67208
(316) 688-1888

Quantification of Human Performance
Massachusetts Institute of Technology
Harvard-MIT Rehabilitation Engineering Center
77 Massachusetts Avenue
Cambridge, MA 02139
(617) 253-0460

Technological Aids for Deaf and Hearing Impaired
The Lexington Center, Inc.
Research and Training Division
30th Avenue and 75th Streets
Jackson Heights, NY 11370
(718) 899-800, Ext. 230

Functional Electrical Stimulation for Restoration of Neural Control
Case Western Reserve University
School of Medicine
2119 Abingdon Road
Cleveland, OH 44106

Quantification of Human Performance
Ohio State University Research Foundation
1314 Kinear Road
Columbus, OH 43212
(614) 293-8710

Service Delivery
South Carolina Vocational Rehabilitation Department
Office of the Commissioner
P.O. Box 15
West Columbia, SC 29171
(803) 734-5301

Low Back Pain
University of Vermont
Department of Orthopedics and Rehabilitation
1 South Prospect Street
Burlington, VT 05405
(802) 656-4067

Improved Wheelchair and Seating Design
University of Virginia
Rehabilitation Engineering Center
Box 3368 University Station
Charlottesville, VA 22903
(804) 977-6730

Access to Computers and Electronic Equipment
University of Wisconsin-Madison
Trace R & D Center
S-151 Waisman Center
1500 Highland Avenue
Madison, WI 53705
(608) 262-6966

Cognitive Rehabilitation Software
Titles and Their Manufacturers

Brain-Link Software
317 Montgomery
Ann Arbor, MI 48103
Memory Pattern
Preposition Recognition
Visual Recognition

Cognitive Rehabilitation
6555 Carrollton Avenue
Indianapolis, IN 46220
Soft Tools '83, '84, '85, 86, 87, 88

Computers to Help People, Inc.
1221 W. Johnson Street
Madison, WI 53715
Maze

Computer Programs for Neuropsychological
8840 Warner Avenue, Suite 301
Fountain Valley, CA 92708
Testing and Cognitive Rehabilitation/Sbordone, Robert

Conover Company
P.O. Box 155
Omro, WI 54963
Concept Formation: Shape Matching

CREATE
P.O. Box 28
Hales Corners, WI 53130
CREATE

Creative Learning, Inc.
P. O. Box 829
North San Juan, CA 95960
Multisensory Curriculum

Dekro, Inc.
4595 Club Drive, N.E.
Atlanta, GA 30319
VISPA

Educational Electronic Techniques, Ltd.
1088 Wantagh Avenue
Wantagh, NY 11793
Brunswick Hospital Cognitive Assessment and Re-training
Rehab Software for Young Adults with Head Injury
Visual/Perceptual Diagnostic Testing and Retraining

Edutek Corporation
415 Cambridge #4
Palo Alto, CA 94306
Hand/Eye Coordination Programs

Greentree Group
RD #1 Box 1044
Leesport, PA 19533
Find It
Purposeful Patterns
Purposeful Symbols
Search !!
Verbal Reasoning
What Belongs

Hartley Courseware, Inc.
133 Bridge Street
Dimondale, MI 48821
Ollie and Seymour

Instructional/Communication Tech.
10 Stepar Place
Huntington Station, NY 11746
Pave
Processing Power Programming
Word Memory Programs

Lambert Software Company
P.O. Box 1257
Ramona, CA 92065
K.L.S. - Cognitive Education System

Life Sciences Associates
1 Fenimore Road
Bayport, NY 11705
Cogrehab Vol. 1, 2, 3, 4
Task Master

Marblesoft
21805 Zumbrota Northeast
Cedar, MN 55011
Mix 'N Match

Network Services
1915 Huguenot Road
Richmond, VA 23235
Captain's Log: Cognitive Training Series

Parrot Software
P. O. Box 1139
State College, PA 16804
Association Pictures
Categorical Reasoning I & II
Cognitive Disorders I, II, III, IV
Cognitive Retraining Function Pictures
Picture Program I, II, III
Rhyming Pictures
Understand Attributes

Psychological Software Services, Inc.
6555 Carrollton Avenue
Indianapolis, IN 46220
Conceptual Skill
Foundation I & II
Memory I, II
Problem Solving
Smart Shaper
Spatial Perceptionals

Southern MicroSystem
716 East Davis Street
Burlington, NC 27215
PII - Personalized Information for Independence

Strawberry Hill Knowledge Software, Inc.
202-11961-88th Avenue
Delta, BC V4C 3C9
CANADA
Surrounding Patterns

Sunset Software
11750 Sunset Boulevard
Suite 414
Los Angeles, CA 90049
Generator

Evaluation Reporting Software

Augmentative Communication Evaluation System (ACES)
Words + , Inc.
P. O. Box 1229
Lancaster, CA 93535
(805) 949-8331

CREATE
Create
P. O. Box 28
Hales Corners, WI 53130

ESS Rehabware
Easter Seal Systems
Rehab Manager
5120 South Hyde Park Boulevard
Chicago, IL 60615
(312) 667-7400

Rehabilitation Report System
Glendale Adventist Hospital and A. J. Weiss and Associates
P. O. Box 404
Pacific Palisades, CA 90272

LADS
Parkside Associates
205 West Touhy Avenue, Suite 204
Park Ridge, IL 60068

Mental Health Assessment System: MHAPS
Glenn Jones
405 Grandville Drive
Daville, VA 24540

RCom
C. Gerald Warren & Associates
4825 Stanford Avenue, NE
Seattle, WA 98105
(206) 527-8844

OT FACT
American Occupational Therapy Association
1383 Piccard Drive
P. O. Box 1725
Rockville, MD 20850-4375

Funding Resources for the Clinician

Many Faces of Funding
Phonic Ear, Inc.
250 Camino Alto
Mill Valley, CA 94941-1490, U.S.A.

Applications for Insurance: Prior Authorization Packet
Prentke Romich Company
1022 Heyl Road
Wooster, OH 44692

Guidelines for Seeking Funding for Communication Aids
Trace Research & Development Center
Reprint Service
S-151 Waisman Center
1500 Highland Avenue
Madison, WI 53705

Funding of Non-Vocal Communication for the Severely Speech and Motor Impaired
Trace Research & Development Center

Reprint Service
1500 Highland Avenue
Madison, WI 53705

Assistive Technology, Volume 1
The Official Journal of RESNA
RESNA
1101 Connecticut Avenue NW
Suite 700
Washington, DC 20036

SPEC Specialized Product/Equipment Council Funding Forms
A Consortium of Organizations Dedicated to Improve Use of and Payment for Specialized Rehabilitation Equipment.

RESNA
1101 Connecticut Avenue NW
Suite 700
Washington, DC 20036

Appendix D
RESOURCE ORGANIZATIONS

Organizational Resources in the United States

AIDS

American Red Cross
18th & E Streets, NW
Washington, DC 20006

Gay Men's Health Crisis
Box 274, 132 West 24th Street
New York, New York 10011
(212) 807-7035

Alcoholism

Alcoholics Anonymous
P.O. Box 459, Grand Central Station
New York, New York 10163
(212) 686-1100

Al-Anon Family Group
   Headquarters, Inc.
P.O. Box 182
Madison Square Station
New York, New York
10159-0182
(212) 683-1771

National Clearinghouse for Alcohol
Information
P.O. Box 2345
Rockville, Maryland 20852
(301) 468-2600

Alzheimer's Disease

Alzheimer's Disease and Related Disorders
   Association, Inc.
70 East Lake Street
Chicago, Illinois 60601
(312) 853-3060

Amputation

National Amputation Foundation, Inc.
12-45 150th Street
Whitestone, New York
11357-1790
(212) 767-0596

Amyotrophic Lateral Sclerosis

The ALS Association
15300 Ventura Boulevard
Sherman Oaks, California 91403
(213) 990-2151

Arthritis

Arthritis Foundation
1314 Spring Street N.W.
Atlanta, Georgia 30309
(404) 872-7100

Autism

National Society for Children and Adults
   with Autism
1234 Massachusetts Avenue N.W.
Washington, DC 20005
(202) 783-0125

Birth Defects

March of Dimes Birth Defects Foundation
1275 Mamaroneck Avenue
White Plains, New York 10605
(914) 428-7100

Blindness

American Foundation for the Blind
15 West 16th Street
New York, New York 10011
(212) 620-2000

National Federation for the Blind
1800 Johnson Street
Baltimore, Maryland 21230
(301) 659-9314

Helen Keller National Center for the Deaf-
Blind Youth and Adults
111 Middle Neck Road
Sands Point, New York 11050
(516) 944-8900

Burn Injuries

Phoenix Society, Inc.
National Organization for Burn Victims
and Their Families
11 Rust Hill Road
Levittown, Pennsylvania 19056
(215) 946-4788

Cancer

American Cancer Society
90 Park Avenue
New York, New York 10016
(212) 599-8200

Cerebral Palsy

United Cerebral Palsy Association, Inc.
66 East 34th Street
New York, New York 10016
(212) 481-6300

National Easter Seal Society
2023 West Ogden Avenue
Chicago, Illinois 60612
(312) 243-8400
TDD: (312) 243-8000

Deafness

National Information Center on Deafness
Gallaudet College
900 Florida Avenue, N.E.
Washington, DC 20002
(202) 651-5109
TDD: (202) 651-5976

Diabetes

National Diabetes Information
Clearinghouse
Box NDIC
Bethesda, Maryland 20892
(301) 468-2162

Epilepsy

Epilepsy Foundation of America
4351 Garden City Drive
Landover, Maryland 20785
(301) 459-3700

Guillain-Barré Syndrome

Guillain-Barré Syndrome National
Foundation
1538 Acacia Road
Akron, Ohio 44313
(216) 666-3053

Head Injury

National Head Injury Foundation
P.O. Box 567
Framingham, Massachusetts 01701
(617) 879-7473

Heart Disease

American Heart Association
7320 Greenville Avenue
Dallas, Texas 75231
(214) 750-5300

Huntington's Disease

National Huntington's Disease Association,
Inc.
1182 Broadway
New York, New York 10001
(211) 684-2781

Learning Disabilities

Foundation for Children with Learning
Disabilities
99 Park Avenue
New York, New York 10016
(212) 687-7211

Mental Illness

National Alliance for the Mentally Ill
1901 North Fort Meyer Drive
Arlington, Virginia 22209-1604
(703) 524-7600

Mental Retardation

Association for Retarded Citizens of the
United States
P.O. Box 6109
2501 Avenue J
Arlington, Texas 76006
(817) 640-0204

Special Olympics
1350 New York Avenue N.W.
Washington, DC 20005
(202) 628-3630

Multiple Sclerosis

National Multiple Sclerosis Society
205 East 42nd Street
New York, New York 10017
(212) 986-3240

Muscular Dystrophy	Muscular Dystrophy Association 810 Seventh Avenue New York, New York 10019 (212) 586-0808		Paralyzed Veterans of America 801 18th Street N.W. Washington, DC 20006 (202) 872-1300
Parkinson's Disease	American Parkinson Disease Foundation 116 John Street New York, New York 10038 (212) 732-9550	**Stroke**	National Stroke Association 1420 Odgen Street Denver, Colorado 80219 (303) 839-1992
Spinal Cord Injury	National Spinal Cord Injury Association 149 California Street Newton, Massachusetts 02158 (617) 964-0521		Stroke Clubs International 805 12th Street EGalveston, Texas 77550 (409) 762-1022

Organizational Resources in Canada

AIDS	Canadian AIDS Society #200 267 Dalhousie Street Ottawa, Ontario K1N 7E3 (613) 230-3580		The War Amputations of Canada (Canadian Amputees Foundation) 2827 Riverside Drive Ottawa, Ontario K1V 0C4 (613) 731-3821
Alcoholism	Alcoholism and Drug Addiction Foundation 33 Russell Street Toronto, Ontario M5S 2S1 (416) 595-6000	**Amyotrophic Lateral Sclerosis**	Amyotrophic Lateral Sclerosis Society of Canada 250 Rogers Road Toronto, Ontario M6E 1R1 (416) 656-5242
	Canadian Addictions Foundation 448 Kildarroch Street Winnipeg, Manitoba R2X 2B5 (204) 582-1709	**Arthritis**	Arthritis Society 250 Bloor Street East, Suite 401 Toronto, Ontario M4W 2PZ (416) 967-1414
Alzheimer Disease	Alzheimer Society of Canada 1320 Yonge Street, Suite 1302 Toronto, Ontario M4T 1X2 (416) 925-3552		Canadian Rheumatism Association 6091 Gilbert Road, Suite 230 Richmond, British Columbia V7C 3V3 (604) 273-8085
Amputation	Canadian Amputees Foundation 2827 Riverside Drive Ottawa, Ontario K1V 0C4	**Autism**	Autism Society Canada 20 College Street, Suite 2 Toronto, Ontario M5G 1K2 (416) 924-4189
	Canadian Amputee Sports Association 1600 James Naismith Drive Gloucester, Ontario K1B 5N4 (613) 748-5630		Society for the Treatment of Autism P.O. Box 8098, Station F Calgary, Alberta T2J 2V2 (403) 253-2291

Birth Defects	Canadian Deaf-Blind and Rubella Association P.O. Box 1625 Meaford, Ontario N0H 1Y0 (519) 538-3431 Easter Seal Society 250 Ferrand Drive, Suite 200 Don Mills, Ontario M3C 3P2 (416) 421-8377	**Deafness**	Canadian Association of the Deaf 271 Spadina Road, Suite 311 Toronto, Ontario M5R 2V3 (416) 928-1350 Canadian Coordination Council on Deafness 116 Kusgar Street, Suite 203 Ottawa, Ontario K2P 0C2 (613) 232-2611
Blindness and Visual Impairment	Canadian Council for the Blind 220 Dundas Street, Suite 610 London, Ontario N6A 1H3 (519) 433-3946 Canadian National Institute for the Blind 1931 Bayview Avenue Toronto, Ontario M4G 4C8 (416) 480-2500	**Diabetes**	Canadian Diabetes Association 78 Bond Street Toronto, Ontario M5B 2J8 (416) 362-4440 Diabetes Canada 44 Victoria Street, Suite 216 Toronto, Ontario M5C 1Y2 (416) 968-4881
Brain Injury	The Head Injury Association of Canada P.O. Box 5283—Station F Ottawa, Ontario K2C 3H5 (613) 723-7798		Juvenile Diabetes Foundation Canada 4652 Yonge Street, Suite 100 Willoowdale, Ontario M2N 5M1 (416) 223-1068
Burns	Burns Survivors Association c/o The Wellesley Hospital 160 Wellesley Street East Toronto, Ontario M4Y 1J3 (416) 486-0541	**Epilepsy**	Epilepsy Canada 2099 Alexandre -De- Seve P.O. Box 1560, Station C Montreal, Quebec H2L 4K8 (514) 876-7455
Cancer	Canadian Cancer Society 77 Bloor Street West, Suite 1702 Toronto, Ontario, M5S 3A1 (416) 961-7223 Cancer Information Service 711 Concession Street Hamilton, Ontario L8V 1C3 (416) 961-7223	**Heart Disease** **Huntington Disease**	Canadian Heart Foundation One Nicholas Street, Suite 1200 Ottawa, Ontario K1N 7B7 (613) 237-4361 Huntington Society of Canada 13 Water Street North, Suite 3 P.O. Box 333 Cambridge, Ontario N1R 5T8 (519) 622-1002
Cerebral Palsy	Canadian Cerebral Palsy Association 40 Dundas Street West, Suite 222 P.O. Box 110 Toronto, Ontario M5G 2C2 (416) 979-7923 Canadian Cerebral Palsy Sports Association 1850 Valley Farm Road, Suite 507 Pickering, Ontario L1V 3W4 (416) 420-6032	**Learning Disabilities**	Canadian Association for Children and Adults with Learning Disabilities P.O. Box 159, Station H Toronto, Ontario M4C 5H9 (416) 363-6681 Learning Disability Association of Canada Maison Kildare House 232 Chapel Street, Suite 200

Ottawa, Ontario K1N 7Z2
(613) 238-5721

Mental Illness Canadian Mental Health Association
2160 Yonge Street, 3rd Floor
Toronto, Ontario M4S 2Z3
(416) 484-7750

Canadian Schizophrenia Foundation
7375 Kingsway
Burnaby, British Columbia V3N 3B5
(604) 521-1728

Mental Retardation International Federation of L'Arche Canada
11339 Yonge Street, RR1
Richmond Hill, Ontario L4C 4X7
(416) 884-3534

Multiple Sclerosis Multiple Sclerosis Society of Canada
250 Bloor Street East, Suite 820
Toronto, Ontario M4W 3P9
(416) 922-6065

Muscular Dystrophy Muscular Dystrophy Association of Canada
150 Eglinton Avenue East, Suite 400
Toronto, Ontario M4P 1E8
(416) 488-0030

Society for Muscular Dystrophy
Information (International)
P.O. Box 479
Bridgewater, Nova Scotia B4V 2X6
(902) 634-3485

Parkinson Disease Parkinson Foundation of Canada
Manulife Centre
55 Bloor Street West, Suite 232
Toronto, Ontario M4W 1A5
(416) 964-1155

Spina Bifida Spina Bifida Association of Canada
633 Wellington Circle
Winnipeg, Manitoba R3M 0A8
(204) 452-7580

Spinal Cord Injury Canadian Paraplegic Association
1500 Don Mills Road, Suite 201
Don Mills, Ontario, M3B 3K4
(416) 391-0203

Stroke (CVA) Canadian Stroke Recovery Foundation
170 The Donway West, Suite 122A
Don Mills, Ontario M3C 2G3
(416) 446-1580

Organizations Providing Resource Information

Clearinghouse on the Handicapped
U.S. Department of Education
Switzer Building, Room 3132
Washington, DC 20202-2319
Telephone: (202) 732-1241

HEALTH Resource Center (Higher Education
and the Handicapped)
One DuPont Circle
Washington, DC 20036

National Handicapped Sports and
Recreation Association
P.O. Box 33141, Farragut Station
Washington, DC 20033
Telephone: (202) 783-1441

National Library Service for the Blind and
Physically Handicapped
The Library of Congress
Washington, DC 20542
Telephone: (202) 287-5100

National Organization on Disability
2100 Pennsylvania Avenue, N.W.
Washington, DC 20037
Telephone: (202) 293-5960

National Rehabilitation
Information Center
Catholic University of America
4407 Eighth Street N.E.
Washington, DC 20017
Telephone or TDD: (202) 635-5826
Toll-free: (800) 346-2742

North American Riding for the
Handicapped Association, Inc.
P.O. Box 100, R.I.B. 218
Ashburn, Virginia 22011
Telephone: (703) 471-1621

P.R.I.D.E. Foundation (Promote
  Real Independence for the Disabled and Elderly)
1159 Poquonnock Road
Groton, Connecticut 06340
Telephone: (203) 445-1448

Scouting for the Handicapped
Boy Scouts of America
1325 Walnut Hill Lane
Irving, Texas 75062-1296
Telephone: (214) 659-2000

Special Recreation, Inc.
362 Koser Avenue
Iowa City, Iowa 52240
Telephone: (319) 337-7578

The American Occupational Therapy
  Association
1383 Piccard Drive
Rockville, Maryland 20850
Telephone: (301) 948-9626

The Association for People with
  Severe Handicaps (TASH)
7010 Roosevelt Way, N.E.
Seattle, Washington 98115
Telephone: (206) 523-8446

General Guidelines for Stages of Practice
(Canadian Association of Occupational Therapists)

The following general guidelines were taken from **GUIDE-LINES FOR THE CLIENT-CENTRED PRACTICE OF OCCUPATIONAL THERAPY**.

a. Referral Guidelines

i. The therapist should receive a referral from an authorized source in accordance with the policy of the service.

ii. The therapist should determine the appropriateness of the referral and the eligibility of the individual for an occupational therapy program. This may be done in an interview or by review of records.

iii. When the referral is received the therapist should document:
- the date of receipt;
- referral source; and
- the kind of services requested.

iv. If the referral is appropriate, the therapist should undertake a general assessment of the individual.

v. If the referral is inappropriate, the therapist should recommend alternatives to the referral source.

vi. The documentation should be done within a time frame that is in accordance with the policy of the service.

b. Assessment Guidelines

i. The therapist should gather data and outline the purposes of the assessment.

ii. The therapist should obtain additional relevant information regarding history, education, work records, family, from the individual and family/significant others.

iii. This global assessment should include an evaluation and documentation of the individual's abilities and deficits in the following areas:

occupational performance areas
- self-care
- productivity
- leisure

performance components
- mental
- physical
- sociocultural
- spiritual

environment
- physical
- social
- cultural

The therapist should document occupational performance and determine if more detailed and specific evaluation is required.

The therapist should ensure complete assessment either within the service or by referral to other professionals.

iv. The therapist should analyse the assessment data, formulate impressions of the presenting problem(s) and make recommendations.

v. This assessment should be documented within a defined time interval following receipt of the referral.

c. Program Planning Guidelines

i. The therapist should determine and document a program plan consistent with the assessment data and the recommendations obtained in the assessment.

ii. The program plan should be developed to include a:

- statement of measurable goals both short-term and long-term;
- selection of a theoretical approach/frame of reference appropriate to the individual's needs;
- selection of methods of intervention;
- schedule for the implementation of the plan;
- tentative discharge plan; and
- evaluation schedule.

iii. The program plan goals and methods must be developed in conjunction with:
- goals of the individual and/or family;
- program plans of other professionals; and
- available resources (institutional and community).

iv. The program plan should be developed within a defined interval following completion of the assessment.

d. Intervention Guidelines

i. The therapist should implement the program according to the program plan.

ii. The therapist should document the occupational therapy services provided and the individual's progress toward the goals at a frequency recommended by the service.

iii. The therapist should regularly (or as determined by the service) reevaluate and document changes in the individual's occupational performance and the performance components of those skills.

iv. The program plan should be modified in accordance with these changes.

v. The therapist should communicate at regular intervals (or as determined by the service) with other involved professionals and family/significant others;

vi. The therapist should review and refine the discharge plan.

e. Discharge Guidelines

i. The therapist should terminate services when the individual has achieved the goals or when maxi-mum benefit has been derived from occupational therapy services.

ii. A discharge plan should be finalized and documented.

iii. The plan should be consistent with:
- the individual's functional abilities and deficits, goals, prognosis, and community resources; and
- the discharge plan of other involved professionals.

iv. Time should be allocated for the coordination and effective implementation of the plan.

v. The therapist should document a discharge summary in accordance with the policies of the service. This could include the individual's functional status, goal attainment, unmet goals, plans for ongoing services and further recommendations.

vi. The client - therapist relationship should be terminated.

f. Follow-up Guidelines

i. The therapist should reevaluate the individual at an appropriate time interval following discharge.

ii. The reevaluation results should be documented.

iii. If the individual requires further service, the therapist should refer to the service needed.

g. Program Evaluation Guidelines

i. The therapist should evaluate the effectiveness and efficiency of the program with respect to:
- adherence to the process guidelines as described above; and
- outcome - i.e., results of intervention.

From Guidelines for the Client-Centred Practice of Occupational Therapy, Report of a Task Force convened by the Canadian Association of Occupational Therapists and the Health Services Directorate, Health Services and Promotion Branch, Department of Health and Welfare, Government of Canada, 1983. *Reprinted with permission of the Canadian Association of Occupational Therapists.*

Canadian Association of Occupational Therapists
Code of Ethics

This code of ethics has been published and distributed by the Canadian Association of Occupational Therapists to guide and assist the members in meeting and maintaining proper standards of professional conduct. The Code of Ethics should be construed as a general guide and not as a denial of the existence of other duties equally imperative and other rights not specifically mentioned.

Certain terms used in the Code require definition as follows: ''Member'' means an Individual or Life Member of the Association and any person eligible for Individual Membership in the Association. ''Patient/client'' means a person to whom a member renders professional services.

Article One

The member should possess the qualities of integrity, loyalty, reliability, and shall maintain a standard of professional competency as required by the profession, and shall at all times demonstrate behavior which reflects the member's professional interest and attitude.

Article Two

The welfare of the patient/client shall be the primary concern of the member. Without limiting the generality of the foregoing, in furtherance of this goal the member shall:

a. provide service at the highest possible level of professional skill;
b. demonstrate respect for the patient and appreciation of the particular need of the patient;
c. respect confidentiality of all patient information;
d. report to the apppropriate authority any alleged unethical conduct or inappropriate practice of occupational therapy of another member.

Article Three

A member shall recognize and accept his responsibility to the relevant employing agency, to other health care colleagues, and to the community at large, and furtherance thereof shall:

a. Co-operate and maintain appropriate communication with other health care colleagues or services dealing with the patient in order that the combined desired results are achieved in the treatment of that patient.
b. Be professionally responsible for all treatment and services rendered by the member, or by other personnel including students, who are under the direct supervision of the member.
c. Respect and uphold the dignity of each individual with whom the member is associated within the profession of occupational therapy.
d. Provide no misrepresentation regarding information relating to the practice of the profession of occupational therapy.
e. Maintain an appropriate relationship with members of the public in order to facilitate the promotion of the goals and functions of the profession of occupational therapy.
f. Refrain from endorsing any goods or services related to the practice of occupational therapy without having made an objective assessment of those goods and services.

Article Four

The members shall endeavor to maintain and improve their professional knowledge and skill, and in this regard shall maintain a progressive attitude.

Article Five

The members shall recognize and accept their responsibilities to the profession and to professional organizations, and shall do everything within their means to provide for the growth and development of occupational therapy.

Adopted from the British Columbia Society of Occupational Therapists' Code of Ethics June 1983. *Reprinted with permission of the Canadian Association of Occupational Therapists.*

Glossary

Abbreviation Expansion Program—software that allows a person to rapidly enter a few defined characters (abbreviation) to print out an expanded long string of characters (expansion) on a computer or communication aid. This system saves the user typing time and effort.

Absolute endurance—muscular endurance when force of contraction tested does not consider individual differences in strength.

Absorption—the process by which a drug is made available to the body fluids for distribution.

Accessibility—the degree to which an exterior or interior environment is available for use, in relation to an individual's physical and/or psychological abilities.

Accommodation—the process whereby the organization of information within a schema must be revised or altered due to the inability to fit new information into any existing mental category.

ACSM—American College of Sports Medicine.

Active stretch—stretch produced by internal muscular force.

Activity pattern analysis—any method for determining the type, amount, and organization of activities which occupy the lives of individuals on a recurring basis.

Activity—productive action required for development, maturation, and use of sensory, motor, social psychological, and cognitive functions. Activity may be productive without yielding an object.

Activity configuration—an evaluation tool which identifies the patient's use of time, the value of one's daily activities and the changes one would like to make in time management and routines.

Acuity—the ability of the sensory organ to receive information.

Adaptation—the satisfactory adjustment of individuals within their environment over time. Successful adaptation equates with quality of life.

ADL—activities of daily living; the typical life tasks required for self-care and self-maintenance, such as grooming, bathing, eating, cleaning the house and doing laundry.

Adverse effects—undesired consequences of chemical agents resulting from toxic doses or allergies.

Aerobic metabolism—energy production utilizing oxygen.

Aerobic power—maximal oxygen consumption; the maximal volume of oxygen consumed per unit time.

Affect—the emotion conveyed in a person's face or body; the subjective experiencing of a feeling or emotion.

Affective state—the emotional or mental state of an individual, which can range from unconscious to very agitated; sometimes referred to as behavioral state.

Agonist—a muscle that resists the action of a prime mover (agonist).

Alarm reaction—the body's immediate response to imposed stress.

American National Standards Institute (ANSI)—a clearinghouse and coordinating body for voluntary standards activity on the national level.

Analgesic—a drug for reducing pain.

Analog—a continuous information system, for example a clock with dials that move continuously on a continuum (as opposed to a digital clock).

Analogue—a contrived situation created in order to elicit specific patient behaviors and allow for their observation.

Anaphylactic shock—a condition in which the flow of blood throughout the body becomes suddenly inadequate due to dilation of the blood vessels as a result of allergic reaction.

ANOVA—a statistical test for comparing groups (analysis of variance).

Antimicrobial—designed to destroy or inhibit the growth of bacterial, fungal or viral organisms.

Antineoplastic agents—drugs used in treating cancer, administered with the purpose of inhibiting the production of abnormal cells.

Anxiolytic—a drug for reducing anxiety.

Aphasia—the absence of cognitive language processing ability which results in deficits in speech, writing, or sign communication. Aphasia occurs most often in people suffering left hemisphere stroke.

Apraxia—inability to motor plan or execute purposeful movement.

Archetypal places—settings in the physical environment that support fundamental human functions, including taking shelter, sleeping, mating, grooming, feeding, excreting, storing, establishing territory, playing, routing, meeting, competing, and working (Spivack, 1973).

Architectural barrier—structural impediment to the approach, mobility, and functional use of an interior or exterior environment.

Arousal—an internal state of the individual characterized by increased responsiveness to environmental stimuli.

Arteriosclerosis—thickening and hardening of the arteries.

ASCII—a standardized coding scheme that uses numeric values to represent letters, numbers, symbols, etc. ASCII is an acronym for American Standard Code for Information Interchange and is widely used in coding information for computers. For example, the letter ''A'' is ''65'' in ASCII.

Assessment—a process by which data are gathered, hypotheses formulated, and decisions made for further action.

Assimilation—the expansion of data within a given category or subcategory of a schema by incorporation of new information within the existing representational structure without requiring any reorganization or modification of prior knowledge.

Atherosclerosis—deposits of fat and cholesterol in arteries.

Augmentative Communication—a method or device which increases a person's ability to communicate. Examples include non-electronic devices such as communication boards, or electronic devices such as portable communication systems which allow the user to speak and print text.

Autistic—a mental disorder characterized by non-communicative, non-interactive behaviors and exclusion from reality.

Autogenic inhibition—the ability to inhibit action in one's own muscle (GTO).

Autogenic facilitation—the ability to stimulate one's own muscle to contract (muscle spindle).

Automatic processes—processes that occur without much attentional effort.

Autonomic nervous system—that part of the nervous system concerned with the control of involuntary bodily functions.

Avoidance—A psychological coping strategy whereby the source of stress is ignored or avoided.

Balance—the ability to maintain a functional posture through motor actions which distribute weight evenly around the body's center of gravity.

Balance of power—complementary functions of brain regions which result in well modulated behavioral responses to environmental stimuli.

Balanced muscle tone—muscle tone that is satisfactory for normal movement.

Ballistic stretch—repeated rhythmic movements at the outer limits of range of motion.

Basic ADL—those ADL tasks which pertain to self-care, mobility and communication.

Battery—an assessment approach or instrument with several parts.

Behavior setting—a physical location in which a standing pattern of behavior occurs irrespective of the particular inhabitants of the setting.

Behavioral assessment—a systematic and quantitative method for observing and assessing behaviors.

Behavioral setting—a milieu in which the specific environment dictates the kinds of behaviors that occur there, independent of the particular individuals who inhabit the setting at the moment.

Bilateral integration—the ability to perform purposeful movement that requires interaction between both sides of the body in a smooth and refined manner.

Bill mark-up—the process in which a legislative committee amends a bill by deleting, modifying, or adding to the bill according to the wishes of lobbyists, the public, or their own inclinations.

Biofeedback—a training program designed to enhance control of the autonomic (involuntary) nervous system by monitoring biological signals or responses and feeding them back to the individual in expanded signals.

Biopsychological assessment—an evaluation used to determine how the central nervous system influences behavior and understand the relationship between physical state and thoughts, emotions and behavior.

Body image—the subjective picture people have of their physical appearance.

Body scheme—the perception of one's physical self through proprioceptive and interoceptive sensations.

Boiler Plates—set paragraphs of narrative information available to modify and use repeatedly in letters or other manuscripts.

Boot Up—to turn on a computer.

Bottom-up processing—when processing starts with the sensory signal and works up from the bottom or is ''data driven.''

Bulletin Board Systems (BBS)—the electronic equal to a common information-sharing bulletin board which is accessed by telephone lines.

Card sort—an approach to gathering information that requires the person being evaluated to consider information contained on separate index cards and to separate or sort the cards according to a specific set of instructions.

Cardiac output—the volume of blood pumped from the heart per unit of time. Cardiac output is the product of heart rate and stroke volume.

Caregiver—one who provides care and support to a dysfunctional person.

Cause and effect—when something occurs as a result of a motion or activity.

Center of gravity—the point at which the downward force created by mass and gravity is equivalent or balanced on either side of a fulcrum.

Centrifugal control—the brain's ability to regulate its own input.

Characteristic behavior—behavior typical of one's performance under everyday conditions.

Checklist—a type of assessment approach whereby a list of abilities, tasks, or interests is presented and those items meeting a designated criterion are checked. An interest checklist, for example, might list a number of activities in varied categories and ask the respondent to check those which are viewed as most interesting.

Classical conditioning—a method of eliciting specific responses through the use of stimuli that occur within a period of time that permits an association to be made between them. Also called Pavlovian conditioning, after the Russian scientist who made the technique famous.

Closed question—a question which asks for a specific response; e.g., one that may be answered with a ''yes'' or a ''no.''

Cocontraction—simultaneous contraction of antagonistic muscle groups which act to stabilize joints.

Cognition—mental processes which include thinking, perceiving, feeling, recognizing, remembering, problem solving, knowing, sensing, learning, judging and metacognition.

Cognitive appraisal—That part of the coping process during which one evaluates a stressor and chooses a strategy for dealing with it.

Cognitive complexity—features of an environment that affect its information-processing demands, such as variety, familiarity, pace, complexity, and responsiveness potential of stimuli.

Colles Wrist Fracture—the transverse fracture of the distal end of the radius (just above the wrist).

Commitment—The degree of importance attached to an event by an individual, based on their beliefs and values. The degree of commitment is an important element in motivation.

Community mental health movement—during the 1960s, government, medical and community organizations supported treatment approaches which would keep patients living in the community rather than confined in long-term hospitals.

Compensatory action of the nervous system—the action that occurs when the central nervous system attempts to respond to stimuli without the usual full complement of information.

Compensatory power—power exercised by giving something of value to the person submitting to that power.

Competence—achievement of skill equal to the demands of the environment.

Competition—rivalry for objects, for resources, facilities or position in an organization.

Comprehensive battery—a battery of tests which measure different components of cognitive functioning and perceptual and motor functioning.

Computerized assessment—an assessment which includes the administration, scoring, and interpretation of test results done by a sophisticated computer program.

Concentric contraction—a muscular contraction during which the muscle fibers shorten in an attempt to overcome resistance.

Condign power—power achieved by imposing an alternative to the unpleasant or painful preference of the individual or group so that such preferences are abandoned.

Conditioned power—power exercised by changing the belief of the individual by education or persuasion causing the individual to submit to the will of others.

Conference committee—committee of senators and representatives with one purpose of working out compromises between different versions of a bill.

Construct—a conceptual structure used in science for thinking about the factors underlying observed phenomena.

Construct validity—in research, the extent to which a test measures the construct (mental representation) variables that it was designed to identify.

Convergence—the ability of the brain to respond only after receiving input from multiple sources.

Coordination—a property of movement characterized by the smooth and harmonious action of groups of muscles working together to produce a desired motion.

Coping—the process through which individuals adjust to the stressful demands of their daily environment.

Corporal potentiality—the ability to screen out vestibular and postural information at conscious levels in order to engage the cortex in higher order cognitive tasks.

Cortically programmed movements—movements that are based on input from structure in the cortex (motor strip or basal ganglia).

Cost benefit analysis—a process used to evaluate the economic efficiency of new policies and programs by comparing an outcome and the costs required to achieve it.

Cost containment—an approach to health care which emphasizes reduced costs.

Crisis interview—following an emergency; an interview used to identify crisis problems and immediate interventions.

Criterion—particular standard or level of performance, or expected outcome.

Criterion validity—in measurement, a test which predicts the specific behaviors required to function in, meet the standards of, and be successful in daily life.

Cultural style—collections of furnishings, objects, and decor with generally accepted cultural connotations of certain life-styles or behavior patterns.

Culture—patterns of behavior learned through the socialization process, including anything acquired by humans as members of society: knowledge, values, beliefs, laws, morals, customs, speech patterns, economic production patterns, etc.

Database—a collection of data organized in information fields in electronic format.

Defense mechanisms—unconscious processes which keep anxiety producing information out of conscious awareness. Some common examples include compensation, denial, rationalization, sublimation and projection.

Dependence—the need to be influenced, nurtured or controlled.

Dermatome—the area on the surface of the skin that is served by one spinal segment.

Dexterity—skill in using the hands, usually requiring both fine and gross motor coordination.

Diagnostic interview—an interview used by a professional to classify the nature of dysfunction in a person under care.

Digital—a discrete form of information, for example a clock that displays only digits at any given moment (as opposed to analog).

Direct Selection—any technique for choosing items that allows a person to point specifically to the desired choice without intermediate steps, generally allowing selections to be made more rapidly. Examples include pointing with a finger, pressing keys on a keyboard, or eye gaze.

Disability behavior—the ways in which people respond to bodily indications and conditions that they come to view as abnormal. It includes how people monitor themselves, define and interpret symptoms, take remedial action, and use sources of help.

Disease—a deviation from the norm of measurable biological variables as defined by the biomedical system. It refers to abnormalities of structure and function in body organs and systems.

Disinhibition—the inability to suppress a lower brain center or motor behavior like a reflex, indicative of damage to higher structures of the brain.

Distractibility—the level at which competing sensory input are able to draw attention away from tasks at hand.

Distribution—refers to manner through which a drug is transported by the circulating body fluids to the sites of action.

Disuse atrophy—the wasting or degeneration of muscle tissue which occurs as a result of inactivity or immobility.

Divergence—the brain's ability to send information from one source to many parts of the central nervous system simultaneously.

Domain—specific occupational performance area; occupational performance domains are work (including education), self-care and self maintenance, and play/leisure.

Domain specificity—a term referring to the specific area of occupational performance to which a given assessment approach is directed.

Dyadic activity—an activity involving another person.

Dynamic flexibility—amount of resistance of a joint(s) to motion.

Dynamic strength—the force of muscular contraction in which joint angle changes.

Dynamometer—device used to measure force produced from muscular contraction.

Dysfunctional hierarchy—the levels of dysfunction including impairment, disability and handicap.

Eccentric contraction—a muscular contraction during which the length of muscle fibers is increased.

Efficacy—having the desired influence or outcome.

Effortful processes—processes which require much attentional effort.

Ego—in psychoanalytic theory, one of three personality structures. It controls and directs one's actions after evaluating reality, monitoring one's impulses and taking into consideration one's values and moral and ethical code. The executive structure of the personality.

Electronic communication system—see Augmentative communication.

Emotion-focused coping—coping strategies that focus on

managing the emotions associated with a stressful episode.

Empathy—while maintaining one's sense of self, the ability to recognize and share the emotions and state of mind of another person.

Empirical base—knowledge based upon the observations and experience of master clinicians.

Emulator—a device which imitates the action of another; for example, a terminal emulator is a system which is not a terminal per se, but is designed to operate like one.

Encoding (cognitive)—those processes or strategies used to initially store information in memory.

Encoding (electronic)—a technique for increasing the number of selections possible from a limited number of input options. Morse code is an example where a full alphabet is encoded to dashes and dots.

Endurance—the ability to sustain effort. A distinction should be made between cardiovascular endurance and muscular endurance.

Enteral—administration of a pharmacologic agent directly into the gastrointestinal tract by oral, rectal or nasogastric routes.

Environment—the external social and physical conditions or factors which have the potential to influence an individual.

Environmental assessment—the process of identifying, describing and measuring factors external to the individual which can influence performance or the outcome of treatment. These can include space and associated objects, cultural influences, social relationships and systems and available resources.

Environmental contingencies—those factors in the environment that influence the patient's performance during an evaluation.

Environmental Control Unit (ECU)—a device that allows those with limited physical ability to operate other electronic devices by remote control.

Environmental press—the tendency of environments to encourage or require certain types of behavior.

Epicritic sensation—the ability to localize and discern fine differences in touch, pain, and temperature.

Epigenesis—the notion that elements of each developmental stage are represented in all developmental stages.

Episodic memory—memory for personal episodes or events that have some temporal reference.

Equipment—a device which usually cannot be held in the hand and is electrical or mechanical (e.g., table or electrical saw or stove); devices can be specifically designed to assist function or compensate for absent function or they can be labor-saving and convenience gadgets.

Ergometer—a device which can measure work done, i.e., bicycle ergometer, arm crank ergometer.

Ergometry—measurement of work.

Ergonomics—the field of study which examines and optimizes the interaction between the human worker and the non-human work environment.

Essential fat—stored body fat that is necessary for normal physiologic function and found in bone marrow, nervous system, and all body organs (also sex characteristic fat deposits in women).

Ethnicity—a component of culture that is derived from membership in a racial, religious, national, or linguistic group or subgroup, usually through birth.

Evaluation—the process of obtaining and interpreting data necessary for treatment.

Excess disability—a disability that occurs above and beyond that which should occur given the person's actual limitations. Excess disability results when the individual is not allowed to do things to retain the skills necessary to perform the tasks.

Exchange relationship—a social concept which views interaction as exchanges of value. For example, the grandfather who teaches his grandson how to fish is exchanging knowledge and experience for the company and affection that the grandson may bring to the interaction.

Excretion—process through which metabolites of drugs (and active drug itself) are eliminated from the body through urine and feces, evaporation from skin, exhalation from lungs, and secretion into saliva.

Exertional angina—paroxysmal thoracic pain due most often to anoxia of the myocardium precipitated by physical exertion (also called angina).

Exhaustion—depletion of energy with consequent inability to respond to stimuli.

Explanatory model—a unique mental model held by an individual about an illness episode, containing knowledge, thoughts, and feelings about etiology, timing and mode of onset of an illness, the pathophysiological process, the natural history and the severity of the illness, ethnoanatomy and ethnophysiology, and appropriate treatments and their rationale.

External stimulation—factors in the area where the activity is being performed which may enhance or impede performance.

Extrinsic motivation—stimulation to achieve or perform that initiates from the environment.

Face validity—the dimension of a test by which it appears to test what it purports to test.

Factor analysis—a statistical test which examines relationships of many variables and their contribution to the total set of variables.

Fatigue—decreased ability to maintain a contraction at a given force.

Federal Register—proposed rules and regulations established by federal agencies in the U.S. that are in a published format.

Figure-ground perception—the person's ability to distinguish shapes and objects from the background in which they exist.

Flexibility—the range of motion at a joint or in a sequence of joints.

Floppy disk—a magnetic storage medium for electronic information of high or low density, single-sided or doubled-sided, and sizes of 5 1/4 inches or 3 1/2 inches.

Frame of reference—a body of theoretical assumptions and principles of practice that give unity and direction to practice and research.

Frequency counts—the process of counting specific behaviors which occur during an identified time period.

Functional assessment—observation of motor performance and behavior to determine if a person can adequately perform the required tasks of a particular role or setting.

Functional electrical stimulation (FES)—the stimulation of nerves from surface electrodes in order to activate specific muscle groups for facilitating function.

Galvanic skin response (GSR)—the change in the electrical resistance of the skin as a response to different stimuli.

General adaptation syndrome (GAS)—the term used by Hans Selye to describe the body's generalized response to noxious stimuli in the environment. This syndrome consists of an alarm reaction, a resistance stage, and an exhaustion stage.

Generalization—skill and performance in applying specific concepts to a variety of related solutions.

Goniometer—instrument for measuring movement at a joint.

Graded activity—an activity which has been modified in one or more of a variety of ways in order to provide the appropriate therapeutic demand or challenge for a patient. The characteristics of activities useful for therapy can be graduated, or incrementally changed, so that a desired level of performance can be attained.

Graded Exercise Test—physical performance of measured, incremental workloads with measurement of physiologic response. Used to assess physiologic response to exercise stress for determination of cardiac and respiratory status.

Graphesthesia—the ability to identify letters or designs on the basis of tactile input to the skin.

Gratification—the ability to receive pleasure, either immediate (immediately upon engaging in activity) or delayed (after completion of the activity).

Group—a plurality of individuals (three or more) who are in contact with one another, who take each other into account, and who are aware of some common goal.

Group roles—patterns of behavior shared by group members and necessary for the group to function and meet its goals. They are often categorized as expressive and instrumental.

Guttman scale—a specific type of behavioral measurement scale which, when scored, results in an inclusive hierarchy of performance. Items on such a scale are ordered in such a way as to assure that if one performs a given item satisfactorily, then one must also have the ability to perform all previous items at a designated criterion level of performance.

Habituate—process of accommodating to a stimulus through diminished response.

Habituation subsystem—a conceptual subsystem in the Model of Human Occupation that houses the ability to organize skills into roles and routines.

Half-life—a measure of the amount of time required for 50% of a drug to be eliminated from the body.

Hallucinations—to sense (e.g., see, hear, smell or touch) something that does not exist externally.

Health policy—the set of initiatives taken by government to direct resources toward promoting and maintaining the health of its citizens.

History—a type of interview, either structured, semi-structured, or unstructured, during which information about specific areas of functional performance is elicited. Historical information can be gathered directly from the patient or client or indirectly through the reports of others who are familiar with one's past performance.

History-taking interview—an interview used to elicit information about the patient's medical, family, marriage, sexual and occupational histories.

Human Factors Engineering—the engineering field which investigates and optimizes function of interactions between humans and machines.

Hydrostatic weighing—underwater weighing to determine body volume; body volume is used to determine body density from which body composition can be calculated.

Hypercard—a software program available for the Apple Macintosh computer which helps in the programming of user-friendly mouse or "push button oriented" applications.

Hypermobility—a condition of excessive motion in joints.

Hyperplasia—increased number of cells.

Hypertonus—a muscular state wherein muscle tension is greater than desired, spasticity; hypertonus increases resistance to passive stretch.

Hypertrophy—increased cell size leading to increased tissue size.

Hypotonicity—a decrease in the muscle tone and stretch reflex of a muscle resulting in decreased resistance to passive stretch and hyporesponsiveness to sensory stimulation.

Hypotonus—a muscular state wherein muscle tension is lower than desired, flaccidity; hypotonus decreases resistance to passive stretch.

Hypoxia—deficiency of oxygen.

Id—in psychoanalysis, the unconscious part of the psyche which is the source of primitive, instinctual drives and strives for self preservation and pleasure. The primary process element of personality.

Illness—the experience of devalued changes in being and in social function. It primarily encompasses personal, interpersonal, and cultural reactions to sickness.

Independence—having adequate resources to accomplish everyday tasks.

Individual Education Plan (IEP)—an interdisciplinary plan required for special education students in the U.S. under the provisions of Public Law 94-142.

Inference—a possible result or conclusion that could be deduced from evaluation data.

Informant interview—an interview in which the therapist gathers information about the patient or environment from significant others.

Institutionalization—the effects of dehumanizing and depersonalizing characteristics of the environment that result in apathy, a significant decrease in motivation and activity and increased passivity of an individual.

Instrumental ADL—Instrumental activities of daily living; originated by Lawton to refer to those essential self-maintenance activities which are necessary for independent living that are not considered as basic ADL or self-care tasks.

Insurance denial—when a third party has denied payment for a service; organizations may appeal denials if they believe the criteria have not been equitably applied.

Intake interview—an interview in which the therapist identifies the patient's needs and his or her suitability for treatment.

Intelligence—the intelligence quotient is the relationship of mental age to chronological age. As commonly used, the potential or ability to acquire, retain and use experience and knowledge to reason and problem solve.

Interface—the program or device that links the way two or more pieces of equipment, or person/machine units work together. There is an interface between the computer and printer, keyboard and computer, persons and wheelchair control, etc.

Internal postural control—the ability of the body to support and control its own movement without reliance on supporting structures in the environment.

International Classification of Diseases—disease classification system developed by the World Health Organization.

Intrinsic motivation—stimulation to achieve or perform that initiates from within oneself.

Inventory—an assessment comprised of a list of items to which the patient gives responses.

Isokinetic strength—force generated by a muscle contracting through a range of motion at a constant speed.

Isometric contraction—contraction of a muscle during which shortening or lengthening is prevented.

Isometric strength—force generated by a contraction in which there is no joint movement and minimal change in muscle length.

Isotonic contraction—contraction of a muscle during which the force of resistance remains constant throughout the range of motion.

Isotonic strength—force of contraction in which a muscle moves a constant load through a range of motion.

Kinesthesia—a person's sense of position, weight and movement in space. The receptors for kinesthesia are located in the muscles, tendons and joints.

Labeling theory—a sociological theory which questions the medical model of psychiatric diagnosis and treatment. The theory suggests that symptoms and illness are deviations from the norm of social behavior and should not be labeled as illness.

Laptop Computer—a portable lightweight computer that can be carried and used on an individual's lap.

Lateral trunk flexion—the ability to move the trunk from side to side without moving the legs which is essential for maintaining balance.

Learning—the enduring ability of an individual to comprehend and/or competently respond to changes in information from the environment and/or from within the self. As one learns about the environment, alterations occur in the definition of the self and possible behaviors; as one learns about the self, alterations occur in the definition of the environment and possible behaviors.

Legislative review—a review of a bill by the legislature when they perceive that an agency has misinterpreted the intent or excessively revised existing regulations.

Levels of processing—the durability of the memory trace is a function of the level to which the information was encoded.

Life roles—daily-life experiences that occupy one's time including roles of student, homemaker, worker (active or retired), sibling, parent, mate, son, daughter, and peer.

Likert scale—a point system which is used to rank a particular level of skill, function or attitude.

Load—To take a program or file from a storage medium such as a disk and place it into current computer memory so that it can be used.

Locus of control—a psychological term referring to one's orientation to the world of events. Persons with an internal locus of control believe they can influence the outcome of events. Those with an external locus of control, conversely, believe that the outcome of events is largely a matter of fate or chance, i.e., that they cannot have influence over the outcome of events.

Long-term memory—permanent memory store for long-term information.

Long-term support system—ensuring that individuals have access to the services that are needed to support independent living.

Lower motor neuron—sensory neuron found in the anterior horn cell, nerve root or peripheral nervous system.

Macro—a single computer instruction that can stand for a group of instructions (e.g., if you had to type occupational therapy 70 times in a paper you might choose to assign a code such as "<alt>OT). Each time you typed <alt>OT the computer would type out occupational therapy, without requiring twenty separate keystrokes.

Mainframe Computer—a term that applies to high capacity, fast computers which also tend to be heavy, large, and expensive. A mainframe system is often a control computer designed to interact with a number of terminals.

Master care plan—the treatment plan, which includes the list of patient problems and identifies the treatment team's intervention strategies and responsibilities.

Mastery—achievement of skill to a criterion level of success.

Maximal Oxygen Consumption (max VO$_2$, maximal oxygen uptake, aerobic capacity)—the greatest volume of oxygen used by the cells of the body per unit time.

Mean—the arithmetic average.

Mechanical efficiency—the amount of external work performed in relation to the amount of energy required to perform the work.

Median—the value or score that most closely represents the middle of a range of scores.

Medicare—a federally funded health insurance program for the elderly, certain disabled people, and most individuals with end-stage renal disease.

Medicare Part A—the Hospital Insurance Program (HI) of Medicare, which covers hospital inpatient care, care in skilled nursing facilities, and home health care.

Medicare Part B—the Supplemental Medical Insurance Program (SMI) of Medicare, which covers hospital outpatient care, physicians fees, home health care, comprehensive outpatient rehabilitation facility fees, and other professional services.

Megabyte—1,000 Kilobytes (K) or 1,000,000 bytes of electronic information. A measure of the capacity of memory, disk storage, etc.

Memory processes—the strategies for dealing with information which are under the individual's control.

Memory structure—the unvarying physical or structural components of memory.

Mental status exam—a standardized diagnostic procedure used to evaluate intellectual, emotional, psychological and personality function.

Metabolism—the process by which the body inactivates drugs (also called biotransformation).

Microchip—an electronic device that consists of thousands electronic circuits such as of transistors on a small sliver, or chip, of plastic. Such devices are the building blocks of computers. Also referred to as an integrated circuit (IC).

Microcomputer—a small computer system usually used by one person (also called personal computer).

Minicomputer—a medium size computer that usually serves as a central computer for many individuals. Used primarily in academic and research settings.

Mobility sphere—a territory within which individuals regularly travel in their daily activity patterns. Its dimensions depend on distances that the person can travel by ambulation or available modes of transportation, as well as on the accessibility features of the environment.

Mode—the value or score in a set of scores that occurs most frequently.

Modem—a device that is most often connected between a telephone line and computer so that the computer can communicate with other computers via the telephone line signals.

Monitoring—determining a patient's status on a periodic or ongoing basis.

Motor planning—the ability to organize and execute movement patterns to accomplish a purposeful activity.

Motor unit—one alpha motor neuron, its axon, and all muscle fibers attached to that axon.

Mouse—a small device that moves on a horizontal plane and controls the cursor on a computer monitor. Mice were named so because they were "palm of the hand size" and had a "tail" which led to the computer. It can have from one to three buttons used to emulate assorted keyboard actions.

Multiaxial evaluation—the five axes of DSM III-R which are used to establish a psychiatric diagnosis that can aid in treatment planning and predicting intervention outcome.

Multidimensional maps—the pictures of self and environment that are created within the central nervous system after receipt and analysis of multisensory input.

Muscle endurance—sustained muscular contraction, measured as repetitions of submaximal contractions (isotonic) or submaximal holding time (isometric).

Muscle strength—a non-specific term relating to muscle contraction, often referring to the force generated by a single maximal isometric contraction.

Muscle tone—the amount of tension or contractibility among the motor units of a muscle; often defined as the resistance of a muscle to stretch or elongation.

MVC—Maximum voluntary contraction.

Narrative documentation—system of documentation which uses summary paragraphs to describe evaluation data and treatment progress.

National health insurance—a form of insurance sponsored by a national government intended to pay for health services used by its citizens.

Naturalistic observation—during an evaluation, the assessor's observation of the patient performing in his/her natural environment.

Network—a communication system between computers, communication between a central computer and users, or any group of computers that are connected in order to send messages to each other.

Networking—a process that links people and information in order to accomplish objectives.

Neuroleptic—a drug or agent that modifies psychotic behavior, antipsychotic.

Neuromuscular re-education—specific treatment regimens carried out by occupational and physical therapists to improve motor strength and coordination in persons with brain or spinal cord injuries.

Neurosis—an emotional disorder in which reality testing is not seriously disturbed; a diagnostic category used prior to DSM III.

Norm-referenced test—any instrument which uses the typical scores of members of a comparison group as a standard for determining individual performance.

Norms—standards of comparison derived from measuring an attribute across many individuals to determine typical score ranges.

Object relations—in psychoanalytic theory, the investment of psychic energy in objects and events in the world; sometimes seen exclusively as the bond(s) between two persons.

Objective measure—a method of assessment which is not influenced by the emotions or personal opinion of the assessor.

Obligatory reflexive response—a reflex which is con-sciously present in a motor pattern; this reflex may dominate all other movement components.

Observer bias—when the previous experiences of the therapist influence his/her observations and interpretation of behaviors being assessed.

Obtrusive observation—when the patient is aware of being observed by the therapist for the purpose of evaluation of cognitive, physical and/or psychosocial performance.

Occupational performance—accomplishment of tasks related to self-care/self-maintenance, work/education, play/leisure, and rest/relaxation.

Occupational performance component—any subsystem that contributes to the performance of self-care/self maintenance, work/education, play/leisure, and rest/relaxation.

Occupational Therapy Uniform Evaluation CheckList—official document of the American Occupational Therapy Association that suggests guidelines for occupational therapy assessment.

On-line—a monitor linked to an off-site computer.

Open-ended question—question which may have multiple responses rather than a definite answer.

Open system—a system of structures that functions as a whole and maintains itself by means of input from the environment and organismic change occurring as needed.

Operant—a form of conditioning in which reinforcement is contingent upon the occurrence of the desired response.

Operant conditioning—a form of conditioning in which reinforcement is contingent upon the occurence of the desired response

Opioid—terminology used to refer to synthetic drugs that have pharmacologic properties similar to opium or morphine.

Optical pointers—devices which sense light and feedback the stimulus to indicate where the device is pointing.

Orthostatic hypotension—lowered blood pressure when a person changes from a horizontal to an erect position.

Osteoporosis—reduction in bone mass associated with loss of bone mineral and matrix occurring when bone resorption is greater than formation.

Outcome measure—an instrument designed to gather information on the efficacy of service programs; a means for determining if goals or objectives have been met.

Overflow—clinical term for unwanted movement in a part of the body inappropriate to the action being performed.

Oxygen consumption—the oxygen used by the mitochondria.

Parallel Interventions—method of applying technology while at the same time providing therapy to maximize abilities for an individual for more powerful technology.

Parasthesia—an abnormal sensation, such as burning or prickling.

Parenteral—administration by subcutaneous, intramuscular or intravenous injection, thereby bypassing the gastrointestinal tract.

Participant-observer—a descriptor which can be applied when a therapist observes and evaluates a patient's performance while engaged in an activity with the patient.

Passive stretch—stretch applied with external force.

Patient management interview—an interview used by multiple professionals to identify the type of intervention or treatment needed.

Patient-related consultation—when the occupational therapist shares information with other professionals regarding patients who are not presently receiving occupational therapy services (AOTA, 1979, p. 6).

Patterns of help-seeking—culturally distinct ways in which people go about finding help at particular times in an illness. It refers to both the range of options (often categorized as the biomedical, popular, and traditional health sectors) and the decision-making process.

Percent body fat—percent of body weight that is fat, includes storage fate (expendable), essential fat, and sex specific fat reserve.

Perception—the ability to interpret incoming sensory information.

Perceptual motor skill—the ability to integrate perceptual (sensory) input with motor output in order to accomplish purposeful activities.

Percutaneous—administration of a drug by inhalation, sublingual, or topical processes.

Performance subsystem—a subsystem in the model of human occupation that includes neuromuscular skills, process skills, and communication/interaction skills.

Perseveration—continued, meaningless repetition of a specific behavior.

Personality trait—a distinguishing feature that reflects one's characteristic way of thinking, feeling and/or adapting.

Person-environment fit—the degree to which individuals have adapted to their unique environments.

Pharmacology—the study of drugs and their actions on living organisms.

Physical environment—that part of the environment which can be perceived directly through the senses. The physical environment includes observable space, objects and their arrangement, light, noise, and other ambient characteristics which can be objectively determined.

Plasticity—the ability of the central nervous system to adapt structurally or functionally in response to environmental demands.

Play/leisure—choosing, performing, and engaging in activities for amusement, relaxation, enjoyment, and/or self-expression.

Policy—laws or decisions that guide one's actions, including the distribution of funds and sources.

Position in space—the person's awareness of the place of his/her body in space.

Postrotary nystagmus—reflexive movement of the eyes that occurs after quick rotational movements have ceased; used as indicator of level of processing of vestibular information.

Power—the ability to impose one's will upon the behavior of other persons.

Praxis—the ability to conceive and organize a new motor act.

Primary appraisal—that part of the appraisal process in coping whereby the individual determines whether a stressful episode poses a situation of potential harm, threat, or challenge.

Prime mover—that muscle with the principal responsibility for a given action. For example, the biceps brachii is the prime mover for flexing the arm at the elbow.

Principle of overload—the concept that repeated imposition of a stress above that normally experienced will produce physiologic adaptation.

Problem-focused coping—coping strategies that are directed at the source of stress itself, rather than at feelings or emotions associated with the stress.

Problem-oriented documentation—a structured system of documentation originated by Weed which has four basic components; subjective and objective data, a problem list and a plan for treatment.

Procedural memory—knowledge for the necessary procedures to perform some activity; the so-called ''knowing how''

Product line—services that are labeled to insure that consumers understand what they are purchasing.

Programming—creating a set of instructions which a computer is able to follow; also a term used to refer to the structuring of activity or influencing of behavior through environmental design, organization or manipulation.

Projective activities—ambiguous stimuli onto which an individual can project inner needs, thoughts, feelings and concerns.

Projective assessment—an evaluation approach which

uses unstructured stimuli to elicit patient responses that suggest personality type, characteristics and unconscious material.

Prophylactic—preventive.

Proprioception—the ability to identify the position of the body and its parts in space, and in relation to each other.

Protective extension response—a reflexive act consisting of extending one's arms in front of the head to protect the face and head during forward falling.

Protopathic sensation—gross sensory abilities in the extremities, allowing one to detect light moving touch, pain and temperature but without the ability to make fine discrimination of extent.

Proxemics—study of humans' use of space.

Psychological constructs—psychological concepts; terms (without universal definitions) commonly used to describe mental states.

Psychometric interview—an interview in which a psychologist does formal psychological testing.

Psychometric techniques (tests)—methods for measuring personality, interest and attitude (frequently used in psychology).

Psychosis—a severe mental disorder causing extreme personality disorganization, loss of reality orientation and poor function in society.

Public good—general welfare or benefit to the majority or large contingent of citizens.

Raw score—an unadjusted score derived from observations of performance; frequently, the arithmetic sum of a subject's responses.

Re-entry programs—rehabilitation programs designed to maximize independence. These programs are usually the final rehabilitation program after hospitalization and rehabilitation programs are completed. Re-entry programs are usually outpatient or community programs.

Reactivity—a characteristic of assessment instruments whereby the act of administering the assessment changes the behavior of the person being evaluated, thus distorting the representativeness of the findings.

Reality testing—the ability to know what is real and what is fantasy, usually accomplished through structured activity.

Reappraisal—in coping, reconsideration of a harm, threat, or loss episode after an initial appraisal has taken place. It is thought that during coping, individuals constantly reassess the stressful episode and their resources and alternatives for dealing with it.

Receptive field—the receptor area served by one neuron.

Receptor—the specific site at which a drug acts through forming a chemical bond.

Reflex—a subconscious, involuntary reaction to an external stimulus.

Relative endurance—muscular endurance when force of contraction tested is based on percentage of measured strength.

Release phenomenon—the ongoing action of one part of the central nervous system without modulation from a complementary functional component.

Reliability—confidence that scores reflect true performance, an index of the amount of measurement error in a test.

Repetitions maximum (R.M.)—maximum weight that can be lifted in isotonic contraction; one R.M. = maximum weight that can be lifted one time, two R.M. = maximum weight that can be lifted twice, etc.

Representative assembly—the policy-making body of the American Occupational Therapy Association.

Re-privatize—to return responsibility to the private sector as opposed to public responsibility.

Resistance development—adaptation which decreases physiologic response to a chronic stressor.

Resource environment—facilities available to an individual within his or her life space that may meet his/her instrumental (survival) or symbolic needs.

Responsivity—the level that the sensory input facilitates reaction or noticing.

Rest/relaxation—performance during time not devoted to other activity and during time devoted to sleep.

Retrospective recording—waiting until the evaluation is completed to record observations of patient function.

RM—Repetition maximum. Maximum weight that can be lifted in isotonic contraction. One RM = maximum that can be lifted one time; two RM = maximum weight that can be lifted twice, etc.

Role—a set of behaviors that have some socially agreed-upon functions and for which there is an accepted code of norms.

RPE—Rating of perceived exertion. Psychophysical scale for subjective rating of exertion during work.

Sample of behavior—selected test items chosen because they constitute a subset of the behaviors that need to be assessed.

Scanning—A technique for making selections on a device such as a communication aid, computer, or environmental control system. Scanning involves moving sequentially through a given set of choices, and making a selection when the desired position is reached. Types of scanning include automatic, manual, row-and-column, and directed.

Schema theory—the notion that standard routine performances occur in given situations in a typical sequence and with typical kinds of participants; within the general framework or structure the details of a given performance may vary but the basic structure remains consistent.

Schemata—the basic units of all knowledge. Each simple organization of experience and knowledge by the mind make up the original ''schema'' or framework which represents our everyday experiences. Each experience, thought and idea is a structural element in an organizational matrix which integrates each person's experiences and history into a meaningful set of categories, each filled with data from one's memory of prior events.

Schemes—structural elements of cognition.

Screening—review of a patient case to determine if occupational therapy services are necessary.

Screening instrument—an assessment device used for purposes of identifying potential problem areas for further in-depth evaluation.

Secondary appraisal—that part of the coping process whereby an individual, having determined the nature of a stressful episode (i.e., harm, threat, or challenge), selects an appropriate strategy for dealing with it.

Self-actualization—the process of striving to achieve one's ultimate purpose in life with accompanying feelings of accomplishment and personal growth.

Self-care activities—personal activities an individual performs to prepare for and maintain a daily routine.

Self-efficacy— the feelings that people have about their ability to be successful in using a particular coping strategy or problem-solving approach.

Self monitoring—a process whereby the patient records specific behaviors or thoughts as they occur.

Self-report—a type of assessment approach where the patient reports on his or her level of function or performance.

Semantic Compaction—A technique for reducing the number of selections a user must make to generate a phrase on a voice-output communication aid. Symbols for semantic units are used rather than number or letter codes (see Encoding).

Semantic memory—memory for general knowledge.

Sensitization—the process of a receptor becoming more susceptible to a given stimulus.

Sensory registration—the brain's ability to receive input and select that which will receive attention and that which will be inhibited from consciousness.

Sensory integration—the ability to organize sensory information to make an adaptive response to the environment.

Sensory or body disregard—a condition characterized by lack of awareness of one side of the body.

Sensory memory—memory store which holds sensory input in its uninterpreted sensory form for a very brief period of time.

Sex identification—the assigning of a masculine or feminine connotation to a given activity.

Short-term memory—a limited capacity memory store which holds information for a brief period of time; the so-called 'working memory'.

Side effect—an effect produced by a drug that is other than its desired action. Most side effects are predictable.

Sign of behavior—patient responses which are viewed as ''indirect manifestations'' (or, signs) of one's underlying personality.

Situation-specific—in psychosocial assessment, those behaviors and tasks which must be mastered to function everyday in a particular environment.

Skin fold measurement—a method for estimating percent body fat by measuring subcutaneous fat with skin fold calipers.

Social climate—the combined variables in the social environment that directly or indirectly influence individual behavior, and that are influenced by individual behavior.

Social environment—those social systems or networks within which a given person operates; the collective human relationships of individuals, whether familial community, or organizational in nature, constitute the social environment of that individual.

Social support—the social relatedness and interactions with others that are perceived by the individual as supplying emotional, physical, and social resources.

Social systems—organized interactions among individuals, as within marriages, families, communities, and organizations, both formal and informal.

Socialization—the development of the individual as a social being and a participant in society that results from a continuing, changing interaction between a person and those who attempt to influence him or her.

Software—Programs that run on computers.

Somatotopic—the organization of cells in the somatosensory system which enables one to identify the exact skin surface touched.

Spasticity—an increase in the muscle tone and stretch reflex of a muscle resulting in increased resistance to passive stretch of the muscle and hyper-responsivity of the muscle to sensory stimulation.

Special interest groups—collectives of individuals and organizations who are bound by beliefs about specific issues and/or populations, and who seek to influence decisions about the allocation of resources.

Specialized battery—a battery of tests which measure a

more specific component of cognitive functioning, such as attention or language.

Specificity—an instrument's ability to accurately identify subjects possessing a specific trait.

Spreadsheet—Type of software used in financial management and accounting systems.

Stabilizer—any muscle that acts to fix one attachment of a prime mover or hold a bone steady to provide a foundation for movement.

Standard deviation—mathematically determined value used to derive standards scores and compare raw scores to a unit normal distribution.

Standard scores—raw scores mathematically converted to a scale that facilitates comparison.

Standardization—a method by which test scores of a typical population are derived thus allowing subsequent test scores to be analyzed in light of that broad population; standardization requires a rigorous process of data collection and comparison.

Standardized assessment—tests and evaluation approaches with specific norms, standards and protocol.

Standardized battery—a battery of tests in which the testing and scoring procedures are well-defined and fixed and the interpretation involves the use of standardized norms.

Static flexibility—range of motion in degrees that a joint(s) will allow.

Static strength—the force of muscular contraction in which there is no change in angle of involved joints.

Static stretch—holding the lengthened position without movement.

Step test—graded exercise test in which subject is required to rhythmically step up and down steps of gradually increasing heights.

Stereognosis—the ability to identify common objects by touch with vision occluded.

Stereotypic behavior—repeated, persistent postures or movements, including vocalizations.

Stimulus-arousal properties—the alerting potential of various sensory stimuli, generally thought to be related to their intensity, their pace, and their novelty.

Storage fat—adipose tissue found primarily subcutaneously and surround the major organs.

Strength—a nonspecific term relating to muscle contraction, often referring to the force generated by a single maximal isometric contraction.

Stress—the individual's general reaction to external demands, or stressors. Stress results in psychological as well as physiological reactions.

Stressors—external events that place demands on an individual above the ordinary.

Stroke volume—the amount of blood pumped out of the heart on each beat.

Structured activities—activities which have rules and can be broken down into manageable steps and which are preplanned and preorganized.

Sub-ASIS Bar—An orthotic bar included in seating and positioning systems placed snugly below the Anterior Superior Iliac Spine of the pelvis to maintain a forward tilt of the pelvis and better postural alignment.

Subjective measure—an assessment designed to identify the patient's own view of problems, performance, etc.

Superego—in psychoanalytic theory, one of three personality components. It houses one's values, ethics, standards and conscience.

Suppression—the ability of the central nervous system to screen out certain stimuli so that others may be attended to more carefully.

Symbolic associations—an object's broader, cultural connotations and its narrower, idiosyncratic associations for individuals or families.

Symbols—abstract representations of perceived reality.

Sympathetic nervous system—that part of the autonomic nervous system that mobilizes the body's resources during stressful situations.

Synergist—any muscle that functions to inhibit extraneous action from a muscle that would interfere with the action of prime mover.

T-Test—Parametric statistical test comparing differences of two data sets.

Target site—desired site for a drug's action within the body.

Task—work assigned to, selected by, or required of a person related to development of occupational performance skills, collection of activities related to accomplishment of a specific goal..

Technology transfer—in occupational therapy, the process by which knowledge is applied; occupational therapy knowledge is technology, which is transferred by administering evaluation and treatment.

Temporal environment—the manner in which social and cultural expectations influence behavior by organizing the time during which activities occur and the amount of time devoted to them.

Tenodesis Splint—Orthosis fabricated to allow pinch and grasp movements through use of wrist extensors in substitution for finger flexors.

Tensiometer—device use to measure force produced from an isometric contraction.

Test protocol—the specific procedures that must be followed when assessing a patient; formal testing procedures.

Test sensitivity—an instrument's ability to detect change in a variable being measured.

Third party payment—payment for services by someone other than the person receiving them.

Thought disorder—disturbance in thinking, including distorted content (ideas, beliefs and sensory interpretation) and distorted written and spoken language (e.g., word salad, loose associations, echolalia).

Threat minimization—a psychological coping strategy whereby emotions are managed through 'playing down' the importance or significance of a stressor.

Threshold—the point at which a stimulus characteristic is identified.

Time-related measures—an assessment in which the patient records the thoughts, feelings and/or behaviors which occur during a specific time period; time sampling and duration are included.

Tolerance—the physiological and physiological accommodation or adaptation to a chemical agent over time.

Tone—state of muscle contraction determined by resistance to stretch.

Tone (tonus)—the status or condition of muscle as characterized by resistance to stretch.

Tonotopic—the organization of cells within the auditory system which enables one to identify the exact sound heard.

Top-down processing—when processing starts with higher order stored knowledge and depends upon contextual information or is 'conceptually driven'.

Topographic—the organization of cells in the visual system which enables one to identify the exact location and features of the stimulus.

Trackball—A control device used to move and operate the cursor on the computer screen.

Transfer appropriate processing—the concept that the cognitive processes used while learning determine the type of criterial task on which one will best perform when evaluated for what has been learned.

Transparent Access—Complete emulation usable with all or an entire major class of software. For example, a successful keyboard emulating interface provides transparent access to standard software using alternate keyboards.

Type A behavior— a cluster of personality traits that includes high achievement motivation, drive, and a fast paced lifestyle.

Unobtrusive observation—observation for assessment which minimizes reactivity.

Unstructured activities— activities which are not preplanned or broken down into steps.

Upper motor neuron— neurons of the cerebral cortex that conduct stimuli from the motor cortex of the brain to motor nuclei of cerebral nerves of the ventral gray columns of the spinal cord.

Validity—the degree to which a test measures what it is intended to measure.

Visual neglect—inattention to visual stimuli occurring in the space on the involved side of the body.

Visual orientation— awareness and location of objects in the environment and their relationship to each other and to oneself.

Visual perception—the brain's ability to understand sensory input to determine size, shape, distance and form of objects.

Volition subsystem—a subsystem in the model of human occupation that includes one's values, interests, and feelings of personal causation.

Weight shift—bearing the body's weight from one leg to another; shifting the center of gravity.

Word Processing—A type of application software that is used to enter, edit, manipulate, and format text.

Word Prediction—Technique used in software to guess the current word or next word when beginning letters or the previous word, respectively, is typed.

Work/education—skill and performance in purposeful and productive activities in the home, in employment, in school, and in the community.

Work setting—any environment in which an individual performs productive activity.

Work space—the physical area in which one performs work.

Index of Assessment Approaches and Instruments

Index